AF838327

Nelson ESSENTIALS OF PEDIATRICS

NOTE TO INSTRUCTORS

Contact your Elsevier Sales Representative for teaching resources, including an image bank, for *Nelson Essentials of Pediatrics*, 10e, or request these supporting materials at: **http://evolve.elsevier.com/Nelson/essentials/**

EDITION
10

Nelson

ESSENTIALS OF PEDIATRICS

ABIGAIL M. SCHUH, MD, MMHPE
Associate Professor of Pediatrics
Medical College of Wisconsin
Milwaukee, Wisconsin

ROBERT M. KLIEGMAN, MD
Professor of Pediatrics
Medical College of Wisconsin
Milwaukee, Wisconsin

KELSEY S. RYAN, MD
Associate Professor of Pediatrics
Medical College of Wisconsin
Milwaukee, Wisconsin

SARAH C. YALE, MD
Associate Professor of Pediatrics
Medical College of Wisconsin
Milwaukee, Wisconsin

MICHELLE L. MITCHELL, MD
Associate Professor of Pediatrics
Medical College of Wisconsin
Milwaukee, Wisconsin

ELSEVIER

Elsevier
1818 Market Street, Suite 3323
Philadelphia, PA 19103-2899

NELSON ESSENTIALS OF PEDIATRICS, TENTH EDITION
INTERNATIONAL EDITION

ISBN: 978-0-443-28702-2
ISBN: 978-0-443-28703-9

Copyright © 2027 by Elsevier Inc. All rights are reserved, including those for text and data mining, AI training, and similar technologies.

For accessibility purposes, images in electronic versions of this book are accompanied by alt-text descriptions provided by Elsevier. For more information, see https://www.elsevier.com/about/accessibility.

Books and Journals published by Elsevier comply with applicable product safety requirements.
For any product safety concerns or queries, please contact our authorized representative, Elsevier B.V., at productsafety@elsevier.com.

Publisher's note: Elsevier takes a neutral position with respect to territorial disputes or jurisdictional claims in its published content, including in maps and institutional affiliations.

No part of this publication may be reproduced or transmitted in any form or by any means, electronic or mechanical, including photocopying, recording, or any information storage and retrieval system, without permission in writing from the publisher. Details on how to seek permission, further information about the Publisher's permissions policies and our arrangements with organizations such as the Copyright Clearance Center and the Copyright Licensing Agency, can be found at our website: www.elsevier.com/permissions.

This book and the individual contributions contained in it are protected under copyright by the Publisher (other than as may be noted herein).

Notice

Practitioners and researchers must always rely on their own experience and knowledge in evaluating and using any information, methods, compounds or experiments described herein. Because of rapid advances in the medical sciences, in particular, independent verification of diagnoses and drug dosages should be made. To the fullest extent of the law, no responsibility is assumed by Elsevier, authors, editors or contributors for any injury and/or damage to persons or property as a matter of products liability, negligence or otherwise, or from any use or operation of any methods, products, instructions, or ideas contained in the material herein.

Previous editions copyrighted 2023, 2019, 2015, 2011, 2006, 2002, 1998, 1994, and 1990.

Senior Content Strategist: Marybeth Thiel
Senior Content Development Specialist: Jennifer Shreiner
Publishing Services Manager: Catherine Jackson
Senior Project Manager: Daniel Fitzgerald
Designer: Renee Duenow

Printed in India.

Last digit is the print number: 9 8 7 6 5 4 3 2 1

ELSEVIER Book Aid International
Working together to grow libraries in developing countries
www.elsevier.com • www.bookaid.org

This book is dedicated to our patients,
who inspire us to learn more; our mentors;
and, now more than ever, our colleagues,
the dedicated medical professionals
whose curiosity and focus on providing excellent care
and who, even in the face of recent adversity,
spur the advancement of our medical practice.

We also dedicate this edition to the memory of
Karen Marcdante,
a former editor of this text,
whose unwavering dedication to pediatric education
continues to inspire our work.

CONTRIBUTORS

Melissa Azul, DO
Assistant Professor of Pediatrics
Section of Hematology and Oncology
Medical College of Wisconsin
Milwaukee, Wisconsin
Hematology

Donald Basel, MD
Professor of Pediatrics
Section Chief, Division of Medical Genetics
Medical College of Wisconsin
Milwaukee, Wisconsin
Metabolic Disorders

Kim Blake, MD, MRCP, FRCPC
Professor of Medicine
Department of General Pediatrics
IWK Health
Dalhousie University
Halifax, Nova Scotia, Canada
Adolescent Medicine

Latasha Bogues, MD, FAAP
Associate Professor of Pediatrics
Morehouse School of Medicine
Atlanta, Georgia
Growth and Development

Amanda M. Brandow, DO, MS
Professor of Pediatrics
Section of Hematology and Oncology
Medical College of Wisconsin
Milwaukee, Wisconsin
Hematology

April O. Buchanan, MD
Professor of Pediatrics
Senior Associate Dean for Medical Education
Emory University School of Medicine
Children's Healthcare of Atlanta
Atlanta, Georgia
Pediatric Nutrition and Nutritional Disorders

Gray M. Buchanan, PhD
Associate Professor of Family Medicine
Medical University of South Carolina
Charleston, South Carolina;
Director, Behavioral Medicine
Family Medicine Residency Program
Self Regional Healthcare
Greenwood, South Carolina
Psychiatric Disorders

Asriani M. Chiu, MD
Professor of Pediatrics (Allergy and Immunology) and Medicine
Medical College of Wisconsin
Division of Allergy and Clinical Immunology
Director, Asthma and Allergy Clinic
Children's Wisconsin
Milwaukee, Wisconsin
Allergy

Yvonne E. Chiu, MD
Professor and Vice Chair of Dermatology
Professor of Pediatrics
Medical College of Wisconsin
Medical Director, Pediatric Dermatology
Children's Wisconsin
Milwaukee, Wisconsin
Dermatology

Sarah C. Hofman DeYoung, MD
Clinical Assistant Professor of Pediatrics
University of Washington School of Medicine
Division of Pulmonary and Sleep Medicine
Seattle Children's Hospital
Seattle, Washington
The Respiratory System

Alison H. Downes, MD
Medical Director, Arrow Pathways
Developmental and Behavioral Pediatrics
Havertown, Pennsylvania
Psychosocial Issues

Dawn R. Ebach, MD
Clinical Professor of Pediatrics
Stead Family Department of Pediatrics
University of Iowa Carver College of Medicine;
Division of Pediatric Gastroenterology, Hepatology, Pancreatology, and Nutrition
University of Iowa Children's Hospital
Iowa City, Iowa
The Digestive System

Yasaman Fatemi, MD, MSHP
Assistant Professor of Pediatrics
University of Washington School of Medicine
Associate Medical Director of Infection Prevention
Division of Pediatric Infectious Disease
Seattle Children's Hospital
Seattle, Washington
Infectious Diseases

Madeline R. Field, MD
Assistant Professor of Clinical Pediatrics
Perelman School of Medicine at the University of Pennsylvania
Division of Emergency Medicine
Children's Hospital of Philadelphia
Philadelphia, Pennsylvania
The Acutely Ill or Injured Child

Kristine Fortin, MD, MPH
Associate Professor of Clinical Pediatrics
Perelman School of Medicine at the University of Pennsylvania;
Attending Physician
Safe Place: Center for Child Protection and Health
Children's Hospital of Philadelphia
Philadelphia, Pennsylvania
Psychosocial Issues

Rachel J. Gottlieb-Smith, MD, MHPE
Clinical Associate Professor of Pediatrics
Division of Pediatric Neurology
University of Michigan Medical School
Ann Arbor, Michigan
Neurology

Larry A. Greenbaum, MD, PhD
Marcus Professor of Pediatrics
Director, Division of Pediatric Nephrology
Emory University School of Medicine
Children's Healthcare of Atlanta
Atlanta, Georgia
Fluids and Electrolytes

Mary Kathleen Heneghan, MD
Attending Physician
Division of Pediatric Endocrinology
Advocate Children's Hospital
Park Ridge, Illinois
Endocrinology

Rosalind Usher Hill, MD, MPH, FAAP
Assistant Professor of Clinical Pediatrics
Perelman School of Medicine at the University of Pennsylvania
Attending Physician
Division of Developmental and Behavioral Pediatrics
Children's Hospital of Philadelphia
Philadelphia, Pennsylvania
Behavioral Disorders

Patty Huang, MD
Associate Professor of Clinical Pediatrics
Perelman School of Medicine at the University of Pennsylvania
Attending Physician
Division of Developmental and Behavioral Pediatrics
Children's Hospital of Philadelphia
Philadelphia, Pennsylvania
Behavioral Disorders

Erin E. Neil Knierbein, DO
Clinical Associate Professor of Pediatrics
Division of Pediatric Neurology
University of Michigan Medical School
Ann Arbor, Michigan
Neurology

Victoria J.L. Konold, MD
Assistant Professor of Pediatric Infectious Diseases
University of Washington School of Medicine
Attending Physician
Division of Pediatric Infectious Disease
Seattle Children's Hospital
Seattle, Washington
Infectious Diseases

Matthew P. Kronman, MD, MSCE
Professor of Pediatric Infectious Diseases
University of Washington School of Medicine
Attending Physician
Division of Pediatric Infectious Disease
Seattle Children's Hospital
Seattle, Washington
Infectious Diseases

Michael N. Levas, MD, MS
Professor of Pediatrics
Division of Pediatric Emergency Medicine
Director of Social Medicine
Medical Director, Project Ujima
Associate Director, Comprehensive Injury Center
Medical College of Wisconsin
Children's Wisconsin
Milwaukee, Wisconsin
The Profession of Pediatrics

David A. Levine, MD, FAAP
Professor of Pediatrics
Morehouse School of Medicine
Atlanta, Georgia
Growth and Development

Paul A. Levy, MD
Associate Professor of Pediatrics and Pathology
Albert Einstein College of Medicine
Children's Hospital at Montefiore
Bronx, New York
Human Genetics and Dysmorphology

Jackson T. Londeree, DO
Assistant Professor of Pediatrics
Division of Pediatric Nephrology
Emory University School of Medicine
Children's Healthcare of Atlanta
Atlanta, Georgia
Fluids and Electrolytes

Erin W. MacKintosh, MD
Clinical Assistant Professor of Pediatrics
University of Washington School of Medicine
Division of Pulmonary and Sleep Medicine
Seattle Children's Hospital
Seattle, Washington
The Respiratory System

Leanne M. Mansfield, MD
Assistant Professor of Pediatric Rheumatology
Division of Allergy, Immunology, and Rheumatology
Department of Pediatrics
University of Wisconsin School of Medicine and Public Health
Madison, Wisconsin
Rheumatic Diseases of Childhood

Maria L. Marquez, MD
Professor of Pediatrics
Georgetown University School of Medicine
Director of Pediatrics
La Clinica del Pueblo
Washington, DC
Pediatric Nutrition and Nutritional Disorders

Susan G. Marshall, MD
Professor
Department of Pediatrics
University of Washington School of Medicine;
Director of Medical Education
Seattle Children's Hospital
Seattle, Washington
The Respiratory System

Cory A. McFall, MD
Assistant Professor of Pediatrics
Division of Critical Care Medicine
Medical College of Wisconsin
Milwaukee, Wisconsin
The Acutely Ill or Injured Child

Caitlin L. McGrath, MD, MS
Assistant Professor of Pediatric Infectious Diseases
Washington University School of Medicine
Attending Physician
Division of Pediatric Infectious Diseases
St. Louis Children's Hospital
St. Louis, Missouri
Infectious Diseases

Thomas W. McLean, MD
Professor of Pediatrics
Wake Forest University School of Medicine
Winston-Salem, North Carolina
Oncology

Hiren P. Patel, MD
Clinical Professor of Pediatrics
The Ohio State University College of Medicine;
Chief, Section of Nephrology and Hypertension
Medical Director, Kidney Transplant Program
Nationwide Children's Hospital
Columbus, Ohio
Nephrology and Urology

Barry J. Pelz, MD
Associate Professor of Pediatrics
Medical College of Wisconsin
Division of Allergy and Clinical Immunology
Children's Wisconsin
Milwaukee, Wisconsin
Allergy

Erica ElSeed Peterson, MD
Assistant Professor of Pediatrics
Division of Neonatology
University of South Florida Morsani College of Medicine
Tampa, Florida
Fetal and Neonatal Medicine

Jocelyn Huang Schiller, MD
Clinical Professor of Pediatrics
University of Michigan Medical School
Ann Arbor, Michigan
Neurology

Abigail M. Schuh, MD, MMHPE
Associate Professor of Pediatrics
Medical College of Wisconsin
Milwaukee, Wisconsin
The Profession of Pediatrics

Paola Palma Sisto, MD
Associate Professor of Pediatrics
Medical College of Wisconsin
Division of Endocrinology
Children's Hospital of Wisconsin
Milwaukee, Wisconsin
Endocrinology

Thelma Alessandra Sugrañes, MD
Clinical Geneticist
Nicklaus Children's Health System
Miami, Florida
Human Genetics and Dysmorphology

Christopher Sumski, DO, MEd
Assistant Professor of Pediatrics
Washington University School of Medicine in St. Louis
Division of Pediatric Cardiology
St. Louis Children's Hospital
St. Louis, Missouri
The Cardiovascular System

Sarah P. Supples, MD
Assistant Professor of Pediatrics
Wake Forest University School of Medicine
Winston-Salem, North Carolina
Oncology

Grant D. Syverson, MD
Clinical Associate Professor of Pediatrics
University of North Dakota School of Medicine
Department Chair, Pediatric Subspecialties
Sanford Health
Fargo, North Dakota
Rheumatic Diseases of Childhood

Sussette Szachowicz, MD
Clinical Assistant Professor of Pediatrics
Stead Family Department of Pediatrics
University of Iowa Carver College of Medicine;
Division of Pediatric Gastroenterology, Hepatology, Pancreatology, and Nutrition
University of Iowa Children's Hospital
Iowa City, Iowa
The Digestive System

Julie-An M. Talano, MD
Professor of Pediatrics
Medical College of Wisconsin
Medical Director, Blood and Marrow Transplant
Division of Pediatric Hematology-Oncology
Children's Hospital of Wisconsin
Milwaukee, Wisconsin
Chapter 77: Hemophagocytic Lymphohistiocytosis

Matthew T. Tallar, MD
Assistant Professor of Pediatrics
Medical College of Wisconsin
Division of Allergy and Clinical Immunology
Children's Wisconsin
Milwaukee, Wisconsin
Allergy

Chelsea M. Torres, MD
Assistant Professor of Pediatrics
Division of General Pediatrics
University of South Florida Morsani College of Medicine
Tampa, Florida
Fetal and Neonatal Medicine

Nancy Van Eyk, MD, FRCSC
Associate Professor of Obstetrics and Gynaecology
IWK Health
Dalhousie University
Halifax, Nova Scotia, Canada
Adolescent Medicine

James W. Verbsky, MD, PhD
Professor of Pediatrics and Microbiology and Immunology
Medical Director, Clinical Immunology Research Laboratory
Medical Director, Clinical and Translational Research
Medical College of Wisconsin
Division of Pediatric Rheumatology
Children's Hospital of Wisconsin
Milwaukee, Wisconsin
Immunology

Beth A. Vogt, MD
Associate Professor of Pediatrics
The Ohio State University College of Medicine
Medical Director, Dialysis and Acute Care Nephrology
Section of Nephrology and Hypertension
Nationwide Children's Hospital
Columbus, Ohio
Nephrology and Urology

Surabhi B. Vora, MD, MPH
Associate Professor of Pediatric Infectious Diseases
University of Washington School of Medicine
Clinical Director, Division of Pediatric Infectious Disease
Seattle Children's Hospital
Seattle, Washington
Infectious Diseases

Kevin D. Walter, MD, FAAP
Associate Professor of Orthopedic Surgery and Pediatrics
Associate Fellowship Director, Sports Medicine
Medical College of Wisconsin
Medical Director, Sports Medicine Outreach and Sports Physical Therapy
Children's Wisconsin
Milwaukee, Wisconsin
Orthopedics

Tanner Wright, MD
Associate Professor of Pediatrics
Division of Neonatology
University of South Florida Morsani College of Medicine
USF Center for Families Impacted by Substance Use
Tampa, Florida
Fetal and Neonatal Medicine

Hsi Yen, MD
Assistant Professor of Clinical Dermatology
Keck School of Medicine of University of Southern California
Attending Physician
Division of Dermatology
Children's Hospital Los Angeles
Los Angeles, California
Dermatology

PREFACE

This edition was created in a time of significant change within the practice of pediatrics and medical education. Disruptions brought about by the COVID-19 pandemic, the rapid rise of artificial intelligence in medicine, and the political environment have altered the clinical learning environment and reshaped how future pediatricians synthesize knowledge, make medical decisions, and care for our patients. Our goal as the editors and authors of this textbook is not only to provide the classic, foundational knowledge we use every day, but also to include recent advances in a readable, searchable, and concise text for medical learners at all levels. Mastering this knowledge, when combined with mindful experiences in the rapidly changing world of medicine, will allow our readers to develop the practical wisdom needed to serve our patients and their families.

We hope that this text will help you investigate the common and classic pediatric disorders in a time-honored, logical format, helping you to both acquire and apply knowledge needed to provide high value care. We are honored to be part of the journey of the thousands of learners who rotate through pediatrics, those who will become new providers of pediatric care in the years to come, and those who continue to build on their knowledge.

Abigail M. Schuh, MD, MMHPE
Robert M. Kliegman, MD
Kelsey S. Ryan, MD
Sarah C. Yale, MD
Michelle L. Mitchell, MD

ACKNOWLEDGMENTS

The editors profusely thank Marybeth Thiel, Jennifer Shreiner, and Dan Fitzgerald, as well as their teams, for their assistance and attention to detail. We also again thank our colleague, Carolyn Redman, whose prompting, organizing, and overseeing of the process helped us create this new edition. Finally, we thank our spouses for their patient support throughout the process.

CONTENTS

SECTION 1

THE PROFESSION OF PEDIATRICS

Abigail M. Schuh | Michael N. Levas

CHAPTER 1

Population and Culture: The Care of Children in Society

CARE OF CHILDREN IN SOCIETY

Health care professionals must appreciate the interactions between medical conditions and social, economic, and environmental influences associated with the provision of pediatric care. New technologies and treatments improve morbidity, mortality, and the quality of life for children and their families, but the costs may exacerbate disparities in medical care. The challenge for pediatricians is to deliver care that is socially equitable; integrates psychosocial, cultural, and ethical issues into practice; and ensures that health care is available to all children.

CURRENT CHALLENGES

Challenges that affect children's health outcomes include access to health care; health disparities; supporting their social, cognitive, and emotional lives in the context of families and communities; and addressing environmental factors, especially poverty. Early experiences and environmental stresses interact with the genetic predisposition of every child and, ultimately, may lead to the development of diseases seen in adulthood. Pediatricians have the unique opportunity to address not only acute and chronic illnesses but also environmental and toxic stressors to promote wellness and health maintenance in children.

Many scientific advances have an impact on the growing role of pediatricians. Newer genetic technologies allow the diagnosis of diseases at the molecular level, aid in the selection of medications and therapies, and may provide information on prognosis. Prenatal diagnosis and newborn screening improve the accuracy of early diagnosis and treatment, even when a cure is not yet possible

Challenges persist due to the increasing incidence and prevalence of chronic illness. Chronic illness contributes to nearly two thirds of pediatric acute care hospitalizations (excluding trauma and newborn admissions). In older children, hospitalizations for mental health diagnoses have continued to increase over the past decade. Political unrest, terrorism, and a global pandemic have caused an increased level of anxiety and fear for many families and children. Pediatricians must also address concerns about environmental toxins and the prevalence of physical, emotional, and sexual abuse and violence.

To address these ongoing challenges, many pediatricians now practice as part of a multidisciplinary health care team that includes psychiatrists, psychologists, nurses, and social workers. This **patient-centered medical home model** of care is designed to provide continuous and coordinated care to maximize health outcomes. Other models, such as school-based health and retail medical facilities, may improve access but may not support continuity and coordination of care.

Childhood antecedents of adult health conditions, such as alcoholism, depression, obesity, hypertension, and hyperlipidemia, are increasingly recognized. Infants who are relatively underweight at birth due to maternal malnutrition are at higher risk of developing certain health conditions later in life, including diabetes, heart disease, hypertension, metabolic syndrome, and obesity. Improved neonatal care results in greater survival of preterm, low birthweight, or very low birthweight newborns, increasing the number of children with chronic medical conditions and developmental delays with their lifelong implications. Exposure to **adverse childhood experiences** (ACEs) such as abuse, household dysfunction, bullying, and community violence increases the risk of diabetes, cardiovascular disease, and mental health disorders in adulthood; ACEs are common, with 64% of adults in the United States reporting that they had experienced at least one ACE before age 18.

LANDSCAPE OF HEALTH CARE FOR CHILDREN IN THE UNITED STATES

Complex health, economic, and psychosocial challenges greatly influence the well-being and health outcomes of children. National reports from the Centers for Disease Control and Prevention (CDC) (e.g., https://www.cdc.gov/nchs/data/hus/hus20-21.pdf) provide information about many of these issues. Some of the key issues include the following:

- **Health insurance coverage.** Because of programs like Medicaid and the State Children's Health Insurance Program, children are more likely than adults to have health insurance coverage. For example, in 2023, 39% of children were covered by Medicaid. The continued decline in uninsured children nationally over the past decade left 5.3% of U.S. children lacking insurance in 2023. However, differences in state policies and fluctuations in support for these programs call for pediatricians to be aware of access for their patients.
- **Prenatal and perinatal care.** Over 75% of women begin prenatal care in the first trimester, with lower rates noted

in Hispanic, Black, and American Indian/Alaska Native populations. Less than 1 in 10 women had delayed or no prenatal care.

- **Preterm births.** The incidence of preterm births (<37 weeks) was 10.4% in 2023, with continued racial and ethnic disparities. However, the rates of low birthweight infants (≤2,500 g [8.6% of all births]) and very low birthweight infants (≤1,500 g [1.4% of all births]) are essentially unchanged since 2006.
- **Birthrate in adolescents.** The national birthrate among adolescents has been steadily declining since 1990, reaching its lowest rate (13.1 births per 1,000) for 15- to 19-year-old adolescents in 2023.
- **Adolescent abortions.** The rate of abortions among adolescents had been decreasing since its peak in 1988, with adolescents aged 15–19 years accounting for 8.3% of all reported abortions in 2022 (abortion rate of 5.6 abortions per 1,000 adolescents that age). The U.S. Supreme Court's overturning of Roe vs. Wade in 2022 eliminated the federal constitutional right to abortion; although adolescent-specific numbers are not yet available, the Guttmacher Institute estimates that 15.4 abortions were performed per 1,000 women in 2024 (an increase of 12% since 2020).
- **Infant mortality.** In 2024 the overall infant mortality rate in the United States was 5.4 deaths per 1,000 live births. However, disparity remains among ethnic groups. Infant mortality among non-Hispanic Black women is nearly double the national average. U.S. geographic variability persists, with the highest mortality rates in the South.
- **Initiation and maintenance of breast-feeding.** In 2021, 84.1% of newborn infants started breast-feeding after birth. That same year, rates of breast-feeding at 6 and 12 months were 59.8% and 39.5%. Breast-feeding rates vary by ethnicity (higher rates in non-Hispanic White and Hispanic mothers) and education (highest in women with a bachelor's degree or higher).
- **Cause of death in U.S. children.** The overall causes of death in all children (1–24 years of age) in the United States in 2022, in order of frequency, were unintentional injuries, homicide, suicide, malignant neoplasms, congenital anomalies, and heart disease (Table 1.1). After a steady decline in death rates among children for nearly 3 decades, the childhood death rate rose in both 2020 and 2021. In these same years, firearms contributed to the deaths of more children than any other type of injury or illness, surpassing motor vehicle collisions as the leading cause of death among American youth.
- **Hospital admissions for children and adolescents.** Pediatric hospitalizations in the United States have decreased steadily since 2009, yet there were still over 1.7 million non–birth-related hospitalizations for patients aged 20 and younger in 2019. Respiratory illnesses are the predominant cause of hospitalization for children 1–9 years of age, and mental illness is the most common cause of admission for adolescents. Access to care is a concern for patients. A 2025 study showed that hospitals closed nearly 30% of pediatric inpatient units in the United States between 2008 and 2022, with rural areas disproportionately affected.

TABLE 1.1 Causes of Death by Age in the United States, 2022

AGE GROUP (YEAR)	CAUSES OF DEATH IN ORDER OF FREQUENCY
1–4	Unintentional injuries Congenital anomalies Homicide Malignant neoplasms Influenza/pneumonia Heart disease
5–9	Unintentional injuries (accidents) Malignant neoplasms Congenital anomalies Homicide Influenza and pneumonia Heart disease
10–14	Unintentional injuries Suicide Malignant neoplasms Homicide Congenital anomalies Heart disease
15–24	Unintentional injuries Homicide Suicide Malignant neoplasms Heart disease COVID-19

From National Center for Health Statistics (US). Health, United States, 2022. https://wisqars.cdc.gov/lcd/?o=LCD&y1=2022&y2=2022&ct=10&cc=ALL&g=00&s=0&r=0&ry=2&e=0&ar=lcd1age&at=groups&ag=lcd1age&a1=0&a2=199.

- **Significant adolescent health challenges: substance use and abuse.** Overall, substance use among U.S. adolescents has decreased since before the COVID-19 pandemic but remains a significant public health concern as adolescent drug fatalities (primarily fentanyl overdoses) more than doubled between 2018 and 2023. Forty-two percent of 12th-grade students report using alcohol in the past 12 months, and 26% report having been drunk. Marijuana is commonly used, with 26% of 12th graders reporting use in the past 12 months; 7% of students reported using illicit drugs other than marijuana. Narcotics other than heroin and fentanyl (including Vicodin, OxyContin, Percocet, etc.) were used by 0.6% of 12th graders in 2024. Tobacco cigarette use has declined among teens over the past decade, but vaping of both nicotine and marijuana remains a concern because vaping has been proven to pose significant health risks to both users and nonusers.
- **Children in foster care.** In 2022, 368,500 children were in the foster care system; of those children, 52% were reunited with families and 28% were adopted. Children leaving foster care often lack the emotional or financial support necessary to succeed in life and experience homelessness and/or joblessness and frequently do not graduate from high school.

OTHER HEALTH ISSUES THAT AFFECT CHILDREN IN THE UNITED STATES

- **Obesity.** Obesity is the second leading cause of death in the United States (estimated 300,000 deaths annually). Rates of childhood obesity continue to rise. The prevalence of obesity among children aged 2–19 years was 19.7% in 2020. Obesity rates among Hispanic and Black populations were well above 20%.

- **Sedentary lifestyle.** With advancing technology, children spend more time in front of a screen (telephone, television, videogames, computer, etc.); some spend more than 7.5 hours for entertainment per day. This does not include additional time spent on a computer for educational purposes.
- **Motor vehicle accidents and injuries.** In 2022, 1,129 children 14 years of age or younger died in motor vehicle crashes, and more than 156,000 were injured. Thirty-nine percent of those killed were not appropriately restrained. In 2022, 1,919 teens, aged 16–19, were killed in motor vehicle crashes. Drivers aged 16–19 are nearly three times more likely than drivers over age 20 to be involved in a fatal crash.
- **Child maltreatment.** In 2023, 1,968 children died of abuse and neglect in the United States, with at least 1 in 7 children having experienced child abuse and/or neglect in the past year. At least 1 in 4 girls and 1 in 20 boys has experienced child sexual abuse at some point in their lifetime, and approximately 90% of childhood sexual abuse is perpetrated by a person known to the child or their family members. Experiencing physical abuse, neglect, or sexual abuse can lead to short- and long-term physical and mental health complications.
- **Toxic stress in childhood and its effect on adult health.** There is a growing understanding of how biological, developmental, and environmental stressors interact with an individual's genetic makeup to influence health outcomes. Research increasingly shows that toxic stress experienced during childhood can have lasting effects on physical, emotional, and behavioral health well into adulthood. By screening for and addressing factors that support or hinder healthy development early on, we have a critical opportunity to improve lifelong health outcomes. The emerging field of epigenetics further underscores this connection, revealing how environmental stress can alter gene expression and contribute to long-term changes in development, health, and behavior.
- **Social media.** The implications of social media on adolescent health are vast and multifaceted, affecting both physical and mental well-being. Although social media offers opportunities for connection, learning, and self-expression, it also poses significant risks to adolescents' health. Numerous studies have linked excessive social media use with increased feelings of anxiety, depression, and stress in adolescents. Constant exposure to curated, idealized portrayals of others' lives can lead to social comparison, feelings of inadequacy, and low self-esteem. The anonymity of social media can facilitate bullying, which can have severe consequences on adolescents' mental health. Victims of cyberbullying may experience depression, anxiety, and, in extreme cases, suicidal ideation. Social media platforms often emphasize a narrow, idealized standard of beauty, which can contribute to body dissatisfaction. Adolescents, especially those who are highly engaged with platforms like Instagram, may develop poor body image and be more prone to eating disorders like anorexia or bulimia.
- **Telehealth.** Telehealth has become a transformative tool in addressing various health care issues in pediatrics, offering both opportunities and challenges for improving access to care, enhancing the quality of treatment, and ensuring better health outcomes for children. One of the most significant advantages of telehealth is its ability to overcome geographic barriers. For families living in rural or underserved areas where pediatric specialists are scarce, telehealth allows them to access high-quality care without having to travel long distances. This is particularly beneficial for children with chronic conditions who require ongoing care. Parents, especially those with young children, may find it difficult to take time off work or navigate transportation challenges to visit a doctor. Telehealth may decrease the need for in-person visits, reducing stress on families and saving time and money.
- **Military deployment and children.** Armed conflicts and political unrest affect millions of adults and their children worldwide each year. Active duty and National Guard/Reserve servicemen and servicewomen are parents to more than a million children. One third of troops returning from armed conflicts have a mental health condition (alcoholism, depression, and post-traumatic stress disorder) or have experienced a traumatic brain injury. Their children are affected by these morbidities as well as by the psychologic impact of deployment. Child maltreatment is more prevalent in families of U.S.-enlisted soldiers during combat deployment than in non-deployed soldiers.

HEALTH DISPARITIES IN HEALTH CARE FOR CHILDREN

Health disparities are the differences that remain after accounting for patients' needs, preferences, and the availability of health care. Social conditions and inequity, discrimination, social stress, language barriers, and poverty are antecedents to and associated causes of health disparities. Disparities in infant mortality relate to poor access to prenatal care and the lack of access to appropriate health services for women, and disparities that begin in childhood have been linked to chronic illness in adulthood. As such, pediatricians play an important role in promoting health equity in their communities. Some important inequities to be aware of include:

- Infant mortality increases as the mother's level of education decreases.
- Children from poor families are less likely to be immunized and receive dental care at 4 years of age.
- Children with Medicaid/public coverage are less likely to be in excellent health than children with private health insurance.

- Children of ethnic minorities and those from poor families are less likely to have physician office or hospital outpatient visits and more likely to have hospital emergency department visits and higher rates of hospital admission.

MENTAL HEALTH IN CHILDHOOD

Mental health is closely intertwined with children's physical health, and pediatricians play an important role in identifying signs and symptoms of mental health conditions that warrant further evaluation and treatment (see Section 4). An estimated 1 in 5 children, ages 13–18 years, has a mental health condition; half of all lifetime cases of mental illness begin by age 14 years. The average delay between onset of symptoms and intervention is 8–10 years. Suicide is the second leading cause of death for children ages 10–14 years and third leading cause of death for children 15–24, making early recognition of mental health concerns paramount. Nationwide, there is a lack of adequate mental health services for children. In 2021 the American Academy of Pediatrics (AAP), the American Academy of Child and Adolescent Psychiatry (AACAP), and the Children's Hospital Association (CHA) declared a national state of emergency for child and adolescent mental health to raise awareness of this issue and advocate for affordable, comprehensive mental and behavioral health care for all youth.

CULTURE

The diversity of the United States requires that health care workers seek to understand the effect of health, illness, and treatment from the patients' and families' context and perspective. This requires open-ended questions, such as: "What *worries* you the most about your child's illness?" and "What do you *think* has caused your child's illness?" One must address concepts and beliefs about how patients/families interact with health professionals, as well as their spiritual and religious approach to health and health care from a cultural perspective, allowing incorporation of differences in perspectives, values, or beliefs into the care plan. Conflicts that may arise because of religious or cultural practices may lead to the possibility and/or perception of child abuse and neglect, which are required, by law, to be reported to social service authorities (see Chapter 21).

Complementary and alternative medicine (CAM) practices constitute a part of the broad cultural perspective. Therapeutic modalities for CAM include biochemical, lifestyle, biomechanical, and bioenergetic treatments, as well as homeopathy. It is estimated that 20–40% of healthy children and more than 60% of children with chronic illness use CAM and do not always reveal CAM use to their physician. Screening for CAM use can aid the pediatrician's counseling and minimize unintentional adverse interactions.

PEARLS FOR PRACTITIONERS

See The Profession of Pediatrics: Pearls for Practitioners at the end of this section.

REVIEW QUESTIONS

Available online.

CHAPTER 2

Professionalism

CONCEPT OF PROFESSIONALISM

Professions require specialized knowledge, skills, and training, typically acquired through formal education and experience, and are governed by ethical standards, codes of conduct, and a set of recognized responsibilities that practitioners must adhere to. A profession often involves a commitment to providing services that benefit society, and individuals in a profession are typically held to high standards of competence and ethics.

The activities of medical professionals are subject to explicit public rules of accountability. Governmental and other authorities at city, state, and federal levels grant limited autonomy to professional organizations and their membership through regulations, licensing requirements, and standards of service (e.g., Medicare, Medicaid, and the Food and Drug Administration). The Department of Health and Human Services regulates physician behavior in conducting research with the goal of protecting human subjects. The National Practitioner Data Bank contains information about physicians and other health care practitioners who have been disciplined by a state licensing board, professional society, hospital, or health plan or named in medical malpractice judgments or settlements. Hospitals are required to review information in this data bank every 2 years as part of clinician re-credentialing. There are accrediting agencies for medical schools, such as the Liaison Committee on Medical Education (LCME), and postgraduate training, such as the Accreditation Council for Graduate Medical Education (ACGME).

Public trust in physicians is based on the physician's commitment to altruism, a cornerstone of the Hippocratic oath and an important rite of passage and part of medical school commencement ceremonies. The core of professionalism is embedded in the daily healing work of the physician and encompasses the patient-physician relationship. Professionalism includes an appreciation for the cultural and religious/spiritual health beliefs of the patient, incorporating the ethical and moral values of the profession (e.g., justice, courage, and wisdom) and the moral values of the patient. Professionalism also includes the understanding that dire circumstances may require physicians to provide care in uncertain situations, whether due to a natural disaster or a global pandemic. The ability of medical professionals to adapt in an ever-changing environment is a vital component of professionalism within medicine.

PROFESSIONALISM FOR PEDIATRICIANS

The American Board of Pediatrics (ABP) adopted professional standards in 2000, and the American Academy of Pediatrics (AAP) updated the policy statement and technical report on Professionalism in 2007, as follows:

- **Honesty/integrity** is the consistent regard for the highest standards of behavior and the refusal to violate one's personal and professional codes. Maintaining integrity requires awareness of situations that may result in conflict of interest or that may result in personal gain at the expense of the best interest of the patient.

- **Reliability/responsibility** includes accountability to one's patients, their families, society, and the medical community to ensure that all needs are addressed. There also must be a willingness to accept responsibility for errors.
- **Respect for others** requires the pediatrician to treat all persons with respect and regard for their individual worth and dignity; be aware of emotional, personal, family, and cultural influences on a patient's well-being, rights, and choices of medical care; and respect appropriate patient confidentiality.
- **Compassion/empathy** requires the pediatrician to listen attentively, respond humanely to patient/family concerns, and provide appropriate empathy for and relief of pain, discomfort, and anxiety as part of daily practice.
- **Self-improvement** is the pursuit of and commitment to providing the highest quality of health care through lifelong learning and education. This includes learning from errors, aspiring to excellence through self-evaluation, and accepting the critiques of others.
- **Self-awareness/knowledge of limits** includes recognition of the need for guidance and supervision when faced with new or complex responsibilities, the effect of behavior on others, and establishing appropriate professional boundaries.
- **Communication/collaboration** is crucial to providing the best care for patients. Pediatricians must work cooperatively and communicate effectively with patients, their families, and all health care providers involved in the care of their patients.
- **Altruism/advocacy** refers to unselfish regard for and devotion to the welfare of others. It is a key element of professionalism. Self-interest or the interests of other parties should not interfere with the care of one's patients and their families.

PEARLS FOR PRACTITIONERS

See The Profession of Pediatrics: Pearls for Practitioners at the end of this section.

REVIEW QUESTION

Available online.

CHAPTER 3

Ethics and Legal Issues

ETHICS IN HEALTH CARE

The ethics of health care and medical decision-making relies on **values**. Sometimes, ethical decision-making in medicine is a matter of choosing the least harmful option among many adverse alternatives. In the day-to-day practice of medicine, major ethical challenges are infrequent although always possible.

The legal system defines the minimal standards of behavior required of physicians and the rest of society through the legislative, regulatory, and judicial systems. Laws support the principle of **confidentiality** for teenagers who are competent to decide about medical issues. Using the concept of **limited confidentiality**, parents, teenagers, and the pediatrician may all agree to openly discuss serious health challenges, such as suicidal ideation and pregnancy. This reinforces the long-term goal of supporting the developing autonomy and identity of the teenager while encouraging appropriate conversations with parents.

Ethical problems usually derive from **value differences** among patients, families, and clinicians regarding choices and options in the provision of health care. Resolving these value differences involves several important ethical principles. **Autonomy**, based on the principle of **respect for persons**, means that competent adult patients can make choices about their health care after being appropriately informed about their health condition and the risks and benefits of alternative diagnostic tests and treatments. **Paternalism** challenges the principle of autonomy and involves the clinician deciding what is best for the patient. Under certain circumstances (e.g., when a patient has a life-threatening medical condition or a significant psychiatric disorder and is threatening self or others), paternalism is an accepted alternative to autonomy.

Other important ethical principles are those of **beneficence** (doing good), **nonmaleficence** (doing no harm or as little harm as possible), and **justice** (the values involved in the equal distribution of goods, services, benefits, and burdens to the individual, family, or society).

ETHICAL PRINCIPLES RELATED TO INFANTS, CHILDREN, AND ADOLESCENTS

Infants and young children do not have the capacity for making medical decisions; thus decision-making falls onto their parents or legal guardians. Parental decision-making should be guided by what is in the best interest of the child. In certain older children, assent can be obtained for medical decision-making. Obtaining the **assent** of a child is the process in which the child is involved in decision-making with information appropriate to the child's capacity to understand. Most adolescents (<18 years of age) cannot legally provide informed consent for medical decisions; however, they can and should provide assent. Exceptions include medical decisions made by an adolescent for certain medical conditions, notably sexual and mental health. Emancipated minors are legally able to provide informed consent for medical decision-making.

The principle of shared medical decision-making is appropriate, but the process may be limited because of issues of confidentiality. A parent's concern about the side effects of immunization raises a conflict between the need to protect and support the health of the individual and of the public. Parental decisions that are dangerous should be challenged.

LEGAL ISSUES

All competent patients of an age defined legally by each state (usually ≥18 years of age) are autonomous regarding their health decisions. To have decision-making capacity, patients must meet the following requirements:

- Understand the nature of the medical interventions and procedures, understand the risks and benefits of these interventions, and be able to communicate their decision.
- Reason, deliberate, and weigh the risks and benefits using their understanding about the implications of the decision on their own welfare.
- Apply a set of personal values to the decision-making process and show an awareness of the possible conflicts or differences in values as applied to the decisions to be made.

These requirements must be placed within the context of medical care and applied to each case with its unique characteristics. Most young children are not able to meet these requirements; hence, parents or guardians serve as their legal surrogate decision-maker unless circumstances preclude them from making decisions in the child's best interest (e.g., abuse).

It is important to become familiar with state law because it, not federal law, determines when an adolescent can consent to medical care and when parents may access confidential adolescent medical information. In 2003 the Health Insurance Portability and Accountability Act (HIPAA) became effective, requiring a minimal standard of confidentiality protection. The law confers less confidentiality protection to minors than to adults. It is the pediatrician's responsibility to inform minors of their confidentiality rights and help them exercise these rights under the HIPAA regulations.

Under special circumstances, non-autonomous adolescents are granted the legal right to consent under state law when they are considered mature or emancipated minors or because of certain public health considerations, as follows:

- **Mature minors.** Some states recognize adolescents who meet the cognitive criteria and emotional maturity for competence and provide them with legal decision-making capacity. In many states where abortion is legal, mature minors can make decisions about abortion without parental consent.
- **Emancipated minors.** Children who are legally emancipated from their parents may seek medical treatment without parental consent. The definition varies from state to state but generally includes children who have graduated from high school; members of the armed forces; those who are married, are pregnant, or have children; runaways; those who live apart from their parents; and those who are financially independent or declared emancipated by a court.
- **Interests of the state (public health).** State legislatures have concluded that minors with certain medical conditions, such as sexually transmitted infections and other contagious diseases, pregnancy (including prevention through the use of birth control), certain mental illnesses, and drug and alcohol abuse, may seek treatment for these conditions autonomously. States have an interest in limiting the spread of disease that may endanger the public health and in eliminating barriers to access for the treatment of certain conditions.

ETHICAL ISSUES IN PRACTICE

Clinicians should engage children and adolescents based on their developmental capacity in discussions about medical plans so that the child has a good understanding of the nature of the treatments and alternatives, side effects, and expected outcomes. There should be an assessment of the patient's understanding of the clinical situation, how the patient is responding, and the factors that may influence the patient's decisions. Pediatricians should always listen to and appreciate patients' requests for confidentiality and their hopes and wishes. The goal is to help nourish a child's capacity to become as autonomous as is appropriate to their developmental stage.

Confidentiality

Confidentiality is crucial to the provision of medical care and is an important part of the basis for a trusting patient-family-physician relationship. Confidentiality means that information about a patient should not be shared without consent. If confidentiality is broken, patients may experience great harm and may not seek needed medical care. See Chapter 66 for a discussion of confidentiality in the care of adolescents.

Ethical Issues in Genetic Testing and Screening in Children

The goal of **screening** is to identify diseases when there is no clinically identifiable risk factor for disease. Screening should take place only when there is a treatment available or when a diagnosis would benefit the child. **Testing** usually is performed when there is some clinically identifiable risk factor. Genetic testing and screening present special problems because test results have important implications. Some genetic screening (sickle cell anemia or cystic fibrosis) may reveal a carrier state, which may lead to choices about reproduction or create financial, psychosocial, and interpersonal problems (e.g., guilt, shame, social stigma, and discrimination in insurance and jobs). Collaboration with, or referral to, a clinical geneticist is appropriate in helping the family with the complex issues of genetic counseling when a genetic disorder is detected or anticipated.

Newborn screening should not be used as a surrogate for parental testing. Examples of diseases that can be diagnosed by genetic screening, even though the manifestations of the disease process do not appear until later in life, are polycystic kidney disease; Huntington disease; certain cancers, such as breast cancer in some ethnic populations; and hemochromatosis. For their own purposes, parents may pressure the pediatrician to order genetic tests when the child is still young. Testing for these disorders should be delayed until the child has the capacity for informed consent or assent and is competent to make decisions, unless there is a direct benefit to the child at the time of testing.

Religious Issues and Ethics

The pediatrician is required to act in the best interests of the child, even when religious tenets may interfere with the health and well-being of the child. When an infant or child whose parents have a religious prohibition against a blood transfusion needs a transfusion to save the child's life, the courts always intervene to allow a transfusion. In contrast, parents with strong religious beliefs may refuse immunizations for their children. States may use the principle of **distributive justice** to require immunization of all during outbreaks or epidemics, including individuals who object on religious grounds.

Children as Human Subjects in Research

The goal of research is to develop new and generalized knowledge. Parents may give informed permission for children to participate in research under certain conditions. Children cannot give consent but may assent or dissent to research protocols, and these decisions should be respected. Special federal regulations have been developed to protect child and adolescent participants in human investigation. These regulations provide additional safeguards beyond those for adult participants while still providing the opportunity for children to benefit from the scientific advances of research.

Many parents with seriously ill children hope that the research protocol will have a direct benefit for their child. The researcher should be sensitive and compassionate in explaining to the parents that research does not guarantee a (better) treatment.

Ethical Issues Surrounding Scarce Resource Allocation

Medical resources are finite and under certain circumstances, notably a global pandemic, risk becoming scarce. In such situations it is possible that allocation strategies need to be developed and implemented. The ethical principles of justice, beneficence, and nonmaleficence serve as guiding pillars to ensure that resources are allocated in a fair manner.

PEARLS FOR PRACTITIONERS

See The Profession of Pediatrics: Pearls for Practitioners at the end of this section.

REVIEW QUESTION

Available online.

CHAPTER 4

Palliative Care and End-of-Life Issues

The death of a child is one of life's most difficult experiences. The **palliative care** approach is defined as patient- and family-centered care that optimizes quality of life by anticipating, preventing, and treating suffering. This approach should be instituted when medical diagnosis, intervention, and treatment cannot reasonably be expected to affect the imminence of death. Central to this approach is the willingness of clinicians to look beyond traditional medical goals of curing disease and preserving life and toward enhancing the life of the child with assistance from family members and close friends. High-quality palliative care is an expected standard at the end of life.

Palliative care in pediatrics is not simply end-of-life care. Children needing palliative care have been described as having conditions that fall into four basic groups based on the goal of treatment. These include conditions of the following scenarios:

- A cure is possible but failure is not uncommon (e.g., cancer with a poor prognosis).
- Long-term treatment is provided with a goal of maintaining quality of life (e.g., cystic fibrosis).
- Treatment that is exclusively palliative after the diagnosis of a progressive condition is made (e.g., trisomy 13).
- Treatments are available for severe, nonprogressive disability in patients who are vulnerable to repeated health complications (e.g., severe spastic quadriparesis with difficulty in controlling symptoms).

These conditions present different timelines and different models of medical intervention while sharing the need to attend to concrete elements affecting the quality of a child's life and possible death and are mediated by medical, psychosocial, cultural, and spiritual concerns.

Palliative care can make important contributions to the end-of-life and bereavement issues for families without time to prepare for an unexpected death. This may become complicated in circumstances where the cause of the death must be fully explored, such as possible child abuse or neglect, because this subjects the family to intense scrutiny and may create guilt and anger directed at the medical team.

PALLIATIVE AND END-OF-LIFE CARE

Palliative treatment is directed toward the relief of symptoms as well as assistance with anticipated adaptations that may cause distress and diminish the quality of life of the dying child. Elements of palliative care include pain management, expertise with feeding and nutritional issues at the end of life, and management of symptoms, such as minimizing nausea and vomiting, bowel obstruction, labored breathing, and fatigue. Psychologic elements of palliative care have profound importance and include sensitivity to bereavement, a developmental perspective of a child's understanding of death, clarification of the goals of care, and ethical issues. Palliative care is delivered through a multidisciplinary approach, giving a broad range of expertise to patients and families as well as providing a supportive network for the caregivers. Caregivers involved may be pediatricians, nurses, mental health professionals, social workers, and pastors.

A model of integrated palliative care rests on the following principles:

- **Respect for the dignity of patients and families.** The clinician should respect and listen to patient and family goals, preferences, and choices. School-age children can articulate preferences about how they wish to be treated. Adolescents can engage in decision-making (see Section 12). **Advanced care** (advance directives) should be discussed with the child and parents to determine what they would like as treatment options as the end of life nears. Differences of opinion between the family and pediatrician should be addressed by identifying the multiple perspectives, reflecting on possible conflicts, and altruistically coming to agreements that validate the patient and family perspectives yet reflect sound practice. **Hospital ethics committees** and consultation services are important resources for the pediatrician and family members.
- **Access to comprehensive and compassionate palliative care.** The clinician should address the physical symptoms,

comfort, and functional capacity, with special attention to pain and other symptoms associated with the dying process; respond empathically to psychologic distress and human suffering; and provide treatment options. Respite should be available at any time during the illness to allow the family and caregivers to rest and recover.

- **Use of interdisciplinary resources.** Because of the complexity of care, no one clinician can provide all needed services. The team members may include primary and subspecialty physicians, nurses in the hospital/facility or for home visits, the pain management team, psychologists, social workers, pastoral ministers, schoolteachers, friends of the family, and peers of the child. The child and family should decide who is involved in care during all phases of the illness process.
- **Acknowledgment and support provisions for caregivers.** The primary caregivers of the child, family, and friends need opportunities to address their own emotional concerns. Team meetings to address thoughts and feelings of team members are crucial. Institutional support may include time to attend funerals, counseling for the staff, opportunities for families to return to the hospital, and scheduled ceremonies to commemorate the death of the child.
- **Commitment to quality improvement of palliative care through research and education.** Hospitals should develop support systems and staff to monitor the quality of care continually, assess the need for appropriate resources, and evaluate the responses of the patient and family members to the treatment program.

Hospice care is a treatment program for the end of life that provides the range of palliative care services by an interdisciplinary team including specialists in the bereavement and end-of-life process. In 2010 legislation was passed allowing children covered under Medicaid or the Children's Health Insurance Program (CHIP) to receive access simultaneously to hospice care and curative care.

BEREAVEMENT

Bereavement refers to the process of psychologic and spiritual accommodation to death on the part of the child and the child's family. **Grief** has been defined as the emotional response caused by a loss, which may include pain, distress, and physical and emotional suffering. It is a normal adaptive human response to death. Assessing the coping resources and vulnerabilities of the affected family before death occurs is central to the palliative care approach.

Parental grief is recognized as being more intense and sustained than other types of grief. Most parents work through their grief. Complicated grief, a pathologic manifestation of continued and disabling grief, is rare. Parents who share their problems with others during the child's illness, who have access to psychologic support during the last month of their child's life, and who have had closure sessions with the attending staff are more likely to resolve their grief. In the era of technology, some parents may find solace in connecting with other parents with similar experiences in an online forum.

A particularly difficult issue for parents is whether to talk with their child about the child's imminent death. Although evidence suggests that sharing accurate and truthful information with a dying child is beneficial, each individual case presents its own complexities based on the child's age, cognitive development, disease, timeline of disease, and parental psychologic state. Parents are more likely to regret not talking with their child about death than having done so.

COGNITIVE ISSUES IN CHILDREN AND ADOLESCENTS: UNDERSTANDING DEATH AND DYING

The pediatrician should communicate with children about what is happening to them while respecting the cultural and personal preferences of the family. A developmental understanding of children's concepts of health and illness helps frame the discussion and can help parents understand how their child is grappling with the situation. Piaget's theories of cognitive development, which help illustrate children's concepts of death and disease, are categorized as sensorimotor, preoperational, concrete operations, and formal operations.

For children up to 2 years of age (sensorimotor), death is seen as a separation, and there is no specific concept of death. The associated behaviors in grieving children of this age usually include protesting and difficulty of attachment to other adults. The degree of difficulty depends on the availability of other nurturing people with whom the child has a good previous attachment.

Children from 3–5 years of age (preoperational; sometimes called *the magic years*) have trouble grasping the meaning of the illness and the permanence of the death. Their language skills at this age make understanding their moods and behavior difficult. Because of a developing sense of guilt, death may be viewed as punishment. If a child previously wished a sibling dead, the death may be seen psychologically as being caused by the child's wishful thinking. They can feel overwhelmed when confronted with the strong emotional reactions of their parents.

In children ages 6–11 years of age (late preoperational to concrete operational), the finality of death gradually comes to be understood. Magical thinking gives way to a need for detailed information to gain a sense of control. Older children in this range have a strong need to control their emotions by compartmentalizing and intellectualizing.

In adolescents older than 12 years of age (formal operations), death is a reality and seen as universal and irreversible. Adolescents handle death issues at the abstract or philosophical level and can be realistic. They may also avoid emotional expression and information, instead relying on anger or disdain. Their wishes, hopes, and fears should be attended to and respected.

CULTURAL, RELIGIOUS, AND SPIRITUAL CONCERNS ABOUT PALLIATIVE CARE AND END-OF-LIFE DECISIONS

Understanding the family's religious/spiritual or cultural beliefs and values about death and dying can help the pediatrician work with the family to integrate these beliefs, values, and practices into the palliative care plan. Cultures vary regarding the roles family members have, the site of treatment for dying people, and the preparation of the body. Some ethnic groups expect the clinical team to speak with the oldest family member or only to the head of the family, outside of the patient's presence, whereas others involve the entire extended family in decision-making. For some families, dying at home can bring the family bad luck; others believe that the patient's spirit will become lost if the death occurs in the hospital. In some traditions, the health care team cleans and prepares the body, whereas in others, family members prefer to complete this ritual. Religious/spiritual or cultural practices may include prayer, anointing, laying on of the hands, an exorcism ceremony to undo a curse, amulets, and other religious objects placed on the child or at the bedside. Families differ in the idea of organ donation and the acceptance of autopsy. Decisions, rituals, and withholding of palliative or lifesaving procedures that could harm the child or are not in the best interests of the child should be addressed. Quality palliative care attends to this complexity and helps parents and families navigate the death of a child while honoring the familial, cultural, and spiritual values.

ETHICAL ISSUES IN END-OF-LIFE DECISION-MAKING

Before speaking with a child about death, the caregiver should assess the child's age, experience, and level of development; the child's understanding and involvement in end-of-life decision-making; the parents' emotional acceptance of death; their coping strategies; and their philosophical, spiritual, and cultural views of death. These may change over time. The use of open-ended questions to repeatedly assess these areas contributes to the end-of-life process. The care of a dying child can create ethical dilemmas involving **autonomy**, **beneficence** (doing good), **nonmaleficence** (doing no harm), truth telling, confidentiality, or the physician's duty. It is extremely difficult for parents to know when the burdens of continued medical care are no longer appropriate for their child and they may, at times, rely on the medical team for guidance. The beliefs and values of what constitutes quality of life, when life ceases to be worth living, and religious/spiritual, cultural, and philosophical beliefs may differ between families and health care workers. The most important ethical principle is what is in the best interest of the child as determined through the process of **shared decision-making**, **informed consent** from the parents, and **assent** from the child. Sensitive and meaningful communication with the family, in their own terms, is essential. The physician, patient, and family must negotiate the goals of continued medical treatment while recognizing the burdens and benefits of the medical intervention plan. There is no ethical or legal difference between withholding treatment and withdrawing treatment, although many parents and physicians see the latter as more challenging. Family members and the patient should agree about what are appropriate **do not resuscitate** (also called **DNR**) orders. Foregoing some measures does not preclude other measures being implemented based on the needs and wishes of the patient and family. When there are serious differences among parents, children, and physicians on these matters, the physician may consult with the **hospital ethics committee** or, as a last resort, turn to the legal system by filing a report about potential abuse or neglect.

ORGAN DONATION IN PEDIATRICS

The gap between supply and demand of transplantable organs in children is widening as more patients need a transplant without a concomitant increase in the organ donor pool. Organ donation can occur one of two ways: after fulfilling criteria for neurologic (brain) death or through a process of donation after circulatory death (DCD). Organ procurement, donation, and transplantation are strictly regulated by governmental agencies to ensure proper and fair allocation of donated organs for transplantation. It is important that pediatric medical specialists and pediatricians be well acquainted with the strategies and methods of organ donation to help acquaint both the donor family and the recipient family with the process and address expectations. Areas of concern within pediatric organ donation include availability of and access to donor organs; oversight and control of the process; pediatric medical and surgical consultation and continued care throughout the transplantation process; ethical, social, financial, and follow-up; insurance coverage; and public awareness of the need for organ donors. Organ donation and organ transplantation can provide significant life-extending benefits to a child who has a failing organ and is awaiting transplant, while at the same time place a high emotional impact on the donor family after the loss of a child.

PEARLS FOR PRACTITIONERS

See The Profession of Pediatrics: Pearls for Practitioners at the end of this section.

REVIEW QUESTION

Available online.

Suggested Readings

American Academy of Pediatrics, Committee on Bioethics, Fallat ME, Glover J. Professionalism in pediatrics: statement of principles. *Pediatrics*. 2007;120(4):895–897.

Committee on Hospital Care, Section on Critical Care, Section on Surgery, Committee on Bioethics. Pediatric Organ Donation and Transplantation: Across the Care Continuum. *Pediatrics*. 2023;152(2):e2023062923.

National Center for Health Statistics. *Health, United States, 2020-2021: Annual Perspective*. Hyattsville, MD; 2023.

National Center for Health Statistics. National Health Interview Survey, 2024. Public-use data file and documentation. https://www.cdc.gov/nchs/nhis/documentation/index.html. 2025.

National Consensus Project for Quality Palliative Care. *Clinical Practice Guidelines for Quality Palliative Care*, 4th edition. Richmond, VA: National Coalition for Hospice and Palliative Care; 2018. https://www.nationalcoalitionhpc.org/ncp.

PEARLS FOR PRACTITIONERS

CHAPTER 1

Population and Culture: The Care of Children in Society

- Pediatricians must continue to address major issues affecting children's health outcomes, including access to care, health disparities, and environmental factors including toxic stressors such as poverty and violence.
- The significant increase in the number of children with a chronic medical condition (e.g., asthma, obesity, attention-deficit/hyperactivity disorder) affects both inpatient and outpatient care.
- Addressing the following as a part of routine health care allows pediatricians to impact health care outcomes:
  - Toxic stressors (e.g., maternal stress, poverty, exposure to violence)
  - The use of electronic nicotine delivery systems or e-cigarettes
  - Sedentary lifestyles as children spend an increased amount of time in front of a screen (television, videogames, computers, cell phones)
  - Early recognition of mental illness (It is estimated that 1 in 5 adolescents has a mental health condition.)
  - Use of complementary and alternative medicine (to minimize unintended interactions)

CHAPTER 2

Professionalism

- The activities of medical professionals are subject to explicit public rules of accountability developed by governmental and other authorities.
- The public trust of physicians is based on the physician's commitment to altruism.
- Extreme circumstances, such as a natural disaster or global pandemic, may necessitate adaptability as physicians expand how they help others by using their medical knowledge and clinical skills in unique and uncertain situations.
- The policy statement on professionalism released by the American Board of Pediatrics emphasizes honesty/integrity, reliability/responsibility, respect for others, compassion/empathy, self-improvement, self-awareness/knowledge of limits, communication/collaboration, and altruism/advocacy.

CHAPTER 3

Ethics and Legal Issues

- Important ethical principles that help guide medical decision-making include autonomy, beneficence, nonmaleficence, and justice.
- The ability to legally make medical decisions for oneself depends on the patient's age, maturity, and determination of competence. Parents (or guardians) serve as medical decision-makers for most children, and these decisions should always be made within the child's best interest.
- Key ethical principles in the care of pediatric patients include autonomy (addressing medical decision-making in children), informed consent by parents, assent by the child, and confidentiality.

CHAPTER 4

Palliative Care and End-of-Life Issues

- Children needing palliative care generally fall into four basic categories: (1) when a cure is possible but unlikely, (2) long-term treatment with a goal of maintaining quality of life (e.g., cystic fibrosis), (3) treatment that is exclusively palliative after the diagnosis of a progressive condition is made (e.g., trisomy 13), and (4) when treatments are available for severe, nonprogressive disabilities.
- Organ donation can occur after fulfilling criteria for neurologic death or through donation after circulatory death.

GROWTH AND DEVELOPMENT

Latasha Bogues | David A. Levine

CHAPTER 5 Normal Growth

HEALTH MAINTENANCE VISITS

Health maintenance visits, also known as *well visits* or *well-child checks,* are recommended at regular intervals to promote optimized growth and development. These visits are more frequent in the first 2 years of life and then should occur on a yearly basis when 3 years and older. Important components of the well visit include not only a history and physical exam, but also discussion of topics such as nutrition, behavior, development, safety, and **anticipatory guidance**.

Disorders of growth and development may be associated with chronic or severe illness or could be the only symptom of neglect or abuse. Normal growth and development do not eliminate the possibility of a serious or chronic illness but rather support a judgment that a child is healthy except for acute, often benign illnesses.

Growth and development are intertwined processes; it is convenient to refer to **growth** as increasing size and **development** as increasing function of processes related to body and mind. Familiarity with normal patterns of growth and development allows for recognition and management of abnormal variations. Growth of the nervous system is most rapid in the first 2 years, correlating with increasing physical, emotional, behavioral, and cognitive development. Rapid change resumes during adolescence.

The genetic makeup as well as the physical, emotional, and social environment determine how a child grows and develops throughout childhood. Helping each child achieve their individual maximum potential through periodically monitoring and screening for the normal progression or abnormalities of growth and development is one goal of pediatrics. The American Academy of Pediatrics recommends routine office visits in the first week of life; by 1 month of age; at 2, 4, 6, 9, 12, 15, 18, 24, and 30 months; and then annually from 3 years old through young adulthood (see Fig. 9.1, "Recommendations for Preventive Pediatric Health Care").

Deviations in growth patterns may be nonspecific or may be important indicators of serious and chronic medical disorders. An accurate measurement of length/height, weight, and head circumference (through age 24 months) should be obtained at every health maintenance visit and compared with statistical norms on growth charts. Table 5.1 summarizes several general benchmarks to evaluate normal growth. Serial measurements establishing a *growth trend* are more useful than single measurements for detecting abnormal growth patterns. A single measurement at a normal percentile could warrant further evaluation for an abnormal growth pattern if it is at a very different percentile than previous measurements.

Growth is assessed by plotting accurate measurements on growth charts and comparing values with measurements from previous health visits. Some example growth charts are in Figures 5.1–5.4. Additional charts can be found at www.cdc.gov/growthcharts. In the United States (US), World Health Organization (WHO) standards are recommended for age 0 to 2 years, and Centers for Disease Control and Prevention (CDC) standards are recommended for 2 years and older. WHO growth charts better describe optimal growth in young children while CDC charts show typical (possibly not ideal) growth in the United States. **Body mass index** (BMI), a measure of adiposity, is body weight in kilograms divided by height in meters squared. BMI is recommended as a screening tool for children and adolescents to identify weight abnormalities. With increasing BMI values in the United States, there are additional CDC growth charts available that extend beyond the 97th percentile to monitor high BMI values. Normal growth patterns have spurts and plateaus, so some shifting in percentile can be normal, but large shifts warrant attention. Large discrepancies in length/height, weight, and head circumference percentiles also deserve investigation.

TABLE 5.1 General Principles for Average Growth

WEIGHT
Weight loss in first few days of life: 5–10% of birthweight Return to birthweight: By 2 weeks of age Double birthweight: By 4 months of age Triple birthweight: By 1 year of age Daily weight gain: 20–30 g for first 3–4 months of life 15–20 g for remainder of the first year
HEIGHT
Average length: 20 in. at birth, 30 in. at 1 year of age Double birth length: By 4 years of age Height increases: 2 in. per year from 4 years of age until puberty
HEAD CIRCUMFERENCE (HC)
Average HC: 35 cm at birth (13.5 in.) HC increases: 1 cm per month for first year (2 cm per month for first 3 months, then slower)

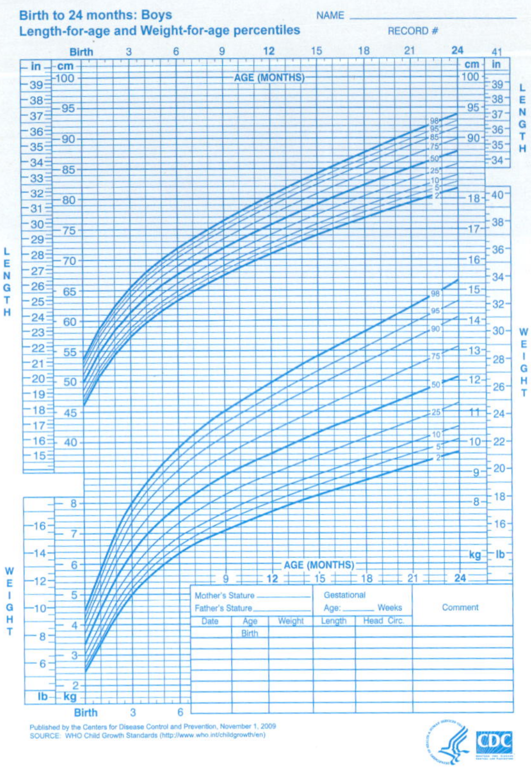

FIGURE 5.1 Birth to 24 months: Males' length-for-age and weight-for-age percentiles. WHO Child Growth Standards. (From Centers for Disease Control and Prevention. *WHO Child Growth Standards.* Atlanta, GA: CDC; 2009. https://www.cdc.gov/growthcharts/data/who/GrChrt_Boys_24LW_100611.pdf from http://www.cdc.gov/growthcharts.)

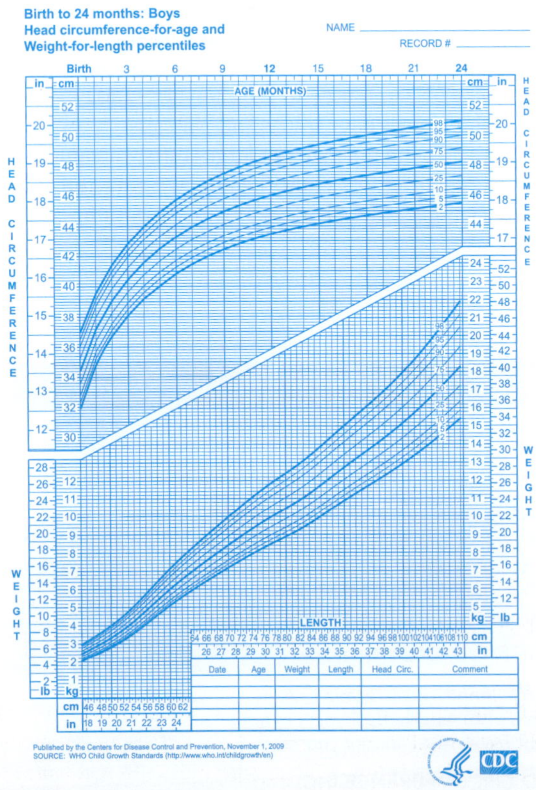

FIGURE 5.2 Birth to 24 months: Males' head circumference-for-age and weight-for-length percentiles. WHO Child Growth Standards. (From Centers for Disease Control and Prevention. *WHO Child Growth Standards.* Atlanta, GA: CDC; 2009. https://www.cdc.gov/growthcharts/data/who/GrChrt_Boys_24HdCirc-L4W_rev90910.pdf from http://www.cdc.gov/growthcharts.)

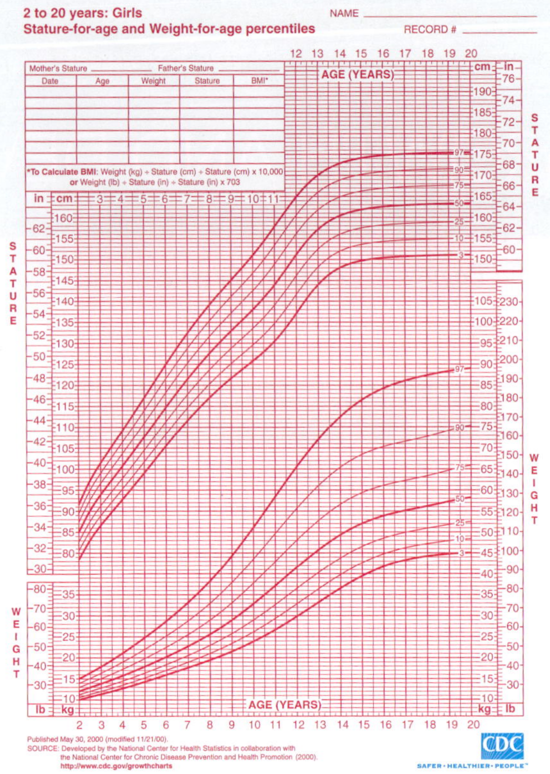

FIGURE 5.3 Two to 20 years: Females' stature-for-age and weight-for-age percentiles. Developed by the National Center for Health Statistics in collaboration with the National Center for Chronic Disease Prevention and Health Promotion. (From Centers for Disease Control and Prevention. Atlanta, GA; 2000. https://www.cdc.gov/growthcharts/data/set1clinical/cj41c022.pdf from http://www.cdc.gov/growthcharts.)

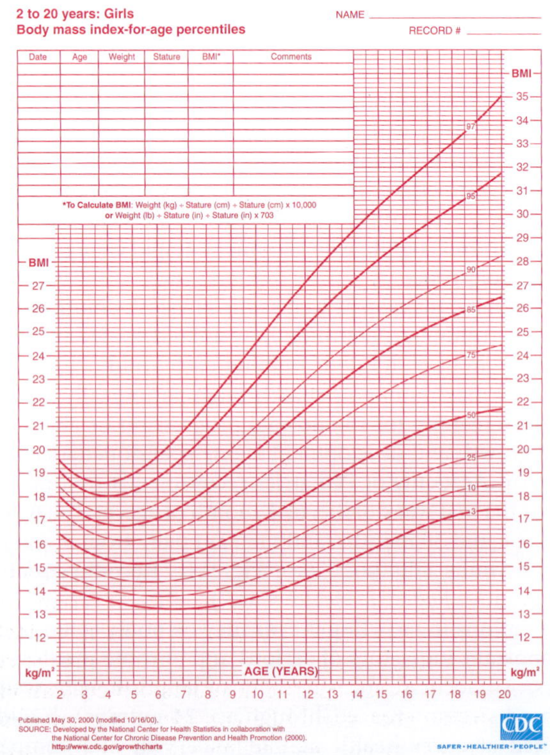

FIGURE 5.4 Two to 20 years: Females' body mass index-for-age percentiles. Developed by the National Center for Health Statistics in collaboration with the National Center for Chronic Disease Prevention and Health Promotion. (From Centers for Disease Control and Prevention. Atlanta, GA; 2000. https://www.cdc.gov/growthcharts/data/set1clinical/cj41c024.pdf from http://www.cdc.gov/growthcharts.)

PEARLS FOR PRACTITIONERS

See Growth and Development: Pearls for Practitioners at the end of this section.

REVIEW QUESTIONS

Available online.

CHAPTER 6
Disorders of Growth

The most common reasons for abnormal measurements of growth are technical (i.e., faulty equipment or operator error); repeating a deviant measurement is the first step. Special growth charts are available and should be used for premature infants and for those with specific disorders (i.e., Turner syndrome, Down syndrome, achondroplasia).

Variability in body proportions occur from fetal to adult life. Newborns' heads are significantly larger in proportion to the rest of their body; this difference gradually disappears. Certain growth disturbances result in characteristic changes in the proportional sizes of the trunk, extremities, and head. Patterns requiring further assessment are summarized in Table 6.1.

Evaluating a child over time, coupled with a careful history and physical examination, helps determine whether the growth pattern is normal or abnormal. Parental heights may be useful when deciding whether to proceed with further evaluation. Though there are exceptions, children generally follow their parents' growth patterns. Calculation of midparental height can provide an estimate of a child's final adult height.

Female midparental height equation:

$$\frac{\text{Paternal height (inches)} + \text{Maternal height (inches)}}{2} - 2.5$$

Male midparental height equation:

$$\frac{\text{Paternal height (inches)} + \text{Maternal height (inches)}}{2} + 2.5$$

Actual growth depends on too many variables to make an accurate prediction solely from midparental height for every child. The growth pattern of a child with low weight, length, and head circumference is commonly associated with **familial short stature** (see Chapter 174). These children are genetically normal but are smaller than most children. A child who starts puberty later than others may have the normal variant called ***constitutional short stature*** (see Chapter 174). Examination for causes of abnormal pubertal development must be completed so as to not miss specific disorders. An evaluation for **primary amenorrhea** should be considered for any female adolescent who has not reached menarche by 15 years or within 3 years of thelarche (beginning of breast development). Lack of breast development by age 13 years also should be evaluated (see Chapter 175). **Bone age**, a measure of skeletal maturity, may be a part of abnormal stature evaluation. Bone age is determined by comparing radiographs of the left hand and wrist to standard images.

TABLE 6.1 Specific Growth Patterns Requiring Further Evaluation

PATTERN	REPRESENTATIVE DIAGNOSES TO CONSIDER	FURTHER EVALUATION TO CONSIDER
Weight, length, head circumference all <5th percentile	• Normal variant (familial or constitutional short stature) • Intrauterine insult • Genetic disorder • Severe caloric insufficiency	• Prenatal and birth records review • Genetic testing • Midparental height • Evaluation of pubertal development
Discrepant percentiles (e.g., weight 5th, length 5th, head circumference 50th, or other discrepancies)	• Normal variant (familial or constitutional short stature) • Endocrine growth failure • Caloric insufficiency	• Midparental height • Bone age • Thyroid hormone • Growth factors, growth hormone testing • Evaluation of pubertal development
Declining percentiles	• Catch-down growth • Caloric insufficiency • Endocrine growth failure	• Midparental height • Complete history and physical examination • Dietary and social history • Growth factors, growth hormone testing

Some children start in high growth percentiles and trend to a lower percentile between 6 and 18 months of age; then they grow along this new, lower percentile. These children usually do not drop more than two major percentiles (lines on growth chart) and have normal developmental, behavioral, and physical examinations. These children with *catch-down growth* should be followed closely, but no further evaluation is warranted.

Through increased oral intake (breast milk or formula), infants born small for gestational age (SGA) or prematurely usually exhibit *catch-up growth* in the first 6 months. These infants should be fed on demand and provided as much as they want unless they are vomiting (not just spitting up [see Chapter 129]). Some infants may benefit from a higher caloric content formula, especially if there are complications that require extra calories. Several psychosocial risk factors that contribute to being born prematurely or SGA may also contribute to nonorganic growth faltering (see Chapter 30). Conversely, infants who recover from being SGA or premature have an increased risk of developing childhood obesity.

When caloric intake is inadequate, the weight percentile falls first, then the height, and the head circumference is last. Caloric intake may be poor due to inadequate feeding or because the child is not receiving adequate attention and stimulation (*nonorganic* growth faltering [see Chapter 30]). Caloric intake also may be inadequate because of increased caloric needs. Children with chronic illnesses (i.e., heart failure or cystic fibrosis) may require a significantly higher caloric intake to sustain growth. An increasing weight percentile in the face of a falling height percentile suggests hypothyroidism. Head circumference may be disproportionately large (macrocephaly) when there is familial megalocephaly, hydrocephalus, or merely *catch-up* growth in a neurologically normal premature infant. A child is considered microcephalic if the head circumference is less than the 3rd percentile, even if length and weight measurements are proportionately low. Serial measurements and plotting of head circumference are crucial during infancy through 2 years of age, a period of rapid brain development. Any suspicion of abnormal growth warrants close follow-up, further evaluation, or both follow-up and evaluation.

PEARLS FOR PRACTITIONERS

See Growth and Development: Pearls for Practitioners at the end of this section.

REVIEW QUESTIONS

Available online.

CHAPTER 7 Normal Development

PHYSICAL DEVELOPMENT

Parallel to the changes in the developing brain (i.e., cognition, language, behavior), the body also undergoes physical development.

NEWBORN PERIOD

The newborn period includes the first 4 weeks of life. Observation of any asymmetric movement or altered muscle tone and function may indicate a central nervous system abnormality or a nerve palsy resulting from the delivery and requires further evaluation. Primitive neonatal reflexes are unique in the newborn period and can further elucidate or eliminate concerns over asymmetric function. A delay in the expected disappearance of the reflexes may also warrant an evaluation of the central nervous system. The most important reflexes to assess during the newborn period are noted below. These reflexes extinguish by 6 months of age; see Chapter 180 for more specific information.

The **Moro reflex** is elicited by allowing the infant's head to gently move back suddenly (from a few inches off the mattress onto the examiner's hand), resulting in a startle with abduction and upward movement of the arms followed by adduction and flexion. The legs respond with flexion.

The **rooting reflex** is elicited by touching the corner of the infant's mouth, resulting in lowering of the lower lip on the same side with tongue movement toward the stimulus. The face also turns toward the stimulus.

The **sucking reflex** occurs with almost any object placed in the newborn's mouth. The infant responds with vigorous sucking. The sucking reflex is replaced later by voluntary sucking.

The **asymmetric tonic neck reflex** is elicited by placing the infant supine and turning the head to the side. This placement results in ipsilateral extension of the arm and the leg into a "fencing" position. The contralateral side flexes.

See Sections 11 and 24 for additional information on the newborn period.

LATER INFANCY

The infant phase lasts until 1 year of age. With the development of gross motor skills, the infant is first able to control posture, then proximal musculature, and lastly, distal musculature. As the infant progresses through these stages, caregivers may notice orthopedic deformities (see Chapters 200–204). The infant also may have deformities that are related to intrauterine positioning. Physical examination should indicate whether the deformity is fixed or can be moved passively into the proper position. When a joint held in an abnormal fashion can be moved passively into the proper position, there is a high likelihood of resolving with the progression of gross motor development. Fixed deformities warrant immediate pediatric orthopedic consultation (see Section 26).

Evaluation of vision and ocular movements is important to prevent serious outcomes of **strabismus** (eye misalignment). The cover test and light reflex should be performed at early health maintenance visits; interventions after age 2 decrease the chance of preserving binocular vision and normal visual acuity (see Chapters 9 and 180).

SCHOOL AGE/PREADOLESCENT

In addition to routine health supervision visits, older school-age children who begin to participate in competitive sports should have a comprehensive sports history and physical examination that includes a careful evaluation of the cardiovascular system. The American Academy of Pediatrics Preparticipation Physical Evaluation form is excellent for documenting cardiovascular and other risks. The patient and parent should complete the history form and be interviewed to assess cardiovascular risk. A history of heart disease or a concerning murmur warrants referral for evaluation by a pediatric cardiologist. A child with a history of dyspnea or chest pain on exertion, irregular heart rate (i.e., skipped beats, palpitations), or syncope should also be referred to a pediatric cardiologist. A family history of a primary (immediate family) or secondary (immediate family's immediate family) atherosclerotic disease (myocardial infarction or cerebrovascular disease) before 50 years of age, hypertrophic cardiomyopathy, or sudden unexplained death at any age also requires additional assessment. Vision should be assessed as a crucial part of the evaluation before participation in sports.

ADOLESCENCE

Adolescents need annual comprehensive health assessments for general health maintenance and to ensure appropriate progression through puberty (see Chapters 66 and 67). All adolescents should be assessed to monitor progression through sexual maturity rating stages. Physical growth and development of adolescents is discussed in Chapter 66. Other issues in physical development include scoliosis (see Chapter 203), obesity (see Chapter 27), and common orthopedic growth issues (e.g., Osgood Schlatter; see Chapter 201). Most scoliosis is mild and requires only observation for resolution. Obesity can first manifest during childhood and is a growing public health concern for adolescents.

DEVELOPMENTAL MILESTONES

The use of **milestones** to assess development focuses on discrete behaviors that the clinician can observe or accept as present by caregiver report. This approach is based on comparing the patient's behavior with that of other children whose behaviors evolve in a uniform sequence within specific age ranges (see Table 8.1). The development of the neuromuscular system, like other organ systems, is determined by genetics with environmental influences.

Although a sequence of specific, easily measured behaviors can adequately represent some areas of development (**gross motor**, **fine motor**, and **language**), other areas, particularly social and emotional development, are not as straightforward to assess. Clearly measured developmental milestones are well established through age 6 years only. Other types of assessment (e.g., intelligence tests, school performance, and personality profiles) that expand the developmental milestone approach are available for older children.

PSYCHOSOCIAL DEVELOPMENT

Bonding and Attachment in Infancy

The terms *bonding* and *attachment* describe the affective relationships between parents and infants. **Bonding** occurs shortly after birth and reflects the feelings of the parents toward the newborn (unidirectional). **Attachment** involves reciprocal feelings between parent and infant and develops gradually over the first year of life.

Attachment of infants outside of the newborn period is crucial for optimal development. Infants who receive extra attention, such as caregivers responding immediately to any crying or fussiness in the first 4 months, show less crying and fussiness at the end of the first year. **Stranger anxiety** develops between 7 and 18 months of age, when infants normally become insecure about separation from the primary caregiver. The infant's new motor skills and attraction to novelty may lead to attraction towards new experiences that result in fright or pain followed by frantic efforts to find and cling to the primary caregiver. The result is dramatic swings from stubborn independence to clinging dependence that can be frustrating and confusing to caregivers. With secure attachment, this period of ambivalence may be shorter and less tumultuous.

Developing Autonomy in Early Childhood

Toddlers begin developing autonomy that allows for separation from caregivers. In times of stress, toddlers often cling to their caregivers, but in their usual activities they may be actively separated. Ages 2–3 years are a time of major accomplishments in fine motor skills, social skills, cognitive skills, and language skills. The dependency of infancy yields to developing independence and the "I can do it myself" age. Limit setting is essential to balance the toddler's emerging independence.

Early Childhood Education

Children who are in high-quality early learning environments are more prepared to succeed in school. Every dollar invested in early childhood education may save taxpayers up to $13 in future costs. These children commit fewer crimes and are better prepared to enter the workforce after school. Early Head Start (<3 years), Head Start (3–4 years), and prekindergarten programs (4–5 years) all demonstrate better educational attainment; the earlier the start, the better the results.

School Readiness

Readiness for preschool depends on the development of autonomy and the ability of the caregiver and the child to separate for hours at a time. Preschool experiences help children develop socialization skills; improve language; and increase skill building in areas such as colors, numbers, letters, and problem solving.

Readiness for school (kindergarten) requires emotional maturity, peer group and individual social skills, cognitive abilities, and fine and gross motor skills (Table 7.1). Other readiness factors include chronological age and gender. Children tend to do better in kindergarten if their fifth birthday is at least 4–6 months before the beginning of school. Females usually are ready earlier than males. If the child is in less than the average developmental range, the child should not be forced into early kindergarten. Holding a child back for reasons of developmental delay, in the false hope that the child will catch up, can also lead to difficulties. The child should enroll on schedule, and educational planning should be initiated to address any deficiencies.

Physicians should be able to identify children at risk for school difficulties, such as those who have developmental delays or physical disabilities. These children may require specialized school services in an individualized education plan and/or environment accommodations in a 504 plan.

TABLE 7.1 Evaluating School Readiness

PHYSICIAN OBSERVATIONS (BEHAVIORS OBSERVED IN THE OFFICE)
Ease of separation of the child from the parent Speech development and articulation Understanding of and ability to follow complex directions Specific preacademic skills • Knowledge of colors • Counts to 10 • Knows age, first and last name, address, and phone number • Ability to copy shapes Motor skills • Stand on one foot, skip, and catch a bounced ball • Dresses and undresses without assistance
PARENT OBSERVATIONS (QUESTIONS ANSWERED BY HISTORY)
Does the child play well with other children? Does the child separate well, such as a child playing in the backyard alone with occasional monitoring by the parent? Does the child show interest in books, letters, and numbers? Can the child sustain attention to quiet activities? How frequent are toilet-training accidents?

Adolescence

One definition of adolescence is 10–25 years of age, but perhaps adolescence is better characterized by the developmental stages (*early, middle*, and *late* adolescence) that all teens must navigate to develop into healthy, functional adults. Different behavioral and developmental issues characterize each stage. The age at which each issue manifests and the importance of these issues vary widely among individuals, as do the rates of cognitive, psychosexual, psychosocial, and physical development.

During **early adolescence**, attention is focused on the present and on the peer group. Concerns are primarily related to the body's physical changes and normality. Strivings for independence are ambivalent. These young adolescents are difficult to interview because they often respond with short, clipped conversation and may have little insight. They are just becoming accustomed to abstract thinking.

Middle adolescence can be a difficult time for adolescents as well as the adults who interact with them. Cognitive processes are more sophisticated. Through abstract thinking, middle adolescents can experiment with ideas, consider things as they might be, develop insight, and reflect on their own feelings and the feelings of others. As they mature, these adolescents focus on issues of identity not limited solely to the physical aspects of their body. They explore their parents' and culture's values, sometimes by expressing the contrary side of the dominant value. Many middle adolescents explore these values in their minds only; others do so by challenging their parents' authority. Some adolescents engage in high-risk behaviors, including unprotected sexual intercourse, substance use, or dangerous driving. The striving of middle adolescents for independence, limit testing, and need for autonomy often distress their families, teachers, or other authority figures. These adolescents are at higher risk for morbidity and mortality from accidents, homicide, or suicide.

Late adolescence usually is marked by formal operational thinking, including thoughts about the future (e.g., educational, vocational, and sexual). Late adolescents are usually more committed to their sexual partners than are middle adolescents. Unresolved separation anxiety from previous developmental stages may emerge at this time as the young person begins to move physically away from the family of origin to college or vocational school, a job, or military service.

PSYCHOSOCIAL BEHAVIOR MODIFICATION

Child behavior is determined by genetics and the environment. **Behavioral theory** postulates that behavior is primarily due to interactions with the external environment, and that external consequences of behavior can be used to modify maladaptive behavior and increase desirable behavior *(operant conditioning)*. The four major methods of operant conditioning are positive reinforcement, negative reinforcement, extinction, and punishment. Common behavioral problems of children may be ameliorated by these methods.

Positive reinforcement increases the frequency of a behavior by following the behavior with a favorable event (e.g., praising a child for excellent school performance). Sometimes this reinforcement may occur unintentionally, increasing the frequency of undesirable behavior. For example, a toddler may purposely try to stick a pencil in a light socket to obtain attention, whether it be positive or negative. **Negative reinforcement** increases the frequency of a behavior by removal, cessation, or avoidance of an unpleasant event (e.g., no longer having to sit at table once vegetables are eaten). **Extinction** occurs when there is a decrease in the frequency of a previously reinforced behavior because the reinforcement is withheld. Extinction is the principle behind the common advice to ignore behavior such as crying at bedtime or temper tantrums, which parents may unwittingly reinforce through attention and comforting. While reinforcement increases behavior frequency, **punishment** decreases the frequency of a behavior through unpleasant consequences. Punishment can be positive (undesired consequence is given) or negative (desired event is taken away).

Positive reinforcement is more effective than punishment. Punishment is more effective when combined with positive reinforcement. A toddler who draws on the wall with a crayon may be punished, but the child learns much quicker when positive reinforcement is given for the proper use of the crayon—on paper, not the wall. Interrupting and modifying behaviors is discussed further in Section 3.

TEMPERAMENT

Significant individual differences exist within the normal development of temperament (behavioral style). Temperament must be appreciated because, if an expected pattern of behavior is too narrowly defined, normal behavior may be inappropriately labeled as *abnormal* or *pathologic*. Three common constellations of temperamental characteristics are as follows:

1. The **easy child** (about 40% of children) demonstrates regularity of biologic functions (consistent, predictable times for eating, sleeping, and elimination), a positive approach to new stimuli, high adaptability to change, mild or moderate intensity in responses, and a positive mood.
2. The **challenging child** (about 10%) demonstrates irregularity of biologic functions, negative withdrawal from new stimuli, poor adaptability, intense responses, and a negative mood.
3. The **slow-to-warm-up child** (about 15%) demonstrates a low activity level, withdrawal from new stimuli, slow adaptability, mild intensity in responses, and a somewhat negative mood.

The remaining 35% of children have more mixed temperaments. The individual temperament of a child has important implications for parenting and for the advice a pediatrician may give in anticipatory guidance or behavioral problem counseling.

Although temperament may be hardwired *(nature)* in each child to some degree, the environment *(nurture)* in which the child grows has a strong effect on the child's adjustment. Social and cultural factors can have marked effects on the child through differences in parenting style, educational approaches, and behavioral expectations.

PEARLS FOR PRACTITIONERS

See Growth and Development: Pearls for Practitioners at the end of this section.

REVIEW QUESTIONS

Available online.

CHAPTER 8
Disorders of Development

DEVELOPMENTAL SURVEILLANCE AND SCREENING

Developmental and behavioral concerns are a common category of pediatric presentations to care. In 2021, 8.5% of U.S. youth aged 3–17 years had a diagnosed developmental disability. Up to 25% of children have psychosocial concerns. Parents often fail to mention these concerns because they think the physician is uninterested or cannot help. It is necessary to screen for the presence of these concerns at health maintenance visits, particularly in the years before preschool or early childhood learning center enrollment.

Development surveillance, done at every office visit, is an informal process comparing skill levels to lists of milestones. In 2019, milestones were updated to reflect ages when 75% of children should achieve a skill. When milestones were previously set at ages when 50% of children would achieve a skill, it was reasonable to wait to see if the skill would be achieved; this led to missed opportunities for earlier intervention. Table 8.1 lists milestones from the U.S. Centers for Disease Control and Prevention's "Learn the Signs. Act Early." program that has helpful resources for parents and clinicians (including checklists, handouts, and milestone videos) that are available at https://www.cdc.gov/act-early/index.html. If developmental or behavioral issues are suspected, further evaluation is warranted. As development surveillance does not have a standard, screening tests are also necessary.

Developmental screening involves the use of standardized screening tests to identify children who require further diagnostic assessment. The American Academy of Pediatrics (AAP) recommends the use of validated standardized screening tools at three of the health maintenance visits: 9 months, 18 months, and 30 months. Clinics and offices that serve a higher-risk patient population often perform a screening test at *every* health maintenance visit. A child who fails to pass a developmental screening test requires more comprehensive evaluation but does not necessarily have a delay; definitive testing must confirm. Developmental evaluations for children with suspected delays and intervention services for children with diagnosed disabilities are available free to families.

Screening tests can be categorized as general screens that cover all behavioral domains or as targeted screens that focus on one area of development. Screening tests may be administered in the office by professionals, while others may be completed prior to or during a visit by caregivers. Effective developmental/behavioral screening instruments have a sensitivity of 70–80% in detecting suspected problems and a specificity of 70–80% in detecting normal development. Although 30% of children screened may be *over-referred* for definitive developmental testing, this group also includes children whose skills are below average and who may benefit from testing to help address relative developmental deficits. The 20–30% of children who have disabilities that are not detected by the single administration of a screening instrument are likely to be identified on repeat screening at subsequent health maintenance visits.

Commonly used developmental screening tools include **Ages and Stages Questionnaires** (developmental milestone driven) and **Parents' Evaluation of Developmental Status (PEDS)**. PEDS is a simple, 10-item questionnaire that caregivers complete at office visits based on concerns with function and progression of development. Caregiver-reported screens have strong validity compared to office-based screening measures. Some offices combine PEDS with developmental surveillance to track milestone attainment.

Autism screening is done for all children at 18 and 24 months of age. Although there are several tools, most clinicians use the **Modified Checklist for Autism in Toddlers—Revised (M-CHAT-R)**. M-CHAT-R is an office-based questionnaire that asks caregivers about typical behaviors, some of which are more predictive than others for autism or other pervasive developmental disorders. If the child demonstrates more than two predictive or three total behaviors, further assessment with an interview algorithm is indicated to distinguish normal variant behaviors from those children needing a referral for definitive testing. The test is freely distributed and is available at https://www.mchatscreen.com/ (see Chapter 20).

Language screening correlates best with cognitive development in the early years. Table 8.2 provides some general principles for language development that focus on speech production *(expressive language)*. Although expressive language is the most obvious language element, the most dramatic changes in language development in the first years actually involve recognition and understanding *(receptive language)*.

Whenever there is a speech and/or language delay, a **hearing deficit** must be evaluated for. If hearing is abnormal and not addressed, speech cannot develop appropriately or appropriately respond to therapy. Universal newborn hearing screening detects most of these children in the newborn period; appropriate early intervention services may be provided. Conditions that present a high risk of an associated hearing deficit are listed in Table 8.3. Dysfluency *(stuttering)* is common in 3–4-year-old children. Unless the dysfluency is severe, is accompanied by tics or unusual posturing, or occurs after 4 years of age, parents should be counseled that it is normal and transient and to accept it calmly and patiently.

After the child's sixth birthday and until adolescence, developmental assessment is initially done by inquiring about school performance (academic achievement and behavior). Inquiring about concerns raised by teachers or other adults who interact with the child (after-school program counselor, coach, religious leader) is prudent. Formal developmental testing of these older children is beyond the scope of the primary care pediatrician. Nonetheless, the health care provider should be the coordinator of the testing and evaluation performed by other specialists (e.g., psychologists, psychiatrists, developmental pediatricians, and educational professionals).

SOCIAL DETERMINANTS OF HEALTH (SDOH) AND ADVERSE CHILDHOOD EXPERIENCES (ACES)

Acknowledgement of the environmental influences on child behavior is crucial to providing effective pediatric care. Adverse childhood experiences (ACEs) are potentially traumatic experiences that occur during childhood and adolescence. These include witnessed or experienced child abuse or neglect, parental substance use disorder, witnessed spousal

TABLE 8.1 Developmental Milestones

AGE	MOVEMENT/PHYSICAL DEVELOPMENT	SOCIAL/EMOTIONAL	LANGUAGE/ COMMUNICATION	COGNITIVE
2 mo	Holds head up prone Opens hands briefly	Calms down when spoken to or picked up Regards face Smiles responsively	Makes sounds other than crying Reacts to loud sounds	Tracks/watches people as they move Looks at a toy for several seconds
4 mo	Holds head steady Holds a toy placed in hand Swings arm at toys Brings hands to mouth	Smiles, looks at you, moves, or makes sounds to get attention Chuckles	Makes sounds like "ooo" and "aahh" Makes sounds back when you talk Turns head to voice	If hungry, opens mouth when sees breast or bottle Looks at own hands
6 mo	Pushes up with straight arms when prone Rolls front to back Tripod sitting (use arms for support)	Knows familiar people Likes to see self in mirror Laughs	Takes turns making sounds with you Blows "raspberries" Squeals	Puts things in mouth Reaches and grabs Closes lips to decline food
9 mo	Transfers objects between hands Sits without support Raking grasp	Is shy or fearful around strangers Many facial expressions Responds to name Reacts when parent leaves Smiles or laughs in peek-a-boo game	Lifts arms up to be picked up Says sounds like "mamama" and "babababa"	Looks for objects when dropped Bangs two things together
12 mo	Pulls up to stand Walks, holding on to furniture Drinks from a cup that someone holds Mature pincer grasp	Plays pat-a-cake	Waves "bye-bye" Says "mama" and "dada," specific Understands "no"	Puts items in container Looks for things they see hidden
15 mo	Takes a few steps Feeds self with fingers	Copies other children Shows an object they like Claps when excited Hugs doll or toy Shows affection	Says one or two words besides "mama" or "dada" Follows directions given with both a gesture and words Points to ask for something or to get help	Tries to use things correctly (phone, cup, book) Stacks two objects
18 mo	Walks Scribbles Drinks from cup Tries to use a spoon Climbs on and off chair	Moves away from parent, but looks to see that they are near Points to show things Looks at a few book pages Helps get dressed	Three words besides "mama" and "dada" Follows one-step command without gesture	Copies doing chores Plays with toys in a simple way
2 yr	Walks up steps Kicks a ball Runs Eats with a spoon	Notices when others are hurt or upset Looks at parent's face to see how to react	Puts two words together Points to pictures in a book Points to two body parts Uses more gestures than waving and pointing (blowing a kiss, nodding "yes")	Holds item in one hand while using other hand Tries to use switches, knobs, or buttons
30 mo	Uses hands to twist things (doorknobs, lids) Takes some clothes off Jumps with both feet Turns book pages, one at a time	Plays next to other children and sometimes plays with them Shows what they can do by saying, "Look at me!" Follows simple routines	Says about 50 words Puts two words together, with one action word ("Doggie run") Names things in a book Uses pronouns	Pretend play Simple problem-solving Follows two-step instructions Knows one color
3 yr	Strings items together Puts on some clothes Uses fork	Calms down within 10 minutes after parent leaves Notices other children and joins play	Converses using at least two back-and-forth exchanges Asks "who," "what," "where," or "why" questions Says what is happening in a picture Says first name Most speech is understood	Draws a circle Avoids touching hot objects after warned

(Continued)

TABLE 8.1 Developmental Milestones—cont'd

AGE	MOVEMENT/PHYSICAL DEVELOPMENT	SOCIAL/EMOTIONAL	LANGUAGE/ COMMUNICATION	COGNITIVE
4 yr	Catches a large ball Serves food to self or pours water Unbuttons some buttons Holds crayon or pencil between fingers and thumb	Pretends to be something else Comforts others who are hurt or sad Avoids danger Likes to be a "helper"	Four-word sentences Repeats words from a song or story Talks about one thing that happened during the day Answers simple questions	Names a few colors Tells what comes next in a known story Draws person with three body parts
5 yr	Buttons some buttons Hops on one foot	Follows game rules, takes turns Sings, dances, or acts for you Does simple chores at home	Tells a story with at least two events Answers questions about a story Holds conversation with more than three back-and-forth exchanges Knows simple rhymes	Counts to 10 Identifies some written numbers 1 to 5 Uses words about time (yesterday, morning, etc.) Pays attention for 5 to 10 minutes (screen time does not count) Writes some letters in name Identifies some written letters

mo, Month; *yr*, year.

TABLE 8.2 General Principles for Speech Screening

AGE (YR)	SPEECH PRODUCTION	ARTICULATION (AMOUNT OF SPEECH UNDERSTOOD BY A STRANGER)	FOLLOWING COMMANDS
1	One to three words	—	One-step commands
2	Two- to three-word phrases	One-half	Two-step commands
3	Routine use of sentences	Three-fourths	—
4	Routine use of sentence sequences; conversational give-and-take	Almost all	—
5	Complex sentences; extensive use of modifiers, pronouns, and prepositions	Almost all	—

yr, Year.

abuse and intimate partner violence, hunger, housing instability, being bullied, experiencing discrimination, and others. **Social determinants of health** (SDOH) are the conditions of where a person is born, grows, works, and lives. Some people prefer the terminology social *drivers* of health as this better represents that these factors exert influence on health outcomes, but they do not fully determine health outcomes. As ACEs and SDOH can greatly impact growth and development, they need to be asked about and addressed. Table 8.4 lists some contextual factors that should be considered in the etiology of a child's behavioral or developmental problem. ACEs are known to trigger "toxic stress" and to stimulate cortisol and the "fight or flight" response. This results in epigenetic DNA activation, leading to a different outcome. Some of these children will later fit the diagnostic criteria for attention-deficit/hyperactivity disorder or other developmental or behavioral issues. Questions to consider using at well-child visits and other relevant visits are in Table 8.5. It is important to have a list of resources for the families that are in need. For example, services that provide housing support, food and clothing banks, school supplies, parental support, and others should be offered to the families that are affected. Most families do not consider this the role of the pediatrician, but a child's health cannot be optimally managed if ACEs and SDOH are not addressed. The AAP has excellent resources on these topics for the pediatric provider (see suggested readings).

BUILDING RAPPORT WITH CAREGIVERS AND THE CHILD

Building rapport with the caregivers and the child is a prerequisite for obtaining the often-sensitive information that is essential for understanding a behavioral or developmental issue. Rapport usually can be established quickly if caregivers sense that the clinician respects them and is genuinely interested in listening to their concerns. The clinician develops rapport with the child by engaging in developmentally appropriate conversation or play, perhaps providing toys while interviewing the parents, and being sensitive to the fears the child may have. Too often, the child is ignored until it is time for the physical examination. Like their parents, children feel more comfortable if they are greeted by name and involved in

TABLE 8.3 Conditions Considered High Risk for Associated Hearing Deficit

Congenital hearing loss in first cousin or closer relative
Bilirubin level of ≥20 mg/dL
Congenital rubella or other nonbacterial intrauterine infection
Defects in the ear, nose, or throat
Birthweight of ≤1,500 g
Multiple apneic episodes
Exchange transfusion
Meningitis
Five-minute Apgar score of ≤5
Persistent fetal circulation (primary pulmonary hypertension)
Treatment with ototoxic drugs (e.g., aminoglycosides and loop diuretics)

TABLE 8.4 Contextual Considerations of Behavioral Problems

CHILD FACTORS
Health (past and current)
Developmental status
Temperament (e.g., challenging, slow to warm up)
Coping mechanisms
PARENTAL FACTORS
Misinterpretations of stage-related behaviors
Mismatch of caregiver expectations and characteristics of child
Mismatch of personality style between caregiver and child
Caregiver characteristics (e.g., depression, lack of interest, rejection, overprotective, coping)
ENVIRONMENTAL FACTORS
Adverse childhood experiences (e.g., marital discord, unemployment, personal loss, racism, hunger, housing instability, child abuse or neglect, bullying, and others)
Support (e.g., emotional, material, informational, child care)
Poverty—including poor housing, poorer education facilities, lack of access to healthy foods (food deserts), unsafe environments, toxic stress, poor access to primary care
Racism

TABLE 8.5 Questions About Social Determinants of Health and Adverse Childhood Experiences

Has any major event that affected your family happened since the last time we met?
If so, how has it had an impact on you and your family?
Do you have adequate funds for housing, clothing, food, and other important expenses?
How are you helping your child through these issues?
Despite any events discussed, what has been going well for you?

pleasant interactions before they are asked sensitive questions or frightened by examinations. Young children can be engaged in conversation on the parent's lap, which provides security and places the child at the eye level of the examiner.

With adolescents, emphasis should be placed on building a physician-patient relationship that is distinct from the relationship with the parents. The parents should not be excluded; the adolescent should have the opportunity to express concerns and ask questions of the physician in confidence. Two intertwined issues must be taken into consideration—consent and confidentiality. Although laws vary from state to state, in general, adolescents who are able to give informed consent (i.e., mature minors) may consent to visits and care related to high-risk behaviors (i.e., depression and mental health issues; substance use; sexual health, including prevention, detection, and treatment of sexually transmitted infections; and pregnancy). Most states support the physician who wishes the visit to be confidential; physicians should become familiar with the governing law in the state(s) where they practice (see https://www.guttmacher.org). Providing confidentiality is crucial and allows for optimal care, especially when obtaining a history of risk behaviors. When assessing development and behavior, confidentiality can be achieved by meeting with the adolescent alone for at least part of each visit. Parents must be informed when the clinician has significant and immediate concerns about the health and safety of the child. Often, the clinician can work with the adolescent to inform the parents directly about a problem or can reach an agreement with the adolescent about how the parents will be informed by the physician (see Chapter 66).

EVALUATING DEVELOPMENTAL AND BEHAVIORAL ISSUES

Responses to open-ended questions often provide clues to underlying and/or unstated problems and identify the appropriate direction for further, more directed questions. Histories about developmental and behavioral problems are often vague and confusing; to reconcile apparent contradictions, the interviewer frequently must request clarification, more detail, or mere repetition. By summarizing an understanding of the information at frequent intervals and by recapitulating at the close of the visit, the interviewer and patient and family can ensure that they understand each other.

If the clinician's impression of the child differs markedly from the caregiver's description, there may be a crucial caregiver concern or issue that has not yet been expressed, either because it may be difficult to talk about (e.g., family problems), because it is unconscious, or because the caregiver overlooks its relevance to the child's behavior. Alternatively, the physician's observations may be atypical, even with multiple visits. The observations of teachers, relatives, and other regular caregivers may be crucial in sorting out this possibility. The caregiver also may have a distorted image of the child, rooted in parental psychopathology. A sensitive, supportive, and noncritical approach to the caregiver is crucial to appropriate intervention. More information about referral and intervention for behavioral and developmental issues is covered in Chapter 10.

PEARLS FOR PRACTITIONERS

See Growth and Development: Pearls for Practitioners at the end of this section.

REVIEW QUESTIONS

Available online.

CHAPTER 9

Evaluation of the Well Child

Health maintenance and supervision visits consist of a comprehensive assessment of the child's health and of the parent's/guardian's role in providing an environment for optimal growth, development, and health. The American Academy of Pediatrics' (AAP) Bright Futures materials standardize each health maintenance visit and provide resources for working with children of different ages (see https://brightfutures.aap.org). Elements of each visit include evaluation and management of caregiver concerns; inquiry about any illness since the last visit; growth, development, and nutrition; anticipatory guidance (including safety information and counseling; Table 9.1); physical examination; screening tests; and immunizations. The Bright Futures/American Academy of Pediatrics Recommendations for Preventive Pediatric Health Care (Fig. 9.1) summarizes requirements and indicates the ages that specific prevention measures should be undertaken. Bright Futures is now the enforced standard for United States Medicaid, the Children's Health Insurance Program, and other insurers, including Patient Protection and Affordable Care Act (ACA) insurances. Health maintenance and immunizations are covered without copays for insured patients per the ACA.

SCREENING TESTS

The following screening tests are recommended for healthy children: newborn metabolic screening with hemoglobin electrophoresis, hearing and vision evaluation, anemia and lead screening, tuberculosis testing, and dyslipidemia screening. On the Bright Futures Recommendations (Fig. 9.1), items marked by a *dot* should be done universally while items marked by a *star* should be performed if a risk factor is found. Sexually active adolescents should be screened for sexually transmissible infections and have an HIV test at least once between 15–21 years. When an infant, child, or adolescent begins with a new provider, there should be close review of the medical record with completion of any missing screening tests and immunizations.

TABLE 9.1 Topics for Health Supervision Visits

FOCUS ON THE CHILD
Concerns (parent's or child's) Past problem follow-up Immunization and screening test update Routine care (e.g., eating, sleeping, elimination, and health habits) Developmental progress Behavioral style and problems
FOCUS ON THE CHILD'S ENVIRONMENT
Family
Caregiving schedule for caregiver who lives at home Parent-child and sibling-child interactions Extended family role Family stresses (e.g., work, move, finances, illness, death, marital, and other interpersonal relationships) Family support (relatives, friends, groups) Screening and intervention in social determinants of health and adverse childhood experiences
Community
Caregivers outside of the family Peer interaction School and work Recreational activities
Physical Environment
Appropriate stimulation Safety

Newborn Screening

Metabolic Screening

Every state in the United States mandates newborn metabolic screening. Each state determines its own priorities and procedures, but the following diseases are usually included in metabolic screening: phenylketonuria, galactosemia, congenital hypothyroidism, maple syrup urine disease, and organic acidemia (see Section 10); most states now screen for cystic fibrosis (CF) by testing for immunoreactive trypsinogen. If that test is positive, then a DNA analysis for the most common CF pathologic variants is performed. This is not a perfect test because many pathogenic variants cause CF (see Chapter 138). Clinical suspicion warrants evaluation even if there were no CF pathogenic variants detected.

Hemoglobin Electrophoresis

Children with hemoglobinopathies are at higher risk for infection and complications from anemia, which early detection may prevent or ameliorate. Infants with sickle cell disease are begun on oral penicillin prophylaxis to prevent sepsis, the major cause of mortality in these infants (see Chapter 151).

Critical Congenital Heart Disease Screening

Newborns with cyanotic congenital heart disease may be missed if the ductus arteriosus is still open; when the ductus closes, these children become profoundly cyanotic, leading to complications and even death. The AAP now mandates screening with pulse oximetry of the right hand and one foot at around 24 hours of life unless discharged earlier. The newborn passes screening if the oxygen saturations are 95% or greater in the foot and right hand with a difference of 3% or less. The screen is failed if the oxygen saturation is less than 90% in the right hand or the foot. Equivocal tests are repeated, or echocardiography and pediatric cardiology consultation are warranted (see Chapters 144 and 145).

Hearing Evaluation

As speech and language are central to a child's cognitive development, a hearing screen is performed before discharge from the newborn nursery. A newborn's hearing can be tested by otoacoustic emissions or auditory brainstem response. These tests are explained in Chapter 10. If the hearing screen is abnormal, further evaluation is indicated. A newborn should have a hearing screen by 1 month of age with follow-up testing for abnormal results by 3 months of age and appropriate intervention by 6 months of age.

Hearing and Vision Screening of Older Children

Infants and Toddlers

Inferences about hearing are drawn both from asking caregivers about responses to sound and speech and by exploring

American Academy of Pediatrics
DEDICATED TO THE HEALTH OF ALL CHILDREN®

Recommendations for Preventive Pediatric Health Care

Bright Futures/American Academy of Pediatrics

Bright Futures. prevention and health promotion for infants, children, adolescents, and their families™

Each child and family is unique; therefore, these Recommendations for Preventive Pediatric Health Care are designed for the care of children who are receiving nurturing parenting, have no manifestations of any important health problems, and are growing and developing in a satisfactory fashion. Developmental, psychosocial, and chronic disease issues for children and adolescents may require more frequent counseling and treatment visits separate from preventive care visits. Additional visits also may become necessary if circumstances suggest concerns.

These recommendations represent a consensus by the American Academy of Pediatrics (AAP) and Bright Futures. The AAP continues to emphasize the great importance of continuity of care in comprehensive health supervision and the need to avoid fragmentation of care.

Refer to the specific guidance by age as listed in the *Bright Futures Guidelines* (Hagan JF, Shaw JS, Duncan PM, eds. *Bright Futures: Guidelines for Health Supervision of Infants, Children, and Adolescents.* 4th ed. American Academy of Pediatrics; 2017).

The recommendations in this statement do not indicate an exclusive course of treatment or serve as a standard of medical care. Variations, taking into account individual circumstances, may be appropriate.

The Bright Futures/American Academy of Pediatrics Recommendations for Preventive Pediatric Health Care are updated annually.

Copyright © 2024 by the American Academy of Pediatrics, updated June 2024.
No part of this statement may be reproduced in any form or by any means without prior written permission from the American Academy of Pediatrics except for one copy for personal use.

	INFANCY								EARLY CHILDHOOD						
AGE[1]	Prenatal[2]	Newborn[3]	3-5 d[4]	By 1 mo	2 mo	4 mo	6 mo	9 mo	12 mo	15 mo	18 mo	24 mo	30 mo	3 y	4 y
HISTORY Initial/Interval	●	●	●	●	●	●	●	●	●	●	●	●	●	●	●
MEASUREMENTS															
Length/Height and Weight		●	●	●	●	●	●	●	●	●	●	●	●	●	●
Head Circumference		●	●	●	●	●	●	●	●	●	●	●			
Weight for Length		●	●	●	●	●	●	●	●	●	●				
Body Mass Index[5]												●	●	●	●
Blood Pressure[6]		★	★	★	★	★	★	★	★	★	★	★	★	●	●
SENSORY SCREENING															
Vision[7]		★	★	★	★	★	★	★	★	★	★	★	★	●	●
Hearing		●[8]	●[9]		→	★	★	★	★	★	★	★	★	★	●
DEVELOPMENTAL/SOCIAL/BEHAVIORAL/MENTAL HEALTH															
Maternal Depression Screening[11]				●	●	●	●								
Developmental Screening[12]								●			●		●		
Autism Spectrum Disorder Screening[13]											●	●			
Developmental Surveillance		●	●	●	●	●	●		●	●		●		●	●
Behavioral/Social/Emotional Screening[14]		●	●	●	●	●	●	●	●	●	●	●	●	●	●
Tobacco, Alcohol, or Drug Use Assessment[15]															
Depression and Suicide Risk Screening[16]															
PHYSICAL EXAMINATION[17]		●	●	●	●	●	●	●	●	●	●	●	●	●	●
PROCEDURES[18]															
Newborn Blood		●[19]	●[20]		→										
Newborn Bilirubin[21]		●													
Critical Congenital Heart Defect[22]		●													
Immunization[23]		●	●	●	●	●	●	●	●	●	●	●	●	●	●
Anemia[24]						★			●	★	★	★	★	★	★
Lead[25]							★	★	● or ★[26]		★	● or ★[26]		★	★
Tuberculosis[27]				★			★		★			★		★	★
Dyslipidemia[28]												★			★
Sexually Transmitted Infections[29]															
HIV[30]															
Hepatitis B Virus Infection[31]		★ ———													
Hepatitis C Virus Infection[32]															
Sudden Cardiac Arrest/Death[33]															
Cervical Dysplasia[34]															
ORAL HEALTH[35]							●[36]	●[36]	★		★	★	★	★	★
Fluoride Varnish[37]							←				●				
Fluoride Supplementation[38]							★	★	★		★	★	★	★	★
ANTICIPATORY GUIDANCE	●	●	●	●	●	●	●	●	●	●	●	●	●	●	●

	MIDDLE CHILDHOOD						ADOLESCENCE										
AGE[1]	5 y	6 y	7 y	8 y	9 y	10 y	11 y	12 y	13 y	14 y	15 y	16 y	17 y	18 y	19 y	20 y	21 y
HISTORY Initial/Interval	●	●	●	●	●	●	●	●	●	●	●	●	●	●	●	●	●
MEASUREMENTS																	
Length/Height and Weight	●	●	●	●	●	●	●	●	●	●	●	●	●	●	●	●	●
Head Circumference																	
Weight for Length																	
Body Mass Index[5]	●	●	●	●	●	●	●	●	●	●	●	●	●	●	●	●	●
Blood Pressure[6]	●	●	●	●	●	●	●	●	●	●	●	●	●	●	●	●	●
SENSORY SCREENING																	
Vision[7]	●	●	★	●	★	●	★	●	★	★	●	★	★	★	★	★	★
Hearing	●	●	★	●	★	●	←		●[10]	→	←	●	→	←		●	→
DEVELOPMENTAL/SOCIAL/BEHAVIORAL/MENTAL HEALTH																	
Maternal Depression Screening[11]																	
Developmental Screening[12]																	
Autism Spectrum Disorder Screening[13]																	
Developmental Surveillance	●	●	●	●	●	●	●	●	●	●	●	●	●	●	●	●	●
Behavioral/Social/Emotional Screening[14]	●	●	●	●	●	●	●	●	●	●	●	●	●	●	●	●	●
Tobacco, Alcohol, or Drug Use Assessment[15]							★	★	★	★	★	★	★	★	★	★	★
Depression and Suicide Risk Screening[16]								●	●	●	●	●	●	●	●	●	●
PHYSICAL EXAMINATION[17]	●	●	●	●	●	●	●	●	●	●	●	●	●	●	●	●	●
PROCEDURES[18]																	
Newborn Blood																	
Newborn Bilirubin[21]																	
Critical Congenital Heart Defect[22]																	
Immunization[23]	●	●	●	●	●	●	●	●	●	●	●	●	●	●	●	●	●
Anemia[24]	★	★	★	★	★	★	★	★	★	★	★	★	★	★	★	★	★
Lead[25]	★	★															
Tuberculosis[27]	★	★	★	★	★	★	★	★	★	★	★	★	★	★	★	★	★
Dyslipidemia[28]		★		★	←	●	→	★	★	★	★	★	←			●	→
Sexually Transmitted Infections[29]							★	★	★	★	★	★	★	★	★	★	★
HIV[30]							★	★	★	★	●						→
Hepatitis B Virus Infection[31]																	→
Hepatitis C Virus Infection[32]														●			→
Sudden Cardiac Arrest/Death[33]							★ ———										
Cervical Dysplasia[34]																	●
ORAL HEALTH[35]	★	★															
Fluoride Varnish[37]	→																
Fluoride Supplementation[38]	★	★	★	★	★	★	★	★	★	★	★	★					
ANTICIPATORY GUIDANCE	●	●	●	●	●	●	●	●	●	●	●	●	●	●	●	●	●

1. If a child comes under care for the first time at any point on the schedule, or if any items are not accomplished at the suggested age, the schedule should be brought up to date at the earliest possible time.
2. A prenatal visit is recommended for parents who are at high risk, for first-time parents, and for those who request a conference. The prenatal visit should include anticipatory guidance, pertinent medical history, and a discussion of benefits of breastfeeding and planned method of feeding, per "The Prenatal Visit" (https://doi.org/10.1542/-peds.2018-1218).
3. Newborns should have an evaluation after birth, and breastfeeding should be encouraged (and instruction and support should be offered).
4. Newborns should have an evaluation within 3 to 5 days of birth and within 48 to 72 hours after discharge from the hospital to include evaluation for feeding and jaundice. Breastfeeding newborns should receive formal breastfeeding evaluation, and their mothers should receive encouragement and instruction, as recommended in "Policy Statement: Breastfeeding and the Use of Human Milk" (https://doi.org/10.1542/peds.2022-057988).Newborns discharged less than 48 hours after delivery must be examined within 48 hours of discharge, per "Hospital Stay for Healthy Term Newborn Infants" (https://doi.org/10.1542/peds.2015-0699).
5. Screen, per "Clinical Practice Guideline for the Evaluation and Treatment of Children and Adolescents with Obesity" (https://doi.org/10.1542/peds.2022-060640).
6. Screening should occur per "Clinical Practice Guideline for Screening and Management of High Blood Pressure in Children and Adolescents" (https://doi.org/10.1542/peds.2017-1904). Blood pressure measurement in infants and children with specific risk conditions should be performed at visits before age 3 years.
7. A visual acuity screen is recommended at ages 4 and 5 years, as well as in cooperative 3-year-olds. Instrument-based screening may be used to assess risk at ages 12 and 24 months, in addition to the well visits at 3 through 5 years of age. See "Visual System Assessment in Infants, Children, and Young Adults by Pediatricians" (https://doi.org/10.1542/-peds.2015-3596) and "Procedures for the Evaluation of the Visual System by Pediatricians" (https://doi.org/10.1542/-peds.2015-3597).
8. Confirm initial screen was completed, verify results, and follow up, as appropriate. Newborns should be screened per "Year 2007 Position Statement: Principles and Guidelines for Early Hearing Detection and Intervention Programs" (https://doi.org/10.1542/peds.2007-2333).
9. Verify results as soon as possible, and follow up, as appropriate.
10. Screen with audiometry including 6,000 and 8,000 Hz high frequencies once between 11 and 14 years, once between 15 and 17 years, and once between 18 and 21 years. See "The Sensitivity of Adolescent Hearing Screens Significantly Improves by Adding High Frequencies" (https://www.sciencedirect.com/science/arti-cle/abs/pii/S1054139X16000483).
11. Screening should occur per "Incorporating Recognition and Management of Perinatal Depression Into Pediatric Practice" (https://doi.org/10.1542/peds.2018-3259).
12. Screening should occur per "Promoting Optimal Development: Identifying Infants and Young Children With Developmental Disorders Through Developmental Surveillance and Screening" (https://doi.org/10.1542/-peds.2019-3449).
13. Screening should occur per "Identification, Evaluation, and Management of Children With Autism Spectrum Disorder" (https://doi.org/10.1542/peds.2019-3447).

(continued)

KEY: ● = to be performed ★ = risk assessment to be performed with appropriate action to follow, if positive ←——★ or ●——→ = range during which a service may be provided

BFNC.2024.PSMAR
3-367/0324

FIGURE 9.1 Recommendations for Preventive Pediatric Health Care. (Copyright 2024 by the American Academy of Pediatrics. Reproduced with permission. https://downloads.aap.org/AAP/PDF/periodicity_schedule.pdf.)

(continued)

14. Screen for behavioral and social-emotional problems per "Promoting Optimal Development: Screening for Behavioral and Emotional Problems" (https://doi.org/10.1542/peds.2014-3716), "Mental Health Competencies for Pediatric Practice" (https://doi.org/10.1542/peds.2019-2757), "Clinical Practice Guideline for the Assessment and Treatment of Children and Adolescents With Anxiety Disorders" (https://pubmed.ncbi.nlm.nih.gov/32439401),"Screening for Anxiety in Adolescent and Adult Women: A Recommendation From the Women's Preventive Services Initiative" (https://pubmed.ncbi.nlm.nih.gov/32510990), and "Anxiety in Children and Adolescents: Screening" (https://www.uspreventiveservicestaskforce.org/uspstf/recommendation/screening-anxiety-children-adolescents). The screening should be family centered and may include asking about caregiver emotional and mental health concerns and social determinants of health, racism, poverty, and relational health. See "Poverty and Child Health in the United States" (https://doi.org/10.1542/peds.2016-0339), "The Impact of Racism on Child and Adolescent Health" (https://doi.org/10.1542/peds.2019-1765), and "Preventing Childhood Toxic Stress: Partnering With Families and Communities to Promote Relational Health" (https://doi.org/10.1542/peds.2021-052582).
15. A recommended tool to assess use of alcohol, tobacco and nicotine, marijuana, and other substances, including opioids is available at http://crafft.org. If there is a concern for substance or opioid use, providers should consider recommending or prescribing Naloxone (see https://www.cdc.gov/ore/search/pages/2018-evidence-based-strategies.html and https://nida.nih.gov/publications/drugfacts/naloxone).
16. Screen adolescents for depression and suicide risk, making every effort to preserveconfidentiality of the adolescent. See "Guidelines for Adolescent Depression in Primary Care (GLAD-PC): Part I. Practice Preparation, Identification, Assessment, and Initial Management" (https://doi.org/10.1542/peds.2017-4081), "Mental Health Competencies for Pediatric Practice" (https://doi.org/10.1542/peds.2019-2757), "Suicide and Suicide Attempts in Adolescents" (https://doi.org/10.1542/peds.2016-1420), and "The 21st Century Cures Act & Adolescent Confidentiality" (https://adolescenthealth.org/press_release/naspag-sahm-statement-the-21st-century-cures-act-adolescent-confidentiality/).
17. At each visit, age-appropriate physical examination is essential, with infant totally unclothed and older children undressed and suitably draped. See "Use of Chaperones During the Physical Examination of the Pediatric Patient" (https://doi.org/10.1542/peds.2011-0322).
18. These may be modified, depending on entry point into schedule and individual need.
19. Confirm initial screen was accomplished, verify results, and follow up, as appropriate. The Recommended Uniform Screening Panel (https://www.hrsa.gov/advisory-committees/heritable-disorders/rusp/index.html), as determined by The Secretary's Advisory Committee on Heritable Disorders in Newborns and Children, andstate newborn screening laws/regulations (https://www.babysfirsttest.org/) establish the criteria for and coverage of newborn screening procedures and programs.
20. Verify results as soon as possible, and follow up, as appropriate.
21. Confirm initial screening was accomplished, verify results, and follow up, as appropriate.See "Clinical Practice Guideline Revision: Management of Hyperbilirubinemia in the Newborn Infant 35 or More Weeks of Gestation" (https://doi.org/10.1542/peds.2022-058859).
22. Screening for critical congenital heart disease using pulse oximetry should be performed in newborns, after 24 hours of age, before discharge from the hospital,per "Endorsement of Health and Human Services Recommendation for Pulse Oximetry Screening for Critical Congenital Heart Disease" (https://doi.org/10.1542/peds.2011-3211).
23. Schedules, per the AAP Committee on Infectious Diseases, are available at https://publications.aap.org/redbook/pages/immunization-schedules. Every visit should be an oppor tunity to update and complete a child's immunizations.
24. Perform risk assessment or screening, as appropriate, per recommendations in the current edition of the AAP Pediatric Nutrition: Policy of the American Academyof Pediatrics (Iron chapter).
25. For children at risk of lead exposure, see "Prevention of Childhood Lead Toxicity" (https://doi.org/10.1542/peds.2016-1493) and "Low Level Lead Exposure Harms Children:A Renewed Call for Primary Prevention" (https://stacks.cdc.gov/view/cdc/11859).
26. Perform risk assessments or screenings as appropriate, based on universal screening requirements for patients with Medicaid or in high prevalence areas.
27. Tuberculosis testing per recommendations of the AAP Committee on Infectious Diseases, published in the current edition of the AAP *Red Book: Report of the Committeeon Infectious Diseases.* Testing should be performed on recognition of high-risk factors.
28. See "Integrated Guidelines for Cardiovascular Health and Risk Reduction in Childrenand Adolescents" (http://www.nhlbi.nih.gov/guidelines/cvd_ped/index.htm).
29. Adolescents should be screened for sexually transmitted infections (STIs) per recommendations in the current edition of the AAP *Red Book: Report of the Committee on Infectious Diseases.*
30. Screen adolescents for HIV at least once between the ages of 15 and 21, making every effort to preserve confidentiality of the adolescent, as per "Human Immunodeficiency Virus (HIV) Infection: Screening" (https://www.uspreventiveservicestaskforce.org/uspstf/recommendation/human-immunodeficiency-virus-hiv-infection-screening); after initial screening, youth at increased risk of HIV infection should be retested annually or more frequently, as per "Adolescents and Young Adults: The Pediatrician's Role in HIV Testing and Pre- and Postexposure HIV Prophylaxis" (https://doi.org/10.1542/peds.2021-055207).
31. Perform a risk assessment for hepatitis B virus (HBV) infection according to recommendations per the USPSTF (https://www.uspreventiveservicestaskforce.org/uspstf/recommendation/hepatitis-b-virus-infection-screening) and in the 2021–2024 edition of the AAP *Red Book: Report of the Committee on Infectious Diseases, making every effort to preserve confidentiality of the patient.*
32. All individuals should be screened for hepatitis C virus (HCV) infection according to the USPSTF (https://www.uspreventiveservicestaskforce.org/uspstf/recommendation/hepatitis-c-screening) and Centers for Disease Control and Prevention(CDC) recommendations (https://www.cdc.gov/mmwr/volumes/69/rr/rr6902a1.htm) at least once between the ages of 18 and 79. Those at increased risk of HCV infection,including those who are persons with past or current injection drug use, should be tested for HCV infection and reassessed annually.
33. Perform a risk assessment, as appropriate, per "Sudden Death in the Young: Informationfor the Primary Care Provider" (https://doi.org/10.1542/peds.2021-052044).
34. See USPSTF recommendations (https://www.uspreventiveservicestaskforce.org/uspstf/recommendation/cervical-cancer-screening). Indications for pelvic examinations prior to age 21 are noted in "Gynecologic Examination for Adolescents in the Pediatric Office Setting" (https://doi.org/10.1542/peds.2010-1564).
35. Assess whether the child has a dental home. If no dental home is identified, performa risk assessment (https://www.aap.org/en/patient-care/oral-health/oral-health-practice-tools/) and refer to a dental home. Recommend brushing with fluoride toothpaste in the proper dosage for age. See "Maintaining and Improving the Oral Health of Young Children" (https://doi.org/10.1542/peds.2022-060417).
36. Perform a risk assessment (https://www.aap.org/en/patient-care/oral-health/oral-health-practice-tools/). See "Maintaining and Improving the Oral Health of Young Children" (https://doi.org/10.1542/peds.2022-060417).
37. The USPSTF recommends that primary care clinicians apply fluoride varnish to the primary teeth of all infants and children starting at the age of primary tooth eruption (https://www.uspreventiveservicestaskforce.org/uspstf/recommendation/prevention-of-dental-caries-in-children-younger-than-age-5-years-screening-and-interventions1). Once teeth are present, apply fluoride varnish to all children every 3 to 6 months in the primary care or dental office based on caries risk. Indications for fluoride use are noted in"Fluoride Use in Caries Prevention in the Primary Care Setting" (https://doi.org/10.1542/peds.2020-034637).
38. If primary water source is deficient in fluoride, consider oral fluoride supplementation. See "Fluoride Use in Caries Prevention in the Primary Care Setting" (https://doi.org/10.1542/peds.2020-034637).

Summary of Changes Made to the Bright Futures/AAP Recommendations for Preventive Pediatric Health Care (Periodicity Schedule)

This schedule reflects changes approved in December 2023 and published in June 2024. For updates and a list of previous changes made, visit www.aap.org/periodicityschedule.

FOOTNOTE CHANGES MADE IN DECEMBER 2023

- **3-5 DAY VISIT**
  (Footnote 4)
  This footnote reflects the AAP "Policy Statement: Breastfeeding and theUse of Human Milk", published June 2022.
- **BODY MASS INDEX**
  (Footnote 5)
  This footnote reflects the AAP "Clinical Practice Guideline for the Evaluation and Treatment of Children and Adolescents with Obesity",published January 2023.
- **BEHAVIORAL/SOCIAL/EMOTIONAL SCREENING**
  (Footnote 14)
  This footnote reflects the USPSTF "Anxiety in Children and Adolescents: Screening" recommendations, published October 2022.
- **TOBACCO, ALCOHOL, OR DRUG USE ASSESSMENT**
  (Footnote 15)
  This footnote reflects the Centers for Disease Control (CDC) and NationalInstitute of Drug Abuse (NIDA) guidance related to recommending and prescribing Naloxone.
- **NEWBORN BILIRUBIN SCREENING**
  (Footnote 21)
  This footnote reflects the AAP "Clinical Practice Guideline Revision: Management of Hyperbilirubinemia in the Newborn Infant 35 or MoreWeeks of Gestation", published August 2022.
- **ORAL HEALTH**
  (Footnotes 35 and 36)
  These footnotes reflect the AAP clinical report, "Maintaining and Improving the Oral Health of Young Children", published December 2022.

CHANGES MADE IN DECEMBER 2022

HIV

The HIV screening recommendation has been updated to extend the upper age limit from 18 to 21 years (to account for the range in which the screening can take place) to align with recommendations of the US Preventive Services Task Force and AAP policy ("Adolescents and Young Adults: The Pediatrician's Role in HIV Testing and Pre- and Postexposure HIV Prophylaxis").

- Footnote 30 has been updated to read as follows: "Screen adolescents for HIV at least once between the ages of 15 and 21, making every effort to preserve confidentiality of the adolescent, as per 'Human Immunodeficiency Virus (HIV) Infection: Screening' (https://www.uspreventiveservicestaskforce.org/uspstf/recommendation/human-immunodeficiency-virus-hiv-infection-screening); after initial screening, youth at increased risk of HIV infection should be retested annually or more frequently, as per 'Adolescents and Young Adults: The Pediatrician's Role in HIV Testing and Pre- and Postexposure HIV Prophylaxis' (https://doi.org/10.1542/peds.2021-055207)"

HRSA
Health Resources & Services Administration
This program is supported by the Health Resources and Services Administration (HRSA) of the U.S. Department of Health and Human Services (HHS) as part of an award totaling $1,766,000 with 0% financed with non-governmental sources. The contents of this document are those of the author(s) and do not necessarily represent the official views of, nor an endorsement, by HRSA, HHS, or the U.S. Government. For more information, please visit HRSA.gov.

FIGURE 9.1, cont'd

speech and language development. Inferences about vision can be made by examining gross motor milestones (children with vision problems may have a delay) and by physical examination of the eye. Photoscreeners (instruments that autodetect some vision abnormalities) are increasingly being used for younger children; they are not recommended over visual acuity screening for older children that can cooperate with testing. Caregiver concerns about vision and hearing should also be elicited. If there are concerns, definitive testing should be pursued. For toddlers and older children who cannot cooperate with formal audiologic testing with headphones, hearing can be screened by auditory evoked responses or with behavioral audiology. Sounds of specific frequencies are provided in a soundproof room and responses are assessed by a trained audiologist. Vision may be assessed by referral to a pediatric ophthalmologist and by visual evoked responses (see Chapter 10).

Children 3 Years of Age and Older

At various ages, hearing and vision should be screened objectively as specified in Bright Futures Recommendations. At 3 years, visual acuity screening is done for the first time if the child is developmentally able. Some 3-year-olds do not have the language or interpersonal skills to do this; these children should have vision re-examined within 6 months. As most of these children do not yet identify letters, using a Snellen eye chart with standard shapes is recommended. When a child can identify letters, the more accurate letter-based chart should be used.

Audiologic testing of sounds with headphones should begin at 4 years. Any suspected audiologic problem should be evaluated by a careful history and physical examination with referral for comprehensive testing. Children who have a documented vision problem, failed screening, or caregiver concern should be referred, preferably to a pediatric ophthalmologist.

Anemia Screening

Anemia can negatively affect development and health. Infants are screened at birth and again at 4 months if there is a documented risk, such as low birthweight or prematurity. All infants are screened at 12 months of age as this is when a high incidence of iron deficiency is noted. Children are assessed at other ages if risk factors for anemia exist. Any abnormalities should be evaluated for underlying etiology. When iron deficiency is strongly suspected, a therapeutic trial of iron may be used (see Chapter 151).

Lead Screening

Lead intoxication can cause developmental and behavioral abnormalities that are irreversible, even if the hematologic and other metabolic complications are treated. The Centers for Disease Control and Prevention (CDC) recommends environmental investigation at blood lead levels of 20 mcg/dL on a single visit or persistent 15 mcg/dL over a 3-month period; levels of 5–10 mcg/dL may cause learning problems. Risk factors for lead intoxication include living in older homes with cracked or peeling lead-based paint, industrial exposure, use of alternative remedies that contain lead (e.g., azarcon for chronic diarrhea), and use of pottery with lead paint glaze. The CDC recommends routine blood lead screening at 12 and 24 months. In addition, standardized screening questions for risk of lead intoxication should be asked for all children between 6 months and 6 years of age (Table 9.2). Any positive response is an indication for obtaining a blood lead level. Capillary blood sampling may produce false-positive results; thus, in most situations, a venous blood sample should be obtained or a process implemented to get children tested with a venous sample if they have an elevated capillary level. County health departments, community organizations, and private companies provide lead inspection and detection services to determine the source of the lead. Standard decontamination techniques should be used to remove the lead while avoiding creation of aerosolized metals that a child might inhale or dust that a child might ingest (see Chapter 151).

Tuberculosis Testing

Children with tuberculosis (TB) can present with serious and multisystem disease (miliary tuberculosis). All children should be assessed for risk of TB at health maintenance visits at 1 month, 6 months, 12 months, and then annually. High-risk groups, as defined by the CDC, are listed in Table 9.3. In general, the standardized purified protein derivative intradermal test is used with evaluation by a health care provider 48–72 hours after injection. The size of induration, not the color of any mark, denotes a positive test; 15 mm of induration is a positive test in anyone. For most patients with risk factors, 10 mm of induration is a positive test. For children with immunosuppressive conditions, recent TB contacts, and other conditions, 5 mm is a positive test. See Chapter 125 for specifics on interpreting TB skin tests. Interferon gamma release assays are blood tests that have the advantage of only needing one office visit, but they cost more.

TABLE 9.2 Lead Poisoning Risk Assessment Questions To Be Asked Between 6 Months and 6 Years

Does the child live in or regularly visit a home built before 1950?
Does the child spend any time in a building built before 1978 with recent or ongoing painting, repair work, remodeling, or damage?
Is there a brother, sister, housemate, playmate, or community member being followed or treated (or even rumored to be) for lead poisoning?
Does the child live with an adult whose job or hobby involves exposure to lead (e.g., lead smelting and automotive radiator repair)?
Does the child live near an active lead smelter, battery recycling plant, or other industry likely to release lead?
Does the family use home remedies or pottery from another country?

TABLE 9.3 Groups at High Risk for TB

Close contact with persons known to have TB, those who have had a positive TB test, or those suspected to have TB
Foreign-born persons from areas with high TB rates (Asia, Africa, Latin America, Eastern Europe, Russia)
Health care workers
High-risk racial or ethnic minorities or other populations at higher risk (Asian, Pacific Islander, Hispanic, Black, Native American, groups living in poverty [e.g., Medicaid recipients], migrant farm workers, individuals experiencing homelessness or substance use disorder)
Children <5 years of age
Immunocompromised individuals

TB, Tuberculosis.

Cholesterol

Children and adolescents who have a family history of cardiovascular disease or have at least one parent with a high blood cholesterol level are at increased risk of having high blood cholesterol levels as adults and increased risk of coronary heart disease. The AAP recommends dyslipidemia screening with fasting lipid panel once between the ages 9–11 years and once between ages 17–21 years. At other ages, screening is done for at-risk populations (Table 9.4). The recommended screening levels are the same for all children 2–18 years. Total cholesterol of less than 170 mg/dL is normal, 170–199 mg/dL is borderline, and 200 mg/dL or greater is elevated.

Sexually Transmitted Infection Testing

Annual office visits are recommended for adolescents. A full adolescent psychosocial history should be obtained in confidential fashion (see Section 12). Part of this evaluation is a comprehensive sexual history that often requires creative questioning. Not all adolescents identify oral sex as sex, and some adolescents misinterpret the term *sexually active* to mean that one has several sexual partners or is very vigorous during intercourse. The straightforward questions, "Are you having sex?" and "Have you ever had sex?" should be asked. In the Bright Futures Guidelines, any child or adolescent who has had any form of sexual intercourse should have at least an annual evaluation (more often if there is a history of high-risk sexual activity) for sexually transmitted infections by physical examination (genital warts, genital herpes, and pediculosis) and laboratory testing (chlamydia, gonorrhea, syphilis, and HIV) (see Chapter 117). Young women should start Papanicolaou testing at 21 years of age to assess for human papillomavirus and precancerous lesions.

Depression Screening

All adolescents, starting at age 11, should have annual depression screening with a validated tool. The Patient Health Questionnaires (PHQ9 and the shorter PHQ2) are commonly used. The Bright Futures Tool and Resource Kit at https://publications.aap.org/toolkits/pages/bright-futures-toolkit includes links to PHQs and other recommended forms for well visits.

Immunizations

Immunization records should be checked at each office visit, regardless of the reason for the visit. Appropriate vaccinations should be administered (see Chapter 95).

TABLE 9.4 Cholesterol Risk Screening Recommendations

Risk screening at ages 2, 4, 6, and 8 years, and annually in adolescence with selective cholesterol screening for:

1. Children and adolescents who have a family history of high cholesterol or heart disease
2. Children whose family history is unknown
3. Children who have other personal risk factors: obesity, high blood pressure, or diabetes

Universal cholesterol screening at ages 9–11 years and ages 17–21 years (once per age range)

DENTAL CARE

Some families in the United States do not have access to or underutilize dental health care. Providers should examine the oral cavity for caries, gingivitis, or malocclusion. All children 1 year and older should have a dental examination by a dentist at least annually plus a dental cleaning every 6 months. Parents should be advised to brush teeth with fluoride toothpaste at first tooth eruption and to floss teeth when teeth begin to touch at 2–3 years old. For prevention of caries, providers need to advise against any overnight beverages other than water in bottles after 1 year. Fluoride topical treatments (dental varnish) and acrylic sealants on the molars are also effective at preventing caries. Bright Futures recommends that pediatricians apply dental varnish every 3–6 months at ages 9 months to 5 years if not done by a dentist. Fluoridation of water or fluoride supplements in communities that do not have fluoridation are important in the prevention of cavities (see Chapter 128).

NUTRITIONAL ASSESSMENT

Plotting a child's growth on standard charts is a vital component of the nutritional assessment. A dietary history should be obtained as the content of the diet may suggest a risk of nutritional deficiency (see Section 6).

ANTICIPATORY GUIDANCE

Anticipatory guidance is information conveyed to caregivers verbally, in written materials, or by directing caregivers to certain websites to assist them in facilitating optimal growth and development for their children. The Bright Futures Tool and Resource Kit includes topics and one-page handouts for families (and for older children) about the highest yield issues for the child's upcoming age. Table 9.5 summarizes representative issues that might be discussed. It is important to give age-appropriate advice and to review topics discussed at previous visits for reinforcement.

Safety Issues

Motor vehicle crashes are a leading cause of accidental death. No newborn should be discharged from a nursery without a properly installed car seat. Automobile dealerships (for their car brand) and fire departments may offer services to caregivers to ensure that safety seats are installed properly. Most states have laws that mandate the use of safety seats until the child reaches 4 years of age or at least 40 pounds in weight. The following are age-appropriate recommendations for car safety:

1. Infants and toddlers should ride in a **rear-facing safety seat** until they are at least 2 years old. It is safest for children to remain rear-facing after 2 years old for as long as possible while within weight and height limits set by the safety seat manufacturer.
2. Toddlers and preschoolers over age 2 who have outgrown the rear-facing car seat should use a **forward-facing car seat** with harness for as long as possible up to the highest weight or height recommended by the manufacturer.
3. School-age children, whose weight or height is above the forward-facing limit for their car seat, should use a **belt-positioning booster seat** until the vehicle seat belt fits properly, when they have reached 4 ft 9 in. in height and are between 8 and 12 years of age.

TABLE 9.5 Anticipatory Guidance Topics Suggested by Age

AGES	INJURY PREVENTION	VIOLENCE PREVENTION	NUTRITIONAL COUNSELING	FOSTERING OPTIMAL DEVELOPMENT
Birth and/or 3–5 days	Crib safety Hot water heaters <120°F Car safety seats Smoke detectors Back to Sleep (safe sleep)	Assess bonding and attachment Identify family strife, lack of support, pathology Educate parents on nurturing	Exclusive breast-feeding encouraged, formula as another option with reminders that "fed is best"	Discuss parenting skills Refer for parenting education
2 weeks or 1 month	Falls Back to Sleep	Reassess* Discuss sibling rivalry Assess if guns in the home	Assess breast-feeding and offer encouragement, problem solving	Recognize and manage postpartum depression Child-care options
2 months	Burns/hot liquids Back to Sleep	Reassess firearm safety		Parent getting enough rest and managing returning to work
4 months	Infant walkers Choking/suffocation Back to Sleep	Reassess	Introduction of solid foods	Discuss central to peripheral motor development Praise good behavior
6 months	Burns/hot surfaces Childproofing	Reassess	Assess status	Consistent limit-setting vs. "spoiling" an infant Praise good behavior
9 months	Water safety Home safety review Ingestions/poisoning Car seat safety (rear-facing until ≥2 yr)	Assess parents' ideas on discipline and "spoiling"	Avoiding juice Begin to encourage practice with cup drinking	Assisting infants to sleep through the night if not accomplished Praise good behavior
12 months	Firearm hazards Auto-pedestrian safety Car seat safety (rear-facing until ≥2 yr)	Discuss time-out vs. corporal punishment Avoiding media violence Review firearm safety	Introduction of whole cow's milk (and constipation with change discussed) Assess anemia, discuss iron-rich foods	Safe exploration Proper shoes Praise good behavior
15 months	Review and reassess topics	Encourage nonviolent punishments (time-out or natural consequences)	Discuss decline in eating with slower growth Assess food choices and variety	Fostering independence Reinforce good behavior Ignore annoying but not unsafe behaviors
18 months	Review and reassess topics	Limit punishment to high yield and major transgressions Parents consistent in discipline	Discuss food choices, portions, "finicky" feeders	Preparation for toilet training Reinforce good behavior
2 years	Falls—play equipment	Assess and discuss any aggressive behaviors in the child	Assess body proportions and recommend low-fat milk Assess family cholesterol and atherosclerosis risk	Toilet training and resistance
3 years	Review and reassess topics	Review, especially avoiding media violence	Discuss optimal eating and the food pyramid Healthy snacks	Read to child Socializing with other children Head Start if possible
4 years	Booster seat vs. seat belts	Reassess	Healthy snacks	Read to child Head Start or pre-K options
5 years	Bicycle safety Water/pool safety	Developing consistent, clearly defined family rules and consequences Avoiding media violence	Assess for anemia Discuss iron-rich foods	Reinforcing school topics Read to child Library card Chores begun at home
6 years	Fire safety	Reinforce consistent discipline Encourage nonviolent strategies Assess domestic violence Avoiding media violence	Assess content, offer specific suggestions	Reinforcing school topics After-school programs Responsibility given for chores (and enforced)

(Continued)

TABLE 9.5 Anticipatory Guidance Topics Suggested by Age—cont'd

AGES	INJURY PREVENTION	VIOLENCE PREVENTION	NUTRITIONAL COUNSELING	FOSTERING OPTIMAL DEVELOPMENT
7–10 years	Sports safety Firearm hazard	Reinforcement Assess domestic violence Assess discipline techniques Avoiding media violence Walking away from fights (either victim or spectator)	Assess content, offer specific suggestions	Reviewing homework and reinforcing school topics After-school programs Introduce smoking and substance abuse prevention (concrete)
11–13 years	Review and reassess	Discuss strategies to avoid interpersonal conflicts Avoiding media violence Avoiding fights and walking away Discuss conflict resolution techniques	Junk food vs. healthy eating	Reviewing homework and reinforcing school topics Smoking, vaping, and substance abuse prevention (begin abstraction) Discuss and encourage abstinence; possibly discuss condoms and contraceptive options Avoiding violence Offer availability
14–16 years	Motor vehicle safety Avoiding riding with substance abuser	Establish new family rules related to curfews, school, and household responsibilities	Junk food vs. healthy eating	Review school work Begin career discussions and college preparation (PSAT) Review substance abuse, sexuality, and violence regularly Discuss condoms, contraception options, including emergency contraception Discuss sexually transmitted infections, HIV Providing "no questions asked" ride home from at-risk situations
17–21 years	Review and reassess	Establish new rules related to driving, dating, and substance abuse	Heart healthy diet for life	Continuation of above topics Off to college or employment New roles within the family

*Reassess *means to review the issues discussed at the prior health maintenance visit.*
PSAT, Preliminary Scholastic Aptitude Test.

4. Older children should always use **lap and shoulder seat belts** for optimal protection. All children younger than 13 years should be restrained in the rear seats of vehicles for optimal protection. This is specifically to protect them from airbags, which may injure children.

The Back to Sleep initiative reduced the incidence of sudden infant death syndrome (SIDS). Before the initiative, infants routinely were placed prone to sleep. Since 1992, when the AAP recommended this program, the annual SIDS rate has decreased by more than 70%. The initiative was expanded to the **Safe to Sleep** campaign in 2022 to address various causes of sleep-related death. SIDS continues to be the leading cause of death at age 28 days to 1 year.

Fostering Optimal Development

See Table 9.5 as well as the Bright Futures Recommendations (Fig. 9.1) for age-appropriate activities that the pediatrician may advise for families.

Discipline means to teach, not merely to punish. The ultimate goal of discipline is the child's self-control. Overbearing punishment to control a child's behavior interferes with the learning process and focuses on external control at the expense of the development of self-control. Parents who set too few reasonable limits may be frustrated by children who cannot control their own behavior. Discipline should teach a child what is expected by supporting and reinforcing positive behaviors and responding appropriately to negative behaviors with proper limits. It is more important and effective to reinforce good behavior rather than just punish bad behavior.

Parenting styles are important because a caregiver's interactions with a child influence the child's growth, development, and eventual adult behavior. Parenting styles vary in the level of expectations and number of rules set for a child (demandingness), and in the level of warmth, communication, and consideration of the child's opinions (responsiveness). There are four recognized parenting styles: authoritative (high demandingness, high responsiveness), authoritarian (high demandingness, low responsiveness), permissive (low demandingness, high responsiveness), and uninvolved (low demandingness, low responsiveness). Authoritative parenting is regarded as the style most likely to result in a child who is happy, successful, and self-disciplined.

Other techniques to control undesirable behaviors in children include scolding, physical punishment, and threats. These techniques have potential adverse effects on children's sense of security and self-esteem. The effectiveness of scolding diminishes the more it is used. Scolding should not be allowed to expand from an expression of displeasure about a specific event to derogatory statements about the child. Scolding also may escalate to the level of psychologic abuse. It is important to educate parents that they have a *good child who does bad things from time to time*, so parents do not think and tell the child that they are "bad."

Frequent mild physical punishment (corporal punishment) may become less effective over time and tempt the parent to escalate the physical punishment, increasing the risk of child abuse. Corporal punishment teaches a child that in certain situations it is proper to strike another person. Commonly, in households that use spanking, older children who have been raised with this technique are seen responding to younger sibling behavioral problems by hitting their siblings.

Threats by caregivers to leave or to give up the child are perhaps the most psychologically damaging ways to control a child's behavior. Children of any age may remain fearful and anxious about loss of the caregiver long after the threat is made. Threatening a mild loss of privileges (no videogames for 1 week or grounding a teenager) may be appropriate, but the consequence must be enforced if there is a violation.

Parenting involves a dynamic balance between **setting limits** and allowing and encouraging freedom of expression and exploration. A child whose behavior is out of control improves when clear limits on the behavior are set and enforced. Parents must agree on where the limit will be set and how it will be enforced. The limit and the consequence of breaking such limit must be clearly presented to the child. Enforcement of the limit should be consistent. Too many limits are difficult to learn and may thwart the normal development of autonomy. The limit must be reasonable in terms of the child's age, temperament, and developmental level. To be effective, all caregivers must consistently enforce limits. Otherwise, children may effectively *split* the parents and seek to test the limits with the more indulgent parent. In all situations, to be effective, punishment must be brief and linked directly to a behavior. More effective behavioral change occurs when punishment is linked to praise of the intended behavior.

Extinction is an effective and systematic way to eliminate frequent, annoying, and relatively harmless behavior by ignoring it. First, parents should note the frequency of the behavior to realistically appreciate the magnitude of the problem and to evaluate progress. Parents must determine what reinforces the child's behavior and what needs to be consistently eliminated. An appropriate behavior is identified to give the child a positive alternative that the parents can reinforce. Parents should be warned that the annoying behavior usually increases in frequency and intensity (and may last for weeks) before it decreases when the parent ignores it (removes the reinforcement). A child who has an attention-seeking temper tantrum should be ignored or placed in a secure environment. This action may anger the child more, and the behavior may get louder and angrier. Eventually, with no audience for the tantrum, the tantrums decrease in intensity and frequency. In each specific instance, when the child's behavior has become appropriate, the child should be praised, and extra attention should be given. This is an effective technique for early toddlers before their capacity to understand and adhere to a time-out develops.

A **time-out** consists of a short period of isolation immediately after a problem behavior is observed. Time-outs interrupt the behavior and immediately link it to an unpleasant consequence. This method requires considerable effort from the parents because the child does not wish to be isolated. A parent may need to physically hold the child in a time-out. In this situation, the parent should become *part of the furniture* and should not respond to the child until the time-out period is over. One effective protocol for the time-out procedure involves interrupting the child's activity when the behavior occurs and having the child sit in a dull, isolated place for a brief period, measured by a portable timer with an alarm to signal the end of the punishment. Time-out is simply punishment and is not a time for a young child to *think* about the behavior (these children do not possess the capacity for abstract thinking) or a time to deescalate the behavior. The amount of time-out should be appropriate to the child's short attention span; 1 minute per year of a child's age is recommended. This inescapable and unpleasant consequence of the undesired behavior motivates the child to learn to avoid the behavior.

PEARLS FOR PRACTITIONERS

See Growth and Development: Pearls for Practitioners at the end of this section.

REVIEW QUESTIONS

Available online.

CHAPTER 10

Evaluation of the Child With Special Needs

Children with disabilities, severe chronic illnesses, congenital defects, and health-related educational and behavioral problems are children with **special health care needs (SHCN)**. These children share a broad group of experiences and encounter similar problems, such as school difficulties and family stress. The term *children with special health care needs* defines the increased service needs of these children without regard to specific diagnoses. Approximately 19% of children in the United States younger than 18 years of age have a physical, developmental, behavioral, or emotional condition requiring services of a type or amount beyond those required by most children.

The goal in managing a child with SHCN is to maximize their potential for meaningful adult functioning by treating the primary diagnosis as well as helping the patient and family deal with the stresses and secondary impairments. Whenever a chronic disease is diagnosed, family members may go through phases of grief, anger, denial, negotiation (in an attempt to forestall the inevitable), and depression. As the child with SHCN is a constant reminder of the object of this grief, it may take family members a long time to accept the condition. A supportive physician can facilitate the process of acceptance by education and by allaying guilty feelings and fear. To minimize denial, it is helpful to confirm the family's observations about the child. The family may not be able to absorb any additional information initially, so written material and the option for delayed further discussion should be offered.

The primary physician should provide a **medical home** that maintains close oversight of care and subspecialty services, provides preventive care, and facilitates interactions with school and community agencies. A major goal of *family-centered care* is for the family and child to feel in control; they should be involved in developing care plans. Treatment plans for routine care at home should allow the greatest degree of normalization of the child's life. As the child matures, self-management programs that provide health education, self-efficacy skills, and techniques such as symptom monitoring help promote good long-term health habits. These programs should be introduced at 6 or 7 years of age or when a child is developmentally able to take on chores and benefit from being given responsibility. Self-management minimizes *learned helplessness* and the *vulnerable child syndrome*, both of which occur commonly in families with chronically ill or disabled children.

MULTIFACETED TEAM ASSESSMENT OF COMPLEX PROBLEMS

When developmental screening and surveillance suggest the presence of developmental delays, the physician should coordinate further assessment of the child by a team of professionals and provide continuity of care. If the child is at high risk for development delay (e.g., prematurity), a structured follow-up program to monitor the child's progress may already exist. Under federal law, all children are entitled to assessments if there is a suspected developmental delay or a risk factor for delay (e.g., prematurity, growth faltering, or parental intellectual developmental disorders [IDD]). **Early intervention programs** for children up to 3 years of age are run by states to implement this policy. Developmental interventions are paid for by local program funding when there is no insurance coverage. After 3 years of age, development programs are usually administered by school districts. Federal laws mandate that special education programs be provided for all children with developmental disabilities from birth through 21 years of age.

Children with special needs may be enrolled in pre-K programs with a therapeutic core, including visits to the facility by therapists. School-age children (kindergarten through secondary school) should be evaluated by the school district and provided with an **individualized education plan (IEP)** to address any deficiencies. An IEP may feature individual tutoring time, special education programming, placement in alternative settings for children with significant emotional or behavioral problems, or other strategies. As part of the comprehensive evaluation of developmental/behavioral issues, all children should receive a thorough medical assessment. A variety of specialists may assist in the assessment and intervention, including subspecialists (e.g., child neurologist, pediatric orthopedist, child and adolescent psychiatrist, developmental/behavioral pediatrician, geneticist), therapists (e.g., occupational, physical, oral-motor), and others (e.g., psychologist, early childhood development specialist).

Medical Assessment

As part of a team assessment, a physician's main goals should be to identify the cause of the developmental delay if possible (often a specific cause is not found) and identify other medical conditions that may have a developmental impact. The comprehensive history (Table 10.1) and physical examination (Table 10.2) include a careful graphing of growth parameters and an accurate description of dysmorphic features; oftentimes, causative diagnoses are rare or unusual diseases or syndromes. Some of these diseases and syndromes are discussed further in Sections 9 and 24.

Motor Assessment

The comprehensive neurologic examination is a foundation for evaluating motor function, but it should be supplemented by observing and evaluating a child's motor skills (see Chapter 180). Observing the child at play aids assessment of function. Specialists in early childhood development, occupational therapists, and physical therapists can provide excellent input into the evaluation of age-appropriate adaptive function.

Psychologic Assessment

Psychologic assessment includes the testing of cognitive ability (Table 10.3) and the evaluation of personality and emotional well-being. The intelligence quotient (IQ) and mental age scores taken in isolation are only partially descriptive of a person's functional abilities, which are a combination of cognitive, adaptive, and social skills. Tests of achievement are subject to variability based on culture, educational exposures, and experience; these must be standardized for social factors. Although a child should not be labeled as having a problem solely based on a standardized test, these tests provide important and reasonably objective data for evaluating a child's progress within a particular educational program.

Educational Assessment

Educational assessment involves the evaluation of specific strengths and weaknesses in reading, spelling, written expression, and mathematical skills. Schools routinely screen children with grouped tests to aid in problem identification and program evaluation. For the child with special needs, this screening should lead to individualized testing and the development of an IEP that would enable the child to progress comfortably in school. Diagnostic teaching, in which the child's response to various teaching techniques is assessed, may also be helpful.

Social Environment Assessment

Assessments of the environment in which the child is living, working, playing, and growing are important in understanding the child's development. A home visit by a social worker, community health nurse, and/or home-based intervention specialist can provide valuable information about the child's social milieu. Often, the home visitor can suggest additional

TABLE 10.1 Information to Elicit During the History Taking of a Child With Suspected Developmental Disabilities

ITEM	POSSIBLE SIGNIFICANCE
Parental concerns	Parents are quite accurate in identifying development problems in their children
Current levels of developmental functioning	Should be used to monitor child's progress
Temperament	May interact with disability or may be confused with developmental delay
PRENATAL HISTORY	
Alcohol ingestion	Fetal alcohol spectrum disorder; index of caregiving risk
Exposure to medication, illicit drugs, or toxin	Development toxin (e.g., phenytoin); may be an index of caregiving risk
Radiation exposure	Damage to CNS
Nutrition	Inadequate fetal nutrition
Prenatal care	Index of social situation
Injuries, hyperthermia	Damage to CNS
Smoking	Possible CNS damage
HIV exposure	Congenital HIV infection
Maternal illness ("**TORCH**" infections)	**T**oxoplasmosis, Syphilis (**O**ther in the mnemonic), **R**ubella, **C**ytomegalovirus, **H**erpes simplex virus infections
PERINATAL HISTORY	
Gestational age, birthweight	Biologic risk from prematurity and small for gestational age
Labor and delivery	Hypoxia or index of abnormal prenatal development
APGAR scores	Hypoxia, cardiovascular impairment
Specific perinatal adverse events	Increased risk of CNS damage
NEONATAL HISTORY	
Illness—seizures, respiratory distress, hyperbilirubinemia, metabolic disorder	Increased risk of CNS damage
Malformations	May represent genetic syndrome or new pathologic variant associated with developmental delay
FAMILY HISTORY	
Consanguinity	Autosomal recessive condition more likely
Cognitive functioning	Increased hereditary and environmental risks
Illnesses (e.g., metabolic diseases)	Hereditary illness associated with developmental delay
Family member died young or unexpectedly	May suggest inborn error of metabolism or storage disease
Family member requires special education	Hereditary causes of developmental delay
SOCIAL HISTORY	
Resources available (e.g., financial, social support)	Necessary to maximize child's potential
Educational level of parents	Family may need help to provide stimulation
Mental health problems	May exacerbate child's conditions
High-risk behaviors (e.g., illicit drugs, sex) in parent(s) or adolescents	Increased risk for HIV infection; index of caregiving risk
Other stressors (e.g., marital discord)	May exacerbate child's conditions or compromise care
OTHER HISTORY	
Sex of child	Important for X-linked conditions
Developmental milestones	Index of developmental delay; regression may indicate progressive condition
Head injury	Even moderate trauma may be associated with developmental delay or learning disabilities
Serious bacterial infections (e.g., meningitis)	May be associated with developmental delay
Toxic exposure (e.g., lead)	May be associated with developmental delay
Physical growth	May indicate malnutrition; obesity, short stature, genetic syndrome
Recurrent otitis media	Associated with hearing loss and abnormal speech development
Visual and auditory functioning	Sensitive index of impaired vision and hearing
Nutrition	Malnutrition during infancy may lead to delayed development
Chronic conditions such as renal disease	May be associated with delayed development or anemia

CNS, Central nervous system.
Modified and updated from Liptak G. Mental retardation and developmental disability. In: Kliegman RM, ed. Practical Strategies in Pediatric Diagnosis and Therapy. *Philadelphia: WB Saunders; 1996.*

TABLE 10.2 Information to Elicit During the Physical Examination of a Child With Suspected Developmental Disabilities

ITEM	POSSIBLE SIGNIFICANCE
General appearance	May indicate significant delay in development or features characteristic of a syndrome
STATURE	
Short stature	Williams syndrome, malnutrition, Turner syndrome; children with severe intellectual developmental disorders often have associated short stature
Obesity	Prader-Willi syndrome
Large stature	Sotos syndrome
HEAD	
Macrocephaly	Alexander syndrome, Sotos syndrome, gangliosidosis, hydrocephalus, mucopolysaccharidosis, subdural effusion
Microcephaly	Conditions that can inhibit brain growth (e.g., malnutrition, Angelman syndrome, Cornelia de Lange syndrome, fetal alcohol effects)
FACE	
Coarse, triangular, round, or flat face; hypotelorism or hypertelorism, slanted or short palpebral fissure; unusual nose, maxilla, and mandible	Specific measurements may provide clues to inherited, metabolic, or other diseases such as fetal alcohol syndrome, cri du chat syndrome (5p- syndrome), Williams syndrome, sialidosis II
EYES	
Prominent	Crouzon syndrome, Seckel syndrome, fragile X syndrome
Cataract	Galactosemia, Lowe syndrome, prenatal rubella, hypothyroidism
Cherry-red spot in macula	Gangliosidosis (GM_1), metachromatic leukodystrophy, Tay-Sachs disease, Niemann-Pick disease, Farber lipogranulomatosis, sialidosis
Chorioretinitis	Congenital infection with cytomegalovirus, toxoplasmosis, or rubella
Corneal cloudiness	Mucopolysaccharidosis I and II, Lowe syndrome, congenital syphilis
EARS	
Pinnae, low set or malformed	Trisomies such as 18, Rubinstein-Taybi syndrome, Down syndrome, CHARGE association, cerebro-oculo-facio-skeletal syndrome, fetal phenytoin effects

(Continued)

TABLE 10.2 Information to Elicit During the Physical Examination of a Child With Suspected Developmental Disabilities—cont'd

ITEM	POSSIBLE SIGNIFICANCE
Hearing	Loss of acuity in mucopolysaccharidosis; hyperacusis in several types of encephalopathy
HEART	
Structural anomaly or hypertrophy	CHARGE association, CATCH-22, velocardiofacial syndrome, glycogenosis II, fetal alcohol spectrum disorder, mucopolysaccharidosis I; chromosomal anomalies such as Down syndrome; maternal phenylketonuria; chronic cyanosis may impair cognitive development
LIVER	
Hepatomegaly	Fructose intolerance, galactosemia, glycogenosis types I to IV, mucopolysaccharidosis I and II, Niemann-Pick disease, Tay-Sachs disease, Zellweger syndrome, Gaucher disease, ceroid lipofuscinosis, gangliosidosis
GENITALIA	
Macro-orchidism (usually not noted until puberty)	Fragile X syndrome
Hypogenitalism	Prader-Willi syndrome, Klinefelter syndrome, CHARGE association
EXTREMITIES	
Hands, feet, dermatoglyphics, and creases	May indicate specific entity such as Rubinstein-Taybi syndrome or be associated with chromosomal anomaly
Joint contractures	Sign of muscle imbalance around joints (e.g., with meningomyelocele, cerebral palsy, arthrogryposis, muscular dystrophy; also occurs with cartilaginous problems such as mucopolysaccharidosis)
SKIN	
Café-au-lait spots	Neurofibromatosis, tuberous sclerosis, Bloom syndrome
Eczema	Phenylketonuria, histiocytosis
Hemangiomas and telangiectasia	Sturge-Weber syndrome, Bloom syndrome, ataxia-telangiectasia
Hypopigmented macules, streaks, facial angiofibromas	Tuberous sclerosis, hypomelanosis of Ito
HAIR	
Hirsutism	Cornelia de Lange syndrome, mucopolysaccharidosis, fetal phenytoin effects, cerebro-oculo-facio-skeletal syndrome, trisomy 18 syndrome

(Continued)

TABLE 10.2 Information to Elicit During the Physical Examination of a Child With Suspected Developmental Disabilities—cont'd

ITEM	POSSIBLE SIGNIFICANCE
NEUROLOGIC	
Asymmetry of strength and tone	Focal lesion, cerebral palsy
Hypotonia	Prader-Willi syndrome, Down syndrome, Angelman syndrome, gangliosidosis, early cerebral palsy
Hypertonia	Neurodegenerative conditions involving white matter, cerebral palsy, trisomy 18 syndrome
Ataxia	Ataxia-telangiectasia, metachromatic leukodystrophy, Angelman syndrome

CATCH-22, Cardiac defects, Abnormal face, Thymic hypoplasia, Cleft palate, Hypocalcemia, defects on chromosome 22; *CHARGE,* Coloboma, Heart defects, Atresia choanae, Retarded growth, Genital anomalies, Ear anomalies (deafness).
Modified and updated from Liptak G. Mental retardation and developmental disability. In: Kliegman RM, Greenbaum LA, Lye PS, eds. Practical Strategies in Pediatric Diagnosis and Therapy. *2nd ed. Philadelphia: Saunders; 2004:540.*

adaptive equipment or renovations if there are challenges at home. If there are suspicions of inadequate parenting, neglect, or abuse (including emotional abuse), the child and family must be referred to the local child protection agency (see Chapter 21). Information about reporting hotlines and local child protection agencies can be found at https://www.childwelfare.gov/organizations/.

MANAGEMENT OF DEVELOPMENTAL/ BEHAVIOR PROBLEMS

Intervention in the Primary Care Setting

The clinician must decide whether a problem can be managed in the primary care setting or if referral for further diagnostic evaluation and management is needed. Counseling roles required in caring for these children are listed in Table 10.4. When a child is young, much of the counseling interaction takes place between the parents and the clinician, and as the child matures, counseling increasingly shifts directly toward the child.

The assessment process may itself be therapeutic. By assuming the role of a nonjudgmental, supportive listener, the clinician creates a climate of trust, allowing the family to express difficult or painful thoughts and feelings. Expressing emotions may allow the parent or caregiver to move on to the work of understanding and resolving the problem.

Interview techniques can facilitate clarification of the problem for the family and for the clinician. The family's ideas surrounding the causes of the problem and attempts at coping can provide a basis for developing strategies for problem management. When approached in this manner, these strategies are more likely to be implemented successfully as they emanate, in part, from the family. The clinician shows respect by endorsing the parent's ideas when appropriate; this can increase self-esteem and sense of competency.

Educating parents through anticipatory guidance about normal and abnormal development and behavior may prevent problems through early detection and communicates the physician's interest in hearing parental concerns. Early detection allows for intervention before the problem becomes entrenched and associated problems develop.

The severity of developmental and behavioral problems ranges from slight variations of normal to problematic responses to stressful situations to frank disorders. The clinician must try to establish the severity and scope of the patient's symptoms so that appropriate intervention can be planned.

Counseling Principles

For the child, behavioral change must be learned, not simply imposed. It is easiest to learn when the lesson is simple, clear, consistent, and presented in an atmosphere free of fear or intimidation. Parents often try to impose behavioral change in an emotionally charged atmosphere, most often at the time of a behavioral *violation*. Similarly, clinicians may try to *teach* parents with hastily presented advice when the parents are distracted by other concerns or not engaged in the suggested behavioral change.

Apart from management strategies directed specifically at the problem behavior, regular times for positive parent-child interaction should be instituted. Frequent, brief, affectionate physical contact over the day provides opportunities for positive reinforcement of desirable child behaviors and for building a sense of competence in the child and the parent.

Some parents feel guilty when their children have a developmental/behavioral problem. Guilt may be caused by the fear that the problem was caused by inadequate parenting or by previous angry responses to the child's behavior. If possible and appropriate, the clinician should find ways to alleviate guilt, which may be a serious impediment to problem solving.

Interdisciplinary Team Intervention

A team of professionals is required to provide the breadth and quality of services needed to appropriately serve the child with SHCN. The primary care physician should monitor the progress of the child and continually reassess that the requisite therapy is being accomplished.

Educational intervention for a young child begins as home-based infant stimulation, often with an early childhood specialist (e.g., nurse/therapist), providing direct stimulation for the child and training the family to provide the stimulation. As the child matures, a center-based early learning center program may be indicated. For the school-age child, special services may range from extra attention in the regular classroom to learning in a separate special education classroom.

Psychologic intervention may be directed to the parent or family or, with an older child, primarily the child. Examples of therapeutic approaches are guidance therapies such as directive advice giving, counseling to create their own solutions to problems, psychotherapy, behavioral management techniques, psychopharmacologic treatment (involving a psychiatrist), and cognitive-behavioral therapy.

Motor intervention may be performed by a physical or occupational therapist. *Neurodevelopmental therapy* (NDT) is the most commonly used method. NDT is based on the concept that nervous system development is subject to some plasticity; with therapeutic handling of the child during activities, their nervous system receives input to develop desired skills. NDT is used for gait training and motor development

TABLE 10.3 Tests of Cognition

TEST	AGE RANGE	SPECIAL FEATURES
INFANT SCALES		
BSID-4	16 days–42 mo	5 domains: cognitive, language, motor, social-emotional, and adaptive behavior
Cattell Infant Intelligence Scale	2–30 mo	Used to extend Stanford-Binet downward
GDO-R	2.5–9 yrs	Used frequently by pediatricians
Ordinal Scales of Infant Psychologic Development	Birth–24 mo	Six subscales; based on Piaget's stages; weak in predicting later intelligence
PRESCHOOL AND SCHOOL-AGE SCALES		
SBI-5	2 yr–adult	Four area scores, with subtests and composite IQ score
McCarthy Scales of Children's Abilities	2–8 yr	6–18 subtests; good at defining learning disabilities; strengths/weaknesses approach
WPPSI-IV	2 yr 6 m–7 yr 7 m	11 subtests; verbal, performance IQs; long administration time; good at defining learning disabilities
Merrill-Palmer Scale of Mental Tests	18 mo–4 yr	19 subtests cover language skills, motor skills, manual dexterity, and matching ability
DAS-II	2½–<18 yr	Special nonverbal composite; short administration time
WISC-V	6–16 yr	See comments on WPPSI-R
Leiter-3	2–20 yr	Nonverbal measure of intelligence; ideal for use with those who are cognitively delayed, non-English speaking, hearing impaired, speech impaired, or autistic
WAIS-IV	16 yr–adult	See comments on WPPSI
ADAPTIVE BEHAVIOR SCALES		
Vineland-3	Birth–90 yr	Interview/questionnaire; typical persons and blind, deaf, developmentally delayed, and intellectually disabled
American Association on Intellectual and Developmental Disabilities DABS	4–21 yr	Measures conceptual, social, and practical skills needed for daily functioning. Significant limitations in these domains is needed to diagnose ID

BSID-4, Bayley Scales of Infant Development, 4th ed.; *DABS,* Diagnostic Adaptive Behavior Scale; *DAS-II,* Differential Abilities Scale, 2nd ed.; *GDO-R,* Gesell Developmental Observation-Revised; *ID,* intellectual disability; *IQ,* intelligence quotient; *Leiter-3,* Leiter International Performance Scale, 3rd ed.; *SBI-5,* Stanford-Binet Intelligence Scale, 5th ed.; *Vineland-3,* Vineland Adaptive Behavior Scale, 3rd ed.; *WAIS-IV,* Wechsler Adult Intelligence Scale, 4th ed.; *WISC-V,* Wechsler Intelligence Scale for Children, 5th ed.; *WPPSI-IV,* Wechsler Primary and Preschool Test of Intelligence, 4th ed.

including daily living skills, perceptual abilities such as eye-hand coordination, and spatial relationships. *Sensory integration therapy* is also used by occupational therapists to structure sensory experience from the tactile, proprioceptive, and vestibular systems to allow for adaptive motor responses; this can be helpful for children with autism spectrum disorders, attention-deficit/hyperactivity disorder, and other conditions.

Speech-language intervention by a speech and language therapist/pathologist (oral-motor therapist) is often part of the overall educational program and is based on the tested language strengths and weaknesses of the child. Children needing this type of intervention may show difficulties in reading and other academic areas and develop social and behavioral problems because of their difficulties in being understood and in understanding others. **Hearing intervention**, performed by an audiologist (or an otolaryngologist), includes monitoring hearing acuity and providing amplification via hearing aids when necessary.

Social and environmental intervention generally includes nursing or social work involvement with the family. Social workers and case managers may be involved in coordinating services.

Medical intervention for a child with a developmental disability involves providing primary care as well as specific treatment of conditions associated with the disability. Although curative treatment often is not possible, functional impairment can be minimized through thoughtful medical management. Certain general medical problems are found more frequently in delayed and developmentally disabled people (Table 10.5), especially if the delay is part of a known syndrome. Some children may have a limited life expectancy; supporting the family through palliative care, hospice, and bereavement is another important role of the primary care pediatrician.

SELECTED CLINICAL PROBLEMS: THE SPECIAL NEEDS CHILD

Intellectual Developmental Disorder

Intellectual Developmental Disorder (IDD) is a disorder with onset during the developmental period that includes both intellectual and adaptive functioning deficits in conceptual, social, and practical domains (see Table 10.6). The replacement of the term *intellectual disability* with *IDD* helps to clarify the relationship with the World Health Organization's International

TABLE 10.4 Primary Care Counseling Roles

Create safe space for patients/families to express frustrations
Facilitate clarification
Support patient problem solving
Provide specific reassurance
Provide education
Provide specific parenting advice
Suggest environmental interventions
Provide follow-up
Facilitate appropriate referrals
Coordinate care and interpret reports after referrals

Classification of Diseases-11 classification system, which uses the term *disorders of intellectual development.* The prevalence of developmental disabilities in children aged 3–17 years is approximately 8.5%. The specifiers (mild, moderate, severe, and profound) for IDD are defined on the basis of adaptive functioning rather than simple IQ scores; it is adaptive functioning that determines the level of support required for children.

The etiology of a central nervous system insult resulting in IDD may involve genetic disorders, teratogenic influences, perinatal insults, acquired childhood disease or injury, and environmental and social determinants of health (Table 10.7). Mild IDD correlates with socioeconomic status, profound IDD does not. Although a single organic cause may be found, each individual child's performance should be considered a function of the interaction of environmental influences with the individual's organic substrate. Behavioral difficulties resulting from IDD itself and from the family's reaction to the child and the condition are common. More severe forms of IDD may be traced to biologic factors. The earlier the cognitive slowing is recognized, the more severe the deviation from normal is likely to be.

The first step in the diagnosis and management of a child with IDD is to identify functional strengths and weaknesses for purposes of medical and rehabilitative therapies. A history and physical examination may suggest a diagnosis that can be confirmed by laboratory testing (e.g., chromosomal analysis, genetic testing) and/or imaging (e.g., magnetic resonance imaging of the brain). Almost one third of individuals with IDD do not have readily identifiable reasons for their disability.

TABLE 10.5 Recurring Medical Issues in Children With Developmental Disabilities

PROBLEM	ASK ABOUT OR CHECK
Motor	Range of motion examination; scoliosis check; assessment of mobility; interaction with orthopedist, physical medicine and rehabilitation, and physical therapist/occupational therapist as needed
Diet	Dietary history, feeding observation, growth parameter measurement and charting, supplementation as indicated by observations, oro-motor therapist as needed
Sensory impairments	Functional vision and hearing screening; interaction as needed with ophthalmologist, audiologist
Dermatologic	Examination of *all* skin areas for decubitus ulcers or infection
Dentistry	Examination of teeth and gums; confirmation of access to dental care (preferably with ability to use sedation)
Behavioral problems	Aggression, self-injury, pica; sleep problems; psychotropic drug levels and side effects
Seizures	Seizure activity (frequency, length); monitoring of anticonvulsant levels and side effects
Infectious diseases	Ear infections, diarrhea, respiratory illnesses, immunizations (including COVID-19 and influenza)
Gastrointestinal problems	Constipation, vomiting, gastroesophageal reflux, gastrointestinal bleeding
Sexuality	Sexuality education, preventing abuse, contraception, menstrual suppression, genetic counseling
Other syndrome-specific problems	Ongoing evaluation of other "physical" problems as indicated by known intellectual developmental disorder etiology
Advocacy for services and enhancing access to care	Educational program, family support, financial support, legislative advocacy to support programs

Vision Impairment

Visual impairment is a common problem in children. **Partial vision** (defined as visual acuity between 20/70 and 20/200) occurs in 1 in 500 school-age children in the United States. **Legal blindness** is defined as distant visual acuity of 20/200 or worse and affects about 35,000 children in the United States. Such impairment can be a major barrier to optimal development.

The most common cause of **severe visual impairment** in children is retinopathy of prematurity (see Chapter 60). Congenital cataracts may lead to significant amblyopia. Cataracts also are associated with other ocular abnormalities and developmental disabilities. **Amblyopia** is a reduction in visual acuity in one or both eyes. Amblyopia is due to a distortion of the normal clearly formed retinal image (from congenital cataracts or severe refractive errors), abnormal binocular interaction between the eyes (strabismus) with one eye competitively inhibiting the other, or a combination of both mechanisms. Albinism, hydrocephalus, congenital cytomegalovirus infection, and birth asphyxia are other significant contributors to blindness in children.

Children with **mild-to-moderate visual impairment** usually have an uncorrected refractive error. The most common presentation is myopia (nearsightedness). Other causes are hyperopia (farsightedness) and astigmatism (alteration in the shape of the cornea leading to visual distortion). In children younger than 6 years, high refractive errors in one or both eyes may cause amblyopia, aggravating visual impairment.

The diagnosis of severe visual impairment often occurs at 4–8 months of age. Clinical suspicion is based on parental concerns aroused by unusual behavior, such as lack of smiling in response to appropriate stimuli, the presence of nystagmus, wandering eye movements, or motor delays in reaching

TABLE 10.6 Diagnostic Criteria for Intellectual Developmental Disorder

INTELLECTUAL DEVELOPMENTAL DISORDER (INTELLECTUAL DISABILITY)
Diagnostic Criteria
Intellectual developmental disorder (intellectual disability) is a disorder with onset during the developmental period that includes both intellectual and adaptive functioning deficits in conceptual, social, and practical domains. The following three criteria must be met:
A. Deficits in intellectual functions, such as reasoning, problem solving, planning, abstract thinking, judgment, academic learning, and learning from experience, confirmed by both clinical assessment and individualized, standardized intelligence testing.
B. Deficits in adaptive functioning that result in failure to meet developmental and sociocultural standards for personal independence and social responsibility. Without ongoing support, the adaptive deficits limit functioning in one or more activities of daily life, such as communication, social participation, and independent living, across multiple environments, such as home, school, work, and community.
C. Onset of intellectual and adaptive deficits during the developmental period.
Specify current severity;
(F70) **Mild**
(F71) **Moderate**
(F72) **Severe**
(F73) **Profound**

Reprinted with permission from the Diagnostic and Statistical Manual of Mental Disorders, Fifth Edition, Text Revision (Copyright © 2022). American Psychiatric Association. All Rights Reserved.

for objects. Fixation and visual tracking behavior should be seen in most infants by 6 weeks of age. This behavior can be assessed by moving a brightly colored object (or the examiner's face) across the visual field of a quiet but alert infant at a distance of 1 ft. The eyes also should be examined for red reflexes and pupillary reactions to light. Optical alignment (binocular vision with both eyes consistently focusing on the same spot) should not be expected until the infant is beyond the newborn period. Persistent nystagmus is abnormal at any age. If ocular abnormalities are identified, referral to a pediatric ophthalmologist is indicated.

During the newborn period, vision may be assessed by physical examination and by **visual evoked response**. This test evaluates the conduction of electrical impulses from the optic nerve to the occipital cortex of the brain. The eye is stimulated by a bright flash of light or with an alternating checkerboard of black-and-white squares, and the resulting electrical response is recorded from electrodes strategically placed on the scalp, similar to an electroencephalogram.

There are several developmental implications of visual impairment. Perception of body image is abnormal, and imitative behavior, such as smiling, is delayed. Delays in mobility may occur in children who are visually impaired from birth, although their postural milestones (ability to sit) usually are achieved appropriately. Social bonding with the parents is also often affected.

Visually impaired children can be assisted in various ways. Classroom settings may be augmented with resource-room assistance to present material in a nonvisual format. Fine motor activity development, listening skills, and Braille reading and writing are intrinsic to successful educational intervention for a child with severe visual impairment.

TABLE 10.7 Potential Causes of Intellectual Developmental Disorders*

EARLY ALTERATIONS OF EMBRYONIC DEVELOPMENT
Sporadic events affecting embryogenesis, usually a stable developmental challenge
Chromosomal changes (e.g., trisomy 21)
Prenatal influences (e.g., substance abuse, teratogenic medications, intrauterine TORCH infections)†
UNKNOWN CAUSES
No definite issue is identified, or multiple elements present, none of which are diagnostic (may be multifactorial)
ENVIRONMENTAL AND SOCIAL PROBLEMS
Dynamic influences, commonly associated with other challenges
Deprivation (neglect)
Parental mental illness
Environmental intoxications (e.g., significant lead intoxication)*
PREGNANCY PROBLEMS AND PERINATAL MORBIDITY
Impingement on normal intrauterine development or delivery
Fetal malnutrition and placental insufficiency
Perinatal complications (e.g., prematurity, birth asphyxia, birth trauma)
HEREDITARY DISORDERS
Preconceptual origin, variable expression in the individual infant, multiple somatic effects, frequently a progressive or degenerative course
Inborn errors of metabolism (e.g., Tay-Sachs disease, Hunter disease, phenylketonuria)
Single-gene abnormalities (e.g., neurofibromatosis or tuberous sclerosis)
Other chromosomal aberrations (e.g., fragile X syndrome, deletion pathogenic variants such as Prader-Willi syndrome)
Polygenic familial syndromes (pervasive developmental disorders)
ACQUIRED CHILDHOOD ILLNESS
Acute modification of developmental status, variable potential for functional recovery
Infections (all can lead to brain damage, but most significant are encephalitis and meningitis)
Cranial trauma (accidental and child abuse)
Accidents (e.g., near-drowning, electrocution)
Environmental intoxications (prototype is lead poisoning)

**Some health problems fit in several categories (e.g., lead intoxication may be involved in several areas).*
†*This also may be considered as an acquired childhood disease.*
TORCH, Toxoplasmosis, Other (congenital syphilis), Rubella, Cytomegalovirus, and Herpes simplex virus.

Hearing Impairment

The clinical significance of hearing loss varies with type (conductive vs. sensorineural), frequency, and severity as measured in the number of decibels heard or the number of decibels of hearing lost. The most common cause of mild-to-moderate hearing loss in children is a conduction abnormality caused by acquired middle ear disease (acute and chronic otitis media). Severe hearing impairment is more commonly caused by sensorineural hearing loss. Causes of sensorineural deafness include congenital infections (e.g., rubella and cytomegalovirus), meningitis, birth asphyxia, kernicterus, ototoxic drugs (especially aminoglycoside antibiotics), and tumors (including their treatment). There are several genetic causes of deafness (i.e., *GJB2*, *GJB6*, *STRC*); these are the most common cause of hearing impairment in schools for the deaf. With Down syndrome, there is a predisposition to conductive loss caused by middle-ear infection and sensorineural loss caused by cochlear disease. Any hearing loss may have a significant effect on a child's speech and language development. Delayed communication skills subsequently affect all areas of the child's cognitive and skills development (Table 10.8).

It is sometimes quite difficult to accurately determine the presence of hearing in infants and young children. Inquiring about a child's response to sounds or even observing the response to sounds in the office is unreliable for identifying hearing-impaired children. Universal screening of newborns is required prior to nursery discharge and includes the following:

1. **Auditory brainstem response (ABR)** measures how the brain responds to sound. Clicks or tones are played through soft earphones into the child's ears. Three electrodes placed on the child's head measure the brain's response.
2. **Otoacoustic emissions** measure sound waves produced in the inner ear. A probe is placed inside the child's ear canal. It plays clicks or tones into the ears and measures the response (echo) from the cochlea.

These tests are both quick (5–10 minutes), painless, and may be performed while the infant is sleeping or lying still. The tests are sensitive but not as specific as more definitive tests. Infants who do not pass these tests are referred for more comprehensive testing; early diagnosis and intervention is important.

For children not screened at birth or children with suspected acquired hearing loss, testing may allow early appropriate intervention. Hearing can be screened with an office audiogram for older children, but other techniques are needed (ABR, behavior audiology) for young, neurologically immature or impaired, and behaviorally difficult children. The typical audiologic assessment includes pure-tone audiometry over a variety of sound frequencies (pitches), especially over the range of frequencies in which most speech occurs. **Pneumatic otoscopic** examination and **tympanometry** are used to assess middle ear function and tympanic membrane compliance for pathology in the middle ear, such as fluid, ossicular dysfunction, and eustachian tube dysfunction (see Chapter 106).

Conductive hearing loss is largely due to otitis media and middle ear effusions; treatment of these conditions is discussed in Chapter 106. Treatment of sensorineural hearing impairment may be medical or surgical. If amplification is indicated, hearing aids can be tuned preferentially to amplify the frequency ranges in which the patient has decreased acuity. Educational intervention includes speech-language therapy and teaching American Sign Language. Even with amplification, hearing-impaired children can show deficits in processing auditory information, requiring special educational services for help reading and for other academic skills. **Cochlear implants** are surgically implantable devices that provide hearing sensation to individuals with severe-to-profound hearing loss. The implants are designed to substitute for the function of the middle ear, cochlear mechanical motion, and sensory cells, transforming sound energy into electrical energy that initiates impulses in the auditory nerve. Cochlear implants are indicated for children older than 12 months with profound bilateral sensorineural hearing loss who have limited benefit from hearing aids, have failed to progress in auditory skill development, and have no radiologic or medical contraindications. Implantation in children as young as possible provides them with the most advantageous auditory environment for speech-language learning.

Speech-Language Impairment

Parents often bring the concern of speech delay to the physician's attention when they compare their young child with others of the same age (Table 10.9). The most common causes of speech delay are IDD, hearing impairment, social deprivation, autism spectrum disorder, and oral-motor abnormalities. If a problem is suspected, often based on screening tests such as Ages and Stages Questionnaires, the Parents' Evaluation of Developmental Status test (see Chapter 8), or other standard screening test (Early Language Milestone Scale), a referral to a specialized hearing and speech center is indicated. While awaiting the results of testing or initiation of speech-language therapy, parents should be advised to speak slowly and clearly to the child (and avoid *baby talk*). Caregivers should read frequently to the speech-delayed child.

Speech disorders include **articulation**, **fluency**, and **resonance disorders**. Articulation disorders include difficulties producing sounds in syllables or saying words incorrectly to the point that other people cannot understand what is being said. Fluency disorders include problems such as **stuttering**, the condition in which the flow of speech is interrupted by abnormal stoppages, repetitions *(st-st-stuttering)*, or prolonged sounds and syllables *(ssssstuttering)*. Resonance or voice disorders include problems with the pitch, volume, or quality of a child's voice that distract listeners from what is being said.

Language disorders can be either receptive or expressive. Receptive disorders refer to difficulties understanding or processing language. Expressive disorders include difficulty putting words together, limited vocabulary, or inability to use language in a socially appropriate way.

Speech-language pathologists (also called *speech* or *oral-motor therapists*) assess the speech, language, cognitive communication, and swallowing skills of children; determine what types of communication problems exist; and identify the best way to treat these challenges. Speech-language pathologists skilled at working with infants and young children are also vital in training parents and infants in other oral-motor skills, such as how to feed an infant born with a cleft lip and palate.

Speech-language therapy involves having a speech-language specialist work with a child on a one-on-one basis, in a small group, or directly in a classroom using a variety of therapeutic strategies. Language intervention activities involve a speech-language specialist interacting with a child by playing and talking to the child using pictures, books, objects, or ongoing events to stimulate language development. Articulation therapy involves having the therapist model correct sounds and syllables for a child, often during play activities.

Children enrolled in therapy early (<3 years of age) have better outcomes than children who begin therapy later. Older children can make progress in therapy, but progress may occur more slowly as these children often have learned patterns that need to be modified or changed. Caregiver involvement is crucial to the success of a child's progress in speech-language therapy.

TABLE 10.8 Neurodevelopmental-Behavioral Complications of Hearing Loss

SEVERITY OF HEARING LOSS	POSSIBLE ETIOLOGIC ORIGINS	COMPLICATIONS			TYPES OF THERAPY
		SPEECH-LANGUAGE	EDUCATIONAL	BEHAVIORAL	
Slight 15–25 dB (ASA)	Chronic otitis media/middle ear effusions	Difficulty with hearing distant or faint speech	Possible auditory learning dysfunction	Usually none	May require favorable class setting, speech therapy, or auditory training
	Perforation of tympanic membrane		May reveal a slight verbal deficit		Possible value in hearing aid, surgery
	Sensorineural loss				Favorable class setting
	Tympanosclerosis				Favorable class setting
Mild 25–40 dB (ASA)	Chronic otitis media/middle ear effusions	Difficulty with conversational speech over 3–5 ft	May miss 50% of class discussions	Psychologic problems	Special education resource help, surgery
	Perforation of tympanic membrane	May have limited vocabulary and speech disorders	Auditory learning dysfunction	May act inappropriately if directions are not heard well	Hearing aid, surgery
	Sensorineural loss			Acting out behavior	Favorable class setting, hearing aid, cochlear implant
	Tympanosclerosis			Poor self-concept	Lip reading instruction Speech therapy
Moderate 40–65 dB (ASA)	Chronic otitis media/middle ear effusions	Conversation must be loud to be understood	Learning disability	Emotional and social problems	Special education resource or special class, surgery
	Middle ear anomaly	Defective speech	Difficulty with group learning or discussion	Behavioral reactions of childhood	Special help in speech-language development
	Sensorineural loss	Deficient language use and comprehension	Auditory processing dysfunction	Acting out	Hearing aid and lip reading
			Limited vocabulary	Poor self-concept	Speech therapy
Severe 65–95 dB (ASA)	Sensorineural loss	Loud voices may be heard 2 ft from ear	Marked educational disability	Emotional and social problems that are associated with handicap	Full-time special education for deaf children, cochlear implant
	Severe middle ear disease	Defective speech and language No spontaneous speech development if loss present before 1 yr	Marked learning disability, limited vocabulary	Poor self-concept	Full-time special education for deaf children, hearing aid, lip reading, speech therapy, surgery, cochlear implant
Profound ≥95 dB (ASA)	Sensorineural or mixed loss	Relies on vision rather than hearing Defective speech and language Speech and language will not develop spontaneously if loss present before 1 yr	Marked learning disability because of lack of understanding of speech	Congenital and prelingually deaf may show severe emotional problems	Full-time special education for deaf children, hearing aid, lip reading, speech therapy, surgery, cochlear implant

ASA, Acoustical Society of America.

Modified and updated from Gottlieb MI. Otitis media. In: Levine MD, Carey WB, Crocker AC, et al., eds. Developmental-Behavioral Pediatrics. *Philadelphia: WB Saunders; 1983.*

TABLE 10.9 Clues to When a Child With a Communication Disorder Needs Help

0–11 MONTHS
Before 6 months, the child does not startle, blink, or change immediate activity in response to sudden, loud sounds.
Before 6 months, the child does not attend to the human voice and is not soothed by mother's voice.
By 6 months, the child does not babble strings of consonant and vowel syllables or imitate gurgling or cooing sounds.
By 10 months, the child does not respond to own name.
At 10 months, the child's sound-making is limited to shrieks, grunts, or sustained vowel production.
12–23 MONTHS
At 12 months, the child's babbling or speech is limited to vowel sounds.
By 15 months, the child does not respond to "no," "bye-bye," or "bottle."
By 15 months, the child does not imitate sounds or words.
By 18 months, the child is not consistently using at least six words with appropriate meaning.
By 21 months, the child does not respond correctly to "Give me...," "Sit down," or "Come here" when spoken without gestural cues.
By 23 months, two-word phrases that are spoken as single units (e.g., "whatszit," "thankyou," "allgone") have not emerged.
24–36 MONTHS
By 24 months, at least 50% of the child's speech is not understood by familiar listeners.
By 24 months, the child does not point to body parts without gestural cues.
By 24 months, the child is not combining words into phrases (e.g., "go bye-bye," "go car," "want cookie").
By 30 months, the child does not show understanding of spatial concepts: on, in, under, front, and back.
By 30 months, the child is not using short sentences (e.g., "Daddy went bye-bye").
By 30 months, the child has not begun to ask questions (using "where," "what," "why").
By 36 months, the child's speech is not understood by unfamiliar listeners.
ALL AGES
At any age, the child is consistently dysfluent with repetitions, hesitations; blocks or struggles to say words. Struggle may be accompanied by grimaces, eye blinks, or hand gestures.

Modified and updated from Weiss CE, Lillywhite HE. Communication Disorders: A Handbook for Prevention and Early Detection. *St Louis: Mosby; 1976.*

Cerebral Palsy

Cerebral palsy (CP) refers to a group of nonprogressive, but often changing, motor impairment syndromes secondary to anomalies or lesions of the brain arising before or after birth. The prevalence of CP at age 8 in the United States is 1.5–4 per 1,000; prevalence is much higher in premature and twin births. Prematurity and low birthweight infants (leading to perinatal asphyxia), congenital malformations, and kernicterus are causes of CP noted at birth. Ten percent of children with CP have acquired CP, developing at later ages. Meningitis and head injury (accidental and nonaccidental) are the most common causes of acquired CP (Table 10.10). Nearly 50% of children with CP have no identifiable risk factors. As genomic medicine advances, numerous causes of idiopathic CP are being identified.

Most children with CP, except in its mildest forms, are diagnosed in the first 18 months of life when they fail to attain motor milestones or show abnormalities such as asymmetric gross motor function, hypertonia, or hypotonia. CP can be characterized further by the affected parts of the body (Table 10.11) and descriptions of the predominant type of motor disorder (Table 10.12). Comorbidities in these children often include epilepsy, learning difficulties, behavioral challenges, and sensory impairments; some children have an isolated motor deficit.

Treatment of CP depends on the pattern of dysfunction. Physical and occupational therapy can facilitate optimal positioning and movement patterns, increasing function in affected parts. Spasticity management may include muscle relaxants (dantrolene, benzodiazepines, and baclofen), botulinum toxin injections, and implantation of intrathecal baclofen pumps. Management of seizures, spasticity, orthopedic impairments, and sensory impairments may help improve educational attainment. CP cannot be cured, but a host of interventions can improve functional abilities, participation in society, and quality of life. Like all children, an assessment and reinforcement of strengths are important.

TABLE 10.10 Risk Factors for Cerebral Palsy

PREGNANCY AND BIRTH
Low socioeconomic status
Prematurity
Low birthweight/fetal growth restriction (<1,500 g at birth)
Maternal seizures/seizure disorder
Maternal treatment with thyroid hormone, estrogen, or progesterone
Pregnancy complications
Polyhydramnios
Eclampsia
Third-trimester bleeding (including threatened abortion and placenta previa)
Multiple births
Abnormal fetal presentation
Maternal fever
Congenital malformations/syndromes
Newborn hypoxic-ischemic encephalopathy
Bilirubin (kernicterus)
ACQUIRED AFTER THE NEWBORN PERIOD
Meningitis
Head injury
Motor vehicle accidents
Child abuse
Drowning
Stroke

TABLE 10.11 Descriptions of Cerebral Palsy by Site of Involvement

Hemiparesis (hemiplegia): predominantly unilateral impairment of the arm and leg on the same (e.g., right or left) side
Diplegia: motor impairment primarily of the legs (often with some limited involvement of the arms; some authors challenge this specific type as not being different from quadriplegia)
Quadriplegia: all four limbs (whole body) are functionally compromised

TABLE 10.12 Classification of Cerebral Palsy by Type of Motor Disorder

Spastic cerebral palsy: most common form of cerebral palsy, accounting for 70–80% of cases. It results from injury to the upper motor neurons of the pyramidal tract. It may occasionally be bilateral. It is characterized by at least two of the following: abnormal movement pattern, increased tone, or pathologic reflexes (e.g., Babinski response, hyperreflexia).
Dyskinetic cerebral palsy: occurs in 10–15% of cases. It is dominated by abnormal patterns of movement and involuntary, uncontrolled, recurring movements.
Ataxic cerebral palsy: accounts for <5% of cases. This form results from cerebellar injury and features abnormal posture or movement or loss of orderly muscle coordination or both.
Dystonic cerebral palsy: uncommon. It is characterized by reduced activity, stiff movement (hypokinesia), and hypotonia.
Choreoathetotic cerebral palsy: rare now that excessive hyperbilirubinemia is aggressively prevented and treated. This form is dominated by increased and stormy movements (hyperkinesia) and hypotonia.
Mixed cerebral palsy: accounts for 10–15% of cases. This term is used when more than one type of motor pattern is present and when one pattern does not clearly dominate another. It is associated with more complications, including sensory deficits, seizures, and cognitive-perceptual impairments.

PEARLS FOR PRACTITIONERS

See Growth and Development: Pearls for Practitioners at the end of this section.

REVIEW QUESTIONS

Available online.

Suggested Readings

Centers for Disease Control and Prevention. Learn the Signs. Act Early. *National Center on Birth Defects and Developmental Disabilities*, Centers for Disease Control and Prevention. Atlanta, Georgia. https://www.cdc.gov/ncbddd/actearly/index.html.

Duffee J, Szilagyi M, Forkey H, Kelly ET; Council on Community Pediatrics, Council on Foster Care, Adoption, and Kinship Care, Council on Child Abuse and Neglect, Committee on Psychosocial Aspects of Child and Family Health. Trauma-Informed Care in Child Health Systems. *Pediatrics*. 2021;148(2):e2021052579.

Gardner HG. American Academy of Pediatrics Committee on Injury, Violence, and Poison Prevention. Office-based counseling for unintentional injury prevention. *Pediatrics*. 2007;119(1):202–206.

Ghandour RM, Hirai AH, Kenney MK. Children and Youth With Special Health Care Needs: A Profile. *Pediatrics*. 2022;149(Suppl 7):e2021056150D.

Hagan JF, Shaw JS, Duncan PM, eds. *Bright Futures: Guidelines for Health Supervision of Infants, Children, and Adolescents*. 4th ed. Elk Grove Village, IL: American Academy of Pediatrics; 2017.

Kliegman R, Geme J St. *Nelson Textbook of Pediatrics*. 22nd ed. Philadelphia: Elsevier; 2024.

Li Q, Li Y, Zheng J, et al. Prevalence and trends of developmental disabilities among US children and adolescents aged 3 to 17 years, 2018-2021. *Sci Rep*. 2023;13(1):17254.

Loveday S, Hall T, Constable L, et al. Screening for Adverse Childhood Experiences in Children: A Systematic Review. *Pediatrics*. 2022;149(2):e2021051884.

Stewart J, McCallin T, Martinez J, Chacko S, Yusuf S. Hyperlipidemia. *Pediatr Rev*. 2020;41(8):393–402.

Zubler JM, Wiggins LD, Macias MM, et al. Evidence-Informed Milestones for Developmental Surveillance Tools. *Pediatrics*. 2022;149(3):e2021052138.

PEARLS FOR PRACTITIONERS

CHAPTER 5

Normal Growth

- Health maintenance visits, also known as *well visits* or *well-child checks*, are recommended at regular intervals to promote optimized growth and development.
- Standard growth charts are used to monitor growth.
  - For 0–2 years, use WHO growth charts to follow weight, recumbent length, head circumference, and weight for length.
  - For ≥2 years, use CDC growth charts to follow weight, height, and BMI.
- General principles for average growth
  - Double birthweight by age 4 months
  - Triple birthweight by age 1 year
  - Double birth length by age 4 years

CHAPTER 6

Disorders of Growth

- Error from equipment or operator failure is the most common cause of abnormal growth measurements; repeat measurement to verify accuracy of value before pursuing further evaluation.
- Disease-specific growth charts should be used for prematurity and for specific disorders such as achondroplasia, Down syndrome, and Turner syndrome.
- Specific patterns of abnormal growth can suggest diagnoses and guide the evaluation.
  - Weight decreases first, then length, then head circumference: caloric inadequacy
    - May be organic (e.g., increased work of breathing with congestive heart failure) or nonorganic (neglected child, parental depression)

- Increasing weight percentile with decreasing height percentile: hypothyroidism
- All growth parameters less than the 5th percentile
  - Normal variants: familial short stature, constitutional delay
  - Intrauterine insult
  - Genetic disorder
- Declining percentiles at 6–18 months but otherwise normal development: "catch-down growth"

CHAPTER 7
Normal Development

- Neonatal reflexes including the Moro, rooting, sucking, and asymmetric tonic neck reflexes assist in evaluation of the newborn.
- Specific issues to address vary by age:
  - During infancy, joint contractures that are fixed deformities require pediatrics orthopedic evaluation. Joint contractures that can be moved to the proper position can just be followed as they are likely to resolve.
  - By no later than 1 year, examine for binocular vision with the light reflex and cover test.
  - Older children and adolescents who play sports need a preparticipation physical that includes cardiovascular and orthopedic risk assessments.
- Developmental milestones
  - Gross motor, fine motor, speech, and personal-social milestones are used to assess development as delayed, appropriate, or advanced.
  - Selected age-appropriate issues
    - Bonding and attachment in infancy are critical for optimal outcomes.
    - As autonomy develops in early childhood, children explore but need quick access to their caregivers.
      - Stranger anxiety begins around 9 months: support the infant when the child is exploring and when others are present.
      - "Terrible twos": reinforce desired behaviors and try extinguishing the undesired behaviors (by not responding to the behavior).
      - Early childhood education, as early as 3 years, increases educational achievement and success as an adult.
  - School readiness should be assessed, not assumed, to have optimal educational outcomes.
  - In modifying behaviors, punishment (consequences for unwanted behaviors) is less effective than positive reinforcement (rewarding wanted behaviors); punishment can be combined with positive reinforcement to improve results.

CHAPTER 8
Disorders of Development

- Developmental surveillance should be addressed at every office visit with more careful attention at health maintenance visits.
- Developmental screening is completed using validated tools.
  - Done at 9, 18, and 30 months at a minimum
  - Most common tools are Ages and Stages and Parents' Evaluation of Developmental Status
  - Abnormalities require definitive testing.
- Autism screening using a validated tool is done at 18 and 24 months.
  - Most common is the Modified Checklist for Autism in Toddlers—Revised (M-CHAT-R)
  - Abnormalities require definitive testing.
- Language development is critical in early childhood.
  - Highly correlates with cognitive development
  - Even with newborn hearing test, may need to re-test hearing at any age
  - Speech therapy is more effective the younger it is started.
- After age 6, school performance is assessed; if there are academic or behavioral issues, there should be further testing by psychologists, psychiatrists, developmental pediatricians, or educational experts.
- Context of behavioral problems
  - Caregiver factors: mismatch in temperament or expectations between parent and child, depression, other health issues
  - Adverse childhood experiences
  - Witnessed or experienced abuse and neglect, domestic violence, substance use disorder, incarceration, or death of relative
- Social determinants of health
  - Stress, lack of parental support, perceived prejudice, and racism
  - Poverty: housing with environmental exposures, poor access to quality education, poor access to healthy nutrition (food deserts), toxic stress
- Developing rapport and open communication with adolescents is critical.
- Adolescents can usually consent for sexual health, mental health, and substance abuse services although local laws may vary.
  - Confidentiality is critical unless there is information that would seem to allow harm to come to the individual or others.

CHAPTER 9
Evaluation of the Well Child

- The Bright Futures/American Academy of Pediatrics Recommendations for Preventive Pediatric Health Care (Fig. 9.1) summarizes standardized recommendations for preventive measures and screening by age.
- Elements of the visits
  - Measurements: growth, blood pressure, sensory screening (vision and hearing)
  - Developmental/behavioral assessment
    - Depression screening should start at age 11; PHQ2 and PHQ9 are available in Bright Futures resources.

- Physical examination
- Procedures
  - Newborn screening, screening for critical congenital heart disease
  - Hemoglobin, lead, and TB testing universally at certain ages and more frequently if risks are present at other ages
  - Lipid screening once at age 9–11 and 17–21 years; also at other ages if risk factors
  - STI/HIV risk assessment and screening at ages 15 and 21 years (or earlier if sexually active)
  - Oral health: dental referral starting at age 1 year; fluoride varnish every 3–6 months from age 9 months to and including age 5 years
- Anticipatory guidance that is age and developmentally appropriate
  - Bright Futures has age-appropriate one page handouts for each health maintenance visit by age in the Tool and Resource Kit.

- Promoting optimal development
  - Discipline means to teach, not just to punish.
  - Reinforcing positive behaviors and activities is more effective than punishment.
  - Time-out technique is optimal for altering undesired behaviors; corporal punishment teaches children it is okay to hit.
  - Setting limits that are agreed upon by all caregivers leads to optimal outcomes.

CHAPTER 10
Evaluation of the Child With Special Needs

- Children with special health care needs share broad experiences in school difficulties and family stress; 19% of U.S. children have a special health care need.
- Treatment goals are to maximize potential by treating the primary issue and helping the family and patient deal with the stresses and secondary impairments.
- Optimal care
  - Primary care pediatrician in a medical home—provides big picture oversight, evaluates the concern and provides diagnosis, provides preventive care, and facilitates:
    - Pediatric subspecialists
    - Pediatric therapists—OT, PT, speech
    - Social work or health navigator may assist by finding needed community services (e.g., medically fragile childcare).
  - Developmental assessments under age 3 are mandated to happen with no charge to the family or insurance through early intervention programs; over age 3, they are performed by school districts.
  - Psychology, education, and social environment assessments
- Selected special health care needs
  - Intellectual developmental disorders—myriad causes that should be investigated; children may often "outperform" their expected intelligence with excellent support.
  - Vision impairment
    - Can be tested as early as newborn using visual evoked response
    - Diagnosed between 4 and 8 months; clues: the child does not respond to the parent's smile, has wandering eye movements, or has motor delays in reaching for objects.
  - Hearing impairment
    - Newborns have their hearing tested but may need additional testing later if there is a clinical suspicion.
    - A newborn should have a hearing screen by 1 month of age with follow-up testing for abnormal results by 3 months of age. If follow-up test is abnormal, interventions should be implemented by 6 months of age. (Test by 1 month, repeat by 3 months, intervene by 6 months.)
    - Hearing impairment can be conductive or sensorineural, each has different available treatment.
  - Speech disorders
    - For ages 2–4 years, a stranger should be able to understand a percentage of a child's language that correlates with age in years divided by 4. (For age 2, 2/4 = 50% of speech should be easily understood.)
    - Several causes: ID, hearing impairment, deprivation and poor use of language with caregivers, autism, oral-motor abnormalities
    - Immediate speech-language evaluation and hearing evaluation
    - Commence speech therapy as soon as a true deficit is found; outcomes are better the earlier speech therapy is started.
    - Articulation, fluency, stuttering, and resonance disorders may be discovered and are amenable to speech-language therapy.
- Cerebral palsy: nonprogressive motor impairment syndrome
  - Myriad causes: 50% of cases have no cause identified.
    - Congenital: prematurity, low birthweight, congenital malformations, kernicterus in the past
    - Acquired: meningitis/encephalitis, head injury (crashes or child abuse)
  - May be associated with other deficits depending on the causes, but this is a motor deficiency by definition; some children are intellectually gifted.
  - Team approach for optimal outcomes
    - Physicians provide spasticity treatments
    - Home health care and durable medical equipment
    - OT/PT/speech therapy as needed
    - Social work/health navigator

SECTION 3

BEHAVIORAL DISORDERS

Patty Huang | Rosalind Usher Hill

CHAPTER 11

Crying and Colic

Crying is one of the first ways an infant learns to communicate their wants and needs to those around them. For caregivers, trying to understand what their child may need while they are crying can be a source of stress and concern. Crying can be described by the characteristics of timing, duration, frequency, intensity, and modifiability. Most infants cry little during the first 2 weeks of life. Crying duration gradually increases to a mean duration of 117–133 minutes per day during the first 6 weeks of life. Crying duration decreases to 68 minutes per day by 10–12 weeks, although this can vary widely from infant to infant.

Duration of crying can differ by infant care practices and culture. Understanding patterns of crying can help the clinician determine the etiology of crying, as well as how to guide the caregiver to cope with the infant's crying. Crying behavior in former premature infants also may be influenced by ongoing medical conditions. The duration of crying is often modifiable by caregiving strategies.

Frequency of crying is less variable than duration. At 6 weeks of age, the mean frequency of combined crying and fussing is 10 episodes in 24 hours. *Diurnal variation* in crying is the norm, with crying concentrated in the late afternoon and evening.

The **intensity** of infant crying varies, ranging from fussing to screaming. An intense infant cry (pitch and loudness) is more likely to elicit concern or alarm from caregivers than an infant who fusses more quietly. Pain cries of newborns are remarkably loud: 80 dB at a distance of 30.5 cm from the infant's mouth. Although pain cries can have a higher frequency than hunger cries, when not attended to for a protracted period, hunger cries become acoustically similar to pain cries. Fortunately, most infant crying is of a lesser intensity, consistent with fussing.

COLIC

Infantile colic is defined as episodes of uncontrollable crying or fussing in an otherwise healthy infant. Colicky crying is often described as paroxysmal and may be characterized by facial grimacing, leg flexion, and passing flatus. Infantile colic has been associated with abusive head trauma, postpartum depression, parental guilt, and multiple physician visits.

The 2016 Rome IV criteria can be used for the diagnosis of colic. The criteria are as follows:

1. Infant is ≤5 months when the symptoms start and stop.
2. Recurrent and prolonged periods of crying, fussing, or irritability that start and stop without obvious cause and cannot be prevented or resolved by caregivers.
3. No evidence of poor weight gain, fever, or illness.
4. Caregiver reports of crying/fussing for ≥3 hours per day on ≥3 days/week in a telephone or face-to-face interview.
5. Total daily crying confirmed to be ≥3 hours when measured by at least one prospectively kept 24-hour diary.

Epidemiology

The rates of colic vary from 10–40%, peaking at approximately 6 weeks of age. There is no known association with gender, gestational age, breast versus bottle feeding, season of year, or socioeconomic status. Concern about infant crying also varies by culture, and this may influence what is recorded as crying or fussing.

Etiology

Fewer than 5% of infants evaluated for excessive crying have an organic etiology. The etiology of colic is unknown; cow's milk protein intolerance, changes in the gut microbiome, increase in serotonin secretion, poor feeding technique, and maternal smoking may be associated. Higher levels of fecal calprotectin, a marker of colonic inflammation, have been reported. Because colic is a diagnosis of exclusion, a thorough evaluation of infants with excessive crying is necessary to evaluate for other serious diagnoses.

Clinical Manifestations

A thorough history and physical examination to assess for underlying medical disorders and to determine the need for further testing are necessary; serious diseases and injuries that can mimic the symptoms of colic must be ruled out. The **history** should include a description of the crying (i.e., onset, duration, frequency, diurnal pattern, intensity, periodicity, and relieving or exacerbating factors) as well as associated symptoms such as leg flexion, facial grimacing, vomiting, or back arching. The history should also elicit any presence of fevers and any acute or subtle changes in the infant. Review of systems may identify or reassure against other serious conditions such as nonaccidental trauma. Birth history may identify perinatal problems that could increase the likelihood of neurologic causes of crying. A detailed feeding history assesses for feeding-related problems including hunger, air swallowing (worsened by crying), gastroesophageal reflux, and feeding intolerance. The social history, including a family's ability to handle stress and their knowledge of infant soothing strategies, can assist in assessing risk for parental mental health comorbidities and developing an intervention plan suitable for the family.

The diagnosis of colic is made only when the **physical examination** reveals no organic cause for the infant's excessive crying. An infant who is not able to be consoled is considered to be irritable and warrants further investigation. The physical examination needs to include a full general exam as well as vital signs, weight, length, and head circumference, looking for effects of systemic illness on growth trends. A thorough inspection may identify possible sources of pain, including skin lesions, **corneal abrasions, hair tourniquets**, anal fissures, or signs of nonaccidental trauma such as **bruising** or **fractures** (see Chapters 21 and 199). A neurologic examination may reveal previously undiagnosed neurologic conditions. Abdominal masses, hepatosplenomegaly, and signs of an acute abdomen (e.g., volvulus, intussusception) should be ruled out. Observing the infant during a crying episode (or reviewing a recording of an episode) can be invaluable in assessing the infant's potential for calming and the parents' skills in soothing the infant.

Further evaluation, including potential laboratory and imaging studies, is warranted when the history or physical examination findings suggest an organic cause for excessive crying.

Differential Diagnosis

The differential diagnosis for colic is broad and includes any condition that can cause pain or discomfort in an infant as well as conditions associated with *nonpainful* distress, such as fatigue or sensory overload. It is important to evaluate for emergent conditions such as intracranial pathology, acute infection (i.e., meningitis, bacteremia, urinary tract infection), hypoglycemia, cardiac conditions (i.e., tachyarrhythmias, congenital heart disease, congestive heart failure), nonaccidental trauma, and the acute abdomen.

Cow's milk protein intolerance, gastroesophageal reflux disease, constipation, maternal substance use including nicotine, and anomalous left coronary artery all have been reported as causes of persistent crying. In addition, situations associated with poor infant regulation, including fatigue, hunger, need for attention, parental anxiety, and chaotic and disruptive environmental conditions, may increase the risk of excessive crying.

Anticipatory Guidance and Management

The management of colic begins with education (including features of colic), demystification, and a discussion of its natural course. Anticipatory guidance should also be provided regarding atypical crying that warrants further medical attention. Helping families develop caregiving strategies for the infant's fussy periods is critical to overall outcomes. Techniques for calming infants include Dr. Harvey Karp's **"5 Ss"**: swaddling, side or stomach holding, soothing noises (such as shushing, singing, or white noise), swinging or slow rhythmic movement (such as rocking, walking, or riding in a car), and sucking on a pacifier. Giving caregivers permission to allow the infant to rest or leave the infant alone in a safe place when soothing strategies are not working may alleviate overstimulation in some infants. It is important to encourage parents to seek help and support from others when they are becoming overwhelmed and to advise against harmful methods to soothe an infant (such as placing the infant on a vibrating clothes dryer). Parents should be specifically educated about the dangers of shaking babies. A deliberate approach in management provides access to resources and follow-up of caregivers given the stressors and challenges that accompany colic. Educating parents regarding variable hunger cues, avoiding excessive caffeine and any use of alcohol in nursing mothers, ensuring adequate yet not excessive bottle nipple flow, and cautioning against overfeeding may be helpful.

Therapeutic modalities such as chiropractic manipulation and acupuncture have insufficient evidence to support their use. Similarly, while some herbal medications (such as chamomile, fennel, vervain, licorice, and balm-mint teas) have been suggested, there is no evidence of effectiveness, and they may result in side effects such as hyponatremia and anemia.

In most circumstances, **dietary changes** are not effective in reducing colic but should be considered in certain specific circumstances such as when there is concern for cow's milk protein allergy/intolerance or lactose deficiency.

Medications, including phenobarbital, diphenhydramine, alcohol, simethicone, dicyclomine, and lactase, have no benefit, and some can cause serious side effects. The use of probiotics such as *Lactobacillus reuteri* has been shown to decrease crying time in the infant with colic without adverse effects and can be considered after careful evaluation, certainty of diagnosis, and close follow-up.

Prognosis

Infants with colic do not have adverse long-term outcomes in health or temperament after the affected period. Similarly, infantile colic does not have untoward long-term effects on maternal mental health, as parental distress tends to resolve as colic subsides. The most serious complication of colic is nonaccidental trauma.

PEARLS FOR PRACTITIONERS

See Behavioral Disorders: Pearls for Practitioners at the end of this section.

REVIEW QUESTIONS

Available online.

CHAPTER 12

Temper Tantrums

Temper tantrums are a common childhood behavioral condition, prompting presentation to primary care providers and referrals to behavioral consultants. Temper tantrums are brief episodes of extreme or unpleasant behavior that appear disproportionate to the situation and are in response to being denied access or being told "no" and/or having difficulty communicating wants, needs, or feelings, resulting in secondary emotions of frustration or anger. The median duration of a tantrum is 3 minutes. Behaviors vary and may include whining, crying, screaming, stomping, flailing, head banging, hitting, scratching, throwing objects, and biting. Tantrums can instigate **breath-holding spells** in some children (see Chapter 135), which can be particularly frightening for caretakers.

ETIOLOGY

Temper tantrums are a normal human developmental behavior. Children between 1–4 years old have an increasing desire for independence but are often unable to effectively communicate physical needs and emotions. Common triggers of temper tantrums include fatigue, hunger, discomfort, and frustration.

EPIDEMIOLOGY

Temper tantrums usually begin around the age of 12–18 months, worsen until 3 years of age, and taper off as children develop increased ability to control their emotions and communicate their wants and needs and as they begin to gain independence. Ninety percent of 2- to 3-year-old children have temper tantrums, and 20% have them daily. Approximately 20% of 4-year-olds still have regular tantrums. They usually resolve by the age of 5 years. Tantrums can be more frequent, as well as more aggressive, in children with language delays or underlying neurodevelopmental or genetic conditions. Children with intellectual disability may exhibit tantrums when their developmental age is comparable to 3–4 years. There are no gender or heritage differences in tantrum occurrence.

CLINICAL MANIFESTATIONS

The evaluation of a child with tantrums should include a comprehensive medical and developmental **history** to evaluate for other behavioral, psychologic, or physiologic conditions. Social history should include past or ongoing family stressors (including parental well-being, changes in living situation or school, financial difficulty, barriers to care, and recent changes to the family), as these factors can exacerbate or prolong the normal developmental trajectory of tantrums. The coexistence of sleep disturbances, enuresis, aggression, social communication deficits, repetitive behaviors, or learning problems may suggest the possibility of underlying conditions such as attention-deficit/hyperactivity disorder (ADHD), autism spectrum disorder (ASD), anxiety, or depression.

It is important to differentiate between normal and abnormal temper tantrums (Table 12.1); abnormal tantrums may be indicative of more serious neurodevelopmental, behavioral, mood, or other medical problems. Duration of tantrums should be reviewed; 5–7% of children 1–3 years old have temper tantrums that last more than 15 minutes.

To help caregivers understand the function behind their child's tantrum, it can be helpful to think about them from the perspective of the "ABC's" of behavior. When obtaining a tantrum history from caregivers, include the circumstances surrounding tantrums, including triggers (**A**ntecedent); careful attention should be paid to the child's daily routines, which may reveal triggers such as hunger, fatigue, inadequate physical activity, or overstimulation. A description of the tantrum (**B**ehavior) should include the child's actions, duration, severity, and alleviating and aggravating factors. Then, a description of the caregiver's response (**C**onsequence) to their child's tantrum episodes is needed.

TABLE 12.1 Normal and Abnormal Tantrums

	NORMAL TEMPER TANTRUM	ABNORMAL TEMPER TANTRUM
Age	12 months up to age 4	Continuing past age 4
Behavior during tantrum	Crying, flailing arms or legs, falling to the floor, pushing, pulling, or biting	Injury to themselves or others during the tantrum
Duration	Up to 15 min	Lasting longer than 15 min
Frequency	Less than five times a day	More than five times a day
Mood	Should return to normal between tantrums	Persistent negative mood between tantrums

From Daniels E, Mandleco B, Luthy KE. Assessment, management, and prevention of childhood temper tantrums. J Amer Acad Nurse Pract. 2012;24(10):569–573 [Table 1].

The **physical examination** should focus on identifying signs of underlying illness as well as vision, hearing, and developmental exams to identify possible causes of increased frustration for the child. Behavioral observations can reveal a child's ability to follow instructions, play with age-appropriate toys, and interact with parents and the clinician; observation of attention may be especially helpful in evaluating for ASD or ADHD. Dysmorphic features may reveal a genetic syndrome, and a full skin exam may reveal signs of anemia, neurocutaneous stigma, or signs of nonaccidental trauma (see Chapter 21). Neurologic exam includes the general disposition of the child, a cognition assessment, and exploration for neurologic findings that could suggest brain tumors or other underlying conditions.

Laboratory studies may include screening for iron-deficiency anemia and lead exposure. Additional laboratory and imaging studies should be reserved for situations where the history and physical examination suggest a possible underlying etiology.

DIFFENTIAL DIAGNOSIS

Most children who have temper tantrums have no underlying medical problem. Children with abnormal tantrums or with concerning signs or symptoms warrant further evaluation. The differential diagnosis for abnormal tantrums includes visual and hearing deficits, language or other developmental delays, sleep disturbances, psychosocial stressors, learning disabilities, neurologic disease or injury, genetic syndromes, and psychiatric conditions such as anxiety, depression, oppositional defiant disorder, conduct disorder, post-traumatic stress disorder, ADHD, and ASD.

ANTICIPATORY GUIDANCE AND MANAGEMENT

Management of normal temper tantrums focuses on parental education and reassurance regarding tantrums as a normal developmental phase. It is important to provide anticipatory guidance regarding tantrums at the 12-, 15-, 18-, and 24-month well-child visits to guide expectations, provide strategies for assisting children with emotional regulation, and emphasize the importance of routines to minimize the negative impact of tantrums.

It is helpful to provide parents with strategies to help prevent tantrums, such as communicating clear, consistent, and developmentally appropriate expectations and consequences; providing appropriate positive reinforcements for good behavior; maintaining routine and structure in a child's environment; using distraction techniques when possible; and avoiding triggers (such as hunger, fatigue, loneliness, or hyperstimulation). Helping children learn to communicate desires, needs, and emotions (verbally or in alternate ways such as signing) can help decrease frustration and prevent tantrums. Another helpful strategy is providing children with choices among acceptable alternatives (instead of "Will you clean up?" try "Do you want to place the blocks in the basket or in the bucket?") and supporting autonomy when safe and appropriate (i.e., "picking your battles" such as allowing a child to wear mismatched clothing). For children who struggle with transitions, providing a short warning prior to a change to an undesired activity can be very helpful.

Resources for managing tantrums when they inevitably occur are useful. Parents should be encouraged to stay calm and meet physical and safety needs without complying with the child's demands. Distraction and physically removing the child from the inciting environment can be an effective means of short-circuiting impending tantrums. Parents should be discouraged from punishing children for having tantrums. Further behavioral intervention therapy may be helpful for families for whom typical management is unsuccessful. During the initial stages of any behavioral intervention, tantrum behavior may increase. While parents are working to extinguish or decrease the tantrums, it is important that they provide positive reinforcement for good behavior and decreased attention/reaction to the negative behaviors.

PEARLS FOR PRACTITIONERS

See Behavioral Disorders: Pearls for Practitioners at the end of this section.

REVIEW QUESTIONS

Available online.

CHAPTER 13

Attention-Deficit/Hyperactivity Disorder

Attention-deficit/hyperactivity disorder (ADHD) is the most prevalent neurobehavioral disorder of childhood and one of the most common chronic conditions in school-age children. ADHD is characterized by symptoms of age-inappropriate inattention, motor restlessness, hyperactivity, distractibility, poor impulse control, or a combination of these symptoms. It is diagnosed in childhood and impacts behavioral, emotional, cognitive, and social domains. Without optimal treatment, ADHD can have long-term implications, including decreased likelihood of high school and postsecondary graduation, anxiety, depression, and poor peer relations.

ETIOLOGY

ADHD is multifactorial in origin with certain prenatal exposures and genetic, neural, and environmental contributions. There are several genes associated with development of ADHD, including *DAT1* and *DRD4.* There is high heritability (77–88%) and greater risk of developing ADHD in first-degree relatives, especially those where ADHD persists into adolescence and adulthood.

There are structural differences on neuroimaging in individuals with ADHD, including smaller cortical volumes, small-volume reduction throughout the brain, and abnormalities of the cerebellum (especially with the midline and vermian elements). These imaging findings overlap with other conditions and therefore imaging is not useful for the diagnosis of ADHD. There are also functional differences in neuroimaging for patients with ADHD, including overall delay in cortical maturation and dysregulation of the frontal subcortical circuits, suggesting that the pathophysiologic features include large-scale neuronal networks including frontal to parietal cortical connections.

Environmental links have been described with prenatal exposure to a variety of substances, including nicotine, alcohol, prescription medications, substances of abuse, lead, organophosphate pesticides, and polychlorinated biphenyls. Additionally, central nervous system injury from trauma or infection (i.e., meningitis) increases the risk of ADHD.

EPIDEMIOLOGY

Worldwide ADHD prevalence in children is 7.2%. Per the Centers for Disease Control and Prevention, 11.4% of children aged 3–17 years in the United States, including 2.4% of children aged 2–5 years, have had a diagnosis of ADHD. Symptoms consistent with motor restlessness and aggression are more commonly seen in preschool children, while symptoms of disorganization and inattention are more often noted in older children and adolescents. The male:female ratio is about 2:1. Females with ADHD are more likely to be diagnosed with comorbid anxiety or depression, while males are more likely to have comorbid oppositional defiant disorder. Symptoms of ADHD, particularly impulsivity and inattention, frequently persist past childhood, with up to 80% of those affected having symptoms into adolescence and 40% into adulthood.

Clinical Symptoms

Symptoms of ADHD mimic typical findings of normal development; it is important to consider the child's symptoms in the context of typical, atypical, and abnormal development. To meet criteria for a diagnosis of ADHD, symptoms must be present for at least 6 months to a degree that is inconsistent with developmental level and that negatively impacts social and academic/occupational activities. Symptoms of inattention (e.g., failing to pay close attention to details, appearing to not listen when spoken to directly, concern over executive functioning skills), hyperactivity (e.g., being fidgety or restless, leaving a seat when expected to remain seated), or impulsivity (e.g., blurting out and interruption) may indicate a diagnosis of ADHD (Table 13.1).

Diagnosis and Evaluation

Universal screening for ADHD is not recommended. ADHD is diagnosed in the clinical setting after a full evaluation with a history and a full physical exam. The **history** should rely on open-ended questions to explore specific behaviors and their impact on academic performance, family and peer relationships, safety, self-esteem, and daily activities. Ultimately, a diagnosis of ADHD requires that the symptoms be measured with valid rating scales to establish the diagnosis. These rating scales should reflect performance in at least two settings such as in school and in home.

Clinical guidelines emphasize the use of the *Diagnostic and Statistical Manual of Mental Disorders (DSM),* with specific criteria to diagnose ADHD (Table 13.1). Several inattentive or hyperactive/impulsive symptoms should be present prior to 12 years of age with evidence of significant impairment per caregiver and teacher rating scales in social, academic, or work settings; other mental health disorders should be considered and may be coexisting. *DSM-5-TR* includes diagnostic criteria to help identify the subset of older children, mainly female, who exhibit predominantly inattentive symptoms, which may not be noted until adolescence.

A **physical examination** is essential to identify medical (e.g., neurologic, genetic) or developmental problems (e.g., cognitive impairment, language disorder, learning disability, autism spectrum disorder) that may underlie, coexist, or provide an alternative explanation for the child's behaviors.

Pertinent laboratory tests to evaluate for other disorders should be considered based on the relevant history and clinical components. Consider thyroid function studies, blood lead levels, genetic testing, anemia screening, or other evaluation if indicated by medical history, environmental history, or physical examination.

DIFFERENTIAL DIAGNOSIS

The differential diagnosis of ADHD can be challenging. The diagnostic process should evaluate for other conditions such as sleep disorders, seizure disorders, substance use disorder, thyroid abnormalities, lead intoxication, sensory processing conditions, and vision or auditory deficits—all of which can cause or exacerbate hyperactivity and distractibility. Migraine headaches, asthma, hematologic disorders, and malignancies can also impact attention span and school performance. Inattention and hyperactivity may also be features of genetic disorders such as fragile X, 22q11.2 deletion syndrome, and neurofibromatosis type 1. Attention must be paid to any medications that could contribute to symptoms of ADHD. Finally, psychologic stress from bullying, abuse, or disruptive surroundings can also lead to symptoms of hyperactivity, impulsivity, and inattention that mimic ADHD. Children who have symptoms of ADHD in only one setting may be having problems due to cognitive disability, level of emotional maturity, or feelings of inadequate well-being in that setting. It is prudent to investigate and ensure overall well-being, including sleep and nutritional hygiene, before embarking on an extensive evaluation of ADHD.

Comorbidities

Comorbidities are present in 80% of children with ADHD, including anxiety (~40%), learning disabilities (~35%), developmental language disorders (15–25%), and mood disorders (15–20%). Other comorbidities and associated conditions include sleep disorders, decreased motor coordination skills, oppositional defiant disorder, conduct disorders, Tourette syndrome, and fragile X syndrome. Close surveillance for comorbidities is necessary not only at the time of diagnosis but also in the longitudinal management of ADHD.

Treatment

Management begins with recognizing ADHD as a chronic condition and educating children and caregivers about the diagnosis, treatment options, and prognosis. A management plan should focus on achievable outcomes (such as improved relationships, increased academic performance, or fewer classroom interruptions) jointly agreed upon by the parent, the school, and the child.

Treatment strategies vary with age. Most children show a response to a multimodal-treatment approach that includes behavior and academic interventions and medications. Anticipatory guidance provides caregivers and children with proactive strategies to mediate adverse effects on learning, school functioning, social relationships, family life, and self-esteem. Formal caregiver training interventions and social skills training can improve ADHD symptomatology. Management of co-occurring conditions (such as sleep disorders, anemia, mood disorders, and learning disabilities) is needed for the optimal management of ADHD. In addition, guidance should be given on general nutrition, engaging in extracurricular activities and/or sports, and the use of screen time.

Behavioral therapy is central to children of all ages with ADHD and is the core of overall treatment. **Behavioral management** includes establishment of structure, routine, consistency in adult responses to behaviors, and appropriate behavioral goals. Children also benefit when parents and clinicians work with teachers to address the child's needs. Regular behavior report cards and other "check-in" aids may be helpful to the child in the respective environments within a classroom or the overall school day. Behavioral management strategies such as organizational skills training for the older child can enhance executive function skills.

The pediatrician should advocate for **optimal educational settings** in the school. Children may qualify for individual education plans where school personnel can establish organizational plans and charts for the individual child as part of a management plan. Social skills training or additional mental health interventions may assist some children with behavior change or preservation of self-esteem, particularly when they have coexisting developmental or mental health conditions also requiring treatment.

Medications

Medication-based treatments (Table 13.2) are effective in combination with developmental psychosocial interventions, especially for the older child and adolescent. The clinician

TABLE 13.1 Criteria for Diagnosis of Attention-Deficit/Hyperactivity Disorder

A. A persistent pattern of inattention and/or hyperactivity-impulsivity that interferes with functioning or development, as characterized by (1) and/or (2):
   1. **Inattention:** Six (or more) of the following symptoms have persisted for at least 6 months to a degree that is inconsistent with developmental level and that negatively impacts directly on social and academic/occupational activities:
   Note: The symptoms are not solely a manifestation of oppositional behavior, defiance, hostility, or a failure to understand tasks or instructions. For older adolescents and adults (age 17 and older), at least five symptoms are required.
      a. Often fails to give close attention to details or makes careless mistakes in schoolwork, at work, or during other activities (e.g., overlooks or misses details, work is inaccurate)
      b. Often has difficulty sustaining attention during tasks or play activities (e.g., has difficulty remaining focused during lectures, conversations, or lengthy reading)
      c. Often does not seem to listen when spoken to directly (e.g., mind seems elsewhere, even in the absence of any obvious distraction)
      d. Often does not follow through on instructions and fails to finish schoolwork, chores, or duties in the workplace (e.g., starts tasks but quickly loses focus and is easily sidetracked)
      e. Often has difficulty organizing tasks and activities (e.g., difficulty managing sequential tasks; difficulty keeping materials and belongings in order; messy, disorganized work; has poor time management; fails to meet deadlines)
      f. Often avoids, dislikes, or is reluctant to engage in tasks that require sustained mental effort (e.g., schoolwork or homework; for older adolescents and adults, preparing reports, completing forms, reviewing lengthy papers)
      g. Often loses things necessary for tasks or activities (e.g., school materials, pencils, books, tools, wallets, keys, paperwork, eyeglasses, mobile telephones)
      h. Is often easily distracted by extraneous stimuli (for older adolescents and adults, may include unrelated thoughts)
      i. Is often forgetful in daily activities (e.g., doing chores, running errands; for older adolescents and adults, returning calls, paying bills, keeping appointments)
   2. **Hyperactivity and impulsivity:** Six (or more) of the following symptoms have persisted for at least 6 months to a degree that is inconsistent with developmental level and that negatively impacts directly on social and academic/occupational activities:
   Note: The symptoms are not solely a manifestation of oppositional behavior, defiance, hostility, or a failure to understand tasks or instructions. For older adolescents and adults (age 17 and older), at least five symptoms are required.
      a. Often fidgets with or taps hands or feet or squirms in seat
      b. Often leaves seat in situations when remaining seated is expected (e.g., leaves their place in the classroom, in the office or other workplace, or in other situations that require remaining in place)
      c. Often runs about or climbs in situations where it is inappropriate (**Note:** In adolescents or adults, may be limited to feeling restless)
      d. Often unable to play or engage in leisure activities quietly
      e. Is often "on the go," acting as if "driven by a motor" (e.g., is unable to be or uncomfortable being still for extended time, as in restaurants, meetings; may be experienced by others as being restless or difficult to keep up with)
      f. Often talks excessively
      g. Often blurts out an answer before a question has been completed (e.g., completes people's sentences; cannot wait for turn in conversation)
      h. Often has difficulty waiting their turn (e.g., while waiting in line)
      i. Often interrupts or intrudes on others (e.g., butts into conversations, games, or activities; may start using other people's things without asking or receiving permission; for adolescents and adults, may intrude into or take over what others are doing)

B. Several inattentive or hyperactive-impulsive symptoms were present prior to age 12 years.

C. Several inattentive or hyperactive-impulsive symptoms are present in two or more settings (e.g., at home, school, or work; with friends or relatives; in other activities).

D. There is clear evidence that the symptoms interfere with or reduce the quality of social, academic, or occupational functioning.

E. The symptoms do not occur exclusively during the course of schizophrenia or another psychotic disorder and are not better explained by another mental disorder (e.g., mood disorder, anxiety disorder, dissociative disorder, personality disorder, substance intoxication or withdrawal).

Specify whether:

(F90.2) **Combined presentation:** If both Criterion A1 (inattention) and Criterion A2 (hyperactivity-impulsivity) are met for the past 6 months.

(F90.0) **Predominantly inattentive presentation:** If Criterion A1 (inattention) is met but Criterion A2 (hyperactivity-impulsivity) is not met for the past 6 months.

(F90.1) **Predominantly hyperactive/impulsive presentation:** If Criterion A2 (hyperactivity-impulsivity) is met and Criterion A1 (inattention) is not met for the past 6 months.

Specify if:

In partial remission: When full criteria were previously met, fewer than the full criteria have been met for the past 6 months, and the symptoms still result in impairment in social, academic, or occupational functioning.

Specify current severity:

Mild: Few, if any, symptoms in excess of those required to make the diagnosis are present, and symptoms result in no more than minor impairments in social or occupational functioning.

Moderate: Symptoms or functional impairment between "mild" and "severe" are present.

Severe: Many symptoms in excess of those required to make the diagnosis, or several symptoms that are particularly severe, are present, or the symptoms result in marked impairment in social or occupational functioning.

Reprinted with permission from the Diagnostic and Statistical Manual of Mental Disorders, Fifth Edition, Text Revision (Copyright © 2022). American Psychiatric Association. All Rights Reserved.

should balance the benefits and risks of initiating medication-based treatment in the preschool-age child as they are at higher risk for medication side effects. Medication-based treatments should be considered for preschool-age children if there is moderate-to-severe continued disturbance (i.e., a history of injury to other children or caregivers), a strong family history of ADHD, underlying or associated neurodevelopmental disorders, lack of evidence-based behavioral treatment availability, or if ADHD symptoms are interfering with the other therapies that the child is receiving.

Stimulant medications (methylphenidate or amphetamine compounds) are the first-line agents for pharmacologic

TABLE 13.2 FDA-Approved Medications for Attention-Deficit/Hyperactivity Disorder

MEDICATION TYPE	GENERIC NAME	BRAND NAME	DURATION OF ACTION
STIMULANTS	METHYLPHENIDATES		
	Methylphenidate IR	Ritalin, Methylin	Short-acting (3–6 hours)
	Methylphenidate ER	Ritalin LA, Metadate CD, Metadate ER, QuilliChew ER	Intermediate-acting (6–8 hours)
	Methylphenidate ER	Concerta, Quillivant XR, Daytrana patch Aptensio XR	Long-acting (8–12 hours)
	Methylphenidate ER/DR	Jornay PM	Long-acting and delayed onset (onset after 10 hours and lasts for 10–12 hours)
	Dexmethylphenidate IR	Focalin	Short-acting (3–6 hours)
	Dexmethylphenidate ER	Focalin XR	Intermediate-acting (6–8 hours)
	Dexmethylphenidate/ Serdexmethylphenidate	Azstarys	Long-acting (8–12 hours)
	AMPHETAMINES		
	Amphetamine/Dextroamphetamine IR	Adderall, Evekeo	Short-acting (3–6 hours)
	Amphetamine/Dextroamphetamine ER	Adderall XR, Mydayis, Adzenys XR-ODT, Dyanavel XR	Long-acting (10–12 hours)
	Lisdexamfetamine	Vyvanse	Long-acting (10–14 hours)
	Dextroamphetamine IR	ProCentra, Zenzedi	Short-acting (4–6 hours)
	Dextroamphetamine ER	Dexedrine, Spansule	Intermediate-acting (6–8 hours)
	D-amphetamine	Xelstrym patch	Intermediate-acting (2 hours to effect then lasts 9 hours)
NONSTIMULANTS	CLONIDINE		
	Clonidine	Catapres	Short-acting (3–6 hours)
	Clonidine ER	Kapvay	Long-acting (10–12 hours)
	GUANFACINE		
	Guanfacine	Tenex	Short-acting (3–6 hours)
	Guanfacine ER	Intuniv	Long-acting (12–24 hours)
	SELECTIVE NOREPINEPHRINE REUPTAKE INHIBITORS (SNRIs)		
	Atomoxetine	Strattera	Long-acting (24 hours)
	Viloxazine	Qelbree	Long-acting (24 hours)

FDA, Food and Drug Administration.

treatment of ADHD. Stimulants improve parent report of quality of life and are associated with improved academic performance and lower rates of comorbidities such as mood disorders. Stimulant medications are associated with a significant clinical benefit including decision-making, handwriting, and schoolwork productivity. Stimulant use is also associated with improved reading and math scores, fewer injuries, and overall reduced morbidity and mortality involving motor vehicle accident. In adolescents, the use of extended-release stimulants has a positive impact on evening driving performance.

Stimulant medications are available in short-acting, intermediate-acting, and long-acting forms. Extended-release and long-acting forms are preferred and are considered as first-line therapy for most children and adolescents with ADHD outside of the preschool-age group. Extended-release forms correlate with improved medication adherence. It is essential to determine the optimal dose to avoid significant side effects or lack of efficacy, both of which can result in poor adherence.

Nonstimulant medications, including atomoxetine and viloxazine (norepinephrine reuptake inhibitors) and guanfacine and clonidine (α-agonists), may be helpful in children and are considered as a second-line medication intervention. They have lower treatment response rates and effect size compared to those of stimulants but may be useful for patients in whom stimulants are contraindicated, not well tolerated, or ineffective (or only partially effective), or in patients who have a history of substance use. Guanfacine chloral hydrate XR can be used as a monotherapy regimen or adjunctively with a stimulant medication, especially when treating for both ADHD and comorbid oppositional symptoms in children and adolescents.

Dosing should be based on the individual's response rather than on the severity of the presentation or the child's age. Close monitoring is needed with surveillance for future dose adjustments. The effects of the initial dose should be followed closely within a few days, and then on a weekly basis during the first month of medication initiation.

When treating ADHD, there are numerous potential medication side effects (Table 13.3), many of which are dose-dependent. The most common side effects include insomnia, loss of appetite, weight loss, jitteriness, and rebound irritability. ADHD medications may exacerbate existing tic conditions. Children who are taking medications must be regularly screened for side effects, including careful monitoring of the child's growth. Providers should titrate medication dosages and timing to minimize side effects and optimize treatment response.

Stimulant medications may be associated with adverse cardiovascular events such as sudden cardiac death in patients with an underlying disorder exacerbated by sympathomimetic agents. While episodes are rare, screening for cardiac disease by history, family history, and physical exam is critical prior to initiation of stimulant medication and with continued surveillance during the ongoing treatment with stimulants.

Complementary Alternative Medicine

Complementary alternative medicines are frequently used by families despite a lack of evidence for their effectiveness in children. Practitioners should explicitly ask about the use of alternative medicines including herbal supplements, chiropractic interventions, and meditation/relaxation techniques.

TABLE 13.3 List of ADHD Medication Side Effects

COMMON SIDE EFFECTS (STIMULANTS)
• Decreased appetite • Weight loss • Insomnia • Increased heart rate • Increased blood pressure • Anxiety • Hyperfocus • Irritability • Agitation • Headaches • Abdominal pain
COMMON SIDE EFFECTS (NONSTIMULANTS)
• Fatigue • Drowsiness (clonidine and guanfacine) • Decreased appetite • Nausea • Dry mouth • Dizziness • Constipation • Low blood pressure • Sedation (clonidine and guanfacine) • Mood swings
LESS COMMON/RARE SIDE EFFECTS
• Psychotic symptoms (hallucinations, paranoia, nightmares) (stimulants) • Liver damage (atomoxetine, viloxazine) • Sudden cardiac death (very rare, usually with underlying heart conditions)

ADHD, Attention-deficit/hyperactivity disorder.

PEARLS FOR PRACTITIONERS

See Behavioral Disorders: Pearls for Practitioners at the end of this section.

REVIEW QUESTIONS

Available online.

CHAPTER 14

Control of Elimination

NORMAL DEVELOPMENT OF ELIMINATION

Control of urination and defecation involves physical, developmental, and cognitive maturation and is influenced by cultural norms and practices within the United States and throughout the world. In the first half of the 20th century, toilet mastery by 18 months of age was the norm in the United States. Brazelton's introduction of the *child-centered approach* and the invention of disposable diapers facilitated later toilet training. Social changes, including increased parental work outside of the home and group childcare, have also influenced the trend to later initiation of toilet training. Between 2–4 years of age, a normally developing child is considered ready to begin toilet training. In general, the control of bowel movement passage is achieved before bladder control.

Prerequisites for achieving elimination in the toilet include the child's ability to recognize the urge for urination and defecation, to get to the toilet, to understand the sequence of tasks required, to avoid oppositional behavior, and to take pride in achievement. The entire process of toilet training can take several months.

ENURESIS

Enuresis is defined as urinary incontinence in a child who is adequately mature to have achieved continence. Enuresis is classified as **monosymptomatic** (intermittent nocturnal incontinence), which is the focus of this chapter, or **non-monosymptomatic** (associated with other urinary tract abnormalities such as frequency, urgency, hesitancy, straining, weak stream, intermittency, postvoid dribbling, dysuria, and daytime wetting; see Chapter 169). Nocturnal enuresis refers to discrete episodes of incontinence during sleep in children over the age of 5 years. Nighttime dryness is usually achieved months after daytime dryness. Nocturnal enuresis is classified as either **primary** (incontinence in a child who has never achieved a period of nighttime dryness) or **secondary** (incontinence in a child who has been dry for at least 6 months).

Etiology

Enuresis results from a child failing to wake before voiding and may be due to a variety of factors. A correlation with slower growth and motor delays suggests a maturational delay in the neurologic ability to recognize bladder fullness and suppress bladder contraction; such delays are likely due to normal variations in development. There is genetic predisposition to enuresis with higher monozygotic (68%) than dizygotic (36%) twin concordance; associated genes include *PRDM13, SIM1, EDNRB,* and *KCNJ10.* A child's likelihood of being affected is strongly linked to parental history of nocturnal enuresis and rises from 15% (if neither parent was affected) to 50% (if one parent was affected) and 75% (if both parents were affected).

Anatomic or physiologic abnormalities can contribute to nocturnal enuresis. **Nocturnal polyuria**, suggested by increased nighttime void volumes, can be a factor in some children and may be due to a decreased nocturnal vasopressin peak or secondary to excessive fluid intake late in the day. Small bladder capacity is more likely functional than anatomic, as affected children have similar bladder capacity as unaffected children under general anesthesia. In children with chronic constipation, a dilated colon can impinge on the bladder, resulting in reduced bladder capacity and higher likelihood of enuresis. A malfunction of the detrusor muscle with a tendency for involuntary contractions even when the bladder contains small amounts of urine is possible; an overactive detrusor muscle generally results in daytime wetting as well. Sleep physiology may play a role in the etiology of nocturnal enuresis, with a high arousal threshold of some affected children.

Psychologic or behavioral concerns may be associated with primary nocturnal enuresis, but they tend to improve after acquisition of bladder control, suggesting they are more likely a result than a cause. Stressful life events are more commonly associated with (and a contributing factor for) secondary nocturnal enuresis, which can also be caused by development of poor daily voiding habits and stool retention from constipation.

Epidemiology

Nocturnal enuresis is common, with a prevalence of 15% at 5 years of age, gradually decreasing to 5% at 10 years. One to two percent of adolescents aged 15 and older are still affected (Fig. 14.1). The spontaneous remission rate is reported to be 15% per year. Nocturnal enuresis is twice as common in males than in females. Primary nocturnal enuresis accounts for 80% of cases.

Clinical Manifestations

The **history** focuses on elucidating daytime and nighttime voiding patterns, frequency, and timing; typical amount and timing of fluid intake; and determining whether enuresis is primary or secondary. It is important to explore the expectations of the family and the impact that enuresis has on the child and family. Many families have already attempted interventions prior to seeking care; identifying such attempts and the effect they had on the child and family are essential in determining the impact of the problem and helping identify potential future interventions.

The history should differentiate between monosymptomatic (intermittent nocturnal incontinence) and non-monosymptomatic enuresis (associated with other abnormalities). The presence of daytime incontinence or any associated urinary tract symptoms (urgency, holding maneuvers, interrupted micturition, weak stream, straining to void, or continual dampness suggesting urine leak) or neurologic symptoms (such as abnormal gait or weakness) is concerning for an underlying urologic or neurologic disorder such as posterior urethral valves, ectopic ureter, or spinal dysraphism. Urinary tract infection (UTI), renal disease, diabetes, and primary/psychogenic polydipsia may be suggested by a history pertinent for symptoms such as dysuria, frequency, anorexia, vomiting, weakness, poor growth, weight loss, polydipsia, or polyuria. A sleep history can help identify obstructive sleep apnea (OSA) or other sleep disorders (see Chapter 15); the history should also elicit symptoms suggesting seizure activity. A stooling history is also essential, as chronic constipation can contribute to enuresis via bladder impingement. Family history frequently reveals other affected family members, and a developmental history is important in identifying comorbidities such as autism spectrum disorder or attention-deficit/hyperactivity disorder (ADHD). A social history must include recent stressful events or changes, which are often associated with secondary nocturnal enuresis.

A complete **physical examination** is usually normal in a child with monosymptomatic nocturnal enuresis. Poor growth, hypertension, and edema may signify renal disease; a head, eyes, ears, nose, and throat (HEENT) exam may help identify findings consistent with OSA; and the abdominal and rectal exam may suggest chronic constipation. A careful neurologic exam is indicated to identify signs such as a sacral tuft or other neurocutaneous stigmata, asymmetric gluteal folds, or lower extremity weakness, which are concerning for an occult spinal cord abnormality. When possible, an observed void may help identify weak stream, intermittency, postvoid dribbling, or other signs that can signal urologic abnormalities such as posterior urethral valves, ectopic ureter, or vesicoureteral reflux.

For most children with enuresis, the only **laboratory** test recommended is a clean catch urinalysis (UA) with specific gravity to screen for UTI, renal disease, and diabetes mellitus. A first-morning void is particularly helpful to best evaluate for possible diabetes insipidus or water intoxication. Further testing, such as a urine culture, is based on the UA. A renal ultrasound and/or voiding cystourethrogram is indicated in children with daytime symptoms, recurrent UTI, or concerns for underlying urologic abnormality. Abnormal neurologic findings warrant imaging such as MRI.

Differential Diagnosis

In most cases, there is no identified underlying cause of enuresis; resolution occurs by adolescence without treatment. Children with monosymptomatic primary nocturnal enuresis are most likely to have a family history, and those with secondary nocturnal enuresis are more likely to have a significant psychosocial stressor. Children with non-monosymptomatic or secondary nocturnal enuresis are more likely to have an identified organic etiology. The differential diagnosis includes constipation, psychiatric or developmental problems, renal disease, chronic or recurrent UTIs, diabetes mellitus, diabetes insipidus, primary polydipsia, posterior urethral valves, ectopic ureter, vesicoureteral reflux, sleep disturbance such as OSA, occult spinal dysraphism, or a mass impinging on the urinary system. Referral to renal, endocrine, urologic, sleep, or neurosurgical specialists is recommended when such an

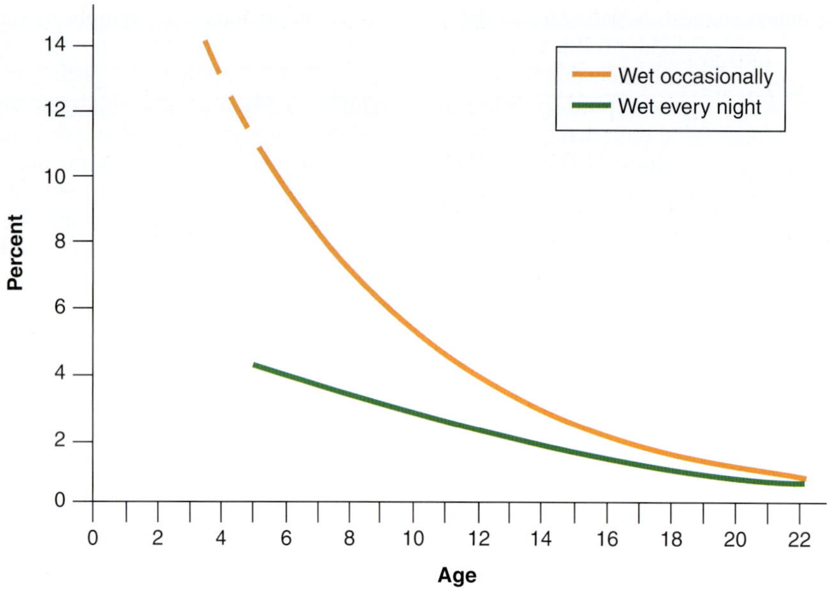

FIGURE 14.1 Epidemiology and prognosis of monosymptomatic enuresis. (From Neveus T, Eggert P, Evans J, et al. Evaluation of and treatment for monosymptomatic enuresis: a standardization document from the International Children's Continence Society. *J Urol.* 2010;183[2]:441–447.)

underlying anatomic or physiologic abnormality is suspected. Constipation may be successfully treated by the primary physician with referral to gastroenterology for refractory cases. Referral to a developmental and behavioral pediatrician, psychologist, or other enuresis specialist is warranted for concerns of underlying developmental or psychiatric problems, children with refractory or nightly enuresis, and for situations where families have unreasonable expectations or blame the child for wetting.

Treatment

Treatment of monosymptomatic enuresis depends on the goals of the child and family (such as fewer wet nights overall or only for occasional sleepovers) and the degree to which it causes distress to the child and family. Treatment success depends largely on the level of motivation for both the child and family, as this requires consistency and close follow-up to be successful. For many families, the only intervention needed is simple reassurance that enuresis is common and generally self-resolves. Caregivers should be educated that nocturnal enuresis is involuntary and should not be punished, which can result in poor self-esteem. Families may benefit from simple tips to help manage enuresis, such as the use of bed protection, room deodorizers, and emollients to protect skin. A plan for handling wet garments and linens in a nonhumiliating and hygienic manner is essential to protect the child's self-esteem. The child should take as much responsibility for cleaning soiled linens as possible, depending on age, development, and family culture.

Minor **behavioral interventions** may be helpful for some highly motivated children and should be considered prior to active therapy. These children may benefit from encouragement to increase the amount of water consumed during the entire day and to drink throughout the day rather than primarily between the time they get home from school and bedtime. They can also be encouraged to void regularly throughout the day (every 2–3 hours), to double void before bed (e.g., the hour before bedtime and then again right before bedtime), as well as to void overnight if they awaken. Refraining from drinks with sugar and caffeine in the evening can be helpful, but limiting the amount of evening fluid intake should only be done when sufficient fluid intake is ensured earlier in the day. Positive reinforcement should be provided for choices made (such as remembering to void before bed), not for remaining dry overnight. Older children are advised to not wear disposable undergarments to sleep (except for occasional use such as sleepovers) as this may decrease motivation to get out of bed when they awaken with a need to void.

In situations where active treatment is desired, recommended first-line therapy consists of either enuresis alarm **conditioning therapy** or desmopressin **pharmacotherapy**. Enuresis alarms consist of a sensor in the undergarment or bed pad and an arousal device clipped to the child's clothing or worn on the wrist. The alarm should wake the child when the probe first senses moisture so that the child can arouse and complete the void in the bathroom. Desmopressin decreases urine production and is taken 1 hour before bed. Fluid intake must be limited prior to dosing and overnight to prevent hyponatremia, and the medication should be held during illness or times of potential fluid and electrolyte imbalance.

Alarm therapy is more time-intensive with high attrition rates, and it takes longer to work, but overall it has a superior response rate and a lower relapse rate and is especially helpful in situations where the patient and family are coping well and adhering to the routine required for success. Desmopressin may work quicker, making it ideal for occasional use such as sleepovers; it may also be indicated when a more rapid effect is needed due to poor coping or when families have difficulty adhering to the routine of an alarm. Desmopressin may be used nightly, in which case trials off the medication should be attempted every few months, and tapering may decrease relapse rate. Desmopressin is contraindicated for children with a history of hyponatremia.

Children with relapse after initial successful treatment often respond to reinitiation of the same treatment regimen. Poor response to either alarm or desmopressin therapy alone may benefit from a combination therapy of both. The addition of an anticholinergic medication to desmopressin may be more effective than desmopressin alone. Tricyclic antidepressants (most commonly imipramine) are reserved for refractory cases due to potential for serious toxicity (particularly cardiac and psychiatric) and should only be prescribed by a specialist. Various other interventions and therapies (including regular waking of the child, bladder training for increased capacity, electrical stimulation therapy, hypnosis, acupuncture, chiropractic, and herbal treatments) have not been studied enough to be considered safe and/or effective.

Complications

Children who experience enuresis often experience social consequences, such as an inability or fear of attending sleepovers or overnight camps with peers. Additionally, the psychologic impact of low self-esteem is a threat, particularly in situations where families misunderstand the cause of enuresis and punish the child, which occurs in up to a third of patients. It is essential to educate families about the etiology and natural course of enuresis regardless of the treatment plan.

FUNCTIONAL CONSTIPATION AND ENCOPRESIS

There are varying definitions of **constipation** and diagnostic criteria are relative to the age of a child. Parental perception of normal and abnormal bowel movements also interplays with the diagnosis of functional constipation. For instance, a young child may have bowel movements every 2 days. An infant who is breast-fed exclusively may have a soft and seedy bowel movement every 4–5 days. These bowel movement patterns can be considered normal depending on the patient's age and developmental stage. An encompassing definition includes the presence of any of the following: infrequent bowel movements, passage of hard stools, difficult passage of large-diameter stool, and voluntary and involuntary fecal evacuation, also called *soiling*. When discussing the presence of hard stools with parents, Bristol stool charts (available online at https://www.continence.org.au/bristol-stool-chart) are helpful when evaluating for constipation.

Epidemiology

In the United States, approximately 30% of children are affected by constipation. Constipation constitutes up to 5% of all outpatient general pediatric visits and accounts for approximately 25% of referrals to pediatric gastroenterology. The peak prevalence is in the preschool child age group.

More than 90% of constipation is considered functional. **Functional constipation** implies that there is no identifiable causative organic condition. Key features of functional constipation are occurrence after infancy, presence of stool-withholding behavior, absence of red flag symptoms, and the episodic passage of large-diameter stools. Red flag symptoms include poor growth, weight loss, growth faltering, emesis, abdominal distention and bloating, perianal disease, blood in stool, abnormal urinary stream, and a history of delayed passage of meconium.

Encopresis (soiling) is the regular, voluntary, or involuntary passage of feces into a place other than the toilet after 4 years of age. This condition should also be considered in an otherwise normally developing 3-year-old who still is not potty-trained with respect to bowel movements. Children with encopresis often leak stool due to underlying constipation or a fecal impaction. Nonretentive encopresis refers to the passage of normal stools into underwear.

Etiology

There are three periods in child development during which children are particularly prone to developing functional constipation. These periods are after the introduction of solids in an infant's diet (>6 months of age), during toilet training (2–3 years of age), and during the start of school (3–5 years of age). In addition, adolescents can develop functional constipation, particularly if associated with eating disorders, school stressors, and ADHD.

The etiology of functional constipation and soiling includes diet, slow gastrointestinal transit time, and chronic withholding of bowel movements. Approximately 95% of children referred to a subspecialist for encopresis have no other underlying pathologic condition. Fifty to ninety percent of children with functional constipation are eventually cured.

Diet

A well-balanced diet of fruits and vegetables with an age-appropriate amount of fiber is recommended for all children and may be useful in preventing or treating mild functional constipation. The addition of extra fiber is not helpful to the child with significant constipation.

Evidence to support a strong link between cow's milk introduction and constipation is lacking. The emergence of constipation with the introduction to cow's milk in the toddler age group has been described anecdotally.

Withholding Behaviors

Withholding of bowel movements can often be traced back to prior painful defecation experiences due to constipation. The child may begin to delay defection due to a history of pain. Stool then accumulates in the rectum and becomes harder or larger, causing even more pain when eventually passed. Thus, it is critical that the underlying primary constipation is addressed to help resolve stool withholding behavior. Parental attempts at early toilet training and coercion to potty train can lead to stool holding behavior with significant sequelae, including severe constipation.

History

The history should include a complete review of systems for gastrointestinal, endocrine, and neurologic disorders to evaluate for organic etiologies. It is also important to obtain a thorough developmental and psychosocial history.

Clinical Manifestations

The presenting clinical symptoms of constipation may vary by age. Children younger than 3 years of age often present with painful defecation, impaction, and withholding. Children may also present with uncontrolled defecation or diarrhea due to leaking of liquid stool around a stool ball. Soiling may be frequent or continuous.

Stool impaction can be felt on abdominal examination in about 50% of patients at presentation. Firm packed stool in the rectum is highly predictive of fecal impaction. A rectal examination allows assessment of sphincter tone and size of the rectal vault. Evaluation of anal placement and existence of any anal fissures also are helpful in considering etiology and severity. A neurologic examination, including lower extremity reflexes, anal wink, and cremasteric reflexes, may reveal underlying spinal cord abnormalities. A complete exam of the lower back should be performed, including examination for any neurocutaneous stigmata.

Abdominal imaging is not required in the diagnosis of functional constipation; it may be helpful to demonstrate the degree of stool load to parents. Other imaging should be considered if an organic cause for the constipation is indicated by history or physical examination (see Chapter 130). Pediatric gastroenterology specialty care should then be sought for consideration of other etiologies such as Hirschsprung disease. Similarly, although endocrinologic conditions such as hypothyroidism can cause chronic constipation, routine laboratory studies are not indicated without the history or physical examination suggesting such a disorder.

Differential Diagnosis

The differential diagnosis for functional constipation and soiling includes organic causes of constipation (e.g., neurogenic, anatomic, endocrinologic, gastrointestinal, and pharmacologic). For instance, a child with chronic constipation with or without soiling who had delayed passage of meconium and has an empty rectum and tight sphincter may have Hirschsprung disease (see Chapter 130). Chronic constipation may be a presenting sign of spinal cord abnormalities, such as a spinal cord tumor or a tethered cord. Physical examination findings of altered lower extremity reflexes, absent anal wink, or a sacral hairy tuft or sacral sinus may be a clue to these anomalies. Hypothyroidism can present with chronic constipation and is accompanied by poor linear growth. Anal stenosis may lead to chronic constipation, as can the use of opiates, phenothiazine, antidepressants, and anticholinergics. Developmental problems, including cognitive impairment and developmental delays, may be associated with chronic constipation.

Treatment

Treatment begins first with education and demystification for the child and family about functional constipation, as well as encopresis. Education should emphasize the chronic nature of this condition, the good prognosis with optimal management, and the time that it can take for full resolution. Explaining the physiologic and behavioral component to the child and the family alleviates blame, enlists cooperation, and avoids the use of inappropriate, negative-reinforcement behavioral interventions. Education may improve adherence to the long-term treatment plan. Treatment plans need to be created for the individual patient considering the physical and developmental status, parental expectations, and the requirement for close surveillance for the appropriate use of medications. More proactive and early approaches to the diagnosis of functional constipation and a keen surveillance of encopresis make the management program more effective and shorter in duration. Treatment involves a combination of behavioral training and use of stool-softening therapy, with the possible addition of laxative therapy (Fig. 14.2).

The next step of treatment is to ensure an effective process for adequate colonic cleanout or disimpaction. Cleanout methods often include higher doses of polyethylene glycol within short windows of administration along with the use of laxatives such as Ex-Lax. It is important that an evidence-based behavioral and medicinal approach is used during both the cleanout and the maintenance phase of functional constipation and encopresis. Choice of disimpaction method depends on the age of the child, family choice, and the clinician's experience with a particular method. The approach for treatment for children with constipation can be seen in Figure 14.3. The child and family should be included in the process of choosing the cleanout method. It is important to educate the parents and child in a developmentally appropriate manner about the need for the cleanout and that the overall goal is to lessen the frequency of cleanouts. Allowing choice and control for the child and praising all signs of cooperation are critical to the overall management plan.

Behavioral training is essential to the treatment of chronic constipation and soiling both in the acute phases of cleanouts and in the maintenance phase of treatment. There are numerous behavioral training plans available for families. A log that monitors and documents the frequency of stool passage and type of stool can be helpful. Most behavioral plans emphasize timed toilet-sitting sessions at scheduled frequencies. It is critical to recognize that often a stepwise, staggered approach is needed to optimize engagement. Every step in the behavioral management plan should feature praise and positive reinforcement for continued behavioral engagement, while punishment and embarrassment must be avoided.

When successful cleanout has been achieved, the child begins the maintenance phase of treatment. This phase promotes regular stool production and prevents re-impaction. It involves attention to diet, medications to promote soft stool regularity, and behavioral training. Attention to any dietary factors that may help the child is particularly helpful in this phase. The use of sorbitol-based juices, including prune, pear, and apple juice, increases the water content of bowel movements. Maintenance medications, including side effects, are listed in Table 14.1 Polyethylene glycol powder is superior to older medications such as lactulose, both in terms of efficacy and compliance. It is well tolerated because the taste and texture are palatable. Treatment failures are often due to problems with adherence, poor recognition of inadequate treatment resulting in re-impaction, or a lack of caregiver understanding of the underlying factors of functional constipation. Referral to pediatric gastroenterology specialty care may be considered for continued persistent or intermittent functional constipation and encopresis.

Prevention

Anticipatory guidance for parents should begin in early infancy regarding typical bowel movements for the different ages and stages of their child. This helps in the early detection of constipation and establishes appropriate parental expectations and behavior approaches to their child's elimination habits. It is very important that complete stool histories are obtained at the regular well-child visits, as well as in detail when a child presents with complaints of other concerns such as UTI, poor appetite, or abdominal pain. Close surveillance is needed for the early detection of functional constipation. Early diagnosis with prompt treatment plans given to families has been shown to decrease the duration and the severity of constipation and help prevent sequelae such as encopresis.

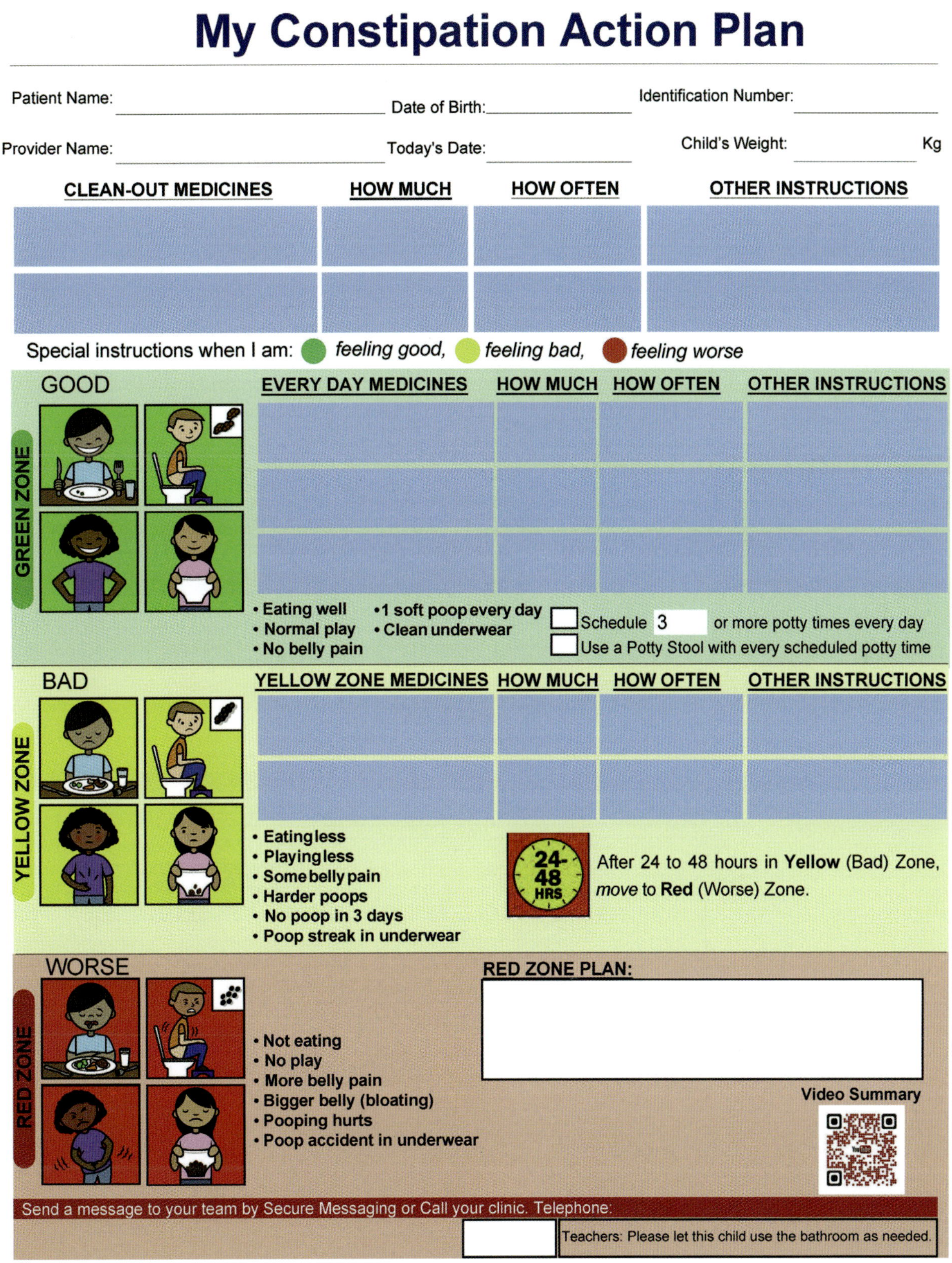

My Constipation Action Plan

Patient Name: ____________ Date of Birth: ____________ Identification Number: ____________

Provider Name: ____________ Today's Date: ____________ Child's Weight: ____________ Kg

CLEAN-OUT MEDICINES	HOW MUCH	HOW OFTEN	OTHER INSTRUCTIONS

Special instructions when I am: *feeling good*, *feeling bad*, *feeling worse*

GREEN ZONE

GOOD

EVERY DAY MEDICINES	HOW MUCH	HOW OFTEN	OTHER INSTRUCTIONS

- Eating well
- Normal play
- No belly pain
- 1 soft poop every day
- Clean underwear

☐ Schedule 3 or more potty times every day

☐ Use a Potty Stool with every scheduled potty time

YELLOW ZONE

BAD

YELLOW ZONE MEDICINES	HOW MUCH	HOW OFTEN	OTHER INSTRUCTIONS

- Eating less
- Playing less
- Some belly pain
- Harder poops
- No poop in 3 days
- Poop streak in underwear

24-48 HRS

After 24 to 48 hours in **Yellow** (Bad) Zone, *move* to **Red** (Worse) Zone.

RED ZONE

WORSE

- Not eating
- No play
- More belly pain
- Bigger belly (bloating)
- Pooping hurts
- Poop accident in underwear

RED ZONE PLAN:

Video Summary

Send a message to your team by Secure Messaging or Call your clinic. Telephone:

Teachers: Please let this child use the bathroom as needed.

FIGURE 14.2 Constipation action plan. (Courtesy the Uniformed Services University of the Health Sciences, Bethesda, MD.)

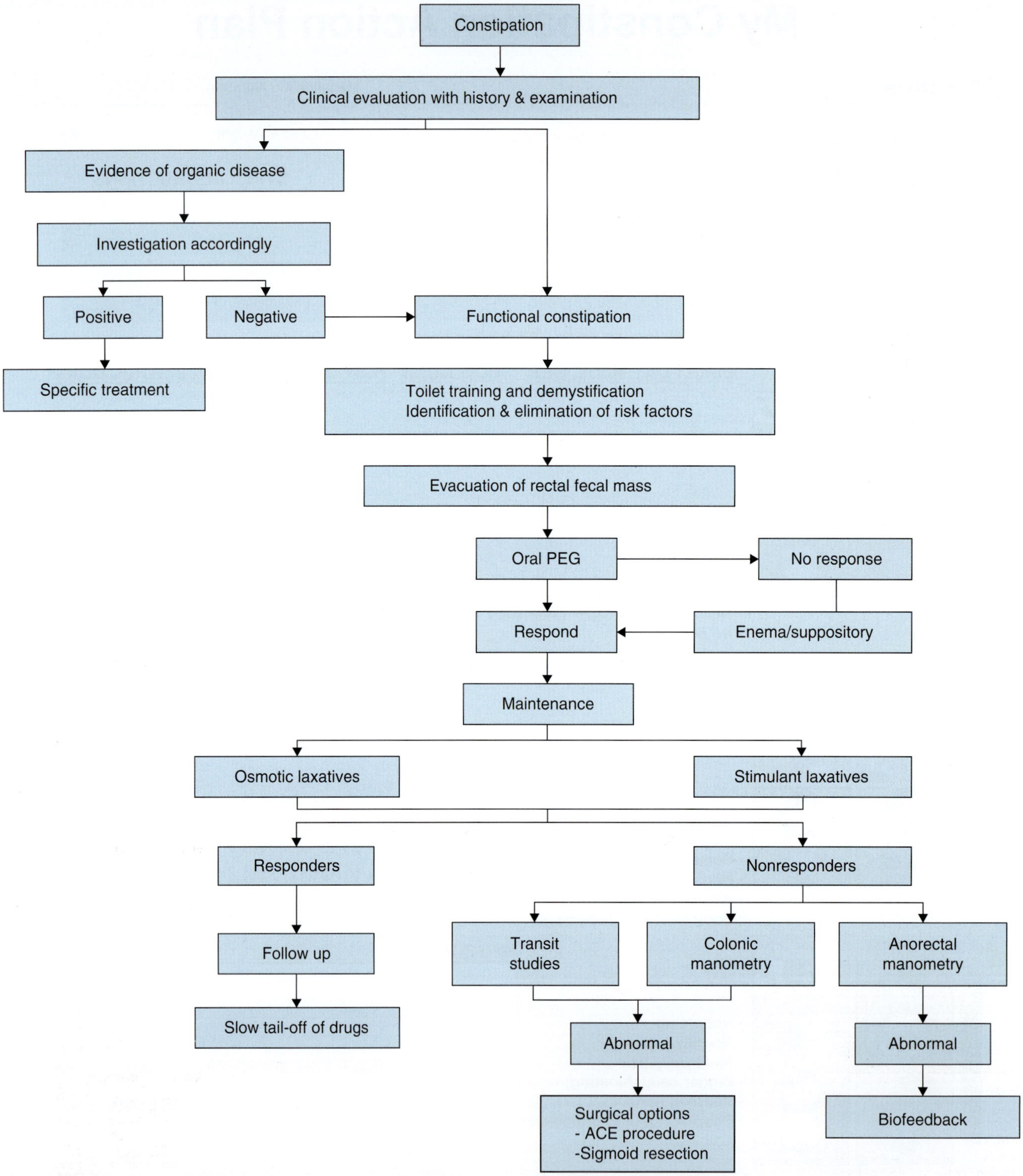

FIGURE 14.3 Algorithm of management of childhood constipation. ACE, Antegrade colonic enema; PEG, polyethylene glycol. (From Rajindrajith S, Devanarayana NM. Constipation in children: novel insight into epidemiology, pathophysiology and management. *J Neurogastroenterol Motil.* 2011;17[1]:35–47.)

TABLE 14.1 Maintenance Therapies for Children With Constipation

THERAPY	DOSAGE	ADVERSE EFFECTS
OSMOTICS		
Polyethylene glycol 3350 (Miralax)*,†	0.4–0.8 g/kg up to 17 g/day	Anaphylaxis, flatulence
Lactulose†	1 mL/kg/day once or twice per day, single dose or in two divided doses	Abdominal cramps, flatulence
Magnesium hydroxide	<2 yr: 0.5 mL/kg/day	Infants are susceptible to magnesium overdose (hypermagnesemia, hyperphosphatemia, hypocalcemia)
	2–5 yr: 5–15 mL/day	
	6–11 yr: 15–30 mL/day	
	≥12 yr: 15–60 mL/day	
	Medication may be given at bedtime or in divided doses	
Sorbitol (e.g., prune juice)†	1–3 mL/kg once or twice per day in infants	Similar to lactulose
STIMULANTS		
Senna (Senokot)†	1 month–2 yr: 1.25–2.5 mL (2.2–4.4 mg) at bedtime (<5 mL/day); 8.8 mg/day	Idiosyncratic hepatitis, melanosis coli, hypertrophic osteoarthropathy, analgesic nephropathy
	2–6 yr: 2.5–3.75 mL (4.4–6.6 mg) or ½ tablet (4.3 mg) at bedtime (<7.5 mL/day or 1 tablet twice daily [maximum dose])	
	6–12 yr: 5–7.5 mL (8.8–13.2 mg) or 1 tablet (8.6 mg) at bedtime (<15 mL/day or 2 tablets twice daily [maximum dose])	
	>12 yr: 10–15 mL (26.4 mg) or 2 tablets (17.2 mg) at bedtime (<30 mL/day or 4 tablets twice daily [maximum dose])	
Bisacodyl (Dulcolax)	Children 3–<10 yr: oral: 5 mg once daily	Abdominal cramps, diarrhea, hypokalemia, abnormal rectal mucosa, proctitis (rare), urolithiasis (case reports)
	Children 10–<12 yr: oral: 5–10 mg once daily	
	Children ≥12 yr and adolescents: oral: 5–15 mg once daily	
LUBRICANTS		
Mineral oil	Children: 5–15 mL/day	Lipoid pneumonia if aspirated, theoretical interference with absorption of fat-soluble substances, foreign body reaction in intestine
	Adolescents: 15–45 mL/day	

*First-line therapy.
†May be used in infants <1 yr.
From Nurko S, Zimmerman LA. Evaluation and treatment of constipation in children and adolescents. Am Fam Physician. 2014;90(2):82–90, with data from Tabbers MM, Dilorenzo C, Berger MY, et al. Evaluation and treatment of functional constipation in infants and children: evidence-based recommendations from ESPGHAN and NASPGHAN. J Pediatr Gastroenterol Nutr. 2014;58(2):265–281; Epocrates. http://www.epocrates.com. Accessed April 3, 2014; Tschudy MM, Arcara KM, Johns Hopkins Hospital. Harriet Lane Handbook: A Manual for Pediatric House Officers. 19th ed. Philadelphia: Elsevier; 2012; Biggs WS, Dery WH. Evaluation and treatment of constipation in infants and children. Am Fam Physician. 2006;73(3):469–477.

PEARLS FOR PRACTITIONERS

See Behavioral Disorders: Pearls for Practitioners at the end of this section.

REVIEW QUESTIONS

Available online.

CHAPTER 15

Normal Sleep and Pediatric Sleep Disorders

Sleep is a universal phenomenon that is critical to child health, development, and daily functioning. Expectations and habits surrounding sleep vary greatly and must be interpreted in the context of each family and culture. Sleep is broadly categorized by polysomnographic patterns into rapid eye movement (REM) sleep and non-REM (NREM) sleep. REM sleep is characterized by an active, awake-like electroencephalography (EEG) pattern and muscle atonia. NREM sleep is further divided into three stages. Stage 1 (N1) is the lightest sleep stage and consists of low-amplitude, high-frequency EEG activity. Stage 2 (N2) is similar to Stage 1, although eye movements stop. Brain waves become slower with occasional bursts of rapid waves (called *sleep spindles* or *K complexes*). Stage 3 (N3), also known as *deep* or *slow-wave* sleep, is characterized by low-frequency, high-amplitude delta waves. REM and NREM sleep alternate in cycles throughout the night. Sleep architecture changes from fetal life through infancy and childhood and parallels physical maturation and development. Newborns require the most sleep and have the most disrupted sleep patterns; newborn sleep cycles last approximately 60 minutes and gradually lengthen to 90 minutes in children and adults. Neonates begin their sleep cycle in REM sleep; older children and adults begin sleep in NREM sleep. REM sleep comprises up to 50% of total sleep time in newborns and gradually decreases to 25–30% by adolescence. Slow-wave sleep is not seen before 3–6 months of age. Starting at 6–12 months and continuing through adulthood, the amount of REM sleep shifts toward the last third of the night, while NREM sleep predominates during the first third of the night. Infants are capable of sleeping through the night without feeds at around 6 months of age; this age varies with factors including gestational age, type of feeding (e.g., breast-fed infants tend to awaken more frequently than formula-fed infants), familial factors, and general cultural contexts.

The timing and duration of sleep also change with age. Sleep duration gradually decreases with age (0–12 years), while longest sleep period increases (0–2 years); number of night awakenings decreases in the first 2 years of life; number of daytime naps decreases (up to age 2). Sleep patterns also become more diurnal. Full-term infants sleep on average 16–18 hours per day in fragmented intervals throughout the day and night, and 1- to 3-year-old children sleep on average 10–16 hours. Naps begin to decrease from two naps to one starting around 15–18 months of age. The biologic need for napping diminishes after age 2; significant consistent napping after age 2 has been associated with later sleep onset and reduced sleep quality and duration. Fifty percent of 3-year-olds still nap. Napping in the older child and adolescent suggests insufficient sleep or a sleep disorder.

ADOLESCENT SLEEP

Adolescents also develop a physiologically based shift toward later sleep onset and wake times relative to those in middle childhood. While experts recommend that adolescents sleep at least 9 hours each night, only about 20% of U.S. adolescents achieve this goal. The average amount of adolescent sleep is 7.5 hours per day; up to 25% of adolescents achieve only 6 hours of sleep a night. For adolescents, insufficient sleep has been associated with morning tiredness, day sleepiness, and negative effects on cognitive function, moods, and motivation. Early school start times have been associated with negative sleep profiles in adolescence. Furthermore, sleep onset latency (the time it takes to fall asleep) in adolescents has been associated with fatigue, mood disorders, and anxiety. Adolescents should be advised to limit or reduce screen time exposure prior to bedtime to optimize sleep hygiene as screen time in the evening is associated with shorter sleep duration among adolescents. Avoiding screen time in the later evening is associated with increased sleep duration and improved daytime vigilance. In addition, excessive social media use is associated with poor sleep quality.

SLEEP DISORDERS

Sleep disorders are a common complaint in pediatrics and can be categorized into organic disorders, parasomnias, behavioral and environmental causes, and circadian rhythm disorders (Table 15.1).

Epidemiology

Sleep disorders occur in up to 80% of children at some point during childhood. Children with comorbid medical conditions, particularly neurodevelopmental and psychiatric disorders, are at higher risk than other children. Behavioral sleep disorders are most prevalent from infancy through preschool age, though they can occur at any age. Overall, behavioral insomnias affect up to 30% of children, with bedtime resistance occurring in 10–15% of toddlers and difficulty falling and/or staying asleep in 20–30% of school-age children and 10% of adolescents. Parasomnias are also common in children, especially children with other sleep disorders that may increase arousal from sleep, such as obstructive sleep apnea (OSA) and restless legs syndrome (RLS). Sleepwalking affects about 15% of children, peaks between 8–12 years of age, has a familial association, and is more common in males. Confusional arousals and sleep terrors (or night terrors) have a prevalence of about 35% and occur most often in young children, usually resolving spontaneously by adolescence. Circadian rhythm disorders occur in up to 16% of adolescents. OSA is reported in up to 5% of children; risk factors include obesity, craniofacial abnormalities, hypotonia, trisomy 21, and second-hand smoke exposure (see Chapter 135). RLS occurs in about 2% of children and up to 4% of adolescents. Narcolepsy is rarely found in children.

TABLE 15.1 Sleep Disorders

	CAUSE	CLINICAL SYMPTOMS	DIAGNOSIS	TREATMENT	SPECIAL CONSIDERATIONS
ORGANIC					
OSA	Adenotonsillar hypertrophy Overweight/obesity Allergic rhinitis Craniofacial abnormalities Neuromuscular diseases	Frequent snoring, unusual sleep positions, enlarged tonsils and adenoids, gasps/snorts, mouth breathing, episodes of apnea, labored breathing, daytime sleepiness, attention and/or learning and/or behavioral problems	PSG	Adenotonsillectomy Weight loss Noninvasive positive pressure support (CPAP/BiPAP)	Detailed history is often needed to detect early symptoms of OSA
Illness	Any chronically irritating disorder (e.g., AOM, atopic dermatitis, URI, GERD, asthma) Triggers can be chronic or acute	Disrupted sleep, variant sleep patterns due to discomfort and pain	Hx and PE	Treat primary illness	Consider when an otherwise normal child presents with acute disruption in sleep Atypical sleep patterns may linger after resolution of instigating illness; behavioral interventions may be needed to restore to normal sleep patterns
Neurodevelopment and CNS disorders	Variable; may need to evaluate for seizures, OSA	Variable sleep disruptions	Hx and PE May need PSG, EEG, and imaging	Evaluate environment Sleep hygiene Depending on disorder, medications may be helpful	Consider use of sleep medicine or neurology specialist, especially when considering medication
Restless leg syndrome	Not fully defined but associated with genetics *(PTPRD, BTBD9, MEIS1)* and iron deficiency	Unpleasant sensation in legs, urge to move legs often starting in the evening or during the night, difficulty falling asleep, lack of focus/hyperactivity, fatigue during the day	Hx, family Hx, PSG, ferritin level	If ferritin is <50 mcg, treat with iron replacement and recheck in 3 mo No other standard medications for children Consider referral to sleep medicine	Diagnosis can be a challenge
PARASOMNIAS					
Sleepwalking, sleep terrors	Stage N3 (deep) sleep instability Genetic predisposition	Awakening 1–3 hr after falling asleep with characteristic behaviors	Hx	Reassurance Protective environment	—
Confusional arousals	Irregular sleep patterns (e.g., nightshift work); stress	Awakening in first 1/3 of night with confused thinking, slow speech	Hx, PSG	Sleep hygiene; treat other sleep disorders	—

(Continued)

TABLE 15.1 Sleep Disorders—cont'd

	CAUSE	CLINICAL SYMPTOMS	DIAGNOSIS	TREATMENT	SPECIAL CONSIDERATIONS
BEHAVIORAL AND ENVIRONMENTAL					
Insomnia of childhood (can have overlap of subtypes) Sleep-onset association subtype Limit setting subtype	10–30% prevalence Inability/unwillingness to fall asleep or return to sleep in absence of specific conditions such as parental rocking Parental anxiety, unwillingness/inability to enforce bedtime rules and limits such as allowing child to sleep in parents' room	Frequent or prolonged night awakenings requiring intervention Bedtime resistance/refusal Excessive expression of "needs" by child	Hx	Prevention and education Put child to bed drowsy but awake; allow to fall asleep independently Minimize nocturnal parental response Modify parental behavior to improve limit setting (provide rewards/positive reinforcement, appropriate consequences)	Careful attention to detailed history and recognition of familial and cultural expectations are needed to negotiate an optimal sleep management plan with caregivers Recognize there are cultural norms for family sleep behavior
Social disruptions	Family stressors	Night waking Refusal to sleep	Hx	Regularize routines Family counseling Family education regarding development and sleep needs of child	Respect family dynamics and refrain from blaming when providing guidance
Nighttime anxiety/fears	Anxiety, stress, traumatic events, disruption in social surrounding such as change in house, bed type, although no specific trigger may be identified	Bedtime resistance Crying, clinging, seeking parental reassurance	Hx	Reassurance of safety Teach coping skills Nightlights, security objects Avoiding "drama" during the night awakening Avoid denial of fears; rather acknowledge and equip child with coping skills	Pay attention to any changes in child's environment and recognize normal development fears
CIRCADIAN RHYTHM DISORDERS					
Irregular sleep-wake pattern	No defined sleep schedule	Variable waking and sleeping	Hx	Regularize schedule	
Delayed sleep phase disorder	A shift in sleep-wake schedule with resetting of circadian rhythm Prevalence is 7–16% in adolescents due to longer circadian rhythm combined with increased social activity (delayed sleep onset)	Not sleepy at bedtime Sleep onset at a consistently late time Morning/daytime sleepiness	Hx	Depends on the trigger that is causing the discrepancy Good sleep hygiene Avoid bright light before bedtime Remove light-emitting devices in bedroom Melatonin	Detailed history and family education are helpful for optimal treatment response Sleep diary is helpful

AOM, Acute otitis media; *BiPAP*, bilevel positive airway pressure; *CNS*, central nervous system; *CPAP*, continuous positive airway pressure; *EEG*, electroencephalography; *GERD*, gastroesophageal reflux disease; *Hx*, history; *OSA*, obstructive sleep apnea; *PE*, physical examination; *PSG*, polysomnography; *URI*, upper respiratory infection.

Clinical Manifestations and Evaluation

Sleep disorders manifest in a variety of ways and are often unrecognized. Some children present with daytime behavioral problems such as inattentiveness, hyperactivity, or irritability rather than overt sleepiness. Screening for sleep disorders is recommended as part of primary care health supervision visits. Clinicians should inquire about problems such as excessive daytime sleepiness, awakenings during the night, and presence of snoring or sleep-disordered breathing. The assessment of sleep complaints begins with a **history** of sleep habits, including typical bedtime, sleep onset and wake times, and schedule variation from day to day. A detailed description of the sleep environment can result in a dynamic understanding of the challenges to and resources for achieving normal sleep; such details include typical bedtime routine, type of bed, household members sharing the bed or room, ambient light, noise, and temperature. Dietary practices (timing of meals, caffeine intake) and household routines (parental work patterns, evening activities) may influence the timing and ease of sleep. A detailed history assessing for symptoms of OSA (snoring, gasping, open-mouth breathing, breathing pauses) should be obtained in all children who snore regularly. Complaints of unpleasant sensations in the legs or frequent urges to move the legs at night may suggest RLS. New-onset sleep disorders may be associated with a psychologic trauma. When the history does not initially reveal the cause of the sleep disorder, a sleep diary can be helpful, especially for adolescents, and should include bedtime routines, timing of food and caffeine intake, electronics use, light or noise in the room, and timing of sleep onset and waking.

A complete **physical examination** is important to evaluate for organic causes of sleep disturbance. A head, eyes, ears, nose, and throat (HEENT) exam may help identify findings consistent with OSA. A careful exam may reveal signs of acute or chronic disorders (such as otitis media or eczema) that cause pain or pruritus, which can disrupt sleep. A neurologic exam may reveal signs of central nervous system disorders.

Evaluation is generally not warranted for children with primary insomnia (difficulty initiating or maintaining sleep), uncomplicated parasomnias, behaviorally based sleep problems, or circadian rhythm disorders. A **polysomnogram**, consisting of an overnight observation and recording in a sleep laboratory, can detect OSA, excessive limb movements, seizure disorder, and other sleep disorders. Low ferritin levels (<50 mcg/L) have been associated with RLS, so obtaining a ferritin level is helpful in the diagnosis of RLS.

Differential Diagnosis

Behavioral insomnia of childhood is divided into two subtypes. *Sleep-onset association subtype* manifests as frequent or prolonged nighttime awakenings that occur in infants or young children. During periods of normal brief arousal with each sleep cycle, the child awakens under conditions different from those experienced as they fell asleep, and they are unable to return to sleep independently. *Limit-setting subtype* is most common in preschool-age and older children and is characterized by bedtime resistance or refusal that stems from a caregiver's unwillingness or inability to enforce bedtime rules and expectations. Nighttime fears are also common causes of bedtime refusal.

Parasomnias include *sleepwalking*, *sleep terrors*, and *confusional arousals*. These occur during NREM sleep and are more likely during the first third of the night. They are most common in preschool children and are likely to resolve with time and developmental maturation. Parasomnias are commonly caused by triggers such as sleep deprivation and fever. Sleepwalking is common and usually benign but is sometimes associated with agitation or dangerous behaviors. Sleep terrors consist of an abrupt awakening with a loud scream or agitation that is unresponsive to caregivers' attempts to console. Sleep terrors are differentiated from nightmares, which occur later in the night and result from arousal in REM or dreaming sleep. Children usually remember their nightmares but have no recollection of sleep terrors. Confusional arousals are similar to sleep terrors but tend to be less dramatic and last longer.

Circadian rhythm disorders are most common during adolescence but can occur at any age. They consist of an exaggerated delayed sleep phase, leading to difficulty arousing in the mornings and failure to meet sleep requirements. The resulting sleep deprivation can lead to problems with cognition and emotional regulation. Some adolescents attempt to recoup lost sleep on the weekends, which has not been found to be effective in preventing the long-term health consequences of sleep deprivation.

Primary organic sleep disorders include OSA and RLS. OSA in childhood is commonly caused by tonsillar or adenoidal hypertrophy. OSA is associated with poor growth in toddlers and can result in neurocognitive, developmental, and behavioral problems in older children. These sequelae can be mitigated by adenotonsillectomy. Primary sleep disorders must be differentiated from sleep disorders associated with psychiatric disorders, including anxiety, depression, psychosis, autism spectrum disorder (ASD), attention-deficit/hyperactivity disorder (ADHD), post-traumatic stress disorder, and substance use. The clinician should also consider medication side effects and other medical problems such as sleep-related epilepsy, neurologic and developmental disorders, and other illnesses that disrupt sleep (such as painful or pruritic conditions) as causes of sleep disorders.

Complications

The most common sequela of suboptimal sleep is daytime sleepiness. Other sequelae include irritability, behavioral problems, learning difficulties, and motor vehicle crashes in adolescents. Clear links between sleep-disordered breathing and academic performance in the school-age child have been firmly established. Children may present with concerns for behavior or emotional lability, which after a careful history is found to be associated with insufficient quantity or quality of sleep.

Prevention and Treatment

Establishing a baseline of healthy sleep habits is essential to both prevention and treatment of sleep disorders at all ages. Recommendations include a consistent and appropriate bedtime and bedtime routine, as well as close attention to sleep hygiene (Table 15.2). A bedtime routine should last no more than 30 minutes and consist of three or four soothing activities that help calm the child and signal that it is time for sleep;

TABLE 15.2 Prevention of Pediatric Behavioral Sleep Disorders

Consistent and appropriate bedtime and wake-up time
Consistent bedtime routine (~30 min) to cue sleep
Consistent ambient noise, light, temperature in bedroom
Adequate food, hydration, socialization, and physical activity during the day
No electronics (television, phones, videogames) or light emission products (e.g., chargers) in bedroom
Avoidance of naps (unless developmentally appropriate)
Caffeine avoidance
Child feels safe and protected
Child allowed to develop self-soothing strategies
Parents are comfortable setting limits/boundaries

activities may include bathing, brushing teeth, reading a story, or singing a song. In older children for whom safe sleep does not require an empty bed, a transitional object such as a blanket or stuffed animal can be used to promote positive sleep associations and encourage self-soothing behaviors. Older children and adolescents also benefit from a consistent prebedtime routine, including use of relaxation techniques. The bedtime should be set early enough to allow for sufficient nighttime sleep, and both bedtime and morning wake time should be consistent, including on weekends. Televisions and other electronic devices should be removed from the bedroom as they lead to delayed sleep onset and maladaptive sleep associations. Children should also restrict the use of the bed to sleeping (not studying, using electronics, etc.), to associate the bed with sleep.

Sleep-onset association disorder in infancy usually can be prevented by parental understanding of infant sleep physiology, developmentally appropriate expectations, and planning the infant sleep environment to coincide with family needs. It is important to recognize and respect cultural and other familial contexts when providing guidance. There is varying guidance regarding "sleep training" itself. Overall, it is recommended that starting around 6 months of age, after feeding, diapering, and comforting measures, infants be put in bed drowsy, but still awake. Some toleration of infant crying is required for the infant to achieve self-regulation of sleep. A safe sleep environment is essential. It is important for parents to understand that it is normal for their infant to wake frequently for the first 6 weeks before settling into a routine of waking every 3–4 hours for feeding. Infants usually do not sleep through the night before 6 months of age, and some do not sleep through the night before 12–18 months of age. Despite *co-sleeping* (infant sleeping with a caregiver) being common and desired by many families for the purposes of convenience and closeness, it is contraindicated due to the increased risk of unexpected death from sudden infant death syndrome or accidental suffocation.

In addition to meticulous attention to sleep hygiene and bedtime practices, **behavioral interventions** comprise the mainstay of treatment for behavioral sleep disorders and circadian rhythm disorders. *Systematic ignoring* consists of not responding to a child's demands for parental attention at bedtime and consists of either *unmodified extinction* ("cry it out"), which involves putting the child to bed and then ignoring the child's demands until the next morning, or *graduated extinction*, which involves waiting successively longer periods of time before briefly checking on the child. Both methods, when consistently applied, are effective in decreasing bedtime resistance and enabling young children to fall asleep independently. *Strategic napping* involves planning the timing and duration of naps to not interfere with bedtime because too much sleep during the day or napping too late in the day can make falling asleep at bedtime difficult. *Positive reinforcement* strategies such as sticker charts can also be used in preschool-age and older children. Rewards should be given for meeting a bedtime goal (such as staying in bed) and should be provided first thing in the morning to increase effectiveness and better link the reward with the positive behavior. Children with nighttime fears may benefit from behavioral therapy aimed at reinforcing feelings of safety. *Bedtime fading* involves gradual resetting of the biologic clock and can assist with circadian rhythm disorders. Bedtime fading involves allowing children or adolescents to go to bed at the time they naturally feel tired and then gradually advancing the bedtime forward over the course of several weeks.

Infrequent or nonintrusive parasomnias do not need treatment beyond education, reassurance, and ensuring a safe environment. Sleep terrors are best managed by minimal intervention as conversation with the child is impossible during the episode, and attempts at calming are unlikely to be successful. Anticipatory brief awakening of the child shortly before the typical occurrence of a parasomnia may be effective in aborting the event. Children with frequent or prolonged parasomnias may need a sleep study to evaluate for possible coexisting sleep disorders or nocturnal seizures. Medications that suppress slow-wave sleep may be indicated in severe cases.

Rarely, children with insomnia are treated **pharmacologically**. There are no U.S. Food and Drug Administration–approved medications for treating insomnia in children, and clinical evidence is lacking for most medications with off-label use. *Melatonin* has soporific properties useful in treating delayed sleep phase syndrome and has been found to be effective in both children with normal development and those with developmental delays, as well as in children with ADHD and ASD. Melatonin should only be used after a full evaluation and with close medical surveillance. Optimal dosing is challenging, particularly because melatonin is not a regulated substance and can vary by manufacturer. Nonprescription *antihistamines* such as diphenhydramine may be used in children with atopic disease and can also be useful for their sedative properties in short-term situations such as illness or travel. They can lead to tolerance and should not be used chronically. Other medications such as clonidine have been used in some situations, but generally should only be used in consultation with a sleep specialist.

PEARLS FOR PRACTITIONERS

See Behavioral Disorders: Pearls for Practitioners at the end of this section.

REVIEW QUESTIONS

Available online.

Suggested Readings

Alonzo R, Hussain J, Stranges S, Anderson KK. Interplay between social media use, sleep quality, and mental health in youth: a systematic review. *Sleep Med Rev*. 2021;56:101414.

Barbaresi WJ, Campbell L, Diekroger EA, et al. Society for Developmental and Behavioral Pediatrics Clinical Practice Guideline for the Assessment and Treatment of Children and Adolescents with Complex Attentio-Deficit/Hyperactivity Disorder. *J Dev Behav Pediatr*. 2020;41 Suppl 2S:S35–S57.

Biagioli E, Tarasco V, Lingua C, et al. Pain-relieving agents for infantile colic. *Cochrane Database Syst Rev*. 2016;9:CD009999.

Brazzelli M, Griffiths PV, Cody JD, et al. Behavioural and cognitive interventions with or without other treatments for the management of faecal incontinence in children. *Cochrane Database Syst Rev*. 2011;12:CD002240.

Bruno A, Celebre L, Torre G, et al. Focus on disruptive mood dysregulation disorder: a review of the literature. *Psychiatry Res*. 2019;279:323–330.

Caldwell PHY, Nankivell G, Sureshkumar P. Simple behavioural interventions for nocturnal enuresis in children. *Cochrane Database Syst Rev*. 2013;7:CD003637.

Elder JS. Enuresis and voiding dysfunction. In: Kliegman RM, Geme J St, eds. *Nelson Textbook of Pediatrics*. Philadelphia: Elsevier; 2020:2816–2820.
Centers for Disease Control and Prevention. *Data and statistics on ADHD*. Centers for Disease Control and Prevention; 2024. https://www.cdc.gov/adhd/data/index.html.
Honaker SM, Meltzer LJ. Sleep in pediatric primary care: a review of the literature. *Sleep Med Rev*. 2016;25:31–39.
Leung AKC, Leung AAM, Wong AHC, et al. Breath-holding spells in pediatrics: a narrative review of the current evidence. *Curr Pediatr Rev*. 2019;15(1):22–29.
Mai T, Fatheree NY, Gleason W, et al. Infantile colic: new insights into an old problem. *Gastroenterol Clin North Am*. 2018;47(4):829–844.
Maqbool A, Liacouras CA. Major symptoms and signs of digestive tract disorders. In: Kliegman RM, Geme J St, eds. *Nelson Textbook of Pediatrics*. Philadelphia: Elsevier; 2020:1902–1911.
Maski K, Owens J. Insomnia, parasomnias and narcolepsy in children; clinical features, diagnosis and management. *Lancet Neurol*. 2016;15:1170–1181.
Paruthi S, Brooks LJ, D'Ambrosio C, et al. Recommended amount of sleep for pediatric populations: a consensus statement of the American Academy of Sleep Medicine. *J Clin Sleep Med*. 2016;12:785–786.
Wolke D, Bilgin A, Samara M. Systematic review and meta-analysis: fussing and crying durations and prevalence of colic in infants. *J Pediatr*. 2017;185:55–61.e4.
Wolraich ML, Hagan JF, Allan C, et al. Clinical practice guideline for the diagnosis, evaluation, and treatment of attention-deficit/hyperactivity disorder in children and adolescents. *Pediatrics*. 2019;144:e20192528.
Zeevenhooven J, Browne PD, L'Hoir MP, et al. Infant colic: mechanisms and management. *Nat Rev Gastroenterol Hepatol*. 2018;15(8):479–496.

PEARLS FOR PRACTITIONERS

CHAPTER 11

Crying and Colic

- Infantile colic is defined as episodes of extreme crying or fussiness in an otherwise healthy infant.
- Infantile colic has been associated with abusive head trauma, postpartum depression, caregiver guilt, and multiple physician visits.
- Infantile colic is a diagnosis of exclusion; it is important to fully evaluate for other conditions.
- Management of colic includes caregiver education regarding its natural and self-limited course, advocacy of caregiver coping mechanisms, and safe maneuvers to soothe baby.
- Symptoms of colic can overlap with the symptoms of gastroesophageal reflux disease and milk protein intolerance.
- Complementary alternative medicine, including herbal therapies, neonatal chiropractor care, and medications, has not been shown to be effective and safe.

CHAPTER 12

Temper Tantrums

- Temper tantrums are part of normal human development during early childhood and are characterized by episodes of extreme frustration and anger, manifesting as a wide range of behaviors that appear disproportionate to the situation.
- Evaluation of tantrums should include a thorough history and physical examination to evaluate for other etiologies and underlying conditions.
- Abnormal tantrums, particularly those that are destructive or injurious, may be indicative of a more serious underlying condition and warrant referral for further work-up.
- Anticipatory guidance for parents should include tips for acute management of temper tantrums, including staying calm, using distraction, cool-down techniques, not giving into the child's demands, and decreasing caregiver's attention to inappropriate behavior.
- Anticipatory guidance should include strategies to mitigate future tantrums such as recognizing triggers, setting and consistently enforcing clear limits, providing routine and structure, teaching communication skills, offering choices, role-modeling, and using positive reinforcement.

CHAPTER 13

Attention-Deficit/Hyperactivity Disorder

- Attention-deficit/hyperactivity disorder (ADHD) is the most prevalent neurobehavioral disorder in children.
- The use of valid screening tools from at least two domains that reflect a child's daily life is needed to establish a diagnosis of ADHD.
- Coexisting conditions (i.e., learning disorders, anxiety, depression, oppositional behaviors, conduct disturbance) must be considered in the initial evaluation as well as the longitudinal management of ADHD.
- Males often present with hyperactivity. Females more often present with inattentive symptoms and are more likely to be underdiagnosed or to receive later diagnoses.
- Treatment for ADHD is outcome-based and should address functional disability. Management plans should include the child, parents, other relevant caregivers, and school personnel.
- Medication-based treatments are effective in combination with developmental psychosocial interventions, especially for the older child and adolescent.

- Behavior management alone, outside of the preschool group, is not as effective as behavior management with medication in reducing core symptoms.
- Stimulant medications are the first-line treatment of ADHD; ongoing close monitoring for medication side effects is needed.

CHAPTER 14

Control of Elimination

- Prerequisites for achieving elimination in the toilet include the child's ability to recognize the urge for urination and defecation, to get to the toilet, to understand the sequence of tasks required, and to take pride in achievement.
- Daytime dryness usually precedes nighttime dryness by at least several months, and often several years.
- Enuresis is classified as non-monosymptomatic (associated with daytime wetting or other urinary tract abnormalities) or monosymptomatic (intermittent nocturnal incontinence), which is further classified as either primary (having never achieved nighttime dryness) or secondary (nocturnal incontinence after having achieved dryness).
- Primary monosymptomatic nocturnal enuresis has a prevalence of 15% at 5 years of age, 5% at 10 years of age, and 1% at 15 years of age.
- A complete history and physical exam are necessary to evaluate for underlying causes of enuresis, and non-monosymptomatic enuresis warrants referral for further evaluation.
- Treatment options for primary enuresis are enuresis alarm conditioning therapy and desmopressin pharmacotherapy.
- Encopresis is the regular, voluntary, or involuntary passage of feces into a place other than the toilet after 4 years of age.
- Encopresis without constipation is uncommon.
- Approximately 95% of children referred to a subspecialist for encopresis have no other underlying pathologic condition.
- Treatment of constipation and encopresis involves a combination of behavioral training and the use of stool softener therapy.

CHAPTER 15

Normal Sleep and Pediatric Sleep Disorders

- Sleep architecture, timing, and duration change from fetal life through infancy and childhood; changes parallel physical maturation and development.
- Establishing a baseline of healthy sleep habits is essential to both prevention and treatment of sleep disorders at all ages.
- Sleep disorders include organic disorders (OSA, RLS), parasomnias (sleepwalking, night terrors), behavioral and environmental causes, and circadian rhythm disorders.
- Evaluation should include a careful history, including a sleep diary, as well as a complete physical examination to evaluate for underlying causes of sleep disorders.
- Adolescents develop a physiologically based shift toward later sleep-onset and wake times relative to those in middle childhood. Insufficient sleep in adolescents is very common and has been associated with negative effects on cognitive function, moods, and motivation.

SECTION 4

PSYCHIATRIC DISORDERS

Gray M. Buchanan

CHAPTER 16

Somatic Symptom and Related Disorders

Somatic symptom and related disorders (SSRDs) are a distinct category in the *Diagnostic and Statistical Manual of Mental Disorders, Fifth Edition Text Revision* (DSM-5-TR). Although prior DSM criteria emphasized medically unexplained symptoms, the DSM-5-TR allows for both unexplained symptoms and symptoms that may accompany diagnosed medical disorders. Disorders in the SSRD group include **somatic symptom disorder**, **functional neurological symptom disorder**, **illness anxiety disorder**, **factitious disorder**, and **psychologic factors affecting other medical conditions**. All SSRDs share a common feature: somatic symptoms and/or illness anxiety associated with significant distress and impairment. Adolescent females tend to report nearly twice as many somatic symptoms compared to adolescent males; prior to puberty the ratio is equal. Children with SSRDs are more likely to have difficulty expressing emotional distress, come from families with a history of marital conflict, have experienced adverse childhood experiences (ACEs), or have a family member with a history of physical illness. Explainable medical conditions and an SSRD can coexist in up to 50% of patients and present difficult diagnostic dilemmas. The most common systemic medical disorders presenting with unexplained physical symptoms include myalgic encephalomyelitis/chronic fatigue syndrome (ME/CFS), multiple sclerosis, myasthenia gravis, systemic lupus erythematous, chronic systemic infections, vocal cord dysfunction, periodic paralysis, acute intermittent porphyria, fibromyalgia, irritable bowel syndrome, polymyositis, and other myopathies. Depression, anxiety, and panic attacks are common co-morbidities and frequently precede the somatic symptoms.

Somatic symptom disorder (SSD) involves one or more somatic symptoms that are distressing or result in significant disruption in daily life. The criteria used to diagnose SSD are listed in Table 16.1. Most individuals previously diagnosed with *somatization disorder* or *hypochondriasis* meet the criteria for SSD. Key symptoms of the disorder often involve excessive thoughts, feelings, or behaviors regarding the somatic complaint (e.g., excessive fatigue or pain). Prevalence estimates for SSD in children are highly variable; between 5 and 7% of adults may be identified with SSD, with a greater proportion being female.

Functional neurological symptom disorder (FNSD), previously *conversion disorder*, involves symptoms affecting voluntary motor or sensory function and is suggestive of a neurologic illness in the absence of a disease process (Table 16.2). A physical condition and a FNSD (e.g., epileptic and nonepileptic seizures) may coexist in the same patient. There are multiple subtypes of FNSD based on the symptoms present, including difficulties with primarily motor, sensory, neurologic, or mixed symptoms. Frequently a significant stressor (acute or chronic) and/or a trauma may precede the presentation of symptoms. Adjustment difficulties, recent stress, unresolved grief reactions, and family psychopathology commonly co-occur with FNSD. Presenting symptoms may follow the psychologic stressor by hours to weeks and often cause more distress for others than for the patient. This seeming absence of concern regarding potentially serious symptoms is referred to as *la belle indifference*. Symptoms are often self-limited but may be associated with chronic sequelae, such as contractures or iatrogenic injury.

Illness anxiety disorder (Table 16.3) involves patients who have a preoccupation with having or acquiring a serious

TABLE 16.1 Criteria for Diagnosis of Somatic Symptom Disorder

A. One or more somatic symptoms that are distressing or result in significant disruption of daily life.
B. Excessive thoughts, feelings, or behaviors related to the somatic symptoms or associated health concerns as manifested by at least one of the following:
   1. Disproportionate and persistent thoughts about the seriousness of one's symptoms
   2. Persistently high level of anxiety about health or symptoms
   3. Excessive time and energy devoted to these symptoms or health concerns
C. Although any one somatic symptom may not be continuously present, the state of being symptomatic is persistent (typically more than 6 months).

Specify if:
With predominant pain (previously pain disorder): This specifier is for individuals whose somatic symptoms predominantly involve pain.
Specify if:
Persistent: A persistent course is characterized by severe symptoms, marked impairment, and long duration (more than 6 months).
Specify current severity:
Mild: Only one of the symptoms specified in Criterion B is fulfilled.
Moderate: Two or more of the symptoms specified in Criterion B are fulfilled.
Severe: Two or more of the symptoms specified in Criterion B are fulfilled, plus there are multiple somatic complaints (or one very severe somatic symptom).

Reprinted with permission from the Diagnostic and Statistical Manual of Mental Disorders, Fifth Edition, Text Revision (Copyright © 2022). American Psychiatric Association. All Rights Reserved.

TABLE 16.2 Criteria for Diagnosis of Functional Neurological Symptom Disorder (Conversion Disorder)

A. One or more symptoms of altered voluntary motor or sensory function
B. Clinical findings provide evidence of incompatibility between the symptom and recognized neurologic or medical conditions.
C. The symptom or deficit is not better explained by another medical or mental disorder.
D. The symptom or deficit causes clinically significant distress or impairment in social, occupational, or other important areas of functioning or warrants medical evaluation.

Specify symptom type: **weakness or paralysis, abnormal movements** (tremor, dystonia, myoclonus, gait disorder), **swallowing symptoms, speech symptom** (dysphonia, slurred speech), **attacks or seizures, anesthesia or sensory loss, special sensory symptom** (visual, olfactory, or hearing disturbance), or **mixed symptoms**

Specify if:
Acute episode: Symptoms present for less than 6 months
Persistent: Symptoms occurring for 6 months or more

Specify if:
With psychological stressor *(specify stressor)*
Without psychological stressor

Reprinted with permission from the Diagnostic and Statistical Manual of Mental Disorders, Fifth Edition, Text Revision (Copyright © 2022). American Psychiatric Association. *All Rights Reserved.*

TABLE 16.3 Criteria for Diagnosis of Illness Anxiety Disorder

A. Preoccupation with having or acquiring a serious illness.
B. Somatic symptoms are not present or, if present, are only mild in intensity. If another medical condition is present or there is a high risk for developing a medical condition (e.g., strong family history is present), the preoccupation is clearly excessive or disproportionate.
C. There is a high level of anxiety about health, and the individual is easily alarmed about personal health status.
D. The individual performs excessive health-related behaviors (e.g., repeatedly checks body for signs of illness) or exhibits maladaptive avoidance (e.g., avoids doctor appointments and hospitals).
E. Illness preoccupation has been present for at least 6 months, but the specific illness that is feared may change over that period of time.
F. The illness-related preoccupation is not better explained by another mental disorder, such as somatic symptom disorder, panic disorder, generalized anxiety disorder, body dysmorphic disorder, obsessive-compulsive disorder, or delusional disorder, somatic type.

Specify whether:
Care-seeking type: Medical care, including physician visits or undergoing tests and procedures, is frequently used.
Care-avoidant type: Medical care is rarely used.

Reprinted with permission from the Diagnostic and Statistical Manual of Mental Disorders, Fifth Edition, Text Revision (Copyright © 2022). American Psychiatric Association. *All Rights Reserved.*

illness. Increased utilization of medical resources is common. Somatic symptoms are not present, and there is a high level of anxiety about health status. Patients commonly seek reassurance from family, friends, and medical staff regarding their health; however, they seldom respond to reassurance regarding their health. Additionally, they are often significantly alarmed by illnesses in others. Approximately 25% of individuals previously diagnosed with *hypochondriasis* meet criteria for this disorder and can be distinguished from those with SSD by their high anxiety and absence of somatic symptoms. Prevalence estimates in children are unknown. There appear to be similar prevalence rates in males and females; the condition appears to worsen in adolescence.

Psychological factors affecting other medical conditions are marked by psychologic or behavioral factors that adversely impact a medical condition by increasing the risk for suffering, death, or disability (Table 16.4). The factors interfere with the treatment of a medical condition (e.g., anxiety exacerbating asthma, poor medication adherence). This diagnosis is more common in young children and may require corroborative history from parents and the child's school. Prevalence of this condition is unclear due to its wide breadth; data suggest that this disorder is more prevalent than SSDs.

Factitious disorder is a condition in which physical or psychologic symptoms are produced intentionally and often with the intent to assume a sick role (Table 16.5). This diagnosis is made via direct observation and by eliminating other possible causes. The falsification of physical and psychologic symptoms may also present as imposing illness or injury on another person (i.e., **factitious disorder imposed on another [FDIA**]; formerly *Munchausen by proxy*). FDIA most commonly occurs following hospitalization of the child or another family member. Many families with FDIA demonstrate improvement when confronted with their behavior or acknowledge the factitious nature of their symptoms. *Approximate answers* (e.g., the patient provides 16 as the answer for 20 – 3) reported during a mental status examination are commonly found in factitious disorders. The prevalence of factitious disorder in children is unknown. Approximately 1% of

TABLE 16.4 Criteria for Diagnosis of Psychological Factors Affecting Other Medical Conditions

A. A medical symptom or condition (other than a mental disorder) is present.
B. Psychologic or behavioral factors adversely affect the medical condition in one of the following ways:
   1. The factors have influenced the course of the medical condition as shown by a close temporal association between the psychological factors and the development or exacerbation of, or delayed recovery from, the medical condition.
   2. The factors interfere with the treatment of the medical condition (e.g., poor adherence).
   3. The factors constitute additional well-established health risks for the individual.
   4. The factors influence the underlying pathophysiology, precipitating or exacerbating symptoms, or necessitating medical attention.
C. The psychological and behavioral factors in Criterion B are not better explained by another mental disorder (e.g., panic disorder, major depressive disorder, post-traumatic stress disorder).

Specify current severity:
Mild: Increases medical risk (e.g., inconsistent adherence with antihypertension treatment)
Moderate: Aggravates underlying medical condition (e.g., anxiety aggravating asthma)
Severe: Results in medical hospitalization or emergency room visit
Extreme: Results in severe, life-threatening risk (e.g., ignoring heart attack symptoms)

Reprinted with permission from the Diagnostic and Statistical Manual of Mental Disorders, Fifth Edition, Text Revision (Copyright © 2022). American Psychiatric Association. *All Rights Reserved.*

TABLE 16.5 Criteria for Diagnosis of Factitious Disorder

FACTITIOUS DISORDER IMPOSED ON SELF
A. Falsification of physical or psychological signs or symptoms, or induction of injury or disease, associated with identified deception. B. The individual presents self to others as ill, impaired, or injured. C. The deceptive behavior is evident even in the absence of obvious external rewards. D. The behavior is not better explained by another mental disorder, such as delusional disorder or another psychotic disorder. *Specify:* **Single episode** or **recurrent episodes** (two or more events of falsification of illness and/or induction of injury)
FACTITIOUS DISORDER IMPOSED ON ANOTHER (PREVIOUSLY FACTITIOUS DISORDER BY PROXY)
A. Falsification of physical or psychological signs or symptoms, or induction of injury or disease, in another, associated with identified deception. B. The individual presents another individual (victim) to others as ill, impaired, or injured. C. The deceptive behavior is evident even in the absence of obvious external rewards. D. The behavior is not better explained by another mental disorder, such as delusional disorder or another psychotic disorder. **Note:** The perpetrator, not the victim, receives this diagnosis. *Specify:* **Single episode** or **recurrent episodes** (two or more events of falsification of illness and/or induction of injury)

Reprinted with permission from the Diagnostic and Statistical Manual of Mental Disorders, Fifth Edition, Text Revision (Copyright © 2022). American Psychiatric Association. All Rights Reserved.

individuals in hospital settings present with such a condition. FDIA is considered a type of **child abuse** and most commonly occurs in neonates and preschool age children.

Evaluation for SSRDs includes the adapted caregiver version of the Patient Health Questionnaire–15 (PHQ-15). Additionally, by also administering the Somatic Symptom Scale–8 (SSS-8), derived from the PHQ-15, and the Somatic Symptom Disorder–B Criteria Scale, the clinician is best able to identify individuals at risk for SSRDs. The Children's Somatic Symptoms Inventory (CSSI) is also available as a self-report measure of somatic distress for children ages 8–17 years.

Treatment for SSRDs should employ an integrated medical and psychiatric approach. The goals are to identify concurrent psychiatric disorders, evaluate for concurrent physical disorders, improve overall functioning, and minimize unnecessary invasive tests and doctor shopping. Treatment is most successful when mental health consultation is presented as part of a comprehensive plan, thereby minimizing stigma and distrust.

Antidepressant medications may be of benefit in the treatment of some conditions such as unexplained headaches, fibromyalgia, body dysmorphic disorder, pain disorder, irritable bowel syndrome, and functional gastrointestinal disorders. Tricyclic antidepressants (e.g., clomipramine) should be avoided in youth with functional abdominal pain (FAP), because it has little proven efficacy in either pain management or mood disorders and is dangerous in overdose. In ME/CFS with co-morbid depression and anxiety, a more activating antidepressant, such as bupropion, may be useful. Stimulants may also be helpful in ME/CFS if concentration concerns are present.

Cognitive-behavioral therapies, which reward health-promoting behaviors and discourage disability and illness behaviors, help in the treatment of recurrent pain, ME/CFS, fibromyalgia, and FAP. Additionally, self-management strategies such as self-monitoring, relaxation, hypnosis, and biofeedback help provide some symptomatic relief and encourage more active coping strategies. Family therapy and family-based interventions may also be useful. School attendance and performance should be emphasized as important indicators of appropriate functioning, and home schooling should be avoided. When addressing pain symptoms (e.g., headaches, abdominal pain), parents should limit attention/reinforcement for pain behavior, strongly encourage normal routines/appropriate schedules (e.g., going to school), help the child identify stress at home and school, provide attention and special activities on days when the child does not have symptoms, and limit rewarding activities and interactions on sick days. Education should be provided for parents and personnel working with the child to limit discussions about excessive discomfort or illness. Mindfulness techniques and relaxation training may also be taught to caregivers and the child to improve control of their physiologic and cognitive responses to discomfort.

Malingering is considered a V code in the DSM-5-TR and involves the purposeful falsification or exaggeration of physical and/or psychologic symptoms for external gain (e.g., money, avoidance of school, work). The key feature of malingering is the seeking of an external reward. Symptoms may not lessen when the reward is attained. Unless the patient is directly observed or confesses to such falsification, malingering is difficult to prove.

PEARLS FOR PRACTITIONERS

See Psychiatric Disorders: Pearls for Practitioners at the end of this section.

REVIEW QUESTIONS

Available online.

CHAPTER 17

Anxiety and Phobias

Anxiety disorders are characterized by uneasiness, excessive rumination, and apprehension about the future. The conditions are often chronic, recurring, and vary in intensity over time. They affect 5–10% of children and adolescents (Table 17.1) and have a lifetime prevalence of approximately 30%. Some conditions (i.e., *obsessive-compulsive disorder [OCD]* and *post-traumatic stress disorder [PTSD]*) are not included in the section on anxiety in the current version of the DSM; these disorders continue to share a close relationship with anxiety disorders.

Panic disorder is the presence of recurrent, unexpected panic attacks. A **panic attack** is a sudden unexpected onset of intense fear associated with a feeling of impending doom in the absence of real danger and may occur in the context of any anxiety disorder. The individual must experience four or

TABLE 17.1 Common Anxiety Disorders: Characteristics

FEATURE	PANIC DISORDER	GENERALIZED ANXIETY DISORDER	SEPARATION ANXIETY DISORDER	SPECIFIC PHOBIA
Epidemiology	Prevalence is 2–3%. Eight times more common and of early onset in family members of affected individuals than in the general population.	Prevalence is 1–3%. Sex ratio equal before puberty but higher in females following puberty. One third of the risk of experiencing GAD is genetic.	Prevalence is 3–7% of children and adolescents. The sex ratio is almost equal. Heritability of SAD is greater for females than for males.	Prevalence is 5% in children and approximately 16% in adolescence. Sex ratio is 2:1 females:males. Increased risk of specific phobias in first-degree relatives of patients with specific phobias.
Onset	Average age at onset is 20–24 years; <0.4% onset before 14 years of age.	Average age at onset is 35 years (later than that of other anxiety disorders).	Average age at onset is 7 years.	Varies
Differential diagnosis	Anxiety disorder due to a general medical condition, substance-related anxiety disorder due to caffeine or other stimulants.	Other anxiety disorders; OCD, PTSD, and depressive, bipolar, and psychotic disorders; substance-related (caffeine and sedative-hypnotic withdrawal).	Other anxiety disorders and conduct, impulse control, and disruptive behavior disorders.	Agoraphobia, panic disorder, OCD, and PTSD.
Co-morbidities	Separation anxiety disorder (common), agoraphobia, substance use disorder, major depression, OCD, and other anxiety disorders. Patients with asthma have a high incidence of panic attacks.	Unipolar depression and other anxiety disorders.	GAD and specific phobia.	Depression and other anxiety disorders.
Prognosis	Frequently chronic with a relative high rate of suicide attempts and completions.	One study showed that 65% of children cease to have the diagnosis in 2 years. GAD is the most frequent anxiety disorder diagnosed in suicides.	Variable; may have periods of exacerbation and remission. Most children with SAD are not diagnosed with significant anxiety disorders as adults.	Social phobia in childhood may be a risk factor for alcohol abuse in adolescence.

GAD, Generalized anxiety disorder; *OCD*, obsessive-compulsive disorder; *PTSD*, post-traumatic stress disorder; *SAD*, separation anxiety disorder.

more symptoms (e.g., sweating, palpitations, feeling of choking, chest pain, trembling/shaking, chills, paresthesias, fear of dying, fear of losing control, derealization, dizziness, nausea, or shortness of breath) during the attack. At least 1 month of persistent worrying about having another panic attack and/or a significant behavioral change following an attack (e.g., attempting to avoid another attack, avoidance of triggers such as exercise) is required to make the diagnosis.

Panic disorder often begins in adolescence or early adulthood. Symptom severity varies greatly. In children, the most common symptoms include shortness of breath, palpitations, chest pain, a choking sensation, and a fear of losing control. Symptoms may be brief or may last for longer periods of time; usually, they last less than 15 minutes. Patients may believe that they are experiencing an acute medical condition (e.g., a heart attack). Adolescents with panic disorder tend to have higher rates of cardiovascular, respiratory, gastrointestinal, and other medical symptoms than adults.

Generalized anxiety disorder (GAD) is characterized by six or more months of persistent, excessive worry and anxiety about a variety of situations or activities. The worries should be multiple, not paroxysmal, not focused on a single theme, and should cause significant impairment. The anxiety must be accompanied by at least one of the following symptoms: restlessness, fatigue, concentration difficulties, irritability, muscle tension, or sleep disturbance. Physiologic signs of anxiety are often present, including shakiness, trembling, and myalgias. Gastrointestinal symptoms (nausea, vomiting, diarrhea) and autonomic symptoms (tachycardia, shortness of breath) are also common. In children and adolescents, symptoms of autonomic arousal are less prominent. Children commonly present as perfectionistic, report symptoms related to school performance or sports, and exhibit concerns about punctuality. Children with GAD are often exceedingly self-conscious, have low self-esteem, and have more sleep disturbance than patients with other anxiety disorders. Care must be taken to elicit internalizing symptoms of negative cognitions about the self (hopelessness, helplessness, worthlessness, suicidal ideation) as well as those concerning relationships (embarrassment, self-consciousness). Inquiry about appetite, weight, energy, and interests should also be performed to eliminate a mood disorder. GAD is more predominant in males prior to puberty, but by adolescence, females outnumber males. The median age of onset for children is 11 years.

Factors such as the presence of stressors, elevated noradrenergic system activity, and low serotonin system activity are believed to influence the development of GAD.

Unspecified anxiety disorder is a common condition in clinical practice. This diagnosis is used when there is impairing anxiety or phobic symptoms that do not meet full criteria for another anxiety disorder.

Separation anxiety disorder (SAD) is marked by excessive distress or concern when separating from a major attachment figure (Table 17.2). Children and adolescents often express vague somatic symptoms (e.g., headaches, abdominal pain, fatigue) to avoid going to school or leaving their home. Children may present with a valid or an irrational concern about a parent or have had an unpleasant experience in school, and the prospect of returning to school provokes extreme anxiety and escalating symptoms. Children may refuse to go to school or leave their home. Children with SAD may seek frequent attention and often struggle with separation at bedtime. SAD is a significant risk factor for developing problems in adulthood, such as panic disorder, agoraphobia, and depression. SAD is highly heritable, with community samples estimating genetic rates as high as 73%. The average age of onset in children is 6 years, and if untreated many children continue to present with this and/or other anxiety disorder. SAD may also present in adulthood, with an adult lifetime prevalence rate of 6.6%.

Social anxiety disorder is a common type of anxiety characterized by a marked and persistent fear of social or performance situations in which one may offend others and/or embarrassment might occur (Table 17.3). There is a 7% prevalence of the disorder; it is more common in females. In children, this apprehension must be present with peers and not just in the presence of adults. Most individuals with this disorder are identified prior to 15 years of age. Children appear to have a lower rate of negative cognitions (e.g., embarrassment, overconcern, self-consciousness) than adults. Left untreated or poorly treated, social anxiety disorder can become immobilizing and result in significant functional impairments.

Selective mutism is present in approximately 1% of children who consistently fail to speak in one or more social settings despite adequate receptive and expressive language skills. Symptoms are present for at least 1 month and interfere with educational or occupational achievement or social communication. Children with selective mutism will often speak at home in the presence of first-degree relatives but may refuse to speak to extended family or others in their environment. Between 25 and 50% of children with selective mutism exhibit

TABLE 17.2 Criteria for Diagnosis of Separation Anxiety Disorder

A. Developmentally inappropriate and excessive fear or anxiety concerning separation from those to whom the individual is attached, as evidenced by at least three of the following:
1. Recurrent, excessive distress when anticipating or experiencing separation from home or from major attachment figures
2. Persistent and excessive worry about losing major attachment figures or about possible harm to them, such as illness, injury, disasters, or death
3. Persistent and excessive worry about experiencing an untoward event (e.g., getting lost, being kidnapped, having an accident, becoming ill) that causes separation from a major attachment figure
4. Persistent reluctance or refusal to go out, away from home, to school, to work, or elsewhere because of fear of separation
5. Persistent and excessive fear of or reluctance about being alone or without major attachment figures at home or in other settings
6. Persistent reluctance or refusal to sleep away from home or to go to sleep without being near a major attachment figure
7. Repeated nightmares involving the theme of separation
8. Repeated complaints of physical symptoms (e.g., headaches, stomachaches, nausea, vomiting) when separation from major attachment figures occurs or is anticipated

B. The fear, anxiety, or avoidance is persistent, lasting at least 4 weeks in children and adolescents and typically 6 months or more in adults.

C. The disturbance causes clinically significant distress or impairment in social, academic, occupational, or other important areas of functioning.

D. The disturbance is not better explained by another mental disorder, such as refusing to leave home because of excessive resistance to change in autism spectrum disorder, delusions or hallucinations concerning separation in psychotic disorders, refusal to go outside without a trusted companion in agoraphobia, worries about ill health or other harm befalling significant others in generalized anxiety disorder, or concerns about having an illness in illness anxiety disorder.

Reprinted with permission from the Diagnostic and Statistical Manual of Mental Disorders, Fifth Edition, Text Revision (Copyright © 2022). American Psychiatric Association. All Rights Reserved.

TABLE 17.3 Criteria for Diagnosis of Social Anxiety Disorder

A. Marked fear or anxiety about one or more social situations in which the individual is exposed to possible scrutiny by others. Examples include social interactions (e.g., having a conversation, meeting unfamiliar people), being observed (e.g., eating or drinking), and performing in front of others (e.g., giving a speech).

Note: In children, the anxiety must occur in peer settings and not just during interactions with adults.

B. The individual fears that they will act in a way or show anxiety symptoms that will be negatively evaluated (i.e., will be humiliating or embarrassing; will lead to rejection or offend others).

C. The social situations almost always provoke fear or anxiety.

Note: In children, the fear or anxiety may be expressed by crying, tantrums, freezing, clinging, shrinking, or failing to speak in social situations.

D. The social situations are avoided or endured with intense fear or anxiety.

E. The fear or anxiety is out of proportion to the actual threat posed by the social situation and to the sociocultural context.

F. The fear, anxiety, or avoidance is persistent, typically lasting for 6 months or more.

G. The fear, anxiety, or avoidance causes clinically significant distress or impairment in social, occupational, or other important areas of functioning.

H. The fear, anxiety, or avoidance is not attributable to the physiological effects of a substance (e.g., a drug of abuse, a medication) or another medical condition.

I. The fear, anxiety, or avoidance is not better explained by the symptoms of another mental disorder, such as panic disorder, body dysmorphic disorder, or autism spectrum disorder.

J. If another medical condition (e.g., Parkinson disease, obesity, disfigurement from burns or injury) is present, the anxiety or avoidance is clearly unrelated or is excessive.

Specify if:

Performance only: If the fear is restricted to speaking or performing in public

Reprinted with permission from the Diagnostic and Statistical Manual of Mental Disorders, Fifth Edition, Text Revision (Copyright © 2022). American Psychiatric Association. All Rights Reserved.

some history of speech delay or speech disorder; diagnosis does not typically occur until kindergarten or first grade when there is an increased demand on speech and social interaction. Children of immigrants (who are non-English speaking) and a parental history of reticence and/or social anxiety are often found in children with selective mutism. There is a relationship between selective mutism and social anxiety disorder in children, with approximately 69% of children presenting with these co-morbidities.

Specific phobias are marked, persistent fears of specific things/objects or situations that often lead to avoidance behaviors. The anxiety is almost always felt immediately when the person is confronted with the feared object or situation, and many patients have had actual fearful experiences with the object or situation (traumatic event). The closer the proximity or the more difficult it is to escape, the higher the anxiety. The response to the fear can range from limited symptoms of anxiety to full panic attacks. Children may not recognize that their fears are out of proportion to the circumstances, unlike adolescents and adults, and express their anxiety as crying, tantrums, freezing, or clinging. Many fears are normal in childhood; therefore only fears lasting greater than 6 months in duration should be considered diagnostically for children. Specific fears may be related to animals/insects, natural events (storms, flooding), blood-related events (injections, needles, medical procedures), situational events (elevator, airplane), or other circumstances/events (loud sounds, clowns).

Agoraphobia is a disorder marked by fear of situations where escape is difficult or would draw unwanted attention to the person. The condition involves two or more of five specific situations: fear/anxiety about the use of public transportation, being in open spaces, being in enclosed spaces, standing in line or being in a crowd, or being outside of the home alone. Agoraphobia is often chronic and can leave people homebound. Although agoraphobia does commonly occur with panic disorder, a substantial number of individuals experience agoraphobia without panic symptoms. First onset of agoraphobia commonly presents in adolescence or young adulthood, with females being twice as likely to experience the disorder. In children, being outside of the home alone as well as worries regarding becoming lost are common complaints.

With **treatment of anxiety disorders**, potential medical conditions should be carefully excluded, including hyperthyroidism, medication side effects, and substance use disorder. Additionally, screening for co-morbid psychiatric disorders such as mood disorders, eating disorders (including avoidant restrictive food intake disorder [ARFID]), tic disorders, and other behavioral disorders should occur. A collaborative history from multiple sources is important because the child may be unable to effectively communicate symptoms.

Multiple broad **screening tools** are available for anxiety disorders in children. Employing a validated screening tool, along with a clinician interview, is recommended. The most commonly employed tools include the Youth Anxiety Measure (YAM), Screen for Child Anxiety–Related Emotional Disorders (SCARED), Anxiety Disorder Interview Schedule (ADIS), and the Pediatric Anxiety Rating Scale (PARS).

Evidence-based **psychotherapies** and **psychoeducation** are first-line for mild to moderate anxiety. Pharmacotherapy is also used to help treat anxiety. Combined therapy demonstrates better efficacy than psychotherapy and psychopharmacology alone. Cognitive and behavioral therapy (e.g., systematic desensitization, exposure techniques, operant conditioning, modeling, and cognitive restructuring) can be beneficial in a variety of anxiety disorders. Psychotherapy may help maintain treatment regimens and increase compliance rates. Care coordination with a patient's school is recommended. Reassurance that the patient does not have a life-threatening illness is important. Other psychosocial treatments that have demonstrated efficacy include stress management, supportive therapies, and biofeedback.

Selective serotonin reuptake inhibitors (SSRIs) are the medications of choice, and the U.S. Food and Drug Administration has approved fluoxetine, sertraline, escitalopram, and fluvoxamine for use in children. SSRIs can initially exacerbate anxiety or even panic symptoms, and their use should be monitored closely. Tricyclic antidepressants have also shown efficacy. Benzodiazepines (alprazolam and clonazepam) may cause disinhibition in children. α_{2a} agonists (guanfacine and clonidine) may be useful if autonomic symptoms are present. Anticonvulsant agents (gabapentin, topiramate, and oxcarbazepine) are used when other agents are ineffective. β blockers help with performance anxiety. Children with anxiety disorders are often less tolerant of medication side effects; careful monitoring should occur.

Co-occurrence of **attention-deficit/hyperactivity disorder** (inattentive type) and an anxiety disorder is common. When using a stimulant, it is advisable to start at a low dose, increasing slowly to minimize the risk of increasing anxiety. Additionally, careful monitoring of sleep and appetite is important.

ARFID may be co-morbid with anxiety disorders in children, and 72% of children with ARFID may also experience an anxiety disorder. These children more commonly present in medical settings, and many anxiety screening tools do not assess for disorders of eating; the clinician may need to directly query families regarding the child's eating.

PEARLS FOR PRACTITIONERS

See Psychiatric Disorders: Pearls for Practitioners at the end of this section.

REVIEW QUESTIONS

Available online.

CHAPTER 18

Depression and Bipolar Disorders

Major depressive disorder (MDD) requires a minimum of 2 weeks of symptoms including either depressed mood or loss of interest or pleasure in nearly all activities. Four additional symptoms must also be present (Table 18.1). In children and adolescents, a new onset of irritability and/or restlessness may be present instead of depressed mood. Many children and adolescents also complain of pervasive boredom. A change in appetite (usually decreased but can be increased), with or

TABLE 18.1 Criteria for Diagnosis of Major Depressive Episode/Disorder

A. Five (or more) of the following symptoms have been present during the same 2-week period and represent a change from previous functioning; at least one of the symptoms is either (1) depressed mood or (2) loss of interest or pleasure.

Note: Do not include symptoms that are clearly attributable to another medical condition.

1. Depressed mood most of the day, nearly every day, as indicated by either subjective report (e.g., feels sad, empty, or hopeless) or observation made by others (e.g., appears tearful). (**Note:** In children and adolescents, can be irritable mood.)
2. Markedly diminished interest or pleasure in all, or almost all, activities most of the day, nearly every day (as indicated by either subjective account or observation)
3. Significant weight loss when not dieting or weight gain (e.g., a change of more than 5% of body weight in a month) or decrease or increase in appetite nearly every day. (**Note:** In children, consider failure to make expected weight gain.)
4. Insomnia or hypersomnia nearly every day
5. Psychomotor agitation or retardation nearly every day (observable by others; not merely subjective feelings of restlessness or being slowed down)
6. Fatigue or loss of energy nearly every day
7. Feelings of worthlessness or excessive or inappropriate guilt (which may be delusional) nearly every day (not merely self-reproach or guilt about being sick)
8. Diminished ability to think or concentrate, or indecisiveness, nearly every day (either by subjective account or as observed by others)
9. Recurrent thoughts of death (not just fear of dying), recurrent suicidal ideation without a specific plan, a specific suicide plan, or a suicide attempt

B. The symptoms cause clinically significant distress or impairment in social, occupational, or other important areas of functioning.

C. The episode is not attributable to the physiological effects of a substance or another medical condition.

Note: Criteria A–C represent a major depressive episode.

Note: Responses to a significant loss (e.g., bereavement, financial ruin, losses from a natural disaster, a serious medical illness or disability) may include feelings of intense sadness, rumination about the loss, insomnia, poor appetite, and weight loss noted in Criterion A, which may resemble a depressive episode. Although such symptoms may be understandable or considered appropriate to the loss, the presence of a major depressive episode in addition to the normal response to a significant loss should also be carefully considered. The decision inevitably requires the exercise of clinical judgment based on the individual's history and the cultural norms for the expression of distress in the context of loss.

D. At least one major depressive episode is not better explained by schizoaffective disorder and is not superimposed on schizophrenia, schizophreniform disorder, delusional disorder, or other specified and unspecified schizophrenia spectrum and other psychotic disorders.

E. There has never been a manic episode or a hypomanic episode.

Note: This exclusion does not apply if all of the manic-like or hypomanic-like episodes are substance-induced or are attributable to the physiological effects or another medical condition.

Specify if: with **anxious distress, mixed features, melancholic features, atypical features, mood-congruent psychotic features, mood-incongruent psychotic features, catatonia, peripartum onset, seasonal pattern** (applies to pattern of recurrent major depressive episodes)

Reprinted with permission from the Diagnostic and Statistical Manual of Mental Disorders, Fifth Edition, Text Revision (Copyright © 2022). American Psychiatric Association. All Rights Reserved.

without accompanying weight changes, and sleep disturbance along with somatic complaints (fatigue, vague aches and pains) may also be present. A key indicator in children may be declining performance in school. **Psychotic symptoms**, seen in severe cases of MDD, are generally mood congruent (e.g., derogatory auditory hallucinations, guilt-associated delusional thinking). **Suicidal** thoughts and attempts are common, with suicide being a leading cause of death in 10- to 19-year-olds. A prior history of suicidal thoughts/attempts and prominent feelings of hopelessness are risk factors that should be closely monitored.

Although most people experience bereavement following a significant loss (e.g., loss of a loved one) without developing depression, many do, in fact, experience depressive symptoms. Treatments for MDD and MDD with bereavement are often likely to help with the remittance of symptoms.

The prevalence of MDD in prepubertal children is approximately 2% with a 1:1 female:male ratio. In adolescence the prevalence is approximately 3 to 7% with a female:male ratio of 2:1 (similar to adults). If untreated, MDD can become chronic in up to 10% of patients.

Genetic predisposition for MDD is present, with twin studies showing 60–70% heritability. Additionally, family studies show a two- to fourfold increased risk for depression in offspring of parents with MDD. Dysregulation of central serotonergic and/or noradrenergic systems, hypothalamic-pituitary-adrenal axis dysfunction, the influence of pubertal sex hormones, and exposure to adverse childhood experiences have been shown to be potential contributing factors for MDD. Additionally, exposure to early maltreatment/neglect and adverse life events in the presence of the serotonin transporter pathogenic variant 5-HTTLPR may further increase the risk for MDD.

Anxiety-related disorders (up to 80% prevalence), **substance-related disorders** (up to 30% prevalence), **conduct/disruptive disorders** (up to 20% prevalence), and **sleep-related disorders** (up to 19% prevalence) frequently present as co-morbid conditions with MDD. Onset of MDD in childhood is also more likely to be related to *bipolar disorder.* This is especially true when a family history of bipolar disorder is present.

Differential diagnoses for MDD are broad. It is always prudent to consider mood disorder due to another medical condition or substance-related mood disorder before considering MDD. In adolescents, a urine toxicology screen may also be useful given the high prevalence of substance use disorder. Dysphoria and concentration concerns related to untreated attention-deficit/hyperactivity disorder (ADHD) may also be misdiagnosed as depression.

Persistent depressive disorder (formerly dysthymia or chronic MDD) is a chronic form of depression characterized by a depressed or irritable mood present for at least 1 year. Two of the following symptoms are also required: changes in appetite, sleep difficulty, fatigue, low self-esteem, poor concentration or difficulty making decisions, and feelings of hopelessness. The prevalence of MDD is 0.5–2.0%, with the highest prevalence in adolescents. Approximately 70% of children and adolescents with persistent depressive disorder eventually develop major depression.

Disruptive mood dysregulation disorder (DMDD) includes children ages 6–18 years who present with a chronic (≥12 months) pattern of severe irritability and behavioral dysregulation. The prevalence rate of DMDD is estimated to be 1.6%, with some studies demonstrating prevalence as high as 9% (up to 31% in community mental health center samples). DMDD typically first presents in school-age children and is more common among males. In distinguishing bipolar disorder in children from DMDD, particular attention should be given to the course of symptoms (DMDD being chronic/persistent and bipolar disorder presenting with episodic mood changes). Co-morbidities with DMDD are common, and conditions such as disruptive behavior disorders should be assessed and are more prevalent in DMDD (around 36%) versus bipolar disorder (around 21%). Children and adolescents with DMDD may also present with other mood concerns, anxiety, and/or autism spectrum disorder symptoms and diagnoses.

Premenstrual dysphoric disorder (PMDD) is marked by repeated irritability, anxiety, and mood lability that presents during the premenstrual cycle and remits near the onset of menses. Approximately 3–8% of adult females are thought to experience PMDD with adolescent rates thought to be at a similar level. At least five physical (e.g., sleep disturbance, breast tenderness, joint/muscle pain, fatigue, appetite changes) and/or behavioral symptoms (e.g., affective lability, irritability, depressed mood, anxiety) must be present. Symptoms peak near the onset of menses. PMDD differs from premenstrual syndrome in the number of symptoms present and regarding the affective symptoms that are present. *MDD is the most commonly presenting co-morbidity.* Adverse childhood experiences, pre-existing anxiety disorder, cigarette smoking, obesity/increased body mass index, and pathogenic variants of $5\text{-}HT_{1A}$ and *ESR1* are risk factors for PMDD. The Premenstrual Symptoms Screening Tool revised for adolescents (PSST-A) is a brief questionnaire available to assist with identifying PMDD in adolescents.

Unspecified depressive disorder is a diagnosis used when patients have functionally impairing depressive symptoms that do not meet criteria for another condition.

Numerous **specifiers for depressive disorders** may also be identified. These include methods of noting additional struggles with anxious distress, mixed features (including elevated mood/hypomanic symptoms), melancholic features (loss of pleasure/lack of reactivity to pleasurable stimuli), psychotic features, and seasonal patterns (symptoms occur in the late fall and early winter when the hours of daylight are shortening).

Treatment of depression involves psychopharmacologic approaches and/or psychotherapy. Regardless of the treatment approach chosen, a thorough diagnostic interview and screening measures should be completed. There are a variety of screening tools such as the Children's Depression Inventory (CDI 2) and the Patient Health Questionnaire Modified for Adolescents (PHQ9-A) that may be helpful. **Medical conditions** such as hypothyroidism, anemia, diabetes, and folate and B_{12} vitamin deficiencies need to be evaluated. Other factors impacting treatment should also be explored including substance use in adolescents (especially alcohol and marijuana), sleep difficulties (e.g., decreased sleep efficiency, shorter REM latency, higher REM density), and medication interactions (e.g., corticosteroids, progestin-releasing implanted contraceptives, and propranolol).

First-line **pharmacologic treatment** involves selective serotonin reuptake inhibitors (SSRIs) that have demonstrated response rates of 50–70% despite high placebo response rates. Fluoxetine is the only medication approved by the FDA for treatment in youth 8 years and older, and escitalopram is approved for youth 12 and older. Many other off-label medications such as citalopram, paroxetine, and venlafaxine have positive clinical effects and have been used off label. An antidepressant should be given an adequate trial (6 weeks at therapeutic doses) before switching or discontinuing unless there are serious side effects. Close follow-up throughout this initial phase should occur because of the increased risk for suicidal ideation (not suicide attempts) and to monitor for the other most common side effects. For a first episode of depression in children and adolescents, treatment for 6–9 months after remission of symptoms is recommended. Patients with recurrent or persistent depression may need to take antidepressants for extended periods (years or even a lifetime). If a patient does not respond to adequate trials of two or more antidepressants, a specialist should be consulted. Following a thorough evaluation, the specialist may use augmentation strategies that include other medications such as lithium, thyroid hormone, lamotrigine, or bupropion.

For acute depression, more frequent office visits and monitoring (e.g., telephone/video check-ins) are indicated, and the risks of medication (including suicidal and self-destructive behaviors) should always be discussed with the patient and caregiver. Psychoeducation about depression and specifically calling if new symptoms occur should be completed with the family. Notable side effects of medication are thoughts of suicide, increased agitation, or restlessness. Other side effects include headache, dizziness, gastrointestinal symptoms, sleep disturbance, sexual dysfunction, akathisia, serotonin syndrome, and risk of increased bruising (due to platelet inhibition).

The FDA has issued warnings regarding the potential for increased suicidal thoughts and/or behaviors when using an antidepressant. The data suggest that antidepressants pose a 4% risk, versus a 2% risk for placebo. An increase in suicides in children and adolescents after that warning has many experts believing that it might be related to lowered prescription rates of antidepressants and resultant untreated depression. Suicide is a fatal complication of MDD. Around 20% of adolescents seriously contemplate suicide and approximately 8% attempt suicide each year. Although the risk of suicide during an MDD episode is high, it can be paradoxically higher during start of treatment, as energy and motivation improve with cognitive recovery from depression. Individual (e.g., substance use, male, impulsivity), familial (e.g., family history of mental illness, history of abuse/neglect, low social support), and community (e.g., high economic distress, rural community, social isolation) factors all increase the risk of suicide. Discussion of safe gun storage and/or the removal of guns from the home should occur given the high frequency of gun-related suicides in adolescents (i.e., 48% gun-related in 2023).

Psychotherapy has good efficacy in mild to moderate depression. In moderate to severe depression, pharmacotherapy has the greatest rate of response, although in severe cases the efficacy was equivalent to medication alone. **Cognitive-behavioral therapy** (CBT) and interpersonal therapies have received the most empirical support. CBT involves a variety of behavioral techniques and skills-building to mitigate cognitive distortions and maladaptive processing. Interpersonal therapy focuses on collaborative decisions between the therapist and patient and is based on the exploration and recognition of precipitants of depression. Family therapy is often used as an adjunct to other treatments for depression. Light therapy is beneficial for seasonal variants of MDD. Electroconvulsive therapy (ECT) is rarely used in children under 11 years but may be considered in older children/adolescents who experience refractory and life-threatening depression.

Treatment is targeted toward decreasing morbidity and suicide. Along with treatments mentioned previously, modalities such as hospitalization, partial hospitalization, therapeutic after-school programs, or group therapies may be needed.

BIPOLAR AND RELATED DISORDERS

Bipolar I disorder (BD) consists of distinct periods of mania (elevated, expansive, or irritable moods and distractibility) and persistent goal-directed activity or energy (Table 18.2) that may alternate with periods of severe depression (see Table 18.1). The prevalence rate in children is relatively low at 0.5% (2–3% for all bipolar-related disorders in children) and often is misdiagnosed, in part because of the large overlap of symptoms with other psychiatric disorders.

To diagnose mania associated with BD, euphoria (elevated or expansive mood) with three additional symptoms or irritable mood with four additional symptoms is required. Children and adolescents with euphoric mood often present as bubbly, giggly, and "over-the-top" happy, to a degree that is socially unacceptable to others. Grandiosity in children is often dramatic, and they may believe they are superior to others in activities, sports, or academics even when it is objectively not true. Racing thoughts and concentration difficulties are common in BD, and speech can be loud and pressured. Periods of extreme rage may also present. Children with BD often present with rapid shifts in mood or lability over brief time frames (e.g., shifting between euphoria and dysphoria or irritability).

A decreased need for sleep without fatigue is a hallmark of mania. There are no other diagnoses where a child has a greatly decreased amount of total sleep (compared with age-appropriate norms) and is not fatigued. Sleep deprivation, substance use disorder, and antidepressants may trigger mania. BD onset often begins with an episode of depression. Mania rarely occurs prior to adolescence. It is estimated that 33% of youth will develop BD within 5 years of a first depressive episode and 20% of all patients with BD will experience their first manic episode during adolescence. *Hypomania* is used to describe a period of more than 4 but fewer than 7 days of manic symptoms. It also is used, less specifically, to describe less intense mania. The prevalence of psychosis in adolescents with BD (most often auditory hallucinations) is 16–60%. Psychosis in children with BD is less than its prevalence in adult BD.

Bipolar II disorder includes at least one current or past full major depressive episode and at least one period of current or past hypomania. It is slightly more prevalent (0.6%) in children than bipolar I disorder. **Unspecified bipolar and related disorder** is used to describe prominent symptoms of BD that do not meet full diagnostic criteria or when historical information is unclear or insufficient to make a specific diagnosis.

Cyclothymic disorder is a chronic (>1 year) mood disorder characterized by several periods of hypomanic symptoms and depressive symptoms (which do not have to meet the full diagnostic criteria for hypomania or a depressive episode, respectively). The lifetime prevalence rate for cyclothymic disorder is around 0.4–1%. Childhood rates are unknown. The male:female ratio for the disorder is equal, and in children the mean age of onset is 6.5 years. ADHD, sleep disorders, and substance-related disorders also show high co-morbidity rates with cyclothymic disorder. Genetic causes of cyclothymic disorder are apparent with a monozygotic twin concordance rate of 57%.

Numerous specifiers for bipolar disorders may also be identified (see Table 18.2). These include methods of noting additional struggles with anxious distress, mixed features (including elevated mood/hypomanic symptoms), melancholic features (loss of pleasure/lack of reactivity to pleasurable stimuli), psychotic features, seasonal patterns, and rapid cycling (four or more mood episodes during a 12-month period).

It is estimated that 60% of BD onset occurs before 20 years of age, although it is often not until adulthood that BD is diagnosed. Although BD in adults tends to be gender neutral, it is estimated that prepubertal BD is almost four times more frequently diagnosed in males.

A family history of mental illness, including MDD, BD, schizophrenia, or ADHD, is common in BD. A first-degree relative with BD leads to a 10-fold increase in a child's chance of developing BD. An earlier onset of BD in a parent increases the risk of early-onset BD in offspring with a more chronic and debilitating course that may be less responsive to treatment.

Patients with BD often have *concurrent conditions* that warrant treatment. ADHD occurs in approximately 60–90% of children with BD. Anxiety disorders also commonly occur with BD and do not respond to antimanic agents. Substance use disorder can precipitate and perpetuate mania and depression. Additionally, the experience of neglect/trauma and exposure to stressful life events (e.g., early parental loss) have been linked with developing BD. The alteration between highs and lows related to some types of substance use disorder often mimics BD. Patients with BD may also self-medicate in attempts to alleviate symptoms (with up to 50% of BD patients presenting with alcohol use disorder). It may be necessary to evaluate a patient in a substance-free state to make an accurate diagnosis of BD. Many patients with BD may meet criteria for conduct disorder (CD) due to aggression and impulsivity. In distinguishing BD from CD, patients with BD generally exhibit reactive aggression, whereas those with CD are more likely to preplan acts/crimes.

No laboratory or imaging studies can diagnose BD. Physical examination, careful history, review of systems, and laboratory testing may be performed to evaluate suspected medical etiologies, including neurologic and substance-related disorders. Self-report scales for depression such as the PHQ9-A and CDI 2 may aid in diagnosis and can be paired with severity rating scales such as the Children's Depression Rating Scale–Revised (CDRS-R) and the Young Mania Rating Scale (YMRS) to guide diagnosis and treatment.

Treatment of BD often initially targets acute symptoms. If suicidal ideation and/or risk-taking behaviors are present, hospitalization may be necessary. Treatment involves a variety of approaches depending upon the developmental level of the child/adolescent. Multiple FDA-approved medications including lithium, divalproex sodium, olanzapine, risperidone, quetiapine, lurasidone, asenapine, and aripiprazole are available for patients with BD. Lithium is used in acute episodes and as a maintenance treatment in children (approved for age >7 years) and adolescents with mania. Common side effects of lithium include hypothyroidism, polyuria, and acne. Anticonvulsants are also a first-line agent (preferable for mixed

TABLE 18.2 Criteria for Diagnosis of Bipolar I Disorder

For a diagnosis of bipolar I disorder, it is necessary to meet the following criteria for a manic episode. The manic episode may have been preceded by and may be followed by hypomanic or major depressive episodes.

MANIC EPISODE

A. A distinct period of abnormally and persistently elevated, expansive, or irritable mood and abnormally and persistently increased goal-directed activity or energy, lasting at least 1 week and present most of the day, nearly every day (or any duration if hospitalization is necessary).
B. During the period of mood disturbance and increased energy or activity, three (or more) of the following symptoms (four if the mood is only irritable) are present to a significant degree and represent a noticeable change from usual behavior:
1. Inflated self-esteem or grandiosity
2. Decreased need for sleep (e.g., feels rested after only 3 hours of sleep)
3. More talkative than usual or pressure to keep talking
4. Flight of ideas or subjective experience that thoughts are racing
5. Distractibility (i.e., attention too easily drawn to unimportant or irrelevant external stimuli), as reported or observed
6. Increase in goal-directed activity (either socially, at work or school, or sexually) or psychomotor agitation (i.e., purposeless non–goal-directed activity)
7. Excessive involvement in activities that have a high potential for painful consequences (e.g., engaging in unrestrained buying sprees, sexual indiscretions, or foolish business investments)

C. The mood disturbance is sufficiently severe to cause marked impairment in social or occupational functioning or to necessitate hospitalization to prevent harm to self or others, or there are psychotic features.
D. The episode is not attributable to the physiological effects of a substance (e.g., a drug of abuse, a medication, other treatment) or to another medical condition.

Note: A full manic episode that emerges during antidepressant treatment (e.g., medication, electroconvulsive therapy) but persists at a fully syndromal level beyond the physiological effect of that treatment is sufficient evidence for a manic episode and, therefore, a bipolar I diagnosis.

Note: Criteria A–D constitute a manic episode. At least one lifetime manic episode is required for the diagnosis of bipolar I disorder.

HYPOMANIC EPISODE

A. A distinct period of abnormally and persistently elevated, expansive, or irritable mood and abnormally and persistently increased activity or energy, lasting at least 4 consecutive days and present most of the day, nearly every day.
B. During the period of mood disturbance and increased energy and activity, three (or more) of the following symptoms (four if the mood is only irritable) have persisted, represent a noticeable change from usual behavior, and have been present to a significant degree:
1. Inflated self-esteem or grandiosity
2. Decreased need for sleep (e.g., feels rested after only 3 hours of sleep)
3. More talkative than usual or pressure to keep talking
4. Flight of ideas or subjective experience that thoughts are racing
5. Distractibility (i.e., attention too easily drawn to unimportant or irrelevant external stimuli), as reported or observed
6. Increase in goal-directed activity (either socially, at work or school, or sexually) or psychomotor agitation
7. Excessive involvement in activities that have a high potential for painful consequences (e.g., engaging in unrestrained buying sprees, sexual indiscretions, or foolish business investments)

C. The episode is associated with an unequivocal change in functioning that is uncharacteristic of the individual when not symptomatic.
D. The disturbance in mood and the change in functioning are observable by others.
E. The episode is not severe enough to cause marked impairment in social or occupational functioning or to necessitate hospitalization. If there are psychotic features, the episode is, by definition, manic.
F. The episode is not attributable to the physiological effects of a substance (e.g., a drug of abuse, a medication, other treatment) or another medical condition.

Note: A full hypomanic episode that emerges during antidepressant treatment (e.g., medication, electroconvulsive therapy) but persists at a fully syndromal level beyond the physiological effect of that treatment is sufficient evidence for a hypomanic episode diagnosis. However, caution is indicated so that one or two symptoms (particularly increased irritability, edginess, or agitation following antidepressant use) are not taken as sufficient for diagnosis of a hypomanic episode nor necessarily indicative of a bipolar diathesis.

Note: Criteria A–F constitute a hypomanic episode. Hypomanic episodes are common in bipolar I disorder but are not required for the diagnosis of bipolar I disorder.

MAJOR DEPRESSIVE EPISODE

A. Five (or more) of the following symptoms have been present during the same 2-week period and represent a change from previous functioning; at least one of the symptoms is either (1) depressed mood or (2) loss of interest or pleasure.

Note: Do not include symptoms that are clearly attributable to another medical condition.
1. Depressed mood most of the day, nearly every day, as indicated by either subjective report (e.g., feels sad, empty, or hopeless) or observation made by others (e.g., appears tearful). (**Note:** In children and adolescents, can be irritable mood.)
2. Markedly diminished interest or pleasure in all, or almost all, activities most of the day, nearly every day (as indicated by either subjective account or observation)
3. Significant weight loss when not dieting or weight gain (e.g., a change of more than 5% of body weight in a month) or decrease or increase in appetite nearly every day. (**Note:** In children, consider failure to make expected weight gain.)
4. Insomnia or hypersomnia nearly every day
5. Psychomotor agitation or retardation nearly every day (observable by others; not merely subjective feelings of restlessness or being slowed down)
6. Fatigue or loss of energy nearly every day
7. Feelings of worthlessness or excessive or inappropriate guilt (which may be delusional) nearly every day (not merely self-reproach or guilt about being sick)
8. Diminished ability to think or concentrate, or indecisiveness, nearly every day (either by subjective account or as observed by others)
9. Recurrent thoughts of death (not just fear of dying), recurrent suicidal ideation without a specific plan, a specific suicide plan, or a suicide attempt

B. The symptoms cause clinically significant distress or impairment in social, occupational, or other important areas of functioning.
C. The episode is not attributable to the physiological effects of a substance or another medical condition.

Note: Major depressive episodes are common in bipolar I disorder but are not required for the diagnosis of bipolar I disorder.

(Continued)

TABLE 18.2 Criteria for Diagnosis of Bipolar I Disorder—cont'd

Note: Responses to a significant loss (e.g., bereavement, financial ruin, losses from a natural disaster, a serious medical illness or disability) may include feelings of intense sadness, rumination about the loss, insomnia, poor appetite, and weight loss noted in Criterion A, which may resemble a depressive episode. Although such symptoms may be understandable or considered appropriate to the loss, the presence of a major depressive episode in addition to the normal response to a significant loss should also be carefully considered. The decision inevitably requires the exercise of clinical judgment based on the individual's history and the cultural norms for the expression of distress in the context of loss.
BIPOLAR I DISORDER
A. Criteria have been met for at least one manic episode (Criteria A–D under "Manic Episode" above). B. At least one manic episode is not better explained by schizoaffective disorder and is not superimposed on schizophrenic, schizophreniform disorder, delusional disorder, or other specified or unspecified schizophrenia spectrum and other psychotic disorder.
Specify if: **with anxious distress**, **mixed features**, **rapid cycling**, **melancholic features**, **atypical features**, **mood-congruent psychotic features** (applies to manic episode and/or major depressive episode), **mood-incongruent psychotic features** (applies to manic episode and/or major depressive episode), **catatonia**, **peripartum onset**, **seasonal pattern**

Reprinted with permission from the Diagnostic and Statistical Manual of Mental Disorders, Fifth Edition, Text Revision (Copyright © 2022). American Psychiatric Association. All Rights Reserved.

or rapid cycling cases) for adults. They have also been used effectively in youth but are not FDA approved in children for BD. Monitoring of blood levels for select medications (lithium and divalproex sodium) can help ensure both treatment safety and an appropriate therapeutic dose of the medication. Neuroleptics (e.g., risperidone, olanzapine, quetiapine, and aripiprazole) have had positive results in youth with BD; the risk of tardive dyskinesia should be considered in using such agents. Benzodiazepines may also be helpful for alleviating insomnia and agitation during acute mania.

Treating co-morbid psychiatric disorders must be done carefully. Stimulants may be used to treat ADHD once the patient has been stabilized on a mood stabilizer. If the patient is depressed or has significant anxiety and is not responsive to other pharmacotherapy, cautious use of antidepressants may be necessary. Careful monitoring for manic reactivation, cycling, and suicidality is needed. Maintenance treatment with medication for years may be necessary and intermittent use of medication is not recommended.

CBT is aimed at initially improving adherence to medication treatments and ameliorating anxiety and depressive symptoms. CBT should not be a monotherapy in acute BD but has demonstrated effectiveness following acute presentations. Psychoeducation and family therapy may also be needed to stabilize the patient's environment and improve prognosis. There should be ongoing safety assessment. Additionally, patients may display struggles with coping skills, impaired social/interpersonal relationships, and developmental deficits due to poor learning while symptomatic; additional skills training and collaboration with the child's school regarding behavior management, special education needs, and an appropriate individualized education plan may also be needed.

When compared with depression, the rates of suicide and suicidal ideation are higher in BD. Forty percent of children and 50% of adolescents with BD attempt suicide with approximately 10–15% completing attempts. High levels of irritability, impulsivity, and poor ability to consider consequences (e.g., substance use disorder) increase the risk of completed suicide. Suicide attempts are more likely to occur in patients who are older, have mixed episodes and psychotic features, have co-morbidities (e.g., substance use, panic disorder), and have a history of physical or sexual abuse. They also commonly have a history of self-harming/self-injurious behaviors, a family history of suicide attempts, and a history of hospitalizations. Legal problems in adolescence are also a strong predictor of suicide attempts, with approximately a fourth of those attempting suicide having experienced legal concerns in the preceding 12 months. Ensuring safety should always be the first goal of treatment. Hospitalization, partial hospitalization, intensive outpatient treatment, and intensive in-home services are used as needed for stabilization and safety.

PEARLS FOR PRACTITIONERS

See Psychiatric Disorders: Pearls for Practitioners at the end of this section.

REVIEW QUESTIONS

Available online.

CHAPTER 19 Obsessive-Compulsive Disorder

Obsessive-compulsive disorder (OCD) is characterized by obsessions, compulsions, or both in the *absence* of another psychiatric disorder that better explains the symptoms (Table 19.1). **Obsessions** involve recurrent intrusive thoughts, images, or impulses. **Compulsions** are repetitive, nongratifying behaviors that a person feels driven to perform to reduce or prevent distress or anxiety. In children, rituals or compulsive symptoms often predominate over worries or obsessions, and the child may attempt to neutralize an obsessive thought by performing compulsions. Symptoms may or may not be recognized as being excessive or unreasonable. The most common obsessions in children involve fears of contamination, fears of dirt/germs, repeated doubts, orderliness or precision, and aggressive thoughts. Common compulsions include grooming (e.g., handwashing, showering), ordering, checking, requesting reassurance, praying, counting, repeating words silently, and touching rituals.

TABLE 19.1 Criteria for Diagnosis of Obsessive-Compulsive Disorder

A. Presence of obsessions, compulsions, or both.
Obsessions are defined by (1) and (2):
1. Recurrent and persistent thoughts, urges, or images that are experienced, at some time during the disturbance, as intrusive and unwanted and that in most individuals cause marked anxiety or distress.
2. The individual attempts to ignore or suppress such thoughts, urges, or images or to neutralize them with some other thought or action (i.e., by performing a compulsion).
Compulsions are defined by (1) and (2):
1. Repetitive behaviors (e.g., handwashing, ordering, checking) or mental acts (e.g., praying, counting, repeating words silently) that the individual feels driven to perform in response to an obsession or according to rules that must be applied rigidly.
2. The behaviors or mental acts are aimed at preventing or reducing anxiety or distress or preventing some dreaded event or situation; however, these behaviors or mental acts are not connected in a realistic way with what they are designed to neutralize or prevent or are clearly excessive.
Note: Young children may not be able to articulate the aims of these behaviors or mental acts.
B. The obsessions or compulsions are time-consuming (e.g., take more than1 hour per day) or cause clinically significant distress or impairment in social, occupational, or other important areas of functioning.
C. The obsessive-compulsive symptoms are not attributable to the physiological effects of a substance (e.g., a drug of abuse, a medication) or another medical condition.
D. The disturbance is not better explained by the symptoms of another mental disorder (e.g., excessive worries, as in generalized anxiety disorder; preoccupation with appearance, as in body dysmorphic disorder; difficulty discarding or parting with possessions, as in hoarding disorder; hair pulling, as in trichotillomania [hair-pulling disorder]; skin picking, as in excoriation [skin-picking] disorder; stereotypies, as in stereotypical movement disorder; ritualized eating behavior, as in eating disorders; preoccupation with substances or gambling, as in substance-related and addictive disorders; preoccupation with having an illness, as in illness anxiety disorder; sexual urges or fantasies, as in paraphilic disorders; impulses, as in disruptive, impulse control, and conduct disorders; guilty ruminations, as in major depressive disorder; thought insertion or delusional preoccupations, as in schizophrenia spectrum and other psychotic disorders; or repetitive patterns of behavior, as in autism spectrum disorder).
Specify if:
With good or fair insight: The individual recognizes that obsessive-compulsive disorder beliefs are definitely or probably not true or that they may or may not be true. **With poor insight:** The individual thinks obsessive-compulsive disorder beliefs are probably true. **With absent insight/delusional beliefs:** The individual is completely convinced that obsessive-compulsive disorder beliefs are true.
Specify if:
Tic related: The individual has a current or past history of a tic disorder.

Reprinted with permission from the Diagnostic and Statistical Manual of Mental Disorders, Fifth Edition, Text Revision (Copyright © 2022). American Psychiatric Association. All Rights Reserved.

Prevalence of OCD in children ranges from 1 to 4%; it increases with age. Males have an earlier age of onset, with approximately 25% of males being diagnosed prior to 10 years of age. OCD is most often diagnosed between the ages of 7 and 12 years. Symptoms have a gradual onset. Obsessive-compulsive symptoms are moderately heritable, with genetic factors accounting for up to 48% of variance. However, some maternal factors, such as prenatal exposure to infection or stress, may significantly reduce heritability estimates.

Up to 50% of youth with OCD have at least one other psychiatric illness. Some of the most common co-morbidities include mood and anxiety disorders (up to 75%), behavioral disorders (attention-deficit/hyperactivity disorder [ADHD] and oppositional defiant disorder) (up to 50%), tic disorders (20–30%), hoarding disorder, developmental disorders, body dysmorphic disorder, hypochondriasis, avoidant/restrictive food intake disorder (ARFID), and **obsessive-compulsive personality disorder (OCPD)**.

OCD has been linked to a disruption in the serotonin, glutamate, and dopamine systems in the brain. Overactivity in neural pathways involving the orbital frontal cortex and caudate nucleus and evidence for a cortico-striato-thalamo-cortical (CSTC) loop have also been implicated in OCD.

Streptococcal infection (i.e., pharyngitis, scarlet fever) causing inflammation in the basal ganglia may account for 10% of childhood-onset OCD and is part of a condition referred to as *pediatric autoimmune neuropsychiatric disorders associated with streptococcal* (PANDAS) infection. PANDAS is a subtype of *pediatric acute-onset neuropsychiatric syndrome* (PANS), which can, in part, be recognized by an abrupt onset of moderate to severe OCD symptoms and is often episodic. Further characteristics that commonly occur in PANS include greater emotional lability and deterioration in handwriting. Antistreptolysin O, antistreptococcal DNAase B titer, group A streptococcal nucleic acid amplification test (NAAT), and throat culture assist in diagnosing a group A β-hemolytic streptococcal infection.

The differential diagnosis for OCD includes depression, other obsessive-compulsive and related disorders (e.g., hoarding, trichotillomania), psychotic disorders, tic disorders, anxiety disorders, and OCPD. Although some children with OCD may have poor insight, they present with clear obsessions/compulsions that distinguish them from delusions. They do not have hallucinations, which helps to distinguish them from schizophrenia spectrum disorders. This may be at times difficult to discern; a delusional fixation on appearance in body dysmorphic disorder and impulsive hair pulling to relieve anxiety or tension in trichotillomania can be confused with OCD. OCPD is a character style involving preoccupation with orderliness, perfectionism, and control. It can be distinguished from OCD in that no true obsessions or compulsions are present in OCPD. If symptoms of both conditions are present, they can be co-morbid, although this is rare.

A thorough history and physical examination is crucial and may reveal rough, cracked skin as evidence of excessive handwashing. Many children also express concerns of persistent fear of illness, concerns regarding the health of family members, and the fear that something bad will happen to someone. The Yale-Brown Obsessive-Compulsive Scale (Y-BOCS) is regarded as the gold standard measure of obsessive-compulsive symptom severity. Although somewhat lengthy, it can be helpful in the clinical setting.

Cognitive-behavioral therapy (CBT) is considered the **treatment** of choice in mild to moderate cases. CBT provides durability of symptom relief and avoidance of potential pharmacotherapy-associated side effects. CBT involves gradually exposing the children to their fear/obsession paired with strategies that target preventing them from performing the unwanted ritual/compulsion. Over time with repeated exposure and response prevention, the urge to repeat the compulsion(s) dissipates. Individual, group, and virtual models have proven effective in ameliorating symptoms. The combination of medications and CBT has shown the best response.

Selective serotonin reuptake inhibitors (SSRIs) are recommended for higher severity of symptoms, with complications or with co-morbidities, when adherence with therapy is low, or when cognitive or emotional ability is insufficient to demonstrate success in CBT. Additionally, if quality CBT is not available, treatment with medications alone while psychotherapy referral is pursued is a reasonable choice.

SSRI (e.g., paroxetine, fluoxetine, fluvoxamine, sertraline, citalopram, and escitalopram) treatment shows a favorable risk:benefit ratio in OCD. An 8- to 12-week trial is recommended; symptom improvement may be seen as early as 2 weeks following the initiation of treatment. Side effects such as activation, akathisia, disinhibition, impulsivity, and hyperactivity may be seen. Monitoring of growth may be advisable due to possible growth suppression associated with the SSRIs.

Common protocols suggest up to three trials of different SSRIs, and, if unsuccessful, clomipramine (tricyclic antidepressant) can be attempted. Careful monitoring for potential anticholinergic side effects (including lowering of blood pressure) and EKG monitoring are necessary. Combination therapy using an SSRI with an antipsychotic medication (risperidone or another atypical antipsychotic) may also be considered, especially with specific co-morbidities (e.g., tic disorders). Antipsychotics may also be useful when the intrusive thoughts associated with OCD become nearly delusional in nature. Patients with both OCD and co-morbid ADHD may benefit from psychostimulants, but there is potential for increased obsessional symptoms and tics with these medications. Suicidal ideation in children can occur and should be closely monitored, especially with increasing symptom severity and depressive co-morbidities.

Most responders exhibit partial response only; as many as 30% of young people with OCD are refractory to treatment. Poor prognostic factors include co-morbid psychiatric illness, high symptom severity, poor adherence with treatment, and a poor initial treatment response.

Deep brain stimulation of the basal ganglia, through surgically implanted electrodes and surgical interventions (anterior capsulotomy, anterior cingulotomy, subcaudate tractotomy, and limbic leucotomy), is reserved for very severe or highly refractory cases. Transcranial magnetic stimulation (TMS) has also shown good promise as a treatment for refractory OCD but is not FDA approved in pediatric patients.

PEARLS FOR PRACTITIONERS

See Psychiatric Disorders: Pearls for Practitioners at the end of this section.

REVIEW QUESTIONS

Available online.

CHAPTER 20

Pervasive Developmental Disorders and Psychoses

Autism spectrum disorder (**ASD**; Table 20.1) involves persistent difficulties with social communication and restricted, repetitive patterns of behavior (RRPB). For ASD there are specifiers of symptom severity in regard to core deficits in the domains of social communication impairments and RRPB. A diagnosis of **social** (pragmatic) **communication disorder (SCD)** may be made in the absence of RRPBs.

Onset of ASD is in infancy and preschool years. Intellectual developmental disorder is common (~40%) in ASD, although approximately 39% demonstrate average to high intelligence scores (however, they often show uneven abilities). About 1 in 36 children in the United States has been identified with ASD according to estimates from the Centers for Disease Control's Autism and Developmental Disabilities Monitoring Network. Although ASD may be identified as young as 1 year, only around 49% of children with ASD are diagnosed by 3 years of age (with a higher percentage of those being identified with a co-morbid intellectual developmental disorder). Males are diagnosed much more frequently than females (4:1 ratio); females with the disorder tend to be more severely affected regarding intellectual abilities and symptom severity.

ASD is often characterized by lifelong impairment in social interaction and social communication in addition to RRPBs. Approximately 20% of parents report relatively normal development until 1–2 years of age, followed by a steady or sudden decline. Many infants with ASD display delayed or absent social smiling. Young children may spend extended time in solitary play and be socially withdrawn with limited responsiveness to attempts at communication. Patients with ASD often struggle to understand nonverbal communication (e.g., eye contact, facial expressions) and do not interact with people as significantly different from objects. Communication and speech are often delayed and, when present, may be marked by echolalia (repetition of language of others), perseveration (prolonged repetition of words or behaviors of others), pronoun reversal, nonsense rhyming, and other abnormalities. Intense interests, ritualistic behavior, and compulsive routines are characteristic, and their disruption may invoke behavioral dysregulation. Self-injurious behaviors (head banging, biting), repetitive motor mannerisms (rocking, lining up objects, simple motor stereotypies), and hyperreactivity/hyporeactivity to their environment (diminished response to pain, adverse reactions to sounds/textures, or unusual visual inspection of objects) are common.

There is an increased risk of ASD in siblings compared to the general population. Twin studies have revealed high concordance rates (60–90%) for identical twins. Family studies reveal prevalence rates of around 20% in siblings, and when absent, there may be increased risk for other language, learning, and social development difficulties.

Although the full etiology of ASD is unknown, it is largely considered a genetic disorder given the high concordance rates. There are several common genes *(SHANK3, CHD8, SYNGAP1)* associated with ASD, and a genetic cause (e.g., chromosomal abnormalities, copy number variants, and

TABLE 20.1 Criteria for Diagnosis of Autism Spectrum Disorder

A. Persistent deficits in social communication and social interaction across multiple contexts, as manifested by the following, currently or by history (examples are illustrative, not exhaustive):
   1. Deficits in social-emotional reciprocity, ranging, for example, from abnormal social approach and failure of normal back-and-forth conversation; to reduced sharing of interests, emotions, or affect to failure to initiate or respond to social interactions
   2. Deficits in nonverbal communicative behaviors used for social interaction, ranging, for example, from poorly integrated verbal and nonverbal communication to abnormalities in eye contact and body language or deficits in understanding and use of gestures to a total lack of facial expressions and nonverbal communication
   3. Deficits in developing, maintaining, and understanding relationships, ranging, for example, from difficulties adjusting behavior to suit various social contexts to difficulties in sharing imaginative play or in making friends to absence of interest in peers

B. Restricted, repetitive patterns of behavior, interests, or activities, as manifested by at least two of the following, currently or by history (examples are illustrative, not exhaustive):
   1. Stereotyped or repetitive motor movements, use of objects, or speech (e.g., simple motor stereotypies, lining up toys or flipping objects, echolalia, idiosyncratic phrases)
   2. Insistence on sameness, inflexible adherence to routines, or ritualized patterns of verbal or nonverbal behavior (e.g., extreme distress at small changes, difficulties with transitions, rigid thinking patterns, greeting rituals, need to take same route or eat same food every day)
   3. Highly restricted, fixated interests that are abnormal in intensity or focus (e.g., strong attachment to or preoccupation with unusual objects, excessively circumscribed or perseverative interests)
   4. Hyperreactivity or hyporeactivity to sensory input or unusual interest in sensory aspects of the environment (e.g., apparent indifference to pain/temperature, adverse response to specific sounds or textures, excessive smelling or touching of objects, visual fascination with lights or movement)

C. Symptoms must be present in the early developmental period (but may not become fully manifest until social demands exceed limited capacities or may be masked by learned strategies in later life).

D. Symptoms cause clinically significant impairment in social, occupational, or other important areas of current functioning.

E. These disturbances are not better explained by intellectual developmental disorder (intellectual disability) or global developmental delay. Intellectual developmental disorder and autism spectrum disorder frequently co-occur; to make co-morbid diagnoses of autism spectrum disorder and intellectual developmental disorder, social communication should be below that expected for general developmental level.

Note: Individuals with a well-established DSM-IV diagnosis of autistic disorder, Asperger disorder, or pervasive developmental disorder not otherwise specified should be given the diagnosis of autism spectrum disorder. Individuals who have marked deficits in social communication but whose symptoms do not otherwise meet criteria for autism spectrum disorder should be evaluated for social (pragmatic) communication disorder.

Specify current severity based on social communication impairments and restricted, repetitive patterns of behavior:
Requiring very substantial support
Requiring substantial support
Requiring support
Specify if:
With or without accompanying intellectual impairment
With or without accompanying language impairment
Specify if:
Associated with a known genetic or other medical condition or environmental factor
Associated with another neurodevelopmental, mental, or behavioral problem
Specify if:
With catatonia (refer to the criteria for catatonia associated with another mental disorder)

Reprinted with permission from the Diagnostic and Statistical Manual of Mental Disorders, Fifth Edition, Text Revision (Copyright © 2022). American Psychiatric Association. All Rights Reserved.

changes in single genes) is identified in approximately 20% of patients. Some environmental factors (e.g., prenatal exposure to some medications, alcohol, heavy metals, and rubella infection) have also been observed.

Brain connectivity in patients with ASD is adversely affected, with abnormalities in the limbic system, temporal, and frontal lobes. Postmortem studies reveal abnormalities in the brain microarchitecture, size, and neuronal packing. Functional magnetic resonance imaging (fMRI) studies show that hypoactivity of the fusiform gyrus of the amygdala, a location involved in face processing tasks and facial expression recognition involved in social and affective judgments, may be impacted in ASD.

There is no definitive lab testing for ASD, but they can help evaluate other diagnoses. A hearing test (may account for the language deficits), genetic testing (to identify fragile X syndrome, tuberous sclerosis, chromosomal duplications or deletions and specific genetic syndromes), and tests for congenital viral infections and metabolic disorders (phenylketonuria) should be performed. Electroencephalography abnormalities may be seen in 20–25% of children with ASD, but they are not diagnostic.

The American Academy of Pediatrics (AAP) recommends screening all children for autism at 18 and 24 months of age. There are numerous screening tools that may be employed (e.g., Childhood Autism Rating Scale, 2nd edition [CARS2], Modified Checklist for Autism in Toddlers–Revised [M-CHAT-R], Gilliam Autism Rating Scale, 3rd edition [GARS3], and Screening Tool for Autism in Toddlers and Young Children [STAT]) to aid in appropriate referral for diagnostic evaluation. Gold standard psychologic measures such as the Autism Diagnostic Observation Schedule–2nd edition (ADOS-2) and Autism Diagnostic Interview–Revised (ADI-R) are commonly recommended to confirm a diagnosis. Additionally, measures of language, adaptive skills, and intelligence are commonly administered if ASD is suspected. Neurocognitive tests in children with ASD often show relative strengths in nonverbal tasks (e.g., puzzles) and weaknesses in verbal abilities. Speech pathology consultation can be helpful in evaluating the communication difficulties.

Common psychiatric co-morbidities with ASD include intellectual developmental disorder, language disorders, anxiety disorders, ADHD, developmental coordination disorder, and depressive disorders. Other medical complexities commonly seen in children with ASD include seizures, sleep disorders, constipation, and food selectivity or ARFID (which may produce nutritional deficiencies of vitamin B_{12}, vitamin C, protein, and iron).

SCD involves struggles with using communication for social purposes (e.g., greeting others, sharing information, conversational rules, inferences, and pragmatic skills). SCD is marked by many of the same communication deficits seen in children with ASD with the absence of RRPBs. SCD is believed to be rare in children prior to 4 years of age. The estimated prevalence in the population is between 7 and 11%. Speech and language therapy and social skills training are employed to treat SCD.

Treatment of ASD is multimodal. There are no pharmacologic treatments for the core symptoms of ASDs. FDA approved antipsychotics (risperidone and aripiprazole) for children ages 5–16 years and 6–17 years, respectively, are used for aggression, agitation, irritability, and self-injurious behavior. Off-label antipsychotics and some anticonvulsants have also been used for aggression. Naltrexone has been used to decrease self-injurious behavior, presumably by blocking endogenous opioids. Selective serotonin reuptake inhibitors are used for anxiety, perseveration, compulsions, depression, and social isolation. Stimulants target hyperactivity and inattention; there are reports of worsening of irritability and aggression in some patients treated with stimulants. α_2 agonists (guanfacine, clonidine) are used for hyperactivity, aggression, and sleep dysregulation, although melatonin is first-line medication for sleep dysregulation.

Most treatments for ASD are nonpharmacologic. The most effective interventions have largely fallen under the classification of behavioral training. Treatment models employ therapies individually tailored for children with ASD and their families/caregivers. Evidence suggests that useful therapies have included techniques from applied behavior analysis (ABA), discrete trial training (DTT), pivotal response training (PRT), functional behavioral analysis (FBA), and structured teaching (TEACCH model). Behavioral management training for caregivers has also demonstrated efficacy in helping with unwanted behaviors. Interventions for building social skills, such as the use of social stories, social skills training, and relationship development interventions (RDI), are often employed. Special education services should be individualized for the child and should be aimed at maximizing functioning. Occupational, speech, and physical therapy are often required. Referrals for disability services, family support groups, and individual supportive counseling for caregivers are useful. The prognosis for ASD varies greatly from child to child. There is a wide range (5–79%) of individuals demonstrating independent living skills with cognitive abilities and language abilities being the strongest predictors of improved long-term prognosis. There are no known methods of primary prevention.

SCHIZOPHRENIA SPECTRUM DISORDERS

Schizophrenia generally presents in adolescence or early adulthood. Diagnostic criteria in children are the same as in adults but must be interpreted in terms of the developmental level of the child (Table 20.2). Schizophrenia requires two or more of the core features of a **psychotic disorder** (delusion, hallucinations, disorganized speech, disorganized/catatonic behavior, negative symptoms) to be present, with at least one of the first three **positive symptoms** also being present. Although not in the diagnostic criteria, patients may also widely experience deficits in executive functioning (e.g., processing speed and working memory).

TABLE 20.2 Criteria for Diagnosis of Brief Psychotic Disorder

A. Presence of one (or more) of the following symptoms. At least one of these must be (1), (2), or (3):
1. Delusions
2. Hallucinations
3. Disorganized speech (e.g., frequent derailment or incoherence)
4. Grossly disorganized or catatonic behavior

Note: Do not include a symptom if it is a culturally sanctioned response.

B. Duration of an episode of the disturbance is at least 1 day but less than 1 month, with eventual full return to premorbid level of functioning.

C. The disturbance is not better explained by major depressive or bipolar disorder with psychotic features or another psychotic disorder such as schizophrenia or catatonia and is not attributable to the physiological effects of a substance (e.g., a drug of abuse, a medication) or another medical condition.

Specify if:

With marked stressor(s) (brief reactive psychosis): If symptoms occur in response to events that, singly or together, would be markedly stressful to almost anyone in similar circumstances in the individual's culture.

Without marked stressor(s): If the symptoms do not occur in response to events that, singly or together, would be markedly stressful to almost anyone in similar circumstances in the individual's culture.

With peripartum onset: If onset is during pregnancy or within 4 weeks postpartum

Specify if:

With catatonia

Specify current severity:

Severity is rated by a quantitative assessment of the primary symptoms of psychosis, including delusions, hallucinations, disorganized speech, abnormal psychomotor behavior, and negative symptoms. Each of these symptoms may be rated for its current severity (most severe in the last 7 days) on a 5-point scale ranging from 0 (*not present*) to 4 (*present and severe*).

Note: Diagnosis of brief psychotic disorder can be made without using this severity specifier.

Reprinted with permission from the Diagnostic and Statistical Manual of Mental Disorders, Fifth Edition, Text Revision (Copyright © 2022). American Psychiatric Association. All Rights Reserved.

Childhood-onset schizophrenia (COS) is rare (<1 in 10,000 children) and usually indicates a more severe form of the disorder. The frequency increases between 13 and 18 years of age, typically with psychotic features presenting initially. The incidence in males is slightly greater than that in females, and the age of onset tends to be later for females. The etiology of schizophrenia is unknown, but there is a substantial genetic predisposition for the disorder (accounting for up to 80% of the risk for schizophrenia). Family studies consistently show a high concordance rate in monozygotic twins (60%) compared with dizygotic twins and siblings. First-degree relatives of patients with schizophrenia have a 10-fold higher risk.

The symptoms of schizophrenia fall into four broad categories:

- Positive symptoms include hallucinations and delusions. Hallucinations are auditory or visual misperceptions that occur without external stimuli. Delusions are fixed false beliefs and can be bizarre or non-bizarre depending on cultural norms.

- Negative symptoms include a lack of motivation, poor social interactions, and flat affect. Negative symptoms are more common in early childhood and later adolescence. Children with high intelligence often show more positive and fewer negative symptoms.
- Disorganization of thoughts and behavior can cause significant impairment.
- Cognitive impairment is common and is perhaps the most disabling feature of schizophrenia, causing marked social and functional impairment.

To meet criteria for schizophrenia, clinical symptoms should be present for at least 6 months. If symptoms are present for less than 1 month, the condition is called a **brief psychotic disorder**. If symptoms are present for more than 1 month but less than 6 months, a diagnosis of **schizophreniform disorder** is made. Psychotic symptoms that do not meet full diagnostic criteria for schizophrenia but are clinically significant are diagnosed as an **unspecified schizophrenia spectrum or other psychotic disorder**. The differential diagnosis of a schizophrenia spectrum disorder commonly includes ASD, neurocognitive disorders, substance-induced psychosis, bipolar disorders, major depressive disorder with psychotic features, post-traumatic stress disorder, organic brain disorders, and autoimmune encephalitis.

There are several disorders that also fall within the spectrum of schizophrenia and other psychotic disorders that should be distinguished from schizophrenia. These include the following:

- **Schizoaffective disorder** is diagnosed when a person has clear symptoms of schizophrenia lasting at least 2 weeks and experiences a major mood episode (major depression/mania) during an uninterrupted period of the illness. These affective episodes occur at other times, even when psychotic symptoms are present. This condition is very rare in children and has a lifetime prevalence that is much lower than schizophrenia (0.3% lifetime prevalence).
- **Psychotic disorder due to another medical condition** describes psychotic symptoms that are the direct result of a general medical condition. There are a variety of potential underlying medical etiologies seen in children with epilepsy, metabolic disorders, and autoimmune encephalitis, and systemic lupus erythematosus being the most common.
- **Substance/medication-induced psychotic disorders** involve psychotic symptoms related to substance intoxication or withdrawal or follow exposure to a medication. Although prevalence is unknown, estimates suggest that between 7 and 25% of first episodes of psychoses are related to substances.

No laboratory tests or imaging studies are diagnostic for schizophrenia; rather, it is a clinical diagnosis based on symptoms. Obtaining a family history with attention to mental illness is critical. Assessing other known risk factors (prenatal complications, childhood trauma, drug use) is also valuable. Synthetic or natural cannabinoids (especially when used at a younger age and in heavy amounts) may induce psychotic effects and are a known risk factor for schizophrenia. Identifying schizophrenia should include a physical and neurologic examination, MRI, substance/drug screening, electroencephalography (temporal lobe epilepsy and autoimmune encephalitis), and metabolic screening. Evaluation for Wilson disease and delirium is also indicated. Psychotic symptoms in younger children must be differentiated from manifestations of normal vivid fantasy life or abuse-related symptoms. Youth with PTSD often have vivid recollections and nightmares related to abuse but sometimes are less specific and can include nightmares with other negative topics. Psychologic testing can also be helpful in identifying psychotic thought processes and cognitive impairments (e.g., executive functioning and memory deficits). Risk factors for poor prognosis include onset at an age younger than 13 years, poor premorbid function, presence of marked negative symptoms, and a family history of schizophrenia. The Brief Psychiatric Rating Scale for Children (BPRS-C) and the Positive and Negative Syndrome Scale for children (Kiddie-PANSS) are also useful in assessing the symptoms and severity changes in children with suspected and/or identified schizophrenia spectrum disorders.

Treatment is multimodal and frequently includes the use of antipsychotic medications. First-line drugs are second-generation antipsychotics (SGA)/atypical antipsychotics (e.g., risperidone, olanzapine, quetiapine, aripiprazole, ziprasidone, and paliperidone). Second-line medications are first-generation antipsychotics (FGA)/typical antipsychotics (e.g., haloperidol, thiothixene, chlorpromazine, trifluoperazine, loxapine, and molindone). Atypical antipsychotics have fewer extrapyramidal side effects and result in less tardive dyskinesia; some (i.e., clozapine and olanzapine) have a higher risk of weight gain or metabolic syndrome.

The U.S. FDA has approved five SGAs (aripiprazole, olanzapine, paliperidone, quetiapine, and risperidone) for use in children with schizophrenia as young as 12 years of age. Antipsychotics can be augmented with lithium or another mood stabilizer. Clozapine is generally reserved for resistant cases. Prepubertal children are less responsive to antipsychotics and adolescents, although demonstrating efficacy with the medications, may not reach the level of full efficacy seen in adults.

Psychosocial treatments, including skills training, supportive psychotherapy, behavior modification, and cognitive-behavioral therapy, are all appropriate and should be considered as needed for individual patients. Attention should be paid to psychoeducation for caregivers and the child about the disease and its treatments. School interventions are needed to ensure that any special learning needs are addressed. Schizophrenia spectrum disorders also carry a high risk for suicidality (5–10% lifetime completion rate), and ideation should be re-evaluated throughout treatment. Co-morbid depressive symptoms increase the risk for suicide.

PEARLS FOR PRACTITIONERS

See Psychiatric Disorders: Pearls for Practitioners at the end of this section.

REVIEW QUESTIONS

Available online.

Suggested Readings

American Psychiatric Association (APA). *Practice Guidelines.* Washington, DC: American Psychiatric Association. Available at http://psychiatryonline.org/guidelines. Accessed 29 August 2024.

Comer JS, Hong N, Poznanski B, Silva K, Wilson M. Evidence base update on the treatment of early childhood anxiety and related problems. *J Clin Child Adolesc Psychol.* 2019;48(1):1–15.

Hirota K, King J. Autism spectrum disorder: a review. *JAMA*. 2023;329(2):157–168.
Melin K, Skarphedinsson G, Thomsen PH, et al. Treatment gains are sustainable in pediatric obsessive-compulsive disorder: three-year follow-up from the NordLOTS. *J Am Acad Child Adolesc Psychiatry*. 2020;59(2):244–253.
Orefici G, Cardona F, Cox CJ, et al. Pediatric autoimmune neuropsychiatric disorders associated with streptococcal infections (PANDAS). In: Ferretti JJ, Stevens DL, Fischetti VA, eds. *Streptococcus Pyogenes: Basic Biology to Clinical Manifestations*. Oklahoma City, OK: University of Oklahoma Health Sciences Center; 2016.
Van Geelen SM, Rydelius PA, Hagquist C. Somatic symptoms and psychological concerns in a general adolescent population: exploring the relevance of DSM-5 somatic symptom disorder. *J Psychosom Res*. 2015;9(4):251–258.
Vassilopoulos A, Mohammad S, Dure L, et al. Treatment approaches for functional neurological disorders in children. *Curr Treat Options Neurol*. 2022;24:77–97.

PEARLS FOR PRACTITIONERS

CHAPTER 16

Somatic Symptom and Related Disorders

- Disorders in the somatic symptom and related disorders (SSRD) group include somatic symptom disorder (SSD), functional neurological symptom disorder (FNSD), illness anxiety disorder, factitious disorder, and psychologic factors affecting other medical conditions.
- All SSRDs share a common feature: somatic symptoms and/or illness anxiety associated with significant distress and impairment.
- Children with SSRDs are more likely to have difficulty expressing emotional distress, come from families with a history of marital conflict, have experienced adverse childhood experiences, or have a family member with a history of physical illness.
- Adolescent females tend to report nearly twice as many somatic symptoms as males; prior to puberty the ratio is equal.
- Common systemic medical disorders presenting with unexplained physical symptoms include myalgic encephalomyelitis/chronic fatigue syndrome (ME/CFS), multiple sclerosis, myasthenia gravis, endocrine disorders, chronic systemic infections, vocal cord dysfunction, periodic paralysis, acute intermittent porphyria, fibromyalgia, irritable bowel syndrome, polymyositis, and other myopathies.
- Somatic symptom disorder (SSD) involves one or more somatic symptoms that are distressing or result in significant disruption in daily life. Key symptoms of the disorder often involve excessive thoughts, feelings, or behaviors regarding the somatic complaint (e.g., excessive fatigue or pain).
- Functional neurological symptom disorder (FNSD), previously conversion disorder, involves symptoms affecting voluntary motor or sensory function and is suggestive of a neurologic illness in the absence of a disease process.
- Psychological factors affecting other medical conditions are marked by psychological or behavioral factors that adversely impact a medical condition by increasing the risk for suffering, death, or disability. The factors interfere with the treatment of a medical condition (e.g., anxiety exacerbating asthma, poor medication adherence).
- Factitious disorder is a condition in which physical or psychologic symptoms are produced intentionally and often with the intent to assume a sick role. The falsification of physical and psychologic symptoms may also present as imposing illness or injury on another person (factitious disorder imposed on another [FDIA]).
- Malingering involves the purposeful falsification or exaggeration of physical and/or psychologic symptoms for external gain (e.g., money, avoidance of school, work). The key feature of malingering is the seeking of an external reward.
- Screening tools for SSRDs include adapted caregiver versions of the Patient Health Questionnaire–15 (PHQ-15), the Somatic Symptom Scale–8 (SSS-8), and the Somatic Symptom Disorder–B Criteria Scale. The Children's Somatic Symptoms Inventory (CSSI) is also available as a self-report measure of somatic distress for children ages 8–17 years.
- Selective serotonin reuptake inhibitors (SSRIs) may benefit SSRDs involving unexplained headaches, fibromyalgia, body dysmorphic disorder, pain disorder, irritable bowel syndrome, and functional gastrointestinal disorders.
- Tricyclic antidepressants should be avoided in youth with functional abdominal pain (FAP); they have little proven efficacy and are very dangerous in overdose.
- Stimulants may also be helpful in myalgic encephalomyelitis/chronic fatigue syndrome (ME/CFS).
- Therapy, such as cognitive-behavioral therapy (CBT), has demonstrated efficacy in treating recurrent pain, ME/CFS, fibromyalgia, and FAP. Self-management strategies (self-monitoring, relaxation, hypnosis, and biofeedback) are also effective.
- For patients with SSRDs, home schooling should be avoided, school attendance and performance should be emphasized, parents should limit attention/reinforcement for pain behavior, and normal routines/appropriate schedules (e.g., going to school) should be emphasized.

CHAPTER 17

Anxiety and Phobias

- Anxiety disorders are characterized by uneasiness, excessive rumination, and apprehension about the future.

  - They tend to be chronic, recurring, and vary in intensity over time.
  - Medical conditions (e.g., hyperthyroidism, medication side effects, and substance use disorder) should be ruled out.
  - The most common co-morbid psychiatric disorders include mood disorders, eating disorders (i.e., avoidant/restrictive food intake disorder [ARFID]), tic disorders, and behavioral disorders.
- Panic disorder is the presence of recurrent, unexpected panic attacks (a sudden unexpected onset of intense fear associated with a feeling of impending doom in the absence of real danger).
  - The most common symptoms in children include shortness of breath, palpitations, chest pain, a choking sensation, and a fear of losing control.
  - Adolescents tend to have higher rates of cardiovascular, respiratory, gastrointestinal, and other medical problems as adults.
- Generalized anxiety disorder (GAD) is characterized by excessive worry and anxiety about a variety of situations or activities. Common symptoms include restlessness, fatigue, concentration difficulties, irritability, muscle tension, or sleep disturbance.
  - Children are often exceedingly self-conscious, have low self-esteem, and have more sleep disturbance than patients with other anxiety disorders.
- Separation anxiety disorder (SAD) is marked by excessive distress or concern when separating from a major attachment figure.
  - Vague somatic symptoms (e.g., headaches, abdominal pain, fatigue) are common and children may refuse to go to school or leave their home.
- Selective mutism is diagnosed for children who consistently fail to speak in one or more social settings despite adequate receptive and expressive language skills.
  - Between 25 and 50% of children exhibit some history of speech delay or speech disorder and a majority also present with social anxiety disorder.
- Social anxiety disorder is characterized by a marked and persistent fear of social or performance situations in which one may offend others and/or embarrassment might occur.
  - Most individuals are identified prior to 15 years of age, and if left untreated or poorly treated, it can become immobilizing and result in significant functional impairments; approximately a third of individuals experience remission of symptoms within 1 year if untreated.
- Specific phobias are marked, persistent fears of specific things/objects or situations that often lead to avoidance behaviors.
- Agoraphobia is a disorder marked by fear of situations where escape is difficult or would draw unwanted attention to the person.
  - Commonly presents in adolescence or young adulthood, with females being twice as likely to experience the disorder. In children, being outside of the home alone and worries regarding becoming lost are common complaints.
- Validated screening tools can be helpful in identifying anxiety disorders and include measures such as the Youth Anxiety Measure (YAM), Screen for Child Anxiety–Related Emotional Disorders (SCARED), Anxiety Disorder Interview Schedule (ADIS), and the Pediatric Anxiety Rating Scale (PARS).
- First-line treatment for mild to moderate anxiety includes evidence-based psychotherapies and psychoeducation. Cognitive-behavioral therapy (e.g., systematic desensitization, exposure techniques, operant conditioning, modeling, and cognitive restructuring) can be beneficial in anxiety disorders.
- SSRIs are the medication of choice for anxiety, and FDA-approved SSRIs for children are fluoxetine, sertraline, escitalopram, and fluvoxamine. They can initially exacerbate anxiety or even panic symptoms. Tricyclic antidepressants have also shown efficacy.
- For children with anxiety, benzodiazepines (e.g., clonazepam) include a risk of causing disinhibition. α2a agonists (guanfacine and clonidine) may be useful with autonomic symptoms. Anticonvulsant agents (e.g., gabapentin) are used when other agents are ineffective. β blockers help with performance anxiety.

CHAPTER 18

Depression and Bipolar Disorders

Depressive Disorders

- Depressive disorders involve the presence of sad/irritable mood along with physical and cognitive impacts on the child's daily functioning.
- In children, depressed mood often presents as irritability and/or restlessness. Furthermore, many children/adolescents complain of pervasive boredom in major depressive disorder (MDD).
- Many depressive disorders demonstrate genetic predispositions. Anxiety disorders, substance use disorder, conduct/disruptive disorders, and sleep disorders frequently present as co-morbidities with MDD.
- Onset of MDD in childhood is more likely to be related to bipolar symptoms versus adult-onset bipolar disorder.
- Disruptive mood dysregulation disorder (DMDD) includes children ages 6–18 years who present with a chronic (≥12 months) pattern of severe irritability and behavioral dysregulation. DMDD exhibits chronic/persistent symptoms and bipolar disorder presents with episodic mood changes.
- Screening tools such as Children's Depression Inventory (CDI 2) and the Patient Health Questionnaire Modified for Adolescents (PHQ9-A) may be helpful.
- Medically, conditions such as hypothyroidism, anemia, diabetes, and folate and B_{12} vitamin deficiencies need to be ruled out.
- SSRIs are first-line pharmacologic treatments. Fluoxetine is the only medication approved by the FDA for treatment in

youth 8 years and older, and escitalopram is approved for youth 12 and older.

- An antidepressant should be given an adequate trial (6 weeks at therapeutic doses) before switching or discontinuing unless there are serious side effects. For a first episode of depression, treatment for 6–9 months after remission of symptoms is recommended.
- Psychotherapy has good efficacy in mild to moderate depression. In moderate to severe depression, combined treatment with psychotherapy and medication has the greatest rate of response, and CBT and interpersonal therapies have received the most empirical support.
- Suicidal ideation and attempts at suicide are high in depressive disorders. Regular assessment of suicidal ideation should occur.
- Although the risk of suicide during an MDD episode is high, it can be paradoxically higher during start of treatment, as energy and motivation improve with cognitive recovery from depression.

Bipolar Disorders (BDs)

- Consist of distinct periods of mania (elevated, expansive, or irritable mood) and persistent goal-directed activity or energy that may alternate with periods of severe depression.
- Often present with rapid shifts in mood or lability over brief time frames (e.g., shifting between euphoria and dysphoria or irritability). A decreased need for sleep is also common.
- A first-degree relative with BD is associated with a 10-fold increase in a child's chance of developing BD.
- Self-report scales for depression such as the PHQ9-A and CDI 2 may aid in diagnosis and can be paired with severity rating scales such as the Children's Depression Rating Scale–Revised (CDRS-R) and the Young Mania Rating Scale (YMRS) to guide diagnosis and treatment.
- FDA-approved medications including lithium, divalproex sodium, olanzapine, risperidone, quetiapine, lurasidone, asenapine, and aripiprazole are available for patients with BD. Lithium is used in acute episodes and as a maintenance treatment in children and adolescents but requires periodic monitoring of blood levels.
- Anticonvulsants are used for mixed or rapid cycling cases in adults. They have also been used effectively in youth, but they are not FDA approved in children for BD.
- Neuroleptics have had positive results in youth with BD; the increased risk of tardive dyskinesia should be considered in using such agents.
- When compared with depression, the rates of suicidal ideation and suicide are higher in BD.

CHAPTER 19

Obsessive-Compulsive Disorder

- Obsessive-compulsive disorder (OCD) is characterized by obsessions, compulsions, or both in the absence of another psychiatric disorder that better explains the symptoms.
- Obsessions (e.g., fears of contamination, fears of dirt/germs, repeated doubts, aggressive thoughts, and orderliness/precision) involve recurrent intrusive thoughts, images, or impulses.
- Compulsions (e.g., grooming, ordering, checking, requesting reassurance, praying, counting, repeating words silently, and touching rituals) are repetitive nongratifying behaviors that a person feels driven to perform to reduce or prevent distress or anxiety.
- Up to 50% of youth with OCD have at least one other psychiatric illness. Rituals/compulsive symptoms often predominate over worries or obsessions, and symptoms may or may not be recognized as being excessive or unreasonable.
- Up to 10% of OCD in children may be a result of pediatric autoimmune neuropsychiatric disorders associated with streptococcal (PANDAS) infection. This subset of diagnoses is characterized by an abrupt onset of moderate to severe OCD symptoms, which are often episodic. PANDAS patients may also display greater emotional lability and deterioration in handwriting.
- The Yale-Brown Obsessive-Compulsive Scale (Y-BOCS) is regarded as the gold standard measure of obsessive-compulsive symptom severity.
- CBT involving exposure and response prevention is considered the treatment of choice in mild to moderate cases of OCD.
- SSRIs are recommended for higher severity of OCD symptoms, with complications with co-morbidities, when adherence with therapy is low, or when cognitive or emotional ability are insufficient to demonstrate success in CBT.
- For treatment of OCD, an 8- to 12-week trial is recommended; symptom improvement may be seen as early as 2 weeks following the initiation of treatment. Side effects include activation, akathisia, disinhibition, impulsivity, and hyperactivity.
- In refractory OCD, up to three trials of an SSRI is common and, if unsuccessful, clomipramine (tricyclic antidepressant) can be attempted. Careful monitoring of potential anticholinergic side effects, lowering of blood pressure, and ECG monitoring is necessary.
- Suicidal ideation in children can occur and should be closely monitored, especially with increasing symptom severity and depressive co-morbidities.

CHAPTER 20

Pervasive Developmental Disorders and Psychoses

Autism Spectrum Disorder (ASD)

- ASD onset is in infancy and preschool years. Core symptoms reflect communication and restricted, repetitive patterns of behavior (RRPB).
- About 1 in 36 children in the United States has been identified with ASD.

- Intellectual disability is common with ASD, and the male:female ratio is 4:1.
- Children with ASD commonly prefer solitary play, are socially withdrawn, struggle to understand nonverbal communication (e.g., eye contact, facial expressions), may demonstrate a delayed/absent social smile, and do not interact with people as significantly different from objects.
- Communication and speech often are delayed with ASD. Intense absorbing interests, ritualistic behavior, and compulsive routines are characteristic.
- Self-injurious behaviors, repetitive motor mannerisms, and hyperreactivity/hyporeactivity to their environment may be noted with ASD.
- Genetic and environmental factors have been found in ASD. Twin concordance rates (60–90%) and sibling rates (20%) suggest the need to obtain a thorough family history.
- No definitive laboratory testing exists for ASD, but they may aid in evaluating other diagnoses. A hearing test, genetic testing, and an electroencephalograph may be useful but are not diagnostic.
- Screening at 18 and 24 months (e.g., CARS2, M-CHAT-R, GARS3, and STAT) and gold standard psychologic measures (i.e., Autism Diagnostic Observation Schedule [ADOS-2] and Autism Diagnostic Interview [ADI-R]) are recommended to confirm ASD.
- Social communication disorder (SCD) is marked by many of the same communication deficits seen in children with ASD with the absence of RRPBs and is rarely diagnosed in children under 4 years of age.
- Nonpharmacologic interventions are first-line for ASD. Therapies have included techniques from applied behavior analysis (ABA), discrete trial training (DTT), pivotal response training (PRT), functional behavioral analysis (FBA), and structured teaching (TEACCH model).
- Occupational, speech, and physical therapy are often required for ASD.
- Interventions for building social skills, such as the use of social stories, social skills training, and relationship development interventions (RDIs) are often employed for ASD.
- There are no pharmacologic treatments for the core symptoms of ASDs. Antipsychotics, anticonvulsants, SSRIs, stimulants, and $\alpha 2$ agonists are commonly used to assist with ameliorating secondary and co-morbid symptoms.

Schizophrenia Spectrum Disorders

- Childhood-onset schizophrenia is rare and involves both positive (hallucinations, delusions) and negative (poor motivation/social interactions, flat affect) symptoms.
- The frequency of schizophrenia increases between 13 and 18 years of age, with psychotic features presenting initially.
- First-degree relatives of patients with schizophrenia have a 10-fold higher risk.
- There are several known risk factors for schizophrenia (prenatal complications, childhood trauma, substance use disorder).
- Synthetic or natural cannabinoids (especially when used at a younger age and in heavy amounts) may induce psychotic effects and are a known risk factor for schizophrenia.
- No diagnostic tests or imaging studies are specific for schizophrenia. It is a clinical diagnosis based on symptoms.
- Work-up for schizophrenia should include a physical and neurologic examination, MRI, electroencephalography. drug screening, and metabolic screening for endocrinopathies. Evaluation for Wilson disease and delirium is also indicated.
- The Brief Psychiatric Rating Scale for Children (BPRS-C) and the Positive and Negative Syndrome Scale for children (Kiddie-PANSS) are also useful in assessing the symptoms and severity changes in children with suspected and/or identified schizophrenia spectrum disorders.
- First-line pharmacologic treatment of schizophrenia includes second-generation antipsychotics (SGAs). Second-line medications are first-generation antipsychotics (FGAs). Antipsychotics can be augmented with lithium or another mood stabilizer.
- SGAs have fewer extrapyramidal side effects and result in less tardive dyskinesia; some (i.e., clozapine and olanzapine) have a higher risk of significant weight gain or metabolic syndrome.
- The U.S. FDA has approved five SGAs (aripiprazole, olanzapine, paliperidone, quetiapine, and risperidone) for use in children with schizophrenia as young as 12–13 years of age.
- Prepubertal children with schizophrenia are less responsive to antipsychotics and adolescents, though demonstrating efficacy, may not reach the level of full efficacy seen in adults.
- Psychosocial treatments (e.g., skills training, supportive psychotherapy, behavior modification, and CBT) are all appropriate for schizophrenia and should be considered as needed.

PSYCHOSOCIAL ISSUES

Kristine Fortin | *Alison H. Downes*

CHAPTER 21
Child Abuse and Neglect

Child maltreatment is a significant public health concern given its prevalence and potential impact on health not only during childhood but also later in life. Each year in the United States, approximately 4 million reports are made to child welfare agencies, of which approximately 2 million are screened for child protective services (CPS) response. CPS reports were substantiated/indicated for over 546,000 U.S. children in 2023. Surveys of adults about their childhood experiences indicate that many cases never come to the attention of authorities. Child maltreatment can cause short- and long-term physical, mental, and developmental health problems and can be fatal. Research on adverse childhood experiences (ACEs) has shown an association between childhood maltreatment and negative adult health outcomes, including physical health problems such as cardiovascular disease and obesity, as well as psychosocial health problems such as depression and substance abuse. A growing body of research demonstrates how toxic stressors in childhood can influence brain development and epigenetics.

Child maltreatment is an act or failure to act by a parent or caretaker that results in death, sexual abuse, harm, or imminent risk of harm. States define child abuse and neglect in civil and criminal statutes. In every state, physicians are mandated by law to report all cases of *suspected* child abuse and neglect. Child abuse and neglect result from a complex interaction of individual, family, and societal risk factors. Risk factors for maltreatment, such as parental substance abuse, parental depression, and domestic violence in the household, can alert physicians to potential risk and guide development of child maltreatment prevention strategies. However, risk factors should not be used to determine whether a specific patient is a victim of abuse. At the societal level, abusive head trauma rates increased in the United States during and after the 2008 economic recession, suggesting that macroeconomic factors impact the incidence of child maltreatment. Increased state spending on public benefits, such as Earned Income Tax Credit and childcare assistance, is associated with decreased child maltreatment reports and substantiation. Bias and structural racism are factors leading to racial disparities throughout the continuum of child welfare involvement. Black and Native American/Alaska Native families are more likely to be reported to CPS, receive an investigation, have a substantiated report, and be involved in foster care. Organizations with resources on addressing disproportionality in the child welfare system include Casey Family Programs (https://www.casey.org/racial-equity-topic-page/) and Chapin Hall (https://www.chapinhall.org/wp-content/uploads/Chapin-Hall_LSA-FSI-Toolkit_October-2023.pdf).

Child abuse and neglect are often considered in broad categories that include physical abuse, sexual abuse, emotional abuse, and neglect.

NEGLECT

Neglect is the most commonly reported form of child maltreatment and is broadly defined as omissions that prevent a child's basic needs from being met. Basic needs include adequate nutrition, shelter, education, emotional needs, adequate supervision, and medical and dental care. Poverty can impact provision of food, shelter, and medical care, and there are state and federal policies aimed at separating poverty from neglect. For example, states such as Washington enacted legislation to prevent children from being separated their families based solely on poverty or lack of housing. Pediatric providers can play a role in identifying and supporting family needs such as food and transportation to medical appointments. Different types of neglect have been described, including dental, emotional, medical, physical, and supervisory neglect.

Regarding medical neglect, the American Academy of Pediatrics outlined factors to consider in the evaluation of medical neglect: (1) whether the lack of health care is causing harm or risk of harm to the child; (2) if the potential benefits of the proposed treatments are greater than its potential harms; (3) if health care is accessible but not used; and (4) if the caregiver received and understood medical advice.

Neglect can impact a child's physical, mental, developmental, and behavioral health. Potential physical health consequences include abnormal growth, poor dentition, injuries, ingestions resulting from lack of supervision or environmental hazards, and poorly controlled health problems. Child neglect can contribute to developmental delays, behavioral problems, school difficulties, emotional problems, and attachment problems. Health care providers play an important role in the multidisciplinary response to neglect. Medical interventions could include treating physical health problems such as growth disturbance or injury, simplifying and clarifying treatment plans for chronic conditions, making referrals to community agencies that can assist with concrete needs such as food or transportation, providing developmental assessments and referrals, and referring patients to mental and behavioral health specialists. The approach to neglect involves identification of both contributing factors and strengths and protective factors. Health care providers can play a role in preventing neglect by screening for and helping with potential precipitating factors such as parental depression as well as by providing anticipatory guidance on topics such as supervision and injury prevention tailored to the child's developmental level.

PHYSICAL ABUSE

Physical abuse is second to neglect as the reason for CPS reports and child maltreatment-related fatality. Physical abuse affects children of all ages. While in some cases children can provide a history of the abuse and present with obvious external injuries, in many cases, the diagnosis is not obvious. Abusive injuries are sometimes occult, and children can present with nonspecific symptoms. The history provided by the parent is often inaccurate because the parent is unwilling to provide the correct history or is a nonoffending parent unaware of the abuse. The child may be too young or ill to provide a history of the assault. An older child may be too scared to do so or may have a strong sense of loyalty to the perpetrator. History that seems incongruent with the clinical presentation of the child raises concern for physical abuse (Table 21.1).

Although injury to any organ system can occur from physical abuse, some injuries are more common. **Bruises** are common findings in healthy ambulatory children but also are commonly identified in abused children. Bruising location, pattern, and the child's age/developmental level are important considerations when evaluating bruising. Bruises suggestive of abuse include those that are patterned, such as a slap mark on the face or looped extension cord marks on the body (Fig. 21.1). Bruises in healthy children generally are distributed over bony prominences; bruises that occur in an unusual distribution, such as isolated to the torso, ears, or neck, should raise concern. Bruises in nonambulatory infants are unusual, occurring in less than 2% of healthy infants seen for routine medical care. **TEN-4-FACESp** is a bruising clinical decision rule validated in children younger than 4 years of age to identify need for further evaluation for potential physical abuse. *TEN* refers to bruising to the torso, ear, or neck; *4* refers to bruising on an infant younger than 4.99 months of age; *FACES* refers to bruising on the frenulum, angle of the jaw, cheek (fleshy part of face cheek), eyelid, and subconjunctivae; and *p* refers to bruising with a pattern. Occasionally, a subtle bruise may be the only external clue to abuse and can be associated with significant internal injury. Previous sentinel injuries, such as bruising, are common among infants presenting with severe physical abuse. Appropriate evaluation and intervention when nonmobile infants present with unexplained bruising could prevent escalating abuse.

Burns are common pediatric injuries and usually represent preventable unintentional trauma (see Chapter 43). Approximately 10% of children hospitalized with burns are victims of abuse. Thermal burns are the most common type of burn and can result from scalding injuries or contact with hot objects (e.g., irons, radiators, or cigarettes) (Fig. 21.2). Features of scald burns that are concerning for inflicted trauma include clear lines of demarcation, uniformity of burn depth, and characteristic pattern. Abusive contact burns tend to have distinct margins (branding of the hot object), while accidental contact burns tend to have less distinctive edges.

Inflicted fractures occur more commonly in infants and young children. Although diaphyseal fractures are most common in abuse, they are nonspecific for inflicted injury. Fractures that should raise suspicion for abuse include fractures that are unexplained, especially in young, nonambulatory children and/or those that involve multiple bones. Certain fractures have a high specificity for abuse, such as rib, classic metaphyseal, scapular, vertebral, or other unusual fractures (Fig. 21.3). **Classic metaphyseal lesions (CML)** are fractures through the immature metaphysis. They are sometimes referred to as *corner fractures* or *bucket handle fractures* given their appearance on radiographs. Some metabolic diseases can be confused with abuse and should be considered in the differential diagnosis when appropriate.

Abusive head trauma is the leading cause of mortality and morbidity from physical abuse. Most victims are young; infants predominate. Caregiver intolerance of infant crying is a common precipitator, and many prevention programs provide education on developmentally normal crying as well as coping techniques. Symptoms at the time of presentation to medical care can range from occult head trauma with no neurologic symptoms to irritability, lethargy, vomiting, seizures, apnea, and coma. Unsuspecting physicians misdiagnose approximately one third of infants initially; of these, more than 25% are reinjured before diagnosis. Subdural hemorrhage is a common intracranial injury in children with abusive head trauma (Fig. 21.4). Secondary brain injury can be due to

TABLE 21.1 Clues to the Diagnosis of Physical Abuse

A child presents for medical care with significant injuries and a history of trauma is denied, especially if the child is an infant or toddler.
The history provided by the caregiver does not explain the injuries identified.
The history of the injury changes significantly over time.
A history of self-inflicted trauma does not correlate with the child's developmental abilities.
There is an unexpected or unexplained delay in seeking medical care.
Multiple organ systems are injured, including injuries of various ages.
The injuries have a high specificity for child abuse.

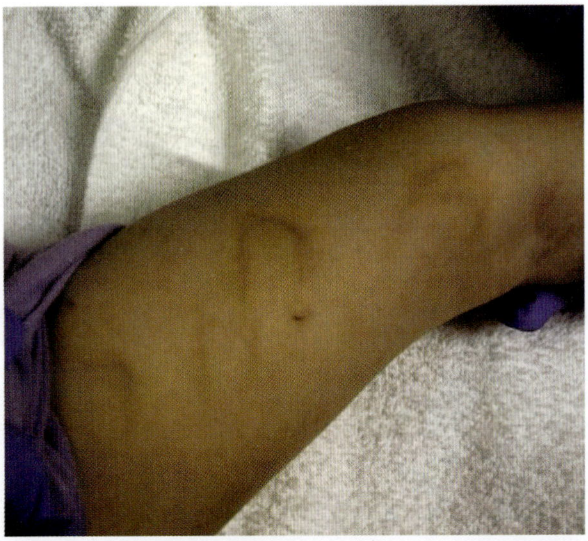

FIGURE 21.1 Multiple looped cord marks on a 2-year-old abused child who presented to the hospital with multiple untreated burns to the back, arms, and feet.

factors such as cerebral edema, hypoxic-ischemic injury, and hypoperfusion. Retinal hemorrhages are seen in many but not all victims. Skeletal trauma, including rib fractures and CMLs, is sometimes present as well. Victims may present with bruising, but often there are no external signs of injury. Survivors are at high risk for permanent neurologic sequelae.

While abdominal injury is not as common as other forms of child physical abuse, it is associated with a high mortality rate. Abdominal trauma is therefore the second leading cause of death from child physical abuse after head injury. Blunt trauma to the abdomen is the primary mechanism of injury; infants and toddlers are the most common victims. Injuries to solid organs such as the liver or pancreas predominate, and hollow viscus injury occurs more commonly with inflicted trauma than accidental. Even in severe cases of trauma, there may be no bruising to the abdominal wall. The lack of external trauma or specific symptoms, along with an inaccurate history, can cause delay in diagnosis. CT scan is the imaging modality of choice in most settings when abusive abdominal trauma is suspected.

The medical evaluation for physical abuse includes taking a detailed history of the events leading up to presentation, presence and timeline of abnormal symptoms, personal and family medical history including birth history and diet for young children, and child development. The physical exam should include a head-to-toe skin examination. Skin injuries to the neck and ears could be missed if these areas are not carefully examined. Attention should be paid to the frenula during the oral exam of young children.

Work-up for physical abuse includes evaluation for occult injury as well as medical conditions that can mimic physical abuse. Children younger than 2 years with suspected physical abuse should undergo a **skeletal survey**

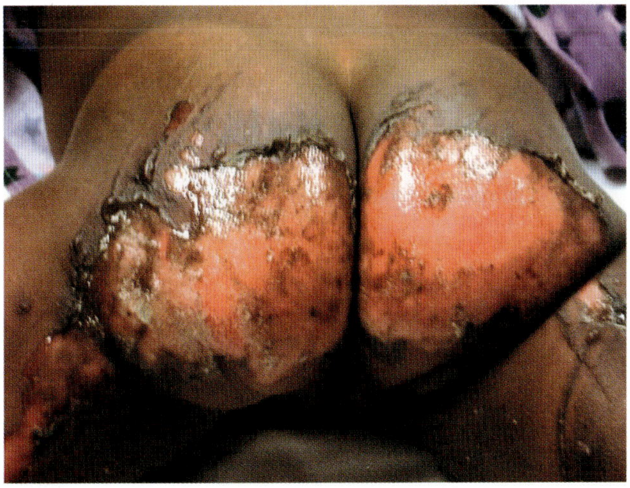

FIGURE 21.2 A 1-year-old child brought to the hospital with a history that the child sat on a hot radiator. Suspicious injuries such as this require a full medical and social investigation, including a skeletal survey to look for occult skeletal injuries and a child welfare evaluation.

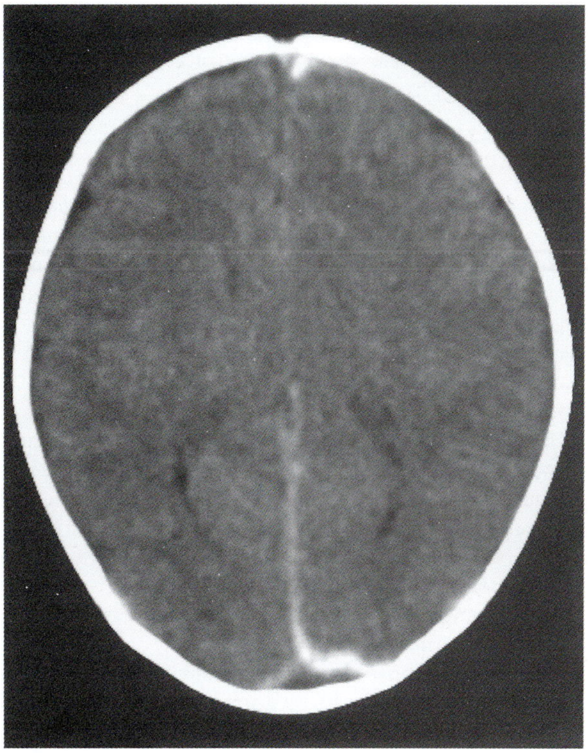

FIGURE 21.4 Acute subdural hemorrhage in the posterior interhemispheric fissure in an abused infant.

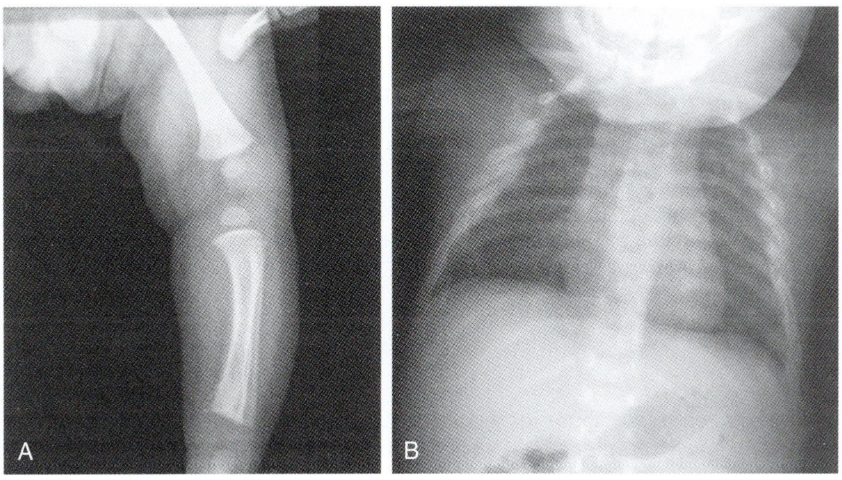

FIGURE 21.3 **(A)** Metaphyseal fracture of the distal tibia in a 3-month-old infant admitted to the hospital with severe head injury. There also is periosteal new bone formation of that tibia, perhaps from a previous injury. **(B)** Follow-up radiograph 2 weeks later showed multiple healing rib fractures. This pattern of fracture is highly specific for child abuse.

per American College of Radiology practice parameters, looking for occult or healing fractures. Infants presenting with extracranial injuries may have occult head trauma, and therefore neuroimaging may be indicated. Laboratory tests including liver transaminases (alanine aminotransferase and aspartate aminotransferase), pancreatic enzymes (amylase and lipase), and urinalysis can be used to screen for occult abdominal injury. The extensive differential diagnosis of physical abuse depends on the type of injury (Table 21.2). For children who present with different types of specific injuries to multiple organ systems, an exhaustive search for medical diagnoses that do not explain the findings is unwarranted. Some medical conditions can be mistaken for abuse, emphasizing the need for careful, objective evaluation of all children. Medical evaluation of household contacts of physically abused children may be useful, including skeletal survey in contacts younger than 2 years as well as physical examination.

MEDICAL CHILD ABUSE

Also referred to as *Munchausen syndrome by proxy, factitious disorder by proxy,* and *caregiver-fabricated illness in a child,* this form of child maltreatment involves a child receiving unnecessary and harmful or potentially harmful medical care at the instigation of a caregiver. Terms proposed to replace *Munchausen syndrome by proxy* shift focus away from the offender to the abuse experienced by the child. Exaggeration, fabrication, and induction of symptoms can lead to unnecessary medical care. *Exaggeration* refers to a pattern of exaggerating the intensity and/or frequency of a child's symptoms. *Fabrication* refers to reporting illness that never occurred (e.g., providing a history of seizure symptoms in a child without these symptoms). *Induction* involves producing signs and symptoms (e.g., by administering medicine that was not prescribed or indicated to produce symptoms or intentionally contaminating a central line to produce infection).

Medical child abuse does not present in a singular way; presenting symptoms can involve any body system. Concerns for medical child abuse may arise when there is a pattern of symptoms only observed or reported by one caregiver, objective findings discordant from reported symptoms, and/or unusual symptoms with an unexpected clinical course. Steps in evaluating for medical child abuse include review of medical records from the different locations care has been sought, noting patterns of misreporting diagnoses or recommendations across care settings, and patterns of inappropriate utilization of care resulting in unnecessary tests and treatments. Discussion with the specialists and primary care providers involved in the child's care is another source of information. Physicians are mandated to report suspected abuse; in addition, harm and risk of harm to the child are important elements to communicate with child welfare professionals. Medical providers can collaborate to deescalate unnecessary care.

TABLE 21.2 Differential Diagnosis of Physical Abuse*

BRUISES
Accidental injury (common in mobile children)
Dermatologic disorders
Dermal melanocytosis (formerly *Mongolian spots*)
Erythema multiforme
Phytophotodermatitis
Hematologic disorders
Idiopathic thrombocytopenic purpura
Leukemia
Hemophilia
Vitamin K deficiency bleeding
Disseminated intravascular coagulopathy
Cultural practices
Cao gio (coining)
Quat sha (spoon rubbing)
Infection
Sepsis
Purpura fulminans (meningococcemia)
Genetic diseases
Ehlers-Danlos syndrome
Familial dysautonomia (with congenital indifference to pain)
Vasculitis
IgA vasculitis
BURNS
Accidental burns (common)
Infection
Staphylococcal scalded skin syndrome
Impetigo
Dermatologic
Phytophotodermatitis
Stevens-Johnson syndrome
Fixed drug eruption
Epidermolysis bullosa
Severe diaper dermatitis, including Ex-Lax ingestion
Cultural practices
Cupping
Moxibustion
FRACTURES
Accidental injury
Birth trauma
Metabolic bone disease
Osteogenesis imperfecta
Copper deficiency
Rickets
Infection
Congenital syphilis
Osteomyelitis
HEAD TRAUMA
Accidental head injury
Hematologic disorders
Vitamin K deficiency (hemorrhagic disease of the newborn)
Hemophilia
Intracranial vascular abnormalities
Infection
Metabolic diseases
Glutaric aciduria type I, Menkes kinky hair syndrome

**The differential diagnosis of physical abuse varies by the type of injury and organ system involved.*
From Christian CW. Child abuse physical. In: Schwartz MW, ed. The 5-Minute Pediatric Consult. *3rd ed. Philadelphia: Lippincott Williams & Wilkins; 2003.*

SEXUAL ABUSE

In 2022, CPS substantiated reports of sexual abuse for more than 60,000 U.S. children. This is likely an underestimate of the true prevalence of sexual abuse, as it does not account for unreported cases. Sexual abuse is more common in females than males, although sexual abuse of males is underrecognized and underreported. Most perpetrators are known to the child through relationships such as family member, neighbor, or member of the community. Most sexual abuse involves manipulation and coercion. Sexual abuse can be a single event but is often recurrent. Sexual abuse can, but does not always, involve physical contact. Examples of abuse not involving physical contact are indecent exposure and deliberately exposing a child to pornography.

Children generally come to attention after they have made a disclosure of abuse, often to a nonoffending parent, sibling, relative, friend, teacher, counselor, health care provider, or other professional. Children commonly delay disclosure for many weeks, months, or years. Children may also present to care with sexual behaviors that raise concern for sexual abuse. Distinguishing between developmentally normal behaviors and sexual behavior problems is a first step in the evaluation. Behaviors that involve children with an age gap (≥4 years), physical or emotional pain, coercion, explicit imitation of intercourse, as well as behaviors that persist despite attempts to redirect are of concern. Hypersexual behaviors are concerning but not pathognomonic for sexual abuse. Alternative considerations include exposure to sexual content or other forms of maltreatment such as neglect. Sexual abuse occasionally is recognized by the discovery of an unexplained vaginal, penile, or anal injury or by the discovery of a sexually transmitted infection. Medical providers may be asked to determine the urgency of medical evaluations. Factors that prompt emergent evaluation include ongoing contact with the alleged perpetrator as well as active physical or psychologic symptoms such as bleeding or suicidal ideation. Timing of the last possible incident of abuse is an important consideration, as there are time windows for collecting forensic evidence and administering sexually transmitted infection prophylaxis, HIV postexposure prophylaxis, and emergency contraception.

In most cases, the diagnosis of sexual abuse is made by the history obtained from the child. Many communities have systems in place, including children's advocacy centers, to ensure quality investigative interviews of sexually abused children. In cases where the child has already undergone an interview prior to the medical visit, medical providers can collaborate with investigative agencies to obtain information needed for medical decision-making. However, in some cases, children may make spontaneous disclosures to the physician, or physicians may evaluate patients prior to investigative interviews and require information for medical decision-making. In these circumstances, open-ended and nonleading questions should be used and carefully documented in the medical record. Information about the medical review of systems, including physical symptoms (e.g., genital discharge, pain) and behavioral/emotional health (e.g., suicidal ideation, depression, sleep problems), should also be obtained from the patient and/or the caregiver, as appropriate for the child's developmental level.

The physical examination includes a head-to-toe examination, with careful external inspection of the genitals and anus. It is important to use a trauma-informed approach when conducting the examination, including respecting the child's autonomy and obtaining assent/consent for the exam as developmentally appropriate, explaining exam procedures and purpose, and asking the child if they would like a support person in the room. Most sexually abused children have a normal genital examination at the time of the medical evaluation; injuries are diagnosed in only approximately 5% of sexually abused children. Many types of sexual abuse (fondling, vulvar coitus, oral genital contact, exhibitionism) do not injure genital tissue or do not even involve contact with the genital tissue. Genital mucosa heals so rapidly and completely that injuries often heal by the time of the medical examination. For children who present within 72 hours of the most recent assault, special attention should be given to identifying acute injury. Guidelines based on research and expert consensus can assist clinicians in differentiating normal variants or nonspecific findings from findings caused by trauma. Examples of the latter include acute, unexplained lacerations or ecchymosis of the hymen and complete transection of the hymen. Injuries to other parts of the body such as the oral mucosa, breasts, or thighs should not be overlooked. Forensic evidence collection is also a consideration when children present acutely. Policies vary by jurisdiction. Forensic evidence collection within 72 hours of an assault that could involve transfer of forensic evidence is recommended in many states, although the time frame is longer in some states. Research showing that forensic evidence is rarely recovered from swabs collected from the bodies of prepubertal children 24 hours after assault may also influence local practice.

The **laboratory evaluation** of a sexually abused child is dictated by the child's age, history, and symptoms. Universal screening for sexually transmitted infections for prepubertal children is unnecessary because the risk of infection is low in asymptomatic young children. The type of assault, identity and known medical history of the perpetrator, and the epidemiology of sexually transmitted infections in the community also are considered. Testing methods for *Chlamydia trachomatis* and *Neisseria gonorrhoeae* have evolved with the advent of nucleic acid amplification tests (NAAT) and the declining use of culture. Local experts, such as specialists in infectious diseases and laboratory medicine, can inform protocols for confirmation of positive NAATs. The diagnosis of most sexually transmitted infections in young children requires an investigation for sexual abuse (see Chapter 117).

Commercial Sexual Exploitation of Children

Commercial sexual exploitation of children (CSEC) refers to abuse or exploitation of a child for financial benefit or in exchange for something of value and includes sex trafficking as well as pornography. CSEC could lead to medical consultation for chief complaints such as injuries, sexual assault, sexually transmitted infections, pregnancy, and treatment of chronic medical conditions. It can be difficult to identify potential victims, but possible indicators include changing demographic information, a child not allowed to speak for oneself, a child accompanied by an unrelated adult, history of multiple sexually transmitted infections, tattoos concerning for branding, and signs of inflicted injury. The American Academy of Pediatrics clinical report related to CSEC provides guidance on questions providers could ask when concerned, including "Has anyone ever asked you to have sex in exchange for something you wanted or needed?" and "Has anyone ever taken sexual pictures of you or posted such pictures on the Internet?" Health care providers are mandated reporters who should comply with local reporting laws. In addition to local resources for assistance in determining procedures and resources, there is a National Human Trafficking Resource Center.

MANAGEMENT

The management of child abuse includes medical treatment for injuries and infections and careful medical documentation of verbal statements and findings. Photographic documentation of physical examination findings can be helpful when possible. Physicians are mandated to report *suspected* child maltreatment to the appropriate authorities (Fig. 21.5). Parents should be informed of the concerns and the need to report to CPS, focusing on the need to ensure the safety and well-being of the child. Crimes that are committed against children are also investigated by law enforcement, so the police become involved in some, but not all, cases of suspected abuse. Physicians should be aware of the potential long-term impacts of maltreatment on child health. Trauma-focused cognitive-behavioral therapy has been shown to improve mental health and behavioral difficulties among children who have experienced trauma. Physicians occasionally are called to testify in court hearings regarding civil issues, such as dependency and custody, or criminal issues. Careful review of the medical records and preparation for court are needed to provide an educated, unbiased account of the child's medical condition and diagnoses.

Medical providers play a role in preventing child abuse and its consequences through interventions and referrals that strengthen and educate families, recognition of abuse and mandated reporting, and trauma-informed management of children who have experienced child maltreatment. Abusive

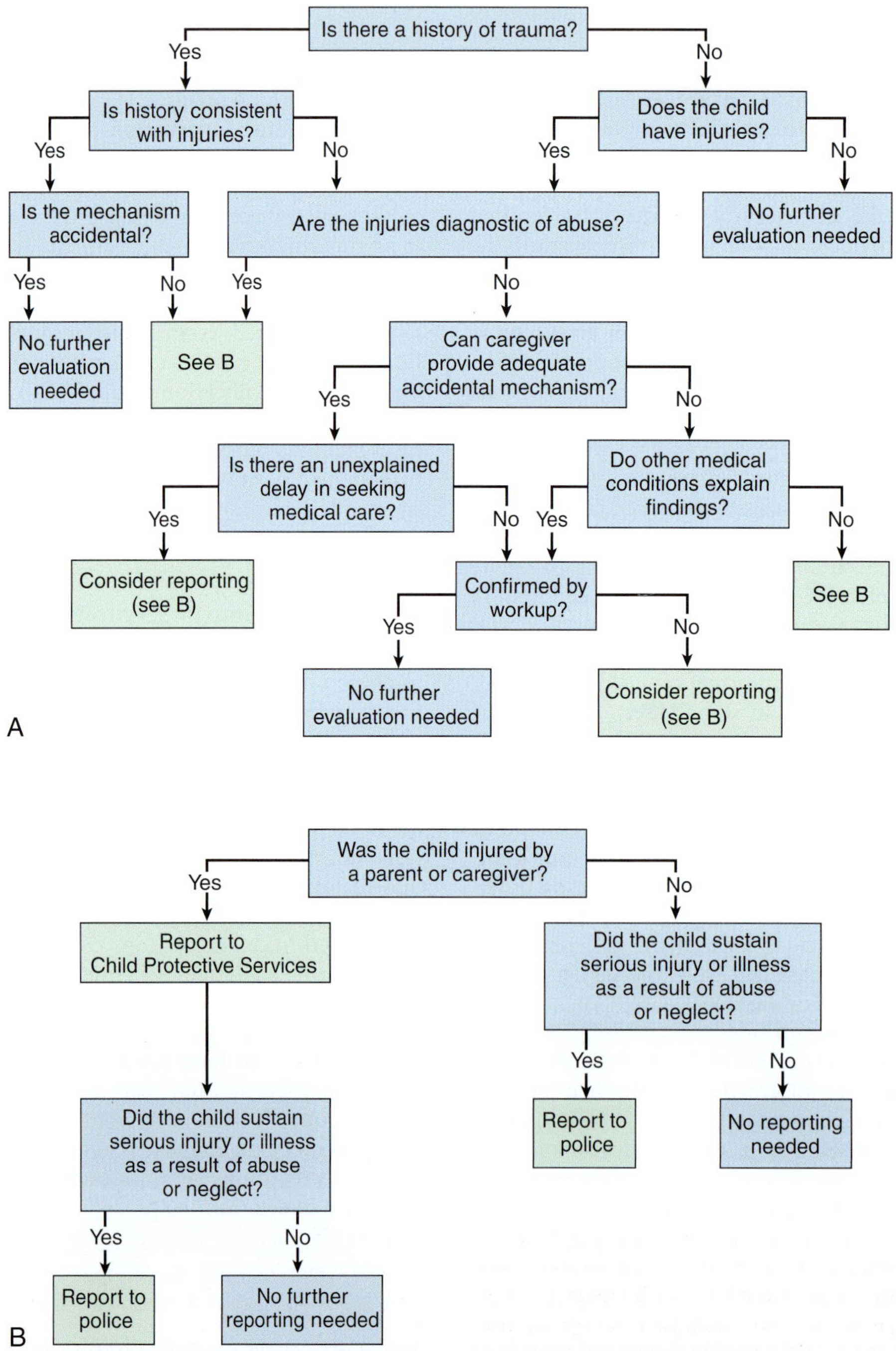

FIGURE 21.5 **(A)** Approach to initiating the civil and criminal investigation of suspected abuse. **(B)** Reporting to child protective services (CPS), law enforcement, or both in child abuse cases. CPS reports are required when a child is injured by a parent, by an adult acting as a parent, or by a caregiver of the child. The police investigate crimes against children committed by any person, including parents or other caregivers. (From Christian CW. Child abuse. In: Schwartz MW, ed. *Clinical Handbook of Pediatrics*. 3rd ed. Baltimore: Lippincott Williams & Wilkins; 2003:192–193.)

head trauma prevention programs consisting of education about the dangers of shaking and strategies to cope with crying are mandated to occur during birth hospital admissions in some states. Programs to address psychosocial factors through provider training and caregiver screening with response to identified needs have shown a reduction in child maltreatment concerns in urban primary care settings. Visiting home nursing programs that begin during pregnancy and continue through early childhood can reduce the risk of abuse and neglect.

Physicians can advocate for individual patients and families, as well as for community prevention programs. Ultimately, physicians need to remain cognizant of the diagnosis, aware of their professional mandates, and willing to advocate on behalf of these vulnerable patients.

PEARLS FOR PRACTITIONERS

See Psychosocial Issues: Pearls for Practitioners at the end of this section.

REVIEW QUESTIONS

Available online.

CHAPTER 22

Family Structure and Function

A family is a continuing system of interactions among biologically, socially, or legally related individuals. As such, families play a crucial role in shaping a child's health, development, and overall well-being. When a family functions well, interactions support the physical and emotional needs of all members and the family can serve as a valuable resource for any individual member in need. Alternatively, the problems of an individual member or the negative interactions between members may interfere with the ability of the family system to satisfy the physical and emotional needs of members and ultimately lead to physical and/or emotional harm. The consequence of a social practice or behavior pattern that undermines the stability of a family unit is referred to as *family dysfunction.*

FAMILY FUNCTIONS

The functions that families carry out in support of their children can be considered within the broad categories of physical needs, emotional support, and education and socialization (Table 22.1). Within these groupings, all families have strengths and weaknesses. The amount of support that an individual child needs in each domain varies with the child's developmental level, personality, temperament, health status, experiences, and stressors. In a healthy family, parents can be counted on to provide consistent and appropriate support for their children. Either too much or too little support can interfere with optimal child health and development. In the case of child neglect, the family underfunctions, providing inappropriate or inadequate support for the child's basic needs. Further, the violation of basic boundaries of appropriate behavior and infringement on safety is considered child abuse. In contrast, a family that overfunctions may limit a child's opportunity for growth and development of independence skills, creating feelings of helplessness and inadequacy. Parental anxiety and perfectionism can create intense pressure on children around achievement and predispose them to become anxious and fearful themselves.

TABLE 22.1 Important Roles Families Play in Supporting Children

PHYSICAL NEEDS
Safety
Food
Shelter
Health and health care
EMOTIONAL SUPPORT
Affection
Stimulation
Communication
Guidance/discipline
EDUCATION AND SOCIALIZATION
Values
Relationships
Community
Formal schooling

Most families have periods of time where functioning is compromised by stressful circumstances (e.g., serious illness, financial difficulties). Healthy families tend to resume normal functioning once the crisis resolves.

FAMILY STRUCTURE

Over the past 50 years, the structure of American family life has changed significantly. Marriages are happening later in life, parents are having fewer children, and the relationship between marriage and parenthood has evolved, with more single parents raising children. The traditional nuclear family, once seen as the dominant cultural ideal, has gradually given way to a wider variety of family forms and social arrangements. According to the U.S. Census Bureau, in 2022, 70% of children aged 0–17 lived with two parents (65% with married parents and 5% with unmarried cohabiting parents), 22% lived with their mothers only, 5% with their fathers only, and 4% lived without either parent. There is little evidence that family structure alone is a significant predictor of child health or development. Instead, the best predictor of secure child health and development is the presence of a loving adult or adults serving in a parental role committed to fulfilling a child's basic needs. Stressful life experiences can test a family's ability to promote optimal developmental outcomes, and different family structures face different challenges. Children thrive in safe, stable, and nurturing environments, which can be found in any family type.

Single-Parent Families

Approximately one-third of families in the United States are led by a single parent. Within single-parent families, most children live in mother-only households, although the share of solo father households has steadily increased. Since the 1980s, the profile of unmarried births has changed: births to younger mothers, particularly teens, have decreased, while births to older mothers, including first-time births, have increased. Children may also live in single-parent families as the result of divorce or the death of a parent (see Chapter 24). Roughly 40–45% of marriages end in divorce, and remarriage is common, often leading to the formation of blended families.

There is a strong link between family structure and socioeconomic status; individuals with higher incomes and education levels are more likely to marry. Additionally, socioeconomic status drives the likelihood of a child in the United States living in a single-parent household. In 2022, nearly 30% of single-parent families lived below the federal poverty line, as opposed to just 6% of married-couple families.

Single parents must rely to a greater extent on other adults for childcare. Fatigue associated with working and raising a child independently contributes to parenting difficulties. Single parents are likely to have less time for a social life or other activities, intensifying feelings of isolation and negatively impacting mental health. These factors may increase the likelihood of developmental and behavioral problems evolving in the child.

Parenting during adolescence brings additional challenges. Being a teenage parent is associated with lower educational attainment, lower paying jobs without much opportunity for autonomy or advancement, and lower self-esteem. Teenage mothers are less likely than adult single mothers to receive support from the child's father. Historically, children born to unmarried mothers face higher risks of adverse birth outcomes, such as low birth weight, preterm birth, and infant mortality, compared to those born to married mothers. Referral to community support programs such as early intervention services or Head Start programs can be impactful.

Many single parents create stable, loving environments for their children. Single parents may have more flexibility to focus on their children's needs, schedules, and interests without the demands of a partner. In some cases, single parents may develop a stronger sense of autonomy, modeling for their children lessons about independence, responsibility, and adaptability. Additionally, ending ongoing conflict before or during a divorce can lead to a calmer home, reducing stress for both parents and children. Single parents who choose to have children through donors or surrogacy may not face the same socioeconomic challenges, lack of support, or parental stress as other single parents. When evaluating family structure, and particularly single-parent households, it's crucial to consider these nuances.

Most children in single-parent households grow up to be resilient adults; however, when compared to kids in married-parent households, children raised in single-parent families are more likely to face emotional and behavioral challenges. These differences in child well-being tend to be small and often disappear when accounting for factors like poverty. Importantly, factors such as strong, stable relationships, parental mental health, socioeconomic status, and access to resources appear to have a greater impact on child well-being than family structure itself. When a single parent has adequate social support, can collaborate well with other care providers, and has sufficient financial resources, they are likely to be successful in raising a child. Pediatricians can improve parental self-esteem through education about child development and behavior, validation of good parenting strategies, positive feedback, and demonstrating confidence in them as parents. Demonstrating empathy and acknowledging the difficulties faced by single parents can have a healing effect and help a parent feel comfortable enough to share concerns that may warrant the need for a referral to other professionals.

LGBTQ+ Parent Families

Lesbian, gay, bisexual, transgender, queer, and other sexual and gender minority (LGBTQ+) parent families may encompass many possible family structures. The number of children living in LGBTQ+ households has likely increased in recent years due to broader societal acceptance, legalization of same-sex marriage, and growing numbers of LGBTQ+ people forming families through biologic children, adoption, or surrogacy. The LGBTQ+ community is also increasingly visible in parenting roles, with both lesbian and gay couples raising children, as well as bisexual and transgender parents becoming more recognized in family structures. While estimates vary, it is generally believed that around 3–4 million children are living in households with LGBTQ+ parents in the United States. According to a 2021 report by the Williams Institute, about 30–40% of children living in LGBTQ+ households were conceived in the context of a heterosexual relationship, particularly for lesbian and bisexual women who may have had children prior to coming out or transitioning to a same-sex relationship.

LGBTQ+ parents and their children face challenges, many of which stem from societal, legal, and health care systems that have historically been structured around heteronormative family models. Many states do not afford joint parenting rights to the nonbiologic, nonadoptive parent. This can impact employer benefits, medical decision-making, tax filing, and the right to custody in the event of death of the legally recognized parent. LGBTQ+ parents can face social discrimination or judgment from extended family, religious communities, schools, or neighbors. Research has demonstrated that children raised in LGBTQ+ families fare just as well as those in heterosexual families. Children of LGBTQ+ parents may experience bullying and discrimination in school and peer groups due to societal stigma, particularly if the family lives in an area with less LGBTQ+ acceptance. There may also be a lack of LGBTQ+ inclusive curricula that reflects the diversity of family structures.

Evidence suggests that having an LGBTQ+ parent does not cause increased problems in the parent-child relationship or impairments in the child's social-emotional development. Gender and gender role behaviors are typical for the child's age.

Adoption

Adoption is a legal and social process in which a person or couple becomes the legal parent(s) of a child who is not biologically theirs, granting the child full membership in the adoptive family. According to the U.S. Department of Health and Human Services, approximately 50,000 children are adopted each year from the foster care system. However, the total number of adoptions each year (including private, international, and blended family adoptions) is higher, with estimates ranging around 135,000–140,000 adoptions annually. A large proportion of legal and informal adoptions are by stepparents or relatives of the child. Most adoptions in the United States involve U.S. parents adopting U.S. children, but shifting cultural trends have increased the diversity in the ways in which adoptions occur (e.g., international adoptions, single-parent adoptions, privately arranged adoptions, and the use of a surrogate). These types of adoption each raise unique considerations for families and health care providers. Open adoptions, an adoption arrangement where there is some level of ongoing contact or communication between the adoptive family and the birth parents, are occurring with increased frequency because there has been a growing recognition of the importance of maintaining connections for the child's sense of identity and understanding of their background.

Pediatricians are in an ideal position to help adoptive parents obtain and evaluate medical information, consider the unique medical needs of the adopted child, and provide a source of advice and counseling beginning in the preadoption period and moving through adolescence. A preadoption visit may allow discussion of medical information that the prospective parents have received about the child and identification of important missing information such as the medical history of the biologic family and the educational and social history of the biologic parents. The preadoption period is the time that families are most likely to be able to obtain this information. Depending on the preadoption history, there may be risks of infections, in utero substance exposure, poor nutrition, or inadequate infant care that should be discussed with adoptive parents.

When the adopted child is first seen, screening for medical disorders beyond the typical age-appropriate screening tests should be considered. If the child has not had the standard newborn screening tests, the pediatrician may need to obtain these tests. Documented immunizations should be reviewed and, if needed, a plan developed to complete the needed immunizations (see Chapter 95). Children may be at high risk for infection based on the birth parent's social history or the country from which the child was adopted, including infection with HIV, hepatitis B, cytomegalovirus, tuberculosis, syphilis, and parasites. A complete blood count may be needed to screen for iron deficiency.

A knowledgeable pediatrician also can be a valuable source of support and advice about psychosocial issues. Talking to an adopted child about their adoption is an important part of helping them understand their identity, build self-esteem, and create a sense of belonging. Discussions will be an ongoing dialogue that will evolve as the child matures, and should be approached with care, honesty, and consideration for the child's developmental stage. Parents should use the term *adoption* around their children during the toddler years and explain the simplest facts first. Children's questions should be answered honestly. It is important to acknowledge the child's unique emotional journey with adoption, giving them space to ask questions and express concerns. As children get older, they may have fantasies of being reunited with their biologic parents, and there may be new challenges as the child begins to interact more with individuals outside of the family. Families may want advice about difficulties created by school assignments such as creating a genealogic chart or teasing by peers. Many adoptees start to show interest in learning about their birth family during adolescence (ages 13–17). However, they might still lack the emotional tools to process the potential outcomes of such a search. Experts often suggest that young adults (18+) are better equipped emotionally to handle the complexities of searching for and possibly meeting their birth parents. By this age, individuals tend to have a stronger sense of their own identity and are generally better prepared to understand the full implications of meeting their birth family. Adoptive parents may need reassurance that these desires do not represent rejection of the adoptive family but rather the child's desire to understand more about their life. Regardless of the child's age, adoptive parents should be involved in the decision, providing emotional support and helping guide the child through the process.

Adopted children may face an increased risk of learning, school, and behavioral problems compared to nonadopted children due to factors like early life experiences or genetic predispositions. However, many adopted children show resilience and thrive academically and socially, especially when provided with early intervention, stable homes, and appropriate support.

By carefully monitoring a child's growth, behavior, and emotional development, pediatricians can help families distinguish between typical developmental variations and signs of potential concerns that may need early intervention, counseling, or other services. **Trauma-informed care** is essential in helping pediatricians recognize how early trauma can affect development. Children who have experienced early adversity may display symptoms such as emotional dysregulation, withdrawal, or difficulties with relationships, which can sometimes be mistaken for typical developmental behaviors like tantrums or social anxiety. Pediatricians should be diligent in monitoring adopted children for signs of attachment disorders, post-traumatic stress, or delays in cognitive, social, and emotional development. This proactive approach can make a significant difference in the child's development and long-term well-being.

Foster Care

Foster care is a temporary arrangement in which children who cannot remain safely with their birth parents are placed with caregivers, known as **foster parents**, in a safe, nurturing environment while effort is made to find a long-term solution. The primary goal in most cases is to reunite children with their biologic parents once they are able to provide a safe and stable environment. If reunification is not possible or appropriate, children may become eligible for adoption or, in some cases, long-term foster care. The most common reasons for children entering foster care are neglect (especially physical and emotional neglect), followed by substance abuse, physical abuse, and domestic violence. These issues often intersect and are compounded by factors like mental illness, parental incarceration, and economic hardship.

From the late 1990s through 2005, over half a million children were in foster care, but since then, the number of children living in foster care has decreased with changes in federal and state policies that have emphasized shortened stays in foster care, promoted more rapid adoptions, and expanded efforts to support families who are struggling. In 2023–2024, there were over 325,000 children in foster care in the United States; about one-third of these children were under the age of 6. Around 40% of children in foster care are school age (6–12 years old), and this age group tends to experience the longest stays in foster care. Black and Native American/Alaska Native children are disproportionately overrepresented in foster care. Black children make up 23–25% of children in foster care, despite being 15% of the general U.S. child population. This is often linked to higher rates of poverty, systemic racism, and historical inequities in child welfare systems. In contrast, White children represent 40–45% of children in foster care, though they make up 50–55% of the general child population.

Approximately 50% of children who exit foster care are reunified with their biologic parents or primary caregivers, and about 25% exit foster care through adoption. Young children (especially infants) are the most likely group to be adopted from foster care, with adoption rates of 60–70% for children under age 6. Roughly 20,000 children each year "age out" of the foster care system without a permanent family.

Children and youth in foster care are at extremely high risk for medical, nutritional, developmental, behavioral, and mental health problems. At the time of placement in foster care, most of these children have received incomplete medical care and have had multiple **adverse childhood experiences (ACEs)**. Comprehensive assessments at the time of placement reveal many untreated acute medical problems, and nearly half of the children have a chronic illness. Developmental delays and serious behavioral or emotional disorders are common. Physical health conditions such as asthma, diabetes, obesity, and neurologic disorders are also more common among children in foster care than in the general child population.

Ideally, foster care provides a healing service for these children and families, leading to reunification or adoption. According to the U.S. Department of Health & Human Services and the Children's Bureau, approximately 25–30% of children in foster care experience three or more placements during their time in the system. This can be disruptive and stressful, further exacerbating the problems foster children may have in forming a secure relationship with adult caregivers. Children may manifest this difficulty by resisting foster parents' attempts to develop a close relationship. This detachment from the foster parent may be difficult for the foster parent to endure, which may perpetuate a cycle of placement failures. The trauma or neglect experienced that led to the need for foster care in combination with instability of placements causes enduring long-term difficulties. Foster care alumni report rates of anxiety disorders, depression, substance abuse, and post-traumatic stress disorder that are two to six times higher than in the general population. Furthermore, although the protections of the foster care system often end at 18 years of age, these adolescents rarely have the skills and maturity needed to allow them to be successful living independently. Approximately 50% of youth who age out of foster care do not have a high school diploma or GED by the time they leave the system, hindering their ability to achieve stable employment or pursue higher education. The Fostering Connections Act of 2008 required states to create comprehensive transition plans for youth aging out of foster care. The Family First Prevention Services Act of 2018 placed even more emphasis on these transitions, requiring more services for older youth in foster care, including extending foster care assistance to age 21 (in many states).

Pediatricians have a unique opportunity to build a trusting relationship with children in foster care. Many of these children have faced trauma, neglect, or abuse, and establishing a consistent and compassionate relationship with a health care provider can help them feel safe and understood. As adolescents approach adulthood, pediatricians can help them transition to adult health care systems, ensuring that they understand how to manage their own health needs, including addressing mental health, sexual health, and chronic conditions.

FAMILY DYSFUNCTION

Physical Needs

Failure to meet a child's physical needs for protection or nutrition results in some of the most severe forms of family dysfunction. There are many other ways in which parental behaviors can interfere with a child having a healthy and safe environment, such as prenatal and postnatal substance use. Prenatal use of alcohol can damage the fetus, resulting in spectrum disorders known as **fetal alcohol spectrum disorders (FASD)**. At the most severe end of the spectrum, this teratogen causes **fetal alcohol syndrome**, characterized by in utero and postnatal growth retardation, microcephaly, intellectual disability, and a characteristic dysmorphic facial appearance. Other manifestations of FASD include birth defects and problems with coordination, attention, hyperactivity, impulsivity, learning, and behavior. Children with these difficulties may be diagnosed with alcohol-related neurodevelopmental disorder, alcohol-related birth defects, or neurobehavioral disorder associated with prenatal alcohol exposure.

Other substances also may affect the fetus, but investigation of these effects is complicated by the fact that often more than one substance is used, and nutrition and prenatal care are not optimal. Cigarette smoking during pregnancy is associated with lower birth weight and increased child behavioral problems. Use of cocaine in the perinatal period has been associated with prematurity, intracranial hemorrhage, and abruptio placentae. Exposure to opiates in utero can result in prematurity and **neonatal opioid withdrawal syndrome**. Investigations of the effects of cocaine and opiates on cognitive development have produced mixed results.

Parental substance abuse after the child's birth is associated with increased family conflict, decreased organization, increased isolation, and increased family stress related to marital and work problems. Family violence may be more frequent.

Parents also may expose children directly to the harmful effects of other substances, such as exposure to **secondhand cigarette smoke**, which is consistently associated with increased rates of childhood respiratory illnesses, otitis media, and sudden infant death syndrome. There are many other ways in which parents may neglect to protect their children. Failing to immunize children, to childproof the home adequately, and to provide adequate supervision are other examples.

Emotional Support, Education, and Socialization

Failure to meet a child's emotional or educational needs can have a severe and enduring negative impact on child development and behavior. Infants need a consistent adult who learns to understand their signals and meets the infant's needs for attention as well as food. As the adult caregiver learns these signals, they respond more rapidly and appropriately to the infant's attempts at communication. Through this process, often referred to as *attachment,* the special relationship between parent and child develops. When affectionate and responsive adults are not consistently available, infants often are less willing to explore the environment and may become unusually clingy, angry, or difficult to comfort.

Appropriate stimulation also is vital for a child's cognitive development. Children whose parents do not read to them and do not play developmentally appropriate games with them have lower scores on intelligence tests and more school problems. In these situations, early intervention has been shown to be particularly effective in improving skill development and subsequent school performance. At the other extreme, there are increasing concerns that some parents may provide too much stimulation and scheduling of the child's day. There may be such emphasis on achievement that children come to feel that parental love is contingent on achievement. There are concerns that this narrow definition of success may contribute to problems with anxiety and self-esteem for some children.

PEARLS FOR PRACTITIONERS

See Psychosocial Issues: Pearls for Practitioners at the end of this section.

REVIEW QUESTIONS

Available online.

CHAPTER 23

Violence

The National Survey of Children's Exposure to Violence found that close to two-thirds of children experienced at least one self- or parent-reported direct exposure to violence in the preceding year. Exposure to violence can impact multiple aspects of well-being including physical, developmental, behavioral, emotional, and social. The landmark Adverse Childhood Experiences (ACE) study conducted in the 1990s demonstrated a graded relationship between ACEs and negative health outcomes later in life. The understanding of the physiologic impact of unmitigated trauma continues to expand, including epigenetic changes, altered immune function, and changes in brain connectivity such as amygdala overactivity. In the context of the high prevalence of exposure to violence and its multifaceted impacts on health, a trauma-informed approach to care is needed.

TRAUMA-INFORMED CARE

Providing trauma-informed medical care involves realizing the prevalence and impact of trauma, recognizing signs and symptoms of trauma, and responding to the impact of trauma on patients, caregivers, and providers. The American Academy of Pediatrics trauma-informed care page links to multiple relevant resources for providers and families (https://www.aap.org/en/patient-care/national-center-for-relational-health-and-trauma-informed-care/). Clinical tools for recognizing and responding to the impact of trauma experiences include the Child Traumatic Stress Care Process Model (CPM) (https://utahpips.org/cpm/). The CPM includes the Pediatric Traumatic Stress Screening tool to assess for trauma exposures and related symptoms (sleep disturbance, hypervigilance, avoidance, negative mood) and guidance on how to respond. Pediatric providers can play an important role in promoting resiliency after trauma by supporting nurturing relationships between children and caregivers, providing anticipatory guidance, and making referrals to community agencies for trauma-informed therapies as needed. Anticipatory guidance for caregivers of children with trauma symptoms includes explaining the relationship between symptoms and the trauma experience and reminding the caregiver not to take the behaviors personally. Examples of anticipatory guidance for specific trauma-related symptoms include developing routines for bedtime and eating, remaining calm when children act out, teaching children calming skills such as breathing exercises, and helping children to verbalize emotions.

It is important to prevent violence, provide timely identification and treatment for violence-related problems, and promote factors associated with resiliency. There are many forms of violence. Physical and sexual abuse were discussed in Chapter 21, and additional types of violence are reviewed in this chapter. Perpetration of violence by youth is also addressed.

INTIMATE PARTNER VIOLENCE AND CHILDREN

Intimate partner violence (IPV) is abuse occurring in a relationship with a current or former intimate partner and can involve physical violence, sexual violence, threats, stalking, and/or psychologic abuse, including humiliation, controlling, social isolation, and deprivation.

Violence may escalate during the perinatal period. IPV in parent relationships affects children. Youth can also experience teen dating violence.

Regarding IPV in caregiver relationships, children experience IPV by seeing or hearing the violence and its aftermath. Children may be injured during violent outbursts, sometimes while attempting to intervene. Children may also be victims of abuse themselves. It is estimated that there is at least a 50% concurrence rate between IPV and child abuse. Exposure to IPV can also impact child development, emotional health, and behavior.

While less than a quarter of women who reported injuries from IPV sought medical care for themselves, almost all sought well care for their children. When caregivers disclose IPV, interventions can include showing support and providing available community resources. It is important to assess the safety of the victim and the children. In some states, physicians are mandated to report IPV to child protective services. In addition to local resources, the National Domestic Violence Hotline can be reached by phone (1-800-799-7233), web (www.thehotline.org), or by texting START to 88788.

DATING VIOLENCE AND DATE RAPE

Teen dating violence includes physical violence, sexual violence, stalking, and/or psychologic abuse (such as name calling, shaming, controlling). Violence can also occur online (e.g., if the perpetrator posts intimate photos, messages constantly, and/or asks for passwords as a way to monitor and control communications). The 2023 United States Youth Risk Behavior Survey found that 10% of high school students experienced physical dating violence and 6% experienced sexual dating violence. Risk factors for dating violence include initiating dating and sexual activity at an early age, prior sexual abuse or victimization, and belief that dating violence is acceptable. Risk factors for perpetrating dating violence include witnessing or experiencing violence in the home, early initiation of sexual activity, and depression or anxiety. Substance use is also a risk factor for harming a partner; alcohol, marijuana, and cocaine may contribute. Flunitrazepam (Rohypnol) and γ-hydroxybutyrate are two commonly implicated drugs that cause sedation and amnesia, especially when used in conjunction with alcohol. Mental health impacts of dating violence can include depression, anxiety, and suicidality. Dating violence can increase the likelihood of unhealthy behaviors such as smoking and substance abuse. It can also have a negative impact on educational outcomes. Experiencing intimate partner violence as a teen can increase risk for victimization later in life.

Relatively few victims of date rape report the assault to law enforcement, and this can decrease the likelihood of timely medical care. It is likely that many sexually assaulted adolescents do not receive medical attention, putting them at risk for physical and mental health consequences. Health care providers can also intervene by screening for adolescent dating violence, counseling about risk factors such as substance abuse, providing routine sexually transmitted infection evaluation, and identifying counseling resources for teens who are victims or perpetrators of dating violence (see Chapter 117). Loveisrespect.org is a project of the National Domestic Violence Hotline focused on preventing and ending abusive relationships among young people; their services include 24/7 support for youth experiencing violence or persons concerned about youth via phone (1-866-331-9474), text, or chat (www.loveisrespect.org). Another resource for teen dating violence prevention is the Centers for Disease Control and Prevention (CDC) Dating Matters, an evidenced-based curriculum for 11- to 14-year-olds to promote healthy relationship skills and decrease risky behaviors.

BULLYING

The CDC defines bullying as repeated unwanted aggressive behavior by another youth or group of youths with a power imbalance (observed or perceived). Bullying can be verbal (name calling, threats), social (spreading rumors, excluding on purpose), or physical (damaging belongings, hitting, pushing, tripping, spitting). Bullying can also occur digitally over social media, games, texts, or apps; this is referred to as *cyberbullying*. The 2023 United States Youth Risk Behavior Survey found that 20% of students experienced bullying on school property, and 16% experienced cyberbullying within the preceding 12 months. Bullied youth can experience negative physical, emotional-social, and educational outcomes such as depression, anxiety, decreased school participation, decreased academic achievement, and physical injuries. Prevention strategies include talking to children about bullying, as well as educating children and families on how they can stand up to it and how to get help. Health care providers can screen for bullying and address it by providing anticipatory guidance, helping to identify school contacts who can help, sharing knowledge of local policies, and providing community referrals. Strategies at the school level include policies and rules, education, and bullying reporting systems. National resources include stopbullying.gov.

ASSAULT

The National Survey of Children's Exposure to Violence found that a third of youth experienced a physical assault within the past year. Peers and siblings were the most common perpetrators of physical assault on youth. Other perpetrators of physical violence on youth include adults, groups, or gangs. Assaults sometimes involve a weapon. Assaults can result in significant physical injury. Homicide is one of the leading causes of death among adolescents. Physical assaults can also have psychosocial consequences.

RACISM

Racism is an organized social system that devalues and disempowers racial groups regarded as inferior; reduces access to resources and opportunities such as employment, housing, education, and health care; and increases exposure to risk factors. Racism has profound impacts on health. *Bias attack* refers to assault of a child because of the child's race, religion, disability, or sexual orientation. Among 14- to 17-year-olds surveyed as part of the National Survey of Children's Exposure to Violence, the lifetime prevalence of experiencing a bias attack was 5%. Pediatricians can recognize and address the effects of racism in patient encounters, health care systems, and their communities. See Chapter 1 (Population and Culture) for further discussion.

COMMUNITY VIOLENCE

Community violence is defined as direct or indirect exposure to intentional violence in public areas. Examples include witnessing shootings, robberies, terrorist attacks, and fights. The National Survey of Children's Exposure to Violence found that 58% of youth aged 14–17 witnessed a community assault, and 13% witnessed a shooting in their lifetime. Community violence can affect psychologic, developmental, and physical health; anxiety, sleep disturbance, somatic pain, and asthma exacerbations are some health issues that could occur after witnessing violence. An example screening question for community violence is, "Has anything violent or frightening happened at school or in the neighborhood?" Anticipatory guidance for families after community violence can include encouraging parental reassurance and finding strategies to get through the crisis period. Pediatricians can also provide referrals to trauma-informed community resources as needed.

VIOLENCE AND TECHNOLOGY

Technology use among youths is prevalent and evolving with the development of new applications and devices. Medical providers, educators, parents, and youth should be aware of the risks for violence, including cyberbullying, through technology. Children can be exposed to violence on television, the Internet including social media, and videogames. Online sexual solicitation involves requests to engage in sexual activities or talk. In some cases, the solicitor attempts to contact the victim offline as well. Negative outcomes of electronic victimization include emotional distress, school absenteeism, and increased risk for in-person victimization. Anticipatory guidance for technology violence prevention includes setting rules for technology use to regulate content, location of use (i.e., common areas of the home), and amount of time spent with technology. Adults should educate children on steps to take if they are victimized, including informing a trusted adult. Children should be advised not to give out personal information online, friend strangers on social media, or meet someone known from the Internet in person without parental supervision.

THE JUVENILE JUSTICE SYSTEM

The majority of confined youth are detained for nonviolent offenses including status offenses (offenses that are illegal for minors but not adults such as truancy, runaway, or drinking), violations of probation, and drug possession. Violent crime index offenses are homicide, aggravated assault, robbery, and sexual assault. After peaking in the 1990s, the annual number of arrests of youth younger than 18 years in the United States was an estimated 424,300 in 2020. There are racial disparities including overrepresentation of Black youth. Health care providers can play a role in preventing youth violence and in addressing the health care needs of youth involved in the juvenile justice system. Youth in the juvenile justice system have high rates of unmet health needs. Physical health needs can include dental, injuries, vision, reproductive health, and chronic illnesses that have been unrecognized or undertreated. There is also an increased prevalence of unmet mental health needs such as untreated substance use disorders, depression, and post-traumatic stress disorder. Pediatric health care providers can also play a role in promoting successful re-entry for youth after release. Pediatricians can request prior medical records to ensure continuity of care and treatment of ongoing health needs. Pediatricians can also support academic and social needs. Finally, pediatric health care providers can play a role in preventing juvenile justice involvement by screening for and addressing risk behaviors such as substance use. Offering parenting support and community referrals is another avenue for prevention. Providers can also support protective factors; educational attainment is a key protective factor.

PEARLS FOR PRACTITIONERS

See Psychosocial Issues: Pearls for Practitioners at the end of this section.

REVIEW QUESTIONS

Available online.

CHAPTER 24

Divorce, Separation, and Bereavement

Each year, approximately 1.3 to 1.4 million children in the United States experience some form of separation from a parent due to divorce, death, and/or deployment. Although the context, sequence, length of separation, and advance knowledge vary across these situations, disruption of the family structure in this way may influence child development, cause stress, and contribute to long-term adverse consequences. The child's adaptation to stress is affected by the reasons for the separation and the child's age, temperament, and available support systems. Stable, responsive relationships are the predominant defense against stress-related adverse outcomes.

DIVORCE

Few events in childhood are as dramatic and challenging for the child as divorce. In the United States, around 40–45% of first marriages end in divorce. The rate varies depending on factors such as age, education, and socioeconomic status, with younger people and those with lower education or income facing higher risks of divorce. Additionally, the divorce rate tends to increase with each subsequent marriage. Most divorces in first-time marriages occur in the first 7 years, and about 20–25% of all divorces happen within the first 5 years of marriage, so there are often young children in the family when divorce occurs. Approximately 40–50% of children in the United States will experience the divorce or separation of their parents before they turn 18, and roughly 1 million children in the United States experience parental divorce each year.

While divorce rates are high, the emotional and behavioral impact on children varies. Some adjust well and develop resilience, while others face challenges; common issues include anxiety, depression, behavioral problems, and difficulties with self-esteem or academic performance. Younger children (under 10) may struggle with confusion, behavioral regression, and adjusting to family changes, while adolescents are more likely to show anger, rebellion, and risky behaviors and have feelings of loss, confusion, and identity struggles due to the divorce. Research from the National Institute of Mental Health suggests that about 20–40% of children in divorced families may experience enough distress to benefit from professional mental health support at some point. Factors like parental conflict, involvement, social support, and parenting style significantly influence whether a child will need therapeutic intervention. Long-term studies suggest that, in the absence of ongoing stressors, most children (75–80%) demonstrate good adjustment a few years after the divorce, but some have enduring difficulties.

Divorce is not a singular event but a process that evolves over time. In most cases, marital conflict begins long before the physical or legal separation, and this ongoing conflict can be emotionally taxing for children. Divorce then leads to permanent changes in the family structure. These adjustments often involve shifts in living arrangements, reductions in economic resources, and decreases in the time and attention parents can devote to their children. Together, these consequences contribute to increased stress and conflict for children.

The child's relationship with each parent is changed by divorce. In the short term, parents may face new burdens and feelings of guilt, anger, or sadness that disrupt their parenting and family routines, leading children to perceive them as unaware of the child's distress during the divorce. Pediatricians should look for maladaptive adult coping responses and encourage parents to seek assistance. Some parents may respond to their increased burdens and distress by treating their children as friends with whom they share their distress. Alternatively, they may place excessive responsibilities on the child or leave the child unsupervised for long periods of time. A child's relationship with the primary custodial parent often becomes more emotionally dependent, as this parent typically becomes the main source of care and stability. While this can strengthen the bond, it may also create feelings of guilt or pressure, especially if the child feels responsible for supporting the custodial parent emotionally. Conversely, the relationship with the noncustodial parent is often impacted by reduced time together, making it harder for the child to maintain a strong emotional connection. Limited contact can sometimes lead to idealization of the noncustodial parent, but in other cases, if the noncustodial parent is less involved, the child may feel neglected or abandoned. These shifts can create emotional challenges, especially when the child feels torn between the two parents. Pediatricians can guide parents on how to reassure their child during a divorce. Maintaining contact with both parents, familiarizing the child with the noncustodial parent's living situation, and, especially, preserving familiar routines can provide comfort and stability amid the upheaval of separation and divorce. Predictability in daily life, including consistent bedtimes, school activities, and parental involvement, fosters a sense of security. A strong support system, including extended family, friends, and school counselors, can buffer the negative effects of divorce, providing emotional support and helping children adapt more easily to the changes.

Reaction to Divorce at Different Ages

The child's reaction to the divorce is influenced by the child's age and developmental level. Although infants do not react directly to the divorce, they require special considerations in relation to custody and visitation to sustain a stable daily routine and regular contact with a primary caregiver to develop secure attachment. Separations from a primary caregiver should be brief. Consequences of stress in infants and toddlers can include irritability and disturbance in sleep and feeding patterns.

Preschool children may have magical beliefs about cause and effects and an egocentric view of the world. They may believe that something they did caused the divorce, leading them to be particularly upset. They may engage in unusual behaviors that they believe will bring the parents back together again. At this age, parents need to deliver a clear message that the divorce was related to disagreements between the parents, that nothing the child did caused the divorce, and that nothing the child could do would bring the parents back together again. Preschool children may reason that if the parents left each other they also might leave the child. To counteract this fear of abandonment, children may need to be reassured that although parents separated, they will not abandon the child and that the child's relationship with both parents will endure.

School-age children have a concrete understanding of cause and effect; if something bad happened, they understand that something caused it to happen. They are not likely to understand fully the subtleties of parental conflict or the idea that multiple factors contribute to a conflict. Children at this age may still worry that something they did caused the divorce. They may express more anger than younger children and often feel rejected. Many young school-age children worry about what will happen to one or both parents. School performance often deteriorates. Older elementary school–age children may believe that one parent was wronged by the other. This belief, in conjunction with their concrete understanding of cause and effect, allows children to be easily co-opted by one parent to take sides against the other. Parents need to understand this vulnerability and resist supporting their child in taking sides.

Adolescents may respond to the divorce by acting out, developing anxiety and/or depression, or by experiencing somatic symptoms. Adolescents are developing a sense of autonomy, a sense of morality, and the capacity for intimacy, and divorce may lead them to question previously held beliefs. They may be concerned about what the divorce means for their future and whether they, too, will experience marital failure. Questioning of previous beliefs in conjunction with decreased supervision may set the stage for risk-taking behaviors, such as truancy, sexual behaviors, and alcohol or drug use.

Outcome of Divorce

Parental conflict and cooperation are key factors in a child's adjustment to divorce. Children fare better when parents minimize conflict, maintain civil communication, and collaborate to provide consistent routines, clear boundaries, and emotional support. High conflict, however, increases stress and confusion, as children may feel torn between parents or exposed to hostility, undermining their sense of safety and stability. For example, if one parent allows the child to stay up much later than the other parent, sleep problems may arise. Similarly, when children feel caught in the middle of ongoing conflicts between their divorced parents, they are more likely to develop behavioral or emotional issues.

Regardless of any anger or frustration between parents, it is crucial that parents understand the importance of shielding their child from this animosity. Children should not be exposed to parental conflict, as it can severely impact their emotional well-being. Ideally, parents should establish clear, consistent rules regarding schedules, discipline, and other parenting roles. However, in cases of conflict, it is also important for parents to recognize that they can only control their own actions and decisions concerning the child, and they cannot control the other parent's behavior. In situations where resolving these issues becomes particularly challenging, mediation can be a valuable tool, providing a neutral space for parents to work through their disagreements and find mutually agreeable solutions for the child's well-being. By focusing on the child's needs and maintaining respect for one another, parents can mitigate the negative impact of divorce on their child. Pediatricians need to be wary of parents' attempts to recruit them into custody battles to substantiate claims of poor parenting, unless the pediatrician has first-hand knowledge that the concerns are valid.

Historically, courts favored mothers in custody decisions, but there has been a shift toward a more balanced approach in recent years. While primary physical custody is still often awarded to mothers, particularly for younger children, there is now greater emphasis on the importance of both parents' involvement in the child's life. Courts increasingly prioritize the child's best interests, which includes fostering strong relationships with both parents when possible, as long as there are no concerns about abuse or neglect. This shift reflects changing societal views on gender roles and parenting, leading to a more gender-neutral approach in custody decisions. Most states now encourage or allow joint physical or legal custody in divorce cases, as long as it's in the child's best interest and there are no concerns about abuse or neglect. Some states presume joint custody, while others decide based on individual circumstances, prioritizing the child's well-being and the parents' ability to cooperate. Legal custody involves decision-making authority over key aspects like education and health care and can be joint or sole, with sole custody granted if a parent is deemed unfit. Physical custody refers to where the child lives; joint physical custody means time with both parents, while sole physical custody means the child primarily lives with one parent. These custody types can be combined in various ways.

Divorce often leads to financial strain, with family income typically declining in the first year as two households need to be supported. These financial changes can have several adverse effects on the child, including disruptions in living arrangements and schooling, such as a move to a new house that requires switching schools and losing peer support. Additionally, if parents increase their work hours to cope with financial pressures, the child may spend more time in childcare.

Role of the Pediatrician

Pediatricians may be confronted with issues related to marital discord before the divorce, may be consulted around the time of the divorce, or may be involved in helping the family manage issues in the years after the divorce. The pediatrician can be an important voice in helping the parents understand and meet the child's needs (Table 24.1). Before a divorce, it is important for parents to decide what to tell their children. Children should be informed about the separation before it happens, with the explanation that it is a necessary step in managing marital conflict. The discussion should prepare the child for the upcoming changes. Parents should be ready to answer questions, knowing that these questions may be repeated over the coming months. Continuing to live together after telling the child about the separation can be confusing and may create false hopes that the parents will reconcile. Clear, consistent communication is key to helping the child understand and adjust to the situation.

Many parents report not feeling emotionally stable for 2–3 years or longer after a divorce, and for some, the divorce remains a painful issue even 10 years later. A child's emotional adjustment to divorce is closely linked to how well the parents adjust. Therefore, it is important for parents to seek support. Additionally, parents in high-conflict situations may benefit from the assistance of a mediator or family therapist to help prioritize the child's needs. In particularly contentious cases, a guardian ad litem—typically a lawyer or mental health professional—may be appointed to investigate the family dynamics and make a recommendation to the court on the child's best interests.

TABLE 24.1 General Recommendations for Pediatricians to Help Children During Separation, Divorce, or Death of a Close Relative

Acknowledge and provide support for grief that the parent/caregiver is experiencing.
Help parent/caregiver consider child's needs and validate feelings.
Encourage parent/caregiver to maintain routines familiar to the child.
Encourage continued contact between child and friends.
If primary residence changes, the child should take transitional objects, familiar toys, and other important objects to the new residence.
Minimize frequent changes in caregivers, and for infants, keep the times spent away from primary caregiver brief.
Have parent/caregiver reassure the child about continued care.
Have parent/caregiver reassure the child that the child did not cause the separation, divorce, or death.
Encourage parent/caregiver to create times or rituals that allow the child to discuss questions and feelings if the child wishes.
Encourage parental self-care. Ensuring that parents are addressing their own mental health needs will have a positive impact on the child's emotional well-being.

SEPARATIONS FROM PARENTS

Children experience separations from their primary caregiver for a variety of reasons. Brief separations, such as those to attend school, camp, or other activities, are nearly a universal experience. Many children experience longer separations for a variety of reasons, including parental business trips, military service, or hospitalization. Child adjustment to separation is affected by child factors, such as the age of the child and the child's temperament; factors related to the separation, such as the length of and reason for the separation and whether the separation was planned or unplanned; and factors related to the caregiving environment during the separation, such as how familiar the child is with the caregiver and whether the child has access to friends and familiar toys and routines.

Children between 6 months and 3–4 years often struggle the most with separation from their primary caregiver, as they lack the cognitive ability to understand the reasons for the change and they don't understand the concept of time, leading to confusion and anxiety. In contrast, older children have better-developed emotional and cognitive skills, allowing them to understand the situation, express their feelings, and anticipate the parent's return. Their ability to verbalize their needs and ask questions helps them process the separation with greater clarity and emotional resilience. For older children, the period just before a planned separation can be especially difficult, as they may fully grasp the impending change and experience heightened anxiety about the uncertainty of what lies ahead. In cases of military deployment, stress is highest during the deployment itself and the subsequent reintegration, when both the absence and the adjustment to the parent's return can be challenging for the child.

If parents anticipate a separation, they should explain the reasons clearly and, when possible, provide concrete details about when they will be in contact with the child and when they will return. Keeping the child in a familiar, supportive environment with a trusted caregiver can help ease the adjustment. If staying at home isn't possible, children should be encouraged to bring transitional objects, such as a favorite blanket, stuffed animal, or a picture of the parent, to provide comfort. Maintaining familiar routines and connections with friends should also be prioritized to help the child feel secure.

DEATH OF A PARENT OR FAMILY MEMBER AND BEREAVEMENT

The death of a close family member is a deeply sad and difficult experience, and when a child loses a parent, the impact can be devastating. This type of loss is not uncommon; by the age of 18, about 1 in 25 children in the United States experience the death of a parent. The emotional and psychologic effects can be profound, particularly if the loss occurs at a young age or under traumatic circumstances. Such a loss often reshapes a child's perception of the world, challenging their sense of security and safety. As with other separations, a child's cognitive development, temperament, and the availability of support systems play key roles in their adjustment to the death of a parent. Many of the recommendations in Table 24.1 are helpful. The death of a parent or close family member also brings up some unique issues.

Explaining Death to a Child

Children's understanding of death and expressions of grief evolve with age and cognitive development (see Chapter 7). Preschoolers (ages 3–5 years) may not grasp that death is permanent and often develop magical thinking about its cause. As a result, they may experience confusion, fear, and anxiety, and exhibit regressive behaviors as they cope with the loss. As children grow, they begin to understand death as permanent, though the full comprehension of its biologic nature—its impact on the body—doesn't typically occur until adolescence. Elementary-aged children (6–11 years) begin to understand that death is irreversible, but they may still struggle with feelings of guilt, worry about the surviving parent, or fear that they caused the death. At this stage, clear explanations and emotional support are key. Adolescents (12–18 years) understand death as an adult does, but their grief can be intense, with feelings of abandonment, anger, and isolation. They may also struggle with identity and social changes, making peer support and professional counseling particularly valuable. The rise of social media and digital memorialization has changed the way children and adolescents grieve. While some find solace in connecting with others online or sharing memories, others may face challenges like cyberbullying or being overwhelmed by digital tributes. In all stages, grief is individual, and age-appropriate interventions are crucial for helping children process their loss.

Death should not be hidden from the child. It should be explained in simple and honest terms that are consistent with the family's beliefs. The explanation should help the child to understand that the dead person's body stopped functioning and that the deceased person will not return. Preschool children should be reassured that nothing they did caused the individual to die. One should be prepared to answer questions about where the body is and let the child's questions help determine what information the child is prepared to hear. False or misleading information should be avoided. Comparisons of death to sleep may contribute to sleep problems in the child.

There are many possible reactions of children to the death of a parent or close relative. Sadness and a yearning to be with the dead relative are common. Sometimes a child might express a wish to die and visit the dead relative, but a plan or desire to commit suicide is uncommon and would need immediate evaluation. A decrease in academic functioning, lack of enjoyment with activities, and changes in appetite and sleep can occur. Research indicates that about half of children experience their most severe symptoms within the first month after the death of a parent. However, for many children, the most intense emotional reactions or severe symptoms may not occur until 6–12 months later. This delayed response is often due to the child's evolving understanding of the loss. Initially, children may be in shock or numb, but as they fully grasp the permanence of the death, grief symptoms may resurface or intensify over time.

Should the Child Attend the Funeral?

Children often find it helpful to attend the funeral, as it provides a clear understanding of the death and offers a chance to say goodbye. Research highlights that participation in rituals, including funerals, can be a valuable part of the grieving process, especially for children old enough to understand what's happening. Children can benefit from "symbolic closure" and from seeing the mourning process modeled by adults. Witnessing others express grief can also help children process and express their own emotions. It can prevent the child from developing fears or misconceptions about the event. If the child attends, they should be informed about what to expect. For preschool-age children who express reluctance, they should not be pressured to go. For older children, attending may be encouraged, but if the child strongly resists, they should not be forced to attend.

PEARLS FOR PRACTITIONERS

See Psychosocial Issues: Pearls for Practitioners at the end of this section.

REVIEW QUESTIONS

Available online.

Suggested Readings

American Academy of Pediatrics. (n.d.). *Health care of children in foster care*. American Academy of Pediatrics. Retrieved January 17, 2025, from https://www.aap.org/en/patient-care/foster-care/.

Arthur JD. Helping children cope with divorce, death, and deployment. *Pediatr Rev*. 2020;41(2):93–95.

Forkey H, Szilagyi M, Kelly ET, Duffee J, Council on Foster Care Adoption and Kinship Care, Council on Community Pediatrics. Council on child abuse and neglect, committee on psychosocial aspects of child and family health. Trauma-informed care. *Pediatrics*. 2021;148(2):e2021052580.

Greenbaum J, Crawford-Jakubiak JE, Committee on Child Abuse and Neglect. Child sex trafficking and commercial sexual exploitation: health care needs of victims. *Pediatrics*. 2015;135(3):566–574.

Jones VF, Schulte EE, Council on Foster Care, Adoption, and Kinship Care. Comprehensive health evaluation of the newly adopted child. *Pediatrics.* 2019;143(5):e20190657.
Kellogg ND, Farst KJ, Adams JA. Interpretation of medical findings in suspected child sexual abuse: an update for 2023. *Child Abuse Negl.* 2023;145:106283.
Lane WG, Seltzer RR. How should clinicians and health care organizations promote equity in child abuse and neglect suspicion, evaluation, and reporting? *AMA J Ethics.* 2023;25(2):E133–E140.
Narang SK, Haney S, Duhaime AC, et al. Abusive head trauma in infants and children: technical report. *Pediatrics.* 2025;155(3):e2024070457.
Schonfeld DJ, Demaria T, Nasir A, Kumar S, Committee on Psychosocial Aspects of Child and Family Health; Council on Children and Disasters. Supporting the grieving child and family: clinical report. *Pediatrics.* 2024;154(1):e2024067212.
Stirling J, Gavril A, Brennan B, Sege RD, Dubowitz H, American Academy of Pediatrics, Council of Child Abuse and Neglect. The pediatrician's role in preventing child maltreatment: clinical report. *Pediatrics.* 2024;154(2):e2024067608.
Trent M, Dooley DG, Dougé J, Section on Adolescent Health; Council on Community Pediatrics; Committee on Adolescence. The impact of racism on child and adolescent health. *Pediatrics.* 2019;144(2):e20191765.

PEARLS FOR PRACTITIONERS

CHAPTER 21
Child Abuse and Neglect

- In all states, physicians and other health care providers are mandated by law to report child abuse and neglect.
- Neglect is the most common form of child maltreatment and can impact physical, mental, developmental, and behavioral health in both the short and long term.
- The bruising clinical decision rule TEN-4-FACESp highlights bruising characteristics that raise concern for inflicted injury. *TEN* refers to bruising to the torso, ear, or neck; *4* refers to bruising on an infant younger than 4.99 months of age; *FACES* refers to bruising on the frenulum, angle of the jaw, cheek (fleshy part of face cheek), eyelid, and subconjunctivae; and *p* refers to bruising with a pattern.
- Children with significant internal abdominal injuries may present without any external bruising.
- Abusive head trauma is the leading cause of mortality and morbidity from child physical abuse. Prevention programs often emphasize coping with crying techniques and education.
- Factors to consider when determining the urgency of medical evaluations for sexual abuse include timing of last abuse within window for forensic evidence collection per local practices; need for emergency contraception, HIV prophylaxis, and sexually transmitted infection prophylaxis; physical symptoms (bleeding, pain), psychologic symptoms (suicidal ideation); and safety concerns.

CHAPTER 22
Family Structure and Function

- The key predictor of secure child health and development is the presence of a loving adult or adults in a parental role committed to meeting a child's basic needs. While stressful life experiences can challenge families, children thrive in safe, stable, and nurturing environments, regardless of family structure.
- Children raised by LGBTQ+ parents do not experience increased problems in the parent-child relationship or impairments in social-emotional development. In fact, they demonstrate resilience in social, psychologic, and sexual health, despite facing economic, legal, and social challenges.
- Pediatricians can enhance parental self-esteem by educating parents about child development and behavior, providing validation for effective parenting strategies, offering positive feedback, and expressing confidence in their abilities as parents. Additionally, demonstrating empathy and acknowledging the challenges parents face can be both healing and help them feel comfortable sharing their concerns.
- Trauma-informed care recognizes the impact of early adversity on development, identifying symptoms such as emotional dysregulation or attachment difficulties and ensuring timely support to improve the child's long-term well-being.
- Children and adolescents in foster care are at extremely high risk for medical, nutritional, developmental, behavioral, and mental health problems.

CHAPTER 23
Violence

- Direct and/or indirect exposure to violence is prevalent among youth. Traumatic experiences impact health outcomes not only in childhood but also into adulthood.
- Violence through technology such as online solicitation, cyberbullying, or exposure to violent materials is a growing concern. Anticipatory guidance could include setting rules for technology use (e.g., location of use, amount of time of allowable use, social media–related rules), advising children not to give out personal information or meet someone known from the Internet in person, and educating children on steps to take if they are bullied.

CHAPTER 24
Divorce, Separation, and Bereavement

- A child's reaction to divorce, separation from a parent, or the death of a loved one is influenced by the child's age, cognitive development, and previous experiences.
- Parental conflict and cooperation are key factors in a child's adjustment to divorce. Children fare better when parents minimize conflict, maintain civil communication, and collaborate to provide consistent routines, clear boundaries, and emotional support.
- In times of family disruption, it is important that children are assured of continued safety and care, their feelings are validated, any concerns of personal responsibility are nullified, consistency of routine is maintained, and time is appropriated for questions and open communication without punitive judgment.

SECTION 6

PEDIATRIC NUTRITION AND NUTRITIONAL DISORDERS

April O. Buchanan | Maria L. Marquez

CHAPTER 25

Diet of the Healthy Infant

Ensuring optimal nutrition during infancy is crucial. Infancy is a period of rapid growth, making optimal nutrition essential for proper growth and organ development. Healthy nutrition contributes to metabolic programming during infancy, influencing lifelong trajectories of health and disease. It is essential to provide nutrients that are critical for brain development and growth in adequate amounts. Weight, length, weight-for-height, and head circumference (HC) are the primary markers used to measure growth rates in infants and children. Trends in growth patterns over time provide more valuable insights than a single measurement. Establishing healthy dietary patterns in childhood can influence eating behaviors and health throughout life. For more details visit https://www.dietaryguidelines.gov/.

HUMAN MILK

Human milk is considered the gold standard for infant feeding and nutrition. Human milk contains antimicrobial, anti-inflammatory, and immunoregulatory agents that support the child's developing immune system. Exclusively feeding human milk is associated with reduced rates of lower respiratory tract infections, severe diarrhea, otitis media, and obesity. For lactating parents, breast-feeding also offers protective effects, lowering risks of postpartum hemorrhage, depression, heart disease, breast cancer, and ovarian cancer.

Medical organizations worldwide recommend exclusively human milk for the first 6 months, breast-feeding for as long as both parent and child mutually desire (up to 2 years or beyond), and introducing appropriate complementary foods around 6 months of age.

Disparities in breast-feeding rates exist across geographic, socioeconomic, and ethnic groups. In the United States, many infants initiate breast-feeding, but most families do not continue for the duration they intend, and a minority of U.S. infants are exclusively breast-feeding at 6 months of age. Support strategies such as peer encouragement, prenatal and postnatal breast-feeding education, paid family leave, and lactation resources in hospitals, clinics, workplaces, and communities may help increase breast-feeding duration. Targeted interventions, such as the World Health Organization's Ten Steps to Successful Breastfeeding, have narrowed disparities in breast-feeding initiation and duration across locations worldwide (Fig. 25.1).

Adequacy of Early Milk Intake

Appropriate milk intake is assessed by infant feeding, voiding, stooling and weight patterns. In the first week, full-term infants typically breast-feed 8–12 times in 24 hours, with at least one feeding every 4 hours. By 4 weeks, they generally feed 7–9 times a day. Infants getting enough milk will urinate 6–8 times daily by day 5 of life. Stooling patterns are more variable, but stools will have transitioned from **meconium** (dark, thick stool formed prenatally and passed in the first 1–3 days after birth) to loose yellow stools.

Term and near-term infants initially experience diuresis resulting in weight loss in the first few days of life and then regain their birth weight within 1–2 weeks. Method of delivery (vaginal vs cesarean section) and mode of feeding (breast-feeding, bottle feeding) affect the expected weight trajectory after birth (see newbornweight.org).

Common Challenges of Breast-Feeding

Inadequate milk intake can result from insufficient milk production, insufficient milk extraction by the infant, or a combination of both.

- **Inadequate milk production** is often caused by infrequent breast-feeding or pumping, because frequent feeding stimulates milk production. Other less common causes include underdeveloped milk-producing tissue, previous breast surgery or radiation, hormonal imbalances, or medications that interfere with milk production.
- **Poor milk extraction** occurs when the infant struggles to latch or suck effectively. Many medical conditions such as prematurity, ankyloglossia (tongue-tie), and hypotonia (such as in Trisomy 21) require specific lactation support.

Nipple and breast pain is also a common challenge and requires nuanced evaluation (Table 25.1).

Breast-Feeding Contraindications

Few absolute contraindications to human milk exist. Some situations, such as when the breast-feeding person has a contagious infectious disease, warrant temporary interruption of direct latching at the breast, but expressing milk may still be possible. Physicians should assess on a case-by-case basis whether breast-feeding should be interrupted or avoided and when resumption is possible (see Table 25.2). During a temporary pause in direct latching, milk expression can maintain milk production. Feeding alternatives include pasteurized donor human milk, previously expressed breast milk,

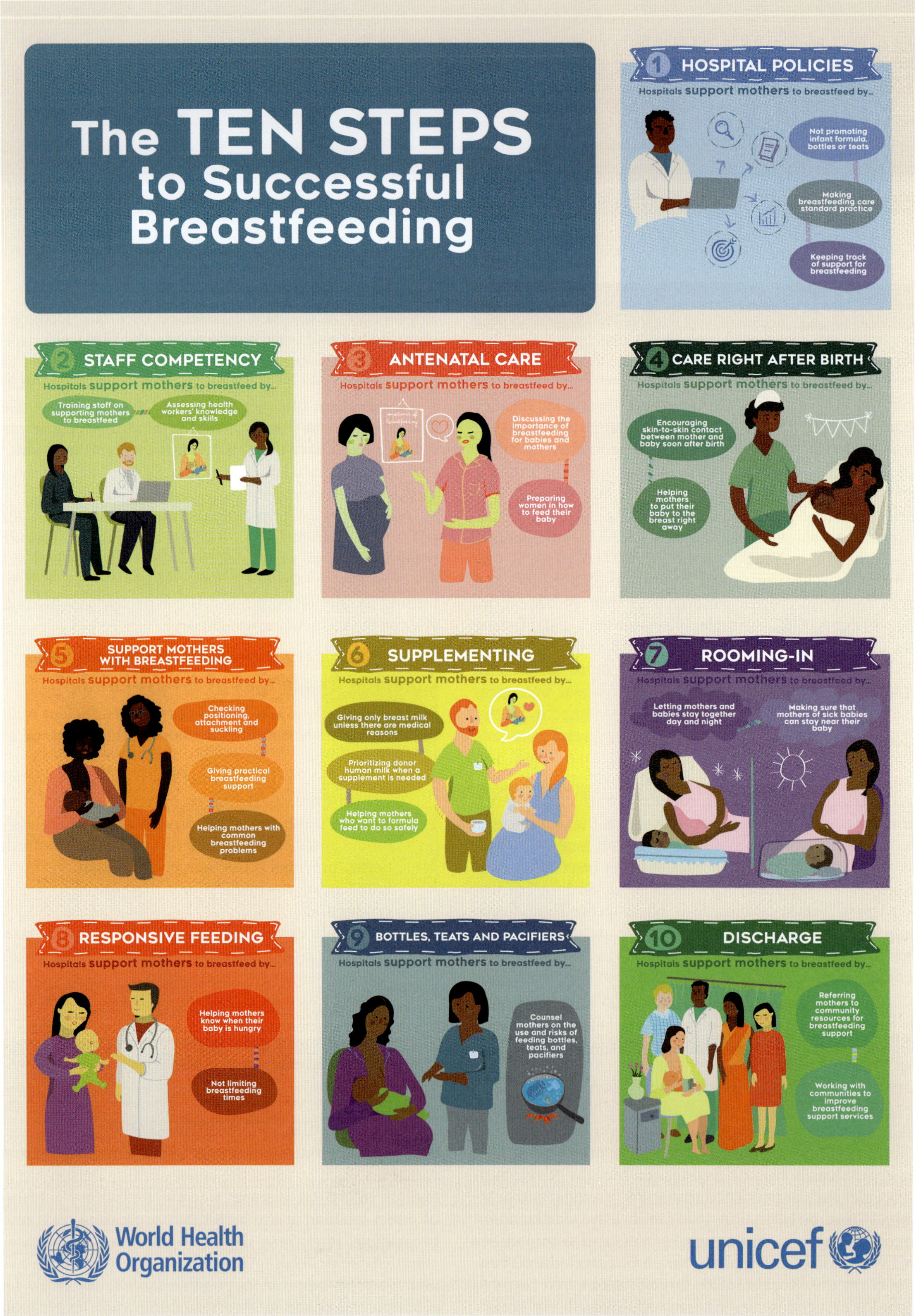
The TEN STEPS to Successful Breastfeeding
1 HOSPITAL POLICIES
Hospitals support mothers to breastfeed by...
Not promoting infant formula, bottles or teats
Making breastfeeding care standard practice
Keeping track of support for breastfeeding
2 STAFF COMPETENCY
Hospitals support mothers to breastfeed by...
Training staff on supporting mothers to breastfeed
Assessing health workers' knowledge and skills
3 ANTENATAL CARE
Hospitals support mothers to breastfeed by...
Discussing the importance of breastfeeding for babies and mothers
Preparing women in how to feed their baby
4 CARE RIGHT AFTER BIRTH
Hospitals support mothers to breastfeed by...
Encouraging skin-to-skin contact between mother and baby soon after birth
Helping mothers to put their baby to the breast right away
5 SUPPORT MOTHERS WITH BREASTFEEDING
Hospitals support mothers to breastfeed by...
Checking positioning, attachment and suckling
Giving practical breastfeeding support
Helping mothers with common breastfeeding problems
6 SUPPLEMENTING
Hospitals support mothers to breastfeed by...
Giving only breast milk unless there are medical reasons
Prioritizing donor human milk when a supplement is needed
Helping mothers who want to formula feed to do so safely
7 ROOMING-IN
Hospitals support mothers to breastfeed by...
Letting mothers and babies stay together day and night
Making sure that mothers of sick babies can stay near their baby
8 RESPONSIVE FEEDING
Hospitals support mothers to breastfeed by...
Helping mothers know when their baby is hungry
Not limiting breastfeeding times
9 BOTTLES, TEATS AND PACIFIERS
Hospitals support mothers to breastfeed by...
Counsel mothers on the use and risks of feeding bottles, teats, and pacifiers
10 DISCHARGE
Hospitals support mothers to breastfeed by...
Referring mothers to community resources for breastfeeding support
Working with communities to improve breastfeeding support services
World Health Organization
unicef

FIGURE 25.1 Ten steps for successful breast-feeding, an initiative from the World Health Organization that has improved breast-feeding rates worldwide. (From World Health Organization. Ten steps to successful breastfeeding. Poster. 23 December 2019. https://www.who.int/multi-media/details/ten-steps-to-successful-breastfeeding.)

TABLE 25.1 Common Causes of Nipple/Breast Discomfort When Breast-Feeding

ETIOLOGY	DESCRIPTION	MITIGATION
Normal sensitivity	Typically peaks around 4 days after birth and subsides within the first week. It usually diminishes after the first 30 seconds of suckling and resolves after a week.	"Chapped" sensation when latching or "pins and needles" sensation during milk let-down, usually fades in the first weeks of breast-feeding
Nipple injury	Causes more severe pain that persists or worsens after feeding begins Nipple may appear pinched, bruised, blistered, bleeding, or discolored after infant detaches Often due to suboptimal latch mechanics	If latch is painful, break infant seal by gently inserting finger into corner of the infant's mouth. Lactation evaluation may identify strategies to improve latch (e.g., deepen infant's latch to include areola) and protect nipple integrity (e.g., nipple shield).
Nipple eczema (atopic dermatitis)	Can cause itching, burning, and a red, scaly rash around the nipple More common in individuals with history of eczema	Evaluate use of soaps, fragrances, lanolin creams, breast pads. May result from a topical reaction to foods the baby has consumed before breast-feeding.
Nipple vasoconstriction	Occurs when blood vessels in the nipple tighten, reducing blood flow and causing pain, burning, or numbness Often triggered by cold, nursing, or injury Nipples may change color, turning white or blue before returning to pink	Keep the body warm, breast-feed in warm conditions, avoid nicotine and caffeine.
Engorgement	Occurs when the breasts become overly full of milk, causing them to feel firm, painful, and tender. This can make it difficult for the baby to latch properly, worsening the condition as the breast remains unemptied.	Increased feeding or milk expression frequency, massage, heat.
Blocked milk duct	Occurs when swelling or pressure causes a tender lump in the breast. If the ducts near the nipple are blocked, a white dot or "bleb" can be visible on the nipple. Causes include poor feeding technique, wearing tight clothing or an ill-fitting bra, abrupt decreases in feeding, engorgement, and infections	Increased feeding or milk expression frequency, massage, heat.
Galactoceles	Milk-filled cysts caused by a blocked milk duct. They are usually painless but can grow large.	Can be surgically drained and/or excised; any persistent breast lump requires careful evaluation, because breast cancer can occur during lactation.
Mastitis	Inflammation and swelling of the breast (usually unilateral), often occurring during the first few months of breast-feeding Swelling puts pressure on the milk ducts, narrowing them and causing pain due to restricted milk flow	Milk flow blocked for more than 1–2 days can lead to bacterial mastitis (symptoms include fever, aches, or fatigue) and require antibiotics. Continued breast-feeding is therapeutic and does not risk infection to the infant.
Oversupply (milk production exceeds the infant's demand)	Can lead to engorgement; difficulty with sustaining latch (infants may have difficulty with rapid let-down or strong flow) Infants receive less high-calorie hindmilk	The breast-feeding mother's production may calibrate to the infant's needs over time; hormonal imbalances or medications may contribute.
Yeast infections of the nipple or breast	Disproportionate breast pain; a history of yeast infections in the mother or thrush in the infant's mouth; shiny or flaky skin on the nipple; yeast visible on microscopy or in breast milk culture	Antifungal treatment for breast-feeding mother and infant, including sterilization of all accessories (breast pump, bottles, pacifiers, etc.)
Bloody nipple discharge, often called "rusty pipe syndrome"	Milk color ranging from pink to red or brown; occurs in the first days to weeks of lactation, especially during the first pregnancy; caused by increased blood flow to the breasts and ducts as milk production begins	Breast-feeding should continue; does not harm infant; typically resolves within a few days. If the discharge lasts more than a week, consult health care provider. Persistent bloody nipple discharge may be a symptom of breast cancer.
Dysphoric milk ejection reflex	Abrupt undesirable feeling that occurs with the milk ejection reflex and then dissipates within minutes	No approved treatments; emphasis on self-care.

TABLE 25.2 Maternal Contraindications and Recommendations for Breast-Feeding

MATERNAL CONTRAINDICATIONS	RECOMMENDATIONS
Classic galactosemia	Breast-feeding and human milk are contraindicated.
Active tuberculosis	Should not directly latch; expressed milk may be provided to child. Latching may resume once breast-feeding person is no longer contagious (often after appropriate treatment for 2 weeks), and any ongoing pharmacotherapy is compatible with breast-feeding.
Varicella or zoster infection	Should not directly latch; expressed milk may be provided to the child if there are no active lesions on the breast. Latching may resume once the breast-feeding person is no longer contagious (all lesions have scabbed, no new lesions).
Active measles	Should not directly latch; expressed milk may be provided to the child. Latching may resume once the breast-feeding person is no longer contagious (all lesions have scabbed, no new lesions).
Human T-cell lymphotropic virus type I or type II (HTLV-1 or -2)	Should not breast-feed or provide expressed breast milk to the infant.
Herpes simplex infection of the breast	Do not bring the infant into contact with lesions. Parent may latch infant on an unaffected breast if lesions on the affected breast are covered. Expressed milk may be provided to the child, but care must be taken to ensure that breast pump parts do not contact active lesions.
Mpox infection	Breast-feeding should be delayed until criteria for discontinuation of isolation have been met, including all lesions have resolved, the scabs have fallen off, and a fresh layer of intact skin has formed. Presence of virus in expressed human milk is unknown, and parents are advised to discard expressed milk until breast-feeding can resume.
Active substance use	Breast-feeding and expressed breast milk are not recommended. Parents who have discontinued substance use by time of delivery and those with substance use disorder in remission on medication (such as methadone, buprenorphine) may breast-feed and provide expressed breast milk.
HIV infection	Mothers with HIV should not breast-feed if they are not on antiretroviral therapy (ART) or have not achieved sustained viral suppression during pregnancy or after giving birth.

Data from "Breastfeeding and human milk." In Kimberlin DW, Banerjee R, Barnett ED, Lynfield R, Sawyer MH (eds). Red Book: 2024–2027 Report of the Committee on Infectious Diseases. Itasca, IL: American Academy of Pediatrics, 2024:135–144.

or formula. Most medications are safe to take while breast-feeding, because they typically have no adverse effect on milk supply or the infant. However, health care providers should carefully weigh the risks and benefits when prescribing medications. For detailed information on medications and breast-feeding, consult resources such as the Drugs and Lactation Database (LactMed).

Exposures to Avoid While Breast-Feeding

Marijuana Use

There is insufficient data to assess the effects of maternal marijuana use during breast-feeding, so it is discouraged. Parents should be informed of the potential risks and encouraged to abstain from marijuana use and avoid second-hand marijuana smoke exposure while breast-feeding.

Alcohol Use

Alcohol levels in breast milk mirror blood alcohol levels, peaking 30 to 60 minutes after consumption. Moderate alcohol consumption (up to 1 drink per day) is generally not harmful to the infant, especially if the mother waits at least 2 hours after drinking before nursing or expressing milk.

Smoking

Breast-feeding parents should be strongly encouraged to quit smoking and minimize second-hand smoke exposure. Smoking and nicotine use can reduce milk production and shorten lactation, and second-hand smoke increases the risk of sudden unexplained infant death (SUID), asthma, and respiratory illnesses in infants. If a parent chooses to smoke or vape, they should minimize their use, avoid smoking while feeding, and never smoke inside the home or car. It is preferable to smoke or vape immediately after breast-feeding to reduce nicotine transmission. Nicotine cessation products can be used while breast-feeding.

Radiologic Procedures

Radiologic procedures using gadolinium or iodinated contrast are not contraindications to breast-feeding, according to the American College of Radiology. Only minimal amounts of contrast enter breast milk, and less than 1% of that is absorbed by the infant. Therefore parents do not need to stop breast-feeding or discard their milk after receiving these contrast agents.

Breast-Feeding and Human Milk for the Very Low Birthweight Infants

Human milk offers multiple benefits for very low birthweight (VLBW) infants (≤1,500 g), such as reducing necrotizing enterocolitis, sepsis, chronic lung disease, and improving neurodevelopment. Expressed milk is considered medical therapy, with higher doses offering greater benefits. Pasteurized human donor milk is an alternative if the parent's milk is unavailable or contraindicated. Fortifying milk with human or bovine milk fortifiers can optimize VLBW infant growth. Pediatricians are encouraged to emphasize early and frequent milk expression.

Late Preterm and Early Term

Late preterm (34–36 weeks) and early term (37–38 weeks) infants have lower breast-feeding rates compared to full-term newborns due to factors such as delayed maternal lactation, infant immaturity, poor milk transfer, and parent-infant separation. Inadequate milk intake can lead to longer hospital stays and higher readmission rates. Expressed maternal milk, pasteurized donor milk, or formula may be used as supplemental milk.

USE OF INFANT FORMULA

Many infants rely on formula for some or all of their nutrition. Most commercial infant formulas are cow's milk–based and typically iron-fortified. Manufacturers have added nutrients like long-chain polyunsaturated fatty acids, prebiotics, and probiotics to mimic the benefits of breast milk. The caloric density of standard formulas is 20 kcal/oz (0.67 kcal/mL), similar to that of human milk. Formula-fed infants often experience different growth patterns compared to breast-fed infants, with higher fat mass and fat-free mass observed up to 6 months of age. Rapid weight gain in the first 2 years of life can also increase the likelihood of becoming overweight or obese later in childhood and adulthood.

Routine formulas are designed for healthy, full-term infants and may include cow's milk, goat's milk, or soy. Some address specific digestive needs, such as:

- Partially hydrolyzed formulas contain cow's milk protein that has already been partially hydrolyzed, or broken down, for easier digestion.
- Formulas for reflux are thickened with the aim of reducing acid reflux.
- Lactose-free options are marketed to infants with digestive concerns.

Specialty formulas address specific medical conditions and may be available only by prescription.

- Hypoallergenic formulas are extensively hydrolyzed formulas, with proteins broken down for easier digestion. They are effective in treating milk protein allergy.
- Amino acid–based formulas use amino acids as their protein source and are suitable for infants with severe milk allergies, short-gut syndrome, or other medical conditions.
- Infant formulas for premature infants contain additional nutrients and calories to meet their increased nutritional needs.
- Formulas for specific medical conditions, like inborn errors of metabolism, are specially designed. For example, formulas for individuals with phenylketonuria (PKU) do not contain the amino acid phenylalanine.

Formula may be sold in powder, liquid concentrate, or ready-to-feed bottles. Preparation requires a safe water source, clean equipment, and attention to appropriate mixing.

VITAMIN AND MINERAL SUPPLEMENTS

All infants should receive intramuscular vitamin K_1 on the first day of life to prevent vitamin K deficiency bleeding (VKDB). Vitamin K is not sufficiently secreted in breast milk to prevent VKDB. Oral vitamin K given to the infant is not recommended due to limited efficacy in preventing VKDB. Infants receiving human milk or consuming less than 28 oz of formula per day should receive 400 IU of vitamin D daily. Iron supplementation is recommended for preterm infants and may also benefit term infants, though delayed cord clamping increases iron stores in newborns.

COMPLEMENTARY FEEDINGS

The AAP recommends exclusive human milk feeding for about 6 months, with the introduction of complementary solids when the child is developmentally ready (Table 25.3). Breast milk should remain the primary source of nutrition as complementary foods are introduced, with appropriate texture adjustments and avoidance of added sugar and fat. For breast-fed infants, it is particularly important to include iron- and zinc-rich complementary foods. Potentially allergenic foods, such as peanuts, eggs, milk products, tree nuts, wheat, shellfish, fish, and soy, should be introduced when other complementary foods are added to an infant's diet. Delaying the introduction of allergenic foods does not prevent food allergies. Grains, including iron-fortified infant cereals like oat, barley, multigrain, and rice, are important for meeting infants' nutrient needs. Although iron-fortified rice cereal is beneficial, it should not be the only cereal offered.

Families can introduce yogurt and cheese, including soy-based yogurt, before 12 months, but cow's milk and fortified soy beverages should not be given as a replacement for human milk or formula before that age. After 12 months, when calcium needs increase, dairy products such as milk, yogurt, cheese, and fortified soy options are good sources of calcium and vitamin D. Dairy products offered to children under 2 should be free of added sugars.

To ensure nutrient adequacy and promote acceptance of healthy foods, it is important to introduce a variety of foods from all food groups to infants. Because young children are trying new textures and flavors, it may take 8–10 exposures for them to accept a new food. A diverse, nutrient-dense diet from 6 to 23 months should include a variety of foods from each group. Key dietary components to limit are fruit juice, added sugars, and high sodium content. Unpasteurized foods and beverages carry increased risk of exposure to pathogenic bacteria. Honey should not be given to infants less than 1 year of age due to the risk of botulism. Plant-based milk alternatives often have added sugars, and most have significantly less

TABLE 25.3 Developmental Readiness for Solid Foods
DEVELOPMENTAL SKILLS NECESSARY
• Controlling head and neck • Sitting up alone or with support • Bringing objects to the mouth • Grasping small objects, such as toys or food • Swallowing food rather than pushing it back out
FOOD TEXTURE AND THICKNESS
Choking Prevention
• Offer age- and developmentally appropriate food sizes and textures. • Ensure that the infant is seated upright in a high chair or supervised space. • Supervise feeding during mealtimes. • Avoid putting solid foods, like cereal, in bottles.
Foods That Can Pose Choking Risks
• Hot dogs, candy, nuts, seeds, raw carrots, grapes, popcorn, peanut butter chunks

Additional Resources: *USDA at https://wicworks.fns.usda.gov/resources/reducing-risk-choking-young-children-mealtimes.*

protein, calcium, and vitamin D than cow milk. There is no need for toddler milks or drinks, because necessary nutrients can be obtained from cow milk, fortified soy beverages, and solid foods.

WATER INTAKE

Free water should not be provided to infants less than 6 months of age because it can cause hyponatremia. With the introduction of complementary foods, small amounts of plain, fluoridated water (up to 4–8 oz per day) can be offered. After age 1, water intake can gradually increase to support hydration and fluoride needs.

PEARLS FOR PRACTITIONERS

See Pediatric Nutrition and Nutritional Disorders: Pearls for Practitioners at the end of this section.

REVIEW QUESTIONS

Available online.

CHAPTER **26**

Diet of the Healthy Child and Adolescent

For a discussion of nutrient needs for children and adolescents, see https://medlineplus.gov/childnutrition.html.

NUTRITION ISSUES FOR TODDLERS AND OLDER CHILDREN

Learning healthy eating behaviors at an early age is an important preventive measure because of the association of diet with several chronic diseases including obesity, diabetes, and cardiovascular disease. These diseases share risk factors that can be modified by lifestyle changes. Diets high in fruits and vegetables together with increased physical activity reduce metabolic risk factors. The first 1,000 days of life are an important time to engage in healthy nutrition behaviors that will promote well-being, including teaching healthy feeding behaviors. Excessively accelerated postnatal growth in infants and young children is an important risk factor for obesity.

MILK

Cow's milk is ideally not introduced until approximately 1 year of age. Low-fat (2%) or whole milk is recommended until 2 years of age, after which fat-free or 1% milk is recommended. Excessive milk intake (>24 oz/day for children less than age 2; >16 oz/day for children greater than age 2) should be avoided because larger intakes may reduce the intake of a good variety of nutritionally important solid foods and result in iron-deficiency anemia; large intakes also may contribute to excessive caloric intake.

JUICES

Juice should not be given to children under 1 and intake for children ages 1–4 should be limited to 4 oz; children ages 4–6 should drink no more than 4–6 oz per day, and children older than 6 should drink no more than 8 oz per day. If juices are provided to children, they should be only natural fruit juices with no added sugar (sugar, fructose, or honey). Children younger than 2 years should not have any added sugars. Young people between the ages of 2 and 18 years should get no more than 25 g of added sugar each day. This is the equivalent of six white sugar packets or 6 teaspoons of serving sugar. The typical American child consumes approximately triple the recommended amount of added sugars. Food products sold in many countries are required to list the amount of added sugars. Water and milk are the recommended drinks instead of soda, sports drinks, sweet tea, fruit drinks, etc.

GENERAL RECOMMENDATIONS

Many people in the United States do not eat a healthy diet. Healthy People 2030 focuses on helping people get the recommended amounts of healthy foods (e.g., fruits, vegetables, whole grains) and key nutrients (e.g., calcium, potassium) to reduce risk for chronic diseases and improve their health. A diet high in unhealthy foods such as saturated fat and added sugars increases risk for obesity, heart disease, type 2 diabetes, and other health problems. Choosing healthy foods can help reduce the risk of chronic diseases and improve overall health. Lack of information needed to choose healthy foods, lack of access to healthy foods, or inability to purchase enough healthy food are key issues. Public health interventions that focus on helping everyone get healthy foods are key to reducing food insecurity and hunger and improving health.

"MyPlate" by the U.S. Department of Agriculture provides parents with general guidelines for the types of foods and the volume to be offered on a regular basis. In addition, a specific MyPlate Plan calculator is available based on age, sex, and physical activity. A child should eat three meals a day and two healthy snacks. A general rule is to offer a child one tablespoon per year of age for each food provided per meal, with more given if the child requests. In general, children should not be eating more than the size of an adult palm per serving. By 1 year of age, infants should be eating meals with the family, have a regular schedule of meals and snacks, and be encouraged to self-feed with appropriate finger foods. The "plate" image is divided into five sections: fruits, grains, vegetables, protein, and dairy (Fig. 26.1). The image portrays that half the "plate" should be vegetables and fruits and the other half grains and proteins, with dairy on the side. Table 26.1 outlines serving size examples for the various food groups. Other suggestions include the following: provide low-fat 2% milk starting at 12 months of age and switch to fat-free or low-fat (1%) milk after age 2 years; make at least half of the grains whole (all would be ideal) instead of refined grains; avoid oversize portions; compare sodium (salt) in foods such as soup, bread, and frozen meals and choose foods with lower sodium content; drink water (fluoridated as possible) instead of sugary drinks; and replace proteins from red meat with a mix of fish, chicken, nuts, and legumes.

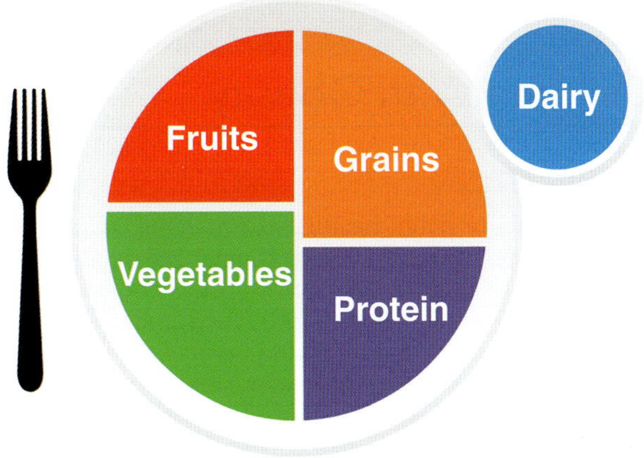

FIGURE 26.1 "MyPlate" guidelines. (From U.S. Department of Agriculture. MyPlate. www.MyPlate.gov.)

TABLE 26.1 Examples of Suggested Serving Sizes

Cup of fruit	1 cup of fresh, frozen, or canned fruit ½ cup of dried fruit 1 cup of 100% fruit juice
Cup of vegetables	1 cup of raw, cooked, frozen, or canned vegetables 2 cups of raw leafy salad greens 1 cup of 100% vegetable juice
Grain portions equal to 1 oz	1 slide of bread 1 cup of ready-to-eat cereal ½ cup of cooked rice, cooked pasta, or cooked cereal
1 oz-equivalent from protein foods group	1 oz of meat, poultry, or fish ½ cup cooked beans 1 egg 1 tablespoon of peanut butter ½ oz of nuts or seeds ¼ cup (about 2 oz) of tofu 1 oz tempeh, cooked
1 cup from the dairy group	1 cup of milk, yogurt, or soy milk 1½ oz of natural cheese

Adapted from MyPlate. U.S. Department of Agriculture. www.MyPlate.gov.

Conflicts between parents and toddlers about eating are common. The parent's role is to decide the what, when, and where of the meals. The child's role is to decide whether and how much to eat.

Recommendations for a nutritious diet for a child are based on the following nutrient-dense foods:

Protein. Provide seafood and fish, lean meat and poultry, eggs, beans, peas, soy products, and unsalted nuts and seeds.

Fruits. Fruits are recommended as essential and help prevent obesity and many other chronic diseases. Using more than one strategy to promote healthy diet (nutrition counseling, school- and workplace-based programs, school healthy nutrition policies) can help people eat more fruits. Current fruit consumption is ~0.51 cup equivalents of fruits per 1,000 calories as the mean daily intake by persons age 2 years and older. The target is to increase the consumption to 0.56 cup-equivalents of fruit per 1,000 calories by 2030.

Vegetables. One of the Healthy People 2030 goals is to increase vegetable consumption from a baseline of 0.76 cup-equivalents of total vegetables per 1,000 calories as the mean daily intake by persons age 2 years and older to a target in 2030 of 0.84 cup-equivalents of vegetables per 1,000 calories. Also, Healthy People 2030 targets an increase in consumption of dark green vegetables, red and orange vegetables, and beans and peas by age 2 years and older. At baseline, the mean daily intake by persons 2 years and older was 0.31 cup-equivalents of dark green vegetables, red and orange vegetables, and beans and peas per 1,000 calories with a target of 0.33 cup-equivalents of dark green vegetables, red and orange vegetables, and beans and peas per 1,000 calories by 2030.

Grains. Choose whole grains, such as whole-wheat bread, oatmeal, popcorn, quinoa, or brown or wild rice. Limit refined grains.

Dairy. Encourage the child to eat and drink fat-free or low-fat dairy products such as milk, yogurt, or cheese.

Aim to limit the child's calories from:

Added sugar. Added sugars in food and drinks can make it hard for people to get the nutrients they need without getting too many calories. People who eat too much added sugar may be at higher risk for tooth decay and obesity. Pricing strategies and education intervention in schools may help people limit foods and drinks with added sugars. Use of the Nutrition Facts label can help people track their consumption. Examples of added sugars include serving sugar, brown sugar, corn sweetener, corn syrup, honey, and others.

Saturated and trans-fats. Saturated fat is a type of fat that has fatty acid chains with all or predominantly single bonds and no double bonds between carbons. Recommendations are to limit saturated fats, which are those that come from animal sources of food such as red meat, poultry, and full-fat dairy products. Healthier fats are also naturally present in olives, nuts, avocados, and seafood. Limit trans-fats by avoiding foods that contain partially hydrogenated oil. People who replace saturated fat in their diet with unsaturated fat are likely to have lower cholesterol, which may reduce the risk of chronic heart disease. Many people in the United States eat too much saturated fat. Nutrition counseling and behavioral interventions can help people eat less saturated fat, and use of the Nutrition Facts label can also help them track their consumption of saturated fat. Healthy People 2030 recommends reduction in saturated fat intake from the baseline of 11.4% as the mean percentage of calories consumed by persons age 2 years and older to a target of 8.4%.

SALT INTAKE

Recommended salt intake for children varies from 1,200 to 2,300 mg a day, depending on age. Nearly 90% of children in the United States consume more than the recommended amount of salt for their age. About 1 in 9 children has elevated blood pressure, a major risk factor for heart disease and stroke. Sodium-heavy breads, pizza, cold cuts, sandwiches, cured meats, processed snacks (chips, pretzels, popcorn, crackers), and soups are among the major high salt products. Healthy People 2030 recommends lowering sodium consumption from baseline of 3,414 mg of sodium from foods and beverages to a target of 2,731 mg.

IRON INTAKE

Iron intake may be inadequate in some children between 1 and 3 years of age in the United States. Toddlers with excessive milk intake (>24 oz/day) and/or those who consume little meat, iron-rich green vegetables, or grains are at risk for iron deficiency. Iron-deficient children are at higher risk for developmental problems. Iron-rich foods and adding iron to more foods in general can help reduce iron deficiency. Supplemental iron is recommended if the child is iron deficient.

NUTRITION ISSUES FOR ADOLESCENTS

Teen nutrition can be a challenge. Advertisements for processed food and images of incredibly thin adolescents provide conflicting and unhealthy ideas about what they should eat. Females age 14–18 years need anywhere from 1,800 to 2,400 calories per day, depending on their activity level and stage of development. Males of the same age group need 2,000–3,200 calories daily. Poor eating habits may develop during adolescence. Skipping meals (especially breakfast), binge eating with friends or alone, dieting, and consumption of nutrient-poor, calorically dense foods are common problems. Excessive consumption of sugar from soda, fruit drinks, and specialty coffee and tea drinks may contribute to excess weight gain, as well as tooth decay, and may displace other needed nutrients. Bones increase in size and mass during periods of growth in childhood and adolescence; peak bone mass is reached around age 30. The greater the peak bone mass, the longer one can delay serious bone loss with aging. Poor calcium intake during adolescence may predispose the adult to future osteoporotic hip fracture. Only 1 of 10 teenage females and 1 of 4 teenage males get enough calcium every day. Adolescents age 9–18 years need 1,300 mg of calcium daily. Good sources include milk, yogurt, fortified orange juice, cheese, soybeans, and tofu.

Inadequate iron intake may result in symptoms of fatigue and iron-deficiency anemia. Iron needs increase during growth spurts, which is why teens are more likely to have iron-deficiency anemia. Teenage females are especially prone to anemia from menstrual blood loss. Student athletes are also vulnerable to inadequate iron intakes, severely restrictive eating patterns, and use of inappropriate nutritional and vitamin supplements.

PEARLS FOR PRACTITIONERS

See Pediatric Nutrition and Nutritional Disorders: Pearls for Practitioners at the end of this section.

REVIEW QUESTIONS

Available online.

CHAPTER 27

Children With Obesity

INTRODUCTION

Obesity is a major public health concern in the United States and many other countries. Once stigmatized as a personal choice, obesity is now understood to have complex genetic, physiological, socioeconomic, and environmental causes. The understanding of obesity within the scientific and medical community continues to evolve, recognizing the role of social determinants of health and the chronic nature of obesity-related co-morbidities. This has led to a more comprehensive view of obesity risk and treatment. Despite its complexity, multiple randomized controlled trials and comparative studies show that effective treatment strategies for obesity exist.

Childhood obesity is the result of a complex interplay of factors affecting both children and their families. Exposure to adversity can lead to changes in immunologic, metabolic, and epigenetic processes that disrupt energy regulation and increase the risk of obesity. These influences are more common among children experiencing negative **social drivers of health (SDoHs)**, such as racism, poverty, living in under-resourced communities, or facing discrimination or stigma. Obesity disproportionately affects these populations, emphasizing the need to address SDoHs and the social contexts of children and their families in the causes and treatment of overweight and obesity.

Children with overweight and obesity benefit from a child-focused, family-centered treatment approach within a patient-centered medical home. This multidisciplinary model, involving various health care professionals, addresses obesity as a chronic condition with significant long-term effects. Early identification and ongoing intervention from childhood through adulthood are crucial for effective management.

DEFINITIONS

BMI (body mass index) is a common measure used to screen for excess body fat. It is calculated by dividing a person's weight in kilograms by the square of their height in meters. For children and teens, BMI is interpreted differently from adults because it is adjusted based on age and sex-specific percentiles. This means that instead of fixed categories like in adults, a child's BMI category (such as healthy weight or overweight) is determined by where they fall on a percentile chart specific to their age and gender (Table 27.1). Annual BMI assessment is recommended during well child visits, starting at age 2 years, to monitor and manage pediatric overweight and obesity. BMI helps identify children who may benefit from interventions. However, caution is needed when interpreting high BMI values beyond the 97th percentile because the Centers for Disease Control and Prevention (CDC) Growth Charts were not intended for extreme BMI ranges.

Child and adolescent with obesity is defined as a BMI at or above the gender-specific 95th percentile on the CDC BMI-for-age growth charts.

TABLE 27.1 Body Mass Index (BMI) Interpretation

BMI/AGE PERCENTILE	INTERPRETATION
<5th	Underweight
5th–85th	Normal
85th–95th	Overweight
>95th	Obese

From Centers for Disease Control and Prevention. Healthy Weight, Nutrition, and Physical Activity. www.cdc.gov/healthyweight.

Childhood with severe obesity is defined as a BMI ≥120% of the gender-specific 95th percentile on the CDC BMI-for-age growth chart.

Child and adolescent with overweight is defined as a BMI between the 85th and 95th percentiles on the CDC BMI-for-age growth charts. Overweight and obese children are more likely to stay obese into adulthood and to develop noncommunicable diseases such as diabetes and cardiovascular diseases (CVDs) at a younger age.

EPIDEMIOLOGY

Obesity is a prevalent and complex chronic disease because it is estimated to affect 14 million children and adolescents and is one of the most common pediatric chronic diseases in the United States. Approximately 1 in 5 children and adolescents are affected by obesity, which leads to significant health care costs for both patients and the health care system. The prevalence of childhood obesity has nearly quadrupled since the 1960s, affecting 19% of children in 2020, with severe obesity increasing significantly as well. Socioeconomic disparities, such as lower parental education, income, and access to healthy food and physical activity, contribute to obesity risk. Children with disabilities and adverse childhood experiences (ACEs) are also at increased risk.

Tracking obesity throughout the life span highlights the critical need for early primary and secondary prevention and treatment efforts. These include evaluating obesity using BMI, identifying children and adolescents at high risk, addressing SDoHs, and providing or referring families to evidence-based obesity treatments.

An elevated BMI tends to track from childhood through adolescence and predicts high adult BMI. Children and adolescents with obesity have increased risk of short- and long-term serious health outcomes later in life, such as cardiovascular disease, hypertension, dyslipidemia, insulin resistance, type 2 diabetes, and nonalcoholic fatty liver disease (NAFLD). Obesity during childhood and adolescence not only is linked to physical and metabolic consequences but is also associated with poor psychological and emotional health, including increased stress, depressive symptoms, and low self-esteem.

Families benefit from understanding the genetic (Table 27.2), biological, environmental, and social determinants of obesity (Table 27.3). Providers serve as trusted advocates in this process, enabling both independent and guided changes.

EVALUATION OF THE PEDIATRIC PATIENT WITH OVERWEIGHT OR OBESITY

Effective obesity treatment in pediatric patients requires a comprehensive evaluation, including medical history, physical examination, and assessment of readiness for behavior changes. Early identification is crucial because both patients and caregivers may overlook abnormal weight gain. Routine well child visits present an opportunity for nonstigmatizing discussions that can lead to practical health plans.

A thorough **medical and social history** is essential to evaluate pediatric overweight and obesity. Creating a safe, empathetic environment for families to explore the complexities of obesity is key to gaining an accurate history. Clinicians should:

1. Ask permission to discuss the patient's BMI or weight.
2. Use person-first language (e.g., "child with obesity" rather than "obese child").
3. Consider using terms such as "evaluation" rather than "screening"; the term "evaluation" is used to emphasize a personalized approach rather than generalized screening.

The medical history should encompass concerns about weight, growth patterns, and family predispositions, including genetics, co-morbidities, and medication history. A comprehensive social history assesses family dynamics, eating habits, and the effect of SDoHs. Trauma-informed care (TIC) should be also integrated, recognizing how ACEs increase obesity risk. A thorough review of systems aids in identifying disease severity and co-morbidities (Table 27.4).

Assessing **nutrition and physical activity** is critical, often facilitated through pre-visit surveys or tools such as food diaries and wearable monitors. A nutrition and physical activity history is often gathered through a pre-appointment healthy habits survey, using tools like 24-hour recalls, food diaries, apps, and activity monitors. Cultural habits, language barriers, and literacy can affect the accuracy of these assessments, and evaluating physical activity in children is particularly challenging due to unreliable recall, requiring sensitivity to cultural and economic factors.

Pediatricians and health care providers should assess the **emotional and behavioral health** of children with overweight and obesity because these issues are more common in this population. Weight-based bullying is frequent, and resources like counseling and stopbullying.gov can help (see Chapter 23). Tools such as the Pediatric Symptom Checklist, Pediatric Symptom Checklist and Patient Health Questionnaire (PHQs), Generalized Anxiety Disorder (GAD) assessment, Screen for Child Anxiety Related Disorders (SCARED) assessment, and Vanderbilt ADHD Rating Scales can evaluate mental health concerns. Providers should also monitor for disordered eating and unhealthy weight loss behaviors during routine visits.

The **physical examination** should include vital signs, with proper equipment used to ensure accurate measurements, especially for blood pressure (BP). Vital signs such as heart rate, pulse, and blood pressure should be assessed, with an appropriately sized cuff used for accurate BP measurements, especially in children with obesity. Severe obesity may require ambulatory BP monitoring to evaluate hypertension and detect abnormal patterns. Key physical signs include short stature, mood indicators, skin conditions, and features that may suggest genetic or endocrinologic causes. Comprehensive

TABLE **27.2** Endocrine and Genetic Causes of Obesity

DISEASE	SYMPTOMS	LABORATORY
ENDOCRINE		
Cushing syndrome	Central obesity, hirsutism, moon face, hypertension	Dexamethasone suppression test
Growth hormone deficiency	Short stature, slow linear growth	Evoked GH response, IGF-1
Hyperinsulinism	Nesidioblastosis, pancreatic adenoma, hypoglycemia, Mauriac syndrome	Insulin level
Hypothyroidism	Short stature, weight gain, fatigue, constipation, cold intolerance, myxedema	TSH, FT_4
Pseudohypoparathyroidism	Short metacarpals, subcutaneous calcifications, dysmorphic facies, intellectual disability, short stature, hypocalcemia, hyperphosphatemia	Urine cAMP after synthetic PTH infusion
GENETIC		
Albright hereditary osteodystrophy	Short stature, skeletal defects, PTH resistance	*GNAS* gene, in syndromic but also in isolated nonsyndromic obesity
Alstrom syndrome	Cognitive impairment, retinitis pigmentosa, insulin-resistant diabetes mellitus, hearing loss, hypogonadism, cardiomyopathy	*ALMS1* gene
Bardet-Biedl syndrome	Retinitis pigmentosa, kidney abnormalities, polydactyly, syndactyly, hypogonadism	~21 different genes
BDNF/TrkB deficiency	Hyperactivity, impaired concentration, limited attention span, impaired short-term memory and pain sensation	*BDNF/TrkB* gene
Carpenter syndrome	Polydactyly, syndactyly, cranial synostosis, intellectual disability	*RAB23* gene, located on chromosome 6
Cohen syndrome	Mid-childhood-onset obesity, short stature, prominent maxillary incisors, hypotonia, cognitive impairment, microcephaly, decreased visual activity, neutropenia, joint laxity	*VPS13B* gene (often called the *COH1* gene) at locus 8q22
Deletion 9q34	Early-onset obesity, intellectual disability, brachycephaly, synophrys, prognathism, behavior and sleep disturbances	Deletion 9q34
Down syndrome	Short stature, dysmorphic facies, cognitive impairment	Trisomy 21
ENPP1 gene	Insulin resistance, childhood obesity	Gene on chromosome 6q
Fröhlich syndrome	Hypothalamic tumor	—
FTO gene polymorphism	Dysregulation of orexigenic hormone acyl-ghrelin, poor postprandial appetite suppression	Homozygous for *FTO* AA allele
KSR2 deficiency	Mild hyperphagia and reduced basal metabolic rate, insulin resistance often with acanthosis nigricans, irregular menses, early development of type 2 diabetes	*KSR2* gene
Leptin or leptin receptor gene deficiency	Early-onset severe obesity, infertility (hypogonadotropic hypogonadism), hyperphagia, infections	Leptin
Melanocortin 4 receptor gene mutation	Early-onset severe obesity, increased linear growth, hyperphagia, hyperinsulinemia **Most common known genetic cause of obesity** Homozygous worse than heterozygous	*MC4R* mutation
Prader-Willi syndrome	Neonatal hypotonia, slow infant growth, small hands and feet, intellectual disability, hypogonadism, hyperphagia leading to severe obesity, paradoxically elevated ghrelin	Partial deletion of chromosome 15 or loss of paternally expressed genes: *MKRN3, ZNF127, MAGEL2, SNRPN*
Proopiomelanocortin (POMC) deficiency	Obesity, red hair, pale skin, adrenal insufficiency due to ACTH deficiency, hyperproinsulinemia, hyperphagia, cholestatic jaundice	Loss of function of *POMC* gene
Rapid-onset obesity with hypothalamic dysfunction, hypoventilation, and autonomic dysregulation (ROHHAD)	Often confused with congenital central hypoventilation syndrome, presentation ≥1.5 years with weight gain, hyperphagia, hypoventilation, cardiac arrest, central diabetes insipidus, hypothyroidism, growth hormone deficiency, pain insensitivity, hypothermia, precocious puberty, neural crest tumors	Unknown genes May be a paraneoplastic disorder
Turner syndrome	Ovarian dysgenesis, lymphedema, web neck, short stature, cognitive impairment	XO chromosome

cAMP, Cyclic adenosine monophosphate; *FT_4,* free thyroxine; *IGF,* insulin-like growth factor; *PTH,* parathyroid hormone; *TSH,* thyroid-stimulating hormone.
Adapted from Gahagan S. Overweight and obesity. In Kliegman RM, St. Geme JW, eds. Nelson Textbook of Pediatrics. 22nd ed. Philadelphia: Elsevier; 2025 (Table 65.1).

TABLE 27.3 Risk Factors for Childhood Obesity

CATEGORY	RISK FACTORS
Policy factors	Marketing unhealthy foods
	Under-resourced communities
	Food insecurity
Neighborhood/community environmental factors	School environment
	Lack of fresh food access
	Fast food proximity
	Access to safe physical activity
	Environmental health
Family and home	Parental feeding style
	Sugar sweetened beverages
	Portion sizes, snacking and restaurant meals
	Family meals
	Screen time
	Sedentary behavior
	Sleep duration
	Environmental smoke exposure
	Psychosocial factors
	Adverse childhood experiences (ACEs)
Individual factors	Genetic factors
	Epigenetics
	Prenatal risk factors
	Postnatal risk factors
	Childhood medical, behavioral health, and neurodiversity
	Medication use

exams, including head, cardiopulmonary, liver, neurological, and orthopedic evaluations, help identify obesity-related co-morbidities like sleep apnea, heart failure, and musculoskeletal issues. Special attention should be given to evaluating skin for conditions linked to insulin resistance, assessing liver size, and performing cardiopulmonary, orthopedic, and neurological evaluations to identify co-morbid conditions. In severe obesity, ambulatory blood pressure monitoring (ABPM) may be needed (Table 27.5).

For body composition evaluation, dual-energy x-ray absorptiometry (DXA) is considered the gold standard, though BMI is more practical for routine use. BMI is used to classify overweight (85th–95th percentile) and obesity (≥95th percentile), though it has limitations in accurately measuring body fat, particularly in children with high muscle mass.

The laboratory evaluation of obesity-related co-morbidities in children with overweight and obesity should include a thorough history, physical examination, and lab tests to assess both the causes and complications of obesity. Conditions such as dyslipidemia, prediabetes, diabetes, hypertension, and NAFLD should be considered, with testing recommendations based on age and risk factors.

TREATMENT OF CHILDHOOD OBESITY

For children and adolescents with a BMI at or above the 95th percentile for age and sex, the U.S. Preventive Services task Force (USPSTF) recommends that primary care providers connect families to comprehensive, family-based weight management programs. Additionally, Bright Futures advises primary care providers to screen for excess weight and provide dietary and physical activity counseling for all children and adolescents with overweight or obesity (BMI between the 85th and 95th percentiles for age and sex). The CHILD 1 diet is the first step in management for children with elevated cardiovascular risk, such as elevated lipid levels (Table 27.6).

Obesity is a chronic disease requiring intensive, long-term care strategies, including ongoing medical monitoring and treatment of associated co-morbidities such as abnormal lipids, glucose dysregulation, liver enzyme abnormalities, and elevated blood pressure. Successful obesity treatment relies on the chronic care model, which takes into account individual patient factors such as family, household influences, access to healthy food and activity spaces, and SDoHs. The medical home model is recommended as the standard for coordinating care between specialists and community resources.

Concerns have been raised about whether diagnosing and treating pediatric obesity might inadvertently increase focus on eating habits and body image, leading to disordered eating as children grow into adulthood. Although self-guided dieting may heighten the risk for disordered eating, professionally run weight management programs decrease symptoms such as emotional eating, binge eating, and bulimic behaviors up to 6 years after treatment. These programs focus on healthy food choices, enjoyable physical activity, and boosting self-esteem and have been shown to lower the prevalence and risk of eating disorders in children.

Motivational interviewing (MI) is a patient-centered counseling method that helps individuals identify and strengthen their own motivation for behavior change. Unlike traditional methods where a provider prescribes change, MI focuses on the patient or family's priorities. MI does not impose specific goals but supports the patient in choosing a behavior to change, such as reducing intake of sugary drinks, increasing physical activity, or improving sleep. Pediatricians focus on parent motivation for younger children and shift toward adolescent motivation as the child grows.

Motivational interviewing involves four processes: engaging, focusing, evoking, and planning. **Engaging** builds on the relationship between the pediatrician and the family, allowing for discussions about readiness to change. **Focusing** emphasizes the family's autonomy in deciding which behaviors to address, with the patient increasingly taking control as they age. **Evoking** highlights the importance of understanding patient values and motivations, and **planning** helps establish concrete steps and support for change. Pediatricians play a key role in guiding, supporting, and adapting plans, particularly when setbacks occur. MI is a collaborative, flexible approach, empowering patients and families to make sustainable changes.

Comprehensive obesity treatment (COT) involves providing intensive, ongoing care within the medical home, with

TABLE 27.4 Key Elements in the Review of Systems for Patients With Overweight or Obesity

SYSTEM	SYMPTOMS	POSSIBLE OBESITY-RELATED CAUSES
General	Poor growth velocity	Endocrinologic contributors (Cushing, hypothyroidism)
	Hyperphagia	Various genetic etiologies including Prader-Willi Syndrome
	Developmental delay	Various genetic etiologies
Respiratory	Shortness of breath	Obesity-related asthma phenotype, deconditioning
	Snoring, apnea	Obstructive sleep apnea (OSA)
Gastrointestinal	Asymptomatic vague abdominal pain	Nonalcoholic fatty liver disease, nonalcoholic steatohepatitis
	Heart burn, dysphagia, chest pain, regurgitation	Gastroesophageal reflux disease (GERD)
	Abdominal pain, enuresis, encopresis, anorexia	Constipation
	Right upper quadrant abdominal pain	Gallbladder disease
Endocrine	Polyuria, polydipsia	Diabetes
Gynecologic	Oligomenorrhea, dysfunctional uterine bleeding	Polycystic ovarian syndrome (PCOS)
Orthopedic	Hip, thigh, or groin pain, uneven gait	Slipped capital femoral epiphysis (SCFE), Blount disease
	Knee pain	SCFE, Blount disease
	Foot pain	Increased weight bearing
	Back pain	Increase weight bearing, sedentary activity
Mental health	Sadness, anhedonia, school avoidance, flat affect	Depression, anxiety, bullying
	Purging, restricting intake, binge-eating, night eating	Eating disorder
	Impulsivity, distractibility, hyperactivity	ADHD
Urinary	Nocturia, enuresis	Diabetes, OSA
Dermatologic	Rash	Intertrigo
	Darkened skin of flexural areas	Acanthosis nigricans
	Pustules, abscesses	Hidradenitis suppurative
	Hirsutism	PCOS
	Flesh-colored striae	Rapid weight gain
	Purplish striae	Cushing syndrome
	Skinfold irritation	Candidiasis
Neurologic	Morning headaches, daytime sleepiness	OSA
	Persistent headaches	Idiopathic intracranial hypertension (IIH)

Data from Krebs NF, Himes JH, Jacobson D, Nicklas TA, Guilday P, Styne D. Assessment of child and adolescent overweight and obesity. Pediatrics. 2007;120(Suppl 4):S193–S228.

a focus on evaluating and managing both medical and psychological co-morbidities related to obesity. It addresses social determinants of health and employs nonstigmatizing, individualized treatment approaches. COT incorporates motivational interviewing to promote evidence-based changes in nutrition, physical activity, and health behaviors. Treatment goals extend beyond BMI stabilization, focusing on improving co-morbidities, quality of life, and self-image. Multidisciplinary strategies, including behavior modification, pharmacotherapy, and potentially surgery, are tailored to the child's evolving needs and family context.

Intensive health behavior and lifestyle treatment (IHBLT) aims to educate and support families in making nutritional and physical activity changes to improve weight, manage co-morbidities, and promote long-term health. It is most effective when delivered face-to-face, involving the entire family, with at least 26 hours of instruction over 3–12 months. IHBLT is a key part of comprehensive obesity treatment and may be combined with pharmacotherapy or surgery. Programs can be offered in pediatric care, medical centers, or community settings.

Medications

The AAP Clinical Guidelines recommend considering weight loss pharmacotherapy for children ages 8–11 with obesity, as an adjunct to health behavior and lifestyle treatment, based on the risks and benefits. Although IHBLT has the strongest evidence for effectiveness, pharmacotherapy may be needed for children with severe obesity or life-threatening

TABLE 27.5 Physical Examination Findings in Children and Adolescents With Obesity

SYSTEMS	PHYSICAL EXAM FINDINGS	DEFINITION
Vital signs	Hypertension	Blood pressure ≥95th percentile on more than three readings
	Increased heart rate	Heart rate above upper limits of normal range
Anthropometrics	Changes in height velocity	Early height velocity increase, earlier onset of peak height velocity
	Changes in weight gain	Early weight gain before age 5 years
Head, eye, ear, nose and throat	Papilledema	Edema of the optic disc
	Dental caries	White or brown stains or eroded areas of enamel or dentin
	Tonsillar hypertrophy	Tonsils occupy >50% of the oral pharynx
Chest	Gynecomastia	>2 cm of breast tissue in biological males
	Cervicodorsal hump	Fatty tissue over the upper back and lower neck
Gastrointestinal	Liver enlargement	Liver span >5 cm in 5-year-olds and 15 cm in adults by age 15 years. Liver palpable below the right costal margin by >3.5 cm in adults and >2 cm in children
Genitourinary	Buried penis	Suprapubic fat obscuring penile shaft
Musculoskeletal	Gait abnormalities	Side-to-side motion ("waddle")
	Hip pain	Antalgic gait
	Knee pain	Antalgic gait, swelling, tenderness, erythema
	Genu varum/valgum	Seen in children and adolescents with obesity Genu varum: bowlegs Genu valgum: knock-knees
	Pes planus	"Flat feet," where the arches of the feet flatten
Skin	Acanthosis nigricans	Characterized by thickened, darkened skin that may be itchy. It most commonly appears on the nape area (99%), the underarms (73%), and less frequently on areas like the groin, eyelids, and hands. The condition usually occurs in areas exposed to friction and is often linked to insulin resistance, obesity, or endocrine disorder.
	Hirsutism	Abnormal growth of coarse, dark hair in women on body areas where men typically grow hair, such as the face, chest, and back
	Acne	Clogged hair follicles with oil (sebum) and dead cells, forming pimples, blackheads, or cysts
	Striae	"Stretch marks" commonly linear, smooth, or atrophic. Rapid weight gain may cause tearing of the dermis.
	Intertrigo	Macerated, erythematous plaques in skinfolds, where friction and moisture accumulate, often leading to irritation and secondary infections
	Pannus	Overhanging excess skin and subcutaneous fat, located in the lower abdomen

Adapted from Armstrong S, Lazorick S, Hampl S, et al. Physical examination findings among children and adolescents with obesity: an evidence-based review. Pediatrics. 2016;137(2):e20151766 (Table 1).

co-morbidities. Currently, there is insufficient evidence to recommend pharmacotherapy solely for obesity in children under 12 (Table 27.7).

Weight Loss Surgery

Weight loss surgery, such as laparoscopic Roux-en-Y gastric bypass and vertical sleeve gastrectomy, may offer severely obese adolescents who have been unable to lose weight through lifestyle changes with significant and sustained weight loss as well as improvements in obesity-related conditions like hypertension, type 2 diabetes, and dyslipidemia. The process of determining eligibility for pediatric metabolic and bariatric surgery involves a comprehensive, multidisciplinary assessment of the patient's BMI, co-morbidities, and physiological and psychosocial factors. This includes evaluating potential contraindications, such as treatable causes of obesity, substance use, and pregnancy.

Adolescents who undergo surgery tend to experience better remission of cardiometabolic conditions compared to adults, suggesting that early intervention may offer long-term advantages. Although most complications after surgery are minor (e.g., nausea and dehydration), major complications occur in about 8% of cases, and some patients may require additional procedures within 5 years. Micronutrient deficiencies also highlight the importance of long-term monitoring

TABLE 27.6 Summary of Cardiovascular Health Integrated Lifestyle Diet (CHILD 1) Recommendation for Children Aged 2–10 Years and 11–21 Years

NUTRITION	2–10 YEARS	11–21 YEARS
Primary beverage	Fat-free milk	Fat-free milk
	Limit sugar-sweetened beverages	Limit sugar-sweetened beverages
	Encourage water	Encourage water
Fat content	Total fat: 25–30% of daily calories	Total fat: 25–30% of daily calories
	Saturated fat: 8–10% of daily calories (red meats, poultry skin, full fat dairy products, butter, deep fried food, margarine, shortening, lard, pastries, processed foods)	Saturated fat: 8–10% of daily calories
	Avoid trans fats as much as possible (fried and processed foods, shortening, pastries, donuts, baking mixes)	Avoid trans fats as much as possible
	Monounsaturated, polyunsaturated fats up to 20% of daily calories (vegetable oils, avocados, peanut butter)	Monounsaturated, polyunsaturated fats up to 20% of daily calories
Cholesterol	Less than 300 mg/day	Less than 300 mg/day
Dietary fiber	Encourage high dietary fiber intake from foods: goal +5 g/day	Encourage high dietary fiber intake from foods: goal 14 g/day

TABLE 27.7 Medicines Approved by the U.S. Food and Drug Administration for Treating Children and Adolescents With Obesity

MEDICATION	INDICATED AGE	ROUTE	DESCRIPTION
Orlistat	≥12 years	Oral capsules	Gastric and pancreatic lipase inhibitor that limits the absorption of dietary cholesterol
Liraglutide (Saxenda)	≥12 years	Injection	GLP-1 agonist Approved for treatment of obesity
Phentermine/topiramate (Qsymia)	≥12 years	Oral capsules	May increase GABA (γ-aminobutyric acid) in the brain Approved for chronic weight management
Phentermine monotherapy	≥16 years	Oral capsules	Increases norepinephrine brain levels, suppressing appetite and increasing metabolic rate Used short term for adolescents with obesity
Semaglutide (Wegovy, Ozempic)	≥12 years	Injection	GLP-1 agonist Approved to treat obesity and diabetes

GLP-1, Glucagon-like peptide-1.

postsurgery. Families should be fully informed about the risks and benefits of surgery, and insurance coverage should extend to all phases of treatment, from referral and surgery to postoperative care.

TRANSITION TO ADULT PRIMARY CARE PROVIDERS

A transition of care plan for children and adolescents with obesity to adult primary care providers is essential as they age. Although the literature on transition plans for childhood obesity is still emerging, such plans are known to improve self-efficacy and help integrate young adults into new care settings in conditions like diabetes and congenital heart disease. Transition plans for obesity should include specific goals and timelines, beginning discussions as early as age 12. Regular communication between pediatric and adult providers is key, as is peer support for both the patient and family. Given the complexity of obesity management, including behavioral strategies, community program connections, medication, and potential surgery, a well-coordinated transition plan is critical.

PEARLS FOR PRACTITIONERS

See Pediatric Nutrition and Nutritional Disorders: Pearls for Practitioners at the end of this section.

REVIEW QUESTIONS

Available online.

CHAPTER 28

Pediatric Undernutrition

Pediatric undernutrition is usually the result of inadequate food supply, access (food insecurity), or utilization; poor access to health and sanitation; chronic health conditions; and/or inappropriate feeding, behavioral issues, or child-care practices. There are four categories of undernutrition including **stunting** (low height for age), **wasting** (low weight for height), **underweight** (low weight for age), and **deficiencies** in vitamins and minerals. The greatest risk of undernutrition occurs when the child is in utero through age 2 years, a period of rapid growth (Table 28.1). International references standardize anthropometric measures using ***z* scores**. The 2006 World Health Organization (WHO) charts are recommended for children up to 2 years of age who are measured supine for length. The Centers for Disease Control and Prevention (CDC) 2000 growth charts are recommended for children and adolescents (age 2–20 years) when measured with a standing height. Indicators that can be used to diagnose and document undernutrition in the pediatric population ages 1 month to 18 years are *z* scores for weight for height/length, body mass index for age, length/height for age, or mid-upper arm circumference when a single data point is available. When two or more data points are available, indicators may also include weight gain velocity (younger than 2 years of age), weight loss (2–20 years of age), deceleration in weight for length/height *z* score, and inadequate nutrient intake (Table 28.2).

Protein-energy malnutrition (PEM) is a spectrum of conditions caused by varying levels of protein and calorie deficiencies. Primary PEM is caused by social or economic factors that result in a lack of adequate intake. Secondary PEM occurs in children with various conditions associated with increased caloric requirements (infection, trauma, cancer) (Fig. 28.1), increased caloric loss (malabsorption), reduced caloric intake (anorexia, cancer, oral intake restriction, social factors), or a combination of these three variables. Resulting nutrient deficiencies may be evident on physical examination (Table 28.3). Given the complex interplay of chronicity, etiology, and severity, a parenteral and enteral nutrition (ASPEN) working group developed a proposed classification scheme for malnutrition for hospitalized children (Fig. 28.2).

TABLE 28.1 Weight Gain Velocity (0–2 Years of Age, g/day)

AGE (MONTHS)	EXPECTED GROWTH (g/day)	CATCH-UP GROWTH (g/day)
Preterm infant	30–40	
0–3	20–30	30–45
3–6	15–20	20–30
6–9	10–15	15–20
9–12	10	15
12–24	6	10

From Diab LK, Gilley SP, Krebs NF. Malnutrition in High-Resource Settings. In: Kliegman RM, St. Geme J, eds. Nelson Textbook of Pediatrics. 22nd ed. Philadelphia: Elsevier, 2025 (Table 64.6).

Pediatric **undernutrition** in the United States is often termed **growth faltering** (formerly failure to thrive) and describes circumstances in which a child fails to gain weight appropriately or, in more severe cases, experiences failure in linear growth or head circumference (see Chapter 30).

MARASMUS

Marasmus results from the body's physiologic response to inadequate calories and nutrients. Loss of muscle mass and subcutaneous fat stores can be confirmed by inspection or palpation and quantified by anthropometric measurements. The head may appear large but generally is proportional to the body length. Edema usually is absent. The skin is dry and thin, and the hair may be thin, sparse, and easily pulled out. Children with marasmus may be apathetic and weak and may be irritable when touched. Bradycardia and hypothermia signify severe and life-threatening malnutrition. Inappropriate or inadequate human milk weaning practices and chronic diarrhea are common contributing factors. Stunting (impaired *linear* growth) results from a combination of malnutrition, especially micronutrients, and recurrent infections.

KWASHIORKOR

Kwashiorkor results from inadequate protein intake in the presence of fair to good caloric intake. The hypoalbuminemic state results in pitting edema that starts in the lower extremities and ascends with increasing severity. Other factors, such as acute infection, toxins, and possibly specific micronutrient or amino acid imbalances, are likely to contribute to the etiology. The major clinical manifestation of kwashiorkor is that the body weight is near normal for age; weight alone does not accurately reflect the nutritional status because of edema. Physical examination reveals a relative maintenance of subcutaneous adipose tissue and a marked atrophy of muscle mass. Edema varies from a minor pitting of the dorsum of the foot to generalized edema with involvement of the eyelids and scrotum. The hair is sparse, easily plucked, and appears dull brown, red, or yellow-white. Nutritional repletion restores hair color, leaving a band of hair with altered pigmentation followed by a band with normal pigmentation (flag sign). Skin changes are common and range from hyperpigmented hyperkeratosis to an erythematous macular rash (pellagroid) on the trunk and extremities. In the most severe form of kwashiorkor, a superficial desquamation occurs over pressure surfaces ("flaky paint" rash). Angular cheilosis, atrophy of the filiform papillae of the tongue, and monilial stomatitis are common. Enlarged parotid glands and facial edema result in moon facies; apathy and disinterest in eating are typical of kwashiorkor. Examination of the abdomen may reveal an enlarged, soft liver with an indefinite edge. Lymph node and tonsils are commonly atrophic. Chest examination may reveal basilar rales. The abdomen is distended, and bowel sounds tend to be hypoactive.

MIXED MARASMUS-KWASHIORKOR

Children with mixed marasmus-kwashiorkor often have concurrent wasting and edema in addition to stunting. These children exhibit features of dermatitis, neurologic abnormalities, and fatty liver.

TABLE 28.2 Comprehensive Malnutrition Indicators

INDICATORS*	SEVERE MALNUTRITION	MODERATE MALNUTRITION	MILD MALNUTRITION
Weight-for-length *z* score	≥3 *z* score or worse	−2.0 to 2.99 *z* score	−1.0 to −1.99 *z* score†
BMI-for-age *z* score	≥3 *z* score or worse	−2.0 to 2.99 *z* score	−1.0 to −1.99 *z* score†
Weight-for-length/height *z* score	≥3 *z* score or worse	No data available	No data available
Mid-upper arm circumference (<5 years of age)	≥3 *z* score or worse	−2.0 to 2.99 *z* score	−1.0 to −1.99 *z* score
Weight gain velocity (≤2 years of age)	≤25% of norm	26–50% of norm	51–75% of the norm
Weight loss (2–20 years of age)	>10% of UBW	>7.5% UBW	>5% UBW
Deceleration in weight-for-length/height or BMI-for-age	Deceleration across 3 *z* score lines	Deceleration across 2 *z* score lines	Deceleration across 1 *z* score line
Inadequate nutrient intake	≤25% of estimated energy-protein need	26–50% of estimated energy-protein need	51–75% of estimated energy-protein need

**It is recommended that when a child meets more than one malnutrition acuity level, the provider should document the severity of the malnutrition at the highest acuity level to ensure that an appropriate treatment plan and appropriate intervention, monitoring, and evaluation are provided.*
†Needs additional positive diagnostic criteria to make a malnutrition diagnosis.
BMI, Body mass index; *UBW*, usual body weight. Use clinical judgment when applying these diagnostic criteria.
Adapted from Becker PJ, Carney LN, Corkins MR, et al. Consensus statement of the Academy of Nutrition and Dietetics/American Society for Parenteral and Enteral Nutrition: indicators recommended for the identification and documentation of pediatric malnutrition (undernutrition). J Acad Nutr Diet. 2014;114(12):1988–2000.

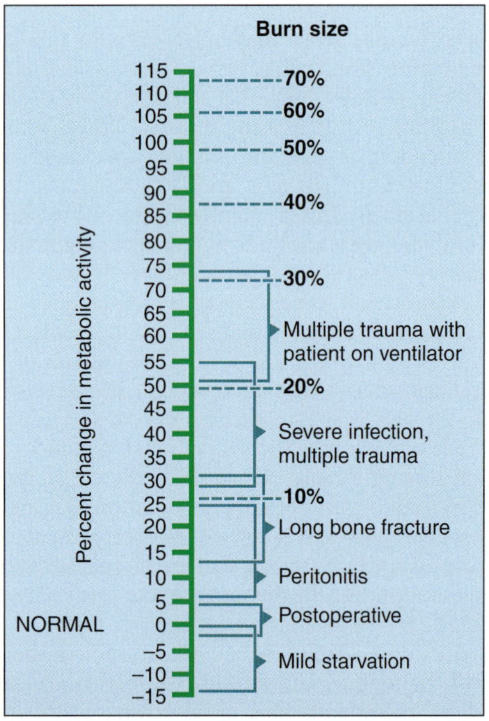

FIGURE 28.1 Increased energy needs with stress. (Modified from Wilmore D. *The Metabolic Management of the Critically Ill*. New York: Plenum Publishing; 1977. Revised in Walker W, Watkins J, eds. *Nutrition in Pediatrics: Basic Science and Clinical Application*. Boston: Little, Brown; 1985.)

TREATMENT OF MALNUTRITION

The basal metabolic rate and immediate nutrient needs decrease in cases of malnutrition. When nutrients are provided, the metabolic rate increases, stimulating anabolism and increasing nutrient requirements. The body of the malnourished child may have compensated for micronutrient deficiencies with lower metabolic and growth rates, and re-feeding may unmask these deficiencies. Nutritional rehabilitation should be initiated and advanced *slowly* to minimize these complications. The initial approach involves correction of dehydration and antimicrobial (bacteria, parasites) therapy if indicated. Oral rehydration is recommended over intravenous fluid to avoid excessive fluid and solute load and resultant heart or kidney failure.

When nutritional rehabilitation is initiated, calories can be safely started at 20% above the child's recent intake. If no estimate of the caloric intake is available, 50–75% of the normal energy requirement is safe. High-calorie oral solutions or ready-to-use therapeutic foods (a mixture of powdered milk, peanuts, sugar, vitamins, and minerals) may be used. Nutritional rehabilitation can be complicated by **re-feeding syndrome**, which is characterized by fluid retention, hypophosphatemia, hypomagnesemia, and hypokalemia. Careful monitoring of laboratory values and clinical status with severe malnutrition is essential.

When nutritional rehabilitation has begun, caloric intake can be increased 10–20% per day, monitoring for electrolyte imbalances, poor cardiac function, edema, or feeding intolerance. If any of these occur, further caloric increases are not made until the child's status stabilizes. Caloric intake is increased until appropriate regrowth or catch-up growth is initiated. **Catch-up growth** refers to gaining weight at greater than 50th percentile for age and may require 150% or more of the recommended calories for an age-matched, well-nourished child. A general rule of thumb for infants and children up to 3 years of age is to provide 100–120 kcal/kg based on *ideal* weight for height. Protein needs also are increased as anabolism begins and are provided in proportion to the caloric intake. Vitamin and mineral intake in excess of the daily recommended intake is provided to account for the increased requirements; this is frequently accomplished by giving an age-appropriate daily multivitamin with other individual micronutrient supplements as warranted by history, physical examination, or laboratory studies. Iron supplements are not

TABLE 28.3 Physical Signs of Nutritional Deficiency Disorders

SYSTEM	SIGN	DEFICIENCY
General appearance	Reduced weight for height	Calories
Skin and hair	Pallor	Anemias (iron, vitamin B_{12}, vitamin E, folate, and copper)
	Edema	Protein, thiamine
	Nasolabial seborrhea	Calories, protein, vitamin B_6, niacin, riboflavin
	Dermatitis	Riboflavin, essential fatty acids, biotin
	Photosensitivity dermatitis	Niacin
	Acrodermatitis	Zinc
	Follicular hyperkeratosis (sandpaper-like)	Vitamin A
	Depigmented skin	Calories, protein
	Purpura	Vitamins C, K
	Scrotal, vulval dermatitis	Riboflavin
	Alopecia	Zinc, biotin, protein
	Depigmented, dull hair, easily pluckable	Protein, calories, copper
Subcutaneous tissue	Decreased	Calories
Eye (vision)	Adaptation to dark	Vitamins A, E, zinc
	Color discrimination	Vitamin A
	Bitot spots, xerophthalmia, keratomalacia	Vitamin A
	Conjunctival pallor	Nutritional anemias
	Fundal capillary microaneurysms	Vitamin C
Face, mouth, and neck	Moon facies	Kwashiorkor
	Sunken eyes	Marasmus
	Angular stomatitis	Riboflavin, iron
	Cheilosis	Vitamin B_6, niacin, riboflavin
	Bleeding gums	Vitamins C, K
	Atrophic papillae	Riboflavin, iron, niacin, folate, vitamin B_{12}
	Smooth tongue	Iron
	Red tongue (glossitis)	Vitamins B_6, B_{12}, niacin, riboflavin, folate
	Parotid swelling	Protein
	Caries	Fluoride
	Anosmia	Vitamins A, B_{12}, zinc
	Hypogeusia	Vitamin A, zinc
	Goiter	Iodine
Cardiovascular	Heart failure	Thiamine, selenium, nutritional anemias
Genital	Hypogonadism	Zinc
Skeletal	Costochondral beading	Vitamins D, C
	Subperiosteal hemorrhage	Vitamin C, copper
	Cranial bossing	Vitamin D
	Wide fontanel	Vitamin D
	Epiphyseal enlargement	Vitamin D
	Craniotabes	Vitamin D, calcium
	Tender bones	Vitamin C
	Tender calves	Thiamine, selenium, vitamin C
	Spoon-shaped nails (koilonychia)	Iron
	Transverse nail line	Protein
Neurologic	Sensory, motor neuropathy	Thiamine, biotin, vitamins E, B_6, B_{12}
	Ataxia, areflexia	Vitamin E
	Ophthalmoplegia	Vitamin E, thiamine
	Tetany	Vitamin D, Ca^{2+}, Mg^{2+}
	Intellectual disability	Iodine, niacin
	Dementia, delirium	Vitamin E, niacin, thiamine
	Poor position sense, ataxia	Thiamine, vitamin B_{12}

recommended during the *acute* rehabilitation phase, especially for children with kwashiorkor, for whom ferritin levels are often high. Additional iron may pose an oxidative stress; iron supplementation at this time is associated with higher morbidity and mortality.

In most cases, cow's milk–based formulas are tolerated and provide an appropriate mix of nutrients. Other easily digested foods, appropriate for the age, also may be introduced slowly. If feeding intolerance occurs, lactose-free or semi-elemental formulas should be considered.

COMPLICATIONS OF MALNUTRITION

Malnourished children are more susceptible to **infection**, especially sepsis, pneumonia, and gastroenteritis. Hypoglycemia is common after periods of severe fasting but may

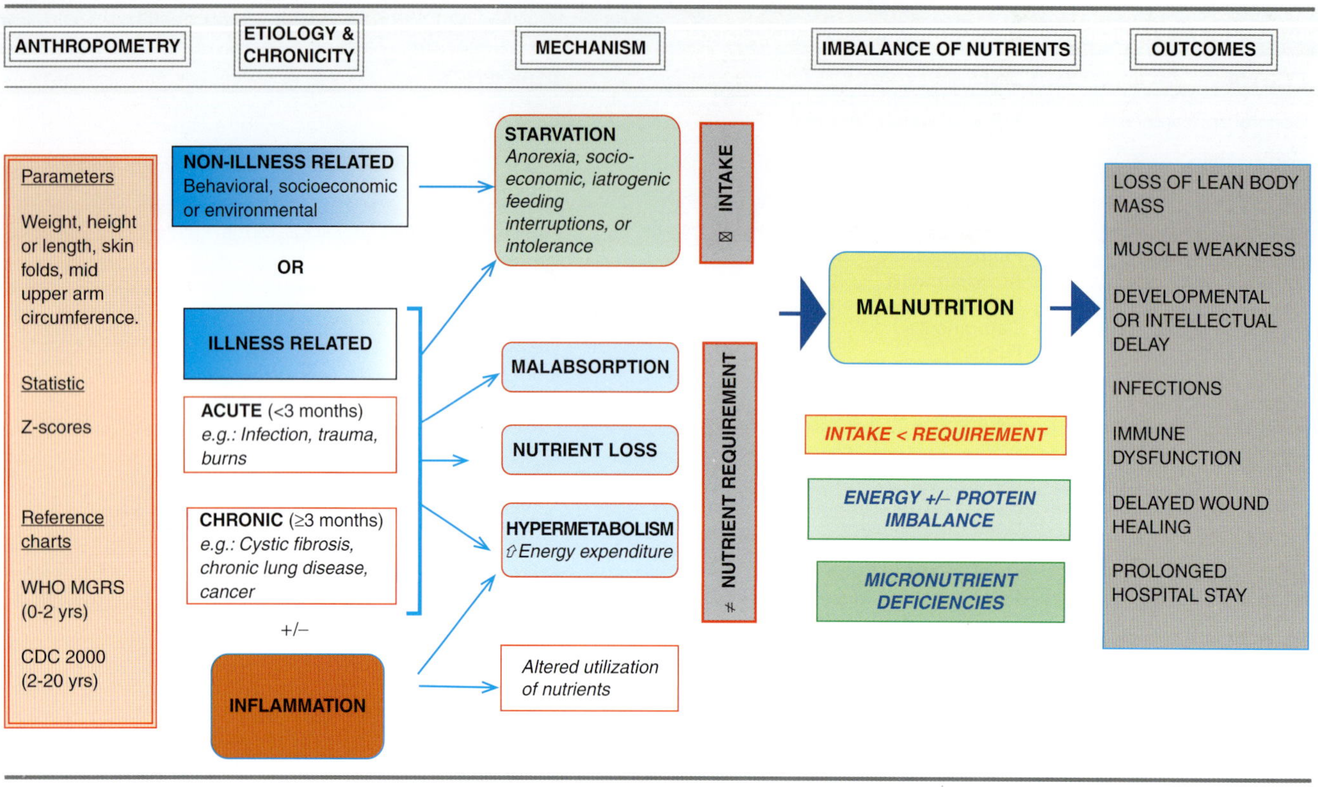

FIGURE 28.2 Defining malnutrition in hospitalized children (A.S.P.E.N.). *CDC,* Centers for Disease Control and Prevention; *MGRS,* Multicenter Growth Reference Study; *WHO,* World Health Organization. (From Mehta NM, Corkins MR, Lyman B, et al. Defining pediatric malnutrition: a paradigm shift toward etiology-related definitions. *JPEN.* 2013;37[4]:460–481.)

also be a sign of sepsis. Hypothermia may signify infection or, with bradycardia, may signify a decreased metabolic rate to conserve energy. Bradycardia and poor cardiac output predispose the malnourished child to heart failure, which is exacerbated by acute fluid or solute loads. **Micronutrient deficiencies** also can complicate malnutrition. Vitamin A and zinc deficiencies are an important cause of altered immune response and increased morbidity and mortality. Depending on the age at onset and the duration of the malnutrition, malnourished children may have permanent growth stunting (from malnutrition in utero, infancy, or adolescence) and delayed development (from malnutrition in infancy or adolescence). Environmental (social) deprivation may interact with the effects of the malnutrition to impair further development and cognitive function.

PEARLS FOR PRACTITIONERS

See Pediatric Nutrition and Nutritional Disorders: Pearls for Practitioners at the end of this section.

REVIEW QUESTIONS

Available online.

CHAPTER 29
Vitamin and Mineral Deficiencies

Micronutrients include vitamins and trace elements. In industrialized societies, frank clinical deficiencies are unusual in healthy children, but they can and do occur in certain high-risk circumstances. Risk factors include diets that are consistently limited in variety (especially with the exclusion of entire food groups), malabsorption syndromes, and conditions causing high physiologic requirements. Various common etiologies of vitamin and nutrient deficiency states are highlighted in Table 29.1, and characteristics of vitamin deficiencies are outlined in Table 29.2.

WATER-SOLUBLE VITAMINS

Water-soluble vitamins are not stored in the body, except for vitamin B_{12}; intake therefore alters tissue levels. Absorption from the diet is usually high, and the compounds exchange readily between intracellular and extracellular fluids. Excretion is via the urine. Water-soluble vitamins typically function as coenzymes in energy, protein, amino acid, and nucleic acid metabolism; as co-substrates in enzymatic reactions; and as structural components.

TABLE 29.1 Etiology of Vitamin and Nutrient Deficiency States

ETIOLOGY	DEFICIENCY
DIET	
Vegans (strict)	Protein, vitamins B_{12}, D, riboflavin, iron
Breast-fed infant	Vitamins K, D
Cow's milk–fed infant	Iron
Bulimia, anorexia nervosa	Electrolytes, other deficiencies
Parenteral alimentation	Essential fatty acids, trace elements
Alcoholism	Calories, vitamins B_1, B_6, folate
MEDICAL PROBLEMS	
Malabsorption syndromes	Vitamins A, D, E, K, zinc, essential fatty acids
Cholestasis	Vitamins E, D, K, A, zinc, essential fatty acids
MEDICATIONS	
Sulfonamides	Folate
Phenytoin, phenobarbital	Vitamins D, K, folate
Mineral oil	Vitamins A, D, E, K
Antibiotics	Vitamin K
Isoniazid	Vitamin B_6
Antacids	Iron, phosphate, calcium
Digitalis	Magnesium, calcium
Penicillamine	Vitamin B_6
SPECIFIC MECHANISMS	
Transcobalamin II or intrinsic factor deficiency	Vitamin B_{12}
Other digestive enzymes	Carbohydrate, fat, protein deficiencies
Menkes kinky hair syndrome	Copper
Acrodermatitis enteropathica	Zinc
Reduced exposure to direct sunlight	Vitamin D

Ascorbic Acid

The principal forms of vitamin C are ascorbic acid and the oxidized form, dehydroascorbic acid. Ascorbic acid accelerates hydroxylation reactions in many biosynthetic reactions, including hydroxylation of proline in the formation of collagen. The needs of full-term infants for ascorbic acid and dehydroascorbic acid are calculated by estimating the availability in human milk.

A deficiency of ascorbic acid results in the clinical manifestation of **scurvy**. Infantile scurvy is manifested by irritability, bone tenderness with swelling, and pseudoparalysis of the legs. The disease may occur if infants are fed unsupplemented cow's milk in the first year of life or if the diet is devoid of fruits and vegetables. Subperiosteal hemorrhage, bleeding gums, petechiae, hyperkeratosis of hair follicles, and a succession of mental changes characterize the progression of the illness. Anemia secondary to bleeding, decreased iron absorption, or abnormal folate metabolism are also seen in chronic scurvy.

B Vitamins

The B vitamins thiamine, riboflavin, and niacin are routinely added to enriched grain products; deficiencies in those following an unrestricted diet are rare in the United States. Levels from human milk reflect maternal intake, and deficiency can develop in breast-fed infants of deficient mothers.

Thiamine

Vitamin B_1 functions as a coenzyme in biochemical reactions related to carbohydrate metabolism, decarboxylation of α-keto acids and pyruvate, and transketolase reactions of the pentose pathway. Thiamine also is involved in the decarboxylation of branched-chain amino acids. Thiamine is lost during milk pasteurization and sterilization.

Thiamine deficiency occurs in alcoholics and has been reported in adolescents who have undergone bariatric surgery for severe obesity. **Infantile beriberi** occurs between 1 and 4 months of age in breast-fed infants whose mothers have a thiamine deficiency, in infants with protein-calorie malnutrition, in infants receiving unsupplemented hyperalimentation fluid, and in infants receiving boiled milk. Acute **wet beriberi** with cardiac symptoms and signs predominates in infantile beriberi. Anorexia, apathy, vomiting, restlessness, and pallor progress to dyspnea, cyanosis, and death from heart failure. Infants with beriberi have a characteristic aphonic cry; they appear to be crying but no sound is uttered. Other signs include peripheral neuropathy and paresthesias.

Riboflavin

Vitamin B_2 is a constituent of two coenzymes, riboflavin 5′-phosphate and flavin-adenine dinucleotide, essential components of glutathione reductase and xanthine oxidase, which are involved in electron transport. A deficiency of riboflavin affects glucose, fatty acid, and amino acid metabolism. Riboflavin and its phosphate are decomposed by exposure to light and by strong alkaline solutions.

Ariboflavinosis is characterized by an angular stomatitis, glossitis, cheilosis, seborrheic dermatitis around the nose and mouth, and eye changes that include reduced tearing, photophobia, corneal vascularization, and the formation of cataracts. Subclinical riboflavin deficiencies have been found in people with diabetes, children in families with low socioeconomic status, children with chronic cardiac disease, and infants undergoing prolonged phototherapy for hyperbilirubinemia.

Niacin

Niacin consists of the compounds nicotinic acid and nicotinamide (niacinamide). Nicotinamide, the predominant form of the vitamin, functions as a component of the coenzymes nicotinamide adenine dinucleotide (NAD) and nicotinamide adenine dinucleotide phosphate (NADP). Niacin is involved in multiple metabolic processes, including fat synthesis, intracellular respiratory metabolism, and glycolysis.

In determining the needs for niacin, the content of tryptophan in the diet must be considered because tryptophan is

TABLE 29.2 Characteristics of Vitamin Deficiencies

VITAMIN	PURPOSE	DEFICIENCY	COMMENTS	SOURCE
WATER SOLUBLE				
Thiamine (B_1)	Coenzyme in ketoacid decarboxylation (e.g., pyruvate → acetyl-CoA transketolase reaction)	*Beriberi:* polyneuropathy, calf tenderness, heart failure, edema, ophthalmoplegia	Inborn errors of lactate metabolism; boiling milk destroys B_1	Liver, meat, milk, cereals, nuts, legumes
Riboflavin (B_2)	FAD coenzyme in oxidation-reduction reactions	Anorexia, mucositis, anemia, cheilosis, nasolabial seborrhea	Photosensitizer	Milk, cheese, liver, meat, eggs, whole grains, green leafy vegetables
Niacin (B_3)	NAD coenzyme in oxidation-reduction reactions	*Pellagra:* photosensitivity, dermatitis, dementia, diarrhea, death	Tryptophan is a precursor	Meat, fish, liver, whole grains, green leafy vegetables
Pyridoxine (B_6)	Cofactor in amino acid metabolism	Seizures, hyperacusis, microcytic anemia, nasolabial seborrhea, neuropathy	Alcoholism	Meat, liver, whole grains, peanuts, soybeans
Pantothenic acid	CoA in Krebs cycle	None reported	—	Meat, vegetables
Biotin	Cofactor in carboxylase reactions of amino acids	Alopecia, dermatitis, hypotonia, death	Bowel resection, biotinidase deficiency, and ingestion of raw eggs	Yeast, meats; made by intestinal flora
B_{12}	Coenzyme for 5-methyltetrahydrofolate formation; DNA synthesis	Megaloblastic anemia, peripheral neuropathy, posterior lateral spinal column disease, vitiligo	Vegans; fish tapeworm; short gut syndrome; transcobalamin or intrinsic factor deficiencies	Meat, fish, cheese, eggs
Folate	DNA synthesis	Megaloblastic anemia; neural tube defects	Goat milk deficient; drug antagonists; heat inactivates	Liver, greens, vegetables, cereals, cheese
Ascorbic acid (C)	Reducing agent; collagen metabolism	*Scurvy:* irritability, purpura, bleeding gums, periosteal hemorrhage, aching bones	May improve tyrosine metabolism in preterm infants	Citrus fruits, green vegetables; cooking destroys it
FAT SOLUBLE				
A	Epithelial cell integrity; vision	Night blindness, xerophthalmia, Bitot spots, follicular hyperkeratosis; immune defects	Common with protein-calorie malnutrition; malabsorption	Liver, milk, eggs, green and yellow vegetables, fruits
D	Maintain serum calcium, phosphorus levels	*Rickets:* reduced bone mineralization	Prohormone of 25- and 1,25-vitamin D	Fortified milk, cheese, liver; sunlight
E	Antioxidant	Hemolysis in preterm infants; areflexia, ataxia, ophthalmoplegia	May benefit patients with G6PD deficiency	Seeds, vegetables, germ oils, grains
K	Post-translation carboxylation of clotting factors II, VII, IX, X and proteins C, S	Prolonged prothrombin time; hemorrhage; elevated protein induced in vitamin K absence (PIVKA)	Malabsorption; exclusively breast-fed infants	Liver, green vegetables; made by intestinal flora

CoA, Coenzyme A; *FAD,* flavin adenine dinucleotide; *G6PD,* glucose-6-phosphate dehydrogenase; *NAD,* nicotinamide adenine dinucleotide.

converted to niacin. Niacin is stable in foods and withstands heating and prolonged storage. Approximately 70% of the total niacin equivalents in human milk are derived from tryptophan. **Pellagra**, or niacin-deficiency disease, is characterized by weakness, lassitude, dermatitis, photosensitivity, inflammation of mucous membranes, diarrhea, vomiting, dysphagia, and, in severe cases, dementia.

Vitamin B_6

Vitamin B_6 refers to three naturally occurring pyridines: pyridoxine (pyridoxol), pyridoxal, and pyridoxamine. The phosphates of the latter two pyridines are metabolically and functionally related and are converted in the liver to the coenzyme form, pyridoxal phosphate. The metabolic functions of vitamin B_6 include interconversion reactions of amino acids, conversion of tryptophan to niacin and serotonin, metabolic reactions in the brain, carbohydrate metabolism, immune development, and the biosynthesis of heme and prostaglandins. The pyridoxal and pyridoxamine forms of the vitamin are destroyed by heat; heat treatment was responsible for vitamin B_6 deficiency and seizures in infants fed improperly processed formulas. *Goat's milk is deficient in vitamin* B_6.

Dietary deprivation or malabsorption of vitamin B_6 in children results in hypochromic microcytic anemia, vomiting, diarrhea, growth faltering, listlessness, hyperirritability, and seizures. Children receiving isoniazid or penicillamine may require additional vitamin B_6 because the drug binds to the vitamin. Vitamin B_6 is unusual as a water-soluble vitamin, in that very large doses (≥500 mg/day) have been associated with a sensory neuropathy.

Folate

A variety of chemical forms of folate are nutritionally active. Folate functions in transport of single-carbon fragments in synthesis of nucleic acids and for normal metabolism of certain amino acids and in conversion of homocysteine to methionine. Food sources include green leafy vegetables, oranges, and whole grains; folate fortification of grains is routine in the United States.

Folate deficiency, characterized by **hypersegmented neutrophils**, **macrocytic anemia**, and **glossitis**, may result from a low dietary intake, malabsorption, or vitamin-drug interactions. Deficiency can develop within a few weeks of birth because infants require 10 times as much folate as adults relative to body weight but have scant stores of folate in the newborn period. Folate is particularly heat labile. Heat-sterilizing home-prepared formula can decrease the folate content by half. *Evaporated milk and goat's milk are low in folate.* Patients with chronic hemolysis (sickle cell anemia, thalassemia) may require extra folate to avoid deficiency because of the relatively high requirement of the vitamin to support erythropoiesis. Other conditions with risk of deficiency include pregnancy, alcoholism, and treatment with anticonvulsants (phenytoin) or antimetabolites (methotrexate). First occurrence and recurrence of **neural tube defects** are reduced significantly by maternal supplementation during embryogenesis. Because closure of the neural tube occurs before usual recognition of pregnancy, all women of reproductive age are recommended to have a folate intake of at least 400 mcg/day as prophylaxis.

Vitamin B_{12}

Vitamin B_{12} is one of the most complex vitamin molecules, containing an atom of cobalt held in a *corrin ring* (similar to that of iron in hemoglobin). The cobalt ion is at the active center of the ring and serves as the site for attachment of alkyl groups during their transfer. The vitamin functions in single-carbon transfers and is intimately related to folate function and interconversions. Vitamin B_{12} is essential for normal lipid and carbohydrate metabolism in energy production and in protein biosynthesis and nucleic acid synthesis.

In contrast to other water-soluble vitamins, absorption of vitamin B_{12} is complex, involving cleavage of the vitamin from dietary protein and binding to a glycoprotein called *intrinsic factor,* which is secreted by the gastric mucosa (parietal cells). The cobalamin–intrinsic factor complex is efficiently absorbed from the distal ileum.

When vitamin B_{12} is absorbed into the portal circulation, it is transported bound to a specific protein, transcobalamin II. Its large stores in the liver also are unusual for a water-soluble vitamin. Efficient enterohepatic circulation normally protects from deficiency for months to years. Dietary sources of the vitamin are animal products only. Strict vegetarians should take a vitamin B_{12} supplement.

Vitamin B_{12} deficiency in children is rare. Early diagnosis and treatment of this disorder in childhood are important because of the danger of irreversible neurologic damage. Most cases in childhood result from a specific defect in absorption (see Table 29.2). Such defects include **congenital pernicious anemia** (absent intrinsic factor), **juvenile pernicious anemia** (autoimmune), and deficiency of transcobalamin II transport. Gastric or intestinal resection and small bowel bacterial overgrowth also cause vitamin B_{12} deficiency. Exclusively breast-fed infants ingest adequate of vitamin B_{12} unless the mother is a strict vegetarian without supplementation.

Depression of serum vitamin B_{12} and the appearance of hypersegmented neutrophils and macrocytosis (indistinguishable from folate deficiency) are early clinical manifestations of deficiency. Vitamin B_{12} deficiency also causes **neurologic manifestations**, including depression, peripheral neuropathy, posterior spinal column signs, dementia, and eventual coma. The neurologic signs do not occur in folate deficiency, but administration of folate may mask the hematologic signs of vitamin B_{12} deficiency, while the neurologic manifestations progress. Patients with vitamin B_{12} deficiency also have increased urine levels of methylmalonic acid. Most cases of vitamin B_{12} deficiency in infants and children are not of dietary origin and require treatment throughout life. Maintenance therapy consists of repeated monthly intramuscular injections, although a form of vitamin B_{12} is administered intranasally.

FAT-SOLUBLE VITAMINS

Fat-soluble vitamins (A, D, E, K) generally have stores in the body, and dietary deficiencies typically develop more slowly than for water-soluble vitamins. Absorption of fat-soluble vitamins depends on normal fat intake, digestion, and absorption. The complexity of normal fat absorption and the potential for perturbation in many disease states explains the more common occurrence of deficiencies of these vitamins.

Vitamin A

The basic constituent of the vitamin A group is retinol. Ingested plant carotene or animal tissue retinol esters release retinol after hydrolysis by pancreatic and intestinal enzymes. Chylomicron-transported retinol esters are stored in the liver as retinol palmitate. Retinol is transported from the liver to target tissues by retinol-binding protein, releasing free retinol to the target tissues. The kidney then excretes the retinol-binding protein. Diseases of the kidney diminish excretion of retinol-binding protein, whereas liver parenchymal disease or malnutrition lowers the synthesis of retinol-binding protein. Specific cellular binding proteins facilitate the uptake of retinol by target tissues. In the eye, retinol is metabolized to form **rhodopsin**; the action of light on rhodopsin is the first step of the visual process. Retinol also influences the growth and differentiation of epithelia. The clinical manifestations of vitamin A deficiency in humans appear as a group of ocular signs termed **xerophthalmia**. The earliest symptom is **night blindness**, which is followed by **xerosis** of the conjunctiva and cornea. Untreated, xerophthalmia can result in ulceration, necrosis, keratomalacia, and a permanent corneal scar. Clinical and subclinical vitamin A deficiencies are associated with **immunodeficiency**; increased risk of infection, especially measles; and increased risk of mortality. Xerophthalmia and vitamin A deficiency should be urgently treated. *Hypervitaminosis A* also has serious sequelae, including headaches, pseudotumor cerebri, hepatotoxicity, and teratogenicity. Any child with measles infection, regardless of geographic location or nutritional status, can benefit from vitamin A supplementation once daily, either orally or parenterally, for 2 days.

Vitamin E

Eight naturally occurring compounds have vitamin E activity. The most active of these, α-tocopherol, accounts for 90% of the vitamin E present in human tissues and is commercially available as an acetate or succinate. Vitamin E acts as a biologic **antioxidant** by inhibiting the peroxidation of polyunsaturated fatty acids present in cell membranes. It scavenges free radicals generated by the reduction of molecular oxygen and by the action of oxidative enzymes.

Vitamin E deficiency occurs in children with fat malabsorption secondary to liver disease, untreated celiac disease, cystic fibrosis, and abetalipoproteinemia. In these children, without vitamin E supplementation, a syndrome of progressive **sensory and motor neuropathy** develops; the first sign of deficiency is loss of deep tendon reflexes. Deficient preterm infants at 1–2 months of age have hemolytic anemia characterized by an elevated reticulocyte count, an increased sensitivity of the erythrocytes to hemolysis in hydrogen peroxide, peripheral edema, and thrombocytosis. All the abnormalities are corrected after oral, lipid, or water-soluble vitamin E therapy.

Vitamin D

Cholecalciferol (vitamin D_3) is the mammalian form of vitamin D and is produced by ultraviolet irradiation of inactive precursors in the skin. Ergocalciferol (vitamin D_2) is derived from plants. Vitamin D_2 and vitamin D_3 require further metabolism to become active. They are of equivalent potency. Clothing, lack of sunlight exposure, and skin pigmentation decrease generation of vitamin D in the epidermis and dermis.

Vitamin D (D_2 and D_3) is metabolized in the liver to calcidiol, or 25-hydroxyvitamin D (25[OH]D); this metabolite, which has little intrinsic activity, is transported by a plasma-binding globulin to the kidney, where it is converted to the most active metabolite calcitriol, or 1,25-dihydroxyvitamin D (1,25[OH_2]D). The action of 1,25(OH_2)D results in a decrease in the concentration of messenger RNA (mRNA) for collagen in bone and an increase in the concentration of mRNA for vitamin D–dependent calcium-binding protein in the intestine (directly mediating increased intestinal calcium transport). The antirachitic action of vitamin D probably is mediated by provision of appropriate concentrations of calcium and phosphate in the extracellular space of bone and by enhanced intestinal absorption of these minerals. Vitamin D also may have a direct anabolic effect on bone. 1,25(OH_2) D has direct feedback to the parathyroid gland and inhibits secretion of parathyroid hormone.

Vitamin D deficiency appears as **rickets** in children and as **osteomalacia** in postpubertal adolescents. Inadequate direct sun exposure and vitamin D intake are sufficient causes, but other factors, such as various drugs (phenobarbital, phenytoin) and malabsorption, may increase the risk of development of vitamin-deficiency rickets. Breast-fed infants are at risk for vitamin D deficiency.

The pathophysiology of rickets results from defective bone growth, especially at the epiphyseal cartilage matrix, which fails to mineralize. The uncalcified osteoid results in a wide, irregular zone of poorly supported tissue, the rachitic metaphysis. This soft, rather than hardened, zone produces many of the skeletal deformities through compression and lateral bulging or flaring of the ends of bones.

The **clinical manifestations** of rickets are most common during the first 2 years of life and may become evident only after several months of a vitamin D–deficient diet. **Craniotabes** is caused by thinning of the outer table of the skull, which when compressed feels like a ping-pong ball to the touch. Enlargement of the costochondral junction **(rachitic rosary)** and thickening of the wrists and ankles may be palpated. The anterior fontanel is enlarged, and its closure may be delayed. In advanced rickets, scoliosis and exaggerated lordosis may be present. Bowlegs or knock-knees may be evident in older infants, and greenstick fractures may be observed in long bones.

The **diagnosis** of rickets is based on a history of poor vitamin D intake and little exposure to direct ultraviolet sunlight. The serum calcium usually is normal but may be low; the serum phosphorus level usually is reduced, and serum alkaline phosphatase activity is elevated. When serum calcium levels decline to less than 7.5 mg/dL, tetany may occur. Levels of 24,25(OH_2)D are undetectable, and serum 1,25(OH_2)D levels are commonly less than 7 ng/mL, although 1,25(OH_2) D levels also may be normal. The best measure of vitamin D status is the level of 25(OH)D. Characteristic **radiographic** changes of the distal ulna and radius include widening, concave cupping, and frayed, poorly demarcated ends. The increased space seen between the distal ends of the radius and ulna and the metacarpal bones is the enlarged, nonossified metaphysis.

Breast-fed infants born of mothers with adequate vitamin D stores usually maintain adequate serum vitamin D levels for at least 2 months, but rickets may develop subsequently if these infants are not exposed to the sun or do not receive supplementary vitamin D. Vitamin D supplementation is recommended for all breast-fed infants in the amount of 400 IU/day, started soon after birth and given until the infant is taking more than 1,000 mL/day of formula or vitamin D–fortified milk (for age >1 year). Toxic effects of excessive chronic vitamin D may include hypercalcemia, muscle weakness, polyuria, and nephrocalcinosis.

Vitamin K

The plant form of vitamin K is phylloquinone, or vitamin K_1. Another form is menaquinone, or vitamin K_2, one of a series of compounds with unsaturated side chains synthesized by intestinal bacteria. Plasma factors II (prothrombin), VII, IX, and X in the cascade of blood coagulation factors depend on vitamin K for synthesis and for post-translational conversion of their precursor proteins. The post-translational conversion of glutamyl residues to carboxyglutamic acid residues of a prothrombin molecule creates effective calcium-binding sites, making the protein active.

Other vitamin K–dependent proteins include proteins C, S, and Z in plasma and γ-carboxyglutamic acid–containing proteins in several tissues. Bone contains a major vitamin K–dependent protein, osteocalcin, and lesser amounts of other glutamic acid–containing proteins.

Phylloquinone is absorbed from the intestine and transported by chylomicrons. The rarity of dietary vitamin K deficiency in humans with normal intestinal function suggests that the absorption of menaquinones is possible. Vitamin K deficiency has been observed in subjects with impaired fat absorption caused by obstructive jaundice, pancreatic insufficiency, and celiac disease; often these problems are combined with the use of antibiotics that change intestinal flora.

Vitamin K deficiency bleeding (**VKDB**, also known as **hemorrhagic disease of the newborn**), may be characterized as early-onset (first 24 hours of life), classic (between 2 days and 1 week of life), or late-onset (1 week to 6 months of age). VKDB usually is marked by generalized ecchymoses, gastrointestinal hemorrhage, or bleeding from a circumcision or umbilical stump; intracranial hemorrhage can occur but is uncommon. It is recommended that parenteral vitamin K (0.5–1 mg) be given to all newborns shortly after birth to prevent VKDB (see Chapter 61).

MINERALS

The *major minerals* are those that require intakes of more than 100 mg/day and contribute at least 0.1% of total body weight. There are seven essential major minerals: calcium, phosphorus, magnesium, sodium, potassium, chloride, and sulfur. Ten *trace minerals,* which constitute less than 0.1% of body weight, have essential physiologic roles. Characteristics of trace mineral deficiencies are listed in Table 29.3.

Calcium

Calcium is the most abundant major mineral. Ninety-nine percent of calcium is in the skeleton; the remaining 1% is in extracellular fluids, intracellular compartments, and cell membranes. Non-skeletal calcium has a role in nerve conduction, muscle contraction, blood clotting, and membrane permeability. There are two distinct bone calcium phosphate pools: a large, crystalline form and a smaller, amorphous phase. Bone calcium constantly turns over, with concurrent bone reabsorption and formation. Approximately half of **bone mineral accretion** occurs during adolescence. Bone mineral density peaks in early adulthood and is influenced by prior and concurrent dietary calcium intake, exercise, and hormone status (testosterone, estrogen).

Calcium intake can come from a variety of sources, with dairy products providing the most common and concentrated source. The calcium equivalent of 1 cup of milk (about 300 mg of calcium) is ¾ cup of plain yogurt, 1.5 oz of cheddar cheese, 2 cups of ice cream, ⅘ cup of almonds, or 2.5 oz of sardines. Other sources of calcium include some leafy green vegetables (broccoli, kale, collards), lime-processed tortillas, calcium-precipitated tofu, and calcium-fortified juices, cereals, and breads.

There is no classic calcium deficiency syndrome because blood and cell levels are closely regulated. The body can mobilize skeletal calcium and increase the absorptive efficiency of dietary calcium. **Osteoporosis** that occurs in childhood is related to protein-calorie malnutrition, vitamin C deficiency, steroid therapy, endocrine disorders, immobilization and disuse, celiac disease, osteogenesis imperfecta, or calcium deficiency (in premature infants). It is believed that the primary method of prevention of **postmenopausal osteoporosis** is to ensure maximum peak bone mass by providing optimal calcium intake during childhood and adolescence. Bone mineral status can be monitored by dual-energy x-ray absorptiometry.

No adverse effects are observed in adults with dietary calcium intakes of 2.5 g/day. There is concern that higher intakes may increase the risk of urinary stone formation, constipation, and decreased kidney function and may inhibit intestinal absorption of other minerals (iron, zinc).

Iron

Iron, the most abundant trace mineral, is used in the synthesis of hemoglobin, myoglobin, and enzyme iron. Body iron content is regulated primarily through modulation of iron absorption, which depends on the state of body iron stores, the form and amount of iron in foods, and the mixture of foods in the diet. There are two categories of iron in food. The first is **heme iron**, present in hemoglobin and myoglobin, which is supplied by meat and rarely accounts for more than one fourth of the iron ingested by infants. The absorption of heme iron is relatively efficient and is not influenced by other constituents of the diet. The second category is **non-heme iron**, which represents the preponderance of iron intake consumed by infants and exists in the form of iron salts. The absorption of non-heme iron is influenced by the composition of consumed foods. Enhancers of non-heme iron absorption are ascorbic acid, meat, fish, and poultry. Inhibitors are bran, polyphenols (including the tannates in tea), and phytic acid, a compound found in legumes and whole grains. The percent intestinal absorption of the small amount of iron in human milk is 10%; 4% is absorbed from iron-fortified cow's milk formula and from iron-fortified infant dry cereals.

In a normal term infant, there is little change in total body iron and little need for exogenous iron before 4 months of age. Iron deficiency is rare in term infants during the first 4 months, unless there has been substantial blood loss. After about 4 months of age, iron reserves become marginal, and, unless exogenous sources of iron are provided, the infant becomes progressively at risk for anemia as the iron requirement to support erythropoiesis increases. Premature or low birthweight infants have a lower amount of stored iron because significant amounts of iron are transferred from the mother in the third trimester. In addition, their postnatal iron needs are greater because of rapid rates of growth and other medical needs (i.e., frequent phlebotomy). Iron needs can be met by supplementation (ferrous sulfate) or by iron-containing complementary foods. Under normal circumstances, iron-fortified formula should be the only alternative to breast milk in infants younger than 1 year of age. Premature infants fed human milk may develop iron-deficiency anemia earlier unless they receive

TABLE 29.3 Trace Elements

ELEMENT	PHYSIOLOGY	EFFECTS OF DEFICIENCY	EFFECTS OF EXCESS	DIETARY SOURCES
Chromium	Potentiates the action of insulin	Impaired glucose tolerance, peripheral neuropathy, and encephalopathy	Unknown	Meat, grains, fruits, and vegetables
Copper	Absorbed via specific intestinal transporter Circulates bound to ceruloplasmin Enzyme cofactor (superoxide dismutase, cytochrome oxidase, and enzymes involved in iron metabolism and connective tissue formation)	Microcytic anemia, osteoporosis, neutropenia, neurologic symptoms, depigmentation of hair and skin	Acute: nausea, emesis, abdominal pain, coma, and hepatic necrosis Chronic toxicity (liver and brain injury) occurs in Wilson disease and secondary to excess intake	Vegetables, grains, nuts, liver, margarine, legumes, corn oil
Fluoride	Incorporated into bone	Dental caries	Chronic: dental fluorosis	Toothpaste, fluoridated water
Iodine	Component of thyroid hormone	Hypothyroidism	Hypothyroidism and goiter; maternal excess can cause congenital hypothyroidism and goiter	Saltwater fish, iodized salt
Iron	Component of hemoglobin, myoglobin, cytochromes, and other enzymes	Anemia, decreased alertness, impaired learning	Acute: nausea, vomiting, diarrhea, abdominal pain, and hypotension Chronic excess usually secondary to hereditary disorders; causes organ dysfunction.	Meat, fortified foods Deficiency can also result from blood loss (hookworm infestation, menorrhagia, GI bleeding)
Manganese	Enzyme cofactor	Hypercholesterolemia, weight loss, decreased clotting proteins*	Neurologic manifestations, cholestatic jaundice	Nuts, meat, grains, tea
Molybdenum	Enzyme cofactor (xanthine oxidase and others)	Tachycardia, tachypnea, night blindness, irritability, coma*	Hyperuricemia and increased risk of gout	Legumes, grains, liver
Selenium	Enzyme cofactor (prevents oxidative damage)	Cardiomyopathy (Keshan disease), myopathy	Nausea, diarrhea, neurologic manifestations, nail and hair changes, garlic odor	Meat, seafood, whole grains, garlic
Zinc	Enzyme cofactor Constituent of zinc-finger proteins, which regulate gene transcription	Decreased growth, dermatitis of extremities and around orifices, impaired immunity, poor wound healing, hypogonadism, diarrhea Supplements are beneficial in diarrhea and improve neurodevelopmental outcomes	Abdominal pain, diarrhea, vomiting Can worsen copper deficiency	Meat, shellfish, whole grains, legumes, cheese

*These deficiency states have been reported only in case reports associated with parenteral nutrition or highly unusual diets.
GI, Gastrointestinal.
From Greenbaum LA. Micronutrient mineral deficiencies. Kliegman RM, St. Geme J, eds. Nelson Textbook of Pediatrics. 22nd ed. Philadelphia: Elsevier, 2025 (Table 72.1).

iron supplements. Formula-fed preterm infants should receive iron-fortified formula.

In older children, iron deficiency may result from inadequate iron intake with excessive cow's milk intake or from intake of foods with poor iron bioavailability. Iron deficiency also can result from blood loss from such sources as cow milk protein allergic colitis, menses, gastric ulceration, or inflammatory bowel disease. Iron deficiency affects many tissues (muscle and central nervous system) in addition to producing anemia. **Iron deficiency** and **anemia** have been associated with lethargy and decreased work capacity and **impaired neurocognitive development**, the deficits of which may be irreversible when onset is in the first 2 years of life.

The diagnosis of iron-deficiency anemia is established by the presence of low serum ferritin levels, low serum iron levels, a microcytic hypochromic anemia, reduced transferrin saturation, normal to elevated red blood cell width distribution, and enhanced iron-binding capacity. The mean corpuscular volume and red blood cell indices are reduced, and the reticulocyte count is low. Iron deficiency may be present without anemia. Clinical manifestations include anemia, decreased alertness, and impaired learning.

Treatment of iron-deficiency anemia includes changes in the diet to provide adequate iron and the administration of 3–6 mg iron/kg per 24 hours (as ferrous sulfate) divided three times daily. Reticulocytosis is noted within 3–7 days of starting treatment. Oral treatment should be continued for 5 months. Intravenous iron therapy is needed if oral iron cannot be given. Parenteral iron therapy should be administered according to a strict protocol, including a test dose.

Zinc

Zinc is the second most abundant trace mineral and is important in protein metabolism and synthesis, in nucleic acid metabolism, and in stabilization of cell membranes. Zinc functions as a cofactor for more than 200 enzymes and is essential to numerous cellular metabolic functions. Adequate zinc status is especially crucial during periods of growth and for tissue proliferation (immune system, wound healing, skin, and gastrointestinal tract integrity); physiologic functions for which zinc is essential include normal growth, sexual maturation, and immune function.

Dietary zinc is absorbed (20–40%) in the duodenum and proximal small intestine. The best dietary sources of zinc are animal products, including human milk, from which it is readily absorbed. Whole grains and legumes also contain moderate amounts of zinc, but phytic acid inhibits absorption from these sources. On a global basis, poor bioavailability secondary to phytic acid is thought to be a more important factor than low intake in the widespread occurrence of zinc deficiency. Excretion of zinc occurs from the gastrointestinal tract. In the presence of ongoing losses, such as in chronic diarrhea, requirements can drastically increase.

Zinc deficiency dwarfism syndrome was first described in a group of children in the Middle East with low levels of zinc in their hair, poor appetite, diminished taste acuity, hypogonadism, and short stature. Zinc supplementation reduces morbidity and mortality from **diarrhea** and **pneumonia** and enhances growth in low resource settings. Mild to moderate zinc deficiency is considered to be highly prevalent in low resource settings, particularly in populations with high infectious burden and high rates of **stunting**. Mild zinc deficiency occurs in older breast-fed infants without adequate zinc intake from complementary foods or in young children with poor total or bioavailable zinc intake in the general diet. Acute, acquired severe zinc deficiency occurs in patients receiving total parenteral nutrition without zinc supplementation and in premature infants fed human milk without fortification. **Clinical manifestations** of mild zinc deficiency include anorexia, growth faltering, and immune impairment. Moderately severe manifestations include delayed sexual maturation, rough skin, and hepatosplenomegaly. The signs of severe deficiency include acral and periorificial erythematous scaling dermatitis, growth and immune impairment, diarrhea, mood changes, alopecia, night blindness, and photophobia.

Diagnosis of zinc deficiency is challenging. Plasma zinc concentrations are most commonly used, but levels are frequently normal in conditions of mild deficiency; levels in moderate to severe deficiency are typically less than 60 mcg/dL. Acute infection also can result in depression of circulating zinc levels. The standard for the diagnosis of deficiency is response to a trial of supplementation, with outcomes such as improved linear growth or weight gain, improved appetite, and improved immune function. Because there is no pharmacologic effect of zinc on these functions, a positive response to supplementation is considered evidence of a preexisting deficiency. Clinically, an empirical trial of zinc supplementation (1 mcg/kg/day) is a safe and reasonable approach in situations in which deficiency is considered possible.

Acrodermatitis enteropathica is an autosomal recessive disorder that begins 2–4 weeks after infants have been weaned from breast milk. It is characterized by an acute perioral and perianal dermatitis, alopecia, and growth faltering. The disease is caused by severe zinc deficiency from a specific defect of intestinal zinc absorption. Plasma zinc levels are markedly reduced, and serum alkaline phosphatase activity is low. **Treatment** is with high-dose oral zinc supplements. A relatively uncommon condition associated with presentation of severe zinc deficiency is due to a defect in the secretion of zinc from the mammary gland, resulting in abnormally low milk zinc concentrations. Breast-fed infants, especially those born prematurely, present with classic signs of zinc deficiency: growth failure, diarrhea, and dermatitis. Because there is no defect in the infant's ability to absorb zinc, treatment consists of supplementing the infant with zinc for the duration of breast-feeding, which can be successfully continued. Subsequent infants born to the mother will also need zinc supplementation if breast-fed. Zinc is relatively nontoxic. Excess intake produces nausea, emesis, abdominal pain, headache, vertigo, and seizures.

Fluoride

Dental enamel is strengthened when fluoride is substituted for hydroxyl ions in the hydroxyapatite crystalline mineral matrix of the enamel. The resulting fluoroapatite is more resistant to chemical and physical damage. Fluoride is incorporated into the enamel during the mineralization stages of tooth formation and by surface interaction after the tooth has erupted. Fluoride is similarly incorporated into bone mineral and may protect against osteoporosis later in life.

Because of concern about the risk of **fluorosis**, infants should not receive fluoride supplements before 6 months of age. Commercial formulas are made with defluoridated water and contain small amounts of fluoride. The fluoride content of human milk is low and is not influenced significantly by maternal intake. Practitioners should evaluate all potential fluoride sources and conduct a caries risk assessment before prescribing fluoride supplementation.

PEARLS FOR PRACTITIONERS

See Pediatric Nutrition and Nutritional Disorders: Pearls for Practitioners at the end of this section.

REVIEW QUESTIONS

Available online.

CHAPTER 30
Growth Faltering

Growth faltering (previously known as failure to thrive) is a descriptive term used when growth is inadequate compared to expected standards. To date, there is no universally accepted definition; objective definitions of malnutrition and undernutrition are more specific. Anthropometric criteria that have been used to define growth faltering include weight below the 3rd or 5th percentile for age; weight decreasing, crossing two major percentile lines on the growth chart over time; or weight less than 80% of the median weight for the height of the child. Caveats to these definitions exist. According to growth chart standards, 3% of the population naturally falls below the 3rd percentile. Children who have constitutional delay of growth usually are proportional (normal weight for height). Additionally, in the first few years of life, fluctuations in percentile position can occur in normal children. For example, children with familial short stature who are born large or appropriate for gestational age can experience catch-down growth. *Z* scores are another way to express anthropometric measures, reflecting the number of standard deviations above or below the population median. A commonly used cut point for undernutrition is a *z* score below −2. *Z* scores can provide more detailed information than percentiles, especially when following growth over time. Given the limitations of anthropometric measurements alone to define growth faltering, clinical diagnosis tools such as the Subjective Global Nutritional Assessment (SGNA) and the Semi-Objective Failure to Thrive (SOFTT) have been studied.

ETIOLOGY

There are multiple possible causes of growth faltering (Table 30.1). In the past, etiologies were sometimes categorized as organic (underlying medical condition diagnosed) and nonorganic (no underlying medical cause). This dichotomous classification can be problematic because, in many cases, the cause of growth faltering is multifactorial with interaction between multiple biologic and psychosocial factors. Growth faltering can be caused by inadequate nutritional intake (e.g., neurologic condition impeding feeding, improper mixing of formula, food insecurity), malabsorption (e.g., celiac disease, milk protein allergy), and/or increased metabolic demands (e.g., cardiac disease, chronic infection). Studies suggest that clinically unsuspected major organic diseases are detected in a minority of patients worked up for growth faltering. Approximately half of children hospitalized for growth faltering have known complex chronic conditions, a reflection of the overall increasing prevalence of children with complex care conditions.

TABLE 30.1 Factors That May Contribute to Growth Faltering

INADEQUATE INTAKE
• Improper formula preparation • Neglect • Food insecurity • Ineffective feeding techniques • Parental depression • Breast-feeding difficulties • Lack of knowledge of dietary needs • Behavioral issues in toddlers • Neurologic condition impeding feeding • Congenital condition such as cleft lip or palate impeding feeding • Upper airway obstruction • Gastroesophageal reflux • Malrotation, volvulus
MALABSORPTION/INCREASED NUTRIENT LOSSES
• Protein allergy • Protein-losing enteropathy • Inborn errors of metabolism • Biliary atresia • Short bowel syndrome • Celiac disease • Cystic fibrosis and other causes of pancreatic insufficiency • Other malabsorption syndromes
INCREASED METABOLIC DEMAND
• Congenital heart disease • Infections (HIV, tuberculosis, urinary tract infection, chronic sinusitis, parasitic infection, TORCH) • Chronic lung disease • Thyroid disease • Adrenal or pituitary disease • Sickle cell disease • Kidney disease (chronic kidney failure, renal tubular acidosis)

HIV, Human immunodeficiency virus; *TORCH,* toxoplasmosis, other, rubella, cytomegalovirus, herpes simplex virus.

DIAGNOSIS AND CLINICAL MANIFESTATIONS

A careful history and physical examination are the cornerstone of growth faltering evaluations. A medical history should include prenatal history, gestational age and perinatal history, birth size (weight, length, and head circumference), family history, and travel history. Indicators of medical diseases, such as vomiting, diarrhea, fever, respiratory symptoms, and fatigue, should be noted. A thorough and detailed diet history is essential including various foods and beverages consumed, amount, timing, and location, including any potential distractions; it is also important to ask about any specific parental dietary beliefs and practices. Lactation problems in breast-fed infants and improper formula preparation are frequent causes of growth faltering early in infancy. A complete psychosocial assessment of the child and family is required. Child factors (temperament, development), parental factors (depression, domestic violence, social isolation, cognitive deficits, substance use), and environmental and societal factors (poverty, unemployment, illiteracy, lead toxicity) all may contribute to growth faltering.

A complete physical examination should be completed starting with vital signs and growth parameters. Growth charts provide important information. Changes in weight should be assessed in relation to height (length) and head circumference. Allowances must be made for prematurity; weight corrections are needed until 24 months of age, height corrections until 40 months of age, and head circumference corrections until 18 months of age. There are specific growth charts for genetic conditions such as Down syndrome and Turner syndrome that should be used when assessing growth for children with these conditions. Although some growth variants can be difficult to distinguish from growth faltering, growth velocity and height-for-weight determinations can be useful in distinguishing the cause. In children with growth faltering, malnutrition initially results in wasting (deficiency in weight gain). Stunting (deficiency in linear growth) generally occurs after months of malnutrition, and head circumference is spared except with chronic, severe malnutrition. Growth faltering that is symmetric (proportional weight, height/length, and head circumference) suggests long-standing malnutrition, chromosomal abnormalities, congenital infection, or teratogenic exposures. Short stature with preserved weight suggests an endocrine etiology. Physical examination should also assess for signs of inflicted injury; oral or dental problems; indicators of pulmonary, cardiac, or gastrointestinal disease; and dysmorphic features that may suggest a genetic or teratogenic cause for growth failure. A complete neurologic examination may reveal spasticity or hypotonia, which can have untoward effects on feeding and growth. Physical findings related to malnutrition include decreased subcutaneous fat, decreased muscle mass, dermatitis, hepatomegaly, cheilosis, or edema (see Chapter 28). Additionally, children with growth faltering have more otitis media, respiratory, and gastrointestinal infections than age-matched controls; severely malnourished children are at risk for a variety of serious infections. Observation during feeding and home visitation, if possible, is of great diagnostic value in assessing feeding problems, food preferences, mealtime distractions, unusual or disruptive parent-child interactions, and the home environment. Feeding evaluation by a speech therapist could also be helpful.

The history and physical examination findings should guide the laboratory evaluation. Routine extensive laboratory and radiology studies are not indicated; rather, tests should be ordered based on findings from the clinical evaluation. Simple screening tests could be used to identify common illnesses that cause growth faltering and to search for medical problems resulting from malnutrition. Initial tests may include a complete blood count, screening for iron-deficiency anemia and lead toxicity, and urinalysis, urine culture, and serum electrolytes to assess renal infection or dysfunction. A review of the child's newborn screen may also be warranted. Additional testing can be ordered as needed, based on the child's signs and symptoms. For example, a stool sample for culture and ova and parasites may be indicated in children with diarrhea, abdominal pain, or malodorous stools.

TREATMENT

Identified biopsychosocial etiologies will inform the treatment plan. Most children with growth faltering can be treated in the outpatient setting. Children with severe malnutrition, with underlying diagnoses that require hospitalization for evaluation or treatment, or whose safety is in jeopardy because of maltreatment require hospitalization. Admitting children to the hospital to induce and document weight gain is not recommended unless intensive outpatient evaluation and intervention has failed or the social circumstances are a contraindication for attempting outpatient management. Potential multidisciplinary treatment team members include pediatricians, nutritionists, speech and occupational therapists, developmental specialists, nurses, and social workers.

Nutritional management is the cornerstone of treatment. Children with growth faltering who are anorexic or picky eaters may have difficulty consuming the amount of calories and protein needed for catch-up growth and require calorie-dense foods. For formula-fed infants, the concentration of formula can be adjusted appropriately. For healthy term infants, formulas are prepared to provide 20 kcal/oz. Powder and liquid concentrates can be mixed with less water to provide a higher caloric density if needed. Final concentrations are reached by adding formula to the specific amount of water needed to reach the desired caloric density. Breast milk can also be fortified if needed. For toddlers, dietary changes should include increasing the caloric density of foods. High-calorie oral supplements (30 cal/oz) are often well tolerated by toddlers. In some cases, specific carbohydrate, fat, or protein additives are used to boost calories by increasing calories without increasing volume requirements. Nasogastric tube feedings are used when children cannot take adequate calories safely by mouth. Vitamin and mineral supplementation can be required, especially during catch-up growth. In general, the simplest and least costly approach to dietary change is warranted.

Treatment must also address the **psychosocial needs** of the family. Families may need concrete resources. Parents of malnourished children may feel personally responsible and/or threatened by the diagnosis. Parents may have their own health and economic concerns and thus cannot focus on their child's needs; they may not immediately recognize the psychosocial and family contributors to malnutrition. These issues can have a profound effect on the success of treatment and need to be addressed.

COMPLICATIONS

Malnutrition causes defects in host defenses. Children with growth faltering may experience a **malnutrition-infection cycle**, in which recurrent infections exacerbate malnutrition, leading to greater susceptibility to infection.

During starvation, the body slows metabolic processes and growth to minimize the need for nutrients and uses its stores of glycogen, fat, and protein to maintain normal metabolic requirements. The body also generally maintains homeostasis and normal serum concentrations of electrolytes. With the rapid reinstitution of feeding after starvation, fluid and electrolyte homeostasis may be lost. Changes in serum electrolyte concentrations and the associated complications are collectively termed **re-feeding syndrome**. These changes typically affect phosphorus, potassium, calcium, and magnesium and can result in life-threatening cardiac, pulmonary, or neurologic problems. Infants and children with marasmus, kwashiorkor, and anorexia nervosa and those who experience prolonged fasting are at risk for re-feeding syndrome. Re-feeding syndrome can be avoided by slow institution of nutrition, close monitoring of serum electrolytes during the initial days of feeding, and prompt replacement of depleted electrolytes.

PSYCHOSOCIAL SHORT STATURE

Occasionally, children who live in psychologic deprivation develop short stature with or without concomitant growth faltering or delayed puberty, a syndrome called **psychosocial short stature**. The signs and symptoms include polyphagia, polydipsia, hoarding and stealing of food, gorging and vomiting, and other notable behaviors. Affected children are typically depressed and socially withdrawn. Endocrine dysfunction including decreased growth hormone and muted response to exogenous growth hormone is often identified in affected children. Removal of the child from the adverse environment typically results in rapid improvement in endocrine function and subsequent rapid somatic and pubertal growth of the child. The prognosis for children with psychosocial short stature depends on the age at diagnosis and the degree of psychologic trauma. Early identification and removal from the environment portends a healthy prognosis. Those diagnosed in later childhood or adolescence may not reach their genetic potential for growth and have a poorer psychosocial prognosis.

ACKNOWLEDGEMENT

The author is grateful to Drs. Kristin Fortin and Allison Downes, whose chapter on this topic appeared in the previous edition and much of their work is retained here.

PEARLS FOR PRACTITIONERS

See Pediatric Nutrition and Nutritional Disorders: Pearls for Practitioners at the end of this section.

REVIEW QUESTIONS

Available online.

Suggested Readings

Andes LJ, Cheng YJ, Rolka DB, Gregg EW, Imperatore G. Prevalence of Prediabetes Among Adolescents and Young Adults in the United States, 2005-2016. *JAMA Pediatr*. 2020;174(2):e194498.

Armstrong S, Lazorick S, Hampl S, et al. Physical Examination Findings Among Children and Adolescents With Obesity: An Evidence-Based Review. *Pediatrics*. 2016;137(2):e20151766.

Buoncristiano M, Williams J, Simmonds P, et al. Socioeconomic inequalities in overweight and obesity among 6- to 9-year-old children in 24 countries from the World Health Organization European region. *Obes Rev*. 2021;22(suppl 6):e13213.

Centers for Disease Control and Prevention. *About social determinants of health (SDOH)*. Available at: https://www.cdc.gov/socialdeterminants/about.html. Accessed October 5, 2022.

Centers for Disease Control and Prevention. *Body mass index (BMI)*. Accessed October 5, 2022. Available at: https://www.cdc.gov/healthyweight/assessing/bmi/index.html.

Centers for Disease Control and Prevention. *Physical Activity Facts*. Available at: https://www.cdc.gov/healthyschools/physicalactivity/facts.htm.

Centers for Disease Control and Prevention. *Prevalence of childhood obesity in the United States*; 2021. Accessed October 5, 2022. Available at: https://www.cdc.gov/obesity/data/childhood.html.

Finkelstein EA, Graham WC, Malhotra R. Lifetime direct medical costs of childhood obesity. *Pediatrics*. 2014;133(5):854–862.

Fryar CD, Carroll MD, Afful J. *Prevalence of overweight, obesity, and severe obesity among children and adolescents aged 2–19 years: United States, 1963–1965 through 2017–2018*. NCHS Health E-Stats; 2020. Available at: https://www.cdc.gov/nchs/data/hestat/obesity-child-17-18/obesity-child.htm. Accessed October 5, 2022.

Ghandour RM, Grason HA, Schempf AH, et al. Healthy people 2010 leading health indicators: how children with special health care needs fared. *Am J Public Health*. 2013;103(6):e99–e106.

Guthold R, Stevens GA, Riley LM, Bull FC. Worldwide trends in insufficient physical activity from 2001 to 2016: a pooled analysis of 358 population-based surveys with 1·9 million participants [published correction appears in Lancet Glob Health. 2019 Jan;7(1):e36.]. *Lancet Glob Health*. 2018;6(10):e1077–e1086.

Hales CM, Fryar CD, Carroll MD, Freedman DS, Ogden CL. Trends in Obesity and Severe Obesity Prevalence in US Youth and Adults by Sex and Age, 2007-2008 to 2015-2016. *JAMA*. 2018;319(16):1723–1725.

Hampl SE, Hassink SG, Skinner AC, et al. Executive Summary: Clinical Practice Guideline for the Evaluation and Treatment of Children and Adolescents With Obesity. *Pediatrics*. 2023;151(2):e2022060641.

Health Resources and Services Administration. *Chronic care model*. Accessed October 5, 2022. Available at: https://www.hrsa.gov/behavioral-health/chronic-care-model.

Hornberger LL, Lane MA, COMMITTEE ON ADOLESCENCE. Identification and Management of Eating Disorders in Children and Adolescents. *Pediatrics*. 2021;147(1):e2020040279.

Jung HW. Current Options in Obesity Pharmacotherapy for Children and Adolescents. A Narrative Review. *Precis Future Med*. 2024;8(2):38–49.

Krebs NF, Himes JH, Jacobson D, Nicklas TA, Guilday P, Styne D. Assessment of child and adolescent overweight and obesity. *Pediatrics*. 2007;120(suppl 4):S193–S228.

Kyle TK, Dhurandhar EJ, Allison DB. Regarding Obesity as a Disease: Evolving Policies and Their Implications. *Endocrinol Metab Clin North Am*. 2016;45(3):511–520.

Lange SJ, Kompaniyets L, Freedman DS, et al. Longitudinal Trends in Body Mass Index Before and During the COVID-19 Pandemic Among Persons Aged 2-19 Years—United States, 2018-2020 [published correction appears in MMWR Morb Mortal Wkly Rep. 2021 Sep 24;70(38):1355]. *MMWR Morb Mortal Wkly Rep*. 2021;70(37):1278–1283.

Li X, Keown-Stoneman CDG, Lebovic G, et al. The association between body mass index trajectories and cardiometabolic risk in young children. *Pediatr Obes*. 2020;15(8):e12633.

Lynch BA, Agunwamba A, Wilson PM, et al. Adverse family experiences and obesity in children and adolescents in the United States. *Prev Med*. 2016;90:148–154.

Maïano C, Hue O, Morin AJ, Moullec G. Prevalence of overweight and obesity among children and adolescents with intellectual disabilities: a systematic review and meta-analysis. *Obes Rev*. 2016;17(7):599–611.

Medvedyuk S, Ali A, Raphael D. Ideology, obesity and the social determinants of health: a critical analysis of the obesity and health relationship. *Crit Public Health*. 2017;28(5):573–585.

Moradi M, Mozaffari H, Askari M, Azadbakht L. Association between overweight/obesity with depression, anxiety, low self-esteem, and body dissatisfaction in children and adolescents: a systematic review and meta-analysis of observational studies. *Crit Rev Food Sci Nutr*. 2022;62(2):555–570.

National Center for Chronic Disease Prevention and Health Promotion. *About chronic diseases*. Accessed October 5, 2022. Available at: https://www.cdc.gov/chronicdisease/about/index.htm.

National Center on Birth Defects and Developmental Disabilities. *Communicating with and about people with disabilities*. Accessed October 5, 2022. Available at: https://www.cdc.gov/ncbddd/disabilityandhealth/materials/factsheets/fs-communicating-withpeople.html.

National Institutes of Health. *Obesity Research Task Force. Strategic Plan for NIH Obesity Research*. Bethesda, MD: US Department of Health and Human Services, National Institutes of Health; 2011.

O'Connor EA, Burda BU, Eder M, Walsh ES, Evans CV, Kaiser Permanente Research Affiliates Evidence-based Practice Center. *Multicomponent Behavioral Interventions for Weight Management in Children and Adolescents Who Are Overweight or With Obesity: A Systematic Evidence Review for the American Psychological Association*. Portland, OR: Kaiser Permanente Center for Health Research; 2016.

O'Connor EA, Evans CV, Burda BU, Walsh ES, Eder M, Lozano P. *Screening for Obesity and Interventions for Weight Management in Children and Adolescents: A Systematic Evidence Review for the U.S. Preventive Services Task Force*. Rockville (MD): Agency for Healthcare Research and Quality (US); 2017.

Ogden CL, Fryar CD, Martin CB, et al. Trends in Obesity Prevalence by Race and Hispanic Origin-1999-2000 to 2017-2018. *JAMA*. 2020;324(12):1208–1210.

Regis A. The CHILD 1 diet: from strategy to practicality. *Pediatr Ann*. 2013;42(9):178–180.

Rogers R, Eagle TF, Sheetz A, et al. The Relationship between Childhood Obesity, Low Socioeconomic Status, and Race/Ethnicity: Lessons from Massachusetts. *Child Obes*. 2015;11(6):691–695.

Sokol R, Austin A, Chandler C, et al. Screening Children for Social Determinants of Health: A Systematic Review. *Pediatrics*. 2019;144(4):e20191622.

Song Z, Wan L, Wang W, et al. Daily stair climbing, disease susceptibility, and risk of atherosclerotic cardiovascular disease: A prospective cohort study. *Atherosclerosis*. 2023;386:117300.
U.S. Department of Agriculture and U.S. Department of Health and Human Services. *Dietary Guidelines for Americans, 2020-2025*. 9th ed. 2020. Available at: DietaryGuidelines.gov.
US Department of Health and Human Services, Office of Disease Prevention and Health Promotion. Healthy people 2030. Available at: https://health.gov/healthypeople/objectives-and-data/social-determinants-health. Accessed October 5, 2022.
US Preventive Services Task Force, Grossman DC, Bibbins-Domingo K, et al. Screening for Obesity in Children and Adolescents: US Preventive Services Task Force Recommendation Statement. *JAMA*. 2017;317(23):2417–2426.
Ward ZJ, Long MW, Resch SC, Giles CM, Cradock AL, Gortmaker SL. Simulation of Growth Trajectories of Childhood Obesity into Adulthood. *N Engl J Med*. 2017;377(22):2145–2153.
Zhang X, Ma N, Lin Q, et al. Body Roundness Index and All-Cause Mortality Among US Adults [published correction appears in JAMA Netw Open. 2024 Jul 1;7(7):E2426540]. *JAMA Netw Open*. 2024;7(6):E2415051.

Pearls for Practitioners

CHAPTER 25

Diet of the Healthy Infant

- **Importance of nutrition in infancy:** Proper nutrition during infancy is crucial for rapid growth, brain development, and establishing healthy dietary habits that can influence lifelong health.
- **Breast-feeding provides optimal infant nutrition:** Breast-feeding is recommended exclusively for the first 6 months, with continued breast-feeding alongside complementary foods up to 2 years or beyond, because it provides vital medical and neurodevelopmental benefits for both infants and breast-feeding parents.
- **Monitoring growth:** Key indicators like weight, length, weight-for-height, and head circumference should be tracked over time to assess infant growth, rather than relying on single measurements.
- **Complementary feeding and developmental readiness:** Around 6 months, nutrient-dense complementary foods, particularly those rich in iron and zinc, should be introduced alongside breast milk or formula to meet increasing nutritional needs. It is important to assess developmental readiness before starting solids; infants should be able to control their head and neck, sit up with support, bring objects to their mouth, and grasp small items. Introducing age-appropriate food textures and avoiding choking hazards helps ensure safe feeding as infants transition to solid foods.
- **Vitamin D and iron supplementation:** Vitamin D supplementation of 400 IU daily is recommended for all infants beginning soon after birth. Iron-rich foods or supplements are crucial after 6 months, especially for breast-fed infants, to support healthy growth and development.
- **Allergenic foods introduction:** Introducing potentially allergenic foods like peanuts, eggs, and milk products early (around 6 months) can help reduce the risk of food allergies, especially for infants at high risk.
- **Safe formula feeding:** For formula-fed infants, iron-fortified formulas are recommended. Parents should be counseled on safe preparation to prevent consequences of improper mixing like hyponatremia or infection.
- **Limiting added sugars and sodium:** Infants' diets should be free of added sugars and low in sodium.
- **Avoid unsafe foods and beverages:** Infants should not consume honey, unpasteurized foods, caffeinated drinks, or sugary beverages due to risks like botulism, infection, and potential choking hazards.
- **Role of pediatricians:** Pediatricians are essential in supporting families with breast-feeding education, introducing complementary foods, and helping to ensure that infants receive the healthiest start in life.

CHAPTER 26

Diet of the Healthy Child and Adolescent

- A healthy diet helps children grow, thrive, and learn and helps prevent obesity and weight-related diseases such as diabetes.
- Cow's milk should be introduced at 12 months of age. Low-fat (2%) or whole milk is recommended until 2 years of age, after which fat-free or 1% milk is recommended.
- Excessive milk intake (>24 oz/day for children 1–2 years of age; >16 oz/day for children older than 2) should be avoided in toddlers.
- No juice is recommended during infancy (<1 year). From 1 to 6 years of life, recommend a maximum of 4 oz per day, and a maximum of 6 oz per day after 7 years.
- MyPlate by the U.S. Department of Agriculture can provide parents with a general guideline for the types of healthy food to feed their child.
- American children have high salt intake. Recommended daily salt intake is 1,900–2,300 mg.
- Poor calcium intake during adolescence has significant consequences for long-term bone health. Good sources include milk, yogurt, fortified orange juice, cheese, soybeans, and tofu.
- Iron deficiency may reappear in menstruating teens.

CHAPTER 27

Children With Obesity

- **Complex etiology of obesity:** Obesity rates among U.S. children and adolescents (ages 2–19) have surged to 19%. Childhood obesity is a complex chronic disease shaped by genetic, biological, environmental, and socioeconomic factors. Effective treatment requires understanding this complexity. Adverse social drivers of health (SDoHs), such as racism, poverty, and limited access to nutritious food and safe spaces, play a significant role and must be addressed to reduce disparities and improve outcomes.

- **Role of pediatricians and primary care providers:** Pediatricians and health care providers are essential in early identification, evaluation, and management of childhood obesity. They must approach obesity as a chronic condition and coordinate care within the medical home model, collaborating with specialists and community resources.
- **Comprehensive obesity treatment (COT):** Effective COT requires a multidisciplinary approach that includes nutrition counseling, physical activity, behavior modification, and sometimes pharmacotherapy or surgery. The focus should be on long-term health, co-morbidity management, and patient-centered goals beyond BMI reduction.
- **Parental and family involvement and motivational interviewing (MI) for behavior change:** MI is a patient-centered counseling method that engages families to identify their motivation for change and set achievable health goals, promoting sustainable behavior change. Family-based interventions are more effective than child-only programs because parents play a key role in modeling healthy behaviors and creating supportive environments. However, parental involvement should be adapted for adolescents to respect their growing autonomy.
- **Intensive health behavior and lifestyle treatment (IHBLT):** Programs involving at least 26 hours of comprehensive, face-to-face family-based treatment over 3–12 months have shown significant success. These interventions address nutritional habits, physical activity, and behavioral support.
- **Early and consistent BMI screening:** Annual BMI evaluations beginning at age 2 are recommended to monitor growth and identify children at risk for obesity. Pediatricians should communicate BMI results in a respectful manner, seeking permission and using person-first language to prevent stigmatization.
- **Addressing co-morbidities:** Obesity significantly raises the risk of various serious physical and mental health conditions, including cardiovascular disease, type 2 diabetes, nonalcoholic fatty liver disease (NAFLD), increased mortality, and higher health care costs. Regular assessment and management of these co-morbidities are crucial for comprehensive care.
- **Challenges and gaps in access to care:** Limited access to specialized obesity treatment programs, especially outside urban areas, remains a significant barrier. Pediatricians should leverage local community resources, telemedicine, and partnerships to improve access and support families in need.

CHAPTER 28

Pediatric Undernutrition

- Pediatric undernutrition results from inadequate food supply, access (food insecurity), or utilization; poor access to health and sanitation; chronic health conditions; and/or inappropriate feeding, behavioral issues, or child-care practices.
- International references are established that standardize anthropometric measures in terms of *z* scores.
- Primary protein-energy malnutrition (PEM) is caused by social or economic factors that result in a lack of adequate intake.
- Secondary PEM occurs in children with various conditions associated with increased caloric requirements (infection, trauma, cancer), caloric loss (malabsorption), reduced intake (anorexia, cancer, oral intake restriction, social factors), or a combination of these.
- Marasmus results from the body's physiologic response to inadequate calories and nutrients.
- Kwashiorkor results from inadequate protein intake in the presence of fair to good caloric intake.
- Vitamin A and zinc deficiency often accompany malnutrition.
- Dermatitis may be seen with protein-calorie malnutrition as well as riboflavin, biotin, and essential fatty acid deficiencies.
- Neuropathy may be seen in thiamine and vitamin B_6, B_{12}, and E deficiencies.

CHAPTER 29

Vitamin and Mineral Deficiencies

- Risk factors for micronutrient deficiencies in developed countries include exclusion of entire food groups, malabsorption syndromes, and conditions causing high physiologic requirements.
- Exclusively breast-fed term infants are at higher risk for vitamin D and K deficiencies.
- Vitamin D supplementation (400 IU/day) should be started soon after birth for all infants.
- Parenteral vitamin K (0.5–1 mg) should be given to all newborns shortly after birth.
- Niacin (vitamin B3) deficiency results in pellagra: a combination of weakness, photosensitivity, dermatitis, vomiting, diarrhea, and dementia.
- Deficiency of vitamin B_{12} results in megaloblastic anemia, peripheral neuropathy, posterior column disease, and vitiligo.
- Folate deficiency results in hypersegmented neutrophils, macrocytic anemia, and neural tube defects.
- Scurvy, a combination of irritability, purpura, bleeding gums, periosteal hemorrhage, and aching bones, results from a deficiency of ascorbic acid (vitamin C).
- Vitamin D deficiency appears as rickets in children and osteomalacia in postpubertal adolescents.
- The diagnosis of iron-deficiency anemia is established by the presence of a microcytic hypochromic anemia, low serum ferritin levels, low serum iron levels, reduced transferrin saturation, normal to elevated red blood cell width distribution, and enhanced iron-binding capacity.
- Because of concern about the risk of fluorosis, infants should not receive fluoride supplements before 6 months of age.

CHAPTER 30

Growth Faltering

- There is no single, universally accepted anthropometric criterion for growth faltering or failure to thrive. Commonly used criteria include weight below the 3rd or 5th percentile for age; weight decreasing, crossing two major percentile lines on the growth chart over time; a *z* score below −2; or weight less than 80% of the median weight for the height of the child.
- Growth faltering can be caused by inadequate intake, malabsorption, or increased metabolic demands.
- History and physical examination to assess for biologic and psychosocial etiologies are the cornerstone of growth faltering evaluations.
- A thorough and detailed diet history is essential including various foods and beverages consumed, amount, timing, and location, including any potential distractions; it is also important to ask about any specific parental dietary beliefs and practices.
- Children with growth faltering have more otitis media, respiratory, and gastrointestinal infections than age-matched controls; severely malnourished children are at risk for a variety of serious infections.

FLUIDS AND ELECTROLYTES

Jackson T. Londeree | Larry A. Greenbaum

CHAPTER 31
Maintenance Fluid Therapy

BODY COMPOSITION

Water is the most plentiful constituent of the human body. **Total body water (TBW)** as a percentage of body weight varies with age. The fetus has a high TBW, which gradually decreases to about 75% of birthweight for a term infant; TBW is higher in premature infants. During the first year of life, TBW decreases to about 60% of body weight and remains at this level until puberty. During puberty, the fat content of females increases more than that of males, who acquire more muscle mass than females. As fat has low water content and muscle has high water content, by the end of puberty, TBW in males remains at 60%, but it decreases to 50% of body weight in females. During dehydration, TBW decreases and is a smaller percentage of body weight.

TBW has two main compartments: **intracellular fluid (ICF)** and **extracellular fluid (ECF)**. In the fetus and newborn, the ECF volume is larger than the ICF volume. The normal postnatal diuresis causes an immediate decrease in the ECF volume, which is then followed by continued expansion of the ICF volume because of cellular growth. By 1 year of age, the ratio of the ICF volume to the ECF volume approaches adult levels. The ECF volume is 20–25% of body weight, and the ICF volume is 30–40% of body weight (Fig. 31.1). With puberty, the increased muscle mass of males results in a higher ICF volume than in females.

The ECF is divided further into **plasma water** and **interstitial fluid** (Fig. 31.1). Plasma water is about 5% of body weight. The blood volume, given a hematocrit of 40%, is usually 8% of body weight, although it is higher in newborns and young infants. The interstitial fluid, normally 15% of body weight, can increase dramatically in diseases associated with edema, such as heart failure, liver failure, and nephrotic syndrome.

The composition of solutes in the ICF and ECF is different. Sodium and chloride are the dominant cation and anion in the ECF. Potassium is the most abundant cation in the ICF, and proteins, organic anions, and phosphate are the most plentiful anions in the ICF. The dissimilarity between the anions in the ICF and the ECF is determined largely by the presence of intracellular molecules that do not cross the cell membrane, the barrier separating the ECF and the ICF. In contrast, the difference in the distribution of cations—sodium and potassium—is due to the activity of the Na^+, K^+-ATPase pump, which extrudes sodium from cells in exchange for potassium.

REGULATION OF INTRAVASCULAR VOLUME AND OSMOLALITY

Proper cell functioning requires close regulation of plasma osmolality and intravascular volume; these are controlled by independent systems for water balance, which determines **osmolality**, and sodium balance, which determines **volume status**. Maintenance of a normal osmolality depends on control of water balance. Control of volume status depends on regulation of sodium balance.

The plasma osmolality is tightly controlled between 285 and 295 mOsm/kg through regulation of water intake and urinary water losses. A small increase in the plasma osmolality stimulates thirst. Urinary water losses are regulated by the secretion of **antidiuretic hormone (ADH)**, which increases in

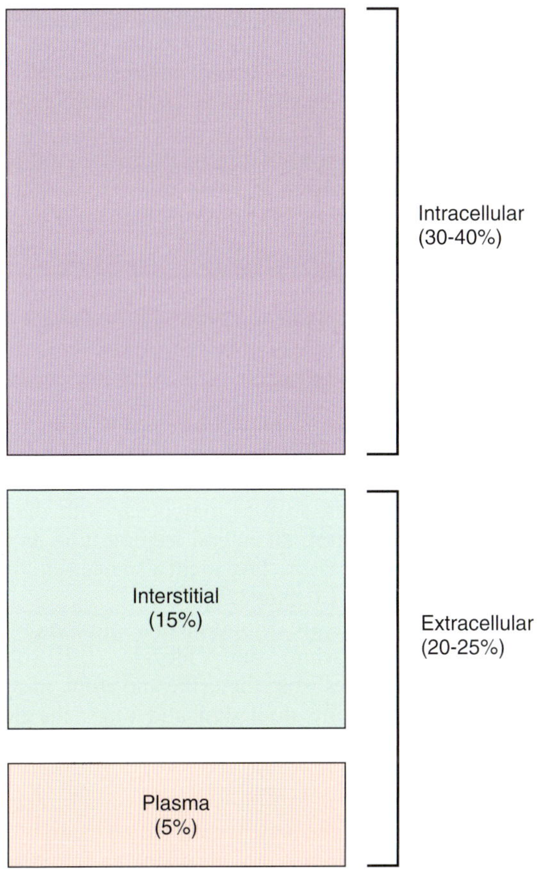

FIGURE 31.1 Compartments of total body water, expressed as percentage of body weight, in an older child or adult. (From Greenbaum LA. Pathophysiology of body fluids and fluid therapy. In: Kliegman RM, St. Geme JW, eds. *Nelson Textbook of Pediatrics*. 22nd ed. Philadelphia: Elsevier; 2025:485.)

TABLE 31.1 Body Weight Method for Calculating Maintenance Fluid Volume and Rate

BODY WEIGHT (kg)	VOLUME PER DAY	HOURLY RATE
0–10	100 mL/kg	4 mL/kg/hr
11–20	1,000 mL + 50 mL/kg for each 1 kg >10 kg	40 mL/hr + 2 mL/kg/hr × (wt − 10)
>20	1,500 mL + 20 mL/kg for each 1 kg >20 kg*	60 mL/hr + 1 mL/kg/hr × (wt − 20)†

*The maximum total fluid per day is normally 2,400 mL.
†The maximum fluid rate is normally 100 mL/hr.

response to an increasing plasma osmolality. ADH, by stimulating renal tubular reabsorption of water, decreases urinary water losses. Control of osmolality is subordinate to maintenance of an adequate intravascular volume. When significant volume depletion is present, ADH secretion and thirst are stimulated, regardless of the plasma osmolality.

Volume depletion and volume overload can cause significant morbidity and mortality. As sodium is the principal extracellular cation and is restricted to the ECF, adequate body sodium is necessary for maintenance of intravascular volume. The kidney determines sodium balance because there is little homeostatic control of sodium intake, although salt craving occasionally occurs in children with chronic kidney salt loss or adrenal insufficiency. The kidney regulates sodium balance by altering the percentage of filtered sodium that is reabsorbed along the nephron. The **renin-angiotensin system** is an important regulator of kidney sodium reabsorption and excretion. The juxtaglomerular apparatus produces renin in response to decreased *effective* intravascular volume. Renin cleaves angiotensinogen, producing angiotensin I, which angiotensin-converting enzyme converts into angiotensin II. The actions of angiotensin II include direct stimulation of the proximal tubule to increase sodium reabsorption and stimulation of the adrenal gland to increase aldosterone secretion, which increases sodium reabsorption in the distal nephron. In contrast, volume expansion stimulates the synthesis of **atrial natriuretic peptide**, which increases urinary sodium excretion.

MAINTENANCE FLUIDS

Maintenance intravenous (IV) fluids are used in children who cannot be fed enterally. Along with maintenance fluids, children may require concurrent **replacement fluids** if they have excessive **ongoing losses**, such as may occur with diarrhea, vomiting, or drainage from an enteral feeding tube. In addition, if dehydration is present, the patient also needs to receive deficit replacement (see Chapter 32).

Maintenance IV fluids are composed of a solution of water, glucose, sodium, potassium, and chloride. This solution replaces electrolyte losses from the urine and stool, as well as water losses from the urine, stool, skin, and lungs. The glucose in maintenance fluids provides approximately 20% of normal caloric needs. This is enough to prevent the development of starvation ketoacidosis and diminishes the protein degradation that would occur if the patient received no calories.

Maintenance fluids do not provide adequate calories, protein, fat, minerals, or vitamins. Patients should not remain on maintenance therapy indefinitely; parenteral nutrition (see Chapter 33) should be used for children who cannot be fed enterally for more than a few days.

Daily water losses are measurable (urine and stool) and not measurable (*insensible losses* from the skin and lungs). Failure to replace these losses leads to a thirsty child and, ultimately, a dehydrated child. Table 31.1 provides a system for calculating **24-hour maintenance water** needs based on the patient's weight.

After calculation of water needs and electrolyte needs, children over 28 days of life typically receive D5 in normal saline plus 20 mEq/L of KCl as a maintenance solution. This assumes that there is no disease process present that would require an adjustment in either the volume or the electrolyte composition of maintenance fluids. Neonates receive hypotonic fluids such as one-half normal saline. Children with decreased kidney function may be hyperkalemic or unable to excrete potassium and may not tolerate 20 mEq/L of KCl. In children with complicated pathophysiologic abnormalities, it may be necessary to adjust the electrolyte composition and rate of maintenance fluids empirically based on electrolyte measurements and assessment of fluid balance.

PEARLS FOR PRACTITIONERS

See Fluids and Electrolytes: Pearls for Practitioners at the end of this section.

REVIEW QUESTIONS

Available online.

CHAPTER 32

Dehydration and Replacement Therapy

REPLACEMENT THERAPY

There are three sources of normal water loss—the components of maintenance water (see Chapter 31): urine (60%), **insensible losses** from the skin and lungs (35%), and stool (5%) (Table 32.1). Sweating is not insensible and, in contrast to evaporative losses, sweat contains water and electrolytes.

A variety of clinical situations modify normal maintenance water requirements (Table 32.2). Evaporative skin water losses can be higher in neonates, especially premature infants who are under radiant warmers or undergoing phototherapy. Burns can result in massive losses of water and electrolytes (see Chapter 43). Fever increases insensible losses. Tachypnea or a tracheostomy increases evaporative losses from the lungs.

The gastrointestinal tract can be a source of considerable water and electrolyte losses. A child who has large amounts of gastrointestinal losses should have these losses measured and replaced with an appropriate **replacement solution** (Table 32.3).

Urine output is normally the largest cause of *water* loss. Diseases such as kidney failure and the **syndrome of inappropriate antidiuretic hormone** can lead to a decrease in urine volume. Maintenance fluids in a patient with oliguria or anuria may produce fluid overload if the cause is acute kidney injury. In contrast, other conditions produce an increase in urine volume; these include the polyuric phase of acute kidney injury, diabetes mellitus, and arginine vasopressin deficiency or resistance. When the urine output is excessive, the patient must receive more than standard maintenance fluids to prevent dehydration.

The approach to decreased or increased urine output is similar (Table 32.4). Insensible losses are replaced by a solution that is administered at a rate one-third of the normal maintenance rate. Placing the **anuric** child on "insensibles" theoretically maintains an even fluid balance, with the caveat that one-third of maintenance fluid is only an *estimate* of insensible losses. This rate may need to be adjusted based on monitoring of the patient's weight and hydration status. An **oliguric** child needs to receive a urine replacement solution. Most children with **polyuria** (except for children with diabetes mellitus [see Chapter 172]) should be placed on insensible fluids plus urine replacement.

Output from surgical drains and chest tubes, when significant, should be measured and replaced. **Third space losses** manifest with edema and ascites and are due to a shift of fluid from the intravascular space into the interstitial space. Third space losses cannot be quantitated. Nonetheless, these losses can be large and can lead to intravascular volume depletion, despite weight gain from edema or ascites. Replacement of third space fluid is empirical but should be anticipated in patients who are at risk, such as children who have sepsis, shock, burns, or abdominal surgery. Third space losses and chest tube output are isotonic and usually require replacement with an **isotonic fluid**, such as normal saline (NS) or Ringer's lactate. Adjustments in the amount of replacement fluid for third space losses are based on continuing assessment of the patient's intravascular volume status (heart rate, blood pressure, urine output).

DEHYDRATION

Dehydration, most often due to gastroenteritis, is common in children. The first step in caring for a dehydrated child is to assess the degree of dehydration. The degree of dehydration dictates the urgency of the situation and the volume of fluid needed for rehydration. Table 32.5 summarizes the clinical features that are present with varying degrees of dehydration.

TABLE 32.1 Components of Maintenance Water

Urine	60%
Insensible losses (skin and lungs)	35%
Stool	5%

TABLE 32.2 Adjustments in Maintenance Water

SOURCE	CAUSES OF INCREASED WATER NEEDS	CAUSES OF DECREASED WATER NEEDS
Skin	Radiant warmer Phototherapy Fever Sweat Burns Extensive exfoliative dermatitis*	Incubator (premature infants)
Lungs	Tachypnea Tracheostomy	Humidified ventilator
Gastrointestinal	Diarrhea Emesis Nasogastric suction	
Kidney	Polyuria	Oliguria/anuria
Miscellaneous	Surgical drain Third space losses	Hypothyroidism

*Epidermolysis bullosa, toxic epidermal necrolysis.

TABLE 32.3 Adjusting Fluid Therapy for Gastrointestinal Losses

AVERAGE COMPOSITION	APPROACH TO REPLACEMENT
Diarrhea	**Replacement of Ongoing Stool Losses**
Sodium: 55 mEq/L	Solution: 5% dextrose in ¼ normal saline + 20 mEq/L sodium bicarbonate + 20 mEq/L potassium chloride Replace stool mL/mL every 1–6 hr
Potassium: 25 mEq/L	
Bicarbonate: 15 mEq/L	
Gastric Fluid	**Replacement of Ongoing Gastric Losses**
Sodium: 60 mEq/L	Solution: normal saline + 10 mEq/L potassium chloride Replace output mL/mL every 1–6 hr
Potassium: 10 mEq/L	
Chloride: 90 mEq/L	

TABLE 32.4 Adjusting Fluid Therapy for Altered Urine Output

OLIGURIA/ANURIA	POLYURIA
Place the patient on insensible fluids (~1/3 maintenance) Replace urine output mL/mL with half normal saline	Place the patient on insensible fluids (~1/3 maintenance) Measure urine electrolytes Replace urine output mL/mL with a solution that is based on the measured urine electrolytes

A patient with **mild dehydration** has few clinical signs or symptoms. The history may describe decreased intake but more often increased fluid losses. An infant with **moderate dehydration** has demonstrable physical signs and symptoms; they require prompt intervention. A patient with **severe dehydration** is gravely ill and a decrease in blood pressure indicates that vital organs may be receiving inadequate perfusion (shock) (see Chapter 39). Patients with severe dehydration should receive immediate and aggressive intravenous (IV) therapy. Clinical assessment of dehydration is only an estimate; the patient must be continually reevaluated during therapy. The degree of dehydration is underestimated in hypernatremic dehydration because the osmotically driven shift of water from the intracellular space to the extracellular space helps to preserve the intravascular volume.

Laboratory Evaluation

Serum blood urea nitrogen (BUN) and creatinine concentrations are useful in assessing a child with dehydration. Volume depletion without kidney injury may cause a disproportionate increase in the BUN, with little or no change in the creatinine concentration. This is secondary to increased passive reabsorption of urea in the proximal tubule caused by appropriate kidney conservation of sodium and water. This increase in the BUN may be absent or blunted in a child with poor protein intake because urea production depends on protein degradation. Conversely, the BUN may be disproportionately increased in a child with increased urea production, as occurs in a child with a gastrointestinal bleed or a child who is receiving glucocorticoids. A significant elevation of the creatinine concentration suggests kidney injury.

The urine specific gravity is usually elevated (≥1.025) in cases of significant dehydration but decreases after rehydration. With dehydration, a urinalysis may show hyaline and granular casts, a few white blood cells, a few red blood cells, and 30–100 mg/dL of proteinuria. These findings usually are not associated with significant kidney pathology, and they remit with treatment of dehydration. Hemoconcentration from dehydration increases the hematocrit and hemoglobin.

Calculation of Fluid Deficit

A child with dehydration has lost water; there is also a concurrent loss of sodium and potassium. The fluid deficit is the percentage of dehydration multiplied by the patient's weight (for a 10-kg child, 10% of 10 kg = 1 L deficit).

Approach to Dehydration

The child with dehydration requires acute intervention to ensure that there is adequate tissue perfusion (see Chapter 39). This resuscitation phase requires rapid restoration of the circulating intravascular volume, which should be done with an isotonic solution, such as NS or Ringer's lactate. Blood is an appropriate fluid choice for a child with acute blood loss but is not always available at the start of fluid resuscitation. The child is given a fluid bolus, 20 mL/kg of the isotonic solution, over about 20 minutes. A child with severe dehydration may require multiple fluid boluses and may need to receive fluid at a faster rate, such

TABLE 32.5 Assessment of Degree of Dehydration

	MILD	MODERATE	SEVERE
Infant	5%	10%	15%
Child or adolescent	3%	6%	9%
Infants and young children	Thirsty, alert; restless	Thirsty; restless or lethargic; irritable	Drowsy; limp, cold, sweaty, cyanotic extremities; may be comatose
Older children	Thirsty, alert	Thirsty, alert (usually)	Usually conscious (but at reduced level), apprehensive; cold, sweaty, cyanotic extremities; wrinkled skin on fingers and toes; muscle cramps
SIGNS AND SYMPTOMS			
Tachycardia	Absent	Present	Present
Palpable pulses	Present	Present (weak)	Decreased
Blood pressure	Normal	Orthostatic hypotension	Hypotension
Cutaneous perfusion	Normal	Normal	Reduced and mottled
Skin turgor	Normal	Slight reduction	Reduced
Fontanelle	Normal	Slightly depressed	Sunken
Mucous membrane	Moist	Dry	Very dry
Tears	Present	Present or absent	Absent
Respirations	Normal	Deep, may be rapid	Deep and rapid
Urine output	Normal	Oliguria	Anuria and severe oliguria

Data from World Health Organization.

as giving the bolus in the push-pull method. The initial resuscitation and rehydration is complete when signs of intravascular volume depletion resolve. The child will become more alert and has a lower heart rate, normal blood pressure, and improved perfusion.

With adequate intravascular volume, it is now appropriate to plan the fluid therapy for the next 24 hours (Table 32.6). The child's total fluid needs are added together (maintenance + deficit). The volume of isotonic fluids the patient has received as acute resuscitation is subtracted from this total. The remaining fluid volume is then administered over 24 hours. Unless significant hypokalemia is present, potassium usually is not included in the IV fluids until the patient voids. Children with significant ongoing losses also need to receive an appropriate replacement solution.

MONITORING AND ADJUSTING THERAPY

All calculations in fluid therapy are only approximations. The patient needs to be monitored during treatment with therapy modifications based on the clinical situation (Table 32.7).

Hyponatremic dehydration occurs in children who have diarrhea and consume a hypotonic fluid (water or diluted formula). Volume depletion stimulates secretion of antidiuretic hormone, preventing the water excretion that should correct the hyponatremia. Some patients develop symptoms, predominantly neurologic, from the hyponatremia (see Chapter 34). Most patients with hyponatremic dehydration do well with the same general approach outlined in Table 32.6. Overly rapid correction of hyponatremia (>10 mEq/L per 24 hours) should be avoided because of the remote risk of **osmotic demyelination syndrome**.

Hypernatremic dehydration is usually a consequence of an inability to take in fluid because of a lack of access, a poor thirst mechanism (neurologic impairment), intractable emesis, or anorexia. The movement of water from the intracellular space to the extracellular space during hypernatremic dehydration partially limits the intravascular volume losses. Urine output may be preserved longer, and there may be less tachycardia. Children with hypernatremic dehydration are often lethargic and irritable. Hypernatremia may cause fever, hypertonicity, hyperreflexia, and seizures. More severe neurologic symptoms may develop if cerebral bleeding or dural sinus thrombosis occurs.

Overly rapid treatment of hypernatremic dehydration may cause significant morbidity and mortality. **Idiogenic osmoles** are generated within the brain during the development of hypernatremia. Idiogenic osmoles increase the osmolality within the cells of the brain, providing protection against brain cell shrinkage secondary to movement of water out of cells into the hypertonic extracellular fluid. These idiogenic osmoles dissipate slowly during correction of hypernatremia. With rapid lowering of the extracellular osmolality during correction of hypernatremia, a new gradient may be created that causes water movement from the extracellular space into the cells of the brain, producing **cerebral edema**. Possible manifestations of the resultant cerebral edema include headache, altered mental status, seizures, and potentially lethal brain herniation.

To minimize the risk of cerebral edema during correction of hypernatremic dehydration, the serum sodium concentration should not decrease more than 10 mEq/L every 24 hours (Fig. 32.1). The choice and rate of fluid replacement are not nearly as important as vigilant monitoring of the serum sodium concentration and adjustment of the therapy based on the result (see Fig. 32.1). Nonetheless, the initial resuscitation-rehydration phase of therapy remains the same as for other types of dehydration.

Oral Rehydration

Mild-to-moderate dehydration from diarrhea of any cause can be treated effectively using a simple **oral rehydration solution (ORS)** containing glucose and electrolytes (see Chapter 113). The ORS relies on the coupled transport of sodium and glucose in the intestine. Oral rehydration therapy has significantly reduced the morbidity and mortality from acute diarrhea but is underused in developed countries. Oral rehydration therapy should be attempted for most patients with mild-to-moderate diarrheal dehydration as it is less expensive than IV therapy and has a lower complication rate. IV therapy may still be required for patients with severe dehydration; patients with uncontrollable vomiting; patients unable to drink because of extreme fatigue, stupor, or coma; or patients with gastric or intestinal distention. Rapidly absorbed sublingual ondansetron may be used to treat nausea and vomiting, thus facilitating oral rehydration.

As a guideline for oral rehydration, 50 mL/kg of the ORS should be given within 4 hours to patients with mild dehydration, and 100 mL/kg should be given over 4 hours to patients with moderate dehydration. Supplementary ORS is given to replace ongoing losses from diarrhea or emesis. An additional 10 mL/kg of ORS is given for each stool. Fluid intake should be decreased if the patient appears fully hydrated earlier than expected or develops periorbital edema. After rehydration, patients should resume their usual diet (breast milk, formula).

When rehydration is complete, maintenance therapy should be started, using 100 mL of ORS/kg in 24 hours until the diarrhea stops. Breast-feeding or formula-feeding should

TABLE 32.6 Fluid Management of Dehydration

Restore intravascular volume:
Isotonic fluid (NS or LR): 20 mL/kg over 20 min
Repeat as needed
Calculate 24-hr fluid needs: maintenance + deficit volume
Subtract isotonic fluid already administered from 24-hr fluid needs
Administer remaining volume over 24 hr using D5 NS + 20 mEq/L KCl
Replace ongoing losses as they occur

D5, 5% Dextrose; *LR*, Ringer's lactate; *NS*, normal saline.

TABLE 32.7 Monitoring Fluid Therapy

Vital signs
Pulse
Blood pressure
Intake and output
Fluid balance
Urine output and specific gravity
Physical examination
Weight
Clinical signs of fluid volume depletion or overload
Electrolytes

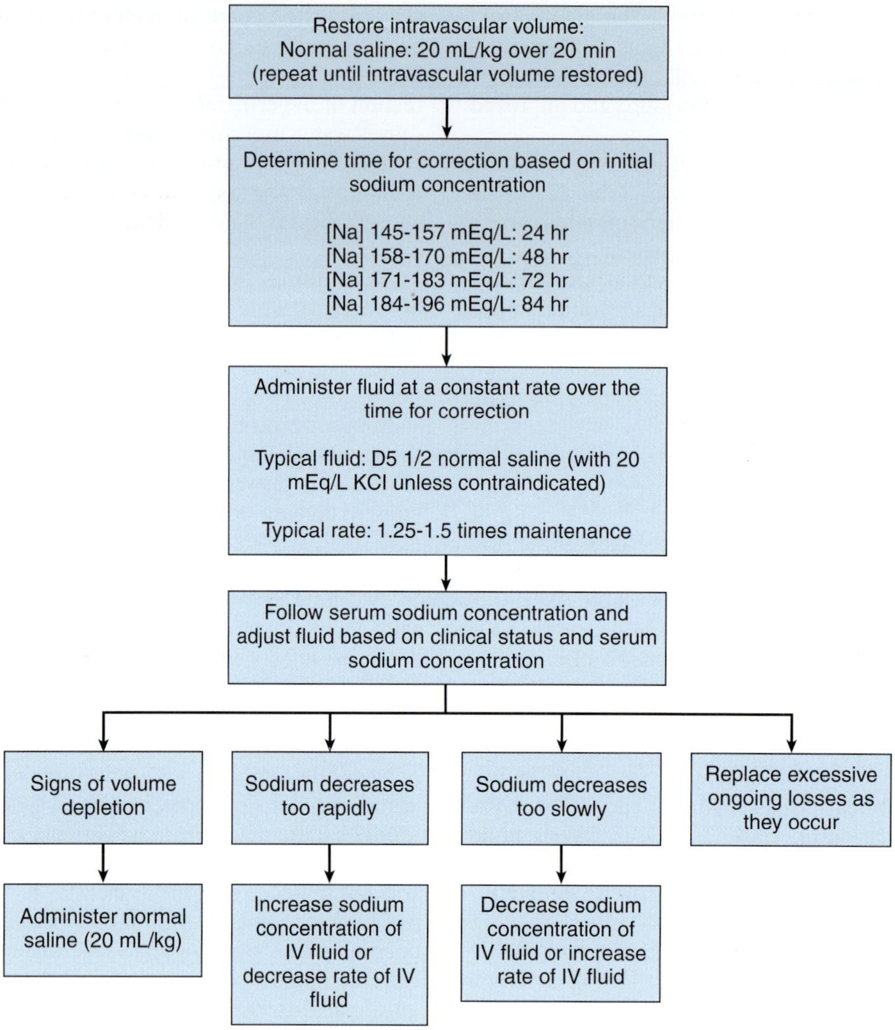

FIGURE 32.1 Algorithm for correcting hypernatremic dehydration.

be maintained and not delayed for more than 24 hours. Patients with more severe diarrhea require continued supervision. The volume of ORS ingested should equal the volume of stool losses. If stool volume cannot be measured, an intake of 10–15 mL of ORS/kg per hour is appropriate.

PEARLS FOR PRACTITIONERS

See Fluids and Electrolytes: Pearls for Practitioners at the end of this section.

REVIEW QUESTIONS

Available online.

CHAPTER 33

Parenteral Nutrition

Parenteral nutrition (PN) is necessary when enteral feeding is inadequate to meet the nutritional needs of a patient. Enteral nutrition is always preferred because it is more physiologic, less expensive, and associated with fewer complications. When possible, providing even some nutrition enterally leads to fewer possible complications.

INDICATIONS

A variety of clinical situations necessitate PN (Table 33.1). Acute PN is frequently given in an intensive care unit when there is poor tolerance of enteral feeds, potentially secondary to a transient ileus, concerns regarding bowel ischemia, or the risk of aspiration pneumonia. **Short bowel syndrome** is the most common indication for long-term PN; this may be caused by a congenital gastrointestinal anomaly or acquired after necrotizing enterocolitis (see Chapter 62). Some patients with a chronic indication for PN eventually may be transitioned to partial or full enteral feedings.

ACCESS FOR PARENTERAL NUTRITION

PN can be given via either a peripheral intravenous (IV) line or a **central venous line (CVL)**. Long-term PN should be given via a CVL. Acute PN may be given peripherally, although a temporary CVL is often used. Most children with cancer or receiving a bone marrow transplant have a CVL. A

TABLE 33.1 Indications for Parenteral Nutrition
ACUTE
Prematurity Trauma Burns Bowel surgery Multiorgan system failure Bone marrow transplantation Malignancy
CHRONIC
Short bowel Intractable diarrhea syndromes Intestinal pseudoobstruction Inflammatory bowel disease Immunodeficiency

peripherally inserted central catheter is an excellent source of central access for acute PN because of the lower risk for complications than with a standard CVL.

A peripheral IV line has two major limitations. First, it frequently fails, necessitating interruption of PN and potentially painful placement of a new line. Second, high-osmolality solutions cause **phlebitis** of peripheral veins; this limits the dextrose and amino acid content of peripheral PN. The dextrose content of peripheral PN cannot be greater than 12%, with a lower limit if the amino acid concentration is high. Lipid emulsion has a low osmolality; it can be administered peripherally via the same IV line as the dextrose and amino acid solution. Patients can receive adequate nutrition via a peripheral IV line, but the volume of PN needs to be higher than is necessary when central access is available because of the limitations on dextrose and amino acid concentration. This situation may be problematic in patients who cannot tolerate larger fluid volumes.

COMPOSITION OF PARENTERAL NUTRITION

PN can provide calories, amino acids, electrolytes, minerals, essential fatty acids, vitamins, iron, and trace elements. The **calories** in PN are from dextrose and fat. The amino acids in PN are a potential source of calories, but they should be used predominantly for protein synthesis. PN is given as two separate solutions: a dextrose plus amino acid solution and a 20% lipid emulsion. The dextrose solution has all the components of PN except for fat.

The dextrose concentration of peripheral PN is 10–12%; central PN has a concentration of about 20%, although it may be increased to 25–30% in patients who are fluid restricted. To avoid hyperglycemia, the dextrose delivery is increased gradually when starting PN. Protein delivery in PN is via amino acids in the dextrose solution. The goal is 0.8–2 g protein/kg per 24 hours for older children, 1.5–3 g/kg per 24 hours for full-term and older infants, and 2.5–3.5 g/kg per 24 hours for preterm infants.

The electrolyte and mineral composition of PN depends on the age and the underlying illness. The 20% lipid emulsion provides essential fatty acids and calories. The lipid emulsion is started at a rate of 0.5–1 g/kg per 24 hours, gradually increasing the rate so that the patient receives adequate calories; this requires 2.5–3.5 g/kg per 24 hours. The lipid emulsion usually provides 30–40% of the required calories; it should not exceed 60%. The serum triglyceride concentration is monitored as the rate of lipid emulsion is increased, with reduction of the lipid emulsion rate if significant hypertriglyceridemia develops.

COMPLICATIONS

There are several potential complications of PN. CVLs are associated with complications during insertion (pneumothorax or bleeding) and long-term issues (thrombosis). **Catheter-related sepsis**, most commonly due to bacteremia with coagulase-negative staphylococci, is common and, on occasion, necessitates catheter removal. Other potential pathogens are *Staphylococcus aureus*, gram-negative bacilli, and fungi. Electrolyte abnormalities, nutritional deficiencies, hyperglycemia, and complications from excessive protein intake (azotemia or hyperammonemia) can be detected with careful monitoring.

The most concerning complication of long-term PN is **cholestatic liver disease**, which can lead to jaundice, cirrhosis, and, occasionally, liver failure. Strategies to decrease the risk of liver disease include PN with reduced amounts of hepatotoxic amino acids and the use of fish-based lipids. The best preventive strategy is early use of the gastrointestinal tract, even if only trophic feeds are tolerated.

PEARLS FOR PRACTITIONERS

See Fluids and Electrolytes: Pearls for Practitioners at the end of this section.

REVIEW QUESTIONS

Available online.

CHAPTER 34

Sodium Disorders

The kidney regulates sodium balance and is the principal site of sodium excretion. Sodium is unique among electrolytes because **water balance**, not sodium balance, usually determines its concentration. When the sodium concentration increases, the resultant higher plasma osmolality causes increased thirst and increased secretion of antidiuretic hormone (ADH), which leads to conservation of water by the kidneys. Both mechanisms increase the water content of the body, and the sodium concentration returns to normal. During hyponatremia, the fall in plasma osmolality decreases ADH secretion, and consequent kidney water excretion leads to an increase in the sodium concentration. Although water balance is usually regulated by osmolality, volume depletion also stimulates thirst, ADH secretion, and kidney conservation of water. In fact, volume depletion takes precedence over osmolality; volume depletion stimulates ADH secretion, even if a patient has hyponatremia.

The excretion of sodium by the kidney is not determined by the plasma osmolality. The patient's effective plasma volume regulates the amount of sodium in the urine through a variety of regulatory systems, including the renin-angiotensin-aldosterone system. In hyponatremia or hypernatremia, the underlying pathophysiology determines the urinary sodium concentration, not the serum sodium concentration.

HYPONATREMIA

Etiology

Different mechanisms can cause hyponatremia (Fig. 34.1). **Pseudohyponatremia** is a laboratory artifact that is present when the plasma contains high concentrations of protein or lipid. It does not occur when a direct ion-selective electrode determines the sodium concentration, a technique that is increasingly used in clinical laboratories. In true hyponatremia, the *measured* osmolality is low; in pseudohyponatremia it is normal. **Hyperosmolality**, resulting from mannitol infusion or hyperglycemia, causes a low serum sodium concentration because water moves down its osmotic gradient from the intracellular space into the extracellular space, diluting the sodium concentration. For every 100 mg/dL increment of the serum glucose, the serum sodium decreases by 1.6 mEq/L. As the manifestations of hyponatremia are due to the low plasma osmolality, patients with hyponatremia caused by hyperosmolality do not have symptoms of hyponatremia and do not require the correction of hyponatremia.

Classification of true hyponatremia is based on the patient's volume status (see Fig. 34.1). In **hypovolemic hyponatremia**, the child has lost sodium from the body. Water balance may be positive or negative, but there has been a higher net sodium loss than water loss; this is often due to oral or intravenous (IV) water intake, with water retention by the kidneys to compensate for the intravascular volume depletion. If the sodium loss is not due to a kidney disease (e.g., diarrhea), the urine sodium concentration is very low, as the kidneys attempt to preserve the intravascular volume by conserving sodium. In kidney diseases, the urine sodium is inappropriately elevated.

Patients with hyponatremia and no evidence of volume overload or volume depletion have **euvolemic hyponatremia**. These patients have an excess of total body water and a slight decrease in total body sodium. Some of these patients have an increase in weight, implying that they are volume overloaded. Nevertheless, they usually appear normal or have only subtle signs of fluid overload. In the **syndrome of inappropriate ADH (SIADH)**, there is secretion of ADH that is not inhibited by either low serum osmolality or expanded intravascular volume. Retention of water causes hyponatremia, and the expansion of the intravascular volume results in an increase in kidney sodium excretion. SIADH is associated with physiologic stress, pneumonia, mechanical ventilation, meningitis, trauma, and other central nervous system disorders. Ectopic production of ADH from tumors is rare in children. SIADH should be distinguished from **cerebral salt wasting**, which is a form of hypovolemic hyponatremia often associated with tuberculosis meningitis or intracranial hemorrhage. Infants can develop euvolemic hyponatremia because of excessive water consumption or inappropriately diluted formula.

In **hypervolemic hyponatremia**, there is an excess of total body water and sodium, although the increase in water is greater than the increase in sodium. In kidney failure, there is an inability to excrete sodium or water; the urine sodium may be low or high, depending on the cause of the decreased kidney function. In other causes of hypervolemic hyponatremia, there is a decrease in the effective blood volume because of

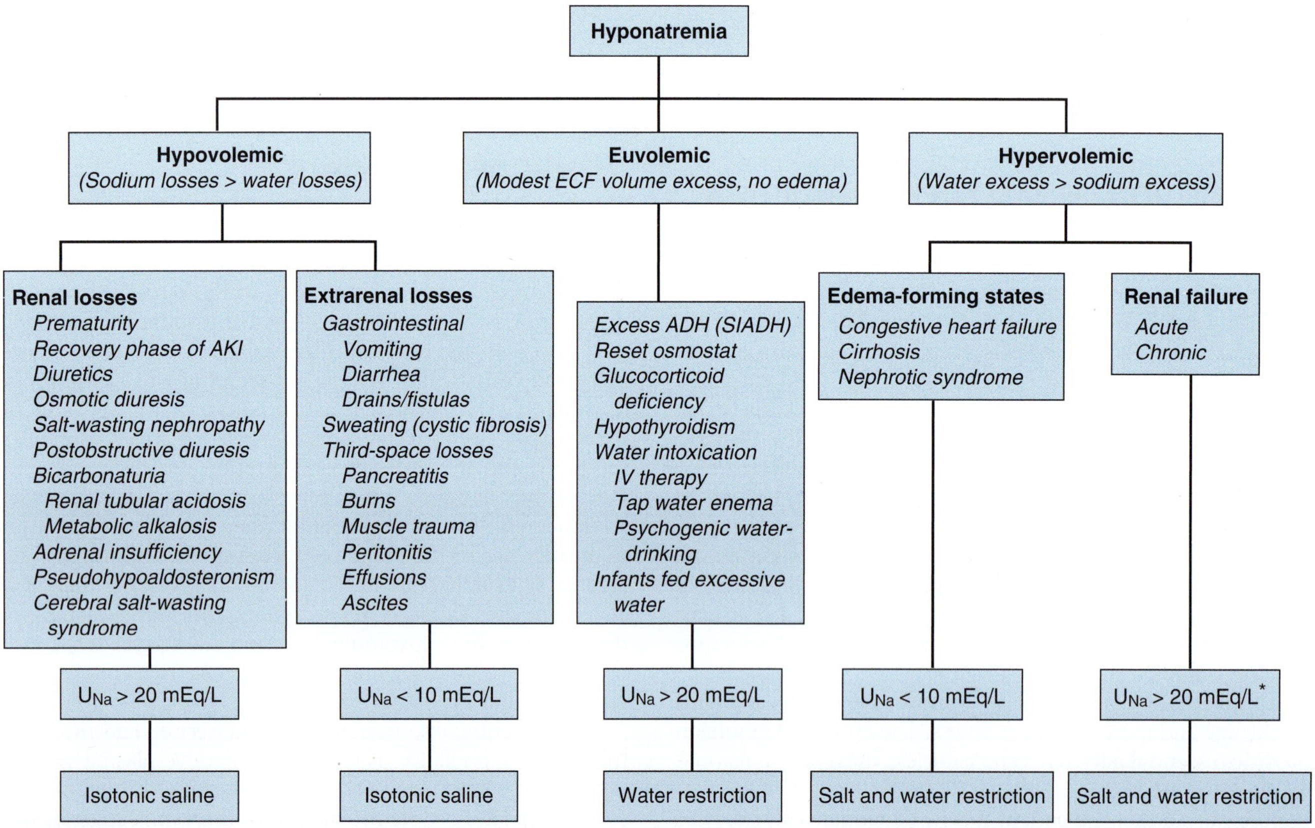

FIGURE 34.1 Classification, diagnosis, and treatment algorithm of hyponatremic states. *In water intoxication the urine sodium is often <20 mEq/L. †Urinary sodium is <10 mEq/L in acute kidney injury secondary to glomerular disease. *ADH*, Antidiuretic hormone; *AKI*, acute kidney injury; *ECF*, extracellular fluid; *IV*, intravenous; *SIADH*, syndrome of inappropriate antidiuretic hormone secretion. (Modified from Berl T, Anderson RJ, McDonald KM, et al. Clinical disorders of water metabolism. *Kidney Int*. 1976;10:117–132. Fig. 2.)

either third space fluid loss or poor cardiac output. In response to the low effective blood volume, ADH causes kidney water retention, and the kidneys also retain sodium, which leads to a low urine sodium concentration. The patient's serum sodium concentration decreases when water intake exceeds sodium intake, and ADH prevents the normal loss of excess water.

Clinical Manifestations

Hyponatremia causes a fall in the osmolality of the extracellular space. Because the intracellular space then has a higher osmolality, water moves from the extracellular space to the intracellular space to maintain osmotic equilibrium. The increase in intracellular water may cause cells to swell. Brain cell swelling is responsible for most of the symptoms of hyponatremia. Neurologic symptoms of hyponatremia include anorexia, nausea, emesis, malaise, lethargy, confusion, agitation, headache, seizures, coma, and decreased reflexes. Patients may develop hypothermia, Cheyne-Stokes respirations, muscle cramps, and weakness. Symptoms are more severe when hyponatremia develops rapidly; chronic hyponatremia can be asymptomatic because of a compensatory decrease in brain cell osmolality, which limits cerebral swelling.

Treatment

Rapid correction of hyponatremia can produce **osmotic demyelination syndrome**. Avoiding more than a 10 mEq/L increase in the serum sodium every 24 hours is prudent, especially in chronic hyponatremia. Treatment of hypovolemic hyponatremia requires administration of IV fluids with sodium to provide maintenance requirements and deficit correction and to replace ongoing losses (see Chapter 32). For children with SIADH, water restriction is the cornerstone of therapy. Additional treatments include oral urea, which causes an osmotic diuresis, or vaptan drugs, which are ADH antagonists. Children with hyponatremia secondary to hypothyroidism or cortisol deficiency need specific hormone replacement. **Acute water intoxication** rapidly self-corrects with the transient restriction of water intake, which is followed by introduction of a normal diet. Treatment of hypervolemic hyponatremia centers on restriction of water and sodium intake, but disease-specific measures, such as dialysis in kidney failure, may also be necessary.

Emergency treatment of **symptomatic hyponatremia** (seizures) uses IV hypertonic saline to rapidly increase the serum sodium concentration, which leads to a decrease in brain edema. One milliliter per kilogram of 3% sodium chloride increases the serum sodium by approximately 1 mEq/L. A child often improves after receiving 4–6 mL/kg of 3% sodium chloride.

HYPERNATREMIA

Etiology

There are three basic mechanisms of hypernatremia (Fig. 34.2). **Sodium intoxication** is frequently iatrogenic in a hospital setting, resulting from correction of metabolic acidosis with sodium bicarbonate. In hyperaldosteronism, there is kidney retention of sodium and resultant hypertension; the hypernatremia is mild.

Hypernatremia resulting from water losses develops only if the patient does not have access to water or cannot drink adequately because of neurologic impairment (adipsia), emesis, or anorexia. Infants are at high risk because of their inability to control their own water intake. Ineffective breast-feeding, often in a primiparous mother, can cause severe hypernatremic dehydration. High insensible losses of water are especially common in premature infants; the losses increase further due to radiant warmers or phototherapy for hyperbilirubinemia. Children with extrarenal causes of water loss have high levels of ADH and very concentrated urine.

Children with arginine vasopressin deficiency or resistance have inappropriately diluted urine. Hereditary **arginine vasopressin resistance** (nephrogenic diabetes insipidus) causes massive urinary water losses. As arginine vasopressin resistance is most commonly an X-linked disorder due to a pathogenic variant in the gene for the ADH receptor *(AVPR2)*, it usually occurs in males, who may have episodes of severe hypernatremic dehydration and growth faltering. *Acquired arginine vasopressin resistance* may be secondary to interstitial nephritis, sickle cell disease, hypercalcemia, hypokalemia, or medications (lithium). If the defect is due to **arginine vasopressin deficiency** (central diabetes insipidus), urine output decreases and urine osmolality increases in response to administration of an ADH analog. Central causes of ADH deficiency include tumor, infarction, or trauma. There is no response to an ADH analog in a child with arginine vasopressin resistance.

Diarrhea results in sodium and water depletion. Most children with gastroenteritis do not develop hypernatremia because they drink enough hypotonic fluid to compensate at least partially for stool water losses. Hypernatremia is most likely in a child with diarrhea who has inadequate intake because of emesis, lack of access to water, or anorexia. Certain kidney diseases (obstructive uropathy, kidney dysplasia, juvenile nephronophthisis) cause losses of sodium and water, potentially producing hypernatremia if the patient consumes insufficient water.

In situations with combined sodium and water deficits, analysis of the urine differentiates kidney and other etiologies. When the losses are extrarenal, the kidney responds to volume depletion with low urine volume, a concentrated urine, and sodium retention (urine sodium <10 mEq/L). With kidney causes, the urine volume is usually high, the urine is not maximally concentrated, and the urine sodium may be inappropriately elevated.

Clinical Manifestations

Most children with hypernatremia are dehydrated and have the typical signs and symptoms of dehydration (see Chapter 32). Children with hypernatremic dehydration tend to have better preservation of intravascular volume owing to the shift of water from the intracellular space to the extracellular space. Hypernatremic infants potentially become more dehydrated before seeking medical attention. Due to intracellular water loss, the pinched abdominal skin of a dehydrated, hypernatremic infant has a *doughy* feel.

Hypernatremia, even without dehydration, causes central nervous system symptoms that tend to parallel the degree of sodium elevation and the acuity of the increase. Patients are irritable, restless, weak, and lethargic. Some infants have a

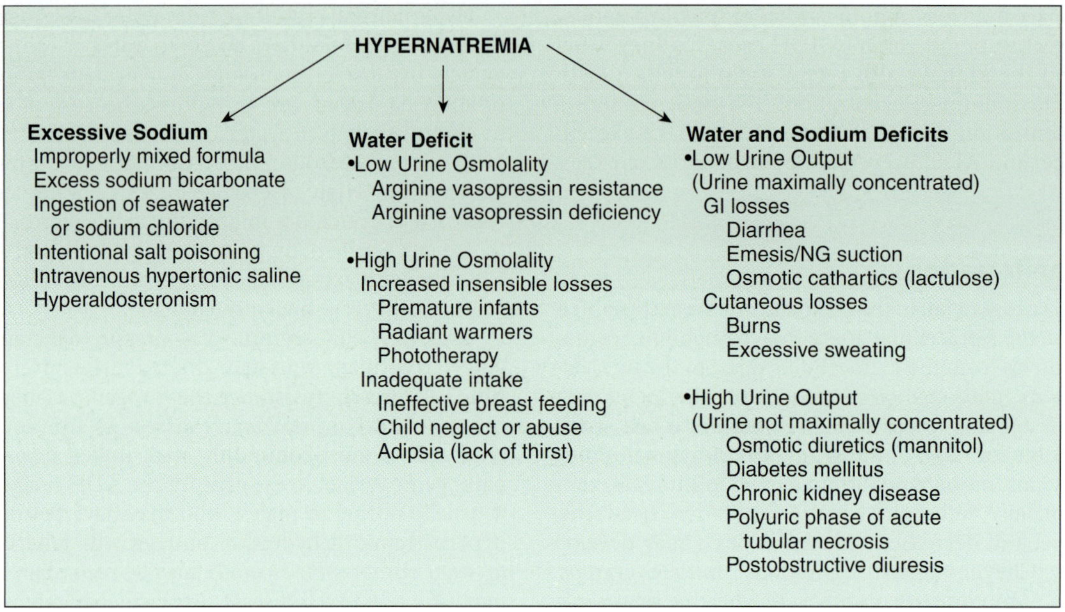

FIGURE 34.2 Differential diagnosis of hypernatremia by mechanism. *GI*, Gastrointestinal; *NG*, nasogastric.

high-pitched cry and hyperpnea; hypernatremia may cause fever. Alert patients are very thirsty, although nausea may be present.

Brain hemorrhage is the most devastating consequence of hypernatremia. As the extracellular osmolality increases, water moves out of brain cells, resulting in a decrease in brain volume. This decrease in volume can result in tearing of intracerebral veins and bridging blood vessels as the brain moves away from the skull and the meninges. Patients may have subarachnoid, subdural, and parenchymal hemorrhage. Seizures and coma are possible sequelae of the hemorrhage.

Treatment

As hypernatremia develops, the brain generates idiogenic osmoles to increase the intracellular osmolality and prevent the loss of brain water. This mechanism is not instantaneous and is most prominent when hypernatremia has developed gradually. If the serum sodium concentration is lowered rapidly, there is movement of water from the serum into the brain cells to equalize the osmolality in the two compartments. The resultant brain swelling manifests as seizures or coma. Due to these dangers, hypernatremia should be corrected slowly. The goal is to decrease the serum sodium by less than 12 mEq/L every 24 hours (see Fig. 32.1). The most important components of correcting moderate or severe hypernatremia are restoring the effective intravascular volume and then frequently monitoring the serum sodium to allow adjustment of fluid therapy and to provide adequate correction that is neither too slow nor too fast.

In a child with hypernatremic dehydration, as in any child with dehydration, the foremost priority is restoration of intravascular volume with isotonic fluid. Figure 32.1 outlines a general approach for correcting hypernatremic dehydration secondary to gastroenteritis. If the hypernatremia and dehydration are secondary to water loss, as occurs with arginine vasopressin deficiency or resistance, a more hypotonic IV fluid is appropriate. A child with arginine vasopressin deficiency should receive an ADH analog to prevent further excessive water loss. A child with arginine vasopressin resistance requires a urine replacement solution to offset ongoing water losses. Chronically, reduced sodium intake, thiazide diuretics, and nonsteroidal antiinflammatory drugs can decrease water losses in arginine vasopressin resistance.

Acute, severe hypernatremia, usually secondary to sodium administration, can be corrected more rapidly because idiogenic osmoles have not had time to accumulate; this balances the high morbidity and mortality from severe, acute hypernatremia with the dangers of overly rapid correction. When hypernatremia is due to sodium intoxication and the hypernatremia is severe, it may be impossible to administer enough water to rapidly correct the hypernatremia without worsening volume overload; some patients require the use of a loop diuretic or dialysis.

PEARLS FOR PRACTITIONERS

See Fluids and Electrolytes: Pearls for Practitioners at the end of this section.

REVIEW QUESTIONS

Available online.

CHAPTER 35

Potassium Disorders

The kidneys are the principal regulator of potassium balance, adjusting excretion based on intake. Factors affecting kidney potassium excretion include aldosterone, acid-base status, serum potassium concentration, and kidney function. The intracellular potassium concentration is approximately 30 times the extracellular potassium concentration. A variety of conditions alter the distribution of potassium between the intracellular and extracellular compartments, potentially causing either hypokalemia or hyperkalemia. The plasma concentration does not always reflect the total body potassium content.

HYPOKALEMIA

Etiology

Hypokalemia is common in children, with the most common etiology being gastroenteritis. Spurious hypokalemia occurs in patients with leukemia and elevated white blood cell counts if plasma for analysis is left at room temperature, permitting the white blood cells to take up potassium from the plasma. There are four basic mechanisms of hypokalemia (Table 35.1). Low intake, nonrenal losses, and kidney losses all are associated with total body potassium depletion. With a **transcellular shift**, total body potassium is normal unless there is concomitant potassium depletion secondary to other factors.

The transcellular shift of potassium after initiation of insulin therapy in children with diabetic ketoacidosis (see Chapter 172) can be dramatic. These patients have reduced total body potassium because of urinary losses, but they often have a normal serum potassium level before insulin therapy from a transcellular shift into the extracellular space secondary to insulin deficiency and metabolic acidosis. Children receiving aggressive doses of β-adrenergic agonists (albuterol) for asthma can develop hypokalemia resulting from the intracellular movement of potassium. Poor intake is an unusual cause of hypokalemia, unless it is also associated with significant weight loss (anorexia nervosa).

TABLE 35.1 Causes of Hypokalemia

TRANSCELLULAR SHIFTS	With metabolic alkalosis
Alkalemia	Low urine chloride
Insulin	Emesis/nasogastric suction
β-adrenergic agonists	Pyloric stenosis
Drugs/toxins (theophylline, barium, toluene)	Chloride-losing diarrhea
Hypokalemic periodic paralysis	Cystic fibrosis
Refeeding syndrome	Low-chloride formula
DECREASED INTAKE	Posthypercapnic
	Previous loop or thiazide diuretic use
EXTRARENAL LOSSES	High urine chloride and normal blood pressure
Diarrhea	Gitelman syndrome
Laxative abuse	Bartter syndrome
Sweating	Loop and thiazide diuretics
KIDNEY LOSSES	High urine chloride and high blood pressure
With metabolic acidosis	Adrenal adenoma or hyperplasia
Distal RTA	Glucocorticoid-remediable aldosteronism
Proximal RTA	Renovascular disease
Ureterosigmoidostomy	Renin-secreting tumor
Diabetic ketoacidosis	17α-hydroxylase deficiency
Without specific acid-base disturbance	11β-hydroxylase deficiency
Tubular toxins (amphotericin, cisplatin, aminoglycosides)	Cushing syndrome
Interstitial nephritis	11β-hydroxysteroid dehydrogenase deficiency
Diuretic phase of acute tubular necrosis	Licorice ingestion
Postobstructive diuresis	Liddle syndrome
Hypomagnesemia	**SPURIOUS**
High urine anions (e.g., penicillin or penicillin derivatives)	High white blood cell count

RTA, Renal tubular acidosis.

Diarrhea has a high concentration of potassium, and the resulting hypokalemia is associated with a metabolic acidosis secondary to stool losses of bicarbonate. With emesis or nasogastric suction, there is gastric loss of potassium, but this is minimal given the low potassium content of gastric fluid (~10 mEq/L). More important is the gastric loss of hydrochloride, leading to a metabolic alkalosis and a state of volume depletion. Metabolic alkalosis and volume depletion increase urinary losses of potassium.

Urinary potassium wasting may be accompanied by a metabolic acidosis (proximal or distal renal tubular acidosis; see Chapter 36). Loop and thiazide diuretics lead to hypokalemia and a metabolic alkalosis. **Bartter syndrome** and **Gitelman syndrome** are autosomal recessive disorders resulting from defects in tubular transporters and are associated with hypokalemia and a metabolic alkalosis. Bartter syndrome is usually associated with hypercalciuria, often with nephrocalcinosis; children with Gitelman syndrome have low urinary calcium losses but hypomagnesemia secondary to urinary losses (Table 35.2).

In the presence of a high aldosterone level, there is urinary loss of potassium, hypokalemia, and a metabolic alkalosis. There also is kidney retention of sodium, leading to hypertension. A variety of genetic and acquired disorders can cause high aldosterone levels. **Liddle syndrome**, an autosomal dominant disorder caused by constitutively active sodium channels, has the same clinical features as hyperaldosteronism, but the serum aldosterone level is low.

Clinical Manifestations

The heart and skeletal muscle are especially vulnerable to hypokalemia. **Electrocardiographic (ECG) changes** include a flattened T wave, a depressed ST segment, and the appearance of a U wave, which is located between the T wave (if still visible) and P wave. Ventricular fibrillation and torsades de pointes may occur, although usually only in the context of underlying heart disease.

The clinical consequences in skeletal muscle include muscle weakness and cramps. **Paralysis** is a rare complication (generally only at potassium levels <2.5 mEq/L) that starts with the legs, followed by the arms. Respiratory paralysis may require mechanical ventilation.

Some patients with hypokalemia develop **rhabdomyolysis**, especially following exercise. Hypokalemia slows gastrointestinal motility; potassium levels less than 2.5 mEq/L may cause an ileus. Hypokalemia impairs bladder function, potentially leading to urinary retention. Polyuria may occur because hyperkalemia causes secondary arginine vasopressin resistance. Chronic hypokalemia may cause kidney damage, including interstitial nephritis and kidney cysts.

Diagnosis

It is important to review the child's diet, history of gastrointestinal losses, and medications. Emesis and diuretic use can be surreptitious. The presence of hypertension suggests excess mineralocorticoids. Concomitant electrolyte abnormalities are useful clues. The combination of hypokalemia and metabolic acidosis is characteristic of diarrhea as well as proximal or distal renal tubular acidosis. A concurrent metabolic alkalosis is characteristic of gastric losses, aldosterone excess, diuretics, Bartter syndrome, or Gitelman syndrome.

TABLE 35.2 Bartter and Gitelman Syndromes

	TYPE 1 BARTTER SYNDROME	TYPE 2 BARTTER SYNDROME	TYPE 3 BARTTER SYNDROME	TYPE 4 BARTTER SYNDROME	TYPE 5 BARTTER SYNDROME	GITELMAN SYNDROME
Inheritance	AR	AR	AR	AR	X-linked	AR
Gene	*SLC12A1*	*KCNJ1*	*CLCNKB*	*BSND* (type 4a) or *CLCNKA* and *CLCNKB* (type 4b)	*MAGED2*	*SLC12A3*
Onset	Prenatal, postnatal	Prenatal, postnatal	Postnatal (prenatal less commonly)	Prenatal, postnatal	Prenatal	Adolescent, adult
Features	Polyhydramnios, prematurity, nephrocalcinosis	Polyhydramnios, prematurity, nephrocalcinosis, transient postnatal hyperkalemia	Term birth (polyhydramnios and premature less commonly), variable nephrocalcinosis and hypomagnesemia	Polyhydramnios, prematurity, sensorineural hearing loss, variable nephrocalcinosis and hypomagnesemia	Massive polyhydramnios, nephrocalcinosis, transient: resolves in infancy	Hypomagnesemia and hypocalciuria

AR, Autosomal recessive.

Treatment

Factors that influence the therapy of hypokalemia include the potassium level, clinical symptoms, kidney function, presence of transcellular shifts of potassium, ongoing losses, and the patient's ability to tolerate oral potassium. Severe, symptomatic hypokalemia requires aggressive treatment. Supplementation is more cautious if kidney function is decreased because of the kidney's limited ability to excrete excessive potassium. The plasma potassium level does not always provide an accurate estimation of the total body potassium deficit because there may be shifts of potassium from the intracellular space to the plasma. Clinically, this shift occurs most commonly with metabolic acidosis and because of the insulin deficiency of diabetic ketoacidosis; the plasma potassium underestimates the degree of total body potassium depletion. When these problems are corrected, potassium moves into the intracellular space, and these patients require more potassium supplementation to correct the hypokalemia. Patients who have ongoing losses of potassium need correction of the deficit and replacement of the ongoing losses.

Due to the risk of hyperkalemia, intravenous (IV) potassium should be used cautiously. Oral potassium is safer in nonurgent situations. The dose of IV potassium is 0.5–1 mEq/kg, usually given over 1 hour. The adult maximum dose is 40 mEq. Conservative dosing is generally preferred with ongoing close monitoring and additional replacement as needed. For patients with excessive urinary losses, potassium-sparing diuretics are effective. When hypokalemia, metabolic alkalosis, and volume depletion are present, restoration of intravascular volume decreases urinary potassium losses.

HYPERKALEMIA

Etiology

Three basic mechanisms cause hyperkalemia (Table 35.3). In the individual patient, the etiology is sometimes multifactorial. **Factitious hyperkalemia** is usually due to hemolysis during phlebotomy, but it can be the result of prolonged tourniquet application or fist clenching during phlebotomy, which causes local potassium release from muscle. Falsely elevated serum potassium levels can occur when serum levels are measured in patients with markedly elevated white blood cell or platelet counts; a promptly analyzed plasma sample usually provides an accurate result.

With the kidney's ability to excrete potassium, it is unusual for excessive intake, by itself, to cause hyperkalemia. This mechanism can occur in a patient who is receiving large quantities of IV or oral potassium for excessive losses that are no longer present. Frequent or rapid blood transfusions can increase the potassium level acutely secondary to the high potassium content of stored blood. Increased intake may precipitate hyperkalemia if there is an underlying defect in potassium excretion.

The intracellular space has a high potassium concentration, so a **shift of potassium from the intracellular space** to the extracellular space can have a significant impact on the plasma potassium. This shift occurs with acidosis, cell destruction (rhabdomyolysis or tumor lysis syndrome), insulin deficiency, medications (succinylcholine, β blockers), malignant hyperthermia, and hyperkalemic periodic paralysis.

Hyperkalemia secondary to decreased excretion occurs with kidney injury. The risk of hyperkalemia secondary to medications that decrease kidney potassium excretion is greatest in patients with underlying decreased kidney function.

Aldosterone deficiency or unresponsiveness to aldosterone causes hyperkalemia, often with associated metabolic acidosis (see Chapter 36) and hyponatremia. A form of congenital adrenal hyperplasia, **21-hydroxylase deficiency**, is the most frequent cause of aldosterone deficiency in children. Untreated patients have hyperkalemia, metabolic acidosis, hyponatremia, and volume depletion.

Renin, via angiotensin II, stimulates aldosterone production. A deficiency in renin, resulting from kidney damage, can lead to decreased aldosterone production. These patients have hyperkalemia and a metabolic acidosis, without hyponatremia. Some patients have impaired kidney function, partially accounting for the hyperkalemia, but the impairment in potassium excretion is more extreme than expected for the degree of kidney injury.

Children with **pseudohypoaldosteronism (PHA) type 1** have hyperkalemia, metabolic acidosis, and salt wasting, leading to hyponatremia and volume depletion; aldosterone levels are elevated. In the autosomal recessive form *(PHA1B)*, there is a defect in the kidney sodium channel that is normally

TABLE 35.3 Causes of Hyperkalemia

SPURIOUS LABORATORY VALUE	DECREASED EXCRETION

Hemolysis
Tissue ischemia during blood drawing
Thrombocytosis
Leukocytosis
	Kidney failure
	Primary adrenal disease
	  Acquired Addison disease
	  21-hydroxylase deficiency
	  3β-hydroxysteroid-dehydrogenase deficiency
	  Lipoid congenital adrenal hyperplasia
	  Adrenal hypoplasia congenita
	  Aldosterone synthase deficiency
	  Adrenoleukodystrophy
	Hyporeninemic hypoaldosteronism
	  Urinary tract obstruction
	  Sickle cell disease
	  Kidney transplant
	  Lupus nephritis
	Renal tubular disease
	  Pseudohypoaldosteronism type 1
	  Pseudohypoaldosteronism type 2
	  Urinary tract obstruction
	  Sickle cell disease
	  Kidney transplant
	Medications
	  ACE inhibitors
	  Angiotensin II blockers
	  Potassium-sparing diuretics
	  Cyclosporine
	  NSAIDs
	  Trimethoprim

INCREASED INTAKE	
IV or PO Blood transfusions	
TRANSCELLULAR SHIFTS	
Acidemia Rhabdomyolysis Tumor lysis syndrome Tissue necrosis Hemolysis/hematomas/gastrointestinal bleeding Succinylcholine Digitalis intoxication Fluoride intoxication β-adrenergic blockers Exercise Hyperosmolality Insulin deficiency Malignant hyperthermia Hyperkalemic periodic paralysis	

ACE, Angiotensin-converting enzyme; *IV*, intravenous; *NSAIDs*, nonsteroidal antiinflammatory drugs; *PO*, oral.

activated by aldosterone. In the autosomal dominant form *(PHA1A)*, patients have a defect in the aldosterone receptor, and the disease is milder, often remitting in adulthood. **PHA type 2**, also called ***Gordon syndrome***, is an autosomal dominant disorder *(PIEZO2)* characterized by hypertension secondary to salt retention and impaired excretion of potassium and acid, leading to hyperkalemia and metabolic acidosis. PHA type 2 responds to a thiazide diuretic.

Clinical Manifestations

The most import effects of hyperkalemia are due to the role of potassium in membrane polarization. The cardiac conduction system is usually the dominant concern. **ECG changes** begin with peaking of the T waves. As the potassium level increases, an increased P-R interval, flattening of the P wave, and widening of the QRS complex occur; this eventually can progress to ventricular fibrillation. Asystole also may occur. Some patients have paresthesias, weakness, and tingling, but cardiac toxicity usually precedes these clinical symptoms.

Diagnosis

The etiology of hyperkalemia is often readily apparent. Spurious hyperkalemia is common in children, so a repeat potassium level is often appropriate. If there is a significant elevation of the white blood cells or platelets, the repeat sample should be from plasma that is evaluated promptly. Initially, the history should focus on potassium intake, risk factors for transcellular shifts of potassium, medications that cause hyperkalemia, and the presence of signs of kidney injury, such as oliguria or an abnormal urinalysis. Initial laboratory evaluation should include serum creatinine and assessment of acid-base status. Some causes of hyperkalemia, such as kidney injury and aldosterone insufficiency or resistance, cause a metabolic acidosis. Cell destruction, as seen in rhabdomyolysis or tumor lysis syndrome, can cause concomitant hyperphosphatemia, hyperuricemia, and an elevated serum lactate dehydrogenase.

TABLE 35.4 Treatment of Hyperkalemia

Rapidly decrease the risk of life-threatening arrhythmias
Cardiac membrane stabilization
IV calcium
Shift potassium intracellularly
Sodium bicarbonate administration (IV)
Insulin and glucose (IV)
β-agonist (albuterol via nebulizer)
Remove potassium from the body
Loop diuretic (IV or PO)
Sodium polystyrene sulfonate and other potassium binding agents (PO or rectal)
Dialysis

IV, Intravenous; *PO*, oral.

Treatment

The plasma potassium level, the ECG, and the risk of the problem worsening determine the aggressiveness of the therapeutic approach. A high serum potassium level with ECG changes requires prompt treatment. An additional source of concern is a patient with increasing plasma potassium despite minimal intake. This situation can occur if there is cellular release of potassium (tumor lysis syndrome), especially in the setting of diminished excretion (kidney injury).

The first action in a child with a concerning elevation of plasma potassium is to stop all sources of additional potassium (oral and IV). If the potassium level is greater than 6.5 mEq/L, an ECG should be obtained to help assess the urgency of the situation. Therapy of hyperkalemia has two basic goals:

1. Prevent life-threatening arrhythmias
2. Remove potassium from the body (Table 35.4)

Treatments that acutely prevent arrhythmias all work quickly (within minutes), but do not remove potassium from the body.

Long-term management of hyperkalemia includes reducing intake via dietary changes and eliminating or reducing medications that cause hyperkalemia. Some patients require medications, such as sodium polystyrene sulfonate and loop or thiazide diuretics, to increase potassium losses. The disorders that are due to a deficiency in aldosterone respond to replacement therapy with fludrocortisone, which is a mineralocorticoid.

PEARLS FOR PRACTITIONERS

See Fluids and Electrolytes: Pearls for Practitioners at the end of this section.

REVIEW QUESTIONS

Available online.

CHAPTER 36

Acid-Base Disorders

Close regulation of pH is necessary for cellular enzymes and other metabolic processes, which function optimally at a normal pH (7.35–7.45). Chronic, mild abnormalities in acid-base status may interfere with normal growth and development; acute, severe changes in pH can be fatal. Control of acid-base balance depends on the kidneys, the lungs, and the intracellular and extracellular buffers.

The lungs and kidneys maintain a normal acid-base balance. Carbon dioxide (CO_2) generated during normal metabolism is a weak acid. The lungs prevent an increase in the partial pressure of CO_2 (Pco_2) in the blood by excreting the CO_2. Production of CO_2 varies depending on the body's metabolic needs. The rapid pulmonary response to changes in CO_2 concentration occurs via central sensing of the Pco_2 and a subsequent increase or decrease in ventilation to maintain a normal Pco_2 (35–45 mm Hg).

The kidneys excrete endogenous acids. A child produces 2–3 mEq/kg per day of hydrogen ions. The hydrogen ions from endogenous acid production are neutralized by bicarbonate, potentially causing the bicarbonate concentration to fall. The kidneys regenerate this bicarbonate by secreting hydrogen ions, maintaining the serum bicarbonate concentration in the normal range (20–28 mEq/L).

CLINICAL ASSESSMENT OF ACID-BASE DISORDERS

Acidemia is a pH below normal (<7.35), and **alkalemia** is a pH above normal (>7.45). **Acidosis** is a pathologic process that causes an increase in the hydrogen ion concentration, and **alkalosis** is a pathologic process that causes a decrease in the hydrogen ion concentration. A **simple acid-base disorder** is a single primary disturbance. During a simple metabolic disorder, there is respiratory compensation; the Pco_2 decreases during metabolic acidosis and increases during metabolic alkalosis. With metabolic acidosis, the decrease in the pH increases the ventilatory drive, causing a decrease in the Pco_2. The fall in the CO_2 concentration leads to an increase in the pH. This **appropriate respiratory compensation** for a metabolic process happens quickly and is complete within 12–24 hours.

During a primary respiratory process, there is metabolic compensation mediated by the kidneys. The kidneys respond to a respiratory acidosis by increasing hydrogen ion excretion, increasing bicarbonate generation, and raising the serum bicarbonate concentration. The kidneys increase bicarbonate excretion to compensate for a respiratory alkalosis; the serum bicarbonate concentration decreases. In contrast to a rapid respiratory compensation, it takes 3–4 days for the kidneys to complete **appropriate metabolic compensation**. There is a small and rapid compensatory change in the bicarbonate concentration during a primary respiratory process. The expected appropriate metabolic compensation for a respiratory disorder depends on whether the process is acute or chronic.

A **mixed acid-base disorder** is present when there is more than one primary acid-base disturbance. An infant with bronchopulmonary dysplasia may have respiratory acidosis from chronic lung disease and metabolic alkalosis from a diuretic used to treat the chronic lung disease. Formulas are available for calculating the appropriate metabolic or respiratory compensation for the six primary simple acid-base disorders (Table 36.1). Appropriate compensation is expected in a simple disorder; it is not optional. If a patient does not have appropriate compensation, a mixed acid-base disorder is present.

METABOLIC ACIDOSIS

Metabolic acidosis occurs frequently in hospitalized children; diarrhea is the most common cause. For a patient with an unknown medical problem, the presence of metabolic acidosis is often diagnostically helpful because it suggests a relatively narrow differential diagnosis (Table 36.2).

Etiology

The plasma **anion gap** is useful for evaluating patients with metabolic acidosis. The anion gap divides patients into two diagnostic groups: normal anion gap and increased anion gap. The formula to calculate the anion gap is:

$$\text{Anion Gap} = Na^+ - (Cl^- + HCO_3^-)$$

A normal anion gap is 9 ± 4 mEq/L.

TABLE 36.1 Appropriate Compensation During Simple Acid-Base Disorders

DISORDER	EXPECTED COMPENSATION*
Metabolic acidosis	$Pco_2 = 1.5 \times [HCO_3^-] + 8 \pm 2$
Metabolic alkalosis	Pco_2 increases by 7 mm Hg for each 10 mEq/L increase in the serum $[HCO_3^-]$
Respiratory acidosis	
Acute	$[HCO_3^-]$ increases by 1 for each 10 mm Hg increase in the Pco_2
Chronic	$[HCO_3^-]$ increases by 3.5 for each 10 mm Hg increase in the Pco_2
Respiratory alkalosis	
Acute	$[HCO_3^-]$ falls by 2 for each 10 mm Hg decrease in the Pco_2
Chronic	$[HCO_3^-]$ falls by 4 for each 10 mm Hg decrease in the Pco_2

*$[HCO_3^-]$ is expressed in mEq/L.

TABLE 36.2 Causes of Metabolic Acidosis

NORMAL ANION GAP
Diarrhea
Renal tubular acidosis
Urinary tract diversions
Posthypocapnia
Ammonium chloride intake
INCREASED ANION GAP
Lactic acidosis (shock or inborn errors of metabolism)
Ketoacidosis (diabetic, starvation, or alcoholic)
Kidney failure
Poisoning (e.g., ethylene glycol, methanol, or salicylates)
Inborn errors of metabolism

Normal anion gap metabolic acidosis occurs in the setting of diarrhea and **renal tubular acidosis (RTA)**. Diarrhea causes a loss of bicarbonate from the body. The amount of bicarbonate lost in the stool depends on the volume of diarrhea and the bicarbonate concentration of the stool, which tends to increase with more severe diarrhea. Diarrhea often causes volume depletion because of losses of sodium and water, potentially exacerbating the acidosis by causing hypoperfusion (shock) and a lactic acidosis.

There are four forms of RTA:

1. Distal (type 1)
2. Proximal (type 2)
3. Mixed type 1 and 2 (type 3)
4. Hyperkalemic (type 4)

In distal RTA (dRTA), children may have accompanying hypokalemia, hypercalciuria, nephrolithiasis, and nephrocalcinosis; rickets is a less common finding. Growth faltering, resulting from chronic metabolic acidosis, is the most common presenting complaint. Autosomal dominant (relatively mild) and autosomal recessive (more severe) forms of dRTA exist (pathogenic variants in *ATP6V0A4*, *ATP6V1B1*, or *FOXI1*). Autosomal recessive dRTA is often associated with deafness secondary to a pathogenic variant for a subunit of an H^+-ATPase that is present in the kidney and the inner ear. dRTA also may be secondary to medications or congenital or acquired kidney disease. Patients with dRTA cannot acidify their urine and can have a urine pH greater than 5.5, despite metabolic acidosis.

Proximal RTA is rarely present in isolation. In most patients, proximal RTA is part of **Fanconi syndrome**, a generalized dysfunction of the proximal tubule. Along with kidney wasting of bicarbonate, Fanconi syndrome causes glycosuria, aminoaciduria, and excessive urinary losses of phosphate and uric acid. The chronic hypophosphatemia is more clinically significant because it ultimately leads to rickets in children. Rickets or growth faltering may be the presenting complaint. Fanconi syndrome is rarely an isolated genetic disorder, with pediatric cases usually secondary to an underlying genetic disorder, most commonly **cystinosis** (pathogenic variant in the *CTNS* gene). Medications, such as ifosfamide, deferasirox, or valproate, may cause Fanconi syndrome. The ability to acidify the urine is intact in proximal RTA, and untreated patients have a urine pH less than 5.5.

In **hyperkalemic RTA**, kidney excretion of acid and potassium is impaired because of either an absence of aldosterone or an inability of the kidney to respond to aldosterone. In severe aldosterone deficiency, as occurs with congenital adrenal hyperplasia secondary to *21α-hydroxylase deficiency*, the hyperkalemia and metabolic acidosis are accompanied by hyponatremia and volume depletion from kidney salt wasting. Incomplete aldosterone deficiency causes less severe electrolyte disturbances; children may have isolated hyperkalemic RTA, hyperkalemia without acidosis, or isolated hyponatremia.

Distal and hyperkalemic RTA are similar in that distal tubular acidification is impaired. Conversely, in proximal RTA, distal tubular acidification is intact but leads to metabolic acidosis due to bicarbonate wasting.

Increased anion gap metabolic acidosis occurs with lactic acidosis, ketoacidosis, chronic kidney disease, and toxic ingestions. Lactic acidosis occurs when inadequate oxygen delivery to the tissues leads to anaerobic metabolism and excess production of lactic acid. Lactic acidosis may be secondary to shock, severe anemia, or hypoxemia. Inborn errors of carbohydrate metabolism produce a severe lactic acidosis (see Chapter 51). In diabetes mellitus, inadequate insulin leads to hyperglycemia and diabetic ketoacidosis (see Chapter 172). Kidney failure (see Chapter 166) causes metabolic acidosis because the kidneys are unable to excrete the acid produced by normal metabolism.

A variety of **toxic ingestions** cause metabolic acidosis. Acute **salicylate** intoxication occurs after a large overdose. Chronic salicylate intoxication is possible because of the gradual buildup of the drug. Patients may also have a respiratory alkalosis. Other symptoms of salicylate intoxication include fever, seizures, lethargy, and coma. Hyperventilation may be particularly marked. Tinnitus, vertigo, and hearing impairment are more likely with chronic salicylate intoxication. **Ethylene glycol**, a component of antifreeze, is converted in the liver to glyoxylic and oxalic acids, causing a severe metabolic acidosis. Excessive oxalate excretion causes calcium oxalate crystals to appear in the urine, and calcium oxalate precipitation in the kidney tubules can cause acute kidney injury. The toxicity of **methanol** ingestion also depends on liver metabolism; formic acid is the toxic end product that causes the metabolic acidosis and other sequelae, which include damage to the optic nerve and central nervous system.

There are several **inborn errors of metabolism** that may cause metabolic acidosis (see Section 10). Metabolic acidosis may be due to excessive production of ketoacids, lactic acid, or other organic anions. Some patients may have accompanying hyperammonemia. In most patients, acidosis occurs only episodically during acute decompensations, which may be precipitated by the ingestion of specific dietary substrates (proteins), the stress of a mild illness (fasting, catabolism), or poor adherence with dietary or medical therapy.

Clinical Manifestations

In children with a mild-to-moderate metabolic acidosis, the underlying disorder is what causes most of the presenting signs and symptoms. The clinical manifestations of the acidosis are related to the degree of acidemia; patients with appropriate respiratory compensation and less severe acidemia have fewer manifestations than patients with a concomitant respiratory acidosis. At a serum pH less than 7.20, there is impaired cardiac contractility and an increased risk of arrhythmias, especially if underlying heart disease or other predisposing electrolyte disorders are present. With acidemia, there is a decrease in the cardiovascular response to catecholamines, potentially exacerbating hypotension in children with volume depletion or shock. Acidemia causes vasoconstriction of the pulmonary vasculature, which is especially problematic in neonates with primary pulmonary hypertension of the newborn (see Chapter 60). The normal respiratory response to metabolic acidosis (compensatory hyperventilation) may be subtle with mild metabolic acidosis, but it causes discernible increased respiratory effort with worsening acidemia. Chronic metabolic acidosis causes growth faltering.

Diagnosis

Calculating the anion gap will narrow the differential diagnosis for acidosis. The anion gap should not be interpreted in dogmatic isolation; consideration of other laboratory abnormalities and the clinical history improves the diagnostic utility. A decrease in the albumin concentration of 1 g/dL decreases the anion gap by roughly 4 mEq/L. Similarly, albeit less commonly, an increase in unmeasured cations, such as calcium, potassium, or magnesium, decreases the anion gap. Conversely, a decrease in unmeasured cations is a rare cause of an increased anion gap. Due to these variables as well as the broad range of a normal anion gap and other factors, the presence of a normal or increased anion gap is not always reliable in differentiating the causes of a metabolic acidosis, especially when the metabolic acidosis is mild. Some patients have more than one explanation for their metabolic acidosis, such as a child with diarrhea and lactic acidosis secondary to shock.

Treatment

The most effective therapeutic approach for patients with a metabolic acidosis is correction of the underlying disorder, if possible. The administration of insulin in diabetic ketoacidosis or restoration of adequate perfusion in lactic acidosis from shock eventually results in normalization of acid-base balance. The use of bicarbonate therapy is indicated when the underlying disorder is irreparable; examples include RTA and chronic kidney disease. In salicylate poisoning, alkali administration increases kidney clearance of salicylate and decreases the amount of salicylate in brain cells. Short-term base therapy is often necessary in other poisonings and inborn errors of metabolism.

METABOLIC ALKALOSIS

Etiology

The causes of a metabolic alkalosis are divided into two categories based on the urinary chloride (Fig. 36.1). Alkalosis in patients with a low urinary chloride is maintained by volume depletion. These patients are **chloride responsive** because volume repletion with fluid containing sodium chloride and potassium chloride is necessary to correct the metabolic alkalosis. Emesis, which causes loss of hydrochloride and volume depletion, is the most common cause of a metabolic alkalosis. Diuretic use increases chloride excretion in the urine. Consequently, while a patient is receiving diuretics, the urinary chloride is high (>20 mEq/L). After the diuretic effect resolves, the urinary chloride is low (<15 mEq/L) because of appropriate kidney chloride retention in response to volume depletion. Categorization of diuretics based on urinary chloride depends on the timing of the measurement. The metabolic alkalosis from diuretics is clearly chloride responsive; it corrects after adequate volume repletion. This is the rationale for including it among the chloride-responsive causes of a metabolic alkalosis.

The **chloride-resistant** causes of metabolic alkalosis can be subdivided based on blood pressure. Patients with the rare disorders that cause metabolic alkalosis and hypertension

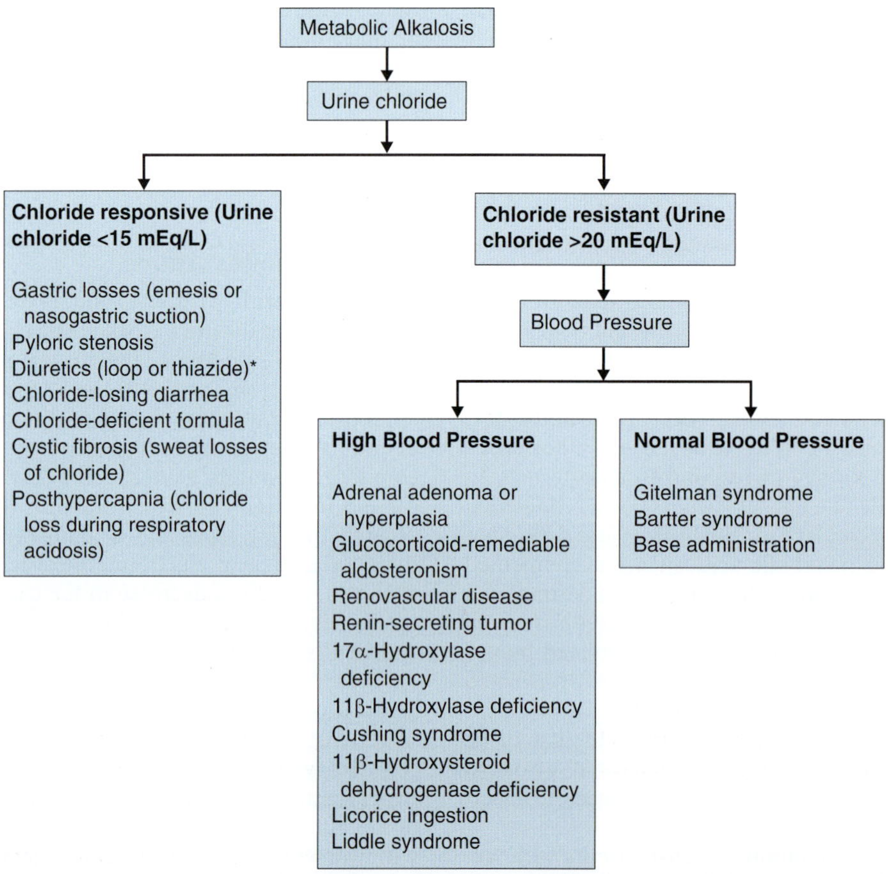

FIGURE 36.1 Causes of a metabolic alkalosis. *Diuretics are associated with an elevated urinary chloride (>20 mEq/L) when the patient is receiving the diuretic but a low urinary chloride (<15 mEq/L) when the effect has worn off but are chloride-responsive and hence grouped with these disorders.

either have increased aldosterone or act as if they have increased aldosterone. Patients with Bartter syndrome or Gitelman syndrome (see Chapter 35) have metabolic alkalosis, hypokalemia, and normal blood pressure secondary to kidney tubular defects, which cause continuous urinary losses of chloride.

Clinical Manifestations

The symptoms in patients with metabolic alkalosis often are related to the underlying disease and associated electrolyte disturbances. Hypokalemia is often present and occasionally severe (see Chapter 35). Children with chloride-responsive causes of metabolic alkalosis often have symptoms related to volume depletion (see Chapter 32). In contrast, children with chloride-unresponsive causes may have symptoms related to hypertension. Severe alkalemia may cause arrhythmias, hypoxia secondary to hypoventilation, or decreased cardiac output.

Diagnosis

Measurement of the urinary chloride concentration is the most helpful test in differentiating among the causes of metabolic alkalosis. The history usually suggests a diagnosis, although no obvious explanation may be present in the patient with bulimia or surreptitious diuretic use. Patients with Bartter syndrome or Gitelman syndrome usually have a history of polyuria and may have salt craving.

Treatment

Treatment of metabolic alkalosis depends on the severity of the alkalosis and the underlying etiology. In children with mild metabolic alkalosis ($[HCO_3^-] < 32$ mEq/L), intervention is often unnecessary. Patients with chloride-responsive metabolic alkalosis respond to the correction of hypokalemia and volume repletion with sodium and potassium chloride, but aggressive volume repletion may be contraindicated if mild volume depletion is medically necessary in the child receiving diuretic therapy. In children with chloride-resistant causes of metabolic alkalosis that are associated with hypertension, volume repletion is contraindicated because it exacerbates the hypertension and does not repair the metabolic alkalosis. Treatment focuses on eliminating or blocking the action of the excess mineralocorticoid. In children with Bartter syndrome or Gitelman syndrome, therapy includes oral sodium and potassium supplementation.

RESPIRATORY ACID-BASE DISTURBANCES

During respiratory acidosis, there is a decrease in the effectiveness of CO_2 removal by the lungs. The causes of respiratory acidosis are either pulmonary or nonpulmonary (Table 36.3). A respiratory alkalosis is an inappropriate reduction in the blood CO_2 concentration. A variety of stimuli can increase the ventilatory drive and cause respiratory alkalosis (Table 36.4). Treatment of respiratory acid-base disorders focuses on correction of the underlying disorder. Mechanical ventilation may be necessary in a child with refractory respiratory acidosis.

TABLE 36.3 Causes of Respiratory Acidosis
Central nervous system depression (encephalitis or narcotic overdose)
Disorders of the spinal cord, peripheral nerves, or neuromuscular junction (botulism or Guillain-Barré syndrome)
Respiratory muscle weakness (muscular dystrophy, myasthenia gravis)
Pulmonary disease (pneumonia or asthma)
Upper airway disease (laryngospasm)

TABLE 36.4 Causes of Respiratory Alkalosis
Hypoxemia or tissue hypoxia (carbon monoxide poisoning or cyanotic heart disease)
Lung receptor stimulation (pneumonia or pulmonary embolism)
Central stimulation (anxiety or brain tumor)
Mechanical ventilation
Hyperammonemia

PEARLS FOR PRACTITIONERS

See Fluids and Electrolytes: Pearls for Practitioners at the end of this section.

REVIEW QUESTIONS

Available online.

Suggested Readings

Albuquerque ALB, Dos Santos Borges R, Conegundes AF, et al. Inherited Fanconi syndrome. *World J Pediatr.* 2023;19(7):619–634.
Brown DH, Paloian NJ. Hypokalemia/Hyperkalemia and Hyponatremia/Hypernatremia. *Pediatr Rev.* 2023;44(7):349–362.
Büyükkaragöz B, Bakkaloğlu SA. Serum osmolality and hyperosmolar states. *Pediatr Nephrol.* 2023;38(4):1013–1025.
Didsbury M, See EJ, Cheng DR, Kausman J, Quinlan C. Correcting Hypernatremia in Children. *Clin J Am Soc Nephrol.* 2023;18(3):306–314.
Feld LG, Neuspiel DR, Foster BA, et al. Subcommittee on Fluid and Electrolyte Therapy. Clinical Practice Guideline: Maintenance Intravenous Fluids in Children. *Pediatrics.* 2018;142(6):e20183083.
Florez ID, Sierra J, Pérez-Gaxiola G. Balanced crystalloid solutions versus 0.9% saline for treating acute diarrhoea and severe dehydration in children. *Cochrane Database Syst Rev.* 2023;5(5):CD013640.
Greenbaum LA. Fluid and electrolyte disorders. In: Kliegman RM, Geme JW, Blum NJ, et al., eds. *Nelson Textbook of Pediatrics.* 22nd ed. Philadelphia: Elsevier; 2025:485–533.
Groh-Wargo S, Barr SM. Parenteral Nutrition. *Clin Perinatol.* 2022;49(2):355–379.
Lehtiranta S, Honkila M, Kallio M, et al. Risk of Electrolyte Disorders in Acutely Ill Children Receiving Commercially Available Plasmalike Isotonic Fluids: A Randomized Clinical Trial. *JAMA Pediatr.* 2021;175(1):28–35.
Yee J, Frinak S, Mohiuddin N, Uduman J. Fundamentals of Arterial Blood Gas Interpretation. *Kidney360.* 2022;3(8):1458–1466.

PEARLS FOR PRACTITIONERS

CHAPTER 31

Maintenance Fluid Therapy

- Maintenance of normal plasma osmolality within the extracellular compartment depends on the regulation of water balance, which is controlled by antidiuretic hormone (ADH); water intake due to thirst has a key role when the osmolality is elevated.
- Control of plasma osmolality is subordinate to the maintenance of an adequate intravascular volume. As such, significant volume depletion stimulates ADH secretion and thirst, regardless of the plasma osmolality.
- Control of volume status depends on the regulation of sodium balance by the kidneys. Effective plasma volume determines the amount of sodium excretion by the kidneys through the renin-angiotensin-aldosterone axis; it is not determined by serum sodium or osmolality.
- Maintenance intravenous fluids should be utilized in patients who cannot be fed enterally to replace insensible, stool, and urinary losses of water, as well as urinary and stool losses of electrolytes.
- The glucose in maintenance fluids provides approximately 20% of normal caloric needs to prevent the development of starvation ketoacidosis and diminish the protein degradation that would occur if the patient received no calories, but maintenance fluids are not a long-term replacement for nutrition.
- The standard maintenance solution is D5 in normal saline plus 20 mEq/L KCl. Exceptions include neonates, where hypotonic fluids are recommended, and disease processes that necessitate changing the rate or electrolyte content of the fluids.

CHAPTER 32

Dehydration and Replacement Therapy

- Insensible water losses from the skin and lungs are about 35% of normal water losses.
- An anuric child who is not dehydrated and is not being fed enterally only requires insensible fluids to maintain euvolemia.
- Children with excessive losses (stool, urine, other) need a replacement solution to avoid volume depletion.
- A 20 mL/kg IV bolus of an isotonic fluid (normal saline, Ringer's lactate) is given over 20 minutes in a child with significant dehydration.
- The blood urea nitrogen (BUN) is elevated out of proportion to the serum creatinine in patients with volume depletion.
- Hyponatremic dehydration occurs when gastrointestinal losses are replaced with hypotonic fluids such as water or diluted formula in a child with gastroenteritis.
- Hypernatremic dehydration occurs in children with poor thirst, poor fluid intake, or excessive urine water losses (arginine vasopressin deficiency or resistance).
- Mild-to-moderate diarrheal dehydration can be treated with oral rehydration solution.

CHAPTER 33

Parenteral Nutrition

- Parenteral nutrition (PN) is necessary when enteral feeding is inadequate to meet nutritional needs.
- Short bowel syndrome is the most common disorder requiring chronic PN.
- Calories from PN are predominantly from dextrose and fat. Amino acids are used for protein synthesis.
- The most concerning complication of long-term PN is cholestatic liver disease, but the risk is reduced by utilization of the gastrointestinal tract even if just for trophic feeds. Other complications of PN include thrombosis and bacteremia.

CHAPTER 34

Sodium Disorders

- Disorders of sodium are secondary to abnormalities in water balance as opposed to sodium balance.
- The symptoms of hyponatremia, such as seizures, are principally due to water movement into brain cells (cerebral edema).
- The symptoms of hypernatremia are due to water movement out of brain cells, which may lead to brain hemorrhage if the hypernatremia is severe.
- Symptoms of hyponatremia are much more likely if the hyponatremia develops rapidly.
- Diagnosing the etiology of hyponatremia should begin by assessing a patient's volume status (hypovolemic, euvolemic, or hypervolemic).
- Most cases of hyponatremia are due to gastroenteritis, but the syndrome of inappropriate antidiuretic hormone secretion (SIADH) or hypervolemic causes (heart failure, cirrhosis) should be considered.
- Most cases of hypernatremia are due to gastroenteritis, but arginine vasopressin deficiency or resistance must be considered.
- Overly rapid correction of hyponatremia can lead to osmotic demyelination syndrome; it is optimal to increase the serum sodium less than 10 mEq/L per 24 hours.

- Due to the presence of idiogenic osmoles, overly rapid correction of hypernatremia can lead to cerebral edema; the target decrease in serum sodium is less than 12 mEq/L per 24 hours.
- Acute water intoxication producing hyponatremia often self-corrects once excessive water intake has stopped.
- The emergency treatment of symptomatic hyponatremia involves the use of intravenous hypertonic saline to decrease brain edema.

CHAPTER 35

Potassium Disorders

- The kidneys are the principal regulator of potassium balance.
- Hypokalemia is secondary to kidney losses, nonrenal losses (diarrhea), low intake, or transcellular shifts.
- Transcellular potassium shifts causing hypokalemia are seen in patients receiving insulin plus dextrose for diabetic ketoacidosis and patients receiving albuterol for asthma.
- Severe hypokalemia causes muscle cramps and muscle weakness, which may proceed to paralysis.
- Hypokalemia with a metabolic acidosis suggests diarrhea or renal tubular acidosis.
- Hypokalemia with a metabolic alkalosis is most commonly due to emesis or nasogastric losses but may also be due to Bartter or Gitelman syndrome or diuretic use.
- Arrhythmias, which may be fatal, can be the initial clinical manifestation of hyperkalemia.
- Hyperkalemia is most commonly due to decreased excretion or a transcellular shift, although increased intake may cause it or contribute to it.
- Hyperkalemia is seen in disorders with decreased renin, decreased aldosterone (congenital adrenal hyperplasia), or lack of response to aldosterone (decreased aldosterone effect).
- Hyperkalemia is associated with peaked T waves and may produce paresthesias and muscle weakness.
- The two goals of treating hyperkalemia, which require different therapeutic approaches, are to prevent cardiac toxicity and to decrease total body potassium.
- Total body potassium may be reduced by loop or thiazide diuretics, dialysis, or potassium-binding resins.

CHAPTER 36

Acid-Base Disorders

- Acute, severe changes in pH can be fatal; chronic, mild abnormalities may interfere with growth and development.
- The lungs and the kidneys maintain normal acid-base balance. The lungs (respiratory) regulate CO_2 concentration, and the kidneys (metabolic) regulate bicarbonate concentration.
- During a primary respiratory process, the kidneys compensate, but full compensation takes a few days.
- During a primary metabolic process, the lungs compensate rapidly (within hours).
- Appropriate compensation is expected in a simple acid-base disorder; it is not optional. If a patient does not have appropriate compensation, a mixed acid-base disorder is present.
- The plasma anion gap divides patients with metabolic acidosis into two categories: normal anion gap and increased anion gap.
- Normal anion gap metabolic acidosis occurs in the setting of diarrhea and renal tubular acidosis.
- Increased anion gap metabolic acidosis occurs with lactic acidosis, ketoacidosis, chronic kidney disease, and toxic ingestions.
- The differential diagnosis of metabolic alkalosis begins by measuring the urine chloride and separating patients based on whether the urinary chloride is low or high.
- Patients with a metabolic alkalosis and a low urine chloride are volume depleted, and the alkalosis responds to administration of sodium or potassium chloride (chloride-responsive).
- Patients with chloride-resistant metabolic alkalosis (urine chloride not low) are subdivided based on the presence of a normal or elevated blood pressure.

SECTION 8

THE ACUTELY ILL OR INJURED CHILD

Madeline R. Field | Cory A. McFall

CHAPTER 37

Assessment and Resuscitation

INITIAL ASSESSMENT

Initial assessment of an acutely ill or injured child includes rapid identification of physiologic derangements in **tissue perfusion and oxygenation**. Once identified, immediate resuscitation must be implemented before pursuing the usual information needed to develop a differential diagnosis. Initial resuscitation measures are directed at achieving and maintaining adequate tissue perfusion and oxygenation. **Oxygen delivery** depends on cardiac output, hemoglobin concentration, and hemoglobin-oxygen saturation. The latter depends on air movement, alveolar gas exchange, pulmonary blood flow, and hemoglobin-oxygen binding characteristics.

HISTORY

In the initial assessment of an acutely ill or traumatically injured child, access to historical information may be limited. Characterization of the onset of symptoms, event details, and a brief identification of underlying medical problems should be sought by members of the team not actively involved in the resuscitation. The mnemonic **AMPLE** can be employed to help direct a focused history during this time: A, Allergies; M, Medications; P, Past medical history; L, Last meal; and E, Events leading up to patient presentation. Attempts at identifying historical issues that affect the physiologic derangements are useful but should not delay intervention if tissue oxygenation and perfusion are markedly impaired.

PHYSICAL EXAMINATION

Initial examination must focus on the responsiveness of a patient followed by assessment of the airway, breathing, and circulation (Table 37.1) to systematically address the issues of oxygen delivery to tissues. The American Heart Association (AHA) Basic Life Support (BLS) guidelines recommend a **CAB sequence (circulation, airway, breathing)** of cardiopulmonary resuscitation for all pulseless patients to decrease the time to the initiation of chest compression and reduce "no blood flow" time. In situations in which a pulse is felt but respirations are ineffective, the traditional sequence of **ABC (airway, breathing, circulation)** may be more appropriate. It is important to note that the leading cause of cardiopulmonary arrest in children is most often of *respiratory etiology* (compared to a cardiac etiology in adults), and thus rapid initial assessment of the airway and breathing is vital. Regardless of the sequence approach utilized, it is best to use a consistent, algorithmic method to ensure effective and efficient cardiopulmonary assessment.

Assessment of airway patency should include evaluation of the injured child's ability to protect the airway. Protection of the cervical spine should be initiated at this step in any child with traumatic injury or who presents with altered mental status of uncertain etiology or distracting injury. Assessment of breathing includes observation of respiratory effort, rate, and chest rise, plus the auscultation of air movement and the application of a pulse oximeter (when available) to identify current oxygenation status. Circulatory status is assessed by palpation for distal and central pulses, focusing on the presence and quality of the pulses. Bounding pulses and a wide pulse pressure are often the first sign of the vasodilatory phase of shock and require immediate resuscitation measures. Weak, thready, or absent pulses are indicators for fluid resuscitation, initiation of chest compressions, or both. When assessment of the ABCs is complete and measures have been taken to achieve an acceptable level of tissue oxygenation, a more complete physical examination is performed. The sequence of this examination depends on whether the situation involves an acute medical illness or trauma. In trauma patients, the examination follows the **xABCDE pathway**. **X** stands for identifying and controlling any life-threatening external bleeding. **D** stands for disability and prompts assessment of the neurologic system (specifically via the Glasgow Coma Scale) and evaluation for major traumatic injuries. **E** stands for exposure; the child is disrobed and examined for evidence of any life-threatening or limb-threatening problems. For the acutely ill and the injured child, the physical examination should seek to identify evidence of organ dysfunction, starting with areas suggested in the chief complaint and progressing to a thorough and systematic investigation of the entire patient.

COMMON MANIFESTATIONS

The physiologic responses to acute illness and injury are mechanisms that attempt to correct inadequacies of tissue oxygenation and perfusion. When initial changes, such as increasing heart and respiratory rates, fail to meet the body's needs, other manifestations of impending cardiopulmonary failure occur (Table 37.2). **Respiratory failure**, the most common cause of acute deterioration in children, may result in inadequate tissue oxygenation and respiratory acidosis. Signs and symptoms of respiratory failure (tachypnea, tachycardia, increased work of breathing, abnormal mentation) progress as tissue oxygenation

TABLE 37.1 Rapid Cardiopulmonary Assessment

AIRWAY PATENCY
Able to be maintained independently Maintainable with positioning, suctioning Unmaintainable, requires assistance
BREATHING
Rate Mechanics • Retractions • Grunting • Use of accessory muscles • Nasal flaring Air movement • Chest expansion • Breath sounds • Stridor • Wheezing • Paradoxical chest motion Color
CIRCULATION
Heart rate Peripheral and central pulses • Present/absent • Volume/strength Skin perfusion • Capillary refill time • Skin temperature • Color • Mottling Blood pressure Regional oximetry
CENTRAL NERVOUS SYSTEM PERFUSION
Responsiveness (AVPU) Recognition of parents or caregivers Pupillary response to light Posturing

AVPU, Alert, responds to voice, responds to pain, unresponsive.

becomes more inadequate. Inadequate perfusion (shock) leads to inadequate oxygen delivery and a resulting metabolic acidosis. **Shock** is characterized by signs of inadequate tissue perfusion (pallor, cool skin, poor pulses, delayed capillary refill, oliguria, and abnormal mentation). The presence of any of these symptoms demands careful assessment and intervention to correct the abnormality and to prevent further deterioration.

INITIAL DIAGNOSTIC EVALUATION

Screening Tests

During the initial phase of resuscitation, monitoring vital signs and physiologic status is the key screening activity. Continuous monitoring with attention to changes may indicate response to therapy or further deterioration requiring additional intervention. During the initial rapid assessment, diagnostic evaluation often is limited to pulse oximetry, heart rate monitoring, and bedside measurement of glucose levels. The latter is important in any child with altered mental status or at risk for inadequate glycogen stores (infants, malnourished patients). Other evaluations including blood pressure measurement and regional oximetry via near-infrared spectroscopy should be sought when available to aid in categorization of type of shock. After resuscitation measures, further diagnostic tests and imaging are often necessary.

TABLE 37.2 Warning Signs and Symptoms Suggesting the Need for Resuscitation*

SYSTEM	SIGNS AND SYMPTOMS
Central nervous system	Lethargy, agitation, delirium, obtundation, confusion, coma, status epilepticus
Respiratory	Apnea, grunting, nasal flaring, dyspnea, retracting, tachypnea, poor air movement, stridor, wheezing
Cardiovascular	Arrhythmia, bradycardia, tachycardia, weak pulses, poor capillary refill, hypotension
Skin and mucous membranes	Mottling, pallor, cyanosis, diaphoresis, poor membrane turgor, dry mucous membranes

**Action would seldom be taken if only one or two of these signs and symptoms were present, but the occurrence of several in concert foreshadows grave consequences. Intervention should be directed at the primary disorder.*

Diagnostic Tests and Imaging

The choice of appropriate diagnostic tests and imaging is determined by the mechanism of injury/disease and the results of evaluation after initial resuscitation. The initial evaluation of major trauma patients is focused on identifying evidence of hemorrhage and organ and tissue injury; labs including complete blood count (CBC) and coagulation studies should be obtained. For an acutely ill child with respiratory distress, a chest x-ray is important. In the setting of traumatic injuries, an **extended focused assessment with sonography in trauma (eFAST)** exam can be used as a quick bedside screening test for blood around the heart or abdominal organs and signs of pneumothorax or hemothorax. Appropriate cultures (such as blood, urine, cerebrospinal fluid, and/or wound) should be obtained when sepsis is suspected. Children with historical or physical evidence of inadequate intravascular volume should have serum electrolyte levels obtained, including bicarbonate, blood urea nitrogen, and creatinine.

RESUSCITATION

Resuscitation is focused on correcting identified abnormalities of oxygenation and perfusion and preventing further deterioration. **Oxygen supplementation** may improve oxygen saturation but may not completely correct tissue oxygenation. When oxygen supplementation is insufficient or air exchange is inadequate, assisted ventilation must be initiated. Inadequate perfusion is usually best managed initially by providing a fluid bolus. **Isotonic crystalloids** (normal saline or a balanced crystalloid solution such as lactated Ringer) are the initial fluids of choice. A bolus of 10–20 mL/kg should be delivered in monitored conditions. Improvement, but not correction, after an initial bolus should prompt repeated boluses until circulation has been reestablished. Because most children with shock have noncardiac causes, fluid administration of this magnitude is well tolerated. If hemorrhage is known or highly suspected, administration of packed red blood cells is appropriate. Monitoring for deteriorating physiologic status during fluid resuscitation (increase in heart rate, decrease in blood pressure, or increased work of breathing) identifies children who may have diminished cardiac function. In these cases, as fluid resuscitation increases the preload, impaired cardiac function may worsen, and pulmonary edema can result. If deterioration occurs, fluid administration should be interrupted, and further resuscitation should be aimed at improving cardiac function.

When respiratory support and fluid resuscitation are insufficient, introduction of **vasoactive substances** is the next step. The choice of which agent to use depends on the type of shock present. Hypovolemic shock (when further volume is contraindicated) and distributive shock benefit from drugs that increase systemic vascular resistance (drugs with α-agonist activity, such as epinephrine or norepinephrine). The treatment of cardiogenic shock is more complex. To improve cardiac output by increasing the heart rate, drugs with positive chronotropy are used (epinephrine, norepinephrine, and dopamine). Afterload reduction, using drugs such as dobutamine, nitroprusside, or milrinone, also may be needed. Measuring central mixed venous oxygen saturation, central venous pressure, and regional oxygen saturations can also guide therapy.

CARDIOPULMONARY ARREST

The outcome of cardiopulmonary arrest in children is poor; survival to hospital discharge is ~10% for out-of-hospital arrest and ~38% for in-hospital arrest, with most survivors having some degree of permanent neurologic disability. The ability to anticipate or recognize pre-cardiopulmonary arrest conditions and initiate prompt and appropriate therapy is not only lifesaving but can also preserve functional status (see Table 37.2).

Children who require cardiopulmonary resuscitation (CPR) usually suffered a primary respiratory arrest. Hypoxia can initiate a cascade of further physiologic deterioration with subsequent organ dysfunction or damage (Table 37.3). The approach to cardiopulmonary arrest extends beyond CPR and includes efforts to preserve vital organ function. The goal in resuscitating a pediatric patient following a cardiopulmonary arrest should be to optimize **cardiac output** and tissue oxygen delivery, which may be accomplished by using artificial ventilation, chest compressions, and judicious administration of pharmacologic agents.

Pediatric Advanced Life Support and Cardiopulmonary Resuscitation

The 2025 AHA guidelines reiterated previous recommendations for resuscitation of adults, children, and infants to initiate chest compressions immediately, rather than beginning with airway and breathing (i.e., compressions-airway-breathing/ventilation [C-A-B]) (Fig. 37.1).

Circulation

Chest compressions should be initiated if a pulse cannot be palpated or if the heart rate is less than 60 beats/min with concurrent signs of poor systemic perfusion. Chest compressions should be performed immediately by one person while a second person prepares to begin ventilation. **Ventilation** is extremely important in pediatric arrests given the high likelihood of a primary respiratory cause; however, ventilation requires equipment and is therefore sometimes delayed. For this reason, the recommendation is to start chest compressions first while preparing for ventilation.

TABLE 37.3 Target Organs for Hypoxic-Ischemic Damage

ORGAN	EFFECT
Brain	Seizures, cerebral edema, infarction, herniation, anoxic damage, SIADH, diabetes insipidus
Cardiovascular	Heart failure, myocardial infarct
Lung and pulmonary vasculature	Acute respiratory distress syndrome, pulmonary hypertension
Liver	Infarction, necrosis, cholestasis
Kidney	Acute kidney injury
Gastrointestinal tract	Gastric ulceration, mucosal damage
Hematologic	Disseminated intravascular coagulation

SIADH, Syndrome of inappropriate antidiuretic hormone secretion.

For optimal chest compressions, the child should be supine on a flat, hard surface. Effective CPR requires a compression depth of one third to one half of the anterior-posterior diameter of the chest with complete recoil after each compression. The compression rate should be at least 100/min with a compression to ventilation ratio of 30 to 2 for single-responder CPR and a ratio of 15 to 2 for two-responder CPR. If an advanced airway is in place, compressions should not pause for ventilation; both should continue simultaneously with a breath given every 2–3 seconds (20–30 breaths/minute). In infants, compressions should be performed with the 2-thumb-encircling hands technique to ensure adequate compression depth.

Airway

Ventilation requires a **patent airway**. In children, airway patency often is compromised by a loss of muscle tone, allowing the mandibular block of tissue, including the tongue, bony mandible, and the soft surrounding tissues, to rest against the posterior pharyngeal wall. The head tilt–chin lift maneuver should be used to open the airway in children with no sign of head or neck trauma. In children with signs of head or neck trauma, the jaw thrust maneuver should be used.

Bag-mask ventilation can be as effective as, and possibly safer than, endotracheal intubation for short periods of time in an out-of-hospital setting. If skilled personnel and proper equipment are available, pediatric patients requiring resuscitation should be endotracheally intubated. Before intubation, the patient should be ventilated with 100% oxygen using a bag and mask. Many conscious patients may benefit from the use of induction medications (sedatives, analgesics, and neuromuscular blockade) to assist intubation, but caution is necessary to prevent further cardiovascular compromise from vasodilating effects of many of these agents. The correct size of an uncuffed endotracheal tube may be estimated according to the size of the child's mid-fifth phalanx or the following formula: 4 + (patient age in years/4). Typically, half a size is subtracted if using a cuffed tube (i.e., 3.5 + [patient age in years/4]).

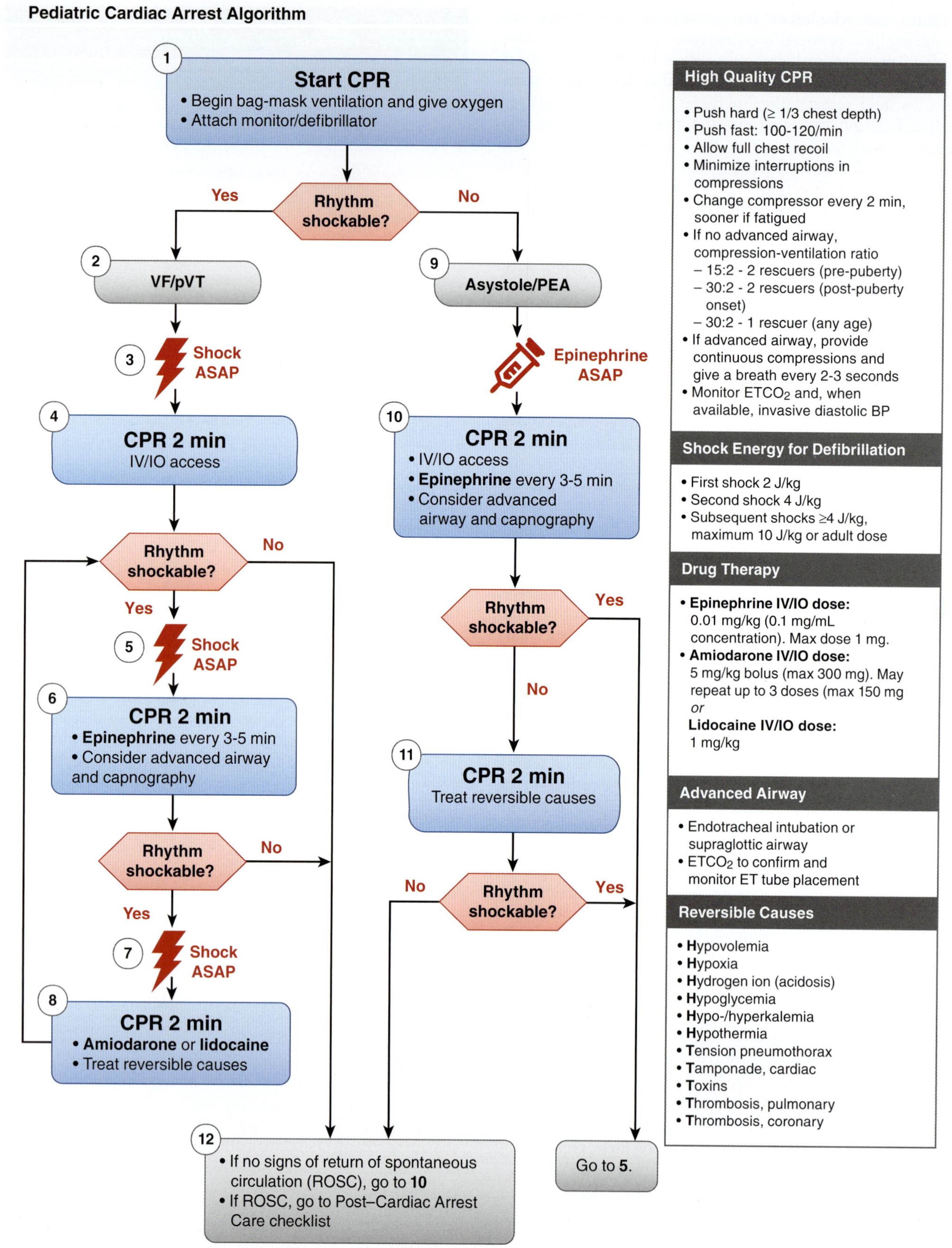

© 2025 American Heart Association and American Academy of Pediatrics

FIGURE 37.1 Pediatric Advanced Life Support cardiac arrest algorithm. *CPR,* Cardiopulmonary resuscitation; *ET,* endotracheal; *HR,* heart rate; *IV,* intravenous; *IO,* intraosseous; *PEA,* pulseless electrical activity; *pVT,* pulseless ventricular tachycardia; *VF,* ventricular fibrillation. (Reprinted with permission Circulation.2025;S479-S537 ©2025 American Heart Association, Inc.)

When the endotracheal tube is in place, the adequacy of ventilation and the position of the tube must be assessed. Use of both clinical assessment and confirmatory devices is recommended. Clinical assessment includes visualizing the tube passing through the vocal cords, looking for adequate chest wall movement, and auscultation of the chest to detect bilateral and symmetric breath sounds. Confirmatory devices, such as end-tidal carbon dioxide (CO_2) monitoring devices, are useful for the validation of endotracheal placement. AHA guidelines recommend utilization of capnography when possible in shockable and non-shockable cardiac arrest rhythms, which can also be an indicator of CPR quality. However, low levels of detected CO_2 may be seen secondary to lack of pulmonary circulation. If the patient's condition fails to improve or deteriorates, consider the possibilities of tube **D**isplacement or **O**bstruction, **P**neumothorax, or **E**quipment failure (mnemonic DOPE).

Breathing

The major role of endotracheal intubation is to protect or maintain the airway and ensure the delivery of adequate oxygen to the patient. Because hypoxemia is the final common pathway in pediatric cardiopulmonary arrests, providing oxygen is more important than correcting the respiratory acidosis. The clinician should deliver 100% oxygen via bag-valve-mask ventilation or an advanced airway; the rate of breaths is determined by the number of CPR responders and the presence of an advanced airway as previously described. Use only the tidal volume necessary to produce visible chest rise. Care should be taken not to hyperventilate the patient.

Medications

When mechanical means fail to reestablish adequate circulation, pharmacologic intervention is essential (Table 37.4). If intravascular access is not present or rapidly established, administration through an intraosseous route is recommended. Some drugs can also be administered effectively through the endotracheal tube or intramuscularly.

Epinephrine, a catecholamine with mixed α-agonist and β-agonist properties, constitutes the mainstay of drug therapy for CPR. The α-adrenergic effects are most important during acute phases of resuscitation, causing an increase in systemic vascular resistance that improves coronary blood flow. For infants and children with non-shockable rhythms, initial doses of epinephrine should be administered as early as possible. Standard dose therapy is recommended for the first and subsequent boluses. There is no benefit offered by high-dose epinephrine. Vasopressin, an endogenous hormone, causes constriction of capillaries and small arterioles and may be useful. Data are insufficient to support its routine use; however, vasopressin may be considered in children failing standard medication administration.

The routine use of **sodium bicarbonate** is currently not recommended. Sodium bicarbonate may be judiciously used to treat toxidromes or hyperkalemic arrest; however,

TABLE 37.4 Drug Doses for Cardiopulmonary Resuscitation

DRUG	INDICATION	DOSE
Adenosine	Supraventricular tachycardia	IV/IO: 0.1 mg/kg (maximum 6 mg); second dose: 0.2 mg/kg (maximum 12 mg)
Amiodarone	Pulseless VF/VT	IV/IO: 5 mg/kg bolus (max 300 mg); may repeat up to 3 doses (max 150 mg subsequent doses)
	Perfusing tachyarrhythmias	Dose as above but administer slowly over 20–60 min. Expert consultation strongly recommended
Atropine	Supraventricular or junctional bradycardia	IV/IO/IM: 0.02 mg/kg; ET: 0.04–0.06 mg/kg; minimum dose 0.1 mg and maximum single dose 0.5 mg (may repeat once); higher doses needed in organophosphate poisoning
Bicarbonate	Hyperkalemia, some toxidromes	IV/IO: 1 mEq/kg bolus; ensure adequate ventilation; monitor ABGs; can repeat every 10 min
Calcium chloride (10%)	Hypocalcemia, calcium channel blocker overdose, hypermagnesemia, hyperkalemia	IV/IO: 20 mg/kg; maximum single dose 2 g; slow push during arrest
Dextrose	Hypoglycemia	IV/IO: Newborns: 5–10 mL/kg of 10% dextrose; infants and children: 2–4 mL/kg of 25% dextrose; adolescents: 1–2 mL/kg of 50% dextrose
Epinephrine	Hypotension, chronotropy, inotropy	IV/IO: 0.01 mg/kg (0.1 mL/kg 1:10,000); ET: 0.1 mg/kg (0.1 mL/kg 1:1,000); may repeat every 3–5 min; may promote arrhythmias
Fluid	Hypovolemia, sepsis	IV/IO: Administer crystalloid in 20 mL/kg boluses titrated to patient's physiologic needs
Lidocaine	VF/pulseless VT, wide-complex tachycardia (with pulses)	IV/IO: 1 mg/kg/bolus followed by 20–50 mcg/kg/min continuous infusion; ET: Loading dose: 2–3 mg/kg/dose; flush with 5 mL of NS and follow with five assisted manual ventilations

ABG, Arterial blood gas; *ET*, endotracheal tube; *IM*, intramuscular; *IO*, intraosseous; *IV*, intravenous; *NS*, normal saline; *VF*, ventricular fibrillation; *VT*, ventricular tachycardia.

Data from the American Heart Association. Web-Based Integrated Guidelines for Cardiopulmonary and Emergency Cardiovascular Care—Part 12. Pediatric Advanced Life Support. https://eccguidelines.heart.org/index.php/circulation/cpr-ecc-guidelines-2/part-12-pediatric-advanced-life-support/.

TABLE 37.5 Recommendations for Defibrillation and Cardioversion in Children

DEFIBRILLATION
Place self-adhesive defibrillation pads or paddles with electrode gel at the apex of the heart and the upper right side of the chest. • Use infant paddles or self-adhesive pads for children <10 kg; adult size for children >10 kg. Notify all participating personnel before discharging paddles so that no one is in contact with the patient or bed. Begin with 2 J/kg; resume chest compressions immediately. If unsuccessful, increase to 4 J/kg and repeat. Higher energy levels may be considered, not to exceed 10 J/kg or the adult maximum dose.
CARDIOVERSION
Consider sedation if possible. For symptomatic supraventricular tachycardia* or ventricular tachycardia with a pulse, synchronize signal with ECG. Choose paddles, position pads, and notify personnel as above. Begin with 0.5–1 J/kg. If unsuccessful, use 2 J/kg.

*Consider adenosine first (see Table 37.4).
ECG, Electrocardiogram.

oxygen delivery and elimination of CO_2 must be established first. Side effects include hypernatremia, hyperosmolality, hypokalemia, metabolic alkalosis (shifting the oxyhemoglobin curve to the left and impairing tissue oxygen delivery), reduced ionized calcium level, and impaired cardiac function.

Routine administration of **calcium** is not recommended. It may be useful in cases of documented hypocalcemia, calcium channel blocker overdose, hypermagnesemia, or hyperkalemia but is otherwise not beneficial and is potentially harmful.

Hypoglycemia is common in infants and children who sustain cardiac arrest. Blood glucose should be checked, and hypoglycemia should be promptly treated with **glucose**.

Prompt electrical **defibrillation** is indicated when ventricular fibrillation or pulseless ventricular tachycardia is noted (Table 37.5). Ensure minimization of perishock pauses in chest compressions which can result in decreased blood flow and oxygen delivery to vital organs. If a second attempt at defibrillation is necessary, it should be followed by a dose of epinephrine. Children failing two episodes of defibrillation may benefit from administration of amiodarone or lidocaine. Defibrillation should be distinguished from **cardioversion** of supraventricular tachycardias (which can also cause cardiovascular compromise). Cardioversion requires a lower starting dose and synchronization of the discharge to the electrocardiogram to prevent discharging during a susceptible period, which may convert supraventricular tachycardia to ventricular tachycardia or fibrillation.

PEARLS FOR PRACTITIONERS

See The Acutely Ill or Injured Child: Pearls for Practitioners at the end of this section.

REVIEW QUESTIONS

Available online.

CHAPTER 38

Respiratory Failure

ETIOLOGY

Acute respiratory failure occurs when the pulmonary system is unable to maintain adequate gas exchange to meet metabolic demands. The resulting failure can be classified as hypercarbic ($Paco_2$ > 50 mm Hg in previously healthy children), hypoxemic (Pao_2 < 60 mm Hg in previously healthy children without an intracardiac shunt), or both. **Hypoxemic respiratory failure** is frequently caused by ventilation-perfusion mismatch (perfusion of lung that is not adequately ventilated) and shunting (deoxygenated blood bypasses ventilated alveoli). **Hypercarbic respiratory failure** results from inadequate alveolar ventilation secondary to decreased minute ventilation (tidal volume × respiratory rate) or an increase in dead space ventilation (ventilation of areas receiving no perfusion).

Respiratory failure may occur with **acute respiratory distress syndrome (ARDS)**. The pediatric-specific definition for acute respiratory distress syndrome (PARDS) builds on the adult-based Berlin definition but has been modified to account for differences between adults and children with ARDS. Pediatric ARDS, and its severity, is defined by (1) timing: onset within 7 days of known clinical insult; (2) respiratory failure not fully explained by cardiac failure or fluid overload; (3) chest imaging findings of new infiltrate(s) consistent with acute pulmonary parenchymal disease; and (4) impairment in oxygenation (as described in Table 38.1). Pediatric ARDS can be triggered by a variety of insults including sepsis, pneumonia, shock, burns, toxins, or traumatic injury, all resulting in inflammation and increased vascular permeability leading to pulmonary edema. Numerous mediators of inflammation (tumor necrosis factor, interferon-γ, nuclear factor kappa B [NF-κB], and adhesion molecules) as well as decreased surfactant action may be involved in the development of ARDS.

EPIDEMIOLOGY

Acute respiratory failure has many etiologies including bronchiolitis (often caused by respiratory syncytial virus [RSV]), asthma, pneumonia, upper airway obstruction, and systemic inflammation resulting in ARDS. Notably, bronchiolitis and asthma are the most common causes of acute respiratory failure in pediatric patients. RSV infects 90% of children within the first 2 years of life and frequently reinfects older children and adults. The World Health Organization estimates that RSV is responsible for ~33 million lower respiratory tract illnesses, 3 million hospitalizations, and up to 199,000 childhood deaths each year. Asthma is the most common chronic condition among children, affecting an estimated 4.7 million children under 18 years in the United States, of which 1.8 million (38.7%) experienced an asthma attack or episode in 2021 according to the Centers for Disease Control and Prevention. Environmental factors (exposure to cigarette smoke) and prior disease characteristics (severity of asthma, exercise intolerance, delayed start of therapy, and previous intensive care unit admissions) affect the rate of hospitalization and near-fatal episodes.

TABLE 38.1 Pediatric Acute Respiratory Distress Syndrome (PARDS) Severity Based on Oxygenation

NONINVASIVE MECHANICAL VENTILATION	INVASIVE MECHANICAL VENTILATION
PARDS (No Severity Stratification)	**PARDS (Severity Per OI or OSI)**
Full face mask: bilevel positive airway pressure or continuous positive airway pressure ≥5 H_2O: PF ratio ≤300 SF ratio ≤264	Mild: 4 ≤ OI < 8; 5 ≤ OSI < 7.5 Moderate: 8 ≤ OI < 16; 7.5 ≤ OSI < 12.3 Severe: OI > 16; OSI ≥ 12.3

PF ratio = Pao_2:Fio_2; if Pao_2 is not available, wean Fio_2 to maintain Spo_2 ≤ 97% to calculate the SF ratio = Spo_2:Fio_2. OI = oxygenation index = [Fio_2 × mean airway pressure × 100]/Pao_2; if Pao_2 is not available, wean Fio_2 to maintain Spo_2 ≤ 97% to calculate the oxygen saturation index (OSI; [Fio_2 × mean airway pressure × 100]/Spo_2).
PARDS, Pediatric acute respiratory distress syndrome.
Modified from Khemani RG, Smith LS, Zimmerman JJ, et al. Pediatric acute respiratory distress syndrome: definition, incidence and epidemiology: proceeding from the Pediatric Acute Lung Injury Consensus Conference. Pediatr Crit Care Med. *2015;16(5 suppl 1):S23–S40 (fig. 2).*

Chronic respiratory failure (with acute exacerbations) is often due to chronic lung disease (bronchopulmonary dysplasia, cystic fibrosis), neurologic or neuromuscular abnormalities, and congenital anomalies.

CLINICAL MANIFESTATIONS

Early signs of hypoxic respiratory failure include **tachypnea and tachycardia**, which are physiologic compensatory mechanisms to improve minute ventilation and cardiac output to maintain delivery of oxygenated blood to the tissues. Further progression of disease may result in dyspnea, nasal flaring, grunting, use of accessory muscles of respiration, and diaphoresis. Late signs of inadequate oxygen delivery include **cyanosis** and **altered mental status** (initially confusion and agitation). Signs and symptoms of hypercarbic respiratory failure include signs of increased minute ventilation (tachypnea and increased depth of breathing) and altered mental status (somnolence).

LABORATORY AND IMAGING STUDIES

A chest radiograph may show evidence of the etiology of respiratory failure. The detection of atelectasis, hyperinflation, infiltrates, or pneumothoraces assists with ongoing management. Diffuse infiltrates or pulmonary edema may suggest ARDS. The chest radiograph may be normal when upper airway obstruction or impaired respiratory controls are the etiology. In patients presenting with stridor or other evidence of upper airway obstruction, a lateral neck film or CT may delineate anatomic defects. Direct visualization through flexible bronchoscopy allows the identification of dynamic abnormalities of the anatomic airway. Helical (spiral) CT helps diagnose a pulmonary embolus.

Pulse oximetry allows noninvasive, continuous assessment of oxygenation but is unable to provide information about ventilation abnormalities. Determination of CO_2 levels requires a blood gas measurement (venous, capillary, or arterial). An **arterial blood gas** is the gold standard for measurement of serum CO_2 levels and allows for analysis of the severity of oxygenation defect through calculation of an alveolar-arterial oxygen difference. A normal $Paco_2$ in a patient who is hyperventilating should heighten concern about the risk of further deterioration. End tidal CO_2 monitors can serve as a proxy for serum CO_2 levels when an arterial blood gas cannot be obtained.

DIFFERENTIAL DIAGNOSIS

Hypoxic respiratory failure resulting from impairment of alveolar-capillary function is seen in ARDS; cardiogenic pulmonary edema; interstitial lung disease; aspiration pneumonia; bronchiolitis; bacterial, fungal, or viral pneumonia; and sepsis. It also can be due to intracardiac or intrapulmonary shunting seen with atelectasis and pulmonary embolism.

Hypercarbic respiratory failure can occur when the respiratory center fails as a result of drug use (opioids, barbiturates, anesthetic agents), neurologic or neuromuscular junction abnormalities (cervical spine trauma, demyelinating diseases, anterior horn cell disease, botulism), chest wall injuries, or diseases that cause increased resistance to airflow (croup, vocal cord paralysis, post-extubation edema). Maintenance of ventilation requires adequate function of the chest wall and diaphragm. Disorders of the neuromuscular pathways, such as muscular dystrophy, myasthenia gravis, and botulism, result in inadequate chest wall movement, development of atelectasis, and respiratory failure. Scoliosis can result in significant chest deformity that leads to restrictive pulmonary function, although rarely. Similar impairments of air exchange may result from distention of the abdomen (postoperatively or due to ascites, obstruction, or a mass) and thoracic trauma (flail chest).

Mixed forms of respiratory failure are common and occur when disease processes result in more than one pathophysiologic change. Increased secretions seen in asthma often lead to atelectasis and hypoxia, whereas restrictions of expiratory airflow may lead to hypercarbia. Progression to respiratory failure results from peripheral airway obstruction, extensive atelectasis, and resultant hypoxemia and retention of CO_2.

TREATMENT

Initial treatment of patients in respiratory distress includes addressing the ABCs (see Chapter 37). **Bag-mask ventilation** must be initiated for patients with apnea. In other patients, oxygen therapy is administered using appropriate methods (e.g., nasal cannula). In patients with mild distress, oxygen therapy administered by nasal cannula or simple mask may be appropriate. However, administration of oxygen by these methods allows the patient to inhale a mixture of room air and supplemental oxygen, making it an insufficient delivery method for most children in respiratory failure. Delivery methods, including intubation and mechanical ventilation, should be employed if there is an inability to increase oxygen saturation or ventilate appropriately.

Patients presenting with hypercarbic respiratory failure are often hypoxic as well. When oxygenation is established, measures should be taken to address the underlying cause of hypercarbia. Patients who are hypercarbic without signs of respiratory fatigue or somnolence may not require intubation based on the P_{CO_2} alone; however, patients with marked increase in the work of breathing or inadequate respiratory effort may require assistance with ventilation.

After identification of the etiology of respiratory failure, specific interventions and treatments are tailored to the needs of the patient. External support of oxygenation and ventilation may be provided by **noninvasive ventilation** methods (heated humidified high-flow nasal cannula, continuous positive airway pressure, biphasic positive airway pressure, or negative pressure ventilation) or through invasive methods (traditional **mechanical ventilation**, high-frequency oscillatory ventilation, or extracorporeal membrane oxygenation [ECMO]). Elimination of CO_2 is achieved through manipulation of minute ventilation (tidal volume and respiratory rate). Oxygenation is improved by altering variables that affect oxygen delivery (fraction of inspired oxygen) or mean airway pressure (positive end-expiratory pressure [PEEP], peak inspiratory pressure, inspiratory time, gas flow). Nitric oxide may be used to aid in oxygenation by improving ventilation/perfusion (V/Q) mismatch.

COMPLICATIONS

The major complication of hypoxic respiratory failure is the development of organ dysfunction. **Multiple organ dysfunction** includes the development of two or more of the following: respiratory failure, cardiac failure, acute kidney injury, gastrointestinal or hepatic insufficiency, disseminated intravascular coagulation, and hypoxic-ischemic brain injury. Mortality rates increase with increasing numbers of involved organs (see Table 37.3).

Complications associated with mechanical ventilation include pressure-related and volume-related lung injury. Both overdistention and insufficient lung distention (loss of functional residual capacity) are associated with lung injury. Pneumomediastinum and pneumothorax are potential complications of both the disease process and iatrogenic overdistention. Inflammatory mediators may play a role in the development of chronic fibrotic lung diseases in ventilated patients.

PROGNOSIS

Prognosis varies with the etiology of respiratory failure. Less than 1% of previously healthy children with bronchiolitis die. Asthma mortality rates are also low, but morbidity and health care costs are significant (see Chapter 79). Population-based studies report a variable mortality rate for pediatric ARDS from 18 to 35% depending on the study population.

PREVENTION

Prevention strategies are explicit to the etiology of respiratory failure. Some infectious causes can be prevented through active immunization against organisms causing primary respiratory disease (pertussis, pneumococcus, *Haemophilus influenzae* type b, seasonal influenza, COVID-19) and sepsis (pneumococcus, *H. influenzae* type b). Passive immunization with respiratory syncytial virus immunoglobulins prevents severe illness in highly susceptible patients (prematurity, bronchopulmonary dysplasia, and all infants in their first RSV season). Primary prevention of traumatic injuries may decrease the incidence of trauma-associated pediatric ARDS. Compliance with appropriate therapies for asthma may decrease the number of episodes of respiratory failure (see Chapter 79).

PEARLS FOR PRACTITIONERS

See The Acutely Ill or Injured Child: Pearls for Practitioners at the end of this section.

REVIEW QUESTION

Available online.

CHAPTER 39
Shock

ETIOLOGY AND EPIDEMIOLOGY

Shock is the inability to provide sufficient perfusion of oxygenated blood and substrate to tissues to meet metabolic demands. **Oxygen delivery** is directly related to the arterial oxygen content (oxygen saturation and hemoglobin concentration) and to cardiac output (stroke volume and heart rate). Changes in metabolic needs are met primarily by adjustments in cardiac output. Stroke volume is related to myocardial end-diastolic fiber length (preload), myocardial contractility (inotropy), and resistance of blood ejection from the ventricle (afterload; see Chapter 146). In a young infant whose myocardium possesses relatively less contractile tissue, increased demand for cardiac output is met primarily by a neurally mediated increase in heart rate. In older children and adolescents, cardiac output is most efficiently augmented by increasing stroke volume through neurohormonally mediated changes in vascular tone, resulting in increased venous return to the heart (increased preload), decreased arterial resistance (decreased afterload), and increased myocardial contractility.

Once the initial assessment of an acutely ill child is completed, the constellation of clinical characteristics can suggest one of the five broad classifications of shock: hypovolemic, distributive, cardiogenic, obstructive, and dissociative.

HYPOVOLEMIC SHOCK

Acute hypovolemia is the most common cause of shock in children. It results from loss of fluid from the intravascular space secondary to inadequate intake or excessive losses (vomiting and diarrhea, blood loss, capillary leak syndromes, or pathologic renal fluid losses) (Table 39.1). Reduced blood volume decreases preload, stroke volume, and cardiac output. Hypovolemic shock results in increased sympathoadrenal activity, producing an increased heart rate and enhanced myocardial contractility. Neurohormonally mediated constriction of the arterioles and capacitance vessels maintains blood pressure, augments venous return to the heart to improve preload, and redistributes blood flow from nonvital to vital organs. If hypovolemic shock remains untreated, the increased heart rate may impair coronary blood flow and ventricular filling, and elevated systemic vascular resistance increases myocardial oxygen consumption, resulting in worsening myocardial function. Ultimately, intense systemic vasoconstriction and hypovolemia produce tissue ischemia, impairing cell metabolism and releasing potent vasoactive mediators from injured cells. Cytokines and other vasoactive peptides can change myocardial contractility and vascular tone and promote release of other inflammatory mediators that increase capillary permeability and impair organ function further.

DISTRIBUTIVE SHOCK

Distributive shock results from a relative inadequacy of intravascular volume caused by venous or arterial vasodilation. This maldistribution of blood flow can result in profound inadequacies in tissue perfusion, even in the presence of a normal or high cardiac output. Septic shock is the most common type of distributive shock in children. Other causes include anaphylaxis, neurologic injury, and ingestion of certain drugs or poisons (see Table 39.1).

Distributive shock may present with the **systemic inflammatory response syndrome** (SIRS), defined as two or more of the following: temperature >38°C or <36°C; heart rate >90 beats/min or more than two standard deviations above normal for age; tachypnea; or white blood cell count >12,000 cells/mm^3, <4,000 cells/mm^3, or with >10% immature forms. Although SIRS is part of the criteria for pediatric sepsis (SIRS + proven or suspected infection = sepsis), it can also be seen in noninfectious states such as trauma or postoperatively.

CARDIOGENIC SHOCK

Cardiogenic shock is caused by an abnormality in myocardial function and is expressed as depressed myocardial contractility and cardiac output with poor tissue perfusion. Compensatory mechanisms may contribute to the progression of shock by depressing cardiac function further. Neurohormonal vasoconstrictor responses increase afterload and add to the work of the failing ventricle. Tachycardia may impair coronary blood flow, which decreases myocardial oxygen delivery. Increased central blood volume is caused by sodium and water retention and by incomplete emptying of the ventricles during systole. This results in elevated left ventricular volume and pressure, which then impairs subendocardial blood flow. As compensatory mechanisms are overcome, the failing left ventricle produces increased ventricular end-diastolic volume and pressure, which leads to increased left atrial pressure, resulting in pulmonary edema. This sequence also contributes to right ventricular failure because of increased pulmonary artery pressure and increased right ventricular afterload.

Primary cardiogenic shock may occur in children who have congenital heart disease. Cardiogenic shock also may occur in previously healthy children secondary to viral myocarditis, dysrhythmias, or toxic or metabolic abnormalities or after hypoxic-ischemic injury (see Chapters 143, 146, and 148; see Table 39.1).

OBSTRUCTIVE SHOCK

Obstructive shock results from mechanical obstruction of the great vessels or of the heart itself. The pathophysiology of obstructive shock can be classified according to the location of the obstruction within the vascular system in relation to the heart. These extravascular, intravascular, or luminal obstructions result in a shock state due to reduced cardiac outflow and the associated critical drop in global oxygen supply. Etiologies of obstructive shock include both congenital lesions

TABLE 39.1 Classification of Shock and Common Underlying Causes

TYPE	PRIMARY CIRCULATORY DERANGEMENT	COMMON CAUSES
Hypovolemic	Decreased circulating blood volume	Hemorrhage Diarrhea Diabetes insipidus, diabetes mellitus Burns Adrenogenital syndrome Capillary leak
Distributive	Vasodilation → venous pooling → decreased preload	Sepsis
	Maldistribution of regional blood flow	Anaphylaxis CNS/spinal injury Drug intoxication
Cardiogenic	Decreased myocardial contractility	Congenital heart disease Arrhythmia Hypoxic/ischemic injuries Cardiomyopathy Metabolic derangements Myocarditis Drug intoxication Kawasaki disease
Obstructive	Mechanical obstruction to ventricular filling or outflow	Cardiac tamponade Massive pulmonary embolus Tension pneumothorax Cardiac tumor
Dissociative	Oxygen not appropriately bound or released from hemoglobin	Carbon monoxide poisoning Methemoglobinemia

CNS, Central nervous system.

(such as coarctation of the aorta, interrupted aortic arch, and severe aortic valvular stenosis) and acquired diseases (such as pulmonary embolus and cardiac tamponade) (see Table 39.1).

DISSOCIATIVE SHOCK

Dissociative shock refers to conditions in which tissue perfusion is normal but cells are unable to utilize oxygen because the hemoglobin has an abnormal affinity for oxygen, preventing its release to the tissues (i.e., carbon monoxide poisoning) (see Table 39.1).

CLINICAL MANIFESTATIONS

All forms of shock produce evidence that tissue perfusion and/or oxygenation are insufficient (increased heart rate, abnormal blood pressure, alterations of peripheral pulses). The etiology of shock may alter the initial presentation of these signs and symptoms.

Hypovolemic Shock

Hypovolemic shock is distinguished from other causes of shock by history and the absence of signs of heart failure or sepsis. In addition to the signs of sympathoadrenal activity (tachycardia, vasoconstriction), clinical manifestations include signs of dehydration (dry mucous membranes, decreased urine output) or blood loss (pallor). Recovery depends on the degree of hypovolemia, the patient's preexisting status, and rapid diagnosis and treatment. The prognosis is good, with low mortality in uncomplicated cases.

Distributive Shock

Patients with distributive shock usually have tachycardia and alterations of peripheral perfusion. In early stages, when cytokine release results in vasodilation, pulses may be bounding and vital organ function may be maintained (an alert patient with rapid capillary refill and some urine output in *warm shock*). As the disease progresses untreated, extremities become cool and mottled with a delayed capillary refill time. At this stage, the patient has hypotension and vasoconstriction.

Cardiogenic Shock

Cardiogenic shock results when the myocardium is unable to supply the cardiac output required to support tissue perfusion and organ function. Because of this self-perpetuating cycle, heart failure progressing to death may be rapid. Patients with cardiogenic shock have tachycardia and tachypnea. The liver is usually enlarged, a gallop is often present, and jugular venous distention may be noted. Because renal blood flow is poor, sodium and water are retained, resulting in edema. Mesenteric edema can develop, resulting in abdominal pain and poor oral intake in subacute presentations.

Obstructive Shock

Restriction of cardiac output results in an increase in heart rate and an alteration of stroke volume. The pulse pressure is narrow (making pulses harder to feel), and capillary refill is delayed. The liver is often enlarged, and jugular venous distention may be evident.

Dissociative Shock

The principal abnormality in dissociative shock is the inability to deliver oxygen to tissues. Symptoms include tachycardia, tachypnea, alterations in mental status, and ultimately cardiovascular collapse.

LABORATORY AND IMAGING STUDIES

Shock requires immediate resuscitation before obtaining comprehensive laboratory or diagnostic studies. Following initial stabilization (including glucose administration if hypoglycemia is present), the type of shock dictates the necessary laboratory studies. Patients with shock may benefit from the determination of a baseline pH via arterial blood gas and blood lactate level to assess the degree of tissue oxygenation impairment. Measurement of a central **mixed venous oxygen saturation** and/or regional oximetry aids in the assessment of the adequacy of oxygen delivery. Notably, in contrast to other forms of shock, patients with vasodilated distributive shock (such as in gram-negative sepsis) often have high mixed venous saturation values due to impairment of mitochondrial function and inability of tissues to extract oxygen. A CBC can reveal altered bone marrow function or provide evidence of disseminated intravascular coagulation (DIC) and may also aid in assessing the severity of blood loss following equilibration in hemorrhagic shock (of note, a CBC may not reveal the true degree of blood loss in the early acute phase of hemorrhagic shock). Electrolyte measurements in patients with hypovolemic shock may identify abnormalities from losses. Patients presenting in septic shock require appropriate bacterial and viral cultures to aid in identification of a causative pathogen. If cardiogenic or obstructive shock is suspected, an echocardiogram assists with the diagnosis and, in the case of tamponade, assists with placement of a pericardial drain to relieve the fluid. Patients with dissociative shock require detection of the causative agent (carbon monoxide, methemoglobin). The management of shock also requires ongoing monitoring of mixed venous oxygen saturations and arterial blood gases for assessment of oxygenation, ventilation (CO_2), and degree of acidosis. Frequent reassessment of serum electrolytes and biochemical markers of end-organ impairment, such as liver and renal function panels as well as coagulation factors and CBC, may aid in subsequent therapeutic interventions.

DIFFERENTIAL DIAGNOSIS

See Table 39.1.

TREATMENT

General Principles

The key to therapy is the recognition of shock in its early, partially compensated state, when many of the hemodynamic and metabolic alterations may be reversible. Initial therapy for shock follows the ABCs of resuscitation (see Chapter 37). Later, therapy can then be directed at the underlying cause. When sepsis is thought to be the etiology of shock, early administration of antibiotics has been shown to improve outcomes. Therapy should minimize cardiopulmonary work, while ensuring cardiac output, adequate perfusion, and gas exchange. Intubation, combined with mechanical ventilation with oxygen supplementation, improves oxygenation and decreases metabolic demand but may impede venous return if distending airway pressures (positive end-expiratory pressure [PEEP] or peak inspiratory pressure) are excessive. Blood pressure support with fluids and/or vasoactive medications is crucial in promoting adequate end-organ perfusion.

Monitoring a child in shock requires maintaining access to the arterial and central venous circulation to record pressure measurements, perform blood sampling, and measure systemic blood pressure continuously. These measurements facilitate the estimation of preload and afterload. Regional oximetry monitoring with near-infrared spectroscopy (NIRS) may allow early noninvasive detection of alterations in perfusion.

Organ-Directed Therapeutics

Fluid Resuscitation

Alterations in preload have a dramatic effect on cardiac output. In hypovolemic and distributive shock, decreased preload significantly impairs cardiac output. In these cases, early and aggressive fluid resuscitation is important and greatly affects outcome. In cardiogenic shock, an elevated preload contributes to pulmonary edema.

Selection of fluids for resuscitation and ongoing use is dictated by clinical circumstances. Crystalloid volume expanders are generally recommended as initial choices because they are effective, inexpensive, and often readily available. Most acutely ill children with signs of shock may safely receive, and usually benefit greatly from, rapid administration of a 10–20 mL/kg bolus of an isotonic crystalloid. This dose may be repeated until a response is noted (usually up to 40–60 mL/kg). Colloids contain larger molecules that may stay in the intravascular space longer than crystalloid solutions and exert oncotic pressure, drawing fluid out of the tissues into the vascular compartment. However, the long-term risks of colloids may exceed the benefits. Care must be exercised in treating cardiogenic shock with volume expansion because the ventricular filling pressures may rise without improvement or with deterioration of cardiac performance. Careful monitoring of cardiac output via vital signs, clinical exam (repeatedly evaluate for development of rales and/or hepatomegaly), and central venous pressure (if available) guides safe volume replacement.

Cardiovascular Support

In an effort to improve cardiac output after volume resuscitation, or when further volume replacement may be dangerous, a variety of inotropic and systemic vascular resistance modulating drugs may be useful (Table 39.2). Therapy is directed first at increasing myocardial contractility and then at decreasing left ventricular afterload and improving end organ perfusion. The hemodynamic status of the patient dictates the choice of the agent.

Epinephrine or norepinephrine may be used as first-line vasoactive medications depending on the patient's hemodynamic profile and desired response; dopamine may be used secondarily. In addition to improving contractility, certain catecholamines cause an increase in systemic vascular resistance. The addition of a vasodilator drug may improve cardiac performance by decreasing the resistance against which the heart must pump (afterload). Afterload reduction may be achieved with dobutamine, milrinone, nitroprusside, nitroglycerin, and angiotensin-converting enzyme inhibitors. The use of these drugs may be particularly important in the later stages of shock, when vasoconstriction is prominent. For patients presenting in cardiogenic shock with fluid overload, diuretics such as furosemide or bumetanide are often used to improve contractility in an overdistended myocardium.

Respiratory Support

The lung is a target organ for inflammatory mediators in SIRS and shock. Respiratory failure may develop rapidly and become progressive. Intervention requires endotracheal intubation and mechanical ventilation accompanied by the use of supplemental oxygen and PEEP. Care must be taken with the process of intubation because a child with compensated shock may suddenly decompensate upon administration of sedative medications that reduce systemic vascular resistance or with converting to positive pressure ventilation. Severe cardiopulmonary failure may require extracorporeal membrane oxygenation (ECMO).

Kidney Support

Poor cardiac output accompanied by decreased renal blood flow may cause prerenal azotemia and oliguria/anuria. Severe hypotension may produce **acute tubular necrosis** and **acute kidney injury (AKI)**. Prerenal azotemia is corrected when blood volume deficits are replaced or myocardial contractility is improved, but acute tubular necrosis does not improve immediately when shock is corrected. Prerenal azotemia is associated with a serum blood urea nitrogen (BUN)-to-creatinine ratio of greater than 10:1 and a urine sodium level less than 20 mEq/L; acute tubular necrosis has a BUN-to-creatinine ratio of 10:1 or less and a urine sodium level between 40 and 60 mEq/L (see Chapter 166). Aggressive fluid replacement is often necessary to improve oliguria associated with prerenal azotemia. Because the management of shock requires administering large volumes of fluid, maintaining urine output greatly facilitates patient management.

Prevention of acute tubular necrosis and the subsequent complications associated with AKI (hyperkalemia, acidosis, hypocalcemia, fluid overload) is important. The use of

TABLE 39.2 Medications Used to Improve Cardiac Output

	POSITIVE INOTROPE	POSITIVE CHRONOTROPE	DIRECT PRESSOR	VASOCONSTRICTOR	VASODILATOR
Dopamine	++	+	±	++ (high dose)	+ (low dose)
Dobutamine	++	±	–	–	+
Epinephrine	+++	+++	+++	++ (high dose)	+ (low dose)
Norepinephrine	+++	+++	+++	+++	–
Milrinone	+	–	–	–	+

pharmacologic agents to augment urine output is indicated when the intravascular volume has been replaced. The use of loop diuretics, such as furosemide, or combinations of a loop diuretic and a thiazide agent, may enhance urine output. Nevertheless, if hyperkalemia, refractory acidosis, hypervolemia, or altered mental status associated with uremia occurs, dialysis or hemofiltration should be initiated.

COMPLICATIONS

Shock results in impairment of tissue perfusion and oxygenation and activation of inflammation and cytokine pathways. The major complication of shock is multiple organ system failure, defined as the dysfunction of more than one organ, including respiratory failure, AKI, liver dysfunction, coagulation abnormalities, or cerebral dysfunction. Patients with shock and multiple organ failure have a higher mortality rate and, for survivors, a longer hospital stay.

PROGNOSIS

Early recognition and **goal-directed intervention** in patients with shock improves survival. Delays in treatment of hypotension, however, increase the incidence of multiple organ failure and mortality.

PREVENTION

Prevention strategies for shock are focused, for the most part, on shock associated with causative exposures (infection, trauma, and ingestion). Some forms of septic shock can be prevented through the use of immunizations (such as *Haemophilus influenzae* type b, meningococcal, pneumococcal vaccines). Decreasing the risk of sepsis in a hospitalized patient requires adherence to strict handwashing, isolation practices, and minimizing the duration of indwelling devices. Measures to decrease pediatric trauma do much to minimize hemorrhage-induced hypovolemic shock. Preventative health measures surrounding environmental toxins (carbon monoxide) and medication storage/administration can aid in the prevention of some forms of dissociative, distributive, and cardiogenic shock (see Table 39.1).

PEARLS FOR PRACTITIONERS

See The Acutely Ill or Injured Child: Pearls for Practitioners at the end of this section.

REVIEW QUESTIONS

Available online.

CHAPTER 40

Injury Prevention

EPIDEMIOLOGY AND ETIOLOGY

Unintentional injury is the leading pediatric cause of death in the developed world. In 2023 unintentional injury accounted for over 18,000 deaths of children, adolescents, and young adults 0–24 years of age in the United States. Between 2018 and 2023 the unintentional injury death rate for children under 19 years increased in the United States from 9 to 11.2 per 100,000. This increase has been attributed to a sharp increase in firearm and overdose-related deaths. Notably, firearm deaths in teenagers rose 50% between 2019 and 2021.

The most common causes of fatal injuries differ among age groups. Suffocation is the most common type of fatal injury among infants (85% of unintentional deaths); however, it accounts for only 1% of unintentional fatalities among 15- to 19-year-olds. Conversely, motor vehicle collisions account for 6% of fatal injuries among infants, whereas they account for 64% of adolescent fatal injuries. Drowning is the most common cause of fatal injury among children ages 1–4 years (35%), and it accounts for 6% of fatal injuries among adolescents. Differences in geography, climate, population density (access to care), and population traits affect the frequency, etiology, and severity of these injuries.

Injury occurs through interaction of the **host** (child) with the **agent** (e.g., car and driver) through a **vector** and an **environment** (e.g., roadways, weather) that is conducive to exposure. The age of the child may determine the exposure to various agents and environments. Most injuries in infants and toddlers occur in the home as the result of exposure to agents found there (water heaters, bathtubs, soft bedding). Gender affects exposure to injury, with males having a fatal injury rate greater than that of females.

EDUCATION FOR PREVENTING INJURIES

The recognition that much of the morbidity and mortality are determined at the scene of an injury has stimulated the development of prevention measures. The **Haddon matrix** combines the epidemiologic components (host, agent, physical and social environments) with time factors (before, during, and after the event) to identify effective interventions focused on different aspects of the injury event. Primary strategies (preventing the event), secondary strategies (minimizing the severity of injury), and tertiary strategies (minimizing long-term impact) can be targeted for each epidemiologic component. Such strategies typically fall into one of three areas: education, enforcement, and environment (including engineering).

Education is often the first strategy considered, but it requires behavioral change and action on the part of people. Most educational strategies are not well evaluated.

Despite the reliance on an action by the individuals involved, some active strategies benefit from **enforcement**. Children wearing bicycle helmets experience a significantly lower incidence of traumatic brain injury and death. The enforcement of seatbelt laws increases seatbelt use and may decrease injuries. Fully enclosed four-sided pool fences and self-closing/latching door locks can reduce the risk of drowning.

Automatic strategies require no action on the part of the population and often change the **environment** (speed bumps) or involve **engineering** (child-resistant pill bottles, air bags). Automatic strategies have more consistently resulted in a significant reduction in injuries. The most successful approaches to preventing injury have combined strategies (education, environmental changes, and engineering changes focused on the host, agent, and environment in all three time phases).

PEARLS FOR PRACTITIONERS

See The Acutely Ill or Injured Child: Pearls for Practitioners at the end of this section.

REVIEW QUESTIONS

Available online.

CHAPTER 41

Major Trauma

ASSESSMENT AND RESUSCITATION

The general goal of **prehospital trauma care** is rapid assessment, support of the ABCs (airway, breathing, and circulation), immobilization, and transportation. Outcomes of patients with major or life-threatening trauma are significantly improved when they receive care in a pediatric trauma center or in an adult center with pediatric trauma certification compared with level I or II adult trauma centers. However, many children live too far from a pediatric trauma center to seek care at those facilities, so it is imperative that all emergency providers understand the unique aspects of pediatric trauma patients.

Once the injured child arrives at the emergency department, the trauma team must initiate an organized and synchronized response. The initial assessment of a seriously injured child should involve a systematic approach, including a primary survey, resuscitation, secondary survey, post-resuscitation monitoring, and definitive care. The **primary survey** focuses on the **xABCDEs** of emergency care, as modified for trauma from the ABCs of cardiopulmonary resuscitation (see Chapter 37). The "**x**" represents an emphasis on identifying and controlling any life-threatening external bleeding. The **airway (A)** and **breathing (B)** assessments should include immobilization of the cervical spine (especially if the patient has an altered mental status or distracting injury); evaluation for injuries to the face, neck, or chest that could impair air entry or gas exchange; and consideration of the patient's aspiration risk based upon last reported or suspected meal. If the airway is not patent or breathing is not spontaneous, measures should immediately be taken to secure an airway with an endotracheal tube prior to further interventions. **Circulation (C)** can be assessed via observation (heart rate, skin color, mental status), palpation (pulse quality, capillary refill, skin temperature), and vital sign assessment (blood pressure). To restore circulation, bleeding should be controlled with direct pressure and two large-bore peripheral intravenous (IV) lines should be placed, when possible, to allow for administration of IV fluids and blood products. Assessment for **disabilities (D)**, particularly neurologic status, includes examination of pupil size and reactivity, a brief mental status assessment, and examination of extremity movement to assess for spinal cord injury. The **Glasgow Coma Scale** (GCS) can direct decisions regarding the initiation of further interventions in patients with suspected closed head injuries including the need for airway stabilization (Table 41.1). **Exposure (E)** requires completely removing the child's clothing for a detailed visual examination of the entire body. The examiner should ensure a neutral thermal environment to prevent hypothermia during this exam.

TABLE 41.1 Glasgow Coma Scales

ACTIVITY	BEST RESPONSE	SCORE
Eye opening	Spontaneous	4
	To verbal stimuli	3
	To pain	2
	None	1
Verbal	Oriented • Infant: coos, babbles	5
	Confused • Infant: irritable, cries	4
	Inappropriate words • Infant: cries to pain	3
	Nonspecific sounds • Infant: moans to pain	2
	None	1
Motor	Follows commands • Infant: spontaneous movement	6
	Localizes pain • Infant: withdraws to touch	5
	Withdraws to pain	4
	Flexion to pain • Infant: abnormal flexion	3
	Extension to pain • Infant: abnormal extension	2
	None	1

On completion of the primary survey, a more detailed head-to-toe examination (the **secondary survey**) should ensue, along with efforts to obtain a more complete history. The purpose of this careful reexamination is to identify life-threatening and limb-threatening injuries, as well as less serious injuries. Coincident with the secondary survey and depending, in part, on the assessed physiologic status of the patient, certain procedures and resuscitative measures are initiated. The prioritization of definitive care needs is determined by the injury findings gathered from the primary and secondary surveys, the child's physiologic response to resuscitation, and the data from continuous monitoring. A **tertiary survey**, including repeat primary and secondary surveys along with a review of the laboratory tests and radiologic studies, should be performed within 24 hours.

ETIOLOGY AND EPIDEMIOLOGY

See Chapter 40.

LABORATORY AND IMAGING STUDIES

Screening laboratory studies during the initial resuscitation often include the tests listed in Table 41.2. Radiographic studies are determined by the pattern of identified potential injuries. A head CT scan should be obtained in patients with GCS of 14 or less or other signs of altered mental status, external evidence of head trauma, or a history of loss of consciousness, vomiting, or severe mechanism of injury. Patients with evidence of abdominal wall trauma including a seatbelt sign or who have significant abdominal tenderness after blunt trauma

TABLE 41.2 Initial Laboratory Evaluation of the Major Trauma Patient

HEMATOLOGY
Complete blood count Coagulation studies (prothrombin time, partial thromboplastin time, international normalized ratio) Type and cross match
URINALYSIS
Gross Microscopic
CLINICAL CHEMISTRY
Basic metabolic panel Amylase/lipase Aspartate aminotransferase/alanine aminotransferase
RADIOLOGY
Cervical spine films Anteroposterior chest radiograph Radiographs of all apparent fractures CT scans as indicated for head, chest, abdominal, and pelvic trauma

may benefit from a CT scan. The extended focused assessment with sonography for trauma (eFAST) has gained popularity because of concerns about radiation exposure but has not yet been shown to decrease rates of CT utilization in pediatric blunt abdominal trauma. eFAST serves as a rapid screening test in the evaluation of the unstable blunt trauma patient or in patients with penetrating trauma with unclear extension into the abdomen that can be performed without moving the patient from the resuscitation area. CT angiography should be performed if there is concern about thoracic aortic injury.

CLINICAL MANIFESTATIONS AND TREATMENT

Head injuries and injuries to the limbs are the most common injuries seen in blunt trauma. Multiple organ system involvement is also common, and penetrating trauma is becoming more prevalent. After initial evaluation and stabilization, the team focuses on the involved organ systems.

Head Trauma

See Chapter 185.

Spinal Cord Trauma

Although spinal cord injury is not common in pediatric trauma patients, it is potentially devastating when it occurs. Cervical spine immobilization should be maintained until a spinal cord injury is ruled out. The Pediatric Emergency Care Applied Research Network (PECARN) has developed screening criteria specific to children who are at risk of cervical spine injury to guide decisions as to who should undergo cervical spine radiographs or advanced imaging. Risk factors include patients with altered mental status as measured by GCS and AVPU scales (see Table 41.1 and Table 37.1); abnormal airway, breathing, or circulation; focal neurologic deficits (paresthesias, numbness, or weakness); patients with neck pain; substantial head injury; substantial torso injury; and midline neck tenderness. However, in patients with continued symptoms, cervical spine radiographs are not sufficient to rule out a spinal cord injury because the immature vertebral column in children may allow stretching of the cord or nerve roots with no radiologic abnormality **(spinal cord injury without radiologic abnormality [SCIWORA])**. When initial imaging is negative but the mechanism of injury and/or clinical presentation is concerning for spinal cord injury, MRI should be performed to evaluate for SCIWORA.

Thoracic Trauma

Thoracic injury is the second leading cause of pediatric trauma death. Although many life-threatening thoracic injuries may be identified clinically during the primary survey, chest radiograph helps to identify other injuries such as pulmonary contusion, pneumothorax, hemothorax, and rib fractures. Patients with pulmonary parenchymal injury should receive supportive treatment to ensure adequate oxygenation and ventilation. Most pediatric blunt thoracic injuries can be managed without surgery. Injury to the heart and great vessels is rare but requires urgent diagnosis and treatment. Great vessel injury should be suspected if a widened mediastinum is seen on chest radiograph with CT angiography used to confirm diagnosis.

Abdominal Trauma

The relative size and closer proximity of intraabdominal organs in children increase the risk of significant injury after blunt trauma. Presentations of children with penetrating traumatic injuries range from no symptoms to hypovolemic shock.

The presence of abdominal pain, visible abdominal wall trauma, tenderness or distention on exam; abnormal chest x-ray; and abnormal laboratory testing including pancreatic enzymes, liver enzymes, hemoglobin/hematocrit, and urinalysis are helpful to risk stratify the presence of intrabdominal injury. Imaging studies such as abdominal CT and serial physical examinations are the primary methods of obtaining information on which to base decisions regarding operative intervention. Abdominal wall bruising, specifically the "seatbelt sign," is an important physical examination finding and is associated with significant intraabdominal injury in more than 10% of patients. Most blunt solid organ injury is handled nonoperatively with close clinical observation. Operative intervention may be required in patients whose vital signs are persistently unstable despite aggressive fluid resuscitation, even in the absence of extravascular volume loss or an enlarging abdomen.

Splenic Trauma

The spleen is the most frequently injured abdominal organ in children. Suspicion of a splenic injury should be heightened if there are left upper quadrant abrasions or tenderness. Pain may also be referred to the left shoulder due to diaphragmatic irritation by the ruptured spleen *(Kehr sign)*. CT scans are used to identify and grade the severity of splenic injury.

Nonoperative management with serial examinations and laboratory studies is the treatment of choice for most serious splenic injuries. If there is continued large blood loss or hemodynamic instability, emergent laparotomy for total or partial splenectomy is indicated. If a splenectomy is performed, patients should receive penicillin prophylaxis as well as pneumococcal, meningococcal, and *Haemophilus influenzae* vaccines due to the increased risk of infection with encapsulated bacteria in the setting of asplenia.

Liver Trauma

Blunt trauma to the liver is a leading cause of mortality. Severe hemorrhage is more common in patients with liver injury than with other abdominal injuries because of its dual blood supply. As with splenic injury, severity is graded based on the pattern of injury, and nonoperative management is recommended but requires close clinical observation for signs of ongoing blood loss or hemodynamic instability.

Kidney Injury

The kidney is less frequently injured than the liver or spleen. Kidney injuries can be seen with high-energy mechanisms or direct blows to the back and are often associated with other injuries. A young child's kidney is more vulnerable to trauma than an adult's because of their more compliant rib cage and relatively immature abdominal muscle development. Diagnosis is based on clinical findings (flank tenderness or ecchymosis) coupled with urinalysis showing blood and increased protein levels. CT with IV contrast is the recommended imaging modality; ultrasound may also be useful. Low-grade kidney injury is usually managed conservatively, but surgery may be required for falling hemoglobin levels, refractory shock, or urinary obstruction caused by clots.

Pancreatic Injury

Injuries of the pancreas are less common in children than in adults. This type of injury is seen in bicycle handlebar injuries, motor vehicle crashes, and nonaccidental trauma. The diagnosis is difficult unless there is obvious injury to overlying structures, such as the stomach or duodenum. Diffuse abdominal tenderness, pain, and vomiting may be accompanied by elevations of amylase and lipase; however, pancreatic enzymes are not sensitive or specific in blunt trauma and may be normal in up to 30% of patients with pancreatic injury. Abdominal CT may not be sufficient to evaluate ductal injury and may miss pancreatic injuries in the initial postinjury period. Nonoperative management is appropriate for contusions, but surgical intervention may be required in patients with ductal injuries. Pancreatic injuries with parenchymal disruption may lead to pseudocyst formation, which often requires surgical drainage as well.

Intestinal Injury

Injury to the intestine occurs less frequently than injury to solid intraabdominal organs. Intestinal injury results from acceleration-deceleration (shearing) forces that occur at points of fixation (the ligament of Treitz, the ileocecal valve, and the ascending and descending peritoneal reflections). These injuries are difficult to diagnose with CT, so pneumoperitoneum should prompt surgical exploration. Serial physical examinations are useful when the clinical picture is uncertain.

Duodenal hematoma can occur in the absence of perforation and may not present until 48–72 hours after the injury. Affected patients often present with persistent pain and bilious emesis. Most hematomas respond to nonoperative management with gastric decompression and parenteral nutrition.

COMPLICATIONS

Patients requiring hospitalization for multiple traumatic injuries are at risk for a variety of complications based on the type and severity of injury. Sepsis and multiple organ failure may occur in children with polytrauma. The presence of ileus can result in delayed initiation of enteral nutrition which may further increase the risk of sepsis secondary to translocation of bacteria across injured or inflamed intestinal mucosa. Acute kidney injury secondary to myoglobinuria may be seen in children who sustain crushing or electrical injuries. Deep venous thrombosis is less common in the pediatric population; however, prophylaxis for children who will be immobilized because of injury should be provided.

PROGNOSIS

Unintentional injury is the leading cause of death for children aged 1–18; however, many of these deaths occur in the field immediately after the injury. Once admitted to the hospital, mortality rates are much lower. Morbidities are numerous and include hypoxic-ischemic brain injury, loss of limbs, and psychologic trauma.

PREVENTION

See Chapter 40.

PEARLS FOR PRACTITIONERS

See The Acutely Ill or Injured Child: Pearls for Practitioners at the end of this section.

REVIEW QUESTIONS

Available online.

CHAPTER 42 Drowning

ETIOLOGY

Drowning is the process of experiencing respiratory impairment from submersion/immersion in liquid. Outcomes may be categorized as death, morbidity, or no morbidity. Other terms such as near drowning, secondary drowning, or dry drowning should not be used.

Initially, submersion or immersion results in aspiration of small amounts of fluid into the larynx, triggering breath holding or laryngospasm. In many cases, the laryngospasm resolves, and larger volumes of water or gastric contents are aspirated into the lungs, destroying surfactant and causing alveolitis and dysfunction of the alveolar-capillary gas exchange. The resulting hypoxemia leads to hypoxic brain injury and cardiovascular injury that is exacerbated by ischemic injury after circulatory collapse.

EPIDEMIOLOGY

In 2021 an estimated 300,000 people died from drowning worldwide; in the United States, drowning was the second leading cause of injury death for children ages 1–14 years in 2022. For every pediatric drowning death, another five receive emergency department care for nonfatal submersion injuries. Males are four times more likely than females to drown. The most common location of drowning varies by age, with drowning in natural bodies of water becoming more frequent in older age groups.

CLINICAL MANIFESTATIONS

Hypoxemia is the result of laryngospasm and aspiration during drowning. Victims may also develop respiratory distress secondary to pulmonary endothelial injury, increased capillary permeability, and destruction of surfactant. Clinical manifestations include tachypnea, tachycardia, increased work of breathing, and decreased breath sounds with or without crackles. The hypoxic-ischemic injury that may occur can lead to depressed myocardial function resulting in tachycardia, impaired perfusion, and, potentially, cardiovascular collapse. After resuscitation, acute respiratory distress syndrome is common. Altered mental status may be present and requires frequent monitoring of neurologic status. Following submersion in cold water, hypothermia may result in relative bradycardia and hypotension and place the child at risk for cardiac dysrhythmias.

LABORATORY AND IMAGING STUDIES

After resuscitation, arterial blood gas measurement assists in assessing pulmonary gas exchange. A chemistry profile may reveal elevated liver enzymes if hypoxemia and ischemia were of long duration and provide baseline kidney function. Electrolytes are often obtained, although alterations of serum electrolytes are minimal, even in freshwater drowning.

Chest x-rays that are normal or with mild pulmonary atelectasis or edema can be useful for predicting patients who are likely to show clinical improvement within 24 hours.

TREATMENT

Resuscitation of a drowning victim includes the basic ABCs (see Chapter 37). Victims of unwitnessed drowning require stabilization of the cervical spine because of the possibility of a fall or diving injury. Optimizing oxygenation and maintaining cerebral perfusion are two of the major foci of treatment. Rewarming the hypothermic patient requires careful attention to detail, including acid-base and cardiac status as well as avoidance of hyperthermia. Further treatment is based on the patient's response to initial resuscitation. Some children begin breathing spontaneously and awaken before arrival at an emergency department. If the episode was significant, these children still require careful observation for pulmonary complications over the subsequent 4–6 hours. Children who have evidence of lung injury, cardiovascular compromise, or neurologic compromise should be monitored in an intensive care unit. Pulmonary dysfunction often results in hypoxemia. Oxygen supplementation should be implemented to maintain normal oxygen saturations. Mechanical ventilation may be needed in patients with significant pulmonary or neurologic dysfunction. Cardiovascular compromise is often the result of impaired cardiac contractility secondary to hypoxic-ischemic injury. The use of intracranial pressure monitoring devices as well as medical management with therapeutic hypothermia and sedation is controversial and has not been shown to improve outcomes. Prophylactic antibiotics have not been shown to be beneficial, but in patients who develop delayed pulmonary infection, broad antibiotic coverage should include *Aeromonas* species. In many cases, cold water can be neuroprotective in children, given that it reduces oxygen demand of the brain; therefore resuscitative measures should be continued until the patient has been warmed to 32°C or greater.

PROGNOSIS

The outcome of drowning is determined by the success of immediate resuscitation efforts and the severity of **hypoxic-ischemic injury** to the brain. Patients who have regained consciousness on arrival at the hospital will likely survive with intact neurologic function. Unfavorable prognostic markers include submersion lasting longer than 5 minutes, delayed resuscitation, the need for continued cardiopulmonary resuscitation (CPR) at the hospital, Glasgow Coma Scale of 5 or less, fixed and dilated pupils, seizures, and coma for more than 72 hours.

PREVENTION

Despite the decreased incidence of drowning since the 1990s, only five major prevention strategies are evidence based. In decreasing order of efficacy, these include installation of four-sided fencing around pools, life jackets, swim lessons, supervision, and lifeguards. Although evidence for other prevention strategies such as pool covers and pool alarms is lacking, these may play a role because experts advocate for multiple layers of environmental protection to prevent drowning.

PEARLS FOR PRACTITIONERS

See The Acutely Ill or Injured Child: Pearls for Practitioners at the end of this section.

REVIEW QUESTIONS

Available online.

CHAPTER 43

Burns

ETIOLOGY

The pathophysiology of burn injury is caused by disruption of the three key functions of the skin: regulation of heat loss, preservation of body fluids, and barrier to infection. Burn injury releases inflammatory and vasoactive mediators resulting in increased capillary permeability, decreased plasma volume, and decreased cardiac output. The body then becomes hypermetabolic with increased resting energy expenditure and protein catabolism. This hypermetabolic state may continue for up to a year after injury.

Burns usually are classified based on four criteria:

- Depth of injury
- Percent of body surface area involved
- Location of the burn
- Association with other injuries

EPIDEMIOLOGY

More than 100,000 children sustain a burn injury requiring emergency department evaluation and/or hospitalization each year. Although most burns are not life-threatening, burns remain a significant cause of morbidity. Males are more likely to sustain a burn injury, as are children age 4 years and under. Scald burns are more common in younger children than in older children. Overall, thermal burns secondary to scald or flame are much more common than electrical or chemical burns. Most fire-related childhood deaths and injuries occur in homes.

CLINICAL MANIFESTATIONS

The depth of injury should be assessed by the clinical appearance. Categories of first degree, second degree, and third degree are commonly used; however, classification by depth (superficial, superficial partial thickness, deep partial thickness, and full thickness) conveys more information about the structures injured and the likely need for surgical treatment and are more clinically useful.

Superficial (first-degree) burns are red, painful, and dry. They are commonly seen with sun exposure or mild scald injuries, and these burns involve injury to the epidermis only. They heal in 5–7 days without scarring and are not included in burn surface area calculations. **Superficial partial-thickness** (second-degree) burns involve the entire epidermis and superficial dermis. These burns have fluid-containing blisters. After debridement, the underlying dermis appears erythematous and wet, is painful, and blanches under pressure. Healing is dependent on the uninjured dermis and usually occurs within 7–21 days without the need for skin grafting and without scarring. **Deep partial-thickness** (also second-degree) burns involve the entire epidermis and deeper portions of the dermis. These burns may also have blistering, but the dermal base is less blanching, mottled pink or white, and less painful than superficial partial-thickness burns. They behave more like full-thickness burns and often require excision and grafting. **Full-thickness** (third-degree and fourth-degree) burns involve all skin layers. They appear dry, white, dark red, brown, or black in color. They do not blanch and are usually insensate. Full-thickness burns require surgical management. Fourth-degree burns involve underlying fascia, muscle, or bone and may require reconstruction in addition to grafting. **Inhalation injuries** should be suspected if there are facial burns, singed nasal hairs, or carbonaceous sputum. Hoarseness on vocalization also is consistent with a supraglottic injury. Inhalation injuries may result in bronchospasm, airway inflammation, and impaired pulmonary function.

One of the multiple methods used for calculating the percentage of skin surface involved in a burn in children of various ages is presented in Figure 43.1. The extent of skin involvement of adolescent and adult patients may be estimated as follows: each upper extremity, 9%; each lower extremity, 18%; anterior trunk, 18%; posterior trunk, 18%; head, 9%; and perineum, 1%.

The location of the burn is important in assessing the risk of disability. The risk is greatest when the face, eyes, ears, feet, perineum, or hands are involved. Inhalation injuries not only cause respiratory compromise but also may result in difficulty in eating and drinking.

LABORATORY AND IMAGING STUDIES

Initial laboratory testing, including complete blood count, type and cross match for blood, coagulation studies, basic chemistry profile, arterial blood gas, and chest radiograph, can be helpful for patients with major burns. A carboxyhemoglobin assessment should be performed for any suspected inhalation exposure (a house or closed-space fire or a burn victim who requires cardiopulmonary resuscitation). Cyanide levels should be considered in children who sustain smoke inhalation and have altered mental status. Unusual patterns of burns may increase suspicion of child abuse and prompt further evaluation to assess for nonaccidental trauma to the skeleton or central nervous system.

TREATMENT

For severe burns, care is best managed by a multidisciplinary team in a qualified burn center. The American Burn Association criteria for patients who should be transferred to a burn center are as follows: partial-thickness burns greater than 10% total body surface area (TBSA); partial- and full-thickness burns involving the face, hands, feet, genitalia, perineum, or major joints; full-thickness burns in any age group; electrical burns (including lightning injury); chemical burns; inhalation injury; burn injury in patients with preexisting medical conditions that could complicate

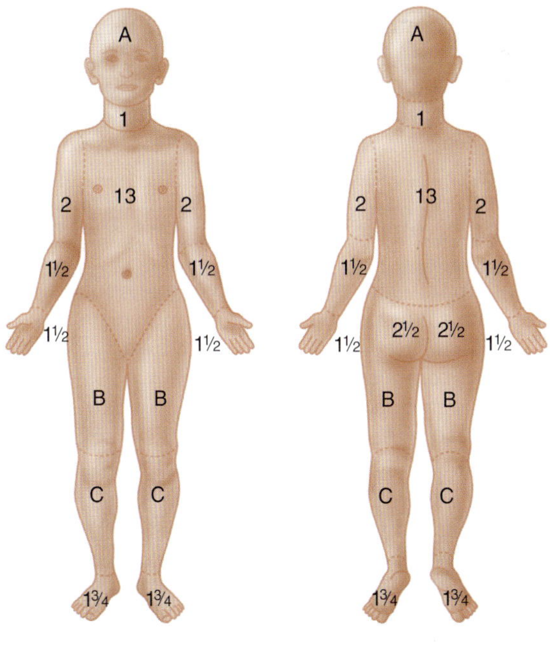

PERCENTAGE OF SURFACE AREA OF HEAD AND LEGS AT VARIOUS AGES

AREA IN DIAGRAM	AGE IN YEARS 0	1	5	10	15
A = ½ of head	9½	8½	6½	5½	4½
B = ½ of one thigh	2¾	3¼	4	4¼	4½
C = ½ of one lower leg	2½	2½	2¾	3	3¼

FIGURE 43.1 This chart of body areas, together with the table inserted in the figure showing the percentage of surface area of head and legs at various ages, can be used to estimate the surface area burned in a child. (From Solomon JR. Pediatric burns. *Crit Care Clin.* 1985;1:159–174.)

management, prolong recovery, or affect mortality; any burn with concomitant trauma in which the burn injury poses the greatest risk; burn injury in children admitted to hospitals without qualified personnel or equipment for pediatric care; and burn injury in patients requiring special social, emotional, or rehabilitative support, including child abuse cases.

Initial treatment should follow the ABCs of resuscitation (see Chapter 37). **Airway management** should include assessment for the presence of airway or inhalation injury, with early intubation if such an injury is suspected. Smoke inhalation may be associated with carbon monoxide toxicity; 100% humidified oxygen should be given if hypoxia or inhalation is suspected.

The systemic capillary leak that occurs after a serious burn makes initial fluid and electrolyte support of a burned child crucial. The first priority is to support the circulating blood volume, which requires the administration of intravenous fluids to provide maintenance fluid and electrolyte requirements and to replace ongoing burn-related losses. Formulas exist to help guide **fluid management**; however, no formula accurately predicts the fluid needs of every burn patient. Children with a significant burn should receive a rapid bolus of 20 mL/kg of crystalloid fluids (Ringer's lactate solution is preferred to avoid hyperchloremic metabolic acidosis). Thereafter the resuscitation formula for fluid therapy is determined by the percentage of body surface burned. Total fluids are 2–4 mL/kg per percentage burn per 24 hours, with half the estimated amount administered during the first 8 hours and the remaining half over the subsequent 16 hours (if resuscitation is delayed, half of the fluid replacement should be completed by the end of the eighth hour postinjury). Fluids should be titrated to achieve adequate perfusion, one marker of which is urine output greater than 1 mL/kg per hour. Controversy exists over whether and when to administer colloid during fluid resuscitation, but colloid therapy may be needed for patients with extensive burns. Additionally, there is ongoing research into the use of vitamin C administration to decrease wound edema.

Because burn injury produces a **hypermetabolic** response, children with significant burns require immediate nutritional support. Enteral feeds should be started early unless there is a specific contraindication. Children with critical burn injury may require parenteral nutrition if unable to tolerate full enteral feeds with supplementation of vitamins and trace elements. Other factors that may improve the hypermetabolic state include pain control, blood glucose control, and the use of medications including anabolic steroids such as oxandrolone and β blockers such as propranolol.

Wound care starts with cleaning and debriding the wound. Effective pain control is important to allow for complete debridement. Topical agents and dressings are then applied to control bacterial colonization, decrease evaporative losses, and aid in pain control. Various grafts, such as cadaver allografts, porcine xenografts, or skin substitutes, have been used initially to cover wounds. For full-thickness burns, skin autografting and skin substitutes are required for eventual closure.

COMPLICATIONS

See Table 43.1.

TABLE 43.1 Complications of Burns

PROBLEM	TREATMENT
Sepsis	Monitor for infection, avoid prophylactic antibiotics
Hypovolemia	Fluid replacement
Hypothermia	Adjust ambient temperature: dry blankets in field
Laryngeal edema	Endotracheal intubation, tracheostomy
Carbon monoxide poisoning	100% oxygen, hyperbaric oxygen
Cyanide poisoning	100% O_2 plus hydroxocobalamin (Cyanokit)
Cardiac dysfunction	Inotropic agents, diuretics
Gastric ulcers	H_2-receptor antagonist, antacids
Compartment syndrome	Escharotomy incision
Contractures	Physical therapy
Hypermetabolic state	Enteral and parenteral nutritional support, pain control, glucose control; consider β blockers and anabolic steroids
Acute kidney injury	Supportive care, dialysis
Transient antidiuresis	Expectant management
Anemia/thrombocytopenia	Transfusions as indicated
Psychologic trauma	Psychologic support
Pulmonary infiltrates	PEEP, ventilation, oxygen
Pulmonary edema	Avoid overhydration, give diuretics
Pneumonia	Antibiotics
Bronchospasm	β-Agonist aerosols

PEEP, Positive end-expiratory pressure.

PROGNOSIS

Most children who sustain burns recover without significant disability, but estimation of morbidity is difficult to ascertain from databases. Physical scarring and emotional impact of disfiguring burns are long-term consequences of burn injuries.

PREVENTION

Most burns occur in the home. Prevention is possible by using smoke and fire alarms, having identifiable escape routes and a fire extinguisher, and reducing hot water temperature to 49°C (120°F). Immersion full-thickness burns develop after 1 second at 70°C (158°F), after 5 seconds at 60°C (140°F), after 30 seconds at 54.5°C (130°F), and after 10 minutes at 49°C (120°F).

PEARLS FOR PRACTITIONERS

See The Acutely Ill or Injured Child: Pearls for Practitioners at the end of this section.

REVIEW QUESTIONS

Available online.

CHAPTER 44
Poisoning

ETIOLOGY AND EPIDEMIOLOGY

The most common agents ingested by young children include cosmetics, personal care products, cleaning solutions, and analgesics. In 2023 fatal childhood poisonings were most commonly caused by analgesics (with opioids being most common), fumes/gases/vapors, and stimulants/street drugs.

More than 2 million human exposures are called into poison control centers in the United States each year. More than half of all exposures are in children (56% in 2023), with a male predominance in children under 13 years but a female predominance in adolescence. Most ingestions in young children are unintentional, with intentional ingestions becoming more common in children 13 years and older.

CLINICAL MANIFESTATIONS

Any child who presents with unexplained symptoms including altered mental status, seizure, cardiovascular compromise, or metabolic abnormality should be considered to have ingested a poison until proven otherwise. A thorough history and physical examination often provide sufficient clues to distinguish between toxic ingestion and organic disease (Table 44.1). Determination of all substances that the child was exposed to, including type of medication, amount of medication, and time of exposure, is crucial in directing interventions. Available data often are incomplete or inaccurate, requiring a careful physical examination and laboratory approach. A complete physical examination, including vital signs, is necessary. Certain complexes of symptoms and signs are relatively specific to a given class of drugs (toxidrome) (Table 44.2).

COMPLICATIONS

A poisoned child can exhibit any one of six basic clinical patterns: coma, direct toxicity to a particular organ system, metabolic acidosis, heart rhythm aberrations, gastrointestinal symptoms, and seizures.

Coma

Coma is perhaps the most striking symptom of a poison ingestion, but it also may be seen as a result of several other causes including trauma, a cerebrovascular accident, asphyxia, or significant infection. A careful history and clinical examination are needed to distinguish among these alternatives.

Direct Toxicity

Hydrocarbon ingestion occasionally may result in systemic toxicity, but more often it leads to pulmonary toxicity. Hydrocarbons with low viscosity, low surface tension, and high volatility pose the greatest risk of producing aspiration pneumonia; however, when swallowed, they pose no risk unless emesis is induced. Emesis or lavage should *not* be initiated in a child who has ingested volatile hydrocarbons.

Caustic ingestions with acids or alkalis may cause dysphagia, epigastric pain, oral mucosal burns, and low-grade fever. Patients with esophageal lesions may have no oral burns or may have significant signs and symptoms. Treatment depends on the agent ingested and the presence or absence of esophageal injury. Alkali agents may be solid, granular, or liquid. Liquid agents are tasteless and produce full-thickness liquefaction necrosis of the esophagus or oropharynx. When the esophageal lesions heal, strictures form. Ingestion of these agents also creates a long-term risk of esophageal carcinoma. Treatment includes antibiotics if there are signs of infection and dilation of strictures that form 2–3 weeks later.

Ingested button batteries also may produce a caustic mucosal injury. Batteries that remain in the esophagus may cause esophageal burns and erosion and should be removed with an endoscope. In addition, acid agents can injure the lungs (with hydrochloric acid fumes), oral mucosa, esophagus, and stomach. Because acids taste sour, children usually stop drinking the solution, limiting the injury. Acids produce a coagulation necrosis, which limits the chemical from penetrating into deeper layers of the mucosa and damages tissue less severely than alkali. The signs, symptoms, and therapeutic measures are similar to those for alkali ingestion.

Metabolic Acidosis

A poisoned child may also have a high anion gap metabolic acidosis (mnemonic, *MUDPILES*) (Table 44.3), which is assessed easily by measuring arterial blood gases, serum electrolyte levels, and urine pH. An osmolar gap, if present, strongly suggests the presence of an unmeasured component such as methanol or ethylene glycol. These ingestions require thorough assessment and prompt intervention.

Dysrhythmias

Dysrhythmias may be prominent signs of a variety of toxic ingestions, although ventricular arrhythmias are rare. Because many drug and chemical overdoses may lead to sinus tachycardia, this is not a useful or discriminating sign; however, sinus bradycardia suggests ingestion of a β blocker, calcium channel blocker, clonidine, opioids, digoxin, or organophosphates. An electrocardiogram is an important study in cases of potential ingestion, and evidence of a prolonged PR interval, QTc prolongation, or widened QRS complex can be a clue to which drug was ingested (Table 44.4).

Gastrointestinal Symptoms

Gastrointestinal symptoms of poisoning include emesis, nausea, abdominal cramps, and diarrhea. These symptoms may be the result of direct toxic effects on the intestinal mucosa or of systemic toxicity after absorption.

Seizures

Children with toxic ingestions may present with seizures. When seizures occur with intoxication, they may be life-threatening and require aggressive therapeutic intervention.

LABORATORY AND IMAGING STUDIES

Laboratory studies helpful in initial management include specific toxin-drug assays; measurement of arterial blood gases and electrolytes, osmoles, and glucose; and calculation of the

TABLE 44.1 Historical and Physical Findings in Poisoning

ODOR	
Bitter almonds	Cyanide
Acetone	Isopropyl alcohol, methanol, paraldehyde, salicylate
Alcohol	Ethanol
Wintergreen	Methyl salicylate
Garlic	Arsenic, thallium, organophosphates, selenium
Rotten eggs	Hydrogen sulfide, sulfur dioxide, methyl mercaptans (additive to natural gas)
OCULAR SIGNS	
Miosis	Opioids, organophosphates, muscarinic mushrooms, clonidine, phenothiazines (typical antipsychotics), chloral hydrate, barbiturates (late)
Mydriasis	Atropine, cocaine, amphetamines, antihistamines, tricyclic antidepressants, PCP, LSD
Nystagmus	Phenytoin, barbiturates, ethanol, carbamazepine, PCP, ketamine, dextromethorphan
Lacrimation	Organophosphates, irritant gas or vapors
Retinal hyperemia	Methanol
Poor vision	Methanol, botulism, carbon monoxide
CUTANEOUS SIGNS	
Needle tracks	Opioids, PCP, amphetamine
Dry, hot skin	Anticholinergic agents, botulism
Diaphoresis	Organophosphates, muscarinic mushrooms, aspirin, cocaine
Alopecia	Thallium, arsenic, lead, mercury
Erythema	Boric acid, mercury, cyanide, anticholinergics
ORAL SIGNS	
Salivation	Organophosphates, salicylate, corrosives, strychnine, ketamine
Dry mouth	Amphetamine, anticholinergics, antihistamine
Burns	Corrosives, oxalate-containing plants
Gum lines	Lead, mercury, arsenic
Dysphagia	Corrosives, botulism
INTESTINAL SIGNS	
Diarrhea	Antimicrobials, arsenic, iron, boric acid, cholinergics
Constipation	Lead, opioids, botulism
Hematemesis	Corrosives, iron, salicylates, NSAIDs
CARDIAC SIGNS	
Tachycardia	Atropine, aspirin, amphetamine, cocaine, cyclic antidepressants, theophylline
Bradycardia	Digitalis, opioids, clonidine, organophosphates, β blockers, calcium channel blockers
Hypertension	Amphetamine, LSD, cocaine, PCP
Hypotension	Phenothiazines, barbiturates, tricyclic antidepressants, iron, β blockers, calcium channel blockers, clonidine, opioids
RESPIRATORY SIGNS	
Depressed respiration	Alcohol, opioids, barbiturates
Increased respiration	Amphetamines, aspirin, ethylene glycol, carbon monoxide, cyanide
Pulmonary edema	Hydrocarbons, organophosphates
CENTRAL NERVOUS SYSTEM SIGNS	
Ataxia	Alcohol, barbiturates, anticholinergics, opioids
Coma	Sedatives, opioids, barbiturates, salicylate, cyanide, carbon monoxide, cyclic antidepressants, alcohol

(Continued)

TABLE 44.1 Historical and Physical Findings in Poisoning—cont'd

Hyperpyrexia	Anticholinergics, salicylates, amphetamine, cocaine
Muscle fasciculation	Organophosphates, theophylline
Muscle rigidity	Tricyclic antidepressants, PCP, phenothiazines, haloperidol
Peripheral neuropathy	Lead, arsenic, mercury, organophosphates
Altered behavior	LSD, PCP, amphetamines, cocaine, alcohol, anticholinergics

LSD, Lysergic acid diethylamide; *NSAID*, nonsteroidal antiinflammatory drug; *PCP*, phencyclidine.

TABLE 44.2 Toxic Syndromes

AGENT	MANIFESTATIONS
Acetaminophen	Nausea, vomiting, pallor, delayed jaundice–hepatic failure (72–96 hr)
Amphetamine, cocaine, and sympathomimetics	Tachycardia, hypertension, hyperthermia, psychosis and paranoia, seizures, mydriasis, diaphoresis, piloerection, aggressive behavior
Anticholinergics	Mania, delirium, fever, red dry skin, dry mouth, tachycardia, mydriasis, urinary retention
Carbon monoxide	Headache, dizziness, coma, weakness, nausea/vomiting, chest pain
Cyanide	Coma, convulsions, hyperpnea, bitter almond odor
Ethylene glycol (antifreeze)	Metabolic acidosis, hyperosmolarity, hypocalcemia, oxalate crystalluria
Iron	Vomiting (bloody), diarrhea, hypotension, hepatic failure, leukocytosis, hyperglycemia, radiopaque pills on abdominal radiograph, late intestinal stricture, *Yersinia* sepsis
Opioids	Coma, respiratory depression, hypotension, pinpoint pupils, bradycardia
Cholinergics (organophosphates, nicotine)	Miosis, salivation, urination, diaphoresis, lacrimation, bronchospasm (bronchorrhea), muscle weakness and fasciculations, emesis, defecation, coma, confusion, pulmonary edema, bradycardia
Salicylates	Tachypnea, fever, lethargy, coma, vomiting, diaphoresis, alkalosis (early), acidosis (late)
Tricyclic antidepressants	Coma, convulsions, mydriasis, hyperreflexia, arrhythmia (prolonged Q-T interval), cardiac arrest, shock

TABLE 44.3 Screening Laboratory Clues in Toxicologic Diagnosis

ANION GAP METABOLIC ACIDOSIS (MNEMONIC = MUDPILES)
Methanol,* metformin Uremia* Diabetic ketoacidosis* Paraldehyde,* phenformin Isoniazid, iron Lactic acidosis (cyanide, carbon monoxide) Ethanol,* ethylene glycol* Salicylates, starvation, seizures
HYPOGLYCEMIA
Ethanol Isoniazid Insulin Propranolol Oral hypoglycemic agents
HYPERGLYCEMIA
Salicylates Isoniazid Iron Phenothiazines Sympathomimetics
HYPOCALCEMIA
Oxalate Ethylene glycol Fluoride
RADIOPAQUE SUBSTANCE ON ABDOMINAL RADIOGRAPH (MNEMONIC = CHIPPED)
Chloral hydrate, calcium carbonate Heavy metals (lead, zinc, barium, arsenic, lithium, bismuth as in Pepto-Bismol) Iron Phenothiazines Play-Doh, potassium chloride Enteric-coated pills Dental amalgam

*Indicates hyperosmolar condition.

anion or osmolar gap. A full 12-lead electrocardiogram should be part of the initial evaluation in all patients suspected of ingesting toxic substances. Urine and serum screens for drugs of abuse or to confirm suspected ingestion of medications in the home may be revealing.

Quantitative toxicology assays are important for some agents (Table 44.5), not only for identifying the specific drug but also for providing guidance for therapy, anticipating complications, and estimating the prognosis. Gas chromatography can be helpful in identifying drugs that are not commonly tested for on urine drug screens but is not always readily available.

TREATMENT

The four foci of treatment for poisonings are supportive care, decontamination, enhanced elimination, and specific antidotes.

Supportive Care

Supportive care is the mainstay of treatment in most cases. Prompt attention must be given to protecting and maintaining the airway, establishing effective breathing, and supporting the circulation. This management sequence takes precedence

TABLE 44.4 Drugs Associated With Major Modes of Presentation

COMMON TOXIC CAUSES OF CARDIAC ARRHYTHMIA	CAUSES OF COMA
QTc Prolongation	Alcohol
Amiodarone	Anticholinergics
Amphetamine	Antihistamines
Antipsychotics	Barbiturates
Antiarrhythmics	Carbon monoxide
Antifungals	Clonidine
Citalopram	Cyanide
Diphenhydramine	Tricyclic antidepressants
Macrolide antibiotics	Hypoglycemic agents
Methadone	Lead
Phenothiazines	Lithium
PR Interval Prolongation	Methemoglobinemia*
β Blockers	Methyldopa
Calcium channel blockers	Opioids
Digoxin	Phencyclidine
Lithium	Phenothiazines
	Salicylates
QRS Prolongation	**COMMON AGENTS CAUSING SEIZURES (MNEMONIC = CAPS)**
Carbamazepine	**C**amphor
Chloroquine, hydroxychloroquine	Carbamazepine
Diphenhydramine	Carbon monoxide
Digoxin	Cocaine
Lamotrigine	Cyanide
Phenothiazines	**A**minophylline
Propranolol	Amphetamine
Quinine, quinidine	Anticholinergics
Tricyclic antidepressants	Antidepressants (cyclic)
	Pb (lead) (also lithium)
	Pesticide (organophosphate)
	Phencyclidine
	Phenol
	Phenothiazines
	Propoxyphene
	Salicylates

**Causes of methemoglobinemia: amyl nitrite, aniline dyes, benzocaine, bismuth subnitrate, dapsone, primaquine, quinones, spinach (infants), sulfonamides.*

TABLE 44.5 Drugs Amenable to Therapeutic Monitoring for Drug Toxicity

ANTIBIOTICS
Aminoglycosides—gentamicin, tobramycin, and amikacin
Chloramphenicol
Vancomycin
IMMUNOSUPPRESSION
Methotrexate
Cyclosporine
ANTIPYRETICS
Acetaminophen
Salicylate
OTHER
Digoxin
Lithium
Theophylline
Anticonvulsant drugs
Serotonin uptake inhibitor agent

over other diagnostic or therapeutic procedures. If the level of consciousness is depressed and a toxic substance is suspected, glucose, 100% oxygen, and naloxone should be administered.

Gastrointestinal Decontamination

The intent of gastrointestinal decontamination is to prevent the absorption of a potentially toxic ingested substance and, in theory, to prevent the poisoning. There has been great controversy about which methods are the safest and most efficacious. Recommendations from the American Academy of Clinical Toxicology (AACT) and the European Association of Poison Centres and Clinical Toxicologists (EAPCCT) follow. **Syrup of ipecac** should not be administered routinely to poisoned patients because of potential complications and lack of evidence that it improves outcome. Likewise, **gastric lavage** should not be used routinely, if ever, in the management of poisoned patients because of the lack of efficacy and potential complications. **Single-dose activated charcoal** decreases drug absorption when used within 1 hour of ingestion; however, it has not been shown to improve clinical outcome; thus it should be used selectively in the management of a poisoned patient. Charcoal is ineffective against caustic or corrosive agents, hydrocarbons, heavy metals (arsenic, lead, mercury, iron, lithium), glycols, and water-insoluble compounds.

The administration of a cathartic (sorbitol or magnesium citrate) alone has no role in the management of the poisoned patient. The AACT has stated that based on available data, the use of a cathartic in combination with activated charcoal is not recommended.

Whole-bowel irrigation using polyethylene glycol (GoLYTELY) as a nonabsorbable cathartic may be effective for toxic ingestion of sustained-release or enteric-coated drugs. The AACT does not recommend the routine use of whole-bowel irrigation. However, there is theoretical benefit in its use for potentially toxic ingestions of iron, lead, zinc, or packets of illicit drugs.

Enhanced Elimination

Multiple-dose activated charcoal should be considered only if a patient has ingested a life-threatening amount of carbamazepine, dapsone, phenobarbital, quinine, or theophylline. **Alkalinization of urine** may be helpful for salicylate or methotrexate ingestion. **Dialysis** may be used for substances that have a low volume of distribution, low molecular weight, low protein binding, and high degree of water solubility, such as methanol, ethylene glycol, salicylates, theophylline, bromide, and lithium.

Specific Antidotes

See Table 44.6.

For recommendations on specific therapy, contact one of the U.S. Poison Control Centers at 1-800-222-1222.

TABLE **44.6** Sample of Specific Antidotes

POISON	ANTIDOTE	PEDIATRIC DOSAGE	COMMENTS
Acetaminophen	*N*-acetylcysteine	Oral regimen: Loading dose 140 mg/kg PO, then 70 mg/kg PO q4h × 17 doses IV regimen: Loading dose 150 mg/kg over 1 hr (max 15 g/dose), then 50 mg/kg over 4 hr (max 5 g/dose), followed by 100 mg/kg over 16 hr (max 10 g/dose)	Most effective within 16 hr of ingestion
Benzodiazepine	Flumazenil	0.2 mg IV, repeat to 1 mg max total dose	Possible seizures, arrhythmias. DO NOT USE FOR UNKNOWN INGESTIONS
β Blockers	Glucagon	0.15 mg/kg bolus IV, followed by infusion of 0.05–0.15 mg/kg/hr	
Carbon monoxide	Oxygen	100% FiO_2; hyperbaric O_2	Half-life of carboxyhemoglobin is 5 hr in room air but 1.5 hr in 100% O_2
Tricyclic antidepressants	Sodium bicarbonate	Bolus 1–2 mEq/kg IV, followed by repeated bolus dosing as needed to keep QRS <110 msec	Follow potassium levels and replace as needed
Iron	Deferoxamine	Infusion of 15 mg/kg/hr IV (max 6 g/24 hr)	Hypotension (worse with rapid infusion rates)
Lead	Edetate calcium disodium (EDTA)	35–50 mg/kg/day IV × 5 days; continuous infusion or divided q12hr	
	British anti-Lewisite (BAL; dimercaprol)	4 mg/kg/dose IM q4hr × 2–7 days	May cause sterile abscesses Prepared in peanut oil; do not use in patients with peanut allergy
	Succimer (2,3-dimercaptosuccinic acid [DMSA])	10 mg/kg/dose PO tid × 5 days, then 10 mg/kg/dose PO bid × 14 days	Few toxic effects, requires lead-free home plus compliant family
Nitrites/ methemoglobinemia*	Methylene blue	1–2 mg/kg IV, repeat every 30–60 min if needed; treat for levels >30%	Exchange transfusion may be needed for severe methemoglobinemia; methylene blue overdose also causes methemoglobinemia
Opioids	Naloxone	0.1 mg/kg IV/IO, IN, IM for full reversal of opioid ingestion (up to 2 mg), repeat as needed.	Naloxone causes no respiratory depression
Organophosphates	Atropine	0.05–0.1 mg/kg IV/IO, repeat every 5–10 min as needed	Physiologic: blocks acetylcholine
	Pralidoxime (2 PAM; Protopam)	25–50 mg/kg IV over 5–10 min (max 2000 mg/dose); may repeat after 1–2 hr, then q10–12hr as needed	Specific: disrupts phosphate-cholinesterase bond

See Table 44.4 footnote for causes of methemoglobinemia.

ET, Endotracheal; *IM*, intramuscular; *IN*, intranasal; *IO*, intraosseous; *IV*, intravenous; *PO*, oral; *SC*, subcutaneous.

Modified from Kliegman RM, St. Geme J, eds. Nelson Textbook of Pediatrics. *22nd ed. Philadelphia: Elsevier; 2024:707–708. Please see this reference for a comprehensive list of antidotes.*

PROGNOSIS

Most poisonings result in minimal or no toxicity or have minor effects. Intentional ingestions result in a much higher rate (5.2%) of major effects or death compared with unintentional ingestions (0.2%). Adolescents are more likely to have a moderate, major, or fatal effect from ingestion compared to younger children (17.3% of teens compared with 1.1% of children under 6 years).

PREVENTION

Properly educating parents regarding safe storage of medications and household toxins is necessary for preventing ingestions. If a child has ingested poison, a poison control center should be called.

PEARLS FOR PRACTITIONERS

See The Acutely Ill or Injured Child: Pearls for Practitioners at the end of this section.

REVIEW QUESTIONS

Available online.

CHAPTER 45

Sedation and Analgesia

An acutely ill pediatric patient may have pain, discomfort, and anxiety resulting from injury, surgery, invasive procedures (intubation, bone marrow aspiration, venous access placement), or during mechanical ventilation. Clear goals should be identified to allow the provision of optimal analgesia or sedation without compromising the physiologic status of the patient. Anxiolysis, cooperation, amnesia, immobility, and lack of awareness are all goals of sedation and can be accomplished with various medications (Table 45.1). Many of these goals can also be achieved with behavioral techniques (preprocedural teaching and the assistance of child life specialists), but sedation is often a necessary adjunct for painful procedures. Pain may be expressed by verbal or visible discomfort, crying, agitation, tachycardia, hypertension, and tachypnea. A variety of scales have been developed to quantify pain and allow more directed therapy. Pain caused by procedural interventions should always be treated with analgesics in addition to sedation (Table 45.2).

ASSESSMENT

Procedural Sedation

A medical evaluation must be performed for any patient receiving procedural sedation to identify underlying medical conditions that may affect the choice of sedative agents. Specific attention must be paid to assessment of the airway (for ability to maintain a patent airway) and respiratory system (chronic lung disease, recent respiratory illness, loose teeth), cardiovascular status (especially adequacy of volume status), factors affecting drug metabolism (kidney or liver disease), and risk of aspiration (adequate nothing-by-mouth status, gastroesophageal reflux). During the administration of procedural sedation, assessment of the patient must include monitoring of oxygen saturation, heart rate, and respiratory rate, as well as some assessment of the effectiveness of ventilation such as capnography. This assessment must be performed by someone who is not involved in the procedure and who will record vital signs and drugs administered on a time-based graph. Monitoring must be continued until the child has returned to baseline. Patients who are receiving long-term sedation (e.g., to maintain endotracheal tube placement) may need only local anesthesia for painful procedures but may benefit from additional sedation or analgesia as well.

Nonprocedural Sedation

Many ventilated pediatric patients require sedation and some analgesia while intubated. Dexmedetomidine, a centrally acting selective α_2-receptor agonist, is a popular choice due to its ability to provide sedation without respiratory depression. Longer acting benzodiazepines and opioids are also commonly used. Avoidance of oversedation is important. Use of appropriate pain and sedation scores allows for titration of medications to achieve the goals of the sedation plan. Long-term use of benzodiazepines and opioids leads to tolerance and subsequent withdrawal, a problematic occurrence that

TABLE 45.1 Agents That Produce Sedation

SEDATIVES	EFFECT	CONCERNS
Midazolam	Anxiolysis, sedation, muscle relaxation, amnesia	Tolerance is possible; apnea, hypotension, depressed myocardial function; short acting
Lorazepam	Anxiolysis, sedation, muscle relaxation, amnesia	Same as midazolam; longer acting
Dexmedetomidine	Sedation without respiratory depression	May cause bradycardia
Ketamine	Anesthesia, analgesia, amnesia	Dissociative reactions, tachycardia, hypertension, increased bronchial secretions, emergent delirium, hallucinations
Chloral hydrate	Sedative	Emesis, hypotension, arrhythmias, hepatic dysfunction
Propofol	Rapid-onset sedative for induction and maintenance of anesthesia	Metabolic acidosis in children; may depress cardiac function

TABLE 45.2 Agents That Produce Analgesia

ANALGESIC	EFFECT	COMPLICATIONS
NON-OPIOIDS		
Acetaminophen and NSAIDs	Moderate analgesia, antipyresis	Ceiling effect NSAIDs—gastrointestinal bleed, ulceration, kidney injury
OPIOIDS		
		No ceiling effect; respiratory depression, sedation, pruritus, nausea/vomiting, decreased gastric motility, urinary retention, tolerance with abuse potential
Morphine	Analgesia	May cause myocardial depression
Codeine	Analgesia	Nausea/vomiting
Fentanyl, alfentanil, sufentanil	Analgesia, sedation	No adverse effects on cardiovascular system; stiff chest syndrome
Methadone	Analgesia	

NSAID, Nonsteroidal antiinflammatory drug.

must be considered as medications are added and weaned. Medications used for sedation and analgesia may also contribute to delirium, a phenomenon that is being increasingly recognized in critically ill patients.

Pain and Analgesia

The subjective aspect of pain requires that self-reporting be used for assessment. The color analog scale (CAS) and Faces Pain Scale–Revised (FPS-R) have been validated for use in older children. Pain scales for younger children such as the Faces, Legs, Activity, Cry, Consolability (FLACC) scale often incorporate behavioral and physiologic parameters, despite the imprecision of physiologic responses.

Local anesthetics, such as lidocaine, can be used for minor procedures. However, lidocaine requires subcutaneous or intradermal injection. The use of topical anesthetic creams such as EMLA (lidocaine and prilocaine) or LMX (lidocaine) is less effective than intradermal lidocaine but is preferred by many pediatric patients.

Patient-controlled analgesia is an effective method for providing balanced analgesia care in older children and adolescents. Children using patient-controlled analgesia have better pain relief and experience less sedation than patients receiving intermittent, nurse-controlled, bolus analgesics. Analgesics can be administered through the patient-controlled analgesia pump with continuous basal infusions, bolus administration, or both. Morphine and hydromorphone are the most frequent opioids used for patient-controlled analgesia. Monitoring of oxygen saturations and respiratory rate are crucial with continuous opioid infusions because of the shift in CO_2 response curve and potential to decrease ventilatory response to hypoxia.

Epidural analgesia decreases the need for inhalation anesthetics during surgery and can provide significant analgesia without sedation in the postoperative period. Decreased costs and length of stay also may be benefits of epidural analgesic approaches. Medications used in epidurals often include a combination of local anesthetics such as bupivacaine and opioids such as morphine. Adverse effects include nausea and vomiting, motor blockade, and technical problems requiring catheter removal. Infection and permanent neurologic deficits are rare.

PEARLS FOR PRACTITIONERS

See The Acutely Ill or Injured Child: Pearls for Practitioners at the end of this section.

REVIEW QUESTIONS

Available online.

Suggested Readings

American Heart Association American Heart Association. CPR and first aid emergency cardiovascular care guidelines. Available at: https://eccguidelines.heart.org/index.php/circulation/cpr-ecc-guidelines-2/part-11-pediatric-basic-life-support-and-cardiopulmonary-resuscitation-quality/.

Coté CJ, Wilson S, American Academy of Pediatrics, American Academy of Pediatric Dentistry. Guidelines for Monitoring and Management of Pediatric Patients Before, During, and After Sedation for Diagnostic and Therapeutic Procedures. *Pediatrics.* 2019;143(6):e20191000.

Henretig FM, Kirk MA, McKay Jr CA. Hazardous Chemical Emergencies and Poisonings. *N Engl J Med.* 2019;380(17):1638–1655.

Kliegman RM, St. Geme J, eds. *Nelson Textbook of Pediatrics.* 22nd ed. Philadelphia: Elsevier; 2025.

PEARLS FOR PRACTITIONERS

CHAPTER 37

Assessment and Resuscitation

- Initial assessment focuses on the ABCs—airway, breathing, and circulation—of an acutely ill or injured child.
- Respiratory failure is the most common cause of acute deterioration in children.
- In cardiopulmonary arrest:
  - The goal should be to optimize cardiac output and tissue oxygen delivery.
  - Begin chest compressions immediately, followed by support of the airway and breathing/ventilation (C-A-B).
- Monitoring vital signs and physiologic status is the key screening activity.
  - The choice of appropriate diagnostic tests and imaging is determined by the mechanism of disease and results of evaluation after initial resuscitation.

CHAPTER 38

Respiratory Failure

- Acute respiratory failure occurs when the pulmonary system is unable to maintain adequate gas exchange to meet metabolic demands.
- Respiratory failure:
  - Can be classified as hypercarbic, hypoxemic, or both.
  - Is frequently caused by bronchiolitis, asthma, pneumonia, upper airway obstruction, and/or systemic inflammation resulting in acute respiratory distress syndrome (ARDS).
- Pediatric ARDS and its severity are defined by (1) onset within 7 days of known clinical insult, (2) respiratory failure not fully explained by cardiac failure or fluid overload, (3) chest imaging findings of new infiltrate(s), and (4) impairment in oxygenation.
- Pulse oximetry allows noninvasive, continuous assessment of oxygenation but is unable to provide information about ventilation abnormalities.

CHAPTER 39

Shock

- Shock is the inability to provide sufficient perfusion of oxygenated blood and substrate to tissues to meet metabolic demands.
  - Acute hypovolemia is the most common cause of shock in children.
  - Other forms of shock include distributive shock, cardiogenic shock, hemorrhagic shock, obstructive shock, and dissociative shock.
- Shock requires immediate resuscitation before obtaining laboratory or diagnostic studies.
- The key to therapy is the recognition of shock in its early compensated/partially compensated state, when many of the hemodynamic and metabolic alterations may be reversible.

CHAPTER 40

Injury Prevention

- Injury occurs through interaction of the host (child) with an agent (e.g., car and driver) through a vector and an environment (e.g., roadways, weather) that is conducive to exposure.
- Unintentional injury is the leading cause of death in children 1–18 years of age.
- The most common causes of fatal injuries differ among age groups.
- The Haddon matrix combines the epidemiologic components with time factors to identify effective interventions focused on different aspects of the injury event.

CHAPTER 41

Major Trauma

- Injury is the leading cause of death in children ages 1–18 years.
- Primary survey is focused on assessment of xABCDE—extreme external bleeding, airway, breathing, circulation, disability (including neurologic status), and exposure (including removing the child's clothing and performing a detailed assessment of the entire body).
- Secondary survey is focused on a more detailed head-to-toe examination along with obtaining more history.
- Resuscitative measures are performed concurrently with primary and secondary surveys.
- Most blunt abdominal organ injuries are managed nonoperatively.

CHAPTER 42

Drowning

- Drowning is defined as respiratory impairment from submersion/immersion in liquid and is the second leading cause of injury-related death for children ages 1–14 years.
- Other terms, including near drowning, secondary drowning, and dry drowning, should not be used.
- Outcomes are categorized as death, morbidity, or no morbidity and are closely linked to the degree of hypoxic-ischemic brain injury.

- Treatment is focused on optimizing oxygenation and perfusion, especially cerebral perfusion.

CHAPTER 43

Burns

- Classification by depth (superficial, superficial partial thickness, deep partial thickness, and full thickness) conveys more information about the structures injured and the likely need for surgical treatment than the commonly used first-degree, second-degree, and third-degree burn designations.
- For severe burns, care is best managed by a multidisciplinary team in a qualified burn center.
- Severe burn injury results in a hypermetabolic state.

CHAPTER 44

Poisoning

- Consider poisoning in any child who presents with unexplained altered mental status, seizure, cardiovascular compromise, or metabolic abnormality.
- A poisoned child can exhibit any one of six basic clinical patterns: coma, toxicity, metabolic acidosis, heart rhythm aberrations, gastrointestinal symptoms, and/or seizures.
- The four foci of treatment for poisonings are supportive care, decontamination, enhanced elimination, and specific antidotes.

CHAPTER 45

Sedation and Analgesia

- Sedation and analgesia are necessary to treat the pain, discomfort, and anxiety experienced by many acutely ill and injured pediatric patients.
- Clear goals should be identified to allow provision of optimal analgesia or sedation without compromising the physiologic status of the patient.
- Long-term use of benzodiazepines and opioids leads to tolerance.

SECTION 9

HUMAN GENETICS AND DYSMORPHOLOGY

Thelma Alessandra Sugrañes | Paul A. Levy

CHAPTER 46

Patterns of Inheritance

TYPES OF GENETIC DISORDERS

Approximately 3% of infants born in the United States have **congenital malformations**, abnormalities of form or function identifiable at birth. The number approaches 7% at 1 year of age because some anomalies may not be identifiable until after the neonatal period. The prevalence of congenital malformations is much greater in inpatient pediatric populations; 30–50% of hospitalized children have congenital anomalies or genetic disorders.

Clinical geneticists attempt to identify the etiology, mode of inheritance, and risk that a disorder might occur in the affected child's siblings. In evaluating children with congenital malformations, the condition's etiology may be classified into one of six different categories:

1. Single-gene abnormalities
2. Chromosomal abnormalities
3. Multifactorially inherited conditions
4. Conditions during pregnancy (infections, phenylketonuria [PKU], thyroid dysfunction, diabetes)
5. Conditions caused by exposure to teratogens
6. Unknown or idiopathic anomalies

INTRODUCTION TO GENETICS AND GENOMICS

DNA is composed of four nucleotide building blocks: adenine, guanine, cytosine, and thymine. Each nucleotide is linked to other nucleotides, forming a chain. The DNA molecule consists of two chains of nucleotides held together by hydrogen bonds. The purine nucleotides, adenine and guanine, cross-link by hydrogen bonds to the pyrimidines, thymine and cytosine. Because of this cross linking, the nucleotide sequence of one strand sets the other strand's sequence. Separating the two strands permits complementary nucleotides to bind to each DNA strand; this copies the DNA and replicates the sequence.

DNA exists as multiple fragments that, together with a protein skeleton (chromatin), form chromosomes. Human cells have 23 pairs of chromosomes, with one copy of each chromosome inherited from each parent. Twenty-two pairs of chromosomes are **autosomes**; the remaining pair consists of **sex chromosomes**. Females have two X chromosomes; males have one X and one Y unless a sex chromosome anomaly is present.

DNA sequences form **genes**, the basic units of heredity. A typical gene contains a promoter sequence, an untranslated region, and an open reading frame. In the open reading frame, every three nucleotides represent a single **codon**, coding for a particular amino acid. In this way, the sequence of bases dictates the sequence of amino acids in the corresponding protein. Some codons, rather than coding for specific amino acids, act as "start" signals; others serve as "stop" signals. Between the start and stop codons, genes consist of two major portions: **exons**, regions containing the code that ultimately corresponds to a sequence of amino acids, and **introns** (intervening sequence), which do not become part of the amino acid sequence but may regulate gene function.

Genes are **transcribed** into messenger RNA (mRNA), then **translated** into proteins. During transcription, RNA is processed to remove introns. The mRNA serves as a template to construct the protein.

Human genetic material contains 3 billion base pairs. Less than 2% of the DNA codes for proteins, comprising the genome's 20,000–24,000 genes. Through a mechanism called ***alternative splicing***, these genes may create more than 100,000 proteins. The remainder of the DNA, the portion not involved in protein formation, was once termed *junk DNA*, but much of this presumed *junk DNA* is functional and likely serves regulatory functions.

Disease may be caused by changes or **pathogenic variants** (previously termed *mutations*) in the DNA sequence, with the **point variant**, a change in a single DNA base, being the most common type. A point variant that changes a codon and the resulting amino acid that goes into the protein is referred to as a **missense variant**. A **nonsense variant** is a point variant that changes the codon to a "stop" signal so that transcription ends prematurely. A **frameshift variant** often stems from the loss or addition of one or more bases; this causes a shift in how the DNA is transcribed and generally leads to premature stop codons.

Pedigree Drawing

To identify specific patterns of inheritance, geneticists construct and analyze **pedigrees**, pictorial representations of a family history. Males are represented by squares and females by circles. A solid line between two symbols indicates that both partners have contributed genetic material to the children, or next generation, represented below. No genetic relationship between parents and children may be represented by a dashed line, and adopted individuals may be denoted by brackets.

Grandparents, uncles, aunts, and cousins are added in similar fashion. Ages or birthdays may be written next to or underneath each symbol. The proband (the patient who is being evaluated) is indicated with an arrow. Affected individuals are indicated by shading or some other technique, which should be explained in a key. Carriers for a disorder (e.g., sickle cell disease) usually are indicated by a dot in the center of their symbol (Fig. 46.1).

Pedigrees should include representatives of at least three generations of family members.

Autosomal Dominant Disorders

If a single copy of a gene bearing a pathogenic variant is sufficient to cause disease and that gene is not on one of the sex chromosomes, that condition is inherited in an autosomal dominant (AD) fashion (Table 46.1). In AD disorders, each child of an affected parent has a 50% chance of inheriting the mutated gene (Fig. 46.2; Table 46.2). Possessing one *working* gene and one *nonworking* gene is termed ***heterozygous***. If both copies are the same, they are referred to as ***homozygous***.

Some people who are obligate carriers of a pathogenic variant known to cause an AD disorder do not show clinical signs of the condition, while other individuals manifest symptoms. This phenomenon is referred to as ***penetrance***. If all individuals who carry a pathogenic variant for an AD disorder show signs of that disorder, the gene is said to have *complete*

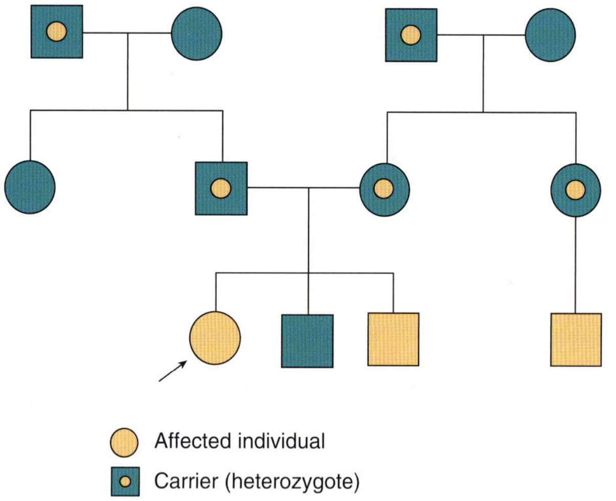

FIGURE 46.1 Pedigree showing affected individuals and carriers.

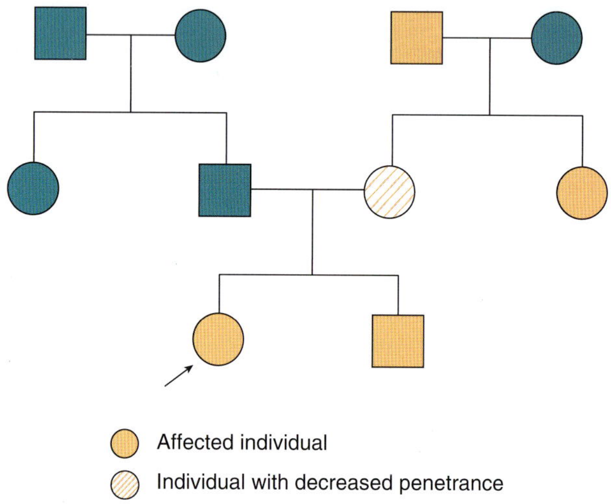

FIGURE 46.2 Pedigree showing decreased penetrance for an autosomal dominant disorder. Proband *(arrow)* is affected. Maternal grandfather also is affected. The individual's mother is presumed to be the carrier of the gene, even though she may show only slight symptoms of disease.

TABLE 46.1 Examples of Autosomal Dominant Diseases

DISEASE	FREQUENCY	COMMENTS
Achondroplasia Thanatophoric dysplasia Crouzon syndrome with acanthosis nigricans Nonsyndromic craniosynostosis	~1:25,000	Pathogenic variants are in the gene for *fibroblast growth factor receptor-3* on chromosome 4p16.3; 80% of cases are de novo variants. Variants in the same gene cause achondroplasia, thanatophoric dysplasia, Crouzon syndrome with acanthosis, and nonsyndromic craniosynostosis.
NF1	1:3,000	About 50% of cases result from de novo variants in the gene for neurofibromin, a tumor suppressor gene located at 17q11.2. Expression is quite variable.
NF2	1:25,000	The *NF2* gene is a tumor suppressor gene located at 22q12.2 that codes for a protein called *Merlin.* Associated with bilateral acoustic neuromas.
HD	Variable in populations, 1:5,000–1:20,000	Caused by a CAG repeat expansion in the Huntington protein gene on chromosome 4p16.3.
DM1, Steinert disease	1:500 in Quebec 1:8,000–20,000 worldwide	Caused by a CTG repeat expansion in the DM protein kinase gene at chromosome 19q13.3. The condition shows genetic anticipation with successive generations.
Marfan syndrome	1:10,000	The syndrome is caused by pathogenic variants in the *FBN1* gene on chromosome 15q21.1; there is variable expression.
HAE (deficiency of C-1 esterase inhibitor that regulates the C-1 component of complement)	1:50,000	The gene is located on chromosome 11q11-q13.2. The phenotype of episodic and variable subcutaneous and submucosal swelling and pain is caused by diminished or altered esterase inhibitor protein, which can result from any one of many pathogenic variants in the gene.

DM1, Myotonic dystrophy type 1; *FBN1,* fibrillin 1; *HAE,* hereditary angioedema; *HD,* Huntington disease; *NF1,* neurofibromatosis 1; *NF2,* neurofibromatosis 2.

TABLE 46.2 Rules of Autosomal Dominant Inheritance

Trait appears in every generation.
Each child of an affected parent has a 1-in-2 chance of being affected.
Males and females are equally affected.
Male-to-male transmission occurs.
Traits generally involve pathogenic variants in genes that code for regulatory or structural proteins (i.e., collagen).

penetrance. Many AD disorders show decreased (or incomplete) penetrance.

Often, AD disorders show variability in symptoms expressed in different individuals carrying the same genetic variant. Some individuals have only mild clinical symptoms, whereas others have more severe disease. This phenomenon is referred to as ***variable expressivity***.

AD disorders sometimes appear in a child of unaffected parents because of a **de novo pathogenic variant** (the variant is new in the child's DNA and not inherited). Known in some cases to be associated with advanced paternal age (>40 years of age), spontaneous pathogenic variants may account for most individuals with some disorders. For instance, 80% of children born with achondroplasia (ACH) have a spontaneous pathogenic variant in the fibroblast growth factor receptor type 3 *(FGFR3)* gene. The following are examples of AD disorders.

Achondroplasia

Caused by a defect in cartilage-derived bone, ACH is the most common skeletal dysplasia in humans. The bony abnormalities lead to short stature, macrocephaly, a flat midface with a prominent forehead, and rhizomelic ("root of the limb") shortening of the limbs. The disorder occurs in approximately 1 in 25,000 births.

ACH is caused by a pathogenic variant in *FGFR3*. Early in development, this gene is expressed during endochondral bone formation. More than 95% of cases of ACH are caused by one of two heterozygous pathogenic variants in the same base pair (site 1138). This site, extremely active for variants, is known as a variant ***hot spot***.

Hydrocephalus and central apnea may occur because of narrowing of the foramen magnum and compression of the brainstem and may present a life-threatening complication in infancy. Bowing of the legs may occur later in childhood because of unequal growth of the tibia and fibula. Dental malocclusion, obstructive apnea, and hearing loss due to middle ear dysfunction are common in later childhood. During later childhood and adolescence, psychologic effects of short stature may manifest. In adulthood, further complications include compression of nerve roots and sciatica. People with ACH have normal life spans and normal intelligence.

The diagnosis of ACH is based on clinical findings, and characteristic x-ray abnormalities confirm the diagnosis. Molecular testing is available, and prenatal diagnosis is possible using fetal cells obtained through amniocentesis or chorionic villus sampling.

Neurofibromatosis Type 1

One of the most common AD disorders, neurofibromatosis type 1 (NF1) is present in 1 in 3,000 individuals. The condition is caused by a heterozygous pathogenic variant in the *NF1* gene, which codes for the protein neurofibromin.

Although the penetrance of NF1 is 100%, the expression is extremely variable, and many affected individuals have features so mild that they are never diagnosed or are diagnosed after another more severely affected family member is diagnosed (see Chapter 187).

Marfan Syndrome

A condition that occurs in approximately 1 in 10,000 individuals, Marfan syndrome (MFS) shows pleiotropy, a condition in which abnormalities in multiple organ systems are caused by a pathogenic variant in a single gene. MFS is caused by a heterozygous pathogenic variant in *FBN1*, the gene for fibrillin (a connective tissue protein). Clinical symptoms mainly involve three systems: **skeletal**, **ophthalmologic**, and **cardiac**.

Skeletal findings include dolichostenomelia (a tall, thin body habitus), long thin fingers and toes (arachnodactyly), abnormalities of the sternum (pectus excavatum or carinatum), scoliosis, pes planus, and joint laxity.

Eye findings include ectopia lentis (dislocation of the lens), early and severe myopia, flat lens, hypoplastic iris, and ciliary muscle hypoplasia. Patients with MFS are at increased risk of retinal detachment. Although cataracts do not occur more frequently in MFS, they tend to occur at a younger age.

Cardiac findings include aortic insufficiency and progressive dilatation of the aortic root, leading to increased risk of aortic dissection, which is a life-threatening complication. Other clinical features include dural ectasia, abnormal pulmonary septation, and striae. Diagnostic criteria for MFS are summarized in Table 46.3.

De novo pathogenic variants in the *FBN1* gene account for approximately 25% of cases of MFS. The gene is large and complex, and more than 3,000 variants have been identified in affected individuals. Many of the symptoms of MFS are caused not by the defect in the fibrillin protein itself but by an excess in transforming growth factor β, a protein usually bound by fibrillin.

Autosomal Recessive Disorders

Disorders that are inherited in an autosomal recessive (AR) manner manifest only when *both* copies of a gene pair located on an autosome (a non–sex chromosome) have a pathogenic variant (Tables 46.4 and 46.5). Children affected with AR disorders are usually born to unaffected parents, each of whom carries one copy of the variant. If both members of a couple are carriers (or heterozygotes) for this variant, each of their offspring has a 25% chance of being affected (Fig. 46.3).

Sickle Cell Disease

See Chapter 151.

Tay-Sachs Disease

See Chapters 55 and 186.

X-Linked Disorders

Approximately 900 genes have been identified on the X chromosome, whereas only 100 are believed to be present on the Y chromosome. Females, whose cells have two X chromosomes, possess two copies of each of these genes, whereas males, who

TABLE **46.3** Revised Ghent Nosology for the Diagnosis of Marfan Syndrome

AORTIC ROOT DILATATION* (Z ≥ 2 SD) OR AORTIC DISSECTION	ECTOPIA LENTIS	SYSTEMIC ≥7 POINTS	*FBN1* PATHOGENIC VARIANT	DIAGNOSIS
WITHOUT FAMILY HISTORY				
+	+	− or +		MFS[†]
+			+	MFS
+	−	+	(unknown or neg)	MFS[†]
−	+		+	MFS
−	+			Ectopia lentis syndrome
−	−	≥5		MASS
Mitral valve prolapse	−	<5		MVPS
WITH FAMILY HISTORY				
	+			MFS
		+		MFS[†]
+ (Z ≥ 2, if >20 yr) (Z ≥ 3, if <20 yr)				MFS[†]
SCORING SYSTEM FOR SYSTEMIC FEATURES[‡]				
Thumb AND wrist sign			3	
Thumb OR wrist sign			1	
Pectus carinatum			2	
Pectus excavatum or chest asymmetry			1	
Hindfoot deformity			2	
Pes planus			1	
Pneumothorax (history)			2	
Dural ectasia			2	
Protrusio acetabuli			2	
Decreased US/LS ratio AND increased arm/height BUT no scoliosis			1	
Scoliosis or thoracolumbar kyphosis			1	
Reduced elbow extension			1	
Facial features (3 of 5)[§]			1	
Skin striae			1	
Myopia >3 diopters			1	
Mitral valve prolapse			1	

Aortic root dilatation (measured at the sinuses of Valsalva).

†*Loeys-Dietz syndrome (LDS), Shprintzen-Goldberg syndrome (SGS), and the vascular form of Ehlers Danlos (vEDS) should be excluded. If clinical features are suggestive, then DNA testing for TGFBR1, TGFBR2 (LDS), COL3A1 (vEDS), or collagen biochemistry should be done to help rule out these disorders.*

‡*Maximum total: 20 points; >7 points indicates systemic involvement.*

§*Facial features: dolichocephaly, enophthalmos, down-slanting palpebral fissures, malar hypoplasia, retrognathia.*

FBN1, Fibrillin-1; *MASS*, phenotype that includes myopia, mitral valve prolapse, borderline aortic root dilatation (Z < 2), striae, skeletal findings; *MFS*, Marfan syndrome; *MVPS*, mitral valve prolapse syndrome; *US/LS*, upper segment/lower segment.

Data from Loeys BL, Dietz HC, Braverman AC, et al. The revised Ghent nosology for the Marfan syndrome. J Med Genet. 2010;47:476–485.

TABLE 46.4 Examples of Autosomal Recessive Diseases

DISEASE	FREQUENCY*	COMMENTS
Classic congenital adrenal hyperplasia (CAH) (21-hydroxylase deficiency)	1:15,000 (classic CAH)	Phenotype variation corresponds roughly to allelic variation. A deficiency causes virilization in females. The gene is located at 6p21.3 within the HLA complex and within 0.005 cM of HLA B.
Phenylketonuria (PKU) (phenylalanine hydroxylase deficiency)	1:25,000	There are hundreds of pathogenic variants in the *PAH* gene located on chromosome 12q22–q24.1. The first population-based newborn screening was a test for PKU because the disease is treatable by diet.
Cystic fibrosis (CF)	1:4,000	The gene *CFTR* is on chromosome 7q31.2. F508del (Δ508) variant is the predominant variant found in those with Northern European ancestry; however, many other variants exist.
Friedreich ataxia (FA)	1:40,000	Frataxin is a mitochondrial protein involved with iron metabolism and respiration. The gene is on chromosome 9q13-q21, and the common pathogenic variant is a GAA-expanded triplet repeat located in the first *intron* of the gene. FA does not show anticipation.
Gaucher disease, all types (glucocerebrosidase deficiency)	1:50,000–1:100,000 1:1,000 Ashkenazi Jews	The gene is located on chromosome 1q21. There are many pathogenic variants; some lead to neuropathic disease, but most are milder in expression.
Sickle cell disease (SCD)	1:300–500 Black Americans 1:13 Black infants in the United States born with sickle cell trait	A single base change results in an amino acid substitution of valine for glutamic acid at position 6 of the β chain of hemoglobin, with resulting hemolytic anemia. The gene is on chromosome 11p15.5 and is associated with multiple sickle cell syndromes (see Chapter 151).

**Frequency estimates in the United States. Frequency of heritable conditions varies by geography, ancestry, newborn screening utilization, diagnostic testing modality, and testing availability.*
cM, Centimorgans; *CTFR*, CF transmembrane conductance regulator; *HLA*, human leukocyte antigen.

TABLE 46.5 Rules of Autosomal Recessive Inheritance

Trait appears in siblings, not in their parents or their offspring.
On average, 25% of siblings of the proband are affected (at the time of conception, each sibling has a 25% chance of being affected).
An unaffected sibling of an affected individual has a two-thirds chance of being a carrier (heterozygote).
Males and females are equally likely to be affected.
Rare traits are likely to be associated with parental consanguinity.
Traits generally involve pathogenic variants in genes that code for enzymes (e.g., phenylalanine hydroxylase–deficient in PKU) and are associated with serious illness and shortened life span.

PKU, Phenylketonuria.

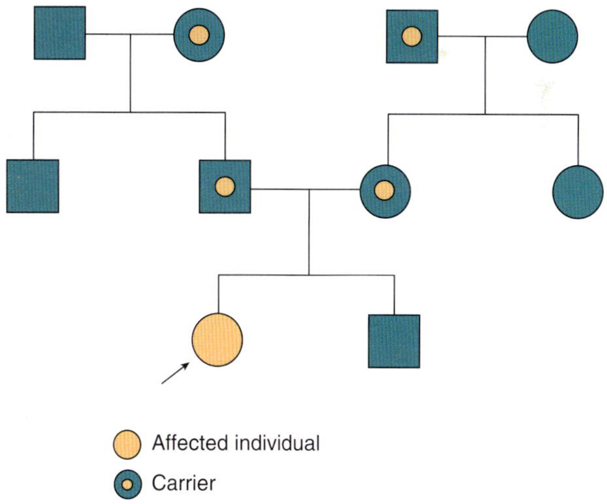

FIGURE 46.3 Pedigree of family showing autosomal recessive inheritance.

have one X chromosome and one Y chromosome, have only one copy. Early in female development, one X chromosome is randomly inactivated in each cell; this is called ***X chromosome inactivation*** **(or lyonization)**, and the inactivated chromosome is called a ***Barr body***. There are many X-linked disorders (colorblindness, Duchenne muscular dystrophy, hemophilia A) in which heterozygous (carrier) females show some manifestations of the disorder due to skewed X chromosome inactivation.

X-Linked Recessive Inheritance

Most disorders involving the X chromosome show recessive inheritance. With only one copy of the X chromosome, males are more likely to manifest these diseases than females. Each son born to a female carrier of an X-linked recessive trait has a 50% chance of inheriting the trait, but none of her daughters would be expected to be affected (each daughter has a 50% chance of being a carrier). An affected father transmits the pathogenic variant to all his daughters, who are carriers, but not to his sons; having received their father's Y chromosome, they would not be affected (thus there is no male-to-male transmission) (Tables 46.6 and 46.7; Fig. 46.4).

Duchenne Muscular Dystrophy

See Chapter 183.

Hemophilia A

See Chapter 152.

TABLE 46.6 Examples of X-Linked Recessive Diseases

DISEASE	FREQUENCY	COMMENTS
Duchenne muscular dystrophy (DMD) (pseudohypertrophic progressive muscular dystrophy (MD), dystrophinopathy, Becker variants)	1:3,500 males	The gene is located at Xp21. The gene is relatively large, with 79 exons, and variants and deletions may occur anywhere. The gene product is called *dystrophin*. Dystrophin is absent in DMD but abnormal in Becker MD.
Hemophilia A (factor VIII deficiency, classic hemophilia)	1:5,000 males	The gene is located at Xq28. Factor VIII is essential for normal blood clotting. Phenotype depends on genotype and the presence of any residual factor VIII activity.
Color blindness (partial deutan series, green color blindness [75%]; partial protan series, red color blindness [25%])	1:12 males	The gene is located at Xq28 (proximal) for deutan color blindness and at Xq28 (distal) for protan color blindness.
Adrenoleukodystrophy (ALD) (XL-ALD)	1:10,000–1:17,000	The gene is located at Xq28. The disease involves a defect in peroxisome function relating to *very long-chain fatty acid CoA synthetase* with accumulation of C-26 fatty acids. Phenotype is variable, from rapid childhood progression to later onset and slow progression.
Glucose-6-phosphate dehydrogenase deficiency (G6PD)	1:10 Black Americans 1:5 Kurdish Jews	The gene is located at Xq28. There are numerous variants in which oxidants cause hemolysis. Variants can confer partial resistance to severe malaria.

TABLE 46.7 Rules of X-Linked Recessive Inheritance

Incidence of the trait is higher in males than in females.
Trait is passed from carrier females, who may show mild expression of the gene, to half of their sons, who are more severely affected.
Each son of a carrier female has a 1-in-2 chance of being affected.
Trait is transmitted from affected males to all their daughters; it is never transmitted father to son.
Because the trait can be passed through multiple carrier females, it may *skip* generations.

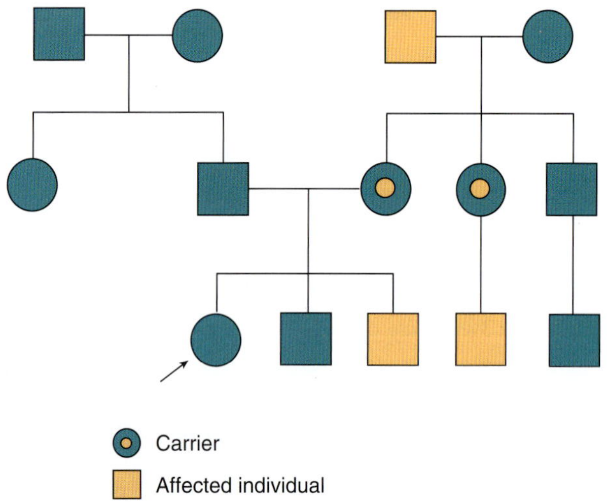

FIGURE 46.4 Pedigree showing X-linked recessive inheritance.

X-Linked Dominant Inheritance

Only a few examples of X-linked dominantly inherited disorders have been described. Both males and females are affected by this group of disorders, but females have less severe symptoms due to X chromosome inactivation. This is the case for **X-linked vitamin D–resistant rickets** (hypophosphatemic rickets), a disorder in which the kidney's ability to reabsorb phosphate is impaired. Phosphate levels and resulting rickets are not as severe in females as in males.

Some X-linked dominant disorders are lethal in males, with death occurring before birth. Affected mothers can have affected or unaffected daughters but only unaffected sons. This is the case in **incontinentia pigmenti**, caused by a pathogenic variant in the *NEMO* or *IKBKG* gene, which has a characteristic swirling skin pattern of hyperpigmentation that develops after a perinatal skin rash with blistering. Affected females also have variable involvement of the central nervous system, hair, nails, teeth, and eyes. In **Rett syndrome**, caused by heterozygous pathogenic variants in the *MECP2* gene, females develop typically after birth but later in the first year of life develop microcephaly, developmental regression, and often a seizure disorder. Females are often diagnosed with autism and, by 2 years of age, adopt stereotypic hand movements (described as hand wringing, or hand washing) that causes them to lose all purposeful hand movements.

OTHER TYPES OF GENETIC DISORDERS

Multifactorial Disorders

Also known as ***polygenic inheritance***, multifactorially inherited disorders result from the interplay of genetic and environmental factors. In addition to 20% of congenital malformations (such as cleft lip and palate and spina bifida), most common disorders of childhood and adult life (such as asthma, atherosclerosis, diabetes, and cancer) result from an interaction between genes and the environment. Though these disorders do not follow simple Mendelian modes of inheritance, affected individuals tend to cluster in families. The disorders occur more often in first- and second-degree relatives than would be expected by chance, and they are more likely to be concordant (although not 100%) in monozygotic twins than in dizygotic twins.

Hypertrophic Pyloric Stenosis

Occurring in 1.5 in 1,000 children in the United States, hypertrophic pyloric stenosis (HPS) is five times more likely to occur in males than in females. When a child with HPS is born, the recurrence risk in future progeny is 5–10% for males and 1.5–2% for females. In adulthood, the risk of an affected male having an affected child is markedly increased over the general population; 4% of sons and 1% of daughters of such males would be likely to be affected. Even more striking is the risk to children born to affected females; 17–20% of sons and 7% of daughters are affected.

The thickness of the pyloric muscle may be distributed across a bell-shaped curve; the position on the bell-shaped curve is determined by many factors, including the expression of multiple, unknown genes. HPS may result when individuals' genetic and environmental influences cause them to fall to an extreme position on this curve, past a certain point called a ***threshold***. In HPS, this threshold is farther to the left for males than it is for females.

Disorders With Unusual Patterns of Inheritance

Mitochondrial Inheritance

Mitochondrial DNA (mtDNA) is nonnuclear DNA contained within human cells. This mtDNA is circular, 16.5 kb in length, and replicates independently of nuclear DNA. Involved in energy production used to run the cell, mtDNA codes for a few respiratory chain proteins (most mitochondrial proteins are coded on **nuclear** DNA) and for a set of transfer RNAs unique to mitochondrial protein synthesis. Virtually all mitochondria are supplied by the oocyte, which means that mtDNA is maternally derived. A female with a variant in mtDNA passes this variant to all her children. More than one population of mitochondria may be present in the oocyte, a phenomenon called ***heteroplasmy***. The mtDNA variant may be present in a few or many mitochondria. When the fertilized egg divides, mitochondria are distributed randomly. The presence of symptoms in the offspring, and their severity, depends on the ratio of variant to wild-type mtDNA present in a particular tissue. If an abundance of variant mitochondria exists in tissue that has high energy requirements (brain, muscle, and liver), clinical symptoms occur (Fig. 46.5). If fewer variant mitochondria are present, few clinical symptoms may be seen.

Mitochondrial encephalomyopathy with lactic acidosis and strokelike episodes (MELAS) is an example of a mitochondrial disorder. Asymptomatic in early childhood, individuals affected with MELAS develop episodic vomiting, seizures, and recurrent cerebral insults that resemble strokes between 5–10 years of age. In 80% of cases, analysis of the mtDNA reveals a specific variant (A3243G) in *MTTL1*, a gene that codes for a mitochondrial transfer RNA.

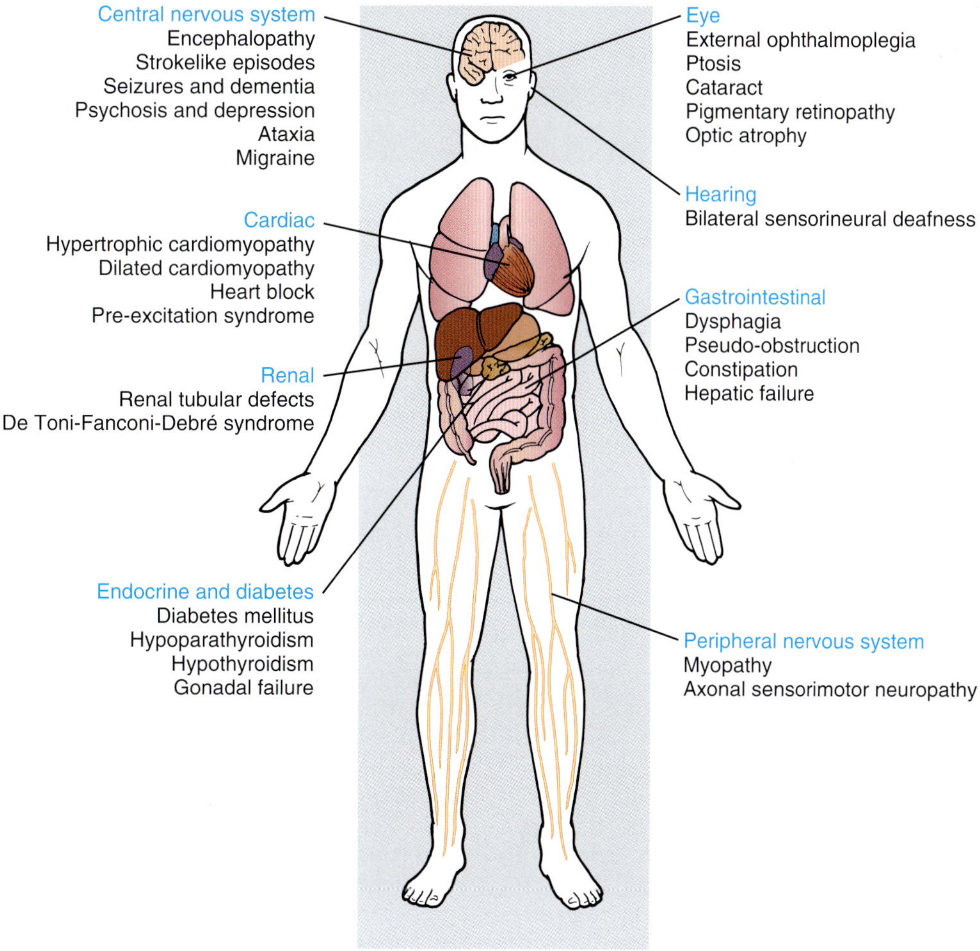

FIGURE 46.5 The range of affected tissues and clinical phenotypes associated with pathologic variants in mitochondrial DNA (mtDNA). (Modified from Chinnery PF, Turnbull DM. Mitochondrial DNA and disease. *Lancet.* 1999;345:SI17–SI21.)

In families in which MELAS occurs, a range of symptoms is seen in first-degree relatives, including **progressive external ophthalmoplegia**, hearing loss, cardiomyopathy, and diabetes mellitus. Although all offspring of a woman who carries a mitochondrial pathogenic variant would be affected, because of heteroplasmy, the severity of disease varies depending on the percentage of mitochondria bearing the variant that is present.

Uniparental Disomy

Evaluation of a child with **uniparental disomy** (UPD) reveals a normal karyotype. However, chromosomal markers will show that the individual has inherited two copies of one parent's chromosome and no copy from the other parent.

UPD probably occurs through multiple mechanisms, but the most common results from a spontaneous *rescue* mechanism. At the time of conception, through nondisjunction, the fertilized egg is trisomic for a particular chromosome, with two copies of one parent's chromosome and one copy of the other parent's chromosome; conceptuses with trisomy often miscarry early in development. Fetuses with UPD survive because they spontaneously lose one of three copies of the affected chromosome. If the single chromosome from one parent is lost, the patient has UPD.

An alternate explanation involves monosomy for a chromosome rather than trisomy. Had the conceptus, at the time of conception, inherited only a single copy of a chromosome, spontaneous duplication of the single chromosome would lead to UPD.

Prader-Willi and Angelman Syndromes

Prader-Willi syndrome (PWS), which occurs in 1 in 20,000–30,000 infants, is characterized by neonatal hypotonia, postnatal growth delay, a characteristic appearance including almond-shaped eyes and small hands and feet, developmental disability, hypogonadotropic hypogonadism, and obesity after infancy. Early in life, affected infants are so hypotonic that they cannot consume enough calories to maintain their weight. Nasogastric feeding is invariably necessary, and growth faltering is common. During the first year of life, muscle tone improves, and children later develop a voracious appetite with resulting obesity. Between 60–70% of individuals with PWS have a small deletion of chromosome 15 (15q11). In individuals without a deletion, 30–40% have UPD of chromosome 15.

Angelman syndrome (AS) is a condition with moderate-to-severe intellectual disability, absence of speech, ataxic movements of the arms and legs, a characteristic craniofacial appearance, seizures, and behavior that includes frequent laughter and smiling often inappropriate to the situation. AS is also characterized by a deletion in the 15q11 region in 70% of affected individuals; UPD for chromosome 15 can be demonstrated in approximately 5% of AS patients.

If the deletion occurs in paternal chromosome 15, the affected individual will develop PWS, whereas AS results from a deletion occurring only in the maternal chromosome 15. When UPD is responsible, maternal UPD results in PWS, whereas paternal UPD results in AS. To summarize, if a copy of paternal chromosome 15q11.2 is lacking, PWS occurs; if maternal chromosome 15q11.2 is lacking, AS results.

This phenomenon is explained by **genomic imprinting**. Imprinting is an **epigenetic** phenomenon, a nonheritable change in the DNA that causes an alteration in gene expression based on parental origin of the gene. PWS is caused by deficiency of the protein product of the gene *SNRPN* (small nuclear ribonucleoprotein). Although present on both maternally and paternally derived chromosome 15, *SNRPN* is expressed only from the paternally derived chromosome. Expression is blocked from the maternal chromosome because of methylation; this physical change in the DNA prevents gene expression. PWS results whenever a paternal chromosome 15 is missing, either through deletion or through UPD.

AS results from a lack of expression of ubiquitin-protein ligase E3A *(UBE3A)*, a second gene in the chromosome 15q11.2 region. *UBE3A* is normally expressed only in the maternally derived chromosome 15. Although present in paternal chromosome 15, *UBE3A* is methylated, and gene expression is blocked. Therefore, if either the critical region of maternal chromosome 15 is deleted or paternal UPD occurs, the individual will manifest symptoms of AS.

Expansion of a Trinucleotide Repeat

More than 50% of human DNA contains repeat sequences, two or three bases repeated over and over again. Disorders caused by expansion of trinucleotide repeats include **fragile X syndrome (FXS)**, **Huntington disease**, **myotonic dystrophy**, **Friedreich ataxia**, and some of the **spinocerebellar ataxias**. Although an increase in the number of the three repeated bases is at the heart of each disorder, the molecular mechanism differs.

FXS, which occurs with a frequency of approximately 1 in 4,000 children, is the most common cause of inherited intellectual disability. Features include characteristic craniofacial findings (large head; prominent forehead, jaw, and ears); macro-orchidism with testicular volume twice the normal size in adulthood; a mild connective tissue disorder, including joint laxity, distended eustachian tubes, and mitral valve prolapse; and a characteristic neurobehavioral profile, including intellectual disability (ranging from mild to profound) and autism spectrum disorders.

Positional cloning in the Xq27 region identified a triplet repeat region composed of one cytosine and two guanine residues (CGG). These repeats occur in the promoter region of the gene *FMR1*. Unaffected individuals who have no family history of FXS have 0–45 CGG repeats (most have 25–35). In individuals with FXS, the number of repeats is greater than 200; such people are said to have a *full mutation*. Between these two categories, a third group has 56–200 repeats; these individuals, known as ***premutation carriers***, have typical development.

FXS results from a failure to express FMRP, the protein product of the *FMR1* gene, which is expressed primarily in the central nervous system and testes during early embryonic development. Although FMRP is produced in unaffected individuals and premutation carriers, in those with the full mutation, FMRP transcription of the protein is blocked because the large number of CGG repeats become methylated (an epigenetic phenomenon). Thus, FXS occurs as a consequence of a **loss-of-function variant**—the failure of expression of FMRP because of methylation of the promoter sequence.

In female premutation carriers, an expansion in the number of repeats from the premutation to the full mutation range may occur during gametogenesis. The cause of this expansion is not understood. Although premutation carriers do not show symptoms and signs of FXS, women may manifest primary ovarian insufficiency and early menopause, and men and women may develop a movement disorder, known as *fragile X tremor/ataxia syndrome*, later in life.

TERATOGENIC AGENTS

Approximately 6–15% of all birth defects are attributed to teratogens—chemical, physical, or biologic agents that have the potential to damage embryonic tissue and result in congenital malformations. Agents known to be teratogenic include drugs (prescription and nonprescription); intrauterine infections (rubella); maternal diseases, such as diabetes mellitus; and environmental substances, such as alcohol and heavy metals. Knowledge of teratogenic agents and their effect on the developing fetus is important because limiting exposure to these agents is an effective way to prevent birth defects (see Chapter 58).

Infections During Pregnancy

See Chapter 65.

Pregnancy Co-Morbidities That Affect the Fetus

See Chapter 58.

Medications and Chemicals

Fetal alcohol spectrum disorders are the most common causes of preventable intellectual disability. Prevalence estimates vary with a range of 0.3–9 cases per 1,000 children in the United States. Features include prenatal and postnatal growth deficiency, developmental disabilities, microcephaly, skeletal and cardiac anomalies, and a characteristic facial appearance. While the amount of alcohol consumed and timing of consumption is often linked to the severity of symptoms, no safe threshold of alcohol consumption in pregnancy has been identified; it is recommended that pregnant women avoid all prenatal alcohol exposure.

Warfarin, retinoic acid, and phenytoin are additional teratogenic agents (see Chapter 58).

Radiation

High-dose radiation exposure during pregnancy in Hiroshima and Nagasaki, Japan, was shown to increase the rate of spontaneous abortion and to result in children born with microcephaly, intellectual disability, and skeletal malformations. Estimates of exposure to cause these effects were approximately 25 rad. *The dose from routine radiologic diagnostic examinations is in the millirad range.*

PEARLS FOR PRACTITIONERS

See Human Genetics and Dysmorphology: Pearls for Practitioners at the end of this section.

REVIEW QUESTIONS

Available online.

CHAPTER 47

Genetic Assessment and Diagnosis

Individuals referred to a geneticist because of suspicion of a genetic disorder are called ***probands***; individuals who come for genetic counseling are **consultands**. Referral for genetic evaluation may be made for a wide variety of reasons and at different stages of life (fetus, neonate, childhood, pregnancy, adulthood).

PRECONCEPTION AND PRENATAL COUNSELING

Familial Factors

Families with relatives affected with genetic disorders may have questions about how a disorder is inherited and whether their progeny may be at risk. The inheritance pattern and the risk of having an affected child can be discussed with a geneticist.

In some cultures, it is common, even desirable, for relatives to marry. This relatedness or **consanguinity** increases the likelihood that offspring may be born with a rare autosomal recessive (AR) condition, as both parents may be carriers of the same pathogenic variant. Generally, the closer the relation between the partners, the greater the chance that the couple shares one or more pathogenic variants in common, increasing the risk that offspring will have an AR disorder. The risk of first cousins having a child with an AR disorder is 1 in 64. In evaluating these couples, it is important to consider which ethnic group they belong to and to test for conditions commonly found in that group.

Screening

It is common for couples to be screened for disorders that may occur more commonly in their ethnic group. People of Ashkenazi Jewish heritage may choose to be screened for heterozygosity for an expanding panel of AR disorders, including Tay-Sachs, Niemann-Pick disease, Bloom syndrome, Gaucher syndrome, Canavan disease, cystic fibrosis, Fanconi anemia, and familial dysautonomia. People whose ancestors originated in the Mediterranean basin may be screened for thalassemia. In addition, many pregnant people are screened for carrier status for sickle cell disease, cystic fibrosis, and spinal muscular atrophy during pregnancy. The American College of Obstetricians and Gynecologists recommends that all pregnant people be provided information about carrier screening.

Historically, prenatal screening has involved invasive and noninvasive testing. Invasive testing includes amniocentesis and chorionic villus sampling (CVS). Noninvasive testing includes sonography, which is utilized routinely throughout pregnancies, and the use of a series of biochemical markers present in the pregnant person's blood.

During the first trimester, measurement of the fetal nuchal fold by sonogram can be used to identify risk for aneuploidy;

increase in the nuchal thickness is a marker not only for fetal chromosomal anomalies but for certain genetic and structural abnormalities as well. The detection rate for aneuploidy using this technique alone is 70%. The addition of testing for abnormalities in free human chorionic gonadotropin (β-HCG) and pregnancy-associated plasma protein increases first trimester screening to a detection rate of almost 90%. However, positive predictive values remain low at less than 5%.

In the second trimester, maternal serum α-fetoprotein (MS AFP), unconjugated estriol, inhibin A, and HCG may be evaluated to create a biochemical profile known as the ***quad screen***, which correctly identifies about 80% of women who are carrying a baby with trisomy 21 (Down syndrome).

Elevated MS AFP is used to identify pregnancies in which the fetus is affected with neural tube defects, omphalocele, or gastroschisis. An additional association between low levels of MS AFP and fetal aneuploidy is known. Approximately 50% of fetuses with autosomal trisomies (trisomy 21 [Down syndrome], trisomy 18, trisomy 13) can be detected by low levels of MS AFP.

Although the risk of nondisjunction resulting in aneuploidy rises with maternal age, all pregnant people should be individually counseled as to their risk for aneuploidy and other fetal abnormalities. A combination of first and second trimester screening together with the pregnant person's age produces an individualized risk factor. *It is important to emphasize that screening tests are just that—tests used to identify individuals who are at increased risk.* If the risk is high or if concerns exist about the presence of a fetal anomaly, a diagnostic test, either CVS or amniocentesis, can be offered as further testing. Fetal cells are usually tested for chromosomal abnormalities by cytogenetic techniques, with the option of chromosomal microarray for increased precision. Biochemical testing for a known family history of an inherited metabolic disorder and molecular screening for known familial pathogenic variants can also be performed on fetal cells.

Noninvasive prenatal screening uses cell-free fetal DNA (cffDNA) in maternal blood to determine the risk of certain trisomies and sometimes microdeletion syndromes in the fetus. The cffDNA allows use of a maternal blood sample without an invasive test (amniocentesis, CVS) and offers predictive values around 50–90% depending on a priori risk; it is important to note that cffDNA is a screening test rather than a diagnostic test and requires confirmatory testing either prenatally (amniocentesis or CVS) or postnatally (testing performed on infant's blood drawn after birth). The cffDNA testing can be done as early as 10 weeks of pregnancy. The utility of cffDNA is reduced in cases of multiple gestation or when the birth parent is affected by a chromosomal anomaly.

Maternal Factors

The presence of either acute or chronic maternal illness during pregnancy may lead to complications in the developing fetus. Chronic conditions may expose the fetus to maternal medications that are potentially teratogenic. Acute illnesses, especially from the TORCH agents (toxoplasmosis, rubella, cytomegalovirus, herpes virus, and "other," including syphilis, varicella, and Zika virus), may cause birth defects. Other factors, such as maternal smoking, alcohol use, and maternal exposure to radiation or chemicals, also may necessitate genetic counseling.

Postnatal—Newborn and Infant

About 3% of newborns have a genetic abnormality or congenital malformation. The broad definition of malformations includes not only visible abnormalities but also functional defects that might not be apparent at birth.

Congenital malformations and genetic disorders have a significant impact on childhood morbidity and mortality. Over 10% of sudden unexplained childhood deaths and 30–50% of neonatal deaths can be traced to a genetic cause. Consultation with a geneticist for a newborn or infant may be prompted by many different findings, including the presence of a malformation, abnormal results on a routine newborn screening test, abnormalities in growth (e.g., failure to gain weight, increase in length, or abnormal head growth), developmental delay, blindness or deafness, the knowledge of a family history of a genetic disorder or chromosomal abnormality, or (as a result of prenatal testing) the presence of a genetic disorder or chromosomal abnormality in the infant.

Adolescent and Adult

Adolescents and adults may be seen by a geneticist for evaluation of a genetic disorder that has later onset. Some neurodegenerative disorders, such as Huntington disease and adult-onset spinal muscular atrophy, present later in life. Some forms of hereditary blindness (retinal degenerative diseases) and deafness (Usher syndrome, neurofibromatosis type 2) may not show significant symptoms until adolescence or early adulthood. Similarly, inherited cardiac disorders such as hypertrophic cardiomyopathy and long QT syndrome may not be identifiable until adulthood. Genetic consultation also may be prompted for a known family history of a **hereditary cancer syndrome** (breast, thyroid, colon, and ovarian cancers). Individuals may wish to have testing done to determine if they carry a pathogenic variant for these syndromes and are at risk for developing certain types of cancers. A known family history or personal history of a genetic disorder or chromosomal abnormality might prompt testing in anticipation of pregnancy planning.

GENERAL APPROACH TO PATIENTS

Family History

A pedigree usually is drawn to help visualize various inheritance patterns. A detailed family history determines if there is an autosomal dominant (AD), AR, X-linked (XL), or sporadic disorder in the family. When a child is affected with the new onset of an AD disorder, it is necessary to closely examine the parents for the presence of manifestations and/or consider targeted testing in parents. If the parents are unaffected, the child's condition is most likely the result of a de novo pathogenic variant, in which case the risk of recurrence is extremely low (although not 0 because of the possibility of gonadal mosaicism in one of the parents). When one parent is affected (even mildly so, due to varying expressivity), the recurrence risk rises to 50% for each subsequent pregnancy. With X-linked disorders, the focus is on the maternal family history to determine if there is a significant enough risk to warrant testing.

Questions about the couple's age are important to ascertain the risk related to maternal age for chromosome abnormalities and paternal age for new pathogenic variants leading to AD and XL disorders. A history of more than two spontaneous abortions increases the risk that one of the parents carries a balanced translocation and the spontaneous abortions are due to chromosomal abnormalities in the fetus.

Pregnancy

During a genetic consultation, it is important to gather information about the pregnancy (see Chapters 57, 58, and 59). A maternal history of a chronic medical condition, such as a seizure disorder or diabetes, has known consequences in the fetus. Medication used in pregnancy can be teratogenic; the pregnant person's exposure to toxic chemicals (work related) or use of alcohol, cigarettes, or substances can have serious effects on the developing fetus. Maternal infection during pregnancy with TORCH agents (see Chapter 65), among others, has been found to cause malformations in the fetus. Follow-up is needed if prenatal testing revealed abnormal results.

Delivery and Birth

An infant born prematurely is likely to have more complications than a term infant. An infant can be small, appropriate, or large for gestational age; each of these has implications for the child (see Chapters 57 and 59).

Medical History

The medical history can provide clues to an underlying disorder. Children with inborn errors of metabolism who have intermittent symptoms often have a history of multiple hospitalizations for dehydration or vomiting, often with encephalopathy. Children with neuromuscular disorders may have a period of typical development followed by increasing weakness or ataxia. Children with lysosomal storage diseases, such as the mucopolysaccharidoses, often have recurrent ear infections and growth issues and can develop sleep apnea.

Development

Many genetic disorders are associated with developmental disabilities. However, the onset of the disability may not always be present from the newborn period; many inborn errors of metabolism, including storage disorders, cause developmental regression after a period of normal development (see Chapters 7 and 8). Some adult-onset disorders have no symptoms until the teen years or later. Assessing school problems is important. The type of learning problem, age at onset, and whether there is improvement with intervention or continued decline all are important for proper assessment.

Physical Examination

A careful and thorough physical examination is necessary for all patients with signs, symptoms, or suspicion of genetic disease. Sometimes subtle clues may lead to an unsuspected diagnosis. Features suggestive of a syndrome are discussed in more detail in Chapter 49.

Laboratory Evaluation

Chromosome Analysis

An individual's chromosome complement, known as the *karyotype*, can be analyzed using cells capable of dividing. In pediatrics, lymphocytes obtained from peripheral blood are the usual source for such cells, but cells obtained from bone marrow aspiration, skin biopsy (fibroblasts), or, prenatally, from amniotic fluid or chorionic villi also can be used. Cells are placed in culture medium and stimulated to grow using a mitogen; their division is arrested in either metaphase or prophase using a spindle poison; slides are made, the chromosomes are stained with Giemsa or other dyes, and the chromosomes are examined and analyzed under a microscope.

Fluorescent in Situ Hybridization

Fluorescent in situ hybridization (FISH) allows the identification of the presence, absence, or rearrangement of a specific region of DNA. A complementary DNA probe specific for the region in question is generated, and a fluorescent marker is attached. The probe is incubated with cells from the subject and viewed under a microscope. The bound probe fluoresces, allowing the number of copies of the DNA segment in question to be counted. Use of FISH has mostly been supplanted by chromosomal microarray testing. However, FISH remains useful in some scenarios including confirming specific deletion disorders or complex chromosomal rearrangements.

Microarray Comparative Genomic Hybridization

Microarray comparative genomic hybridization (array CGH) has essentially replaced prophase analysis and should be ordered in individuals with multiple congenital anomalies without an obvious disorder. DNA from the individual being studied and a control are labeled with fluorescent markers and hybridized to thousands of FISH-like probes for sequences spread around the genome. The probes are derived from known genes and noncoding regions. By analyzing the ratio of intensity of the fluorescent marker at each site, it is possible to determine whether the individual has any difference in copy number compared with the control DNA.

DNA Sequencing

Sequencing technologies allow for examination of DNA for alterations at the nucleotide level. Sanger sequencing and next-generation sequencing (NGS) are two clinically available sequencing technologies. NGS allows for massively parallel sequencing reactions, which has reduced cost and increased efficiency. Despite its many advantages, NGS is not as successful at sequencing repetitive regions as Sanger sequencing. Sanger sequencing examines only a single DNA fragment at a time; it is slower but more accurate. Allele-specific polymerase chain reaction (PCR) and hybridization technologies allow one to detect the presence or absence of a specific allele or pathogenic variants.

Sequencing tests permit targeted approaches that can test for a familial or common variant within a gene, an entire gene or panel of genes, all the exons with exome sequencing (ES), or the entire genome (genome sequencing). The websites https://www.ncbi.nlm.nih.gov/gtr/ (government) and www.concertgenetics.com (commercial) list disorders in which sequencing is available and identify laboratories performing such testing.

Exome Sequencing

ES permits examination of the exonic regions of all 20,000–24,000 genes that compose the human genome (Fig. 47.1).

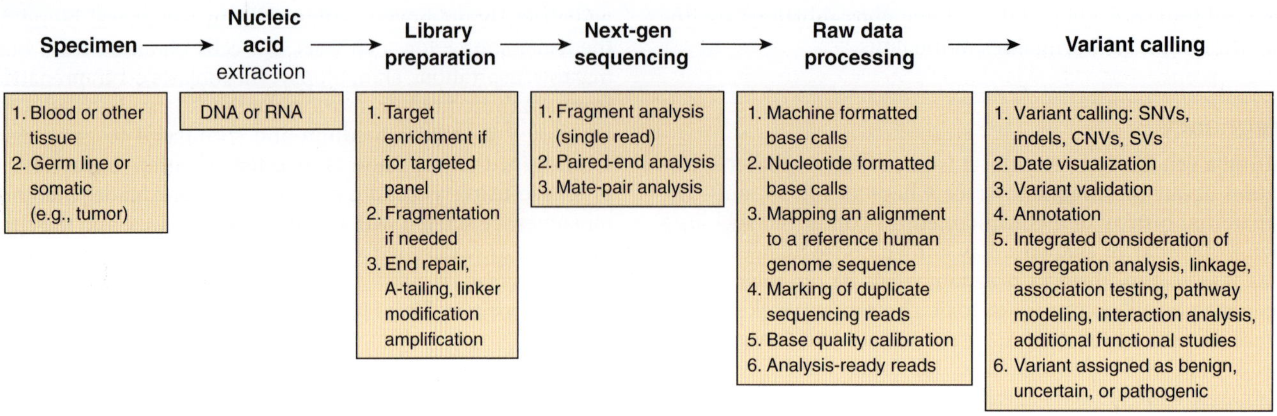

FIGURE 47.1 Overview of the next-generation DNA sequencing workflow. *CNV,* Copy number variant; *Indels,* insertions and deletions; *SNV,* single nucleotide variant; *SV,* structural variant. (Adapted from Casey G, Conti D, Haile R, et al. Next generation sequencing and a new era of medicine. *Gut.* 2013;62[6]:920–932.)

When possible, the test is ordered as a trio (patient plus both parental specimens) so that the proband's results can be further clarified. Using PCR and other techniques developed during the Human Genome Project, ES isolates DNA from an individual, looks for variations in the exomes or coding sequences of the genes, and compares identified variation with the DNA from the individual's parents. Variations are also filtered out based on phenotype and information known about genes and variants. Variation found in the subject that is not present in either parent suggests a spontaneous (de novo) pathogenic variant; two copies of a pathogenic variant in an individual whose parents are each found to be carriers of the variant suggests that the subject is affected with an AR disorder. Despite several shortcomings in ES (it is expensive and the interpretation is complicated with thousands of variations often identified), its impact as a diagnostic tool has been revolutionary.

Whole Genome Sequencing

Whole genome sequencing (WGS) involves analysis of both exonic (coding) and intronic (noncoding) regions of a patient's genome. This results in an ability to detect variants in regulatory regions that may have been missed by ES. WGS can also detect copy number variants (like a chromosomal microarray); newer WGS technologies using longer reads of the sequenced DNA fragments will enable evaluation of trinucleotide repeats, which cannot be done with existing sequencing technology.

PEARLS FOR PRACTITIONERS

See Human Genetics and Dysmorphology: Pearls for Practitioners at the end of this section.

REVIEW QUESTIONS

Available online.

CHAPTER 48 Chromosomal Disorders

Errors that occur in meiosis during the production of gametes can lead to abnormalities of chromosome structure or number. Syndromes caused by chromosomal abnormalities include trisomy 21 (Down syndrome [DS]), trisomy 13, trisomy 18, Turner syndrome (TS), and Klinefelter syndrome (KS), as well as rarer chromosomal duplications, deletions, or inversions.

Fifty percent of spontaneous abortions have a chromosomal abnormality. In newborns and older children, features that suggest the presence of a chromosome anomaly include low birthweight (small for gestational age), growth faltering, neurodevelopmental impairment, and the presence of three or more congenital malformations.

ABNORMALITIES IN NUMBER (ANEUPLOIDY)

During meiosis or mitosis, failure of a chromosomal pair to separate properly results in nondisjunction. **Aneuploidy** is a change in the number of chromosomes that results from nondisjunction. A cell may have one **(monosomy)** or three **(trisomy)** copies of a particular chromosome.

Trisomies

Down Syndrome

DS is the most common abnormality of chromosomal number in liveborn infants. It occurs in approximately 1 of every 700 births. Most cases (~90%) are due to nondisjunction; most often, the nondisjunctional event occurs in maternal meiosis phase I. As a result of nondisjunction, the fertilized egg contains three copies of chromosome 21 (trisomy 21). Using standard cytogenetic nomenclature, trisomy 21 is designated 47,XX,+21 or 47,XY,+21. In 3% of cases, the extra chromosome is part of a **Robertsonian translocation**, which occurs when the long arms (q) of two acrocentric chromosomes (numbers 13, 14, 15, 21, or 22) fuse at the centromeres, and the short arms (p), containing copies of ribosomal RNA, are lost. The most common Robertsonian translocation leading to DS involves chromosomes 14 and 21; standard nomenclature is 46,XX,t(14q21q) or 46,XY,t(14q21q). The parents of infants with DS who have translocations should have a karyotype to exclude a balanced translocation.

In 2% of children with DS, **mosaicism** occurs. These individuals have two populations of cells: one with trisomy 21 and one with a 46 chromosome complement. Mosaicism results either from a nondisjunctional event that occurs sometime after fertilization or from **trisomic rescue**. The loss of this aneuploidy returns the cell to 46,XX or 46,XY. In either case the individual is referred to as a *mosaic* for these two populations of cells and is designated 47,XX, +21/46XX or 47,XY,+21/46,XY. Although it is widely believed that individuals with mosaic DS are more mildly affected, there are wide variations in clinical findings.

Children with DS are usually diagnosed in the newborn period. They tend to have normal birthweight and length, but they are hypotonic. The characteristic facial appearance, with brachycephaly, flattened occiput, hypoplastic midface, flattened nasal bridge, upslanting palpebral fissures, epicanthal folds, and large protruding tongue, is often apparent at birth. Infants also have short broad hands, often with a single transverse palmar crease, and a wide gap between the first and second toes. Hypotonia may cause feeding problems and decreased activity. Intellectual disability is noted in almost all patients with DS.

Almost half of all children with DS have **congenital heart disease**, including atrioventricular canal, ventriculoseptal or atrioseptal defects, and valvular disease. Between 5–15% of newborns with DS have **gastrointestinal tract anomalies**; the three most common defects are duodenal atresia, annular pancreas, and imperforate anus.

Congenital **hypothyroidism** occurs in 2–7% of infants with DS. Acquired hypothyroidism is a more common problem. Thyroid function should be checked at birth, 6 months of age, and then annually.

Polycythemia at birth (hematocrit levels >70%) is common and may require treatment. Some infants with DS show a leukemoid reaction, with markedly elevated white blood cell counts. Although this resembles congenital leukemia, it is a self-limited condition, resolving on its own over the first month of life. Nonetheless, children with DS also have an increased risk of **leukemia**, with a 10- to 20-fold increase in risk compared with individuals without DS. In children with DS who are younger than 2 years of age, the type is generally acute megakaryoblastic leukemia; in individuals older than 3 years of age, the types of leukemia are similar to those of other children, with acute lymphoblastic leukemia being the predominant type.

Children with DS are more susceptible to infection, more likely to develop cataracts, and between 1–2% have *symptomatic* atlantoaxial instability, an increased distance between the first and second cervical vertebrae that can cause spinal cord compression. Many individuals older than 35 years of age develop Alzheimer-like features.

The recurrence risk for parents who have had a child with DS depends on the child's cytogenetic findings. If the child has trisomy 21, the empiric recurrence risk is 1% for women up to 35 years of age; after 35, the age-specific risk alone is used for subsequent pregnancies. If the child has a Robertsonian translocation, chromosomal analysis of both parents must be performed. In approximately 65% of cases, the translocation is found to have arisen de novo (i.e., spontaneously, with both parents having normal karyotypes), and recurrence risk is low. When a parent is identified as having a Robertsonian translocation, the recurrence risk depends on which parent is the carrier: If the mother is the carrier, the risk is 10–15%; if the father is the carrier, the recurrence risk is 2–5%.

Trisomy 18

Trisomy 18 (47,XX,+18 or 47,XY,+18) is the second most common autosomal trisomy, occurring in approximately 1 in 5,000 live births. The majority of cases of trisomy 18 are due to nondisjunction, although de novo mosaic trisomy 18 and heritable partial trisomy 18 (due to a balanced translocation in the parent) can also occur. Infants with trisomy 18 rarely survive; only 13% will reach their first birthday. Most infants with trisomy 18 are small for gestational age. Clinical features include hypertonia, prominent occiput, micrognathia, low-set and malformed ears, short sternum, rocker-bottom feet, hypoplastic nails, and characteristic clenching of fists—the second and fifth digits overlap the third and fourth digits (Table 48.1).

Trisomy 13

Trisomy 13 (47,XX,+13 or 47,XY,+13) occurs in 1 in 12,000 live births. As in trisomy 18, trisomy 13 is usually fatal in the first year of life, with only 11% of infants surviving beyond their first birthday.

As in DS, trisomy 13 can be caused by nondisjunction (seen in 75% of cases) or a Robertsonian translocation (in 20%). The most common translocation involves chromosomes 13 and 14. Counseling regarding recurrence risk for future progeny is similar to that described earlier for trisomy 21.

Infants with trisomy 13 have numerous malformations (see Table 48.1). They are small for gestational age and microcephalic. Midline facial defects such as cleft lip and palate are common, as are midline central nervous system anomalies, such as alobar holoprosencephaly. The forehead is generally sloping, ears are often small and malformed, and microphthalmia or anophthalmia may occur. Postaxial polydactyly of the hands is common, as are overlapping fingers and hyperconvex nails. Hypospadias and cryptorchidism are common in males, whereas females generally have hypoplasia of the labia minora. In addition, most infants with trisomy 13 have congenital heart disease. Many infants with trisomy 13 have a punched-out scalp lesion over the occiput called ***aplasia cutis congenita***; when seen in conjunction with polydactyly and some or all of the facial features, this finding is essentially pathognomonic for the diagnosis of trisomy 13.

Klinefelter Syndrome

Occurring in 1 in 500 newborn males, KS is the most common genetic cause of hypogonadism and infertility in males. It is caused by the presence of an extra X chromosome (47,XXY). The extra chromosome arises from nondisjunction in either the sperm or egg. About 15% of males with features of KS are found to be mosaic, with 46,XY/47,XXY mosaicism being the most common. Before puberty, males with KS are phenotypically indistinguishable from the rest of the population.

The diagnosis is often made in adolescence when the hallmark of the condition, under androgenation with testes that remain infantile in volume, should alert the clinician. Young adults with KS tend to be tall with long limbs. During adolescence or adulthood, gynecomastia may occur.

Because of failure of growth and maturation of the testes, males with KS have hypergonadotropic hypogonadism and **azoospermia** (low or absent sperm in ejaculate). Low production of testicular testosterone results in failure to completely develop secondary sexual characteristics, such as facial hair, deepening of the voice, and libido. In adulthood, osteopenia and osteoporosis develop. Because of these findings, testosterone supplementation is indicated.

Most males with KS are infertile secondary to azoospermia. Through the use of microdissection testicular sperm extraction, a technique in which viable sperm are isolated from

TABLE 48.1 Possible Clinical Findings in Trisomy 13 and Trisomy 18

	TRISOMY 13	TRISOMY 18
Head and face	Scalp defects (e.g., cutis aplasia) Microphthalmia, corneal abnormalities Cleft lip and palate Microcephaly Sloping forehead Holoprosencephaly (arrhinencephaly) Capillary hemangiomas Deafness	Small and premature appearance Tight palpebral fissures Narrow nose and hypoplastic nasal alae Narrow bifrontal diameter Prominent occiput Micrognathia Cleft lip or palate
Chest	Congenital heart disease (e.g., VSD, PDA, and ASD) Thin posterior ribs (missing ribs)	Congenital heart disease (e.g., VSD, PDA, and ASD) Short sternum, small nipples
Extremities	Overlapping of fingers and toes (clinodactyly) Polydactyly Hypoplastic nails, hyperconvex nails	Limited hip abduction Clinodactyly and overlapping fingers; index over third, fifth over fourth Rocker-bottom feet Hypoplastic nails
General	Severe developmental delays, fetal growth restriction, and postnatal growth faltering Renal abnormalities Nuclear projections in neutrophils Approximately 11% live >1 yr	Severe developmental delays, fetal growth restriction, and postnatal growth faltering Premature birth, polyhydramnios Inguinal or abdominal hernias Approximately 13% live >1 year

ASD, Atrial septal defect; *PDA*, patent ductus arteriosus; *VSD*, ventricular septal defect.

testicular tissue, coupled with in vitro fertilization and intracytoplasmic sperm injection, it is possible for men with KS to father children; all children born to these men using this technology have had a normal chromosome complement.

Monosomies

Turner Syndrome

TS is the only condition in which a monosomic conceptus survives to term; however, an estimated more than 90% of embryos with 45,X are spontaneously aborted. TS is seen in up to 10% of first trimester pregnancy losses. Occurring in 1 in 2,000–2,500 liveborn females, TS is notable for its relatively mild phenotype. Affected women tend to have typical intelligence and normal life expectancy.

Females with TS have a characteristic facial appearance with low-set, mildly malformed ears, triangular face, flattened nasal bridge, and epicanthal folds. There may be webbing of the neck, with or without cystic hygroma, a shieldlike chest with widened internipple distance, and puffiness of the hands and feet. Internal malformations may include congenital heart defect in 45% (bicuspid aortic valve is most common followed by coarctation of the aorta; later in life, post-stenotic aortic dilatation with aneurysm may develop). Kidney anomalies, including horseshoe kidney, are seen in more than 50% of affected individuals. Short stature is a cardinal feature of this condition, and acquired hypothyroidism is estimated to occur five times more frequently in women with TS than in the general population.

The presence of **streak gonads** (gonadal dysgenesis) instead of well-developed ovaries leads to estrogen deficiency, which often results in incomplete development of secondary sex characteristics and amenorrhea. Although 10% of females with TS may have normal pubertal development and are even fertile, most affected females require estrogen replacement to complete secondary sexual development.

Infertility in females with TS is not corrected by estrogen replacement. Assisted reproductive technology using donor ova has permitted females with TS to bear children. During pregnancy, these females must be followed carefully because post-stenotic dilatation of the aorta, leading to dissecting aneurysm, may occur.

Females with TS may not be detected during the newborn period because phenotypic features are subtle. Some are diagnosed in childhood during a work-up for short stature (for which they may receive growth hormone therapy); others are diagnosed during adolescence or adulthood when they fail to develop secondary sexual characteristics or during work-ups for infertility.

The karyotypic spectrum in patients with TS is wide. Approximately 50% have a 45,X karyotype; another 30–40% are mosaic (45,X/46,XX or 45,X/46,XY). The remainder have structural X chromosome abnormalities involving a deletion of a portion of one X chromosome. Deletions involving the short (p) arm of the X chromosome (Xp22) produce short stature and congenital malformations, whereas deletions of the long arm (Xq) cause gonadal dysgenesis.

Although monosomy X is caused by nondisjunction, TS is not associated with advanced maternal age. Rather, it is believed that the 45,X karyotype results from a loss of either an X or a Y chromosome after conception; that is, it is a postconceptional mitotic (rather than meiotic) nondisjunctional event.

SYNDROMES INVOLVING CHROMOSOMAL DELETIONS

Cri du Chat Syndrome

A deletion in the short arm of chromosome 5 is responsible for **cri du chat syndrome**, with its characteristic catlike cry during infancy, the result of tracheal hypoplasia. Other clinical features include low birthweight, postnatal growth faltering, hypotonia, developmental disability, microcephaly, and craniofacial dysmorphism, including ocular hypertelorism, epicanthal folds, downward obliquity of the palpebral fissures, and low-set malformed ears. Clefts of the lip and palate, congenital heart disease, and other malformations may be seen.

The clinical severity of cri du chat syndrome depends on the size of the deletion, with larger deletions associated with more severe expression. Most cases arise de novo, with rare cases related to a balanced reciprocal chromosome translocation in a parent. When it arises de novo, the deletion is usually in chromosome 5 inherited from the father.

Williams Syndrome

Caused by a 1.55 megabase deletion in chromosome 7q11.2 that contains at least 28 genes, Williams syndrome is associated with a unique phenotype. Features associated with the condition include congenital heart disease (in 80%), with supravalvar aortic stenosis being the most common anomaly; growth delay with short stature; a distinctive facial appearance, with median flare of the eyebrows, fullness of the perioral and periorbital region, blue irides with a stellate pattern of pigment, and depressed nasal bridge with anteversion of the nares; moderate intellectual disability (average intelligence quotient 57) with strengths in personal social skills and deficiencies in cognitive areas; and hypercalcemia (in ~20%).

Individuals with Williams syndrome often have a striking personality. Loquacious and gregarious, they are often described as having a *cocktail party* personality. However, at least 10% of children with Williams syndrome have features of autism spectrum disorder. Patients occasionally have unusual musical ability. Most children with Williams syndrome have a de novo deletion. In rare cases, the deletion is inherited from a parent in an autosomal dominant pattern.

Aniridia Wilms Tumor Association

WAGR syndrome (**W**ilms tumor, **a**niridia, **g**enitourinary anomalies, and a **r**ange of intellectual disabilities) is caused by a deletion of 11p13. The deletion usually arises de novo, with rare cases being associated with a balanced translocation in one of the parents. Genitourinary abnormalities include cryptorchidism and hypospadias. Patients often have short stature, and 50% have microcephaly. Wilms tumor develops in 50% of patients with WAGR syndrome (see Chapter 160).

Prader-Willi Syndrome

See Chapter 46.

Angelman Syndrome

See Chapter 46.

Chromosome 22q11.2 Deletion Syndrome (22q11DS)

Deletions of chromosome 22q11.2 are responsible for a group of findings that have been called by several names, including ***velocardiofacial syndrome***, ***conotruncal anomaly face syndrome***, ***Shprintzen syndrome***, and ***DiGeorge syndrome***. These conditions represent a continuum of findings, virtually all of which are due to the same chromosomal deletion.

Although 22q11DS can be inherited in an autosomal dominant fashion, most cases arise de novo. Common features include clefting of the palate with velopharyngeal insufficiency, conotruncal cardiac defects (including truncus arteriosus, ventriculoseptal defect, tetralogy of Fallot, interrupted aortic arch, and right-sided aortic arch), and a facial appearance characterized by a prominent nose and broad nasal root. Speech and language difficulties are common, as is mild intellectual impairment. More than 200 additional abnormalities have been identified in individuals with these conditions. About 70% have immunodeficiency, largely related to T-cell dysfunction. A wide spectrum of psychiatric disturbances, including schizophrenia and bipolar disorder, has been seen in at least one-third of affected adults.

Damage to the third and fourth pharyngeal pouches, embryonic structures that form parts of the cranial portion of the developing embryo, leads to abnormalities in the developing face (clefting of the palate, micrognathia), the thymus gland, the parathyroid glands, and the conotruncal region of the heart. This spectrum of findings, called the ***DiGeorge malformation*** sequence, is an important part of 22q11DS.

Confirmation of the deletion requires either fluorescence in situ hybridization or chromosomal microarray analysis. The region, composed of about 3 million bases, contains between 30 and 40 genes. Although many of these deleted genes probably contribute to the phenotype, special attention has been focused on *TBX1* and *COMT*, which are believed to be responsible for many of the features of the condition.

SYNDROMES INVOLVING CHROMOSOME DUPLICATION

Duplications and deletions occur secondary to misalignment and unequal crossing over during meiosis. Small extra chromosomes are found in a small percentage of the population. These "marker" chromosomes may be associated with intellectual disabilities and other abnormalities, but they often have no apparent phenotypic effects.

Inverted Duplication Chromosome 15

Chromosome 15 is the most common of all marker chromosomes, and its inverted duplication accounts for almost 40% of this group of chromosomal abnormalities. Features seen in children with 47,XX,+inv dup (15q) or 47,XY,+inv dup (15q) depend on the size of the extra chromosomal material present: the larger the region, the worse the prognosis. Common features seen include varying degrees of developmental disability, autism spectrum disorders, seizures, and behavioral issues. Minimal dysmorphic features may be seen, including a sloping forehead, short and downward-slanting palpebral fissures, a prominent nose with a broad nasal bridge, a long and well-defined philtrum, a midline crease in the lower lip, and micrognathia.

Cat-Eye Syndrome

Named for the iris coloboma that gives patients' eyes a catlike appearance, cat-eye syndrome is caused by the presence of a small extra chromosome composed of an inversion duplication of 22q11. The two copies of 22q11 on this extra chromosome plus the two normal copies of chromosome 22 result in four copies of this region. Although the colobomas name the syndrome, they occur in fewer than 50% of individuals with the marker chromosome. Other clinical features include mild intellectual disability, behavioral disturbances, ocular hypertelorism, downward-slanting palpebral fissures, micrognathia, preauricular pits and/or tags, anal atresia with rectovestibular fistula, and renal agenesis.

PEARLS FOR PRACTITIONERS

See Human Genetics and Dysmorphology: Pearls for Practitioners at the end of this section.

REVIEW QUESTIONS

Available online.

CHAPTER 49

The Approach to the Dysmorphic Child

Dysmorphology is the study of congenital malformations and the recognition of patterns of malformations that occur in syndromes (Table 49.1).

Syndromes are collections of abnormalities, including **malformations**, **deformations**, dysmorphic features, and abnormal behaviors that result from a unifying, identifiable etiology. This etiology may be the presence of a pathogenic variant in a single gene, as is the case in **Rett syndrome**, a disorder caused by a pathogenic variant in *MECP2*, a gene on Xq28; by the deletion or duplication of genetic material, as in **Prader-Willi syndrome**, caused by the deletion of the paternal copy of the *SNRPN* gene on chromosome 15q11.2; or by exposure to a teratogenic substance during embryonic development, as in fetal alcohol spectrum disorder.

TABLE 49.1 Glossary of Selected Terms Used in Dysmorphology

TERMS PERTAINING TO THE FACE AND HEAD
Brachycephaly: Condition in which head shape is shortened from front to back along the sagittal plane; the skull is rounder than normal
Canthus: The lateral or medial angle of the eye formed by the junction of the upper and lower lids
Columella: The fleshy tissue of the nose that separates the nostrils
Glabella: Bony midline prominence of the brows
Nasal alae: The lateral flaring of the nostrils
Nasolabial fold: Groove that extends from the margin of the nasal alae to the lateral aspects of the lips
Ocular hypertelorism: Increased distance between the pupils of the two eyes
Palpebral fissure: The shape of the eyes based on the outline of the eyelids
Philtrum: The vertical groove in the midline of the face between the nose and the upper lip
Plagiocephaly: Condition in which head shape is asymmetric in the sagittal or coronal planes; can result from in utero or postnatal positioning, asymmetry in suture closure, or from asymmetry of brain growth
Scaphocephaly: Condition in which the head is elongated from front to back in the sagittal plane; most normal skulls are scaphocephalic
Synophrys: Eyebrows that meet in the midline
Telecanthus: A wide space between the medial canthi
TERMS PERTAINING TO THE EXTREMITIES
Brachydactyly: Condition of having short digits
Camptodactyly: Condition in which a digit is bent or fixed in the direction of flexion (a "trigger finger"–type appearance)
Clinodactyly: Condition in which a digit is crooked and curves toward or away from adjacent digits
Hypoplastic nail: An unusually small nail on a digit
Melia: Suffix meaning "limb" (e.g., amelia—missing limb; brachymelia—short limb)
Polydactyly: The condition of having six or more digits on an extremity
Syndactyly: The condition of having two or more digits at least partially fused (can involve any degree of fusion, from webbing of skin to full bony fusion of adjacent digits)

DEFINITIONS

Congenital **malformations** are defined as clinically significant abnormalities in either form or function that are identifiable at birth. About 3% of live births have congenital malformations.

They result from localized **intrinsic** defects in morphogenesis, which were caused by an event that occurred in embryonic or early fetal life. This event may have been a disturbance of development from some unknown cause, but often pathogenic variants in developmental genes lead to the abnormality. **Extrinsic** factors may cause **disruptions** of development resulting from disturbances to the development of apparently normal tissues. These disruptions may include amniotic bands, disruption of blood supply to developing tissues, or exposure to teratogens. A **malformation sequence** is a spectrum of abnormalities, including malformations, deformations, and disruptions that result from the effects of a single malformation. For instance, in the **Pierre Robin sequence**, a primary malformation, the failure of growth of the mandible during the first weeks of gestation results in micrognathia, which forces the normal-sized tongue into an unusual position. The abnormally positioned tongue blocks the fusion of the palatal shelves, which normally come together in the midline to produce the hard and soft palate; this leads to the presence of a U-shaped cleft palate. After delivery, the normal-sized tongue in the smaller-than-normal sized oral cavity leads to airway obstruction, a potentially life-threatening complication.

Malformation sequences can occur alone or may be part of a multiple malformation syndrome. For instance, individuals with Pierre Robin sequence may have it as part of **Stickler syndrome**, an autosomal dominant disorder caused by pathogenic variants in collagen genes. Stickler syndrome also manifests with ocular and musculoskeletal abnormalities.

Deformations arise as a result of environmental forces acting on normal structures. They occur later in pregnancy or after delivery. For instance, **plagiocephaly** (rhomboid-shaped head) may result from intrauterine positioning or from torticollis experienced in the newborn period. Deformations often resolve with minimal intervention, but malformations often require surgical and medical management.

Minor malformations, variants of normal that occur in less than 3% of the population, include findings such as single transverse palmar creases, low-set ears, or ocular hypertelorism (wide-spaced eyes); when isolated, they have no clinical significance. A **multiple malformation syndrome**

is the recognizable pattern of anomalies that results from a single identifiable underlying cause. It may involve a series of malformations, malformation sequences, and deformations. These syndromes often prompt a consultation with a clinical geneticist.

An **association** is a recognizable pattern of anomalies that occur together more often than would be expected by chance alone, but no single underlying etiology has been identified. The **VACTERL** association (**v**ertebral anomalies, **a**nal atresia, **c**ardiac defects, **t**racheo**e**sophageal fistula, **r**enal anomalies, and **l**imb anomalies) is an example of a group of malformations that occur more commonly together than might be expected by chance. No single unifying etiology explains this condition, so it is considered an association.

HISTORY AND PHYSICAL EXAMINATION

Pregnancy History

The history of the pregnancy and birth can reveal multiple factors that may prove helpful to the dysmorphologist. Infants who are small for gestational age may have a chromosome anomaly or may have been exposed to a teratogen. Large for gestational age infants may be infants of diabetic mothers or have an overgrowth syndrome, such as Beckwith-Wiedemann syndrome. When evaluating an older child with intellectual disabilities, complications of extreme prematurity may account for the child's problems. Postmaturity also is associated with some chromosome anomalies (e.g., trisomy 18) and anencephaly. Infants born from breech presentation are more likely to have congenital malformations than those born from vertex presentation.

As a female gets older, there is increased risk of nondisjunction leading to trisomies. Advanced paternal age may be associated with the risk of a new pathogenic variant leading to an autosomal dominant trait. Maternal medical problems and exposures (medications, drugs, cigarette smoking, and alcohol use) are associated with malformations (see Chapters 47 and 58).

An increased amount of amniotic fluid may be associated with intestinal obstruction or a central nervous system anomaly that leads to poor swallowing. A decreased amount of fluid may be the result of a chronic amniotic fluid leak or a congenital anomaly of the kidney and urinary tract that results in a failure to produce urine.

Family History

A pedigree comprising at least three generations should be constructed, searching for similar or dissimilar abnormalities in first- and second-degree relatives. A history of pregnancy or neonatal losses should be documented. For a more detailed discussion of pedigrees, see Chapter 46.

Physical Examination

When examining children with dysmorphic features, the following approach should be used.

Growth

The height (length), weight, and head circumference should be measured carefully and plotted on appropriate growth curves.

The clinician should note if the child is proportionate. Limbs that are too short for the head and trunk imply the presence of a short-limbed bone dysplasia, such as achondroplasia. A trunk and head that are too short for the extremities suggest a disorder affecting the vertebrae, such as spondyloepiphyseal dysplasia. Children who are much taller or much shorter than predicted from their parents' height may suggest a genetic syndrome such as an overgrowth syndrome, skeletal dysplasia, or a genetic syndrome with short stature.

Craniofacial

Careful examination of the head and face is crucial for the diagnosis of many congenital malformation syndromes. Head shape should be carefully assessed; if the head is not normal in size and shape (normocephalic), it may be long and thin (**dolichocephalic**), short and wide (**brachycephalic**), or asymmetric or lopsided (**plagiocephalic**).

Any asymmetry of facial features should be noted. Asymmetry may be due to a deformation related to intrauterine position or a malformation of one side of the face. The face should be divided into four regions, which are evaluated separately. The **forehead** may show overt prominence, as with achondroplasia (often described as a sloping appearance, which occurs in children with primary microcephaly). The **midface**, extending from the eyebrows to the upper lip and from the outer canthi of the eyes to the commissures of the mouth, is especially important. Careful assessment of the distance between the **eyes** (inner canthal distance) and the pupils (interpupillary distance) may confirm the impression of hypotelorism (eyes that are too close together), which suggests a defect in midline brain formation, or **hypertelorism** (eyes that are too far apart). The length of the palpebral fissure should be noted and may help define whether the opening for the eye is short, as is found with fetal alcohol syndrome, or excessively long, as in **Kabuki syndrome** (short stature, intellectual disability, long palpebral fissures with eversion of lateral portion of lower lid).

Other features of the eyes should be noted. The obliquity (slant) of the palpebral fissures may be upward (as seen with Down syndrome) or downward (as in Treacher Collins syndrome). The presence of epicanthal folds (Down syndrome and fetal alcohol syndrome) is also important. Features of the **nose**—especially the nasal bridge, which can be flattened in Down syndrome, fetal alcohol syndrome, and many other syndromes, or prominent as in velocardiofacial (22q11 deletion) syndrome—should be noted.

The **malar** region of the face is examined next. It extends from the ear to the midface. The ears should be checked for size (measured and checked against appropriate growth charts), shape, position (low-set ears are below a line drawn from the inner canthus to the occiput), and orientation (posterior rotation is where the ear appears turned toward the rear of the head). Ears may be low set because they are small (or microtic) or because of a malformation of the mandibular region.

The **mandibular region** is the area from the lower portion of the ears bounded out to the chin by the mandible. In most newborns, the chin is often slightly retruded (i.e., slightly behind the vertical line extending from the forehead to the philtrum). If this retrusion is pronounced, the child may have the Pierre Robin malformation sequence. In addition, the mouth should be examined. The number and appearance of the teeth should be noted, the tongue should be observed for abnormalities, and the palate and uvula checked for defects.

Neck

Examination of the neck may reveal webbing, a common feature in Turner and Noonan syndromes, or shortening, as is seen occasionally in some skeletal dysplasias and in conditions in which anomalies of the cervical spine occur, such as Klippel-Feil syndrome. The position of the posterior hairline also should be evaluated. The size of the thyroid gland should be assessed.

Trunk

The chest may be examined for shape (shieldlike chest in Noonan and Turner syndromes) and for symmetry. The presence of a pectus deformity should be noted and is common in Marfan syndrome. The presence of scoliosis should be assessed; it is common in Marfan syndrome and many other syndromes.

Extremities

Many congenital malformation syndromes are associated with anomalies of the extremities. All joints should be examined for range of motion. The presence of single or multiple joint contractures suggests either intrinsic neuromuscular dysfunction, as in some forms of muscular dystrophy, or external deforming forces that limited motion of the joint in utero. Multiple contractures also are found with **arthrogryposis multiplex congenita** and are due to a variety of causes. **Radioulnar synostosis**, an inability to pronate or supinate the elbow, occurs in fetal alcohol spectrum disorder and in some chromosomal disorders.

Examination of the hands is important. **Polydactyly** (the presence of extra digits) usually occurs as an isolated autosomal dominant trait but also can be seen in trisomy 13. **Oligodactyly** (a deficiency in the number of digits) is seen in Fanconi anemia (see Chapter 151) in which it is generally part of a more severe limb reduction defect or secondary to intrauterine amputation, which may occur with amniotic band disruption sequence. **Syndactyly** (a joining of two or more digits) is common to many syndromes, including Smith-Lemli-Opitz syndrome.

Dermatoglyphics include palmar crease patterns. A transverse palmar crease, indicative of hypotonia during early fetal life, is seen in approximately 50% of children with Down syndrome (and 10% of individuals in the general population). A characteristic palmar crease pattern is also seen in fetal alcohol spectrum disorder.

Genitalia

Genitalia should be examined closely for abnormalities in structure. In males, if the penis appears short, it should be measured and compared with known age-related data. Ambiguous genitalia often are associated with endocrinologic disorders, such as congenital adrenal hyperplasia, or chromosomal disorders such as 45,X/46,XY mosaicism or possibly secondary to a multiple congenital anomaly syndrome (see Chapter 178). Although hypospadias is a common congenital malformation that often occurs as an isolated defect, if it is associated with other anomalies, especially cryptorchidism, there is a strong possibility of a syndrome.

LABORATORY EVALUATION

Chromosome analysis should be ordered for children with multiple congenital anomalies, the involvement of one major organ system and the presence of multiple dysmorphic features, or the presence of intellectual disability. *Microarray comparative genomic hybridization has supplanted routine or high-resolution chromosome analysis in most situations.* For a complete discussion of chromosome analysis, see Chapter 47.

Radiologic imaging plays an important role in the evaluation of children with dysmorphic features. Individuals found to have multiple external malformations should have a careful evaluation to search for the presence of internal malformations. Testing includes **ultrasound exams** of the head and abdomen to look for anomalies in the brain, kidney, bladder, liver, and spleen. **Skeletal radiographs** should be performed if there is concern about a possible skeletal dysplasia. The presence of a heart murmur should trigger a cardiology consultation; an **electrocardiogram** and **echocardiogram** may be indicated. **MRI** may be indicated in children with neurologic abnormalities or a spinal defect. Suspicion of craniosynostosis may warrant a **CT scan** of the head.

For those patients for whom testing does not yield a diagnosis, exome sequencing or whole genome sequencing are powerful tools.

DIAGNOSIS

Although the presence of characteristic findings may make the diagnosis of a multiple malformation syndrome straightforward, in most cases no specific diagnosis is immediately evident. Some constellations of findings are rare and finding a "match" may prove difficult. In many cases, all laboratory tests are normal, and confirmation relies on subjective findings. Clinical geneticists have attempted to resolve this difficulty by developing scoring systems, cross-referenced tables of anomalies that help in the development of a differential diagnosis, and computerized diagnostic programs.

An accurate diagnosis offers an explanation to the family why their child was born with congenital anomalies. This may help allay guilt for parents, who often believe they are responsible for their child's medical problems. A diagnosis facilitates screening for medical problems associated with a particular syndrome and provides reassurance that other medical problems are no more likely to occur than they might with other children who do not have the diagnosis. It permits genetic counseling to be done to identify the risk to future children and permits prenatal testing to be done for the disorders for which it is available. Diagnosis enables the clinician to provide the family with educational materials about the diagnosis and facilitate contact with support groups for particular disorders. The Internet has become an important source for such information. A good site is the National Organization for Rare Disorders (http://www.rarediseases.org), a clearinghouse for information about rare diseases and their support groups.

PEARLS FOR PRACTITIONERS

See Human Genetics and Dysmorphology: Pearls for Practitioners at the end of this section.

REVIEW QUESTIONS

Available online.

Suggested Readings

Bull MJ, Trotter T, Santoro SL, et al. Health Supervision for Children and Adolescents With Down Syndrome. *Pediatrics.* 2022;149(5):e2022057010.

ENCODE Project Consortium. An integrated encyclopedia of DNA elements in the human genome. *Nature.* 2012;489(7414):57–74.

Gjorgioski S, Halliday J, Riley M, Amor DJ, Delatycki MB, Bankier A. Genetics and pediatric hospital admissions, 1985 to 2017. *Genet Med.* 2020;22(11):1777–1785.

Gravholt CH, Andersen NH, Conway GS, et al. Clinical practice guidelines for the care of girls and women with Turner syndrome: proceedings from the 2016 Cincinnati International Turner Syndrome Meeting. *Eur J Endocrinol.* 2017;177(3):G1–G70.

Hersh JH, Saul RA. Committee on Genetics. Health supervision for children with fragile X syndrome. *Pediatrics.* 2011;127(5):994–1006.

Jones KL, Jones MC, del Campo M. *Smith's Recognizable Patterns of Human Malformation.* 8th ed. Philadelphia: Elsevier; 2022.

Miller DT, Freedenberg D, Schorry E, et al. Health Supervision for Children With Neurofibromatosis Type 1. *Pediatrics.* 2019;143(5):e20190660.

Morris CA, Braddock SR. COUNCIL ON GENETICS. Health Care Supervision for Children With Williams Syndrome. *Pediatrics.* 2020;145(2):e20193761.

Online Mendelian Inheritance in Man (website) http://www.ncbi.nlm.nih.gov/sites/entrez?db=omim.PubMed

Óskarsdóttir S, Boot E, Crowley TB, et al. Updated clinical practice recommendations for managing children with 22q11.2 deletion syndrome. *Genet Med.* 2023;25(3):100338.

PEARLS FOR PRACTITIONERS

CHAPTER 46

Patterns of Inheritance

DNA Basics

- The four DNA nucleotides—adenine, guanine, thymine, and cytosine—are linked together to form a DNA strand.
- Two strands form a DNA molecule.
- Pyrimidines (thymine and cytosine) are cross-linked to purines (adenosine and guanine) by hydrogen bonds.
- Chromosomes are strands of DNA wound tightly with a protein skeleton (chromatin) and histones.
- Human cells have 23 pairs of chromosomes, one set of 23 from each parent.
- Twenty-two of the chromosomes are autosomes, and the 23rd pair are the sex chromosomes. Females have two X chromosomes (46,XX), and males have one X chromosome and one Y chromosome (46,XY) unless a sex chromosome anomaly is present.
- Genes are stretches of DNA that code for a protein. A typical gene has a promoter sequence, an untranslated region, and an open reading frame.
- Every three nucleotides represent a single codon that codes for a particular amino acid.
- Some codons act as a start signal and others as a stop signal for transcription.
- Within the gene there are regions—exons—that code for the sequence of the protein, and introns, which are not incorporated into the transcribed messenger RNA (mRNA) but may have important regulatory roles.
- Less than 2% of the 3.1 million DNA bases code for proteins. These regions represent about 20,000–24,000 genes. Alternative splicing of the transcribed mRNA can generate a possible 100,000 proteins.
- Changes in the DNA sequence (variants) can lead to changes in the amino acid in a protein (missense variant) or to a premature stop codon (nonsense variant).
- A third change in the DNA is a frameshift variant, which is the result of the addition or deletion of one or more DNA bases that "shift" the reading frame of the codons, usually resulting in production of a new stop codon that is before the end of the gene and is considered "premature."

Pedigrees

- Pedigrees are symbolic depictions of a family's history with symbols for males (squares) and females (circles).
- Pedigrees permit a quick visual determination of an inheritance pattern in a family.

Autosomal Dominant Disorders

- Results from a nonworking copy of a gene on an autosome.
- Affected individuals have a 50% chance of passing the pathogenic variant on to each child.
- The phenomenon where some affected individuals show clinical symptoms while other affected individuals may not is called *penetrance.* Many autosomal dominant (AD) disorders can show decreased penetrance.
- Variable expressivity describes the phenomenon where different family members may vary in their clinical symptoms and the severity of those symptoms.
- Often, individuals with an AD disorder may have de novo pathogenic variants (they have unaffected parents).

Autosomal Recessive Disorders

- Results from two dysfunctional copies of a gene on an autosome.
- Affected individuals usually have unaffected parents, each of whom is a carrier for the disorder.

X-Linked Disorders (General)

- The X chromosome has approximately 900 genes, the Y about 100.
- Females randomly inactivate one of their X chromosomes (lyonization).

X-Linked Recessive Inheritance

- Most X chromosome disorders show recessive inheritance.
- Males, having one X chromosome, are more likely to manifest disease than females.

- Sons of carrier females have a 50% chance of being affected; daughters have a 50% chance of being a carrier.
- Daughters of affected males have a 50% chance of being a carrier; all sons are unaffected.

X-Linked Dominant

- Females with these disorders show symptoms.
- Females are usually less affected than males due to X chromosome inactivation.
- Some X-linked dominant disorders are lethal in males with death before birth.

Mitochondrial Inheritance

- Mitochondrial DNA (mtDNA) replicates independently from nuclear DNA.
- Virtually all mitochondria are supplied by the oocyte. Thus, disorders involving the mtDNA are maternally inherited.
- mtDNA has a few genes that code for respiratory complex proteins (most are coded on the nuclear DNA) and a set of tRNAs that are needed for protein synthesis within the mitochondria.
- There are many mitochondria in each cell. If the DNA is different in some of these mitochondria (two populations), this is referred to as *heteroplasmy.*
- Some disorders are due to loss or deficiency of mitochondria. This is referred to as *mitochondrial depletion.*

Uniparental Disomy

- Patients with uniparental disomy have a normal karyotype with a normal number of chromosomes.
- Both copies of the affected chromosome will come from one parent—without a copy from the other parent.
- Some genes are methylated ("inactivated") depending on their parental origin. Uniparental disomy might result in both copies of the gene being inappropriately activated or inactivated.

Multifactorial Inheritance

- Result from the interplay of genetic and environmental factors.
- About 20% of congenital malformations are due to multifactorial inheritance.
- Disorders include asthma, atherosclerosis, diabetes, and cancer.
- Do not follow Mendelian rules of inheritance but occur in first- and second-degree relatives more frequently than would be expected by chance and are more likely to be concordant in monozygotic twins than dizygotic twins.

Nucleotide Repeats

- Much of human DNA consists of two or three DNA bases repeated over and over.
- Some disorders are due to expansion of trinucleotide repeats (fragile X syndrome, Huntington disease, myotonic dystrophy, Friedreich ataxia, and the spinocerebellar ataxias).

Exposure to Teratogenic Agents

- Up to 15% of birth defects can be attributed to exposure to teratogens.
- Teratogens can be chemical, physical, or biologic.
- Examples include alcohol, infections, and lead.

CHAPTER 47

Genetic Assessment and Diagnosis

- Individuals referred to a geneticist because of suspicion of a genetic disease are called ***probands.***
- **Consultands** are individuals referred for genetic counseling.
- There are many reasons for referral to genetics. Referral may occur at different stages of life (fetus, neonate, childhood, pregnancy, or adulthood).

Preconception and Prenatal Counseling

- Families with relatives affected with a genetic disorder may wonder if their children are at risk.
- A family history may uncover a pattern of inheritance. A known disorder will have a pattern of inheritance that can be discussed with a geneticist or genetic counselor.
- **Consanguinity** is when couples are related. This increases the likelihood that offspring could be born with a rare autosomal recessive condition.
- Couples may be screened for disorders that affect their particular ethnic group (Western and sub-Saharan African ancestry may suggest screening for sickle cell, Mediterranean ancestry screening for thalassemia, Ashkenazi Jewish ancestry screening for Tay-Sachs, Gaucher).
- Next-generation sequencing has made screening for whole panels of genes relatively inexpensive.

Prenatal Screening and Prenatal Testing

- Screening helps identify an increased risk for an abnormality.
- Many pregnant people are screened to see if they are carriers for diseases such as sickle cell disease, cystic fibrosis, and spinal muscular atrophy (SMA).
- First trimester screening—a maternal blood test to measure PAPP-A (pregnancy-associated plasma protein A) and human chorionic gonadotropin (HCG) together with measurement of the fetus' nuchal (neck) fold by ultrasound—can be used to assess risk for chromosomal abnormality (Down syndrome) and possible cardiac abnormalities.
- Second trimester maternal serum screening (quad screen) measures MS AFP (maternal serum α-fetoprotein), uE3 (unconjugated estriol), inhibin A, and HCG.
- Diagnostic testing on cells from amniocentesis or chorionic villus sampling (CVS) may be suggested after abnormal prenatal screening results.
- Abnormalities on noninvasive prenatal screening (NIPS) with cffDNA from a maternal blood sample require confirmation either prenatally (via chorionic villus sampling or amniocentesis) or postnatally (via testing of infant's blood drawn after delivery).

Postnatal—Newborn and Infant

- Of newborns, 2–4% may have a genetic abnormality or "birth defect."
- This includes malformations (2–3%), inherited disorders (1%), and chromosomal abnormalities (0.5%).
- Consultation with a geneticist may be prompted by the presence of a malformation, abnormal newborn screening results, abnormalities of growth (poor weight gain, poor linear growth, poor head growth), developmental delay,

blindness or deafness, or a family history of a genetic disorder.

Adolescent and Adult

- Adolescents and adults may be referred for evaluation of a later onset genetic disorder. Many neurodegenerative disorders have onset later in life (e.g., Huntington disease, spinocerebellar ataxia, and spinal muscular atrophy).
- A family history of a hereditary cancer (breast, colon, thyroid) may also prompt an evaluation by a geneticist.

General Approach to Patients

- Family History
  - A pedigree is drawn to look for a pattern of inheritance.
  - If there is suspected new onset of an autosomal disorder, examine the parents carefully for signs of the disorder or consider targeted testing in parents.
  - If a de novo pathogenic variant, recurrence risk is about 1% due to gonadal mosaicism.
  - For prenatal counseling, the age of the couple is important. Increased paternal age has an increased risk for certain AD and X-linked disorders. Increased maternal age has an increased risk for chromosomal disorders.
- Pregnancy History
  - Exposure to teratogens (medications, alcohol, infections) can lead to malformations.
  - Poor fetal movement may suggest neurologic abnormalities.
  - A history of low or absent amniotic fluid (oligohydramnios) or high levels of amniotic fluid (polyhydramnios) may suggest neurologic, pulmonary, or kidney problems for the infant.
- Birth History
  - Premature infants have more complications than term infants.
  - The size of the infant—small for gestational age or large for gestational age—has implications for different genetic disorders.
  - Underlying disorders may predispose to a difficult delivery or resuscitation after birth.
- Medical History
  - Children with recurrent hospitalizations for vomiting and dehydration may suggest an inborn error of metabolism.
  - Children with neuromuscular disorders may have a normal period followed by increasing weakness or ataxia.
  - Children with lysosomal storage disorders will have worsening symptoms with increasing age, often having a history of frequent otitis media and growth issues, and they may develop sleep apnea.
  - Evaluation of growth may reveal poor prenatal and postnatal growth, good prenatal and poor postnatal growth, or acquired microcephaly or macrocephaly, all of which suggest different underlying genetic disorders.
- Development
  - Many genetic disorders are associated with delays in development.
  - Sometimes development is typical for a period of time, then slows, and is then followed by regression that can suggest a lysosomal storage disorder, inborn error of metabolism, or other genetic disorders.
- Physical Exam
  - A careful physical exam is necessary for all patients with signs, symptoms, or suspicion of genetic disease.
  - Dysmorphic features may suggest an underlying genetic syndrome.

Laboratory Evaluation

- Chromosome Analysis
  - Routine chromosome analysis during prophase was the standard way of analyzing chromosome number and large chromosome aberrations.
  - It remains the only way to identify balanced chromosome rearrangements.
  - Chromosomal microarray (array CGH) has supplanted routine cytogenetic techniques for chromosome analysis.
  - Fluorescence in situ hybridization (FISH) uses small DNA probes to identify copy number of common chromosome deletions. It is also helpful to determine complex chromosomal rearrangements.
- DNA Sequencing
  - Sequencing of genes involved in many genetic disorders is now often possible. Several websites offer assistance to find labs that do specific gene tests.
  - Sequencing can assess a single gene, a group of genes related to a patient's phenotype (panel testing), or can assess all of the exons contained in the 20,000–24,000 human genes (exome sequencing [ES]).
  - Whole genome sequencing (WGS) involves sequencing both the exonic and intronic regions of a patient's genome.
  - ES and WGS help identify potential causes for undiagnosed genetic disorders; however, analysis and interpretation are complex.

CHAPTER 48

Chromosomal Disorders

- Errors in meiosis lead to abnormalities of chromosome structure or number (aneuploidy).
- Common syndromes caused by abnormalities of chromosome number include the following: Down syndrome, trisomy 13, trisomy 18, Turner syndrome, and Klinefelter syndrome.

Down Syndrome

- Most common chromosome abnormality in liveborn infants.
- About 95% are due to nondisjunction, 3% are due to Robertsonian translocations—a fusion of two acrocentric chromosomes (most commonly chromosomes 21 and 14).
- Characteristic facial features, hypotonia, and congenital heart disease (40%) are noted in the neonatal period.

Trisomy 18

- Second most common autosomal trisomy.
- Most trisomy 18 conceptions end in spontaneous abortion.
- Less than 13% of those born will survive to 1 year of age.

Trisomy 13

- Usually fatal in the first year of life (11% survive).
- Small for gestational age, midline facial defects, postaxial polydactyly, clubfeet, scalp lesions (cutis aplasia).

Klinefelter

- 1:500 males
- Most common cause of infertility in males.
- Hypogonadism results in lack of secondary sexual characteristics.

Turner Syndrome

- Turner syndrome is the only monosomy that survives to term.
- Somewhat characteristic facial features, with webbed neck, shieldlike chest, and short stature. Coarctation of the aorta, horseshoe kidney, hypothyroidism, and infertility are also associated.

Cri du Chat

- Due to the partial deletion of the short arm of chromosome 5. Larger deletions are more severe.
- Catlike cry notable in infancy due to tracheal hypoplasia.

Williams Syndrome

- Deletion of 7q11.2
- Distinctive facial appearance, moderate intellectual disability, verbal skills above their deficiencies in other areas. Supravalvar aortic stenosis is associated.

22q11 Deletion Syndrome (DiGeorge, Velocardiofacial Syndrome)

- Cleft palate, velopharyngeal insufficiency.
- Conotruncal cardiac defects (truncus arteriosus, ventricular septal defect [VSD], tetralogy of Fallot).

CHAPTER 49

The Approach to the Dysmorphic Child

- Dysmorphology is the study of congenital malformations and the patterns of malformations that occur in syndromes.
- Syndromes are collections of abnormalities (malformations, deformations, dysmorphic features, and abnormal behaviors) that are associated with an identifiable etiology.
- Syndromes may be due to a pathogenic variant, a deletion or duplication of a chromosome, or from exposure to a teratogen.
- Congenital **malformations** that are the result of intrinsic defects in morphogenesis are identifiable at birth.
- **Deformations** are due to environmental forces acting on normal structures.
- An **association** is a pattern of anomalies with no clear underlying etiology that occurs more frequently than by chance alone.

History and Physical Examination

- Elements of the history and physical often provide information that leads to a diagnosis.
- Pregnancy
  - Growth of fetus (small or large for gestational age), premature or postmature, fetal movement, amount of amniotic fluid (oligohydramnios or polyhydramnios), exposure to drug and environmental toxins, maternal age
- Family History
  - Important clues about a pattern of inheritance can be determined from the family history.
- Physical Exam
  - Growth
    - Height, weight, and head circumference should be plotted on age-appropriate growth curves.
  - Craniofacial
    - Assess head shape, asymmetry.
    - Face can be divided into four regions (forehead, midface, malar, and mandibular), each of which requires close examination.
  - Neck
    - Length, webbing, posterior hairline, thyroid gland should be assessed.
  - Trunk
    - Chest shape—shieldlike, pectus deformity
    - Scoliosis
  - Extremities
    - Joints should be assessed for range of motion, contractures.
    - Number of fingers and toes, their size, and shape (polydactyly, oligodactyly, syndactyly)
  - Genitalia
    - Male, female, or ambiguous
    - Presence and size of testicles in males.

Laboratory Evaluation

- Chromosome analysis
  - Usually done by chromosomal microarray
- DNA analysis (sequencing)
  - For individual genes or sometimes panels of genes related to a family of disorders
- Exome sequencing and whole genome sequencing
  - Useful for undiagnosed disorders
- Radiologic imaging
  - Individuals with external malformations need a careful evaluation for internal malformations.
  - Ultrasound (head in neonates, abdomen, kidneys)
  - Skeletal radiographs for possible skeletal dysplasias, lysosomal storage disorders
  - MRI for children with possible neurologic abnormalities or spinal defects
  - CT of the skull for craniofacial abnormalities
- A genetic diagnosis is important for the following reasons:
  - Allays guilt of parents
  - Diagnosis with a particular disorder may permit screening for medical problems.
  - May permit treatment for disorder
  - Permits genetic counseling for future pregnancies

SECTION 10

METABOLIC DISORDERS

Donald Basel

CHAPTER 50

Metabolic Assessment

The most significant challenge to diagnosis of patients presenting with inborn errors of metabolism is consideration for the diagnosis itself. Optimal outcomes for children with inborn errors of metabolism (IEMs) depend upon recognition of the signs and symptoms of metabolic disease and prompt evaluation and referral to a center familiar with their management. Delayed diagnosis may result in end-organ damage including progressive neurologic injury or death.

With the exception of phenylketonuria (PKU) and medium-chain acyl-CoA dehydrogenase (MCAD) deficiency, most metabolic disorders are individually rare, with an incidence of less than 1 per 100,000 births in the United States. When considered collectively, the incidence may approach 1 in 800–2,500 births (Table 50.1); the prevalence of a confirmed metabolic disorder detected by newborn screening is 1 in 4,000 live births (about 12,500 diagnoses each year) in the United States. Not all IEMs are detected by newborn screening, which focuses on the relatively more common, treatable disorders.

IEMs are frequent causes of sepsis-like presentations, intellectual disability, seizures, sudden infant death, and neurologic impairment. There are at least 93 identified IEMs that are amenable to therapy targeted to the underlying cause, many of which can present with intellectual disability as a prominent feature. This number constantly evolves as small molecule and gene therapies rapidly advance to target these rare disorders.

Metabolic disorders can be classified using a variety of schemes based on the clinical presentation, including the age of onset, the tissues or organ systems involved, the defective metabolic pathways, or the subcellular localization of the underlying defect. These classification schemes have differing utility when considering the approach to diagnosis, management, and screening strategies. The clinical presentation and long-term prognosis have the most bearing on management of children with genetic metabolic disorders.

Genetic metabolic disorders result from the deficiency (or overactivity) of an enzyme, its cofactors, or biochemical transporters that lead to the deficiency of a required metabolite, the buildup of a toxic compound, or a combination of both processes (Fig. 50.1; Table 50.2). Understanding which of these mechanisms is involved and whether the effects are systemic or restricted to the local tissue enables a rational approach to diagnosis, therapy, and management.

When an IEM is identified or suspected, consultation with a medical geneticist is recommended. Long-term management of patients with IEMs may require frequent surveillance, diet, and medication adjustments and is best conducted by a center with experience treating IEMs.

TABLE 50.1 Estimates of Incidence of Various Classes of Disorders Diagnosed or Followed at Specialized Clinics Per 100,000 Population*

	BRITISH COLUMBIA 1969–1996	WEST MIDLANDS 1999–2003
Amino acid disorders (excluding phenylketonuria)	7.5	19
Lysosomal storage diseases	7.5	19
Phenylketonuria	7.5	8
Organic acidemias	4	12.5
Peroxisomal disorders	3.5	7.5
Mitochondrial diseases	3	20
Glycogen storage diseases	2	7
Urea cycle diseases	2	4.5

*Populations in British Columbia, Canada (a predominantly White population), between 1969 and 1996, and in the West Midlands of the United Kingdom (which has a diverse ethnic breakdown) between 1999 and 2003.

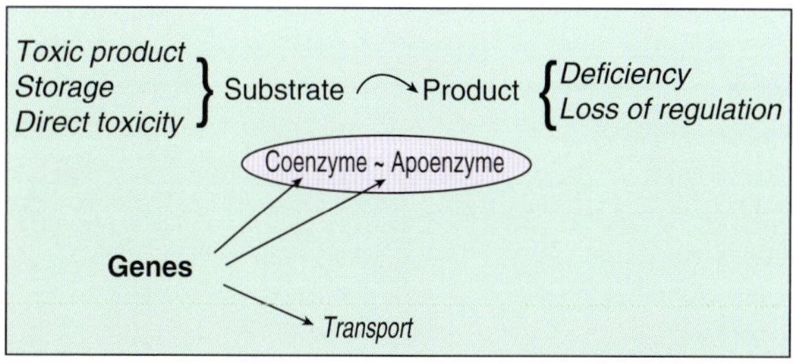

FIGURE 50.1 Depiction of the basic paradigm in inherited disorders of metabolism. Deficiency of an enzyme complex results in accumulation of metabolites proximal to the blocked metabolism and deficiency of the product of the reaction. Sites of genetic control are indicated.

TABLE 50.2 Primary Underlying Pathophysiologic Mechanisms for Select Metabolic Disorders

DISORDER	DEFICIENCY OF A REQUIRED COMPOUND	ACCUMULATION OF TOXIC COMPOUND	RESULT
HYPOGLYCEMIC DISORDERS			
Medium-chain fatty acid oxidation defects	Fat for energy		Use of glucose with consequent hypoglycemia
Long-chain fatty acid oxidation defects	Fat for energy	Long-chain fats	Use of glucose with consequent hypoglycemia; mitochondrial dysfunction in liver, heart, etc., leading to organ dysfunction
Glycogen storage disease	Glucose to prevent fasting hypoglycemia	Glycogen resulting in storage in liver, muscle, heart	Risk of hypoglycemic brain injury and dysfunction of tissue with storage
Ketone utilization disorders	Fat for energy	Ketones	Risk of hypoglycemic brain injury; profound metabolic acidosis and reversible neurologic dysfunction Cyclic vomiting
Galactosemia		Galactose-1-phosphate Galactitol	Elevated galactose leads to severe hepatic dysfunction, neurologic injury, and impaired immune response
INTOXICATING DISORDERS (ENCEPHALOPATHY)			
Urea cycle defects		Ammonia	Central nervous system dysfunction, probably mediated through glutamine
Propionic acidemia, methylmalonic acidemia, other organic acidemias		Organic acids	Systemic or local impairment of mitochondrial function; impaired neurotransmission; impairment of urea cycle
Phenylketonuria	Tyrosine	Phenylalanine	Impairment of tryptophan metabolism leading to serotonin deficiency; defective neurotransmission and white matter damage
Maple syrup urine disease		Leucine	Leucine toxicity leading to cerebral edema
CELLULAR COMPARTMENT DISORDERS			
Mitochondrial disease	Deficiency of ATP (energy) in affected tissues		Failure of affected tissues to carry out normal functions (e.g., muscle weakness, failure of relaxation of blood vessel muscles); failure of Cori cycle leading to lactate accumulation; cardiomyopathy
Peroxisomal disorders	Defect in peroxisomal β-oxidation Deficiency of steroid hormones necessary for signaling	Accumulation of the saturated very long-chain fatty acids	Aberrant embryonic patterning and hormone deficiency, defects in maintenance of myelin and white matter
Lysosomal storage disorders		Tissue-specific accumulation of compound not metabolized by lysosome	Cell type–specific damage and dysfunction as a result of lysosomal failure and reaction to waste product buildup
OTHER			
Disorders of creatine biosynthesis	Deficiency of cerebral creatine	Accumulation of guanidinoacetate in AGAT deficiency leads to seizures	Global brain energy defect leads to severe cognitive delays and seizures
Cholesterol biosynthesis disorders	Deficiency of steroid hormones		Endocrinopathies; disordered cellular signaling leading to aberrant organogenesis

AGAT, Arginine:glycine amidinotransferase deficiency; *ATP*, adenosine triphosphate.

SIGNS AND SYMPTOMS

The signs and symptoms of an inborn error are diverse and can involve any organ system. The presentation varies among age groups. IEMs often present within a few hours to weeks after birth and can mimic late-onset sepsis. Infants who survive the neonatal period without developing recognized symptoms often experience intermittent illness separated by periods of well-being. While pursuing the evaluation of the specific clinical presentations (e.g., the approach to the sick newborn, irritable child, or child with liver dysfunction), the hypoglycemic and intoxicating (encephalopathy) metabolic disorders should be considered in all neonates presenting with lethargy, poor tone, poor feeding, hypothermia, irritability, or seizures. In most cases, these should be evaluated by assessment of plasma ammonia, blood glucose, lactate, and anion gap (Fig. 50.2). Assessment of creatinine, transaminases, urine ketones, and blood counts may also be indicated. Significant ketosis in the neonate is unusual and suggests an organic acid disorder. Similarly, specific metabolic disorders predispose to cardiomyopathy, myopathy, liver dysfunction, developmental delay, seizures, sepsis, and developmental regression; appropriate evaluation should be tailored to the clinical presentation. When multiple organ systems are affected with typical complications, an IEM is more likely.

Figure 50.3 outlines a general diagnostic approach for a patient with unexplained developmental delay/intellectual disability. A useful mobile tool, "Treatable ID," has been developed as an app to aid identification and evaluation of treatable metabolic disorders; this is also accessible through a web interface: http://www.treatable-ID.org.

Obtaining a detailed history of events preceding the onset of symptoms is critical to making a diagnosis. Introduction of new foods or metabolic stress associated with fasting, serious infection, or fever may unmask an IEM during infancy or in older children. The introduction of fructose or sucrose in the diet may lead to decompensation in a child with hereditary fructose intolerance. In older children, increased protein intake may unmask disorders of ammonia detoxification (urea cycle disorders).

TYPES OF CLINICAL PRESENTATION OF INBORN ERRORS

Toxic Presentation

The toxic presentation often presents as an **encephalopathy**. Fever, infection, fasting, or other catabolic stresses may precipitate the symptom complex. **Metabolic acidosis**, vomiting, lethargy, and other neurologic findings may be present. Diagnostic testing is most effective when metabolites are present in highest concentration in blood and urine at presentation. Abnormal metabolism of amino acids, organic acids, ammonia, or carbohydrates may be at fault. **Hyperammonemia** is an important diagnostic possibility if an infant or child presents with features of toxic encephalopathy (see Fig. 50.2). Symptoms and signs depend on the underlying cause of the hyperammonemia, the age at which it develops, and the degree of hyperammonemia. Ammonia is a surrogate marker for metabolites such as CSF glutamine, which are believed to be responsible for the neurological effect of the disorders. The severity of hyperammonemia may provide a clue to the etiology (Tables 50.3 and 50.4). In infants and neonates, IEMs can present as a brief resolved unexplained event (BRUE), sudden infant death syndrome (very rare in general; consider if no newborn screening was performed), or fetal hydrops.

Severe Neonatal Hyperammonemia

Infants with genetic defects in urea synthesis or impaired synthesis of urea and glutamine secondary to genetic disorders of organic acid metabolism can have levels of blood ammonia more than 10 times normal (>1,000 µmol/L) in the neonatal period. Poor feeding, hypotonia, apnea, hypothermia, and vomiting rapidly give way to **coma** and occasionally to intractable seizures. *Respiratory alkalosis is common.* Severe cerebral edema leading to death occurs in hours to days if the condition remains untreated. The duration and severity of untreated hyperammonemia correlate with long-term neurologic outcomes.

Moderate Neonatal Hyperammonemia

Moderate neonatal hyperammonemia (200–400 µmol/L) is associated with depression of the central nervous system, poor feeding, and vomiting. Seizures are not characteristic. Respiratory alkalosis may occur. This type of hyperammonemia may be caused by partial or more distal blocks in urea synthesis and, commonly, is caused by disorders of organic acid metabolism (associated with a more prominent metabolic acidosis) that secondarily interfere with the elimination of nitrogen.

Clinical Hyperammonemia in Later Infancy and Childhood

Infants who are affected by defects in the urea cycle may continue to do well while receiving the low-protein intake of breast milk, developing clinical hyperammonemia when dietary protein is increased, or when catabolic stress occurs. Vomiting and lethargy may progress to coma. Seizures are not typical. During a crisis, the plasma ammonia level is usually 200–500 µmol/L. However, as the ammonia level decreases with decreased protein intake, the condition may go unrecognized for years, especially in the absence of specific central nervous system symptoms. If a crisis occurs during an epidemic of influenza, the child may be mistakenly thought to have **Reye syndrome** (acute noninflammatory encephalopathy with fatty liver failure that follows a viral illness). Older children may have neuropsychiatric or behavioral abnormalities (see Fig. 50.2). Adults may manifest after pregnancy (secondary to increased protein catabolism of placental tissue) or bariatric surgery.

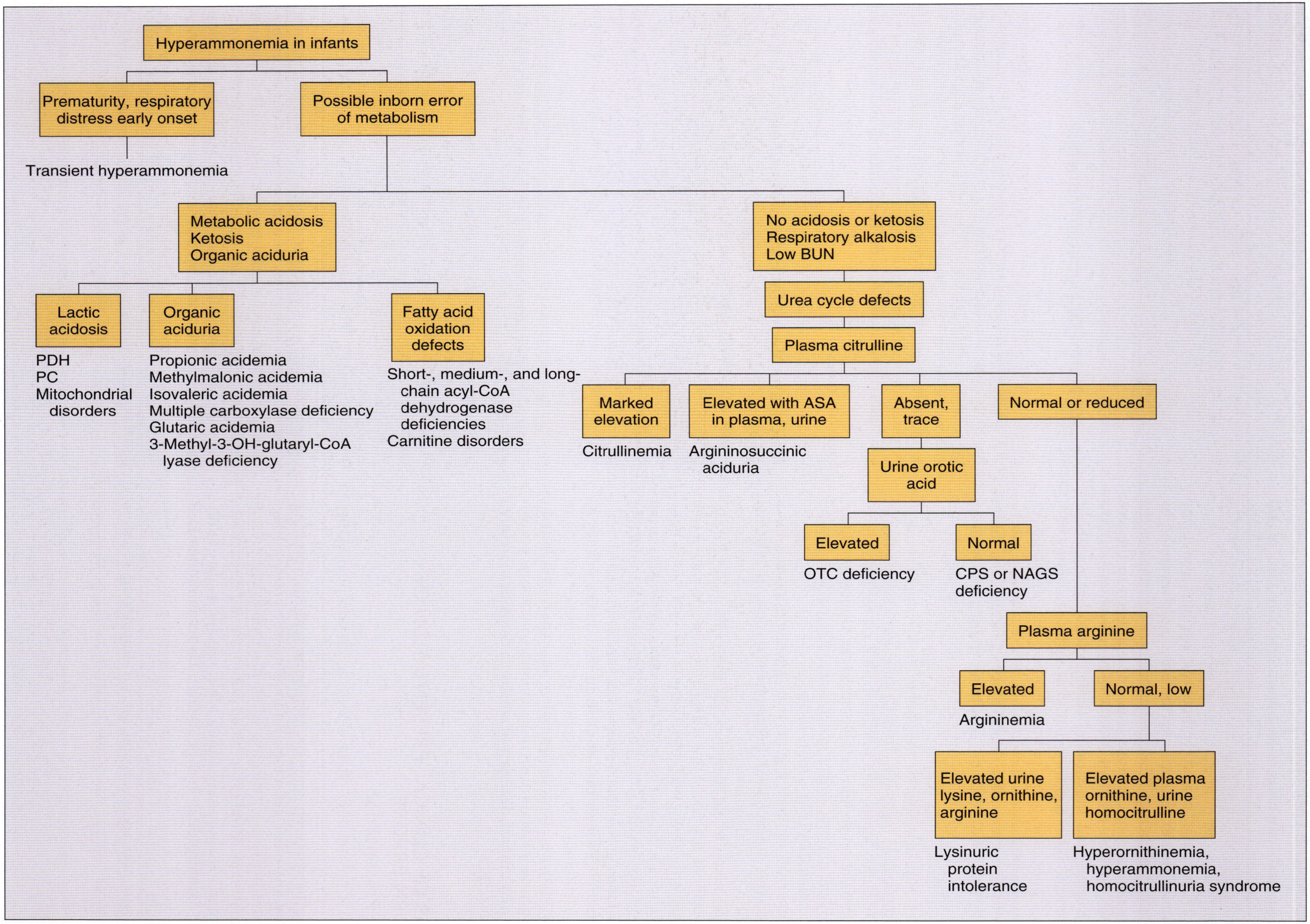

FIGURE 50.2 Algorithm for the approach to hyperammonemia infants. *ASA*, Argininosuccinic acid; *CoA*, coenzyme A; *CPS*, carbamylphosphate synthase; *NAGS*, N-acetylglutamate synthase; *OTC*, ornithine transcarbamylase; *PC*, pyruvate carboxylase deficiency; *PDH*, pyruvate dehydrogenase deficiency.

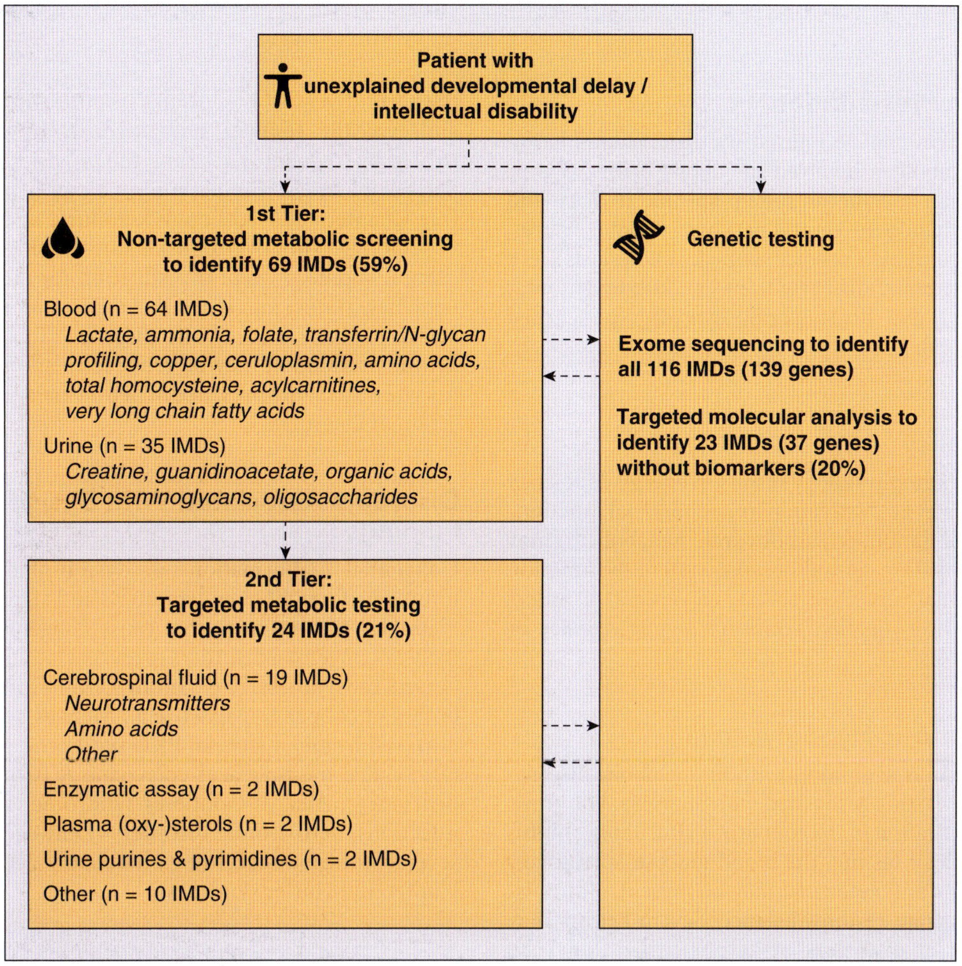

FIGURE 50.3 Diagnostic algorithm for treatable intellectual disabilities. First tier consists of non-targeted metabolic screening tests that are readily available in most developed countries. Second tier consists of targeted metabolic tests, often more invasive and/or less available. Some IMDs are identified by multiple (screening) tests in the first and second tiers. Genetic testing (targeted molecular analysis as well as exome sequencing) can be performed in parallel. *ID,* Intellectual disability; *IMD,* inherited metabolic disorder. (From Hoytema van Konijnenburg EMM, Wortmann SB, Koelewijn MJ, et al. Treatable inherited metabolic disorders causing intellectual disability: 2021 review and digital app. *Orphanet J Rare Dis.* 2021;16[1]:170; fig 1)

TABLE 50.3 Inborn Errors of Metabolism Presenting With Neurologic Signs in Infants Less Than 3 Months of Age

GENERALIZED SEIZURES	ENCEPHALOPATHIC COMA WITH OR WITHOUT SEIZURES
All disorders that cause hypoglycemia: • Most hepatic glycogen storage diseases • Galactosemia, hereditary fructose intolerance • Fructose-1,6-bisphosphatase deficiency • Disorders of fatty acid β-oxidation • Glucose transporter deficiency Disorders of the propionate pathway HMG-CoA lyase deficiency Menkes disease Primary mitochondrial disorders Maple syrup urine disease	Primary mitochondrial disorders Maple syrup urine disease Nonketotic hyperglycinemia Diseases producing extreme hyperammonemia: • Disorders of the urea cycle • Disorders of the propionate pathway Disorders of β-oxidation Congenital lactic acidosis Lysosomal storage disorders Congenital disorders of glycosylation
SEIZURES AND/OR POSTURING	
Nonketotic hyperglycinemia Maple syrup urine disease	

HMG-CoA, 3-hydroxy-3-methylglutaryl-CoA.

TABLE 50.4 Etiologies of Hyperammonemia in Infants

ETIOLOGY OF HYPERAMMONEMIA	COMMENTS
Disorders of the urea cycle	Lethal hyperammonemia is common
Disorders of the propionate pathway	Severe hyperammonemia may precede acidosis
Disorders of fatty acid catabolism and of ketogenesis	Reye-like syndrome possible
Transient neonatal hyperammonemia	Idiopathic, self-limited
Portal-systemic shunting	Thrombosis of portal vein, cirrhosis, hepatitis
Mitochondrial DNA depletion	Typically associated with elevated lactate level and other organ dysfunction
Drug intoxication: salicylate, valproic acid, acetaminophen	Obtain drug levels
Hyperinsulinism/hyperammonemia syndrome	Clinical hypoglycemia, subclinical hyperammonemia
Nonmetabolic liver disease including infections such as herpes, cytomegalovirus	Ensure evaluation of hepatic function and appropriate infectious disease work-up

Specific Organ Presentation

Any organ or system can be injured by toxic accumulation of any of the metabolites involved in inborn errors. Symptoms relate to organ-specific or system-specific toxicity and injury. Examples include the central nervous system (seizures, coma, ataxia), liver (hepatocellular damage, cholestasis), eye (cataracts, optic atrophy, dislocated lenses), kidney (tubular dysfunction, cysts), and heart (cardiomyopathy, pericardial effusion) (Table 50.5).

Energy Deficiency

Disorders whose pathophysiology results in energy deficiency (e.g., disorders of fatty acid oxidation, mitochondrial function/oxidative phosphorylation, or carbohydrate metabolism) may manifest with myopathy; central nervous system dysfunction including intellectual disability, ataxia, movement disorders and seizures; cardiomyopathy; vomiting; hypoglycemia; or renal tubular acidosis.

Ketosis and Ketotic Hypoglycemia

Acidosis is often found in children without metabolic diseases and may be due to fasting associated with anorexia, vomiting, diarrhea, and dehydration in the course of a viral illness. In this physiological result of fasting, the blood glucose is relatively low; a mild acidosis and ketonuria may be present. Administration of carbohydrate restores balance. Severe ketosis may also be the result of **disorders of ketone utilization** such as ketothiolase deficiency or succinyl-CoA:3 ketoacid CoA transferase (SCOT) deficiency. In these conditions, which frequently present in the context of fasting, infection with fever, or decreased intake secondary to vomiting and diarrhea, **hypoglycemia** may be profound; the ketosis resolves slowly. As ketone bodies accumulate, cyclic vomiting may ensue. Permanent ketosis is pathognomonic of SCOT deficiency. These disorders are very rare with fewer than 200 cases reported.

Ketotic hypoglycemia is a more common condition in which tolerance for fasting is impaired. Symptomatic hypoglycemia with seizures or coma occurs when the child encounters a catabolic stress. The hypoglycemia may occur with significant stress (e.g., viral infection with vomiting) or less commonly after minor stress (e.g., a prolongation by several hours of the normal overnight fast). Ketotic hypoglycemia first appears in the second year of life, occurs in otherwise healthy children, and typically resolves spontaneously by adolescence. It is treated by frequent snacks and the provision of glucose during periods of stress. The pathophysiology is poorly understood (see Chapter 173). Although ketonuria is a normal response to prolonged (not overnight) fasting in older infants and children, it should prompt investigation for metabolic disease in neonates. *A high anion gap metabolic acidosis with or without ketosis* suggests a metabolic disorder (Table 50.6). Although ketone production may be reduced in some fatty acid oxidation disorders, the presence of ketonuria does not exclude this group of disorders.

Disorders Associated With Dysmorphic Findings

Congenital malformations or dysmorphic features are not intuitively thought of as symptoms and signs of inborn errors. Examples of conditions that cause congenital malformations include congenital disorders of glycosylation, disorders of cholesterol biosynthesis (e.g., Smith-Lemli-Opitz syndrome), disorders of copper transport (e.g., Menkes syndrome, occipital horn syndrome), maternal PKU syndrome, glutaric aciduria II (also called multiple acyl-coenzyme A [CoA] dehydrogenase deficiency), Aicardi-Goutieres syndrome (mimics congenital infection), peroxisomal disorders (Zellweger syndrome), and several storage diseases (e.g., mucopolysaccharidoses such as Hunter and Hurler syndrome).

Storage Disorders

Storage disorders are caused by accumulation of incompletely metabolized macromolecules. This storage often occurs in subcellular organelles, such as lysosomes. The glycogen storage diseases (GSDs), Niemann-Pick disease, and mucopolysaccharidoses are examples of storage disorders.

CLINICAL ASSESSMENT AND LABORATORY TESTING

The assessment begins with a careful history (family and individual) and clinical evaluation. Clinical laboratory testing can define the metabolic derangement (Table 50.7). The results generate a differential diagnosis and a list of more specific laboratory testing to confirm the diagnosis.

TABLE 50.5 Inborn Errors of Metabolism Presenting With Hepatomegaly or Hepatic Dysfunction in Infants

HEPATOMEGALY	HEPATIC FAILURE	JAUNDICE
GSD I	Citrin deficiency Galactosemia	Citrin deficiency Galactosemia
GSD III	Hereditary fructose intolerance	Hereditary fructose intolerance
Mucopolysaccharidosis I and II	Tyrosinemia type 1 (fumarylacetoacetate hydrolase deficiency)	Infantile tyrosinemia (fumarylacetoacetate hydrolase deficiency)
Gaucher and Niemann-Pick diseases Congenital disorders of glycosylation Other lysosomal storage disorders	GSD IV (slowly evolving) Mitochondrial hepatopathies Congenital disorders of glycosylation Hemochromatosis	Crigler-Najjar disease Rotor, Dubin-Johnson syndromes Peroxisomal disorders Alagille syndrome Bile acid synthesis disorders

GSD, Glycogen storage disease.

TABLE 50.6 Etiologies of Metabolic Acidosis Caused by Inborn Errors of Metabolism in Infants

DISORDER	COMMENT
Methylmalonic acidemia (MMA)	Hyperammonemia, ketosis, neutropenia, thrombocytopenia
Propionic acidemia	Similar to MMA plus cardiomyopathy
Isovaleric acidemia	Odor of sweaty feet
Pyruvate dehydrogenase deficiency	Lactic acidosis, hyperammonemia, encephalopathy, seizures
Pyruvate carboxylase deficiency	Lactic acidosis, hypoglycemia, and ketosis
Respiratory chain (mitochondrial) disorders	Lactic acidosis, ketosis occasionally seen, multisystem dysfunction
Medium-chain acyl-CoA dehydrogenase deficiency (MCAD)	Moderate acidosis, hypoglycemia, decreased/ absent ketones, possible hyperammonemia
Other fatty acid oxidation defects	Similar to MCAD, with potential hepatic and cardiac disease
Galactosemia	Renal tubular acidosis, *Escherichia coli* neonatal sepsis, hypoglycemia
3-Hydroxy-3-methyl-glutaryl-CoA lyase deficiency	Severe lactic acidosis, hyperammonemia, hypoglycemia
Multiple acyl-CoA dehydrogenase deficiency (glutaric aciduria type II)	Metabolic acidosis, hypoglycemia, lethal kidney malformations
Hereditary fructose intolerance	Lactic acidosis, hypoglycemia, central nervous system depression, kidney and hepatic failure

TABLE 50.7 Initial Diagnostic Evaluation for a Suspected Inborn Error of Metabolism*

BLOOD AND PLASMA	URINE
Arterial blood gas	Glucose
Electrolytes—anion gap	pH
Glucose	Ketones
Ammonia	Reducing substances
Liver enzymes	Organic acids
Complete blood count, differential,† and platelet count	Acylglycines‡
Lactate, pyruvate	Orotic acid§
Amino acids	
Acylcarnitines	
Carnitine	

**Organ-specific evaluation is indicated for specific symptoms (e.g., cranial MRI for coma or seizures; echocardiography for cardiomyopathy/poor perfusion; quantitative paired plasma/cerebrospinal fluid amino acids if nonketotic hyperglycemia is suspected).*
†Thrombocytopenia and neutropenia are seen in organic acidurias; vacuolated lymphocytes and metachromatic granules are seen in lysosomal disorders.
‡When disorders of fatty acid oxidation are being considered.
§When urea cycle disorders are being considered.

The combination of symptoms and abnormal clinical laboratory findings demands urgent metabolic evaluation. A metabolic emergency often presents with vomiting, acidosis, hypoglycemia, ketosis (or *lack of appropriate ketosis*), intercurrent infection, anorexia/failure to feed, lethargy proceeding to coma, seizures, and hyperventilation or hypoventilation. Clinical evaluation should focus on the cardiac, kidney, hepatic, hematologic, neurologic, and developmental assessment specifically looking for changes in mental status, seizures, abnormal tone or movements, visual symptoms or presymptomatic retinal disease, global developmental delay, loss of developmental milestones (regression), short stature/ chondrodysplasia, micro- or macrocephaly, cardiomyopathy, cardiac failure, liver failure, bone marrow suppression, hepatosplenomegaly, cystic kidney malformation, and renal tubular dysfunction.

Clinical laboratory testing should begin with tests that are available in most hospital clinical laboratories. Care in the collection and handling of laboratory specimens is crucial to obtaining accurate results. Plasma measurements of lactate and ammonia are particularly subject to false elevations if not handled correctly (prolonged tourniquet time, non–free-flowing sample, sample not stored on ice or not processed immediately). Significant ketosis in the neonate is unusual and suggests an organic acid disorder. Ketosis out of proportion to fasting status in an older child occurs in disorders of ketone utilization. Lack of severe ketosis in an older child under conditions of metabolic stress is a feature of fatty acid oxidation disorders or hyperinsulinemic hypoglycemia syndromes. In some disorders, such as urea cycle disorders, ketone utilization disorders, milder forms of fatty acid oxidation defects, and intermittent maple syrup urine disease (MSUD), the laboratory abnormalities may be absent *except* during an acute presentation. Therefore normal testing in the well state does not rule out a metabolic disorder. In such cases molecular genetic testing may be the best way to make a diagnosis.

GENETIC ASPECTS OF INBORN ERRORS

Mechanisms of Inheritance

Most IEMs are autosomal recessive. Isolation or founder effect may make a specific recessive condition more prevalent in some populations (e.g., MSUD in the Old Order Mennonite population in Pennsylvania, tyrosinemia type 1 in the French-Canadian population in Quebec). X-linked conditions exhibit severe and early presentations in males. In general, carriers of recessive or X-linked diseases are usually asymptomatic. However, in ornithine transcarbamylase (OTC; also known as ornithine carbamoyltransferase) deficiency or Fabry disease, XX heterozygous individuals can be symptomatic if they have a low proportion of unaffected cells (unfavorably skewed X inactivation). Most mitochondrial disorders in children are a result of pathogenic variants in autosomal genes, although there are X-linked forms. Pathogenic variants in the mitochondrial-specific DNA also lead to mitochondrial disease. In this situation, the type and severity of the presentation depend on the specific defects and the tissue-specific ratio of normal to abnormal copies of the mitochondrial DNA *(the degree of heteroplasmy)*.

Identification of Molecular Pathology

Molecular genetic testing is a critical component of the evaluation for IEMs. If the molecular basis of an IEM is known (i.e., the gene or genes have been mapped and disease-causing variants defined), clinical genetic testing should be available. If a category of disorders is suspected but no characteristic metabolites are identified, testing a panel of genes may be the best approach. In some disorders, there is a good correlation between specific disease-causing variants and clinical outcome. Genetic testing for other at-risk family members can provide important information, potentially enabling presymptomatic therapy and alternate decision making throughout the rest of the family.

IDENTIFICATION OF INBORN ERRORS BY NEONATAL SCREENING

Disorders Identified by Neonatal Screening

In the United States, most infants diagnosed with a treatable metabolic disorder will be identified as a result of an abnormal newborn screen. Most states use tandem mass spectrometry to screen for a core panel of metabolic disorders (see Chapter 57).

Strategy of Neonatal Screening

The purpose of neonatal screening is the early detection and rapid treatment of disorders before the onset of symptoms, thus preventing morbidity and mortality. In most states, infants are tested at 24–48 hours (see Chapter 57). A positive test demands prompt evaluation. Specific follow-up testing and treatment of an affected child depends on the disorder. Newborn screening tests are designed to be sensitive rather than specific, and this results in a significant proportion of infants with a positive neonatal screening test that do not have a metabolic disorder. Incorporating elements of genomic sequencing into the newborn screening program may increase specificity and expand the number of potentially screened disorders to include those that do not have an implemented biochemical assay.

Confirmatory Testing Principles

Neonatal screening is designed to maximize detection of affected infants but is not diagnostic. "Cutoff values" for each test are established carefully to identify infants with an elevated concentration of the substance or decreased activity of an enzyme with an acceptable number of false-positive results. A positive screening test must be followed by prompt clinical assessment as recommended by the screening program and/or metabolic specialist. In many cases, children will also be placed on standard of care treatment until the completion of definitive testing.

A positive screening test result causes anxiety for new parents; management of such anxiety is essential to minimize the harm of the program. In addition, definitive testing must be carried out promptly and accurately. If an IEM is excluded, parents need a thorough explanation of the results and reassurance that the infant is well. Such explanations will frequently require the expertise of a metabolic specialist or genetic counselor in the newborn period but may require reassessment of parental understanding by the primary care physician in the long term.

Specialized Laboratory and Clinical Testing

Specialized testing for inherited disorders of metabolism is essential in confirming a diagnosis suspected based on an abnormal newborn screening result or clinical suspicion. The tests that are helpful and examples of diagnoses made using these measurements depend on the deficient pathway in the disorder under consideration (Table 50.8). The most common tests ordered for evaluation of IEMs include plasma amino acids, plasma acylcarnitine, and urine organic acid analyses.

Amino acid analysis may be performed in plasma, urine, or cerebrospinal fluid (CSF). The **plasma amino acid profile** is most useful in identifying disorders of amino acid catabolism. Amino acids may also be abnormal in specific disorders of organic acid degradation but often are normal or not diagnostic. The **urine amino acid profile** is helpful in diagnosing primary disorders of renal tubular function, such as Lowe syndrome and cystinuria, as well as secondary disorders of renal tubular function, such as cystinosis and Fanconi syndrome of any cause. The test may also be useful in screening for several disorders of amino acid transport such as the detection of urinary homocitrulline in hyperornithinemia-hyperammonemia-homocitrullinuria (HHH) syndrome. The urine amino acid profile is **not** the test of choice for diagnosing disorders of amino acid or organic acid metabolism. The **CSF amino acid profile** is most useful in diagnosing errors of amino acid metabolism such as nonketotic hyperglycinemia and serine biosynthesis defects. It is important to obtain plasma amino acids in conjunction with CSF studies to allow for relative comparisons.

Markers of disordered fatty acid oxidation are measured in urine and plasma. Excessive intermediates of fatty acid oxidation and organic acid catabolism are conjugated with glycine and carnitine. The **plasma acylcarnitine profile** and the **urine acylglycine profile** reflect this accumulation. In organic acid disorders and fatty acid oxidation disorders, measurement of free and total plasma carnitine may reveal a secondary deficiency of carnitine and abnormal distribution of free and acylated carnitine. The plasma free fatty acid (nonesterified fatty acid)–to–3-OH-butyrate ratio is helpful in the diagnosis of disorders of fatty acid oxidation. Excessive elevation of 3-OH-butyrate may suggest a disorder of ketone metabolism; absence of ketones or decreased 3-OH-butyrate suggests a fatty acid oxidation disorder. Profiling of fatty acid intermediates in cultured skin fibroblasts may be informative but may not be clinically available as many specialty laboratories have closed.

Many IEMs lead to accumulation of diagnostic metabolites detectable by **urine organic acid analysis**, which is done by tandem mass spectrometry. Disorders of organic acid metabolism, such as propionic acidemia and methylmalonic acidemia, have typical urine organic acid profiles. Although analysis of blood and urine usually suggest the specific diagnosis, more targeted testing by measuring enzymatic activity in the pathway or establishing DNA changes in the gene are typically

TABLE 50.8 Specialized Metabolic Testing

TEST	ANALYTES MEASURED	TEST HELPFUL IN IDENTIFYING DISORDERS
Plasma amino acid profile	Amino acids, including alloisoleucine	PKU, urea cycle defects, tyrosinemias, MSUD, homocystinuria
Plasma total homocysteine	Protein-bound and free homocysteine	Homocystinuria, some forms of methylmalonic acidemia
Urine amino acid profile	Amino acids	Disorders of amino acid renal transport
Plasma acylcarnitine profile	Acylcarnitine derivatives of organic and fatty acid catabolism	Organic acid disorders, fatty acid oxidation disorders
Urine acylglycine profile	Acylglycine derivatives of organic and fatty acid catabolism	Organic acid disorders, fatty acid oxidation disorders
Plasma carnitines	Free, total, and acylated carnitine	Primary and secondary carnitine deficiency; abnormal in many organic acid and fatty acid disorders
Urine organic acid profile	Organic acids	Organic acid disorders, mitochondrial and fatty acid disorders
Urine or blood succinylacetone	Succinylacetone	Tyrosinemia I
Plasma very long-chain fatty acid profile	C22 to C26, pipecolid and phytanic acid	Peroxisomal disorders, X-linked adrenoleukodystrophy
Urine oligosaccharide chromatography	Glycosaminoglycans, mucopolysaccharides	Lysosomal storage disorders

MSUD, Maple syrup urine disease; *PKU*, phenylketonuria.

needed to identify the specific diagnosis. Metabolomic profiling compares multi-sample (urine, CSF and plasma) analytes to generate an artificial intelligence (AI)–driven differential in the quest for diagnosing rare or atypical metabolic disorders.

Disorders of creatine biosynthesis are suggested by abnormalities in creatine and guanidinoacetate levels and/or abnormal ratio of creatine to creatinine in blood, urine, and CSF. Disorders of purine and pyrimidine metabolism are suggested by the presence of an abnormal urinary profile of purines, such as xanthine, hypoxanthine, inosine, guanosine, adenosine, adenine, or succinyladenosine. Similarly, disorders of pyrimidine metabolism are identified by an abnormal profile of pyrimidines, including uracil, uridine, thymine, thymidine, orotic acid, orotidine, dihydrouracil, dihydrothymine, pseudouridine, *N*-carbamoyl-β-alanine, or *N*-carbamoyl-β-aminoisobutyrate, in the urine. Peroxisomal disorders are evaluated by analysis of very long-chain fatty acids, phytanic acid, pristanic acid, and plasmalogens. Congenital disorders of glycosylation are evaluated by isoelectric focusing of carbohydrate-deficient transferrin (detects only N-linked glycosylation defects) or evaluation of both transferrin and N-glycans by tandem mass spectrometry. It is possible to test specifically for the less common O-linked glycosylation defects, but this is not a multiplexed assay and needs to be ordered separately when these disorders are considered within the differential diagnosis.

Some storage disorders show abnormalities in urine glycosaminoglycans (heparan sulfate, dermatan sulfate, or chondroitin sulfate), oligosaccharides, and sialic acid. In several disorders, CSF is the most helpful specimen, including glycine encephalopathy (CSF amino acid profile when compared to concurrent plasma amino acids), disorders of neurotransmitter synthesis (biogenic amine profile), glucose transporter (GLUT1) deficiency (plasma-to-CSF glucose ratio), and serine synthesis defect (amino acid profile).

The correct tissue for enzymatic confirmation depends on the disorder, and in many cases may be measured on white blood cells or cultured skin fibroblasts. Consequently, such samples should only be collected after review of the testing laboratory's requirements.

In many disorders, an abnormal metabolic profile is consistently present during illness and when the child is well. In some cases, it is ***only diagnostic*** *during an episode of illness.*

OVERVIEW OF TREATMENT

There are several basic principles for treatment of IEMs. Syndromes with toxicity often present with encephalopathy; removal of toxic compounds is the first goal of therapy. Strategies for direct removal of the toxic compound include hemodialysis, hemovenovenous filtration, and administration of alternate pathway scavenger agents. A second strategy is to enhance deficient enzyme activity through administration of either the enzyme or cofactors to optimize residual activity (e.g., pyridoxine in homocystinuria, tetrahydrobiopterin in PKU). Small molecule (nanoparticle) therapies such as RNA-based lipid nanoparticles or chaperone therapies along with primary gene therapy are becoming an option for a number of disorders. This allows for a targeted approach to the primary gene defect. If deficiency of a pathway product plays an important role, providing missing products is helpful (e.g., tyrosine in the treatment of PKU). A further principle is to decrease flux through the deficient pathway by restricting precursors in the diet. Examples include the restriction of protein in disorders of ammonia detoxification, phenylalanine in PKU, and specific amino acid precursors in the organic acid disorders.

Preventing and promptly reversing catabolism during times of stress, typically with intravenous glucose, is essential to reducing flux of precursors into deficient pathways for many disorders.

PEARLS FOR PRACTITIONERS

See Metabolic Disorders: Pearls for Practitioners at the end of this section.

REVIEW QUESTIONS

Available online.

CHAPTER 51

Carbohydrate Disorders

GLYCOGEN STORAGE DISEASES

Many glycogen storage diseases are characterized by **hypoglycemia** and **hepatomegaly** (Table 51.1). Glycogen, the storage form of glucose, is found most abundantly in the liver (where it modulates blood glucose levels) and in muscles (skeletal and cardiac, where it facilitates anaerobic work). Glycogen is synthesized from uridine diphosphoglucose through the concerted action of glycogen synthetase and brancher enzyme (Fig. 51.1). The accumulation of glycogen is stimulated by insulin. Glycogenolysis occurs through a cascade initiated by epinephrine or glucagon. It results in rapid phosphorolysis of glycogen to yield glucose-1-phosphate, accompanied by, to a lesser degree, hydrolysis of glucose residues from the branch points in glycogen molecules. In the liver and kidneys, glucose-1-phosphate is converted to glucose-6-phosphate through the actions of phosphoglucomutase; glucose-6-phosphatase hydrolyses glucose-6-phosphate to produce glucose. The latter enzyme is not present in muscles. Glycogen storage diseases (GSD) fall into the following four categories:

1. Diseases that predominantly affect the liver and have a direct influence on blood glucose (types 0, I, VI, and VIII)
2. Diseases that predominantly involve muscles and affect the ability to do anaerobic work (types V and VII)
3. Diseases that can affect the liver and muscles, directly influencing both blood glucose and muscle metabolism (type III)
4. Diseases that affect various tissues but have no direct effect on blood glucose or on the ability to do anaerobic work (types II and IV)

The **diagnosis** of type I GSD is suggested by elevated uric acid, lactate, and triglycerides in blood. Neutropenia is typical of type Ib. Hyperlipidemia is also seen with type III GSD, but lactate and uric acid concentrations are typically normal. For all forms, a diagnosis can normally be confirmed by DNA testing. When this is feasible, invasive procedures, such as muscle and liver biopsy, can be avoided. When DNA testing is not available or is inconclusive, enzyme measurements in tissue from the affected organ confirm the diagnosis. If the diagnosis cannot be established, metabolic challenge and exercise testing may be needed. **Treatment** of hepatic GSD is aimed at maintaining satisfactory blood glucose levels or supplying alternative energy sources to muscle. In glucose-6-phosphatase deficiency (type I), the treatment usually requires nocturnal intragastric feedings of glucose during the first 1–2 years of life. Thereafter, snacks and uncooked cornstarch every 6 hours may be satisfactory. Hepatic tumors (sometimes malignant) are a threat in adolescence and adult life, and cirrhosis may be a long-term complication. Liver transplantation may be indicated in severe cases for some disorders (types I, III, and IV). No specific treatment exists for the diseases of muscle that impair skeletal muscle ischemic exercise, aside from avoidance of strenuous exercise and monitoring of cardiac function. Enzyme replacement early in life is effective in Pompe disease (type II), which involves cardiac and skeletal muscle. Cell-based gene therapies are under development as treatment options for severe GSDs.

GALACTOSEMIA

Galactosemia is an autosomal recessive disease caused by deficiency of galactose-1-phosphate uridyltransferase (Fig. 51.2). Clinical manifestations are most striking in a neonate who, when fed breast or cow's milk, generally exhibits evidence of **liver failure** (hepatomegaly, hyperbilirubinemia, disorders of coagulation, hypoglycemia), disordered renal tubular function (acidosis, glycosuria, aminoaciduria), food intolerance (vomiting, diarrhea, poor feeding), neurologic changes (lethargy, irritability, seizures), and **cataracts**. The neonatal screening test must have a rapid turnaround time because affected infants may die in the first week of life. Affected infants are at increased risk for neonatal sepsis, most commonly from *Escherichia coli*. Major effects on liver and kidney function and the development of cataracts are limited to the first few years of life; older children may have learning disorders despite dietary compliance. Females usually develop premature ovarian failure despite treatment.

Laboratory manifestations of galactosemia depend on dietary galactose intake. When galactose is ingested (as lactose), levels of plasma galactose and erythrocyte galactose-1-phosphate are elevated. Hypoglycemia is frequent, and albuminuria is present. Galactose frequently is present in the urine and can be detected by a positive reaction for reducing substances without a reaction with glucose oxidase on urine strip tests. The absence of urinary reducing substances cannot be relied on to exclude the diagnosis. The diagnosis is made by showing extreme reduction in erythrocyte galactose-1-phosphate uridyltransferase activity. DNA testing for pathogenic variants in galactose-1-phosphate uridyltransferase confirms the diagnosis and may be useful in predicting prognosis. Renal tubular dysfunction may be evidenced by a normal anion-gap hyperchloremic metabolic acidosis. **Treatment** by the elimination of dietary galactose results in rapid correction of abnormalities, but infants who are extremely ill before treatment may die before therapy is effective.

Galactokinase deficiency, an autosomal recessive disorder, also leads to the accumulation of galactose in body fluids (see Fig. 51.2), which results in the formation of galactitol (dulcitol) through the action of aldose reductase. Galactitol, acting as an osmotic agent, can be responsible for cataract formation and, rarely, for increased intracranial pressure. Individuals homozygous for galactokinase deficiency usually develop cataracts

TABLE 51.1 Glycogen Storage Diseases*

DISEASE	AFFECTED ENZYME	ORGANS AFFECTED	CLINICAL SYNDROME	NEONATAL MANIFESTATIONS	PROGNOSIS
Type 0: Glycogen synthase deficiency†	Glycogen synthase	Liver	Early morning drowsiness and fatigue, fasting hypoglycemia and ketosis	Early morning drowsiness, emesis, fatigue, hypoglycemia, ketosis, and occasionally seizures	Good; resolution of hypoglycemia is typical for patients who survive to adulthood.
Type 1a: von Gierke	Glucose-6-phosphatase	Liver, kidney, GI tract, platelets	Hypoglycemia, lactic acidosis, ketosis, hepatomegaly, hypotonia, slow growth, diarrhea, bleeding disorder, gout, hyperlipidemia, hypertriglyceridemia, hyperuricemia, xanthomas	Hypoglycemia, lactic acidemia, liver may not be enlarged	Early death from hypoglycemia, lactic acidosis; do well with early diagnosis and strict adherence to dietary therapy; hepatomas may occur in late childhood.
Type 1b	Glucose-6-phosphate translocase	Liver, kidney, GI tract, platelets, white blood cells	As type 1a but in addition have clinically significant neutropenia, periodontal disease, and inflammatory bowel disease symptoms	As type 1a but also may present with infections	In addition to risks for type 1a, children have significant IBD-like symptoms. Historically, death due to infections has occurred in the second decade.
Type II: Pompe	Lysosomal α-glucosidase	All; notably striated muscle, nerve cells	Symmetric profound proximal limb girdle muscle weakness with early involvement of the diaphragm, cardiomegaly, heart failure, shortened PR interval, hepatomegaly	"Floppy infant" appearance, feeding difficulties, macroglossia, hepatomegaly, hypertrophic cardiomyopathy	Very poor in neonatal form; death in the first year of life is usual; variants exist; therapy with recombinant human α-glucosidase.
Type III: Forbes	Debranching enzyme	Liver and muscles (IIIa), liver only (IIIb)	Hypoglycemia, ketonuria, hyperlipidemia, growth retardation, hepatomegaly that resolves with age; may show muscle fatigue	Usually none	Very good for hepatic disorder; if myopathy present, it tends to be like that of types I and V.
Type IV: Andersen	Branching enzyme	Liver, other tissues	Hypotonia, hepatomegaly or splenomegaly; hepatic cirrhosis beginning at several months of age; early liver failure	Usually none	Very poor; death from hepatic failure in first decade is typical.
Type V: McArdle	Muscle phosphorylase	Muscle	Muscle fatigue beginning in adolescence	None	Good, with sedentary lifestyle
Type VI: Hers	Liver phosphorylase	Liver	Mild hypoglycemia with hepatomegaly, hyperlipidemia, ketonuria	Usually none	Probably good
Type VII: Tarui	Muscle phosphofructokinase	Muscle	Clinical findings similar to type V	None	Similar to that of type V
Type VIII	Phosphorylase kinase	Liver	Clinical findings similar to type III, without myopathy	None	Good

*Except for one form of hepatic phosphorylase kinase, which is X linked, these disorders are autosomal recessive.
†Not a true glycogen storage disease as it is an enzyme deficiency that leads to decreased glycogen stores.
GI, Gastrointestinal; *IBD*, inflammatory bowel disease.

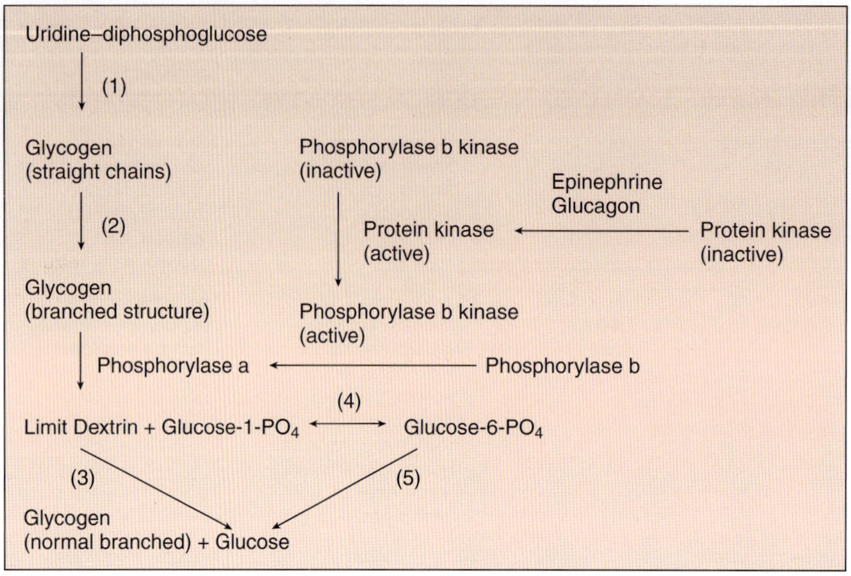

FIGURE 51.1 Glycogen synthesis and degradation. (1) Glycogen synthetase, (2) brancher enzyme, (3) debrancher enzyme, (4) phosphoglucomutase, (5) glucose-6-phosphatase.

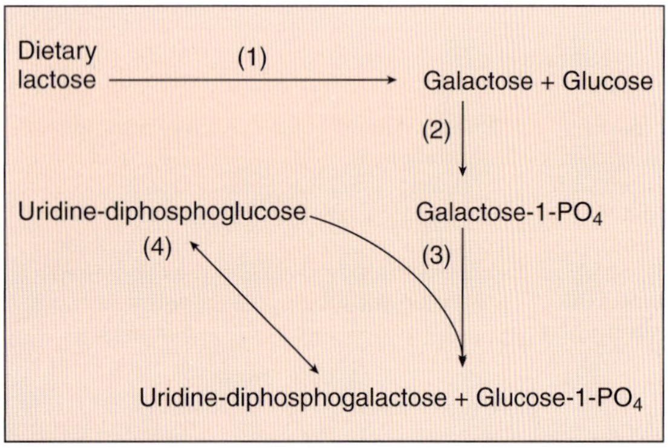

FIGURE 51.2 Pathway of galactose metabolism. (1) Lactase (intestinal), (2) galactokinase, (3) galactose-1-phosphate uridyltransferase, (4) uridine diphosphoglucose-4-epimerase.

after the neonatal period, whereas heterozygous individuals may be at risk for cataracts as adults.

Hereditary fructose intolerance, in many ways, is analogous to galactosemia. When fructose, sucrose, or sorbitol is ingested, deficiency of fructose-1,6-bisphosphate aldolase leads to the intracellular accumulation of fructose-1-phosphate with resultant emesis, hypoglycemia, and severe liver and kidney disease. Elimination of fructose and sucrose from the diet prevents clinical disease. **Fructosuria** is caused by fructokinase deficiency, but its deficiency is not associated with clinical consequences.

PEARLS FOR PRACTITIONERS

See Metabolic Disorders: Pearls for Practitioners at the end of this section.

REVIEW QUESTIONS

Available online.

CHAPTER 52

Amino Acid Disorders

DISORDERS OF AMINO ACID METABOLISM

Disorders of amino acid metabolism are the result of the inability to catabolize specific amino acids derived from protein. Usually a single amino acid pathway is involved. This amino acid accumulates in excess and is toxic to various organs, such as the brain, eyes, skin, or liver. Treatment is directed at the specific pathway and usually involves dietary restriction of the offending amino acid and supplementation with specialized medical foods (formulas) that provide the necessary amino acids and other nutrients at levels that are safe for oral intake. Confirmatory testing includes quantitative plasma amino acid profile, specific gene testing, and enzyme analysis if available.

PHENYLKETONURIA

Phenylketonuria (PKU), an autosomal recessive disease, primarily affects the brain and occurs in 1 in 10,000 persons in the United States; incidence varies throughout the world. Classic PKU is the result of a defect in the hydroxylation of phenylalanine to form tyrosine (Fig. 52.1); the activity of phenylalanine hydroxylase in the liver is absent or greatly reduced. Affected infants are normal at birth, but, if untreated, severe intellectual disability (IQ <35) develops in the first year of life; a musty odor of the breath, skin, or urine may also be noted. A positive newborn screening test must be followed up by performing quantitative plasma amino acid analysis. A plasma phenylalanine value of greater than 360 μM (6 mg/dL) is consistent with the diagnosis of one of the hyperphenylalaninemias and demands prompt evaluation and treatment. Untreated, classic PKU is characterized by blood phenylalanine concentrations higher than 600 μM. Milder forms of hyperphenylalaninemia are indicated by values of plasma phenylalanine lower than this but higher than 360 μM. A significant percentage of premature infants and a few full-term infants have transient elevations in phenylalanine. Short-term follow-up usually identifies these infants promptly. A small percentage of infants diagnosed with PKU (≤2% in the United States) have a defect in the synthesis or metabolism of tetrahydrobiopterin, the cofactor for phenylalanine hydroxylase and for other enzymes involved in the intermediary metabolism of aromatic amino acids. Disorders of biopterin metabolism are diagnosed by measuring dihydrobiopterin reductase in erythrocytes and by analyzing biopterin metabolites in urine. This testing should be carried out in all infants with elevated phenylalanine.

Treatment aims to maintain plasma phenylalanine values in the therapeutic range of 120–360 mM using a diet specifically restricted in phenylalanine but otherwise nutritionally complete. Treatment for life is recommended to reduce the risks of long-term neuropsychiatric problems.

Outcome of treatment in classic PKU is excellent. Most infants with classic PKU who are treated within the first 10 days of life achieve normal intelligence. However, learning problems and problems with executive function are more frequent than in unaffected peers. The safe concentration of phenylalanine in older children and adults with PKU has not been clearly established and thus lifelong attention to phenylalanine levels is recommended. Reversible cognitive dysfunction is associated with acute elevations of plasma phenylalanine in adults and children with PKU. If the elevated level has been sustained, the dysfunction may not be reversible. Treatment with modified preparation of tetrahydrobiopterin (sapropterin) shows good response in individuals with mild to moderate PKU and in 10% of individuals with classic PKU. Enzyme replacement therapy has been shown to maintain reduced phenylalanine levels and frequently allows affected patients to eat a normal protein diet. It is U.S. Food and Drug Administration (FDA) approved for adolescents and adults with PKU. Gene therapy is under investigation.

Anyone who lives with PKU and can become pregnant must be educated on the risks and prevention of "maternal PKU" syndrome. **Hyperphenylalaninemia** during conception and pregnancy requires rigorous management to prevent fetal brain injury, congenital heart disease, and severe microcephaly.

TYROSINEMIAS

Tyrosinemia is identified in neonatal screening programs using tandem mass spectrometry methods to detect elevated tyrosine and/or succinylacetone. Elevated tyrosine levels also occur as a nonspecific consequence of severe liver disease or transient tyrosinemia of the newborn (TTN). TTN is common (1% of live births), more prevalent in premature infants, resolves spontaneously by 2 months of age, and is of uncertain clinical significance. The inherited disorders of tyrosine metabolism are a target of neonatal screening. **Tyrosinemia type I**, which is due to fumarylacetoacetate hydrolase deficiency (see Fig. 52.1), is a rare disease in which accumulated metabolites produce severe liver disease associated with bleeding diathesis, hypoglycemia, hypoalbuminemia, elevated transaminases; defects in renal tubular function; and peripheral neuropathy. Hepatocellular carcinoma may eventually occur. Quantitative measurement of plasma tyrosine and blood or urine succinylacetone is performed after a positive neonatal screen. The **diagnosis** of tyrosinemia I is confirmed by an increased concentration of succinylacetone; DNA testing is available. **Treatment** with nitisinone (NTBC; an inhibitor of the oxidation of parahydroxyphenylpyruvic acid) reduces the production of the toxic succinylacetone. Because nitisinone increases the concentration of tyrosine in the blood, a low-phenylalanine, low-tyrosine diet is important to prevent tyrosine deposition

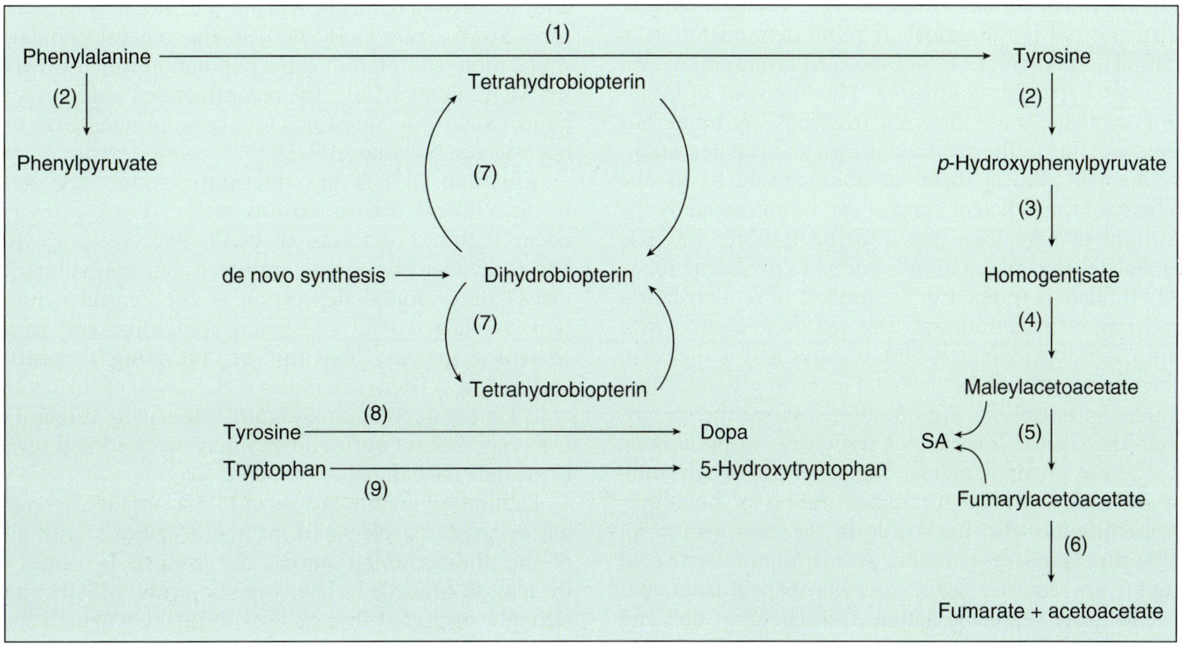

FIGURE 52.1 Metabolism of aromatic amino acids. (1) Phenylalanine hydroxylase, (2) transaminase, (3) *p*-hydroxyphenylpyruvate oxidase, (4) homogentisate oxidase, (5) maleylacetoacetate isomerase, (6) fumarylacetoacetate hydrolase, (7) dihydrobiopterin reductase, (8) tyrosine hydroxylase, (9) tryptophan hydroxylase. *SA*, Succinylacetone.

in the cornea. These treatments have reduced the immediate need for liver transplantation in children identified by neonatal screening. Nitisinone therapy, especially if initiated within 30 days of life, may reduce the risk of hepatocellular carcinoma.

Tyrosinemias II and **III** are less severe forms of hereditary tyrosinemia. Blocked metabolism of tyrosine at earlier steps in the pathway is responsible, and succinylacetone is not produced. The clinical features include **hyperkeratosis** of palms and soles and **keratitis**, which can cause severe visual disturbance. Significant elevations of tyrosine levels are associated with mild cognitive impairment and specific defects in executive function. Diagnosis is made by elevated tyrosine plasma assays in patients with suggestive exam findings; molecular testing may also be performed. Treatment with a phenylalanine- and tyrosine-restricted diet is effective in preventing these complications.

HOMOCYSTINURIA

Homocystinuria, an autosomal recessive disease (1:200,000 live births) affecting connective tissue, the brain, and the vascular system, is caused by a deficiency of cystathionine β-synthase. In the normal metabolism of the sulfur amino acids, methionine gives rise to cystine; homocysteine is a pivotal intermediate (Fig. 52.2). When cystathionine β-synthase is deficient, homocysteine accumulates in the blood and appears in the urine. Another result is enhanced reconversion of homocysteine to methionine, resulting in an increase in the concentration of methionine in the blood. The most commonly used neonatal screening test evaluates for elevated methionine. An excess of homocysteine produces a slowly evolving **clinical syndrome** that includes dislocated ocular lenses; long, slender extremities; malar flushing; and livedo reticularis. Arachnodactyly, scoliosis, pectus excavatum or carinatum, and genu valgum are skeletal features that mimic Marfan syndrome. Intellectual disability, psychiatric illness, or both may be present. Major arterial or venous thromboses are a constant threat.

Confirmation of the **diagnosis** requires demonstration of elevated total homocysteine in the blood. A plasma amino acid profile reveals hypermethioninemia. Measurement of cystathionine β-synthase is not clinically available, but numerous pathogenic variants in the gene are known and can be tested.

There are two clinical forms of homocystinuria. In one form, activity of the deficient enzyme can be enhanced by the administration of large doses of pyridoxine (typically 100–500 mg/day). Folate supplementation is added to overcome folate deficiency if folate is trapped in the process of remethylation of homocysteine to methionine. This pyridoxine-responsive form comprises approximately 50% of cases and is the form more likely to be missed by neonatal screening because the methionine concentrations are not always above the screening cutoff. The second form is not responsive to pyridoxine therapy. The use of supplemental betaine (trimethylglycine), a donor of methyl groups for remethylation of homocysteine to methionine, also has a role in the management of pyridoxine-unresponsive patients. A methionine-restricted diet is frequently required. Some cases may benefit from vitamin B_{12} and folate supplementation. Consequently, diet and betaine are sometimes required to control plasma homocysteine, even in pyridoxine-responsive patients. The prognosis is good for infants whose plasma homocysteine concentration is controlled. Agents and circumstances that raise the risk for thromboembolism (i.e., oral contraceptives) should be avoided.

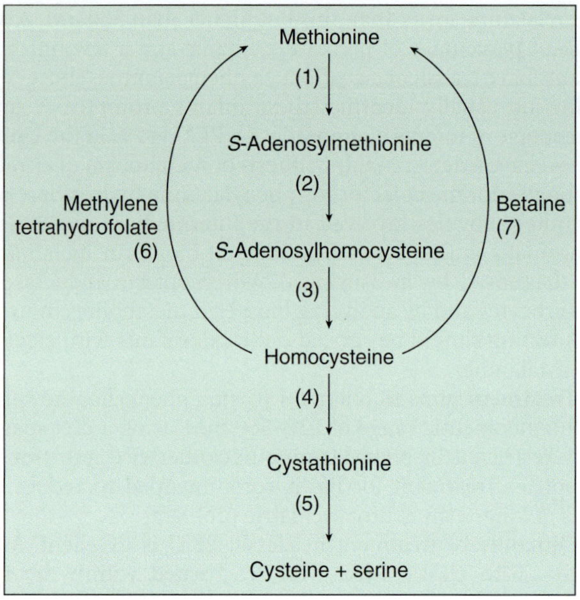

FIGURE 52.2 Metabolism of methionine and homocysteine. (1) Methionine adenosyltransferase, (2) glycine *N*-methyltransferase, (3) *S*-adenosylhomocysteine hydrolase, (4) cystathionine β-synthase, (5) cystathionase, (6) homocysteine methyltransferase, (7) betaine-homocysteine methyltransferase.

MAPLE SYRUP URINE DISEASE

Maple syrup urine disease (MSUD) is an autosomal recessive disease, also called **branched chain ketoaciduria**. It is caused by a deficiency of the decarboxylase that initiates the degradation of the ketoacid analogs of the three branched chain amino acids—leucine, isoleucine, and valine (Fig. 52.3). Classic MSUD is rare (1:185,000) in the general population but much more common in some population isolates (Pennsylvania Mennonites 1:380). The recommended uniform screening panel (RUSP) of conditions for states to include on the newborn screen includes MSUD.

Although MSUD has intermittent-onset and late-onset forms, **clinical manifestations** of the classic form typically occur within 1–4 weeks of birth. Poor feeding, vomiting, and tachypnea commonly are noted, but the hallmark of the disease is profound depression of the central nervous system, associated with alternating hypotonia and hypertonia **(extensor spasms, "fencing," or "bicycling")**, opisthotonos, and seizures. Hyperleucinosis is the cause of the central nervous system depression and may cause acute cerebral edema. Decompensation during illness may be rapid and severe. The urine may have the odor of maple syrup.

Laboratory manifestations of MSUD include hypoglycemia and a variable presence of metabolic acidosis, with elevation of the undetermined anions; the acidosis is caused in part by plasma branched chain organic acids. MSUD should be strongly suspected in a child with positive urine ketones on dipstick with no or low β-hydroxybutyrate. A rapid, more specific test demonstrates the rapid formation of copious white precipitate when 2,4-dinitrophenylhydrazine is added to the

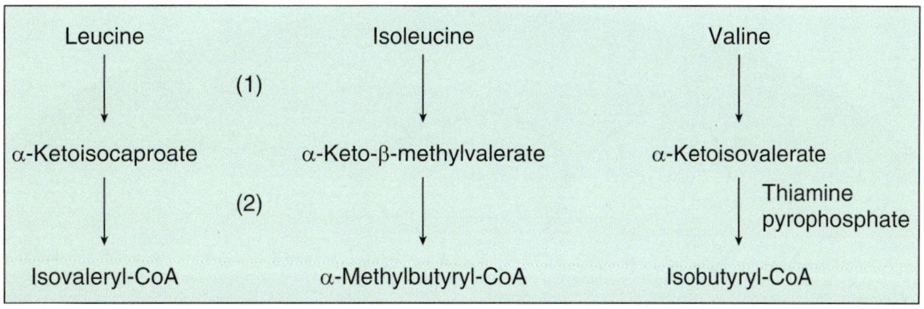

FIGURE 52.3 Metabolism of the branched chain amino acids. (1) Aminotransferases, (2) α-ketoacid dehydrogenase complex.

urine sample. This is because branched chain ketoacids in urine (but not β-hydroxybutyrate or acetoacetate) specifically react with 2,4-dinitrophenylhydrazine.

The **definitive diagnosis** of MSUD generally is made by showing large increases in plasma leucine with fewer increases in isoleucine and valine concentrations and identification of excess alloisoleucine in the plasma; alloisoleucine above 5 μmol/L is considered pathognomonic. The urinary organic acid profile is usually abnormal and shows the ketoacid derivatives of the branched chain amino acids. The diagnosis can be substantiated by detection of pathogenic variants in one of three genes: *BCKDHA,* encoding BCKA decarboxylase (E1) α subunit (MSUD type 1A); *BCKDHB,* encoding BCKA decarboxylase (E1) β subunit (MSUD type 1B); and *DBT,* encoding dihydrolipoyl transacylase (E2) subunit (MSUD type 2). A biochemical mimic of MSUD results from gain of function variants in BCKDK, an enzyme that is an endogenous inhibitor of the BCKD complex. This is a rare disorder that screens positive on MSUD newborn screening and, to date, has no known clinical phenotype. Patients with this phenomenon are managed as mild MSUD without dietary restrictions.

Provision of adequate calories and protein *with restriction of leucine* is crucial for acute and chronic management. Some patients with disease due to *BCKDHB* variants may be responsive to thiamine supplementation. Ordinary catabolic stresses, such as moderate infections or labor and delivery in a pregnant person with MSUD, can precipitate clinical crises. The highest risk complication of metabolic decompensation is cerebral edema. In critically ill patients, hemodialysis should be instituted to rapidly decrease plasma leucine levels. Liver transplantation effectively treats MSUD but does not reverse preexisting cognitive disability, psychiatric illness, and neurologic injury.

DISORDERS OF AMMONIA DISPOSAL

Inherited enzymatic deficiencies have been described for each of the steps of urea synthesis (Fig. 52.4). Collectively, their incidence is estimated to be at least 1:35,000 births. Neonatal screening currently detects the distal urea cycle disorders but does not detect the proximal disorders. Clinically, the two most frequent disorders in the United States are ornithine transcarbamylase (OTC) deficiency and argininosuccinate lyase (ASL) deficiency; these disorders should be suspected in neonates with severe hyperammonemia.

OTC deficiency is X linked. Pathogenic variants range from whole gene deletions to single nucleotide substitutions. If the enzyme is nonfunctional, there is no OTC activity in affected males, who are not likely to survive the neonatal period. Affected females are heterozygous and, because of skewed X inactivation, may have a significant degree of enzyme deficiency; they may become clinically affected at any time in life. **Clinical manifestations** range from lethal disease in the male (coma, encephalopathy) to clinical normalcy in a high percentage of females. Late-onset forms in males also occur. Manifestations in clinically affected females include recurrent emesis, lethargy, seizures, developmental delay, psychosis, or episodic confusion, often following ingestion of a high-protein diet or due to a catabolic state (e.g., infection).

Confirmatory testing for OTC deficiency includes a plasma amino acid profile, which may show low citrulline concentration with increased glutamate and alanine. A urine organic acid profile may show increased excretion of orotic acid after protein loading or with an allopurinol challenge test. Molecular sequencing typically screens the entire coding region of the *OTC* gene and can detect deletions which are a common mechanism of disease in OTC (10–15% of all cases). OTC enzyme activity can be assessed in liver tissue.

ASL deficiency is autosomal recessive, and most children in the United States are detected as a result of an elevated citrulline on newborn screening. In addition to hyperammonemia the disorder is characterized by hepatitis, cirrhosis, neurocognitive deficiencies, hypertension, and trichorrhexis nodosa (coarse, brittle hair). The diagnosis is confirmed by the detection of elevated argininosuccinic acid in the blood, urine, or cerebrospinal fluid.

The proximal urea cycle disorders *N*-acetylglutamate synthase (NAGS) deficiency and carbamoyl phosphate synthetase 1 (CPS1) deficiency (the rarest disorders of urea disposal) present with hyperammonemia, decreased citrulline, and absent orotic acid. NAGS deficiency may respond to supplementation with carglumic acid, an analog of *N*-acetylglutamate.

Treatment of Hyperammonemia

During episodes of symptomatic hyperammonemia, protein intake is reduced and intravenous glucose is given in sufficient quantity to suppress catabolism of endogenous protein. Ammonia can be eliminated by use of the **alternate pathway** agents, **sodium benzoate** and **sodium phenylacetate**, which are excreted in the urine as conjugates of glycine and glutamine. Arginine, which is usually deficient, is supplied. When ammonia levels are very high (>1,000 μM) or refractory to therapy, direct removal of ammonia using hemodialysis or hemofiltration, but not peritoneal dialysis (clearance of ammonia is substantially lower), is required. The neurologic status must be followed closely and cerebral edema treated promptly. Despite successful management of hyperammonemic crises, the long-term outcome for males with severe neonatal OTC deficiency and all children with severe ASL

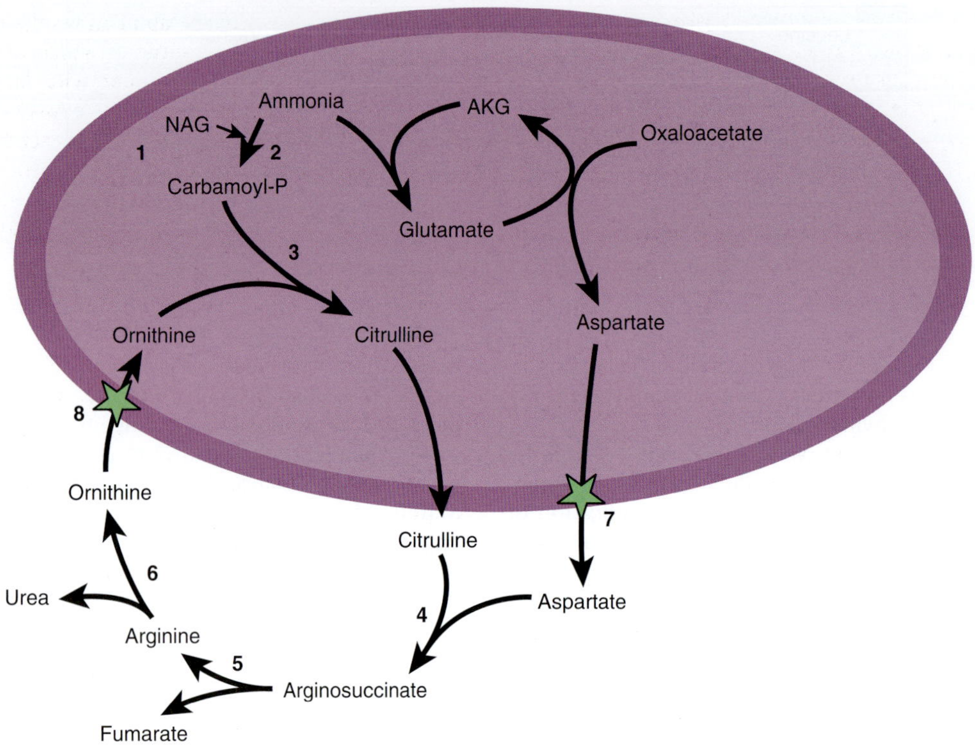

FIGURE 52.4 The urea cycle. Site of enzymatic defects: (1) *N*-acetylglutamate synthase *(NAG)*, (2) carbamoylphosphate synthetase, (3) ornithine transcarbamylase, (4) argininosuccinate acid synthetase, (5) argininosuccinate acid lyase, (6) arginase. Transporters *(star)*: (7) citrin, (8) ornithine translocator *(star)*. *AKG*, α-ketoglutarate.

deficiency is guarded. Early liver transplantation has increased survival, especially in males with severe OTC deficiency.

Restriction of dietary protein intake to daily needs is the mainstay of ongoing treatment for urea cycle defects. Essential amino acids can be supplied in amounts just sufficient to support protein synthesis. Arginine is an essential amino acid when arginine synthesis via the urea cycle is grossly impaired; thus arginine or citrulline must be supplied except in the case of arginase deficiency. Ongoing maintenance treatment with oral phenylbutyrate (which is metabolized to phenylacetate) prevents accumulation of ammonia. Gene therapy is under investigation in clinical trials.

DISORDERS OF AMINO ACID TRANSPORT THAT AFFECT SPECIFIC TRANSPORT MECHANISMS IN THE KIDNEY AND INTESTINE

Cystinuria is a disorder of renal tubular transport of cystine, lysine, arginine, and ornithine. Although intestinal transport is affected in some genetic forms, the symptoms are largely due to the renal transport abnormality. The concentration of cystine exceeds its solubility product and results in significant kidney stones. Evaluation and diagnosis are based on the pattern of amino acid excretion in the urine. DNA testing is likely to be informative. **Treatment** is based on increasing the solubility of cystine by alkalinizing the urine with sodium bicarbonate or sodium citrate and by complexing it with compounds such as penicillamine.

Intestinal transport of tryptophan is impaired in **Hartnup syndrome**; pellagra-like symptoms result from this deficiency as well as psychosis, cerebellar ataxia, and delayed development. Diagnosis is based on elevated excretion of the 10 neutral amino acids in urine. Treatment with niacin or nicotinamide improves outcomes.

PEARLS FOR PRACTITIONERS

See Metabolic Disorders: Pearls for Practitioners at the end of this section.

REVIEW QUESTIONS

Available online.

CHAPTER 53

Organic Acid Disorders

DISORDERS OF ORGANIC ACID METABOLISM

Organic acid disorders result from a block in the pathways of amino acid catabolism. Occurring after the amino moiety has been removed, they result in the accumulation of specific organic acids in the blood and urine. Treatment is directed at the specific abnormality, with restriction of precursor substrates and administration of enzyme cofactors, when available. Outcome is generally poor for children with neonatal-onset propionic or methylmalonic acidemia but is influenced by frequency and severity of crises and is optimal when diagnosis is made before the onset of the first episode. Liver transplantation may be used in cases refractory to standard management but is not curative. Confirmatory testing begins with a urine organic acid profile, plasma amino acid profile, and plasma acylcarnitine profile. These disorders are tested for in most newborn screening laboratories. More specific testing often requires enzyme measurements in appropriate tissues. When abnormal results suggest a specific disorder, DNA testing may identify the pathogenic variants involved.

PROPIONIC ACIDEMIA AND METHYLMALONIC ACIDEMIA

Propionic acidemia and methylmalonic acidemia result from defects in the propionate pathway (Fig. 53.1). Defects in these steps produce **metabolic acidosis, ketosis,** and **hyperglycinemia.** Propionic acidemia and methylmalonic acidemia are identified by neonatal screening with tandem mass spectrometry methods and confirmed with genetic testing. The **clinical manifestations** of both of these disorders in the neonatal period consist of tachypnea, vomiting, lethargy, coma, intermittent ketoacidosis or lactic acidosis, hyperglycinemia, neutropenia, thrombocytopenia, hyperammonemia, and hypoglycemia. Propionic acidemia causes cardiomyopathy. Methylmalonic acidemia causes secondary intellectual disability, tubulointerstitial nephritis, and kidney failure. Both disorders can cause "metabolic stroke" with infarction of the basal ganglia during acute episodes. If these disorders are not identified by neonatal screening, intermittent episodes of metabolic acidosis occur. Crises occur during periods of catabolic stress, such as fever, vomiting, and diarrhea; they also may occur without an apparent precipitating event. During periods of neutropenia, the risk of serious bacterial infection is increased. Growth faltering and impaired development are common.

Propionic acidemia results from deficiency in propionyl coenzyme A (CoA)–carboxylase, an enzyme that has two pairs of identical subunits. All forms of propionic acidemia are inherited in an autosomal recessive manner and are due to pathogenic variants in one of the subunits. **Methylmalonic acidemia** results from deficiency in methylmalonyl mutase; this may be caused by pathogenic variants in the gene for the mutase protein itself or in one of the steps of the synthesis of the cobalamin (B_{12}) cofactors for the enzyme. A complex set of defects in cobalamin metabolism results in other forms of methylmalonic acidemia, some of which are associated with hyperhomocystinemia. **Treatment** with large doses of parenteral hydroxocobalamin (the active form of vitamin B_{12}) is helpful in some cases of methylmalonic acidemia.

For propionic acidemia and the vitamin B_{12}–unresponsive forms of methylmalonic acidemia, management includes the restriction of dietary protein and addition of a medical food deficient in the specific amino acid precursors of propionyl-CoA (isoleucine, valine, methionine, and threonine). Carnitine supplementation is often needed because it is lost in the urine as acylcarnitines. Intestinal bacteria produce a significant quantity of propionate; thus antibacterial treatment with neomycin or metronidazole to reduce the population of bacteria in the gut has some beneficial effect in propionic acidemia and vitamin B_{12}–unresponsive methylmalonic acidemia. Decompensations must be treated with intravenous glucose to provide adequate calories to prevent catabolism. In severe decompensation, hemodialysis or hemofiltration may be required to treat acidosis or hyperammonemia.

ISOVALERIC ACIDEMIA

Isovaleric acidemia results from a block in the catabolism of leucine. Its clinical manifestations are similar to those of defects in the propionate pathway. The strong odor of isovaleric acid results in **sweaty feet odor** in untreated infants, best appreciated in body sweat or cerumen. Therapy is effective in promoting normal development and involves restricting the intake of leucine and providing glycine as an alternate pathway therapy that conjugates isovaleric acid (Fig. 53.2) and is then excreted in the urine.

GLUTARIC ACIDEMIA I

Glutaric acidemia I results from a deficiency at the end of the lysine catabolic pathway. It is an autosomal recessive disease produced by deficiency of glutaryl-CoA dehydrogenase activity (Fig. 53.3). **Clinical manifestations** include **macrocephaly**

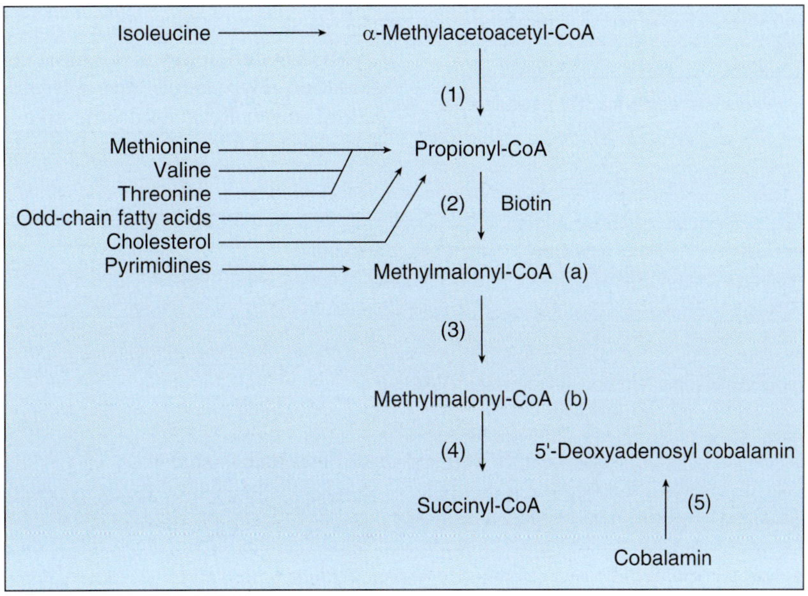

FIGURE 53.1 The propionate pathway. (1) β-Ketothiolase, (2) propionyl-CoA carboxylase, (3) methylmalonyl-CoA isomerase, (4) methylmalonyl-CoA mutase, (5) cobalamin metabolic pathway. *CoA,* Coenzyme A.

(75% of affected individuals), which may be present at birth. Before the advent of newborn screening, more than 70% of children had *metabolic stroke-like episodes* associated with infarction of the basal ganglia and **dystonia**, which characteristically develops after an episode of intercurrent illness or stress but may occur spontaneously. **Treatment** includes a protein-restricted diet accompanied by a medical food deficient in lysine and tryptophan, carnitine supplementation, and aggressive management of intercurrent illness. Despite this treatment, as many as one third of children still develop neurologic symptoms.

BIOTINIDASE DEFICIENCY AND HOLOCARBOXYLASE SYNTHETASE DEFICIENCY

Biotin is a ubiquitous vitamin that is covalently linked to many carboxylases and cannot be recycled from its attachment to the carboxylases. Thus inherited biotinidase deficiency greatly increases the dietary requirement for biotin. Affected individuals become biotin deficient while consuming normal diets. Clinical disease can appear in the neonatal period or be delayed until later infancy, depending on the degree of deficiency. Virtually all infants with biotinidase deficiency are detected by newborn screening of biotinidase activity. Newborn screening for holocarboxylase synthetase deficiency can detect elevated C5-OH-carnitine on tandem mass spectrometry, but biotinidase activity is normal in these patients.

Clinical manifestations of biotin deficiency vary greatly (seizures, hypotonia, sensorineural deafness, vision loss, alopecia, skin rash, metabolic acidosis, hyperammonemia, immune deficits, ataxia, developmental delay) and depend on which enzymes in which tissues have the most biotin depletion. Carboxylation is a crucial reaction in the metabolism of organic acids; most patients with biotinidase deficiency excrete abnormal amounts of several organic acids, among which β-methylcrotonylglycine is prominent. In addition to biotinidase deficiency, an inherited deficiency of holocarboxylase synthetase gives rise to severe disease and to similar patterns of organic aciduria. Both conditions respond well to lifelong **treatment** with large doses of biotin (5–10 mg/day). Early treatment is essential as vision and hearing loss are permanent. Confirmatory testing is accomplished with quantitative measurement of the deficient enzyme.

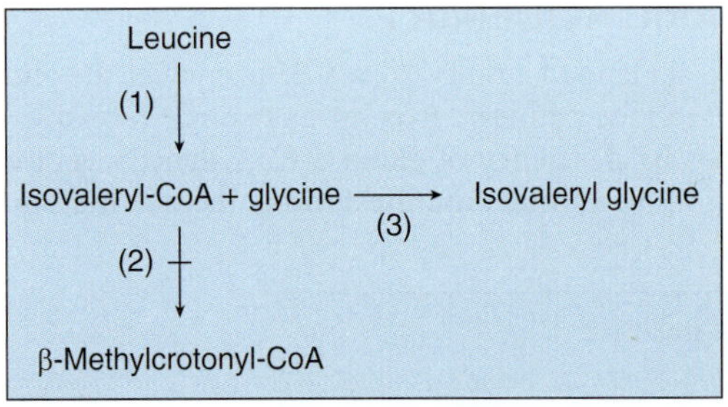

FIGURE 53.2 Metabolism in isovaleric acidemia. (1) Leucine catabolic pathway (transamination and decarboxylation), (2) isovaleryl-CoA dehydrogenase, (3) glycine acyltransferase. *CoA*, Coenzyme A.

PEARLS FOR PRACTITIONERS

See Metabolic Disorders: Pearls for Practitioners at the end of this section.

REVIEW QUESTIONS

Available online.

CHAPTER 54

Fatty Acid Oxidation Disorders

DISORDERS OF FATTY ACID OXIDATION

Fatty acids are derived from hydrolysis of triglycerides and catabolism of fat. The catabolism of fatty acids (Fig. 54.1) proceeds through the serial oxidative removal of two carbons at a time as acetyl groups (each as acetyl-coenzyme A [CoA]). The reactions are catalyzed by a group of enzymes that exhibit specificities related to the chain length and other properties of the fatty acids: very long-chain acyl-CoA dehydrogenase (VLCAD), long-chain hydroxyacyl-CoA dehydrogenase (LCHAD) or trifunctional protein, medium-chain acyl-CoA dehydrogenase (MCAD), and short-chain acyl-CoA dehydrogenase (SCAD). The pattern of plasma acylcarnitine elevations is diagnostic. The prevalence of these disorders is approximately 1:10,000.

MCAD deficiency is the most common inborn error of β-oxidation. Hypoketotic hypoglycemia is a common manifestation, as is a Reye syndrome–like illness with hypoglycemia and elevated liver enzymes. Fatty infiltration of the liver also

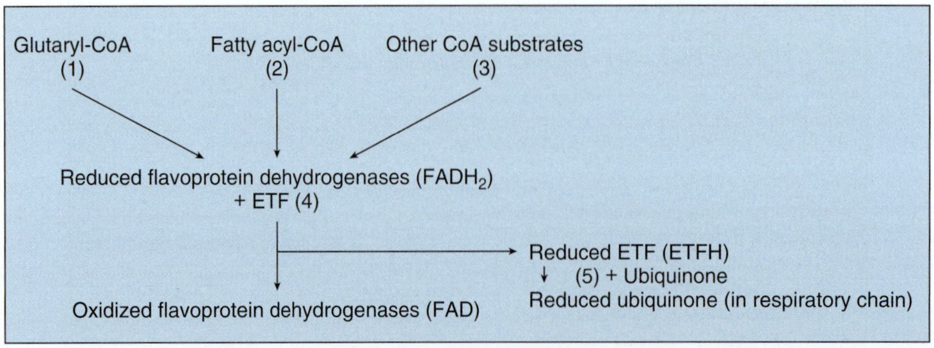

FIGURE 53.3 Scheme of flavoprotein metabolism with reference to glutaric aciduria types I and II. (1) Glutaryl-CoA dehydrogenase (deficient in glutaric aciduria type1), (2) fatty acyl-CoA dehydrogenases, (3) other flavoprotein dehydrogenases, (4) ETF (deficiency results in glutaric aciduria type II), (5) ETF-ubiquinone oxidoreductase (deficiency results in glutaric aciduria type II). *CoA*, Coenzyme A; *ETF*, electron transfer flavoprotein.

occurs. True hepatic failure is rare. Episodes may be recurrent in the patient or the family. **Sudden infant death syndrome** is reported in infants with MCAD deficiency, perhaps related to hypoglycemia.

VLCAD deficiency and LCHAD (trifunctional protein) deficiency result in significant myopathy and cardiomyopathy in addition to hypoglycemia. This cardiomyopathy may be rapidly reversed with appropriate dietary treatment. LCHAD deficiency is accompanied by a retinopathy in later childhood. Female carriers for LCHAD who are carrying affected fetuses are at risk for HELLP syndrome (hemolysis, elevated liver enzymes, and low platelets in pregnant and postpartum patients). In all of the disorders of β-oxidation, carnitine depletion can occur through excessive urinary excretion of carnitine esters of the incompletely oxidized fatty acids. Measurement of plasma carnitine is helpful in monitoring for this deficiency, which results in weakness and muscle pain, along with myoglobinuria in some people. In acute decompensation, patients must be screened for rhabdomyolysis and cardiomyopathy as both are rapidly reversible with appropriate therapy and fluid goals must be adjusted if cardiomyopathy is present.

3-Hydroxy-3-methylglutaryl-CoA lyase deficiency, although not a disorder of β-oxidation, interferes profoundly with hepatic adaptation to fasting by impairing ketogenesis (see Fig. 54.1). The clinical manifestations are those of MCAD deficiency, except that carnitine depletion is less prominent.

The diagnosis of disorders involving a deficiency of β-oxidation is suggested by the clinical picture and by **hypoketotic hypoglycemia**. The diagnosis is suggested by abnormal urinary organic acid and acylglycine profiles, along with plasma acylcarnitine and free fatty acid profiles. DNA testing is required to confirm the diagnosis. The profile of acylcarnitines in cultured skin fibroblasts may be helpful if other testing is not conclusive but is not widely available clinically. In MCAD deficiency a single pathogenic variant c.985 A→G accounts for a significant percentage of cases, especially among children of Northern European ancestry. **Treatment** of all disorders of fatty acid oxidation includes avoidance of fasting, as well as fluid and calorie supplementation (either intravenous or oral) during periods of metabolic stress, such as fever. In MCAD deficiency, medium-chain triglycerides must be avoided. In the long-chain fatty acid oxidation disorders, provision of medium-chain fatty acids improves muscle energy metabolism. The use of a 7-chain fatty acid, heptanoyl-L-carnitine (triheptanoin), which is FDA approved as a treatment in fatty acid oxidation disorders (FAODs), has been shown to have improved long-term outcomes for patients with more severe long-chain fatty acid disorders.

GLUTARIC ACIDURIA TYPE II

Glutaric aciduria type II (multiple acyl-CoA dehydrogenase deficiency) is an autosomal recessive disorder produced by a defect in the transfer of electrons from flavin adenine nucleotides to the electron transport chain (electron transfer flavoprotein [ETF], or ETF dehydrogenase); this defect results in a deficiency of multiple fatty acyl-CoA dehydrogenases (see Fig. 54.1) from variants in one of three genes. It should not be confused with glutaric acidemia type I (see Chapter 53). When the enzyme essentially is nonfunctional, congenital anomalies are common, including kidney cysts, facial abnormalities, rocker-bottom feet, and hypospadias. Severely affected infants have nonketotic hypoglycemia, metabolic acidosis, hepatomegaly, cardiomegaly, and the odor of sweaty feet soon after birth; these infants may die within the neonatal period. Less severely affected infants may have a more episodic, Reye syndrome–like illness. Skeletal and cardiac myopathy with rhabdomyolysis can

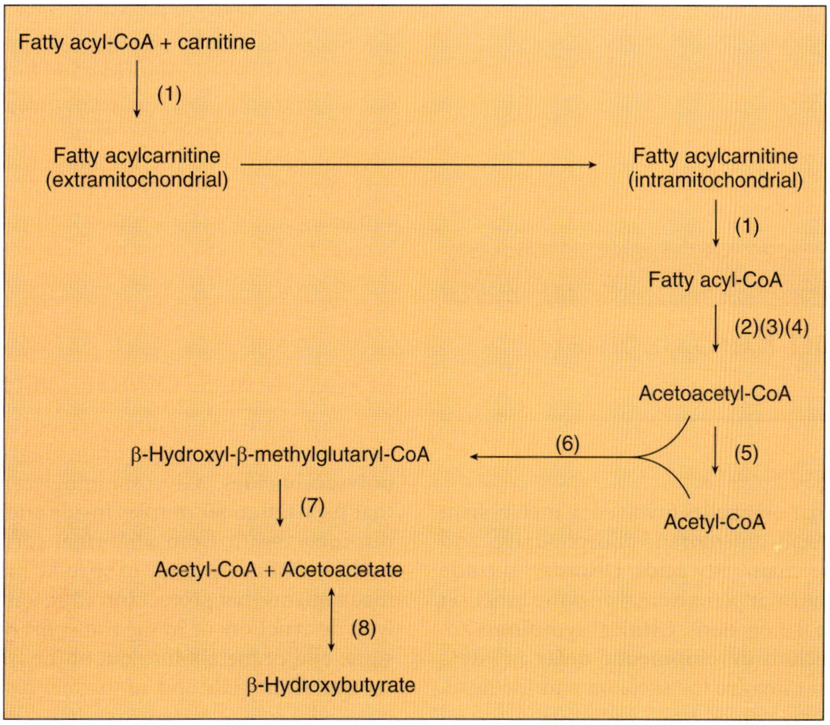

FIGURE 54.1 Scheme of fatty acid and catabolism and ketone body formation. (1) Carnitine acyl-CoA dehydrogenases, (2) long-chain fatty acyl-CoA dehydrogenase (trifunctional protein), (3) medium-chain fatty acyl-CoA dehydrogenase, (4) short-chain fatty acyl-CoA dehydrogenase, (5) β-ketothiolase, (6) β-hydroxy-β-methylglutaryl-CoA synthase, (7) β-hydroxy-β-methylglutaryl-CoA lyase, (8) β-hydroxybutyrate dehydrogenase. CoA, Coenzyme A.

be prominent in this complex, multisystemic disease. Onset in later childhood may be marked by recurrent hypoglycemia and myopathy. **Treatment** has not been effective in infants with complete deficiency. Milder forms respond to avoidance of fasting and caloric support during metabolic stress. Some patients respond to administration of riboflavin. The diagnosis may be suggested by abnormal urine organic acid or plasma acylcarnitine profile. It is typically confirmed through DNA testing.

CARNITINE DEFICIENCY

Carnitine is a crucial cofactor in the transport of long-chain fatty acids across the mitochondrial inner membrane (see Fig. 54.1). It is synthesized from lysine by humans and is present in dietary red meat and dairy products. Carnitine deficiency is either primary (caused by failure of intake, synthesis, or transport of carnitine) or secondary (caused by the excretion of excessive amounts of carnitine as carnityl esters in patients with other inborn errors of metabolism, by treatment with drugs that complex carnitine such as valproic acid, or as a result of kidney replacement therapy). Primary systemic carnitine deficiency is rare and results from inadequate kidney reabsorption of carnitine secondary to pathogenic variants in the sodium-dependent carnitine transporter. It is detected by neonatal screening and responds well to high-dose carnitine supplementation. There are numerous examples of secondary carnitine deficiency among the organic acidurias, most prominently in disorders of the propionate pathway and in disorders of the β-oxidation of long-chain and medium-chain fatty acids. Clinical manifestations of carnitine deficiency include hypoketotic hypoglycemia, lethargy, lassitude, muscle weakness, sudden death, and cardiomyopathy.

PEARLS FOR PRACTITIONERS

See Metabolic Disorders: Pearls for Practitioners at the end of this section.

REVIEW QUESTIONS

Available online.

CHAPTER 55

Lysosomal and Peroxisomal Disorders

PEROXISOMAL DISORDERS

Peroxisomes are subcellular organelles involved in metabolism and biosynthesis of bile acids, membrane phospholipids, and some β-oxidation of long-chain fatty acids. Disorders include conditions caused by abnormal peroxisomal enzyme function and abnormal peroxisomal biogenesis. **Clinical symptoms** are diverse and frequently include **developmental delay** and **dysmorphic features** that can involve the skeleton and the head. Zellweger syndrome, neonatal adrenoleukodystrophy, and infantile Refsum disease are examples of disorders of peroxisome biogenesis. **Zellweger syndrome (aka Zellweger spectrum disorder)**, an autosomal recessive disease (1:100,000 births), is also called *cerebrohepatorenal syndrome*. Peroxisome structure may be disrupted and function is affected, including the oxidation of very long-chain fatty acids (VLCFAs) and a variety of other metabolic pathways. Affected infants have high foreheads, flat orbital ridges, widely open fontanelles, hepatomegaly, bony stippling of the long bones, and hypotonia. Other anomalies are common. Growth faltering, seizures, and nystagmus develop early, and death occurs within the first year. Adult Refsum disease, X-linked adrenoleukodystrophy, and malonic aciduria are examples of peroxisomal single-enzyme disorders. Diagnostic testing includes measurement of VLCFAs in plasma and pipecolic acid in urine. Specific molecular testing, particularly for the disorders involving one in the series of *PEX* genes, is available for some disorders. Most of these conditions are untreatable; however, bone marrow transplant can be helpful in X-linked adrenoleukodystrophy (X-ALD) before the onset of severe symptoms.

X-ALD is recommended to be included in every newborn screening program. This disorder, which affects 1:20,000 males, is caused by a defect in a peroxisomal membrane protein. There are three main ALD phenotypes seen in males with pathogenic variants in the *ABCD1* gene: childhood-onset cerebral form, adrenomyeloneuropathy (AMN), and "Addison disease only"; adolescent and asymptomatic forms are also seen in childhood. Impaired adrenocortical function is variably present in all types. Diagnosis is made by analysis of VLCFAs and DNA testing, but the phenotype of affected males cannot be predicted by VLCFA levels or by genotype. The childhood cerebral form is a severe progressive disease that typically presents between ages 4 and 8 years with inattentive symptoms and can progress from impaired cognition, vision, hearing, and motor function to total disability within 6 months. AMN presents in adulthood with leg weakness as well as decreased sphincter control and sexual dysfunction. Approximately 20% of carrier females will develop a milder form of the AMN phenotype. Hematopoietic stem cell transplantation (HSCT) should be considered for males in the early stages of the cerebral form who have evidence of brain involvement on MRI. Because of the significant risks and limited benefit in symptomatic individuals, HSCT is recommended only for individuals with evidence of brain involvement by MRI and minimal neuropsychologic findings (performance IQ >80) with a normal clinical neurologic examination. Corticosteroid replacement therapy can be lifesaving in individuals with AMN or Addison only presentation. The most sensitive indicators of adrenal dysfunction are elevated plasma adrenocorticotropic hormone (ACTH) and impaired cortisol response to ACTH challenge.

LYSOSOMAL STORAGE DISORDERS

Lysosomes are subcellular organelles that contain degradative enzymes for complex **glycosaminoglycans**, also called **mucopolysaccharides**. Glycosaminoglycans are macromolecules that play a number of roles inside and outside of cells. Genetic disorders result from abnormal formation of the lysosome itself or from deficiency in specific hydrolytic enzymes, in the mechanisms that protect intralysosomal enzymes from hydrolytic destruction, or in the transport of materials into the lysosome and of metabolites out of the lysosome. These materials are stored in cells and ultimately result in their destruction, especially in the nervous system. The clinical disorders are diverse, reflecting tissue specificity of lysosomal function and the intrinsic turnover rates of the compounds whose cycling is affected (Table 55.1). Some disorders are apparent only during

TABLE 55.1 Lysosomal Storage Diseases

DISEASE (EPONYM)	ENZYME DEFICIENCY	CLINICAL ONSET	DYSOSTOSIS MULTIPLEX	CORNEA	RETINA	LIVER, SPLEEN	CNS FINDINGS	STORED MATERIAL IN URINE	WBC/BONE MARROW	COMMENT	MULTIPLE FORMS
MUCOPOLYSACCHARIDOSES (MPS)											
MPS I (Hurler)	α-L-iduronidase	~1 yr	Yes	Cloudy	—	Both enlarged	Profound loss of function	Acid mucopolysaccharide	Alder-Reilly bodies (WBC)	Kyphosis on RUSP	Yes—Scheie and compounds
MPS II (Hunter)	Iduronate-2-sulfatase	1–2 yr	Yes	Clear	Retinal degeneration, papilledema	Both enlarged	Slow loss of function	Acid mucopolysaccharide	Alder-Reilly bodies (WBC)	X linked	Yes
MPS III (Sanfilippo)	One of several degrading heparan SO_4s	2–6 yr	Mild	Clear	—	Liver ± enlarged	Rapid loss of function	Acid mucopolysaccharide	Alder-Reilly bodies (WBC)	—	Several types biochemically
MPS IV (Morquiro)	Galactose-6-sulfatase or β-galactosidase	2 yr	No, dwarfism deformities	Faint clouding	—		Normal	Acid mucopolysaccharide	Alder-Reilly bodies (WBC)	—	Yes
MPS VI (Maroteaux-Lamy)	*N*-acetylgalactosamine-4-sulfatase	2 yr	Yes	Cloudy	—	Both may be enlarged	Normal	Acid mucopolysaccharide	Alder-Reilly bodies (WBC)	—	Yes
MPS VII (Sly)	β-Glucuronidase	Variable neonatal	Yes	± Cloudy	—	Both enlarged	± Affected	Acid mucopolysaccharide	Alder-Reilly bodies (WBC)	Nonimmune hydrops	Yes
LIPIDOSES											
Glucosylceramide lipidosis (Gaucher 1)	Glucocerebrosidase	Any age	No	Clear	Normal	Both enlarged	Normal	No	Gaucher cells in marrow	Bone pain fractures	Variability is the rule
Glucosylceramide lipidosis 2 (Gaucher 2)	Glucocerebrosidase	Fetal life–6 mo	No	Clear	Normal	Both enlarged	Profound loss of function	No	Gaucher cells in marrow	—	Yes
Sphingomyelin lipidosis A (Niemann-Pick A)	Sphingomyelinase	1st mo	No	Clear	Cherry red spots (50%)	Both enlarged	Profound loss of function	No	Foam cells in marrow	—	No
Sphingomyelin lipidosis B (Niemann-Pick B)	Sphingomyelinase	1st mo or later	No	Clear	Cherry red spot possible (~33%)	Both enlarged	Normal	No	Foam cells in marrow	—	Yes
Niemann-Pick C	Lysosomal cholesterol; trafficking (*NPC1* gene)	Variable	No	Clear	Normal	Enlarged	Vertical ophthalmoplegia, dystonia, cataplexy, seizures	No	Foam cells and sea-blue histiocytes in marrow	Pathogenesis not as for NP-A and NP-B	Lethal neonatal to adolescent onset

(Continued)

TABLE 55.1 Lysosomal Storage Diseases—cont'd

DISEASE (EPONYM)	ENZYME DEFICIENCY	CLINICAL ONSET	DYSOSTOSIS MULTIPLEX	CORNEA	RETINA	LIVER, SPLEEN	CNS FINDINGS	STORED MATERIAL IN URINE	WBC/BONE MARROW	COMMENT	MULTIPLE FORMS
GM_2 gangliosidosis (Tay-Sachs)	Hexosaminidase A	3–6 mo	No	Clear	Cherry red spots	Normal	Profound loss of function	No	Normal	Sandhoff disease related	Yes
Generalized gangliosidosis (infantile) (GM_1)	β-Galactosidase	Neonatal to 1st mo	Yes	Clear	Cherry red spots (50%)	Both enlarged	Profound loss of function	No	Inclusion in WBC	—	Yes
Metachromatic leukodystrophy	Arylsulfatase A	1–2 yr	No	Clear	Normal	Normal	Profound loss of function	No	Normal	—	Yes
Fabry disease	α-Galactosidase A (cerebrosidase)	Childhood, adolescence	No	Cloudy by slit lamp	—	Liver may be enlarged	Normal	No	Normal	X linked	No
Krabbe disease	Galactocerebroside β-galactosidase	Infancy	No	Clear	Optic atrophy	Normal	Profound loss of function	No	Normal	Storage not lysosomal	Yes
Wolman disease	Acid lipase	Neonatal	No	Clear	Normal	Both enlarged	Profound loss of function	No	Inclusion in WBC	New therapy recently approved	Yes
Farber lipogranulomatosis	Acid ceramidase	First 4 mo	No	Usually clear	Cherry red spots (12%)	May be enlarged	Normal or impaired	Usually not	—	Arthritis, nodules	Yes
MUCOLIPIDOSES (ML) AND CLINICALLY RELATED DISEASE											
Sialidosis II (formerly ML I)	Neuraminidase	Neonatal	Yes	Cloudy	Cherry red spot	Both enlarged	Yes	Oligosaccharides	Vacuolated lymphocytes	—	Yes (also see galactosialidosis)
Sialidosis I (formerly ML I)	Neuraminidase	Usually second decade	No	Fine opacities	Cherry red spot	Normal	Myoclonus, seizures	Oligosaccharides	Usually none	Cherry red spot/ myoclonus syndrome	Severity varies
Galactosialidosis	Absence of PP/CathA causes loss of neuraminidase and β-galactosidase	Usually second decade	Frequent	Clouding	Cherry red spot	Occasionally enlarged	Myoclonus, seizures, intellectual disability	Oligosaccharides	Foamy lymphocytes	Onset from 1 to 40 yr	Congenital and infantile forms such as sialidosis 2
ML II (I-cell disease)	Mannosyl phosphotransferase	Neonatal	Yes	Clouding	—	Liver often enlarged	Profound loss of function	Oligosaccharides	No	Gingival hyperplasia, cardiac involvement	No
ML III (pseudo-Hurler polydystrophy)	Mannosyl phosphotransferase	2–4 yr	Yes	Late clouding	Normal	Normal in size?	Modest loss of function	Oligosaccharides	No	—	No

(Continued)

DISEASE (EPONYM)	ENZYME DEFICIENCY	CLINICAL ONSET	DYSOSTOSIS MULTIPLEX	CORNEA	RETINA	LIVER, SPLEEN	CNS FINDINGS	STORED MATERIAL IN URINE	WBC/BONE MARROW	COMMENT	MULTIPLE FORMS
Multiple sulfatase deficiency	Many sulfatases	1–2 yr	Yes	Usually clear	Usually normal	Both enlarged	Profound loss of function	Acid mucopolysaccharide	Alder-Reilly bodies (WBC)	Ichthyosis	Yes
Aspartylglycosaminuria	Aspartylglucos-aminidase	6 mo	Mild	Clear	Normal	Early, not late	Profound loss of function	Aspartylglucosamine	Inclusions in lymphocytes	Develop cataracts	No
Mannosidosis	α-Mannosidase	1st mo	Yes	Cloudy	—	Liver enlarged	Profound loss of function	Oligosaccharides	Inclusions in lymphocytes	Cataracts	Yes
Fucosidosis	α-L-fucosidase	1st mo	Yes	Clear	May be pigmented	Both enlarged commonly	Profound loss of function	Oligosaccharides	Inclusions in lymphocytes	—	Yes
STORAGE DISEASES CAUSED BY DEFECTS IN LYSOSOMAL PROTEOLYSIS											
Neuronal ceroid lipofuscinosis (NCL), Batten disease	Impaired lysosomal proteolysis—various specific etiologies	6 mo–10 yr, adult form	No	Normal	May have brown pigment	Normal, distinct	Optic atrophy, seizures, dementia			Clinical picture consistent, time course variable	Etiologies for age-related forms
STORAGE DISEASES CAUSED BY DEFECTIVE SYNTHESIS OF THE LYSOSOMAL MEMBRANE											
Cardiomyopathy, myopathy, intellectual disability, Danon disease	Lamp-2, a structural protein of lysosomes, is deficient	Usually 5–6 yr	No	Normal	Normal	Hepatomegaly	Delayed development, seizures			X-linked pediatric disease in males only	Variability in time course of signs
STORAGE DISEASES CAUSED BY DYSFUNCTION OF LYSOSOMAL TRANSPORT PROTEINS											
Nephropathic cystinosis	Defect in cystine transport from lysosome to cytoplasm	6 mo–1 yr	No	Cystine crystals	Pigmentary retinopathy	Hepatomegaly common	Normal CNS function	Generalized aminoaciduria	Elevated cystine in WBCs	Treatment with cysteamine is effective	Yes
Salla disease	Defect in sialic acid transport from lysosome to cytoplasm	6–9 mo	No	Normal	Normal	Normal	Delayed development, ataxia, nystagmus, exotropia	Sialic aciduria	Vacuolated lymphocytes may be found	Growth retarded in some	Lethal infantile form

CNS, Central nervous system; *RUSP*, recommended uniform screening panel; *WBC*, white blood cell.

adult life. Storage in solid organs results in hepatosplenomegaly and cardiomyopathy. Some disorders affect many tissues but spare the brain, with some having almost exclusive involvement of the musculoskeletal system. In many of these disorders, developmental delay, corneal clouding, and limitation of joint mobility are common features. Storage in tissues of the upper and lower airways may result in respiratory compromise. Nonimmune hydrops fetalis occurs in several lysosomal disorders.

DIAGNOSTIC TESTING

Most cases of Pompe (see Chapter 51) and mucopolysaccharidosis type I (MPS I) will be detected on newborn screening in states that have adopted this testing. However, this testing has a significant false-positive rate. Diagnostic testing includes measurement of glycosaminoglycans in urine and specific assays for lysosomal enzyme activity in white blood cells. If the urine test is positive, it helps direct specific enzyme measurement and gene testing. If it is negative, it does not exclude a lysosomal storage disorder, and other testing modalities are needed if clinical signs are convincing. In disorders in which specific pathogenic variants are known, molecular testing refines the diagnosis and is an important way to resolve disease status in infants with a positive newborn screen. Specific diagnosis, carrier testing, and evaluation of at-risk family members often require a multipronged approach to testing. Making a specific diagnosis is important because treatment for some lysosomal disorders is most effective when started early in the disease course.

TREATMENT STRATEGIES

Treatment directed at the metabolic abnormality is available for several lysosomal disorders. In specific disorders (e.g., Gaucher disease), oral medication may be successful in reducing the accumulation of the metabolite that cannot be catabolized. For some disorders, bone marrow (stem cell) transplantation is the most efficacious mechanism to restore lysosomal function. For others, replacement of the missing hydrolytic enzyme by systemic administration of the enzyme allows degradation of stored material. The disorders caused by deficient α-L-iduronidase (MPS I, Hurler syndrome, Scheie syndrome, and their variants) respond to treatment with intravenous human recombinant α-L-iduronidase (laronidase). Examples of other disorders for which enzyme therapy is available include MPS VI (Maroteaux-Lamy syndrome), Gaucher disease, Fabry disease, and MPS II (Hunter syndrome). Stem cell transplantation or ex vivo gene therapy has been helpful or under investigation in the following disorders: MPS type I (Hurler syndrome), MPS VI (Maroteaux-Lamy syndrome), MPS VII (Sly syndrome), metachromatic leukodystrophy, α-fucosidosis, α-mannosidosis, Gaucher disease, Krabbe disease, and Niemann-Pick disease type B. A discussion of appropriate target therapeutic strategies should be held with patients and their relevant caregivers by an expert in the specific disorder. Nonetheless, treatment for many of these conditions is supportive, with careful attention to respiratory status and physical therapy. As a result of the rapidly changing diagnostic and therapeutic options, providers with a special interest in these disorders should be consulted when a diagnosis is suspected. Treatment decisions should be made by the family in light of the potential therapeutic benefits and burdens of therapy and should be resolved before the onset of central nervous system manifestations, which are typically not improved by these approaches.

PEARLS FOR PRACTITIONERS

See Metabolic Disorders: Pearls for Practitioners at the end of this section.

REVIEW QUESTIONS

Available online.

CHAPTER **56**

Mitochondrial Disorders

MITOCHONDRIAL FUNCTION

Mitochondria are very complex organelles located in virtually all cells of the body. They perform a variety of functions such as intracellular signaling of oxygen tension and key roles in programmed cell death. From a biochemical perspective, mitochondria are the key site of energy production in the cell. They are the site of β-oxidation (see Chapter 54), the Krebs cycle, and parts of the urea cycle (see Fig. 52.4). This complexity requires more than 1,000 proteins localized specifically to the mitochondrion. Only 13 of these are encoded by the mitochondrial DNA (mtDNA); the remainder are nuclear encoded (on the chromosomes) and require import into the mitochondrion. In addition, the mtDNA needs its own set of proteins to allow for its maintenance, transcription, and translation.

Mitochondrial disorders are typically defined as defects in the ability to generate energy from oxidative phosphorylation to produce adenosine triphosphate (ATP) by transferring electrons formed by glycolysis and the Krebs cycle to a cascade that generates nicotinamide adenine dinucleotide hydrogen (NADH) and flavin adenine dinucleotide hydrogen ($FADH_2$) (Fig. 56.1) and are also known as phosphorylation disorders or respiratory chain disorders. The more dependent on energy production an organ is, the more profound the symptoms of deficiency of mitochondrial function in that organ. Certain proteins are only expressed in specific tissues, and defects in these will lead to differing patterns of disease. Although individually rare, taken together mitochondrial disorders may affect as many as 1 in 2,500 people.

SIGNS AND SYMPTOMS OF GENETIC DISORDERS OF MITOCHONDRIAL FUNCTION

The signs and symptoms of mitochondrial disorders are varied. Symptoms depend on how an organ is affected by energy deficiency. Muscle function that is compromised will result in muscle fatigue and weakness. Myopathy is common and may show **ragged red fibers** on a muscle biopsy. **Rhabdomyolysis** can occur. Brain dysfunction may be expressed as encephalopathy, seizures, loss of intellectual function, headache, or signs consistent with stroke. Spastic paraplegia and neuropathy may occur. Ataxia and basal ganglia symptoms are features of some disorders. Vision and eye muscle movement may be compromised, with **progressive external ophthalmoplegia** being almost diagnostic of an oxidative phosphorylation defect. Sensorineural hearing loss may occur. **Cardiomyopathy** is frequent, and cardiac rhythm disturbances occur. Liver dysfunction may be expressed as both synthetic deficiencies and frank liver failure. Diabetes may signal pancreatic involvement. Renal tubular abnormalities and kidney failure both occur. Gastrointestinal symptoms include both diarrhea and constipation that are difficult to treat. Sideroblastic anemia or bone marrow failure are typical of some disorders. **Alpers disease** (cerebral degeneration and liver disease) and **Leigh disease** (subacute necrotizing encephalomyelopathy) show similar brain lesions but in distinctly different areas of the brain. Because the signs and symptoms may involve multiple organs and may seem nonspecific, physicians may not suspect a mitochondrial disorder until significant progression has occurred (Fig. 56.2). Conversely, because there are no reliable tests to exclude a mitochondrial diagnosis, a high degree of confidence should be required before labeling a child as having a mitochondrial disease. Clinical criteria have been developed to classify patients as "definitive," "probable," "possible," or "unlikely" mitochondrial disorders. The criteria combine data from muscle, central nervous system, and multisystem involvement, plus metabolic and imaging studies (Table 56.1, Fig. 56.3).

BIOCHEMICAL ABNORMALITIES IN MITOCHONDRIAL FUNCTION

Although mitochondrial dysfunction produces many biochemical abnormalities, very few are specific for a hereditary disorder due to the frequency of secondary mitochondrial dysfunction (due to sepsis, kidney, cardiac or liver failure, many neurologic disorders). Defects in the mitochondrial respiratory chain may produce **lactic acidosis**. Given the complexity of the respiratory chain, it is not surprising that the described defects are varied as to cause, intensity, and tissues affected. The metabolism of glucose to carbon dioxide and water, with pyruvate as an intermediate (Fig. 56.4), occurs as part of the energy cycle in many tissues. Interference with mitochondrial oxidative metabolism may result in the accumulation of pyruvate. Because lactate dehydrogenase is ubiquitous, and because the equilibrium catalyzed by this enzyme greatly favors lactate over pyruvate, the accumulation of pyruvate results in lactic acidosis. The most common cause of such lactic acidosis is end-organ oxygen deficiency caused by hypoxia or poor perfusion. Lactic acidosis also occurs when specific reactions of pyruvate are impaired. In the liver, pyruvate undergoes carboxylation to form oxaloacetate using the enzyme pyruvate carboxylase; deficiency in this enzyme causes severe lactic acidosis. In an acute hospital setting, iatrogenic lactic acidosis may be induced when a high GIR (glucose infusion rate) is used as a component of therapy; judicious use of insulin assists

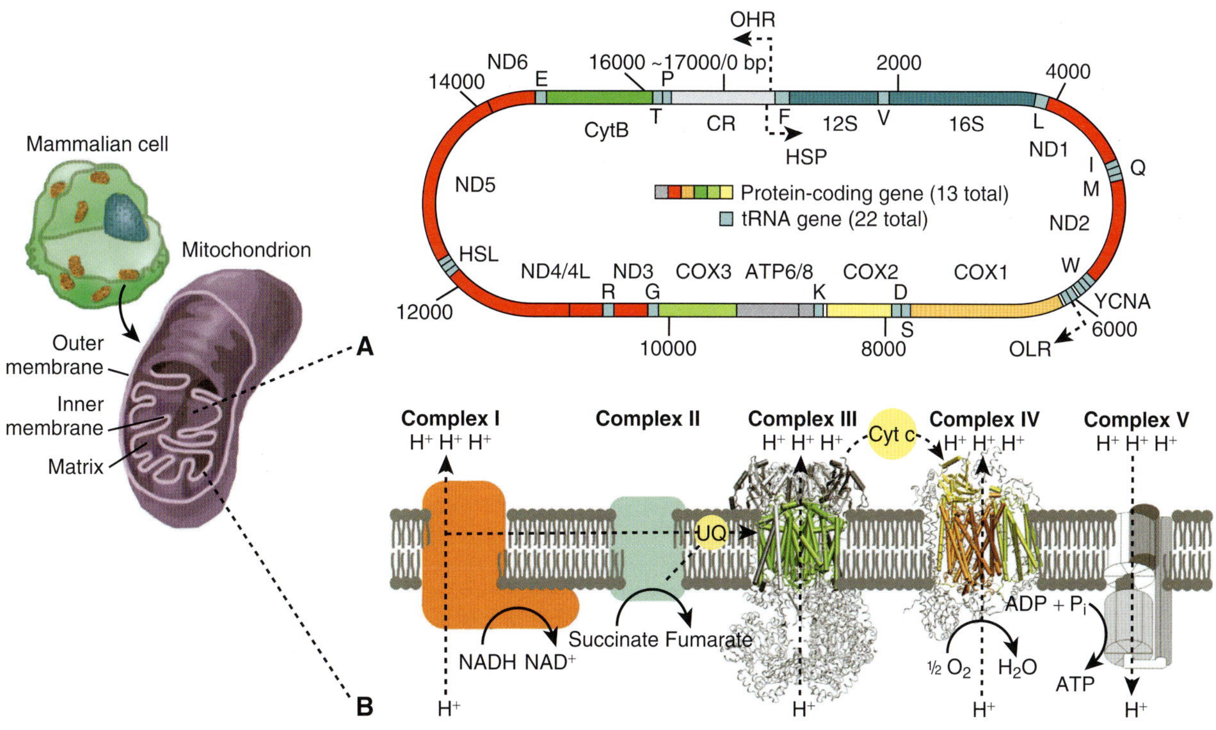

FIGURE 56.1 The mammalian mitochondrial genome and its protein-coding gene repertoire involved in the oxidative phosphorylation pathway. **(A)** Schematic representation of genes within mammalian mitochondrial genome (~7,000 bp). Genes on the outer circle are transcribed from the light strand. Location of the tRNAs *(red boxes)* conforms to the canonical placental mammalian arrangement. **(B)** Simplified view of the mitochondrial oxidative phosphorylation machinery. Complexes I (NADH dehydrogenase) and II (succinate dehydrogenase) receive electrons from either NADH or $FADH_2$. Electrons are then carried between complexes by the carrier molecules coenzyme Q/ubiquinone (UQ) and cytochrome c (CYC). The potential energy of these electron transfer events is used to pump protons against the gradient, from the mitochondrial matrix into the intermembrane space (complexes I and III [cytochrome bc_1] and IV [CYC oxidase]). ATP synthesis by complex V (ATP synthase) is driven by the proton gradient and occurs in the mitochondrial matrix. *HSP,* Putative heavy-strand promoter; *IM,* intermembrane space; *MM,* mitochondrial matrix; *OHR,* origin of heavy-strand replication; *OLR,* origin of light-strand replication. (From da Fonseca RR, Johnson WE, O'Brien SJ, et al. The adaptive evolution of the mammalian mitochondrial genome. *BMC Genomics.* 2008;9:119.)

in limiting the freely available glucose which can be converted to pyruvate and subsequently lactate. In many tissues, lactate is catabolized to form acetyl-coenzyme A (CoA) by the pyruvate dehydrogenase complex; deficiency in pyruvate dehydrogenase also can cause lactic acidosis. Because these reactions also play a role in gluconeogenesis, hypoglycemia can be a feature of these disorders. These disorders comprise forms of **primary lactic acidosis**. They frequently present as intractable, lethal acidosis in the first days or weeks of life and are difficult to treat. Some of the enzymes in this pathway can be measured and specific diagnoses can be made. This may require white blood cells or tissue biopsy. Measurement of growth and differentiation factor 15 (GDF-15) or fibroblast growth factor 21 (FGF-21; not reliable under 2 years of age), cytokines that are elevated when mitochondrial turnover is increased or the respiratory chain is deficient, can be used as quantitative screening tests for mitochondrial disorders. Urine organic acids may show suggestive elevations.

GENETICS OF MITOCHONDRIAL DISORDERS

Mitochondrial function is carried out by proteins that are encoded by both nuclear and mitochondrial genes. The mitochondrial genome encodes 13 subunits of the enzymes involved in mitochondrial oxidative phosphorylation. More than 85 autosomal genes code for the rest of the subunits of these enzymes. In children, only about 15% of cases of mitochondrial disease are caused by pathogenic variants in mtDNA; the rest are due to pathogenic variants in nuclear genes. The most frequent cases in several large series have been pathogenic variants that lead to a reduction in the ability of the mtDNA to maintain itself. Large population studies show carrier rates of about 2% of the population for pathogenic variants in polymerase (DNA directed), gamma *(POLG)*, and deoxyguanosine kinase *(DGUOK)*. Most disorders show autosomal recessive inheritance. A few are autosomal dominant, X linked, or caused by pathogenic variants in the mtDNA inherited from the mother, such as **MELAS** (mitochondrial encephalopathy,

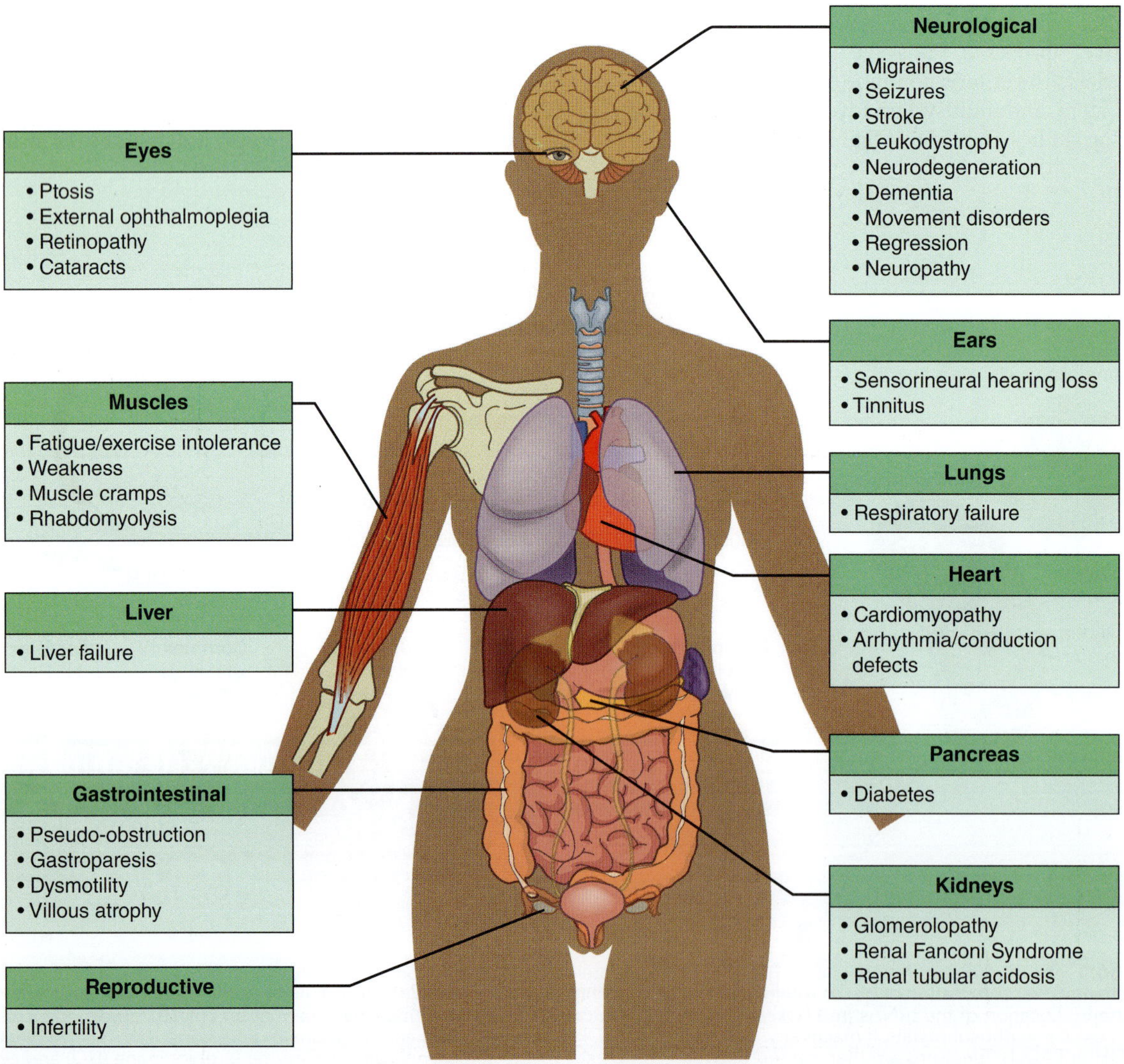

FIGURE 56.2 Clinical features of primary mitochondrial disease. The multisystem nature of mitochondrial disease can affect individuals across the age spectrum. Almost every organ in the body may be involved and often a specific combination of organ dysfunction (e.g., pancreas and cochlea) is the first indication of the diagnosis of mitochondrial disease.

TABLE **56.1** Mitochondrial Disease Criteria (MDC) Score for Assessing Mitochondrial Disease Diagnosis

MITOCHONDRIAL DISEASE CRITERIA (MDC) SCORE		
Clinical		
Muscular	Myopathy Abnormal EMG Motor developmental delay Exercise intolerance	Max score 2
Neurological	Severe hypotonia Dystonia/spasticity Ataxia Regression Neuropathy Seizures or encephalopathy	Max score 2
Multisystem	GI pseudo-obstruction Growth faltering Sensorineural hearing loss Immune dysregulation Ophthalmoplegia Renal tubular acidosis Cardiomyopathy	Max score 3
Total clinical score		**Maximum score for section is 4**
Laboratory/Imaging		
Metabolic	Lactate elevated to at least 2× (score 2) GDF15 elevated 10× Krebs' cycle intermediates elevated Ethyl malonic and methyl malonic acid 3-Methyl glutaconic acid CSF lactate, alanine elevated	
Imaging/other	Leigh disease (score 2) Stroke like episodes (score 2) Basal ganglia/brain stem Lactate peak on MRS	
Total clinical/metabolic/imaging score		**Maximum score for section is 4**
Histology/Morphology		
	Ragged red/blue fibers (score 4) COX-negative fibers (score 4) Reduced SDH staining SDH positive blood vessels (score 2) Abnormal mitochondria on EM (score 2)	
Total histology score		**Maximum score for section is 4**
Total MDC score (clinical, laboratory, imaging, histology)		**Total score is a maximum of 12**

A score of 1 indicates unlikely mitochondrial disorder; score of 2–4, possible mitochondrial disorder; score of 5–7, probable mitochondrial disorder; score of ≥8, definite mitochondrial disorder.
Data from Morava E, van den Heuvel L, Hol F, et al. Mitochondrial disease criteria: diagnostic applications in children. Neurology. *2006;67:1823–1826.*

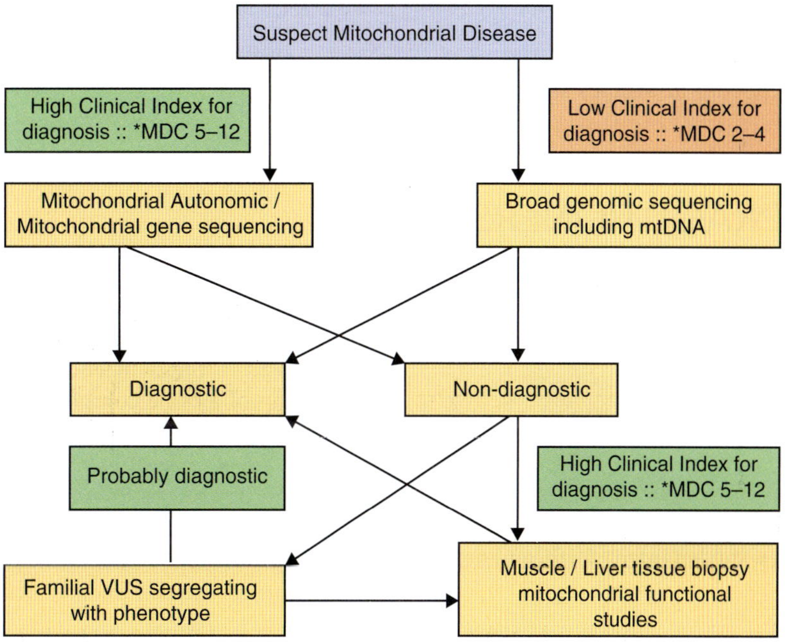

FIGURE 56.3 Diagnostic algorithm for assessing risk for mitochondrial disease. *MDC derived from Table 56.1. *MDC*, Mitochondrial disease criteria score; *mtDNA*, mitochondrial DNA; *VUS*, variant of unknown significance. (Data from Witters P, Saada A, Honzik T, et al. Revisiting mitochondrial diagnostic criteria in the new era of genomics. *Genet Med.* 2018;20[4]:444–451.)

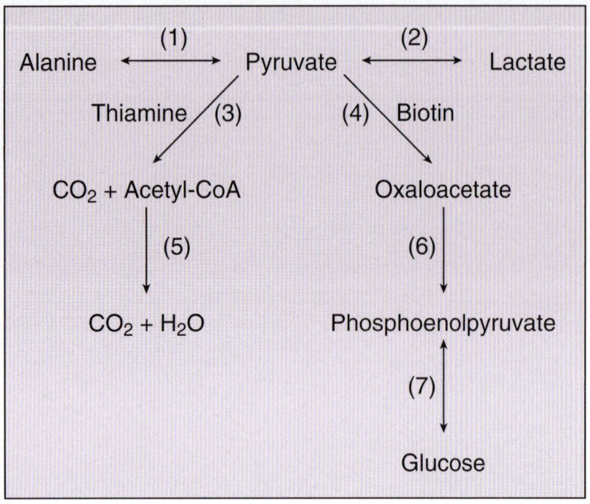

FIGURE 56.4 Metabolism of pyruvate and lactate. (1) Alanine aminotransferase, (2) lactate dehydrogenase, (3) pyruvate dehydrogenase, (4) pyruvate carboxylase, (5) Krebs cycle, (6) phosphoenolpyruvate carboxykinase, (7) reverse glycolysis. *CoA*, Coenzyme A.

lactic acidosis, and stroke-like episodes) and **MERRF** (mitochondrial encephalopathy with ragged red fibers), or deletions such as **MIDD** (maternally inherited diabetes and deafness). Diagnosis of a primary mitochondrial disorder may require sequencing of mtDNA, nuclear mitochondrial genes, and/or exome sequencing.

TREATMENT OF MITOCHONDRIAL DISORDERS

Repairing the basic energy deficit and getting the appropriate therapeutics and cofactors to the appropriate location within the mitochondrion are difficult. Nevertheless, a number of strategies are used, including judicious physical therapy and exercise with adequate rest, adequate nutrition, and cofactors for the deficient pathway. Specific treatment is limited for most mitochondrial defects. Providing adequate calories with intravenous dextrose during acute illness is essential. Vitamin cofactors for the respiratory chain, such as riboflavin and pharmaceutical forms of coenzyme Q, are often used, but evidence for their efficacy alone or in combination is limited. Proven therapies exist for some disorders, such as arginine supplementation for preventing stroke-like episodes in MELAS and idebenone for vision loss in LHON (Leber hereditary optic neuropathy). When a single organ bears most of the damage, organ transplant may be effective. Long-term surveillance and early treatment for complications are recommended. Identification of family members at risk may allow earlier diagnosis and treatment.

PEARLS FOR PRACTITIONERS

See Metabolic Disorders: Pearls for Practitioners at the end of this section.

REVIEW QUESTIONS

Available online.

Suggested Readings

Ah Mew N, Simpson KL, Gropman AL, et al. Urea Cycle Disorders Overview. In: Adam MP, Feldman J, Mirzaa GM, et al., eds. *GeneReviews® [Internet]*. Seattle (WA): University of Washington, Seattle; 2003:1993–2025. https://www.ncbi.nlm.nih.gov/books/NBK1217/.

Bali DS, El-Gharbawy A, Austin S, et al. Glycogen Storage Disease Type I . In: Adam MP, Feldman J, Mirzaa GM, et al., eds. *GeneReviews® [Internet]*. Seattle (WA): University of Washington, Seattle; 2006:1993–2025. https://www.ncbi.nlm.nih.gov/books/NBK1312/. (Updated October 14, 2021).

Chang IJ, Lam C, Vockley J. Medium-Chain Acyl-Coenzyme A Dehydrogenase Deficiency. In: Adam MP, Feldman J, Mirzaa GM, et al., eds. *GeneReviews® [Internet]*. Seattle (WA): University of Washington, Seattle; 2000:1993–2025. https://www.ncbi.nlm.nih.gov/books/NBK1424/. (Updated September 26, 2024).

Clarke LA. Mucopolysaccharidosis Type I. In: Adam MP, Feldman J, Mirzaa GM, et al., eds. *GeneReviews® [Internet]*. Seattle (WA): University of Washington, Seattle; 2002:1993–2025. https://www.ncbi.nlm.nih.gov/books/NBK1162/. (Updated April 11, 2024).

Raymond GV, Moser AB, Fatemi A. X-Linked Adrenoleukodystrophy. In: Adam MP, Feldman J, Mirzaa GM, et al., eds. *GeneReviews® [Internet]*. Seattle (WA): University of Washington, Seattle; 1999:1993–2025. https://www.ncbi.nlm.nih.gov/books/NBK1315/. (Updated April 6, 2023).

Sloan JL, Carrillo N, Adams D, et al. Disorders of Intracellular Cobalamin Metabolism. In: Adam MP, Feldman J, Mirzaa GM, et al., eds. *GeneReviews® [Internet]*. Seattle (WA): University of Washington, Seattle; 2008:1993–2025. https://www.ncbi.nlm.nih.gov/books/NBK1328/. (Updated December 16, 2021).

Strauss KA, Puffenberger EG, Carson VJ. Maple Syrup Urine Disease. In: Adam MP, Feldman J, Mirzaa GM, et al., eds. *GeneReviews® [Internet]*. Seattle (WA): University of Washington, Seattle; 2006:1993–2025. ht tps://www.ncbi.nlm.nih.gov/books/NBK1319/. (Updated April 23, 2020).

PEARLS FOR PRACTITIONERS

CHAPTER 50

Metabolic Assessment

- Metabolic inborn errors of metabolism (IEMs) are individually uncommon but as a group account for a significant disease burden.
- IEMs are frequent causes of sepsis-like presentations, intellectual disability, seizures, sudden infant death, and neurologic impairment.
- Genetic metabolic disorders result from the deficiency of an enzyme, its cofactors, or biochemical transporters that lead to the deficiency of a required metabolite, the buildup of a toxic compound, or a combination of both processes.
- There are at least 93 identified IEMs that are amenable to therapy targeted to the underlying cause and that present with intellectual disability as a prominent feature.
- Hypoglycemic and intoxicating (encephalopathy) metabolic disorders should be considered in all neonates presenting

with lethargy, poor tone, poor feeding, hypothermia, irritability, or seizures.

- All children presenting with altered levels of consciousness, irritability, neurologic impairment, or apparent sepsis-like episodes should have a plasma ammonia, blood glucose, and anion gap tested.
- In general, diagnostic testing for disorders of small molecule metabolism is most effective when metabolites are present in highest concentration in blood and urine, typically at times of catabolism such as during intercurrent illness or prolonged starvation.
- Respiratory alkalosis is frequently seen in the early stages of a hyperammonemic crisis, but this may give way to respiratory failure as the ammonia level increases.
- General clinical laboratory testing can define the metabolic derangement and refine the differential diagnosis in a child suspected to have an IEM.
- In the United States, most infants diagnosed with a treatable metabolic disorder will be identified as a result of an abnormal newborn screen.
- The recommended uniform screening panel (RUSP) is a list of conditions which helps states determine which serious, treatable rare diseases should be included in their newborn screening program. To be added to the RUSP, conditions must have a proven benefit of identification through newborn screening, including potential early intervention(s) that may reduce mortality or improve long-term outcomes.
- Newborn screening tests have a wide range of specificity, with some tests having close to a 90% false-positive rate. Therefore it is essential to perform appropriate confirmatory testing. Counseling of parents throughout the testing process is important due to the potential psychosocial harm of false-positive test results.
- Therapy for metabolic disease may focus on reducing the intake of specific substances that lead to buildup of toxic compounds. In addition, specific medications may prevent the buildup of toxic substances. Therapy may provide supraphysiologic cofactors that enhance residual enzymatic function.
- Catabolism increases the rate of production of these toxic small molecules in many metabolic disorders. Consequently, adequate and, at times, supraphysiologic provision of sources of energy (e.g., parenteral dextrose) is used to create an anabolic state, decreasing production of toxic metabolites.
- In many metabolic disorders, compounds that would otherwise be nonessential need to be provided (e.g., tyrosine in phenylketonuria [PKU], citrulline in ornithine transcarbamylase [OTC]).
- In specific metabolic disorders, the primary pathology is driven by a deficiency of essential compounds. In these disorders ongoing replacement of such factors is essential for prevention of secondary injury.
- Enzyme replacement therapy, organ transplant (e.g., liver transplant in OTC deficiency), or cell-based therapy (e.g., hematopoietic stem cell transplantation [HSCT] in mucopolysaccharidosis type 1 [MPS1]) are methods of providing missing enzymes in some disorders.

CHAPTER 51
Carbohydrate Disorders

- Glycogen storage disease type I manifests with hypoglycemia, hepatomegaly, lactic acidosis, and hypertriglyceridemia.
- Enzyme replacement therapy improves the outcome of Pompe disease (glycogen storage disease type II), which presents with hypotonia and cardiomyopathy.

CHAPTER 52
Amino Acid Disorders

- PKU is an autosomal recessive disorder and will result in severe intellectual disability; patients are normal at birth. Maternal PKU is the disorder that results in severe fetal growth restriction, microcephaly and severe developmental delays in an infant not directly affected by PKU but exposed to teratogenic levels of phenylalanine in the womb due to untreated PKU during pregnancy.
- Tyrosinemia type I manifests with severe hepatic dysfunction, coagulopathy, hypoglycemia, and renal tubular dysfunction.
- Homocystinuria resembles a connective tissue disorder and manifests with dislocated lens, long slender fingers, scoliosis, and arterial or venous thrombosis.
- Maple syrup urine disease (MSUD) presents 1–4 weeks after birth with poor feeding, emesis, coma, and hypotonia alternating with extensor spasms.

CHAPTER 53
Organic Acid Disorders

- Propionic and methylmalonic acidemias may present with tachypnea, emesis, lethargy, coma, neutropenia, thrombocytopenia, ketosis, hypoglycemia, and hyperglycinemia.
- Glutaric acidemia I presents with macrocephaly, dystonia, and metabolic strokes.

CHAPTER 54
Fatty Acid Oxidation Disorders

- Medium-chain acyl-CoA dehydrogenase (MCAD) deficiency is the most common disorder of fatty acid oxidation and presents with hypoketotic hypoglycemia, sudden death, and a Reye syndrome–like illness.

- Glutaric aciduria II may present with structural congenital malformations (kidney cysts, facial abnormalities, rocker-bottom feet, hypospadias), nonketotic hypoglycemia, and myopathy.

CHAPTER 55

Lysosomal and Peroxisomal Disorders

- Peroxisomal disorders often present with developmental delay and dysmorphic features affecting the skeleton or skin.
- Lysosomal storage disorders affect many organ systems and typically involve progressive central nervous system disease. Treatments include enzyme replacement therapy and hematopoietic stem cell transplant.

CHAPTER 56

Mitochondrial Disorders

- Most mitochondrial disorders are due to pathogenic variants in nuclear genes.
- Mitochondrial DNA pathogenic variants are maternally inherited.
- Mitochondrial disorders can produce myopathy, cardiomyopathy, central nervous system dysfunction, or hepatopathy, with or, occasionally, without lactic acidosis.

SECTION 11

FETAL AND NEONATAL MEDICINE

Chelsea M. Torres | Erica ElSeed Peterson | Tanner Wright

The following text focuses on some pregnancy-related or associated events. It makes use of concepts or descriptions that align with the traditional gender definitions by using concepts such as "maternal," "pregnant women," or "women." However, the concepts described are translatable to all persons who experience a pregnancy, regardless of their gender identity or intention to parent. We have used the term *people who are pregnant* to describe the individuals in this section but often refer to prior literature or text that uses noninclusive language.

CHAPTER 57

Assessment of the Birth Parent, Fetus, and Newborn

ASSESSMENT OF THE BIRTH PARENT

Pregnancies associated with perinatal morbidity or mortality are considered high risk. Identification of high-risk pregnancies is essential as they may be caused by maternal and/or fetal conditions. Conditions include fetal growth restriction (FGR, also called *intrauterine growth restriction* [IUGR]) or excessive fetal growth, congenital anomalies, birth asphyxia and trauma, prematurity (birth at <37 weeks) or postmaturity (birth at ≥42 weeks), neonatal disease, and long-term risks of cerebral palsy, intellectual disability, and chronic sequelae of neonatal intensive care. Ten to 20% of pregnancies may be high risk at some point. Although some obstetric complications are first seen during labor and delivery and cannot be predicted, more than 50% of perinatal mortality and morbidity results from problems identified before delivery. After a high-risk pregnancy is identified, measures can be instituted to prevent complications, provide intensive fetal surveillance, and initiate appropriate treatments of the birth parent and fetus.

A history of previous premature birth, intrauterine fetal demise, multiple gestation, FGR, congenital malformation, explained or unexplained neonatal death (e.g., group B streptococcal sepsis), birth trauma, preeclampsia, gestational diabetes, grand multipara status (five or more pregnancies), or cesarean section is associated with additional risk in subsequent pregnancies.

Pregnancy complications that increase the risk of adverse outcomes can be secondary to maternal or fetal conditions or both (Table 57.1). Neonatal complications include conditions of the placenta that tend to cause asphyxia and anemia.

Maternal medical complications associated with increased risk of maternal and fetal morbidity and mortality include diabetes, chronic hypertension, cardiac conditions, and autoimmune diseases (i.e., systemic lupus erythematosus with or without antiphospholipid antibodies). **Obstetric complications** often are associated with increased fetal or neonatal risk. Vaginal bleeding in the first trimester or early second trimester may be caused by a threatened or actual abortion. Painless vaginal bleeding that is not associated with labor and occurs in the late second or (more likely) third trimester can be the result of **placenta previa** (presence of placenta over the cervical os). Bleeding develops when the placental mass overlies the internal cervical os; this may produce maternal hemorrhage, necessitating transfusions. Bleeding also may result in premature delivery. Painful vaginal bleeding is often the result of retroplacental hemorrhage or **placental abruption**. Associated findings include advanced maternal age and parity, maternal chronic hypertension, cocaine or other stimulant use, preterm rupture

TABLE 57.1 Major Causes of Perinatal and Neonatal Mortality

FETUS
Abruptio placentae
Chromosomal anomalies
Congenital malformations (heart, CNS, kidney)
Hydrops fetalis
Intrauterine asphyxia
Intrauterine infection
Maternal underlying disease (chronic hypertension, autoimmune disease, diabetes mellitus)
Multiple gestation
Placental insufficiency
Umbilical cord accident
PRETERM INFANT
Respiratory distress syndrome/bronchopulmonary dysplasia (chronic lung disease)
Congenital anomalies
Infection
Intraventricular hemorrhage
Necrotizing enterocolitis
FULL-TERM INFANT
Birth asphyxia
Birth trauma
Congenital anomalies
Infection
Macrosomia
Meconium aspiration pneumonia
Persistent pulmonary hypertension

CNS, Central nervous system.

of membranes, polyhydramnios, twin gestation, and preeclampsia. Fetal asphyxia ensues as the retroplacental hematoma causes placental separation that interferes with fetal oxygenation. Both types of bleeding are associated with fetal blood loss. Neonatal anemia may be more common with placenta previa.

Abnormalities in the volume of amniotic fluid, oligohydramnios or polyhydramnios, are associated with increased morbidity. **Oligohydramnios** (amniotic ultrasound fluid index ≤2 cm) is associated with FGR and major congenital anomalies (particularly of the fetal kidneys) and with chromosomal abnormalities. Bilateral renal agenesis results in diminished production of amniotic fluid and **Potter syndrome**, which includes clubfeet, characteristic compressed facies, low-set ears, scaphoid abdomen, and diminished chest wall size accompanied by pulmonary hypoplasia. The absence of amniotic fluid restricts lung growth; neonates with this condition often die of respiratory failure rather than renal insufficiency. Twin-to-twin transfusion syndrome (usually affecting monochorionic twin pregnancies with disproportionate blood supply between fetuses) and complications from amniotic fluid leakage also are associated with oligohydramnios. Oligohydramnios increases the risk of fetal distress during labor.

Polyhydramnios may be acute and associated with premature labor, maternal discomfort, and respiratory compromise. More commonly, polyhydramnios is chronic. Polyhydramnios is often the result of unknown causes but can be associated with diabetes, immune or nonimmune hydrops fetalis, multiple gestation, trisomy 18 or 21, and other major congenital anomalies. Conditions that may cause reduced fetal swallowing and may ultimately lead to polyhydramnios are anencephaly, hydrocephaly, meningomyelocele, and intestinal atresias. Additional causes of polyhydramnios include spinal muscular atrophy and Beckwith-Wiedemann syndrome, chylothorax, congenital pulmonary airway malformation, diaphragmatic hernia, gastroschisis, sacral teratoma, placental chorioangioma, and myotonic dystrophy. The recipient of a larger amount of blood flow in twin-to-twin transfusion syndrome also may be associated with polyhydramnios. If severe, polyhydramnios may be managed with serial amniocenteses.

Hydrops fetalis may be a result of Rh or other blood group incompatibilities and anemia caused by intrauterine hemolysis of fetal erythrocytes by maternal immunoglobulin G–sensitized antibodies crossing the placenta. Hydrops is characterized by fetal edema, ascites, hypoalbuminemia, and heart failure. Causes of **nonimmune hydrops** include fetal arrhythmias (supraventricular tachycardia, congenital heart block), fetal anemia (parvovirus infection, bone marrow suppression, nonimmune hemolysis, or twin-to-twin transfusion), severe congenital malformation, intrauterine infections, congenital neuroblastoma, inborn errors of metabolism (storage diseases), fetal hepatitis, nephrotic syndrome, and pulmonary lymphangiectasia.

Premature rupture of the membranes, which occurs in the absence of labor, and **prolonged rupture of the membranes** (>18 hours) are associated with an increased risk of maternal (intraamniotic infection, also termed *chorioamnionitis*) or fetal infection and preterm birth. In the immediate newborn period, group B streptococcus and *Escherichia coli* are the two most common pathogens associated with sepsis. *Listeria monocytogenes* is a less common cause. *Mycoplasma hominis, Ureaplasma urealyticum*, *Chlamydia trachomatis*, and anaerobic bacteria of the vaginal flora also have been implicated in infection of the amniotic fluid. Infection with community-acquired or hospital-acquired methicillin-resistant *Staphylococcus aureus* must be considered for infants with skin infections or with known exposures. The risk of serious fetal infection increases as the duration between rupture and labor (latent period) increases, especially if the period is greater than 24 hours. Intrapartum antibiotic therapy decreases the risk of neonatal sepsis.

Multiple gestations are associated with increased risk resulting from polyhydramnios, premature birth, FGR, abnormal presentation (breech), intrauterine fetal demise, birth asphyxia, and twin-to-twin transfusion syndrome. **Twin-to-twin transfusion syndrome** is associated with high mortality and is seen only in **monochorionic multiple gestations** who share a common placenta and have an arteriovenous connection between their circulations. The fetus on the arterial side of the shunt serves as the blood donor, resulting in fetal anemia, growth restriction, and oligohydramnios for this fetus. The recipient, or venous-side fetus, is larger or discordant in size, is plethoric and polycythemic, and may show polyhydramnios. Ultrasonography in the second trimester reveals discordant amniotic fluid volume with oliguria/oligohydramnios and hypervolemia/polyuria/polyhydramnios with a distended bladder, with or without hydrops and heart failure. Treatment includes attempts to ablate the vascular anastomoses. The birth order of twins also affects morbidity by increasing the risk of the second-born twin for breech position, birth asphyxia, birth trauma, and respiratory distress syndrome.

Overall, twinning occurs in 2–4% of births worldwide. The diagnosis of the type of twins can be determined by placentation, sex, fetal membrane structure, and, if necessary, DNA analysis. Of note, multiple gestation does impact interpretation of routine prenatal screening tests (i.e., first trimester beta human chorionic gonadotropin [hCG] and pregnancy-associated plasma protein A [PAPP-A], second trimester quad screen, and cell free fetal DNA).

Preeclampsia/eclampsia is a disorder of unknown but probably vascular etiology that may lead to maternal hypertension, uteroplacental insufficiency, FGR, intrauterine asphyxia, maternal seizures, and maternal death. Preeclampsia is more common in nulliparous women and in women with multiple gestation, chronic hypertension, obesity, renal disease, positive family history of preeclampsia/eclampsia, systemic lupus erythematosus, or diabetes mellitus. A subcategory of preeclampsia, *HELLP* syndrome (**h**emolysis, **el**evated **l**iver enzyme levels, **l**ow **p**latelets), is more severe and associated with higher rates of maternal morbidity and mortality.

FETUS AND NEWBORN

The late fetal–early neonatal period has the highest mortality rate of any age interval. **Perinatal mortality** refers to fetal deaths occurring from the 20th week of gestation until the 28th day after birth and is expressed as number of deaths per 1,000 live births. Intrauterine fetal death accounts for 40–50% of the perinatal mortality rate. Such infants, defined as **stillborn**, are born without a heart rate and are apneic, limp, pale, and cyanotic. Many stillborn infants exhibit pale, peeling skin; corneal opacification; and soft cranial contents.

Mortality rates around the time of birth are expressed as number of deaths per 1,000 live births. The **neonatal mortality rate** includes all infants dying during the period from after birth to the first 28 days of life. Modern neonatal intensive care allows many newborns with life-threatening diseases to survive the neonatal period, only to die of their original diseases or of complications of therapy after 28 days of life. This delayed mortality and mortality caused by acquired illnesses occurs during the **postneonatal period**, which begins after 28 days of life and extends to the end of the first year of life.

The **infant mortality rate** encompasses the neonatal and the postneonatal periods. In the United States, infant mortality was 5.6 per 1,000 live births in 2023 per the Centers for Disease Control vital statistics report. The rate for Black infants was approximately 10.9 per 1,000 live births. The most common causes of perinatal and neonatal death are listed in Table 57.1. Overall, congenital anomalies and diseases of the premature infant are the most significant causes of neonatal mortality.

Low birthweight (LBW) infants, defined as infants having birthweights of less than 2,500 g, represent a disproportionately large component of the neonatal and infant mortality rates. Although LBW infants make up only 7–8% of all births, they account for more than 70% of neonatal deaths. FGR is the most common cause of LBW in developing countries, whereas prematurity is the more common cause in developed countries.

Very low birthweight (VLBW) infants, weighing less than 1,500 g at birth, represent about 1.5% of all births but account for 50% of neonatal deaths. Compared with infants weighing 2,500 g or more, LBW infants are 40 times more likely to die in the neonatal period; VLBW infants have a 200-fold higher risk of neonatal death. The United States continues to see the proportion of births affected by LBW increase over time. This is one of the major reasons that the U.S. infant mortality rate is high compared with other large, modern, industrialized countries.

Maternal factors associated with LBW caused by premature birth or FGR include a previous LBW birth, low socioeconomic status, low level of maternal education, poor antenatal care, maternal age younger than 16 years or older than 35 years, short interval between pregnancies, cigarette smoking, alcohol and untreated substance use, psychologic (poor social support) stresses, low prepregnancy weight (<45 kg), and poor weight gain during pregnancy (<10 lb). In the United States, LBW and VLBW rates for Black women are twice the rates for White women. The neonatal and infant mortality rates are nearly two-fold higher among Black infants. The difference in prevalence across racial groups is not attributable to a specific genetic predisposition and is only partially explained by socioeconomic status; systemic racism and health care disparities are significant contributors to poor outcomes.

ASSESSMENT OF THE FETUS

Fetal growth can be assessed by determining the fundal height of the uterus through bimanual examination of the gravid abdomen. **Fetal size** can be determined accurately by ultrasound techniques. Ultrasound measurements of the fetal biparietal diameter, femur length, head circumference, and abdominal circumference are used to estimate fetal growth. A combination of these measurements predicts fetal weight. Deviations from the normal fetal growth curve are associated with high-risk conditions.

FGR (also called *IUGR*) is present when estimated fetal weight and/or abdominal circumference is less than the 10th percentile for gestational age. Growth restriction may result from fetal conditions that reduce the innate growth potential, such as fetal infections, skeletal dysplasias, chromosomal abnormalities, and congenital malformation syndromes. Reduced fetal production of insulin and insulin-like growth factor I is associated with fetal growth restriction. Placental causes of FGR include villitis (often caused by congenital infections), placental tumors, chronic abruptio placentae, twin-to-twin transfusion syndrome, multiple gestation, teratogen exposure, uterine abnormalities, and (most commonly) placental insufficiency. Maternal causes include severe peripheral vascular diseases that reduce uterine blood flow (chronic hypertension, diabetic vasculopathy, and preeclampsia/eclampsia), reduced nutritional intake, intractable vomiting, alcohol or untreated substance use, cigarette smoking, uterine constraint (noted predominantly in birth parents of small stature with a low prepregnancy weight), and reduced weight gain during pregnancy. The outcome of FGR depends on the cause of the reduced fetal growth and the associated complications after birth (Table 57.2). Fetuses subjected to chronic intrauterine hypoxia as a result of uteroplacental insufficiency are at an increased risk for the comorbidities of birth asphyxia, polycythemia, and hypoglycemia. Fetuses with reduced tissue mass due to chromosomal, metabolic, or multiple congenital anomaly syndromes have poor outcomes based on the prognosis for the particular syndrome. Fetuses born to small birth parents and fetuses of birth parents with poor nutritional intake usually show catch-up growth after birth.

Fetal size does not always correlate with functional or structural maturity. Determining **fetal maturity** is crucial when deciding to deliver a fetus because of fetal or maternal disease. Fetal gestational age may be determined accurately based on a correct estimate of the last menstrual period (assuming regular menstrual cycles). Clinically relevant landmark dates can be used to determine gestational age; the first audible heart tones by Doppler methods are detected at 12–14 weeks, and quickening of fetal movements usually is perceived at 18–20 weeks. However, it is not always possible to determine fetal

TABLE 57.2 Problems of Fetal Growth Restriction and Small for Gestational Age

PROBLEM*	PATHOGENESIS
Intrauterine fetal demise	Hypoxia, acidosis, infection, lethal anomaly
Temperature instability	Cold stress, ↓ fat stores, hypoxia, hypoglycemia
Perinatal asphyxia	↓ Uteroplacental perfusion during labor with or without chronic fetal hypoxia-acidosis, meconium aspiration syndrome
Hypoglycemia	↓ Tissue glycogen stores; ↓ gluconeogenesis, hyperinsulinism, ↑ glucose needs of hypoxia, hypothermia, large brain
Polycythemia-hyperviscosity	Fetal hypoxia with ↑ erythropoietin production
Reduced oxygen consumption/hypothermia	Hypoxia, hypoglycemia, starvation effect, poor subcutaneous fat stores
Dysmorphology	Chromosomal-genetic disorders, oligohydramnios-induced deformations
Pulmonary hemorrhage	Hypothermia, polycythemia, hypoxia

*Other problems are common to the gestational age–related risks of prematurity if born before 37 weeks.

Modified from Brandsma E, Christ LA, Duncan AF. The high-risk infant. In: Kliegman RM, St. Geme JW, eds. Nelson Textbook of Pediatrics. *22nd ed. Philadelphia: Elsevier; 2024.*

maturity by such dating, especially in a high-risk situation, such as preterm labor or a diabetic pregnancy; in the absence of known last menstrual period, fetal ultrasonography before 22 weeks of gestation provides the most accurate measure of gestational age.

Methods used to assess **fetal well-being** before the onset of labor are focused on identifying a fetus at risk for asphyxia or a fetus already compromised by uteroplacental insufficiency. In certain circumstances (equivocal antenatal testing or when there is question if labor can be tolerated), the **contraction stress test** (historically referred to as the *oxytocin challenge test*) stimulates uterine contractions through an infusion of oxytocin sufficient to produce three contractions in a 10-minute period. The development of periodic fetal bradycardia out of phase with uterine contractions (late deceleration) is a positive test result and predicts an at-risk fetus.

The **nonstress test** examines the heart rate response to fetal body movements. Heart rate accelerations of more than 15 beats/min lasting 15 seconds are reassuring. If two such episodes occur in 20 minutes, the test result is considered reactive (vs. nonreactive), and the fetus is considered low risk. The **biophysical profile** can include the nonstress test with ultrasonography observation of fetal breathing movements, gross body movements, fetal tone, and the presence of amniotic fluid pockets more than 2 cm in size; this offers the most accurate fetal assessment.

Doppler examination of the umbilical arteries in the setting of FGR permits identification of decreased or reversed diastolic blood flow associated with increased peripheral vascular resistance, fetal hypoxia with acidosis, and placental insufficiency. **Cordocentesis** (percutaneous umbilical blood sampling) can provide fetal blood for Pao_2, pH, lactate, and hemoglobin measurements to identify a hypoxic, acidotic, or anemic fetus that is at risk for intrauterine fetal demise or birth asphyxia. While not commonly used to determine fetal well-being, cordocentesis can be used to determine fetal blood type, platelet count, microbial testing, antibody titer, and karyotype, as well as facilitate fetal transfusions if necessary.

In a high-risk pregnancy, the fetal heart rate should be monitored continuously during labor, as should uterine contractions. Fetal heart rate abnormalities may indicate baseline **tachycardia** (>160 beats/min as a result of anemia, β-sympathomimetic drugs, maternal fever, hyperthyroidism, arrhythmia, or fetal distress), baseline **bradycardia** (<120 beats/min as a result of fetal distress, complete heart block, or local anesthetics), or **reduced beat-to-beat variability** (flattened tracing resulting from fetal sleep, tachycardia, atropine, sedatives, prematurity, or fetal distress). Periodic changes of the heart rate relative to uterine contraction help determine the presence of hypoxia and acidosis caused by uteroplacental insufficiency or maternal hypotension (late decelerations) or by umbilical cord compression (variable decelerations). The presence of severe decelerations (late or recurrent variable) that do not resolve with resuscitation efforts may be suggestive of **fetal acidemia**, prompting cesarean delivery.

Fetal anomalies may be detected by ultrasonography. Emphasis should be placed on visualization of the genitourinary tract; the head (for anencephaly or hydrocephaly), neck (for thickened nuchal translucency), and back (for spina bifida); skeleton; gastrointestinal tract; and heart. Four-chamber and great artery views are required for detection of heart anomalies. Certain **chromosomal anomaly syndromes** (T21, T18) can be associated with an abnormal "quadruple screen." Fetal genetic and chromosomal disorders can also be detected by analyzing cell-free fetal DNA that is present in the maternal circulation (often referred to as *noninvasive prenatal testing*). If a fetal abnormality is detected, fetal therapy or delivery with therapy in the neonatal intensive care unit may be lifesaving.

ASSESSMENT OF THE NEWBORN

The approach to the birth of an infant requires a detailed history (Table 57.3). Knowing the birth parent's risk factors enables the delivery room team to anticipate problems that may occur. The history of a woman's labor and delivery can reveal events that might lead to complications affecting either the birth parent or the neonate, even when the pregnancy was previously considered low risk. Anticipating the need to resuscitate a newborn as a result of fetal distress increases the likelihood of successful resuscitation.

Newborn Physiology

The **transition from fetal to neonatal physiology** occurs at birth. Oxygen transport across the placenta results in a gradient between the maternal and fetal Pao_2. Although fetal oxygenated blood has a low Pao_2 level compared with that of adults and infants, the fetus is not anaerobic. Fetal oxygen uptake and consumption are similar to neonatal rates, even though the thermal environments and activity levels of fetuses and neonates differ. The oxygen content of fetal blood is almost equal to the oxygen content in older infants and children because fetal blood has a much higher concentration of hemoglobin.

Fetal hemoglobin (two α and two γ chains) has a higher affinity for oxygen than adult hemoglobin, facilitating oxygen transfer across the placenta. The fetal hemoglobin-oxygen dissociation curve is shifted to the left of the adult curve (Fig. 57.1); at the same Pao_2 level, fetal hemoglobin is more saturated than adult hemoglobin. Fetal hemoglobin functions on the lower end of the oxygen saturation curve resulting in adequate delivery of oxygen to the tissue. In contrast, at the higher oxygen concentrations present in the placenta, oxygen loading is enhanced. In the last trimester, fetal hemoglobin production begins to decrease as adult hemoglobin production begins to increase, becoming the only hemoglobin available to the infant by 3–6 months of life. At this time, the hemoglobin dissociation curve has shifted to the adult position.

A portion of well-oxygenated umbilical venous blood returning to the heart from the placenta partially perfuses the liver. The remainder bypasses the liver through a shunt (the **ductus venosus**) and enters the inferior vena cava. This oxygenated blood in the vena cava constitutes 65–70% of venous return to the right atrium. Venous return from the upper body combines with the remaining two-thirds of the caval blood in the right atrium and is directed to the right ventricle. This mixture of venous low-oxygenated blood from the upper and lower body enters the pulmonary artery. Only 8–10% of it is pumped to the pulmonary circulation; the remaining 80–92% of the right ventricular output bypasses the lungs through the **ductus arteriosus** and enters the descending aorta. Vasoconstriction produced by medial muscle hypertrophy of the pulmonary arterioles and fluid in the fetal lung increases resistance to pulmonary blood flow. Pulmonary artery tone also

TABLE 57.3 Components of the Perinatal History

DEMOGRAPHIC SOCIAL INFORMATION	PRESENT PREGNANCY
Age Ethnicity Sexually transmitted infections, hepatitis, HIV Substance use: nicotine, ethanol, cocaine, stimulants, opiates Laboratory screening: syphilis, rubella, hepatitis B, HIV, blood group Occupational exposure	Single or multiple gestation* Current gestational age* and method of assessing gestational age Fetal surveillance (NST, biophysical profile) Prenatal screening test results, including ultrasonography (anomalies, hydrops, oligohydramnios, polyhydramnios) Amniotic fluid analysis (L/S ratio) Vaginal bleeding
PAST MEDICAL DISEASES	**PRETERM LABOR**
Chronic hypertension Heart disease Diabetes mellitus Thyroid disorders Hematologic/malignancy Autoimmune (SLE) Genetic history: inborn errors of metabolism, bleeding, jaundice	Rupture of membranes (duration, timing) Preeclampsia Urinary tract infection Colonization status (herpes simplex, group B streptococcus) Medications/substance exposures Acute medical illness/exposure to infectious agents Fetal therapy
PRIOR PREGNANCY	**LABOR AND DELIVERY**
Abortion/stillbirths Intrauterine fetal demise Neonatal death Congenital malformation Incompetent cervix Birthweight Prematurity Multiple gestations Blood group sensitization/ neonatal jaundice Hydrops Infertility	Duration of labor Presentation: vertex, breech Vaginal vs. cesarean section Spontaneous labor vs. augmented or induced with oxytocin (Pitocin) Instrumentation at delivery Antibiotics given, if any, and time received Maternal fever/intraamniotic infection Fetal heart rate patterns (distress) Presence of meconium and/or blood in the amniotic fluid* Maternal analgesia, anesthesia Apgar score Methods of resuscitation Postnatal gestational age assessment Growth status (AGA, LGA, SGA) Management of umbilical cord (delayed clamping) and complications (nuchal, knot, prolapse, avulsion)*

Components of Neonatal Resuscitation Program (NRP) "prebirth questions."
AGA, Average for gestational age; *L/S*, lecithin-to-sphingomyelin ratio; *LGA*, large for gestational age; *NST*, nonstress test; *SGA*, small for gestational age; *SLE*, systemic lupus erythematosus.

responds to hypoxia, hypercapnia, and acidosis with vasoconstriction, a response that may increase pulmonary vascular resistance further. The ductus arteriosus remains patent in the fetus because of low $Pa{O_2}$ levels and dilating prostaglandins. In utero, the right ventricle is the dominant ventricle, pumping 65% of the combined ventricular output, which is a high

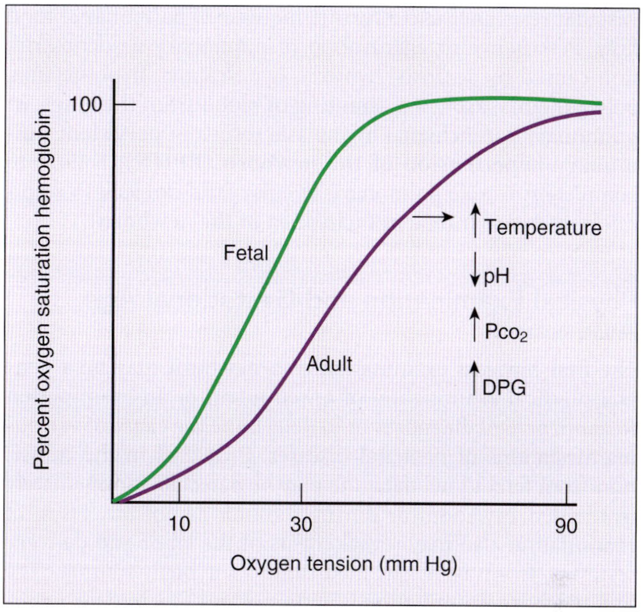

FIGURE 57.1 Hemoglobin-oxygen dissociation curves. The position of the adult curve depends on the binding of adult hemoglobin to 2,3-diphosphoglycerate (DPG), temperature, $P{CO_2}$, and hydrogen ion concentration (pH).

volume (450 mL/kg/min) compared with that pumped by an older infant's right ventricle (200 mL/kg/min).

The **transition of circulation**, occurring between the fetal and neonatal periods, involves the removal of the low-resistance circulation of the placenta, onset of neonatal breathing, reduction of pulmonary arterial resistance, and closure of in utero shunts. Clamping the umbilical cord eliminates the low-pressure system of the placenta and increases systemic blood pressure. Decreased venous return from the placenta decreases right atrial pressure. As breathing begins, air replaces lung fluid, maintaining the functional residual capacity. With normal transition, fluid leaves the lung through pulmonary lymphatic and venous system absorption, and remaining fluid in the oropharynx after delivery is subsequently swallowed.

Most infants require little pressure to spontaneously open the lungs after birth (5–10 cm H_2O). With the onset of breathing, pulmonary vascular resistance decreases, partly a result of the mechanics of breathing and partly a result of the elevated arterial oxygen tensions. The increased blood flow to the lungs increases the volume of pulmonary venous blood returning to the left atrium; left atrial pressure now exceeds right atrial pressure, and the foramen ovale closes. As the flow through the pulmonary circulation increases and arterial oxygen tensions rise, the ductus arteriosus begins to constrict. In a term infant, this constriction functionally closes the ductus arteriosus within 1–2 days after birth. A permanent closure requires thrombosis and fibrosis, a process that may take several weeks. In a premature infant, the ductus arteriosus is less sensitive to the effects of oxygen; if circulating levels of vasodilating prostaglandins are elevated, the ductus arteriosus may remain patent. This patency is a common problem in a premature infant with respiratory distress syndrome.

Ventilation, oxygenation, and normal pH and $P{CO_2}$ levels immediately reduce pulmonary artery vasoconstriction by causing smooth muscle relaxation. Remodeling of the medial muscle hypertrophy begins at birth and continues for the next 3 months, resulting in a further reduction of pulmonary vascular resistance and a further increase of pulmonary blood flow. Persistence or aggravation of pulmonary vasoconstriction caused by acidosis, hypoxia, hypercapnia, hypothermia, polycythemia, asphyxia, shunting of blood from the lungs, or pulmonary parenchymal hypoplasia results in **persistent pulmonary hypertension of the newborn (PPHN)**. Failure to completely excrete pulmonary alveolar fluid can lead to respiratory distress **(transient tachypnea of the newborn)**.

Physical Examination and Gestational Age Assessment

The first physical examination of a newborn may be a general physical examination of a well infant or an examination to confirm fetal diagnoses or to determine the cause of various manifestations of neonatal diseases. Problems in the transition from fetal to neonatal life may be detectable immediately in the delivery room or during the first day of life. Physical examination also may reveal effects of the labor and delivery resulting from asphyxia, medications, or birth trauma. The first newborn examination is an important way to detect congenital malformations or deformations (Table 57.4).

Appearance

Signs such as cyanosis, nasal flaring, intercostal retractions, and grunting suggest an airway or pulmonary issue. Meconium staining of the umbilical cord, nails, and skin suggest possible fetal distress and can be associated with meconium aspiration. The level of spontaneous activity, passive muscle tone, quality of the cry, and apnea are useful screening signs to evaluate the state of the nervous system.

TABLE 57.4 Life-Threatening Congenital Anomalies

NAME	MANIFESTATIONS
Choanal atresia (stenosis)	Respiratory distress/cyanosis that improves with crying, unable to pass nasogastric tube through nares
Pierre Robin (Stickler) syndrome	Micrognathia, cleft palate, airway obstruction
Diaphragmatic hernia	Scaphoid abdomen, bowel sounds present in chest, heart shifted to right, respiratory distress, polyhydramnios
Tracheoesophageal fistula	Polyhydramnios, aspiration pneumonia, excessive salivation, unable to place nasogastric tube in stomach
Intestinal obstruction: volvulus, duodenal atresia, ileal atresia	Polyhydramnios, bile-stained emesis, abdominal distention
Gastroschisis/omphalocele	Polyhydramnios; intestinal obstruction
Renal agenesis/Potter syndrome	Oligohydramnios, anuria, pulmonary hypoplasia, pneumothorax
Hydronephrosis	Bilateral abdominal masses
Neural tube defects: anencephaly, meningomyelocele	Polyhydramnios, elevated α-fetoprotein; decreased fetal activity
Down syndrome (trisomy 21)	Hypotonia, congenital heart disease, duodenal atresia
Ductal-dependent congenital heart disease	Cyanosis, murmur, shock

Vital Signs

The examination should proceed with an assessment of vital signs, particularly heart rate (normal rate, 120–160 beats/minute), respiratory rate (normal rate, 30–60 breaths/minute), temperature, and blood pressure (often reserved for sick infants). Length, weight, and head circumference should be measured and plotted on growth curves to determine whether growth is normal, increased, or decreased for the gestational age.

Gestational Age

Gestational age is determined by an assessment of various physical signs (Fig. 57.2) and neuromuscular characteristics (Fig. 57.3) that vary according to fetal age and maturity. **Physical criteria** mature with advancing fetal age, including increasing firmness of the pinna of the ear; increasing size of the breast tissue; decreasing fine, immature lanugo hair over the back; and appearance of external genitalia. **Neurologic criteria** mature with gestational age, including increasing flexion of the legs, hips, and arms; increasing tone of the flexor muscles of the neck; and decreasing laxity of the joints. These signs can be determined during the first day of life and are assigned scores. The cumulative score is correlated with a gestational age, which is usually accurate to within 2 weeks (Fig. 57.4).

Gestational age assessment can aid in the detection of both prematurity and abnormal fetal growth patterns, both of which contribute to risk of neonatal morbidity and mortality. Infants born at a weight greater than the 90th percentile for age are considered **large for gestational age (LGA)**. **Macrosomia** describes infants born at >4,000 grams regardless of gestational age. Among the risks associated with being LGA are all the risks of the infant of a diabetic mother and risks associated with postmaturity. Infants born at a weight less than 10th percentile for age (some growth curves use <2 standard deviations or the 5th percentile) are **small for gestational age** (SGA) and commonly have a history of FGR prenatally. Problems associated with SGA infants are listed in Table 57.2.

Skin

The skin should be evaluated for pallor, plethora, jaundice, cyanosis, meconium staining, petechiae, ecchymoses, congenital nevi, and neonatal rashes. Vasomotor instability with cutis marmorata, telangiectasia, phlebectasia (intermittent mottling with venous prominence), and acrocyanosis (feet and hands) is normal in a premature infant. Acrocyanosis also may be noted in a healthy term infant in the first days after birth.

The skin is covered with soft lanugo hair, which often disappears by term gestation. **Hair tufts** (thick, coarse hair) over the lumbosacral spine suggest a spinal cord defect. **Vernix caseosa**, a soft, white, creamy protective layer covering the skin in preterm infants, reduces by term. Post-term infants often have peeling, parchmentlike skin. **Congenital dermal melanocytosis** are transient, gray-blue to black pigmented macules more commonly seen in infants with more melanated skin types; they are frequently located over the lower back, buttocks, and

Physical maturity	–1	0	1	2	3	4	5
Skin	Sticky, friable, transparent	Gelatinous, red, translucent	Smooth, pink, visible veins	Superficial peeling or rash, few veins	Cracking, pale areas, rare veins	Parchment, deep cracking, no vessels	Leathery, cracked, wrinkled
Lanugo	None	Sparse	Abundant	Thinning	Bald areas	Mostly bald	
Plantar surface	Heel–toe 40-50 mm: –1 Less than 40 mm: –2	<50 mm, no crease	Faint red marks	Anterior transverse crease only	Creases on anterior 2/3	Creases over entire sole	
Breast	Impercep-tible	Barely perceptible	Flat areola–no bud	Stripped areola, 1-2 mm bud	Raised areola, 3-4 mm bud	Full areola, 5-10 mm bud	
Eye/ear	Lids fused, loosely (–1), tightly (–2)	Lids open, pinna flat, stays folded	Slightly curved pinna; soft, slow recoil	Well-curved pinna, soft but ready recoil	Formed and firm; instant recoil	Thick cartilage, ear stiff	
Genitals male	Scrotum flat, smooth	Scrotum empty, faint rugae	Testes in upper canal, rare rugae	Testes descending, few rugae	Testes down, good rugae	Testes pendulous, deep rugae	
Genitals female	Clitoris prominent, labia flat	Prominent clitoris, small labia minora	Prominent clitoris, enlarging minora	Majora and minora equally prominent	Majora large, minora small	Majora cover clitoris and minora	

FIGURE 57.2 Physical criteria for assessment of maturity and gestational age. Expanded Ballard Score includes extremely premature infants and has been refined to improve accuracy in more mature infants. (From Ballard JL, Khoury JC, Wedig K, et al. New Ballard Score, expanded to include extremely premature infants. *J Pediatr.* 1991;119:417–423.)

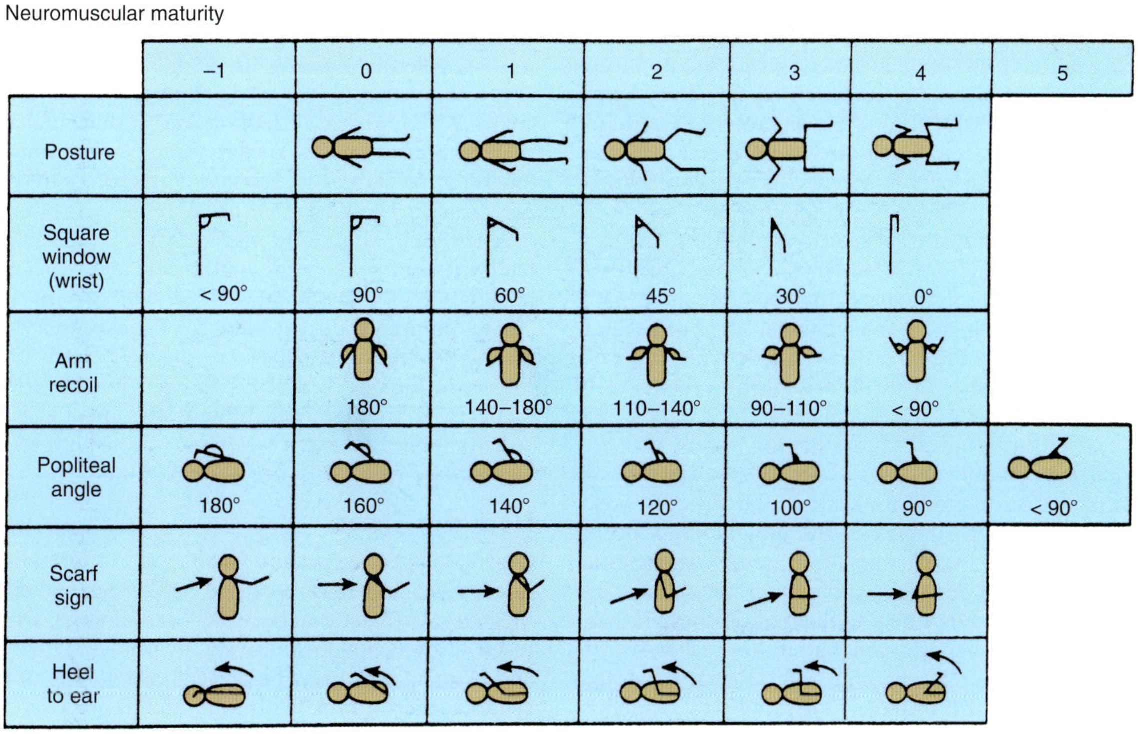

FIGURE 57.3 Neuromuscular criteria for assessment of maturity and gestational age. Expanded Ballard Score includes extremely premature infants and has been refined to improve accuracy in more mature infants. (From Ballard JL, Khoury JC, Wedig K, et al. New Ballard Score, expanded to include extremely premature infants. *J Pediatr.* 1991;119:417–423.)

Maturity rating

Score	Weeks
−10	20
−5	22
0	24
5	26
10	28
15	30
20	32
25	34
30	36
35	38
40	40
45	42
50	44

FIGURE 57.4 Maturity rating as calculated by adding the physical and neurologic scores, calculating the gestational age. (From Ballard JL, Khoury JC, Wedig K, et al. New Ballard Score, expanded to include extremely premature infants. *J Pediatr.* 1991;119:417–423.)

large joints. **Nevus simplex**, or pink macular hemangioma, is common, usually transient, and noted on the back of the neck, eyelids, and forehead. **Nevus flammeus**, or **port-wine stain**, is seen on the face and should cause the examiner to consider multiple congenital syndromes (i.e., Sturge-Weber, Klippel-Trenaunay, Parkes-Weber, Proteus).

Congenital melanocytic nevi are pigmented lesions of varying size noted in 1% of neonates. **Giant pigmented nevi** are uncommon but have malignant potential. **Capillary hemangiomas** are raised, red lesions, whereas **cavernous hemangiomas** are deeper, blue masses. Both lesions increase in size after birth then resolve over 1–4 years. When significantly enlarged or numerous, these hemangiomas may produce high-output heart failure or platelet trapping and hemorrhage. **Erythema toxicum** is an erythematous, papular-vesicular rash common in neonates that develops after birth and involves eosinophils in the vesicular fluid. **Pustular melanosis**, more common in melanated skin types, may be seen at birth and consists of small, dry pustules that slough off to reveal a pigmented brown macular base. Erythema toxicum and pustular melanosis are benign lesions that are often diagnosed clinically. In cases where the appearance may mimic more serious conditions, such as the vesicular rash of disseminated herpes simplex or the bullous eruption of *S. aureus* impetigo, Tzanck smear, Gram stain, Wright stain, direct fluorescent antibody stain, and polymerase chain reaction assays for herpes DNA help to distinguish these rashes. Other common characteristic rashes are **milia** (yellow-white epidermal cysts of the pilosebaceous follicles that are noted on the nose or chin) and **miliaria** ("prickly heat"), which is caused by obstructed sweat glands. Periorbital edema is common in the first 1–2 days after birth. Diffuse edema may be present in preterm infants but could also suggest hydrops fetalis, hypoalbuminemia, or lymphatic disorders.

Skull

The skull may be elongated and molded after a prolonged labor; this resolves 2–3 days after birth. The sutures should be palpated to determine the width and the presence of premature fusion or **craniosynostosis**. The anterior and posterior fontanelles should be soft and nonbulging, with the anterior larger than the posterior. A large fontanelle is associated with hydrocephalus, hypothyroidism, rickets, and other disorders. Soft areas away from the fontanelle are **craniotabes**; these lesions feel like a Ping-Pong ball when they are palpated. The skull should be examined carefully for signs of trauma or lacerations from internal fetal electrode sites; these may become a nidus for infection.

Vaginal delivery or prolonged labor prior to a cesarean section may result in a **caput succedaneum**, a soft edematous subcutaneous scalp swelling that crosses suture lines, or a **cephalohematoma**, a subperiosteal hematoma confined within suture lines.

Face, Eyes, and Mouth

The face should be inspected for dysmorphic features, such as epicanthal folds, hypertelorism, preauricular tags or sinuses, low-set ears, long philtrum, and cleft lip or palate. Facial asymmetry may be a result of seventh nerve palsy; head tilt may be caused by torticollis.

The eyes should open spontaneously, especially in an upright position. Before 28 weeks of gestational age, the eyelids may be fused. Coloboma, megalocornea, and microphthalmia suggest other malformations or intrauterine infections. A cloudy cornea greater than 1 cm in diameter also may be seen in congenital glaucoma, uveal tract dysgenesis, and storage diseases. Conjunctival and retinal hemorrhages are common and usually of no significance. The pupillary response to light is present at 28 weeks of gestation. The **red reflex of the retina** is appreciated by viewing the pupil through the ophthalmoscope. A normal retinal reflex appears a warm yellow-to-red color. A white reflex, or **leukokoria**, is abnormal and may be the result of cataracts, ocular tumor, severe chorioretinitis, persistent hyperplastic primary vitreous, or retinopathy of prematurity.

The mouth should be inspected for the presence of natal teeth, clefts of the soft and hard palate and uvula, and micrognathia. A bifid uvula suggests a submucosal cleft. White, shiny, multiple transient epidermal inclusion cysts (Epstein pearls) on the hard palate are normal. Hard, marble-sized masses in the buccal mucosa are usually transient idiopathic fat necrosis. The **tympanic membranes** are dull, gray, opaque, and immobile in the first 1–4 weeks. These findings should not be confused with otitis media.

Neck and Chest

The neck appears short and symmetric. Abnormalities include midline clefts or masses caused by thyroglossal duct cysts or by goiter and lateral neck masses (or sinuses), which are the result of branchial clefts. Cystic hygromas (lymphangiomas) and hemangiomas may be present. Shortening of the sternocleidomastoid muscle with a fibrous tumor over the muscle produces head tilt and asymmetric facies (neonatal torticollis). Arnold-Chiari malformation and cervical spine lesions also produce torticollis. Edema and webbing of the neck suggest Turner syndrome. Both clavicles should be palpated for fractures.

Examination of the chest includes inspection of the chest wall to identify asymmetry resulting from absence of the pectoralis muscle and inspection of the breast tissue to determine gestational age and detect any breast abscess. Male and female infants may have breast engorgement and produce milk; milk expression should not be attempted. **Supernumerary nipples** can be unilateral or bilateral.

Lungs

Examination of the lungs includes observations of the rate, depth, and nature of intercostal or sternal retractions. Breath sounds should be equal on both sides of the chest, and rales should not be heard after the first 1–2 hours of life. Diminished or absent breath sounds on one side suggest pneumothorax, collapsed lung, pleural effusion, or diaphragmatic hernia. Subcutaneous emphysema of the neck or chest also suggests a pneumothorax or pneumomediastinum, whereas bowel sounds auscultated in the chest in the presence of a scaphoid abdomen suggest a diaphragmatic hernia.

Heart

The position of the heart in infants is more midline than in older children. The first heart sound is normal, whereas the second heart sound may not be split in the first day of life. Decreased splitting of the second heart sound is noted in PPHN, transposition of the great vessels, and pulmonary atresia. Heart murmurs in newborns are common during the first day of life. Most of these murmurs are transient and are due to closure of the ductus arteriosus, peripheral pulmonary artery stenosis, or a small ventral septal defect. Pulses should be palpated in the upper and lower extremities (over the brachial and femoral arteries). Blood pressure in the upper and lower extremities should be measured in all patients with a murmur or heart failure. An upper-to-lower blood pressure extremity gradient of more than 20 mm Hg could suggest coarctation of the aorta.

Abdomen

A normal liver may be palpable up to 2 cm below the right costal margin. The spleen tip is less likely to be palpable. A left-sided liver suggests situs inversus and asplenia syndrome. Both kidneys can be palpated in the first day of life with gentle, deep palpation. The first urination occurs during the first 24 hours of life in more than 95% of normal term infants.

Abdominal masses usually represent hydronephrosis or dysplastic-multicystic kidney disease. Less often, masses indicate ovarian cysts, intestinal duplication, neuroblastoma, or mesoblastic nephroma. Masses should be evaluated immediately with ultrasound. Abdominal distention may be caused by intestinal obstructions, such as ileal atresia, meconium ileus, midgut volvulus, imperforate anus, or Hirschsprung disease. Meconium stool is passed normally within 48 hours of birth in 99% of term infants. The anus should appear patent. An imperforate anus is not always visible. The abdominal wall musculature may be absent, as in prune-belly syndrome, or weak, resulting in diastasis recti. **Umbilical hernias** are commonly noted in neonates; they should be reducible and without signs of strangulation. The umbilical cord should be inspected to determine the presence of two arteries and one vein and the absence of a urachus or a herniation of abdominal contents, as occurs with an **omphalocele**. The latter is associated with extraintestinal problems, such as genetic trisomies (T21, T18, T13), Turner syndrome, and Beckwith-Wiedemann syndrome. Persistent bleeding from the cord suggests a coagulation disorder. Chronic discharge may be a granuloma of the umbilical stump or, less frequently, a draining omphalomesenteric cyst or urachus. Significant erythema around the umbilicus can be a sign of **omphalitis** and can lead to portal vein thrombophlebitis and subsequent extrahepatic portal hypertension if not treated appropriately. The herniation of bowel through the abdominal wall 2–3 cm lateral to the umbilicus is a **gastroschisis**.

Genitalia

At term, the testes should be descended into a well-formed pigmented and rugated scrotum. The testes occasionally are in the inguinal canal; this is more common among preterm infants, as is cryptorchidism. Scrotal swelling may represent a hernia, transient hydrocele, in utero torsion of the testes, or, rarely, dissected meconium from meconium ileus and peritonitis. Hydroceles are clear and readily seen by transillumination, whereas testicular torsion in the newborn may present as a painless, dark swelling. The urethral opening should be at the end of the penis. Epispadias or hypospadias alone should not raise concern about disorders of sexual differentiation. However, if no testes are present in the scrotum and hypospadias is present, disorders of sexual differentiation should be investigated. Circumcision should be deferred with hypospadias because the foreskin may be needed for the repair. The normal prepuce is often too tight to retract in the neonatal period, and families should be counseled that there is no need to retract the neonatal foreskin for hygiene purposes.

The female genitalia normally may reveal a milky white or blood-streaked vaginal discharge as a result of maternal hormone withdrawal. Mucosal tags of the labia majora are common. Distention of an imperforate hymen may produce hydrometrocolpos and a lower midline abdominal mass as a result of an enlarged uterus. Clitoral enlargement with fusion of the labial-scrotal folds (labia majora) suggests excessive androgen exposure, such as from congenital adrenal hyperplasia.

Extremities

Examination of the extremities should involve assessment of length, symmetry, and presence of hemihypertrophy, atrophy, polydactyly, syndactyly, single transverse palmar creases, absent fingers, overlapping fingers, rocker-bottom feet, clubfoot, congenital bands, fractures, and amputations.

Spine

The spine should be examined for evidence of sacral hair tufts, a dermal sinus tract above the gluteal folds, congenital scoliosis (a result of hemivertebra), and soft tissue masses such as lipomas or meningomyeloceles.

Hips

The hips should be examined for congenital dysplasia (noted by dislocation). Gluteal fold asymmetry or leg length discrepancy is suggestive of dysplasia, but the examiner should perform the Barlow test and the Ortolani maneuver to evaluate the stability of the hip joint. These tests determine whether the femoral head can be displaced from the acetabulum **(Barlow maneuver)** or reduced back into the acetabulum **(Ortolani maneuver)**.

NEUROLOGIC ASSESSMENT

The neurologic examination should include assessment of active and passive tone, level of alertness, primary neonatal (primitive) reflexes, deep tendon reflexes, spontaneous motor activity, and cranial nerves (involving retinal examination, extraocular muscle movement, masseter power as in sucking, facial motility, hearing, and tongue function). The Moro reflex, present at birth and gone in 3–6 months, is one of the primary newborn reflexes. It is elicited by sudden, slight dropping of the supported head from a slightly raised supine position, which should elicit opening of the hands and extension and abduction of the arms, followed by upper extremity flexion and a cry. The palmar grasp is present by 28 weeks of gestation and gone by 4 months of age. Deep tendon reflexes may be brisk in a normal newborn; up to 5–10 beats of ankle clonus can be normal. The Babinski sign is expected to be extensor (upgoing) in normal infants. The sensory examination can be evaluated by withdrawal of an extremity, grimace, and cry in response to painful stimuli. The rooting reflex (turning of the head toward light tactile stimulation of the perioral area) is present by 32 weeks of gestation. For further discussion of neonatal reflexes, please see Table 180.1.

Delivery Room Assessment and Care

The **Apgar score**, a rapid standardized assessment based on physiologic responses to the birth process, is a good method for assessing the need to resuscitate a newborn (Table 57.5). At intervals of 1 and 5 minutes after birth, each of the five physiologic parameters is observed or elicited by a qualified examiner. Full-term infants with a normal cardiopulmonary adaptation should score 8–9 at 1 and 5 minutes. Apgar scores of 4–7 warrant close attention to determine whether the infant's status will improve and to ascertain whether any pathologic condition is contributing to the low Apgar score.

An Apgar score of 0–3 represents either a cardiopulmonary arrest or a condition caused by severe bradycardia, hypoventilation, or central nervous system depression. Most low Apgar scores are caused by difficulty in establishing adequate ventilation and not by primary cardiac pathology. Low Apgar scores may be caused by fetal hypoxia or other factors listed in Table 57.6. Most infants with low Apgar scores respond to assisted ventilation by face mask or by endotracheal intubation.

About 80–85% of infants born at term will initiate spontaneous breathing by 10 to 30 seconds; another 10% will begin respirations with stimulation. However, about 3% of infants will establish spontaneous breathing only after positive pressure ventilation (PPV) while another 2% will require endotracheal intubation and less than 1% will require chest compressions and medications.

Resuscitation of the newborn is a process of assessment, intervention, and reassessment. It begins with the initial steps of providing warmth, ensuring that the airway is patent and open, clearing the airway of secretions (as needed), drying, and providing gentle tactile stimulation. Observation of the infant drives the resuscitation. The newborn should be observed for vigor and muscle tone, heart rate, and respirations, including use of a pulse oximeter. If the baby is vigorous with good muscle tone, heart rate is above 100 beats/minute, and breathing is unlabored, no further resuscitation is needed. Alternatively, if the neonate is apneic or hypoventilating and remains cyanotic, PPV should be initiated. Ventilation should be performed with a well-fitted mask attached to a self-inflating bag, a flow-inflating bag, or a T-piece resuscitator. A manometer should be used to prevent extremely high pressures from being given to the newborn; initially 21% oxygen (for infants >35 weeks of gestational age) should be administered through the mask. If the infant's heart rate does not respond to adequate PPV (remains <100 bpm), an endotracheal tube should be placed. Color change on an end tidal carbon dioxide detector, signaling effective ventilation, may not occur immediately when heart rate, perfusion, and gas exchange are low. The usual recovery after a cardiac arrest first involves a return to a normal heart rate, followed by disappearance of cyanosis and noticeably improved perfusion. An infant may remain limp and be apneic for a prolonged time after return of cardiac output and correction of acidosis.

Resuscitation of a newborn with low Apgar score follows a similar systematic sequence as that for resuscitation of older patients, but in the newborn period this simplified ABCD approach requires some qualification (Fig. 57.5).

In the ABCD approach, **A** stands for initial steps to establish an open **airway** through positioning, stimulation of spontaneous respirations, and suctioning of amniotic fluid or meconium if needed.

B represents **breathing**. PPV should be provided to support breathing for newborns with apnea or bradycardia. Infants with labored breathing can benefit from continuous positive airway pressure, while those with low oxygen saturations for age (in minutes) should be trialed with supplemental oxygen.

TABLE **57.5** Apgar Score

	POINTS		
SIGNS	**0**	**1**	**2**
Heart rate	0	<100/min	>100/min
Respiration	None	Slow, gasping, or weak cry	Vigorous cry
Muscle tone*	None	Some extremity tone and flexion	Arms and legs well flexed, active motion
Reflex irritability (grimace)	None	Some motion/grimacing in response to stimulation	Cry, cough, sneezes
Color of body	Pale or blue	Pink body, blue extremities	Pink all over

**Passive tone; assessed compared to level appropriate for estimated gestational age.*

TABLE 57.6 Etiology of Birth Asphyxia

TYPE	EXAMPLE
INTRAUTERINE	
Hypoxia-ischemia	Uteroplacental insufficiency, abruptio placentae, prolapsed cord, maternal hypotension, unknown
Anemia-shock	Vasa previa, placenta previa, fetomaternal hemorrhage, erythroblastosis
INTRAPARTUM	
Birth trauma	Cephalopelvic disproportion, shoulder dystocia, breech presentation, spinal cord transection
Hypoxia-ischemia	Umbilical cord compression, tetanic uterine contraction, abruptio placentae
POSTPARTUM	
Central nervous system	Maternal medication, trauma, previous episodes of fetal hypoxia-acidosis
Congenital neuromuscular disease	Congenital myasthenia gravis, myopathy, myotonic dystrophy
Infection	Sepsis with shock, pneumonia
Airway disorder	Choanal atresia, severe obstructing goiter or tumor, laryngeal webs
Pulmonary disorder	Severe immaturity, pneumothorax, pleural effusion, diaphragmatic hernia, pulmonary hypoplasia
Renal disorder	Pulmonary hypoplasia, pneumothorax

C represents **circulation**. Concurrently, while assessing the pulmonary status of the infant, heart rate is critical to assess. If PPV does not improve bradycardia or if asystole is present, chest compressions should be performed at a rate of 120 compressions/minute with compressions and breaths given at a ratio of 3:1 (3 compressions followed by 1 breath). Most neonates respond to ventilatory intervention without need of chest compressions.

D represents the administration of **drugs**. If bradycardia is unresponsive to ventilation and coordinated chest compressions, epinephrine should be administered. Epinephrine (1:10,000) can be given through an umbilical venous line, via intraosseous route, or injected into the endotracheal tube. However, when epinephrine is administered through the endotracheal tube, the result is uncertain due to unpredictable absorption. Often, effective ventilation and airway support for the persistently apneic newborn are sufficient.

In newborns of more than 35 weeks of gestation with moderate-to-severe hypoxic-ischemic injury at birth, induced **therapeutic hypothermia** (33.0–34.0°C) for 72 hours may reduce the severity of brain injury. Brain hypothermia, whether induced by whole body or selective head cooling, provides neuroprotection against encephalopathy presumably due to hypoxic ischemia.

Newborn Care

All newborn infants benefit from certain standard interventions.

Vitamin K prophylaxis (intramuscular injection) prevents hemorrhagic disease of the newborn. **Erythromycin ocular ointment** is used to prevent gonococcal ophthalmia neonatorum. Before birth hospitalization discharge, infants should be screened for various diseases through the **newborn screening program**, which varies by state or country. Although states can opt to include screenings for additional conditions, in the United States there is a Recommended Uniform Screening Panel that includes core conditions (Table 57.7) that should be included in every newborn screening program and secondary conditions that can be detected in the differential diagnosis of a core disorder. Adjunct components of newborn screening are the newborn hearing screen and critical congenital heart defect (CCHD) screening. **Newborn hearing screening** is conducted via otoacoustic emissions or auditory brain stem response, with further audiology testing if concerns are identified. The aim is for all infants to have a hearing screen by 1 month of age, a diagnosis (made on confirmatory testing) by 3 months of age, and intervention for hearing loss initiated no later than 6 months of age to optimize clinical and developmental outcomes. **CCHD screening** measures oxygen saturation of a preductal and postductal limb to determine if a gradient is present, indicating need for further work-up (echocardiogram) to detect certain critical heart defects (see Chapters 144 and 145). While not all critical congenital heart disease will be detected by this screening test, it can facilitate early identification and intervention. All infants with birthweight greater than 2 kg should receive the **hepatitis B vaccine** in the first 24 hours of life; all infants with birthweight less than 2 kg should receive the hepatitis B vaccine prior to birth hospitalization discharge. All infants should also be assessed for respiratory syncytial virus (RSV) prevention prior to birth hospitalization discharge. Maternal vaccination for RSV during pregnancy or postnatal RSV immunoglobulin injection for the infant reduce the risk of severe RSV disease in the first year of life.

Newborn-Specific Findings and Other Conditions

Cyanosis

Acrocyanosis (blue color of the hands and feet with pink color of the rest of the body) is common in the delivery room and is usually normal. **Central cyanosis** of the trunk, mucosal membranes, and tongue can occur at any time after birth and is always a manifestation of a serious underlying condition. Cyanosis is noted with 4–5 g/dL of deoxygenated hemoglobin, corresponding to <80% SpO_2 in a neonate. The "cyanotic blind spot" refers to the inability to clinically detect hypoxemia in the range of SpO_2 81–93% by assessing appearance alone. Clinicians, and pulse oximeters, have also demonstrated varied ability to detect cyanosis across the spectrum of skin melanin concentrations. Central cyanosis can be caused by problems in many different organ systems, although cardiopulmonary diseases are the most common (Table 57.8). Respiratory distress syndrome, sepsis, and cyanotic heart disease are common causes of cyanosis in infants admitted to a neonatal intensive care unit. A systematic evaluation of these and other causes of cyanosis is required for every cyanotic infant after prompt administration of oxygen, with or without assisted ventilation.

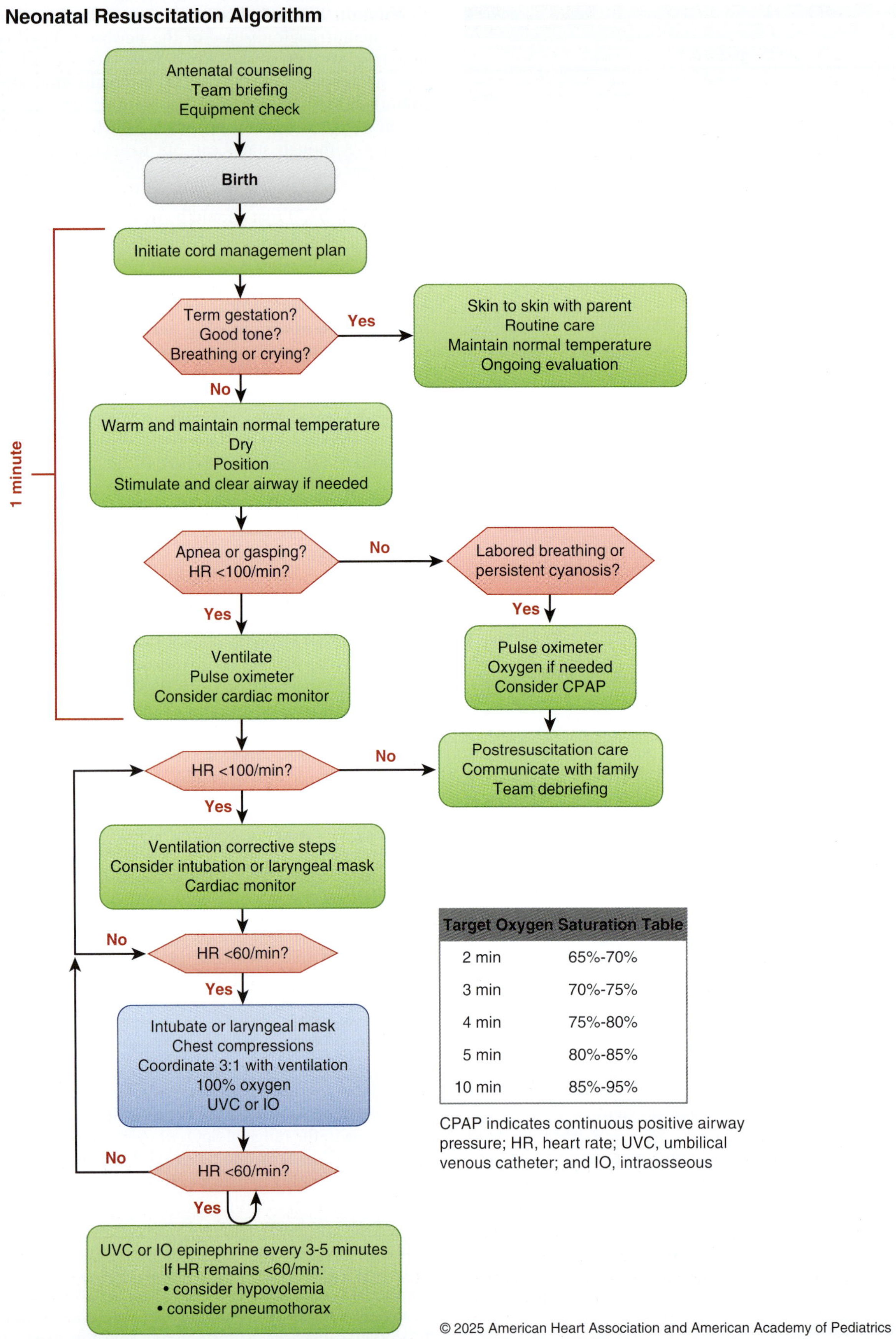

Target Oxygen Saturation Table	
2 min	65%-70%
3 min	70%-75%
4 min	75%-80%
5 min	80%-85%
10 min	85%-95%

FIGURE 57.5 Steps of neonatal resuscitation. *CPAP,* Continuous positive airway pressure; *HR,* heart rate; *IV,* intravenous; *PPV,* positive pressure ventilation; *SpO$_2$,* blood oxygen saturation. (Reprinted with permission *Circulation.*2025;152:S385-S423 ©2025 American Heart Association, Inc.)

TABLE 57.7 Recommended Uniform Screening Panel: Core Conditions

- 3-Hydroxy-3-methyglutaric aciduria
- 3-Methylcrotonyl-CoA carboxylase deficiency
- Argininosuccinic aciduria
- Biotinidase deficiency
- Carnitine uptake defect/carnitine transport defect
- Citrullinemia, type I
- Classic galactosemia
- Classic phenylketonuria
- Congenital adrenal hyperplasia
- Critical congenital heart disease*
- Cystic fibrosis
- Glutaric acidemia type I
- Glycogen storage disease type II (Pompe)
- Guanidinoacetate methyltransferase deficiency
- Hearing loss*
- Holocarboxylase synthase deficiency
- Homocystinuria
- Infantile Krabbe disease (low galactocerebrosidase and psychosine ≥10 nM)
- Isovaleric acidemia
- Long-chain L-3 hydroxyacyl-CoA dehydrogenase deficiency
- Maple syrup urine disease
- Medium-chain Acyl-CoA dehydrogenase deficiency
- Methylmalonic acidemia (cobalamin disorders)
- Methylmalonic acidemia (methylmalonyl-CoA mutase)
- Mucopolysaccharidosis type I
- Mucopolysaccharidosis type II
- Primary congenital hypothyroidism
- Propionic acidemia
- S, β-thalassemia
- S,C disease
- S,S disease (sickle cell anemia)
- Severe combined immunodeficiencies
- Spinal muscular atrophy due to homozygous deletion of exon 7 in SMN1
- β-Ketothiolase deficiency
- Trifunctional protein deficiency
- Tyrosinemia, type I
- Very long-chain Acyl-CoA dehydrogenase deficiency
- X-linked adrenoleukodystrophy

**Indicates testing conducted as part of the universal newborn screening program but not obtained from dried blood spot analysis.*
Newborn metabolic screening is processed from dried blood spot specimens.
From the Advisory Committee on Heritable Disorders in Newborns and Children. Recommended uniform screening panel. Bethesda, MD: U.S. Department of Health and Human Services, updated January 2023. https://www.hrsa.gov/advisory-committees/heritable-disorders/rusp.

Life-Threatening Congenital Malformations

Various congenital anomalies can interfere with vital organ function after birth (see Table 57.4). Some malformations, such as choanal atresia and other lesions obstructing the airway, may complicate ventilation. Intrathoracic lesions, such as cysts or diaphragmatic hernia, interfere with respiration. Other malformations that obstruct the gastrointestinal system at the level of the esophagus, duodenum, ileum, or colon may lead to aspiration pneumonia, intestinal perforation, or necrosis. Gastroschisis and omphalocele are associated with exposed bowel on the abdominal wall. Omphalocele is often associated with other malformations, requiring a thorough work-up to evaluate for other anomalies and underlying genetic abnormalities. Gastroschisis is not usually associated with genetic abnormalities or other anomalies. However, it may be associated with necrotic bowel. Collaboration with pediatric surgeons for management of these patients is imperative.

Perinatal Hypoxia and Asphyxia

Whether in utero or after birth, asphyxia-caused **hypoxic-ischemic brain injury** (encephalopathy) is the result of reduced gas exchange. Asphyxia associated with severe bradycardia or cardiac insufficiency reduces or eliminates tissue blood flow, resulting in ischemia. The fetal and neonatal circulatory systems respond to reduced oxygen availability by shunting the blood preferentially to the brain, heart, and adrenal glands and away from the intestine, kidneys, lungs, and skin.

Metabolic acidosis during asphyxia is caused by the combined effects of poor cardiac output secondary to hypoxic depression of myocardial function, systemic hypoxia, and tissue anaerobic metabolism. With severe or prolonged intrauterine or neonatal asphyxia, multiple vital organs are affected (Table 57.9).

Many conditions that contribute to **fetal or neonatal asphyxia** are the same medical or obstetric problems associated with high-risk pregnancy. Maternal diseases that interfere with uteroplacental perfusion (chronic hypertension, preeclampsia, and diabetes mellitus) place the fetus at risk for intrauterine asphyxia. Medications given during labor to treat these conditions, such as intrapartum magnesium given to someone with preeclampsia to prevent seizures or pain medication given to manage labor pain, may cross the placenta and depress the infant's respiratory center, resulting in apnea at the time of birth.

Fetal conditions associated with asphyxia usually do not manifest until delivery, when the infant must initiate and sustain ventilation. In addition, the upper and lower airways must be patent and unobstructed. Alveoli must be free from foreign material (meconium, amniotic fluid, and infectious exudates), which increases airway resistance, reduces lung compliance, and leads to respiratory distress and hypoxia. Some extremely immature infants weighing less than 1,000 g at birth may be unable to expand their lungs, even in the absence of other pathology. Their compliant chest walls and surfactant deficiency may result in poor air exchange, retractions, hypoxia, and apnea.

The newborn (particularly a preterm infant) responds paradoxically to hypoxia with apnea rather than tachypnea as occurs in adults. Episodes of intrauterine asphyxia also may depress the neonatal central nervous system. If recovery of the fetal heart rate occurs as a result of improved uteroplacental perfusion, fetal hypoxia and acidosis may resolve. Nonetheless, if the effect on the respiratory center is more severe, a newborn may not initiate an adequate ventilatory response at birth and may undergo another episode of asphyxia.

Shock

Shock is often represented by pallor, poor capillary refill time, lack of palpable pulses, hypotonia, cyanosis, and eventually cardiopulmonary arrest. Blood loss before or during labor and delivery is a common cause of shock in the delivery room. Blood loss may be caused by fetal-maternal hemorrhage, placenta previa, vasa previa, twin-to-twin transfusion syndrome, or displacement of blood from the fetus to the placenta *(asphyxia pallida)*. Hemorrhage into a viscus, such as the liver or spleen, may be noted in macrosomic infants, and hemorrhage into the cerebral ventricles may produce shock and apnea in preterm infants. Anemia, hypoalbuminemia, hypovolemia, and shock are common manifestations of Rh immune hydrops, which is less commonly seen now given administration of Rh-D immunoglobulin.

Severe intrauterine bacterial sepsis may present with shock in the delivery room or after the infant is transferred

TABLE 57.8 Differential Diagnosis of Neonatal Cyanosis

SYSTEM/DISEASE	MECHANISM
PULMONARY	
Respiratory distress syndrome	Surfactant deficiency
Sepsis, pneumonia	Inflammation, pulmonary hypertension, ARDS
Meconium aspiration syndrome	Mechanical obstruction, inflammation, pulmonary hypertension
Persistent pulmonary hypertension of the newborn	Pulmonary hypertension
Diaphragmatic hernia	Pulmonary hypoplasia, pulmonary hypertension
Transient tachypnea	Retained lung fluid
CARDIOVASCULAR	
Cyanotic heart disease with decreased pulmonary blood flow	Right-to-left shunt as in pulmonary atresia, tetralogy of Fallot
Cyanotic heart disease with increased pulmonary blood flow	Mixing lesion as in single ventricle or truncus arteriosus
Cyanotic heart disease with congestive heart failure	Pulmonary edema and poor cardiac output as in hypoplastic left heart and coarctation of aorta
Heart failure alone	Pulmonary edema and poor cardiac contractility as in sepsis, myocarditis, supraventricular tachycardia, or complete heart block; high-output failure as in PDA or vein of Galen or other arteriovenous malformations
CNS	
Maternal sedative drugs	Hypoventilation, apnea
Asphyxia	CNS depression
Intracranial hemorrhage	CNS depression, seizure
Neuromuscular disease	Hypotonia, hypoventilation, pulmonary hypoplasia
HEMATOLOGIC	
Acute blood loss	Shock
Chronic blood loss	Heart failure
Polycythemia	Pulmonary hypertension
Methemoglobinemia	Low-affinity hemoglobin or red blood cell enzyme defect
METABOLIC	
Hypoglycemia	CNS depression, congestive heart failure
Congenital adrenal hyperplasia	Shock (salt-losing)

ARDS, Acute respiratory distress syndrome; *CNS*, central nervous system; *PDA*, patent ductus arteriosus.

TABLE 57.9 Effects of Asphyxia

SYSTEM	EFFECT
Central nervous system	Hypoxic-ischemic encephalopathy, intraventricular hemorrhage, periventricular leukomalacia, cerebral edema, seizures, hypotonia, hypertonia
Cardiovascular	Myocardial ischemia, poor contractility, tricuspid insufficiency, hypotension
Pulmonary	Persistent pulmonary hypertension, respiratory distress syndrome
Renal	Acute tubular or cortical necrosis
Endocrine	Adrenal hemorrhage
Gastrointestinal	Perforation, ulceration, necrosis
Metabolic	Inappropriate antidiuretic hormone, hyponatremia, hypoglycemia, hypocalcemia, myoglobinuria
Skin	Subcutaneous fat necrosis
Hematology	Disseminated intravascular coagulation

to the nursery. Typically, these infants are mottled, hypotonic, and cyanotic and have diminished peripheral pulses. They have a normal hemoglobin concentration but may manifest neutropenia, thrombocytopenia, and disseminated intravascular coagulation. Congenital left ventricular cardiac obstruction (critical aortic stenosis or hypoplastic left heart syndrome) also produces shock, although not usually in the delivery room.

Treatment of newborn infants with shock may be anticipated through knowledge of the infant's immune status, evidence of hydrops, or suspicion of intrauterine infection or anomalies. Stabilization of the airway and institution of respiratory support are essential. Hypovolemic shock should be managed with repeated boluses of 10 mL/kg of normal saline or lactated Ringer solution. O negative blood should be available in the delivery room and given to the newborn if signs of anemia and/or hypovolemic shock are present, such as in severe immune hemolysis or neonatal blood loss secondary to trauma. Drugs such as dopamine, epinephrine, or cortisol may improve cardiac output and tissue perfusion.

Birth Injury

Birth injury refers to avoidable and unavoidable injury to the fetus during the birth process. **Caput succedaneum** is a diffuse, edematous, often dark swelling of the soft tissue of the scalp that extends across the midline and suture lines. In infants delivered from a face presentation, soft tissue edema and bruising of the face is an equivalent phenomenon. Caput succedaneum may be seen after prolonged labor in full-term and preterm infants. Molding of the head often is associated with caput succedaneum and is the result of pressure that is induced from overriding the parietal and frontal bones against their respective sutures.

A **cephalohematoma** is a subperiosteal hemorrhage that does not cross the suture lines surrounding the respective bone. Rarely, linear skull fracture may be seen underlying a cephalohematoma. Over days to weeks, the cephalohematoma may resorb, or less frequently, organize, calcify, or form a central depression.

Infants with cephalohematoma and caput succedaneum require no specific treatment. Occasionally, an infant may develop a massive scalp hemorrhage. This **subgaleal bleeding** requires close attention to hemodynamic status and may cause indirect hyperbilirubinemia requiring phototherapy. **Retinal**

and subconjunctival hemorrhages are common but usually are small and insignificant; no treatment is necessary.

Spinal cord or **spine injuries** may occur in the fetus as a result of the hyperextended *star gazing* posture. Injuries also may occur in infants after rotational (at C3–4) or longitudinal (at C7–T1) force is transmitted to the neck during vertex or breech delivery. Fractures of vertebrae are rare; trauma may cause direct damage to the spinal cord, leading to transection and permanent sequelae, hemorrhage, edema, and neurologic signs. Rarely, a snapping sound indicating cord transection rather than vertebral displacement is heard at the time of delivery. Neurologic dysfunction usually involves complete flaccid paralysis, absence of deep tendon reflexes, and absence of responses to painful stimuli below the lesion. Painful stimuli may elicit reflex flexion of the legs. Infants with spinal cord injury often are flaccid, apneic, and asphyxiated, all of which may mask the underlying spinal cord transection.

Injury to the nerves of the **brachial plexus** may result from traction on the neck, producing paresis or complete paralysis. The mildest injury (neurapraxia) is edema; axonotmesis is more severe and consists of disrupted nerve fibers with an intact myelin sheath; neurotmesis, or complete nerve disruption or root avulsion, is most severe. **Erb-Duchenne paralysis** involves the fifth and sixth cervical nerves and is the most common and usually mildest injury. The infant cannot abduct the arm at the shoulder, externally rotate the arm, or supinate the forearm. The usual picture is one of painless adduction, internal rotation of the arm, and pronation of the forearm. The **Moro reflex** is absent on the involved side; the hand grasp is intact. **Phrenic nerve palsy** (C3, C4, and C5) may lead to diaphragmatic paralysis and respiratory distress. Elevation of the diaphragm caused by nerve injury must be differentiated from elevation caused by eventration resulting from congenital weakness or absence of diaphragm muscle. **Klumpke paralysis** is caused by injury to the seventh and eighth cervical nerves and the first thoracic nerve, resulting in a paralyzed hand and, if the sympathetic nerves are injured, an ipsilateral **Horner syndrome** (ptosis, miosis). Complete arm and hand paralysis are noted with the most severe form of damage to C5, C6, C7, C8, and T1. Treatment of brachial plexus injury is supportive and includes physical therapy to avoid contractures. Active and passive range of motion exercises also may be beneficial. If the deficit persists, nerve grafting may be beneficial.

Facial nerve injury may be the result of compression of the seventh nerve between the facial bone and the birth parent's pelvic bones or the physician's forceps. This peripheral nerve injury is characterized by asymmetric facial features, where one side of the face, including the forehead, moves in a regular manner. The affected side is flaccid, the eye does not close, the nasolabial fold is absent, and the side of the mouth droops at rest. If there is a central injury to the facial nerve, only the lower two-thirds of the face (not the forehead) are involved. Complete agenesis of the facial nucleus results in a central facial paralysis; when this is bilateral, as in Möbius syndrome, the face appears expressionless. **Asymmetric crying facies** refers specifically to an infant whose face appears normal and symmetric at rest, but only one corner of the mouth moves downward when crying. While this may be a facial nerve compression injury (which often improves with time), it can also result from hypoplasia or agenesis of the depressor anguli oris muscle (DAOM). Agenesis of the DAOM will not change over time, although other facial muscles compensate as the child grows.

Skull fractures are rare, usually linear, and require no treatment other than observation for very rare, delayed (1–3 months) complications (e.g., leptomeningeal cyst). Depressed skull fractures are unusual but may be seen with complicated forceps delivery and may need surgical elevation. Fractures of the **clavicle** usually are unilateral and are associated with macrosomic infants after shoulder dystocia. A snap may be heard with difficult delivery, but more commonly, the infant will present with an asymmetric Moro response and decreased movement of the affected side. The prognosis is excellent; many infants require no treatment.

Extremity fractures are less common than fractures of the clavicle and involve the humerus more often than the femur. Treatment involves relative immobilization for the humerus fracture and splint or Pavlik harness for a femoral fracture. The prognosis is excellent.

Fractures of the **facial bones** are rare, but dislocation of the cartilaginous part of the nasal septum out of the vomeral groove and columella is more common. Clinical manifestations include feeding difficulty, respiratory distress, asymmetric nares, and a flattened, laterally displaced nose. Treatment reduces the dislocation by elevating the cartilage back into the vomeral groove.

Visceral trauma to the liver, spleen, or adrenal gland occurs in macrosomic infants and in extremely premature infants, with or without breech or vaginal delivery. Rupture of the liver with subcapsular hematoma formation may lead to anemia, hypovolemia, shock, hemoperitoneum, and disseminated intravascular coagulation. Infants with anemia and shock who are suspected to have an intraventricular hemorrhage but with a normal head ultrasound examination should be evaluated for hepatic or splenic rupture. Adrenal hemorrhage may be asymptomatic, detected only by finding calcified adrenal glands in normal infants. Infants with severe adrenal hemorrhage may exhibit a flank mass, jaundice, hematuria, and/or shock.

Temperature Regulation

After birth, a newborn remains covered by amniotic fluid and situated in a cold environment (20–25°C). An infant's skin temperature may decrease 0.3°C/minute, and the core temperature may decrease 0.1°C/minute in the delivery room. In the absence of an external heat source, the infant must increase metabolism substantially to maintain body temperature.

Heat loss occurs through four basic mechanisms. In the cold delivery room, the wet infant loses heat predominantly by **evaporation** (cutaneous and respiratory loss when wet or in low humidity), **radiation** (loss to nearby cold, solid surfaces), and **convection** (loss to air current). When the infant is dry, radiation, convection, and **conduction** (loss to object in direct contact with infant) are important causes of heat loss. After birth, all high-risk infants should be dried immediately to eliminate evaporative heat losses. A radiant or convective heat source should be provided for high-risk infants. Normal term infants should be dried and wrapped in a blanket.

The ideal environmental temperature is the **neutral thermal environment**, where the ambient temperature results in the lowest rate of heat being produced by the infant to maintain normal body temperature. The neutral thermal environmental temperature decreases with increasing gestational and postnatal age. Ambient temperatures less than the neutral thermal environment result in increasing rates of oxygen consumption for heat production. If the ambient temperature decreases further or if oxygen consumption cannot increase sufficiently (due to hypoxia, hypoglycemia, or medications), the core body temperature decreases.

Heat production by a newborn is created predominantly by nonshivering thermogenesis in specialized areas of tissue containing brown adipose tissue. Brown fat is highly vascular, contains many mitochondria per cell, and is situated around large blood vessels, resulting in rapid heat transfer to the circulation. The vessels of the neck, thorax, and interscapular region are common locations of brown fat. These tissues also are innervated by the sympathetic nervous system, which serves as a primary stimulus for heat production by brown adipose cells. Shivering does not occur in newborns.

Severe **cold injury** in an infant is manifested by acidosis, hypoxia, hypoglycemia, apnea, bradycardia, pulmonary hemorrhage, and a pink skin color. The color is caused by trapping of oxygenated hemoglobin in the cutaneous capillaries. Many of these infants appear nonvigorous, but most respond to treatment and recover. Milder degrees of cold injury in the delivery room may contribute to metabolic acidosis and hypoxia after birth. Conversely, hypoxia delays heat generation in cold-stressed infants.

Treatment of severe hypothermia should involve resuscitation and rapid warming of core (e.g., lung and stomach) and external surfaces. Fluid resuscitation also is needed to treat hypovolemia seen in many of these infants. Reduced core temperature (32–35°C) in the immediate newborn period often requires only external warming with a radiant warmer, incubator, or both.

Elevated Temperature

Exposure to ambient temperatures above the neutral thermal environment results in *heat stress* and an elevated core temperature. Sweating is uncommon in newborns and may be noted only on the forehead. In response to moderate heat stress, infants may increase their respiratory rate to dissipate heat.

MISCELLANEOUS DISORDERS

Hypocalcemia

Hypocalcemia is common in sick and premature newborns. Calcium levels are higher in cord blood than in maternal blood because of active placental transfer of calcium to the fetus. Fetal calcium accretion in the third trimester approaches 150 mg/kg/24 hours; fetal bone mineral content doubles between 30 and 40 weeks of gestation. All infants show a slight decline of serum calcium levels after birth, reaching a trough level at 24–48 hours, the point at which hypocalcemia usually occurs.

The etiology of hypocalcemia varies with the time of onset and the associated illnesses of the child. **Early neonatal hypocalcemia** occurs in the first 3 days of life and is often asymptomatic. Transient hypoparathyroidism and a reduced parathyroid response to the usual postnatal decline of serum calcium levels may be responsible for hypocalcemia in premature infants and infants of diabetic mothers. Congenital absence of the parathyroid gland with DiGeorge syndrome is a cause of hypocalcemia. **Hypomagnesemia** may be seen simultaneously with hypocalcemia, especially in infants of diabetic mothers. Treatment with calcium alone does not relieve symptoms or increase serum calcium levels until hypomagnesemia is also treated. Sodium bicarbonate therapy, phosphate release from cell necrosis, transient hypoparathyroidism, and hypercalcitoninemia may be responsible for early neonatal hypocalcemia associated with asphyxia. Early-onset hypocalcemia associated with asphyxia often occurs with seizures as a result of hypoxic-ischemic encephalopathy.

Late neonatal hypocalcemia, or **neonatal tetany**, often is the result of ingestion of high phosphate–containing milk or the inability to excrete the usual phosphorus in commercial infant formula. Hyperphosphatemia usually occurs in infants with hypocalcemia after the first week of life. Vitamin D deficiency states and malabsorption also have been associated with late-onset hypocalcemia.

The clinical manifestations of hypocalcemia and hypomagnesemia include apnea, muscle twitching, seizures, and laryngospasm. The **Chvostek sign** (facial muscle spasm when the side of the face over the seventh nerve is tapped) and **Trousseau sign** (carpopedal spasm induced by partial inflation of a blood pressure cuff) are rare in the immediate newborn period.

Neonatal hypocalcemia may be prevented in high-risk neonates by administration of intravenous (IV) or oral calcium supplementation. Early asymptomatic hypocalcemia of preterm infants and infants of diabetic mothers often resolves spontaneously. Symptomatic hypocalcemia should be treated with calcium gluconate given intravenously slowly over 10–15 minutes, followed by a continuous infusion of elemental calcium. If hypomagnesemia is associated with hypocalcemia, magnesium sulfate should be given.

The treatment of late hypocalcemia includes immediate management plus the initiation of feedings with low-phosphate formula. Subcutaneous infiltration of IV calcium salts can cause tissue necrosis; oral supplements are hypertonic and may irritate the intestinal mucosa.

In Utero Substance Exposure

Consistent fetal exposure to certain medications or other substances (i.e., methadone, buprenorphine, other opioids, barbiturates, benzodiazepines) during pregnancy places infants at risk of neonatal abstinence syndrome. Other exposures such as nicotine or selective serotonin reuptake inhibitors are also associated with characteristic postnatal symptoms in the infant (sometimes termed *poor neonatal adaption syndrome*), which self-resolve with time. A history of IV substance use increases the risk of bloodborne infectious pathogens, such as hepatitis, HIV, and syphilis. Due to many contributing factors, including social determinants of health, chronic stress-related "weathering," adverse childhood/in-utero experiences, and coexposures (i.e., nicotine/smoking), infants with prenatal substance exposure have been associated with higher rates of SGA, as well as a higher rate of sudden unexpected infant deaths (more specifically, sleep-related infant deaths).

Opioids

Chronic prenatal exposure to partial or complete opioid agonists puts an infant at risk of **neonatal opioid withdrawal syndrome (NOWS)**, which usually presents at 1–2 days of life with exposure to short-acting opioids (pain medications, heroin, fentanyl) and at 2–3 days with common exposure to medications for opioid use disorder (methadone and buprenorphine). Natural improvement in symptoms may occur by day 5–7, although mild symptoms may last for weeks. Clinical manifestations of withdrawal can include excessive crying, fragmented sleep, tremors, increased muscle tone, and/or gastrointestinal dysfunction (poor feeding, hyperphagia, feeding intolerance, loose or watery stools). The primary treatment includes nonpharmacologic measures such as swaddling, skin-to-skin, rocking, rooming-in, decreased external stimuli, and so forth. When symptoms are significant enough to interfere with the functional ability of the infant (sleeping, feeding, soothing), pharmacologic treatment may be indicated. Opioids are the first-line pharmacotherapy for NOWS. Support, education, and empowerment of caregivers and the family can improve symptoms and improve hospital outcomes (decreased overall length of stay, decreased need for pharmacotherapy, etc.).

Stimulants

Cocaine use during pregnancy is associated with preterm labor, abruptio placentae, and neonatal irritability. Infants with in utero exposure to stimulants may be SGA and have small head circumferences (including microcephaly). Usually, no treatment is needed.

PEARLS FOR PRACTITIONERS

See Fetal and Neonatal Medicine: Pearls for Practitioners at the end of this section.

REVIEW QUESTIONS

Available online.

CHAPTER 58

Birth Parent Diseases Affecting the Newborn

Diseases affecting the birth parent during pregnancy can affect the fetus directly or indirectly (Table 58.1). Autoantibody-mediated diseases can have direct consequences on the fetus and neonate because antibodies of the immunoglobulin G (IgG) type can readily cross the placenta to the fetal circulation.

ANTIPHOSPHOLIPID SYNDROME

Antiphospholipid syndrome is associated with thrombophilia and recurrent pregnancy loss. Antiphospholipid antibodies are found in 2–5% of the general healthy population, but they also may be associated with systemic lupus erythematosus (SLE) and other rheumatologic diseases. Obstetric complications arise from the prothrombotic effects of the antiphospholipid antibodies on placental function. Vasculopathy, infarction, and thrombosis have been identified in birth parents with antiphospholipid syndrome. Antiphospholipid syndrome can include fetal growth impairment, placental insufficiency, maternal preeclampsia, premature birth, and possible fetal thrombosis.

IDIOPATHIC (IMMUNE) THROMBOCYTOPENIA

Idiopathic thrombocytopenic purpura (ITP) is an immune process in which platelet-associated IgG antibodies directed against platelets cross the placenta and cause thrombocytopenia in the fetus and newborn. The severely thrombocytopenic fetus is at increased risk for intracranial hemorrhage. ITP during pregnancy requires close maternal and fetal management to reduce the risks of life-threatening maternal hemorrhage and trauma to the fetus at delivery. Postnatal management involves observation of the infant's platelet count. For infants who have evidence of hemorrhage, platelet transfusion may be necessary. The infant may benefit from an infusion of intravenous immunoglobulin. Neonatal thrombocytopenia usually resolves within 4–6 weeks.

SYSTEMIC LUPUS ERYTHEMATOSUS

Immune abnormalities in SLE and related autoimmune disorders (Sjögren's, etc.) can lead to the production of anti-Ro (SS-A) and anti-La (SS-B) antibodies that can cross the placenta and injure fetal tissue. The most serious complication is damage to the cardiac conducting system, which results in **congenital heart block**. This heart block tends to be complete (third degree), although less advanced blocks have been observed. The mortality rate is approximately 20%; most surviving infants require cardiac pacing. Neonatal lupus may occur and is characterized by skin lesions (sharply demarcated erythematous plaques or central atrophic macules with peripheral scaling with predilection for the eyes, face, and scalp), thrombocytopenia, autoimmune hemolysis, and hepatic involvement.

NEONATAL HYPERTHYROIDISM

Graves disease is associated with thyroid-stimulating antibodies. The prevalence of clinical hyperthyroidism in pregnancy has been reported to be about 0.1–0.4%; it is the second most common endocrine disorder during pregnancy (after diabetes). Neonatal hyperthyroidism is due to the transplacental passage of thyroid-stimulating antibodies; hyperthyroidism can appear rapidly within the first 12–48 hours. Symptoms may include fetal growth restriction, prematurity, goiter (may cause tracheal obstruction), exophthalmos, stare, craniosynostosis (usually coronal), flushing, heart failure, tachycardia, arrhythmias, hypertension, hypoglycemia, thrombocytopenia, and hepatosplenomegaly. Treatment includes methimazole, propranolol, and iodine, if needed. Autoimmune-induced neonatal hyperthyroidism usually resolves in 2–4 months.

DIABETES MELLITUS

Both diabetes mellitus that develops during pregnancy (*gestational diabetes*, noted in about 5–10% of women) and diabetes that is present before pregnancy adversely affect fetal and neonatal well-being. The effect of diabetes on the fetus depends, in part, on the severity of the diabetic state: age of onset of diabetes, duration of treatment with insulin, and presence of vascular disease. Poorly controlled maternal diabetes leads to maternal and fetal hyperglycemia that stimulates the fetal pancreas, resulting in hyperplasia of the islets of Langerhans. Fetal hyperinsulinemia results in increased fat and protein synthesis, producing a fetus that is large for gestational age. After birth, hyperinsulinemia persists, resulting in fasting neonatal hypoglycemia. Appropriately controlling maternal diabetes

TABLE 58.1 Birth Parent Conditions Affecting the Fetus or Neonate

DISORDER	EFFECT(S)	MECHANISM(S)
Assisted reproductive technology	Beckwith-Wiedemann, Silver-Russel, Angelman syndromes	Altered imprinting
Autoantibody against folate receptors	Neural tube defects	Blockage of cellular uptake of folate
Cervical neoplasia	Preterm premature rupture of membranes, preterm birth	Associated with loop electrosurgical excision procedure or cone therapy
Cholestasis	Preterm delivery, intrauterine fetal demise	Unknown, possibly bile acid–induced fetal arrhythmia
Cyanotic heart disease	IUGR	Low fetal oxygen delivery
Diabetes mellitus		
Mild	LGA, hypoglycemia	Fetal hyperglycemia: produces hyperinsulinemia; insulin promotes growth
Severe	Growth restriction	Vascular disease, placental insufficiency
Graves disease	Transient neonatal thyrotoxicosis	Transplacental passage of IgG TRAb
Hyperparathyroidism	Neonatal hypocalcemia	Maternal calcium crosses to fetus and suppresses fetal parathyroid gland
Hypertension	FGR, intrauterine fetal demise	Placental insufficiency, fetal hypoxia
Idiopathic thrombocytopenic purpura	Thrombocytopenia	Nonspecific maternal platelet antibodies cross placenta
Isoimmune neutropenia or thrombocytopenia	Neutropenia or thrombocytopenia	Specific antifetus neutrophil or platelet antibody crosses placenta after sensitization of birth parent
Kidney transplantation	FGR	Uteroplacental insufficiency
Malignant melanoma	Placental or fetal tumor	Placental metastasis
Myasthenia gravis	Transient neonatal myasthenia	IgG antibody to acetylcholine receptor crosses placenta
Myotonic dystrophy	Neonatal myotonic dystrophy, congenital contractures, respiratory insufficiency	Genetic anticipation
Obesity, insulin resistance	LGA or FGR, hypoglycemia	Unknown, similarities to diabetes
Phenylketonuria	Microcephaly, intellectual disability	Elevated fetal phenylalanine values
Poor nutrition	FGR, adult insulin resistance	Reduced fetal nutrients, nutritional programming
Preeclampsia, eclampsia	FGR, thrombocytopenia, neutropenia, fetal demise	Uteroplacental insufficiency, fetal hypoxia, vasoconstriction
Rhesus or other blood group sensitization	Fetal anemia, hypoalbuminemia, hydrops, neonatal jaundice	IgG crosses placenta and is directed to fetal cells with antigen
Sickle cell anemia	Preterm birth, FGR, stillbirth	Placental insufficiency via maternal sickling, producing fetal hypoxia
Systemic lupus erythematosus	Congenital heart block, rash, anemia, thrombocytopenia, neutropenia	Antibody directed to fetal heart, red and white blood cells, and platelets

FGR, Fetal growth restriction; *IgG*, immunoglobulin G; *IUGR*, intrauterine growth restriction; *LGA*, large for gestational age; *TRAb*, thyroid receptor antibody.
Modified from Triebwasser JE, Dolin CD. High-risk pregnancies. In: Kliegman RM, St. Geme J, eds. Nelson Textbook of Pediatrics. *22nd ed. Philadelphia, Elsevier, 2025. Table 116.3.*

during pregnancy and preventing hyperglycemia during labor and delivery prevent macrosomic fetal growth and neonatal hypoglycemia. Additional problems of the diabetic birth parent and the fetus and newborn are summarized in Table 58.2.

OTHER CONDITIONS

Other maternal illnesses, such as severe pulmonary disease (i.e., cystic fibrosis), cyanotic heart disease, and sickle cell anemia, may reduce oxygen availability to the fetus. Severe hypertensive or diabetic vasculopathy can result in uteroplacental insufficiency. The fetus and the newborn may also be adversely affected by the medications used to treat maternal illnesses. These effects may appear as teratogenesis or as an adverse metabolic, neurologic, or cardiopulmonary adaptation to extrauterine life (Table 58.3). Acquired infectious diseases of the birth parent also may affect the fetus or newborn adversely (see Chapter 65).

TABLE 58.2 Problems of Diabetic Pregnancy

BIRTH PARENT
Ketoacidosis Hyperglycemia/hypoglycemia Nephritis Preeclampsia Polyhydramnios Retinopathy
NEONATAL
Birth asphyxia Birth injury (macrosomia, shoulder dystocia) Congenital anomalies (lumbosacral dysgenesis—caudal regression) Congenital heart disease (ventricular and atrial septal defects, transposition of the great arteries, truncus arteriosus, double-outlet right ventricle, coarctation of the aorta) Hyperbilirubinemia (unconjugated) Hypocalcemia Hypoglycemia Hypomagnesemia Neurologic disorders (neural tube defects, holoprosencephaly) Organomegaly Polycythemia (hyperviscosity) Kidney disorders (double ureter, renal vein thrombosis, hydronephrosis, renal agenesis) Respiratory distress syndrome Small left colon syndrome Transient tachypnea of the newborn/respiratory distress syndrome

TABLE 58.3 Birth Parent Medications and Toxins: Possible Effects on the Fetus and Newborn

MEDICATION	EFFECT ON FETUS AND NEWBORN
ANALGESICS AND ANTIINFLAMMATORIES	
Acetaminophen	Generally safe except with maternal overdose
Aspirin	Hemorrhage, premature closure of ductus arteriosus, pulmonary artery hypertension (effects not seen at ≤100 mg/day)
Opioids	NOWS with chronic use
Ibuprofen	Reduced amniotic fluid volume when used in tocolysis; risk for premature ductus arteriosus closure and pulmonary hypertension
Indomethacin	Closure of fetal ductus arteriosus and pulmonary artery hypertension
Meperidine	Respiratory depression peaks 2–3 hours after maternal dose
ANESTHETICS	
General anesthesia	With prolonged anesthesia prior to delivery, respiratory depression of infant at delivery
Lidocaine	High serum levels cause CNS depression
ANTIBIOTICS	
Aminoglycosides	Ototoxicity reported after use of kanamycin and streptomycin
Cephalosporins	Some drugs in this group displace bilirubin from albumin
Isoniazid	Risk for folate deficiency
Penicillins	Generally, no adverse effect
Tetracyclines	Yellow-brown staining of infant's teeth (when given at ≥5 months of gestation); stillbirth and prematurity due to maternal hepatotoxicity
Sulfonamides	Some drugs in this group displace bilirubin from albumin; can cause kernicterus
Trimethoprim	Folate antagonism
Vancomycin	Potential for ototoxicity

(Continued)

TABLE 58.3 Birth Parent Medications and Toxins: Possible Effects on the Fetus and Newborn—cont'd

MEDICATION	EFFECT ON FETUS AND NEWBORN
ANTICONVULSANTS	
Carbamazepine	Neural tube defects; midfacial hypoplasia
Phenobarbital	Neonatal abstinence syndrome, hemorrhagic disease; midfacial hypoplasia
Phenytoin	Hemorrhagic disease; fetal hydantoin syndrome: growth and mental deficiency, midfacial hypoplasia, hypoplasia of distal phalanges
Valproic acid	Neural tube defects, midfacial hypoplasia
ANTICOAGULANTS	
Warfarin (Coumadin)	Warfarin embryopathy: stippled epiphyses, growth and mental deficiencies, seizures, hypoplastic nose, eye defects, CNS anomalies including Dandy-Walker syndrome, neonatal anticoagulation
Heparin	No direct adverse effects on the fetus
ANTINEOPLASTICS	
Aminopterin	Cleft palate, hydrocephalus, meningomyelocele, fetal growth restriction
Cyclophosphamide	Fetal growth restriction, cardiovascular and digital anomalies
Methotrexate	Absent digits, CNS malformation
ANTIVIRALS	
Acyclovir	No definite adverse effects
Ribavirin	Teratogenic and embryo-lethal in animals
Zidovudine	Potential for fetal bone marrow suppression; combined maternal and neonatal treatment reduces perinatal transmission of HIV
CARDIOVASCULAR DRUGS AND ANTIHYPERTENSIVES	
Angiotensin-converting enzyme inhibitors	Fetal hypocalvaria, oligohydramnios and fetal compression, oliguria, renal failure
β-Blockers (propranolol)	Neonatal bradycardia, hypoglycemia, fetal growth restriction
Diazoxide	Hyperglycemia; decreased placental perfusion with maternal hypotension
Digoxin	Fetal toxicity with maternal overdose
Methyldopa	Mild, clinically insignificant decrease in neonatal blood pressure
DIURETICS	
Furosemide	Increases fetal urinary sodium and potassium levels
Thiazides	Thrombocytopenia, hypoglycemia, hyponatremia, hypokalemia
HORMONES AND RELATED DRUGS	
Androgenics (danazol)	Masculinization of female fetuses
Corticosteroids	Cleft lip/palate
Diethylstilbestrol	DES daughters: vaginal adenosis, genital tract anomalies, increased incidence of clear cell adenocarcinoma, increased rate of premature delivery in future pregnancy DES sons: possible increase in genitourinary anomalies
Estrogens, progestins	Risk for virilization of female fetuses reported with progestins; small, if any, risk for other anomalies
Insulin	No apparent direct adverse effects, uncertain risk related to maternal hypoglycemia
Tamoxifen	Animal studies suggest potential for DES-like effect
SEDATIVES, TRANQUILIZERS, AND PSYCHIATRIC DRUGS	
Barbiturates	Risk for hemorrhage and neonatal abstinence syndrome
Benzodiazepines	Neonatal abstinence syndrome
Selective serotonin reuptake inhibitors	Persistent pulmonary hypertension, jitteriness, irritability, poor delivery room transition, PNAS
Lithium	Ebstein anomaly, diabetes insipidus, thyroid depression, cardiovascular dysfunction
Thalidomide	Limb deficiency, cardiac defects, ear malformations
Tricyclic antidepressants	Jitteriness, irritability

(Continued)

TABLE 58.3 Birth Parent Medications and Toxins: Possible Effects on the Fetus and Newborn—cont'd

MEDICATION	EFFECT ON FETUS AND NEWBORN
SOCIAL AND ILLICIT DRUGS	
Alcohol	FASD, renal and cardiac anomalies
Amphetamines	Irritability, prematurity, decreased birthweight and head circumference
Cocaine	Decreased birthweight, microcephaly, prematurity, abruptio placentae, intrauterine fetal demise
Fentanyl	Neonatal opioid withdrawal syndrome, novel synthetic analogues may be associated with constellation of dysmorphic features and abnormal cholesterol metabolism
Marijuana	Decreased birthweight
Methadone/opioids	Neonatal opioid withdrawal syndrome, possible strabismus and torticollis
Phencyclidine	Irritability, jitteriness, hypertonia, poor feeding
Tobacco smoking (nicotine)	Jitteriness, elevated blood carboxyhemoglobin; decreased birthweight, increased prematurity rate, increased premature rupture of membranes, placental abruption and previa, increased fetal death, possible oral clefts
TOCOLYTICS	
Magnesium sulfate	Respiratory depression, hypotonia, bone demineralization with prolonged (weeks) use for tocolysis
Terbutaline	Neonatal hypoglycemia
VITAMINS AND RELATED DRUGS	
Vitamin A (preformed, not carotene)	Excessive doses (≥10,000 IU/day) may be teratogenic
Acitretin	Activated form of etretinate (see later)
Vitamin D	Megadoses may cause hypercalcemia, craniosynostosis
Etretinate	Limb deficiency, neural tube defect; ear, cardiac, and CNS anomalies
Isotretinoin (13-*cis*-retinoic acid)	Ear, cardiac, CNS, and thymic anomalies
Menadione (vitamin K_3)	Hyperbilirubinemia and kernicterus
Phytonadione (vitamin K_1)	No adverse effect
MISCELLANEOUS	
Anticholinergics	Neonatal meconium ileus
Antiemetics	Doxylamine succinate and/or dicyclomine HCl with pyridoxine reported to be teratogens, but bulk of evidence is clearly negative
Chorionic villus sampling	Limb deficiency with early CVS
Radiation	Adverse effects primarily associated with therapeutic, not diagnostic doses, and is dose-dependent: fetal death, microcephaly, fetal growth restriction
Lead	Decreased IQ (dose-related)
Methimazole	Aplasia cutis
Methylene blue	Hemolytic anemia, hyperbilirubinemia, methemoglobinemia; intraamniotic injection in early pregnancy associated with intestinal atresia
Methylmercury	CNS injury, neurodevelopmental abnormalities, microcephaly
Misoprostol	Moebius sequence
Oral hypoglycemics	Neonatal hypoglycemia
Polychlorinated biphenyls (no longer commercially produced in the U.S.)	Cola skin coloration, minor skeletal anomalies, neurodevelopmental deficits

CNS, Central nervous system; *FASD*, fetal alcohol spectrum disorders; *IQ*, intelligence quotient; *NOWS*, neonatal opioid withdrawal syndrome; *PNAS*, poor neonatal adaptation syndrome.
From Fanaroff AA, Fanaroff JM. Klaus & Fanaroff's Care of the High-Risk Neonate. *6th ed. Philadelphia: Elsevier; 2013. Table 4.2.*

PEARLS FOR PRACTITIONERS

See Fetal and Neonatal Medicine: Pearls for Practitioners at the end of this section.

REVIEW QUESTIONS

Available online.

CHAPTER 59

Diseases of the Fetus

The principal determinants of fetal disease include the fetal genotype and the environment in utero. The ability to assess a fetus genetically, biochemically, and physically is greatly enhanced through the development of amniocentesis, fetoscopy, chorionic villus sampling, fetal blood sampling, genetic testing of circulating fetal DNA in the birth parent's blood, and real-time ultrasonography.

FETAL GROWTH RESTRICTION AND SMALL FOR GESTATIONAL AGE

Fetuses subjected to abnormal maternal, placental, or fetal conditions that restrain growth are a high-risk group and are traditionally classified as having **fetal growth restriction** ([FGR], also termed *intrauterine growth restriction*). The terms *FGR* and *small for gestational age (SGA)* are not synonymous. FGR represents a deviation from expected growth patterns. The decreased fetal growth associated with FGR is usually an adaptation to unfavorable intrauterine conditions that result in permanent alterations in metabolism, growth, and development. FGR most frequently occurs with a variety of maternal conditions that are also associated with preterm delivery. **Small for gestational age** (SGA) describes an infant whose birth weight is statistically less than the 10th percentile or two standard deviations below the mean birthweight for gestational age. The cause of SGA may be pathologic, as in an infant with FGR, or nonpathologic, as in an infant who is small but otherwise healthy (Table 59.1).

Measurement and recording of maternal fundal height in conjunction with serial ultrasound assessment of the fetus (growth rate, amniotic fluid volume, malformations, anomalies, and Doppler velocimetry of uterine, placental, and fetal blood flow) can aid detection. When suspected and identified, FGR and SGA fetuses must be monitored for fetal well-being, and appropriate maternal care should be instituted (see Chapter 57).

At birth, infants who are mildly to moderately SGA appear smaller than normal with decreased subcutaneous fat. More severely affected infants may present with a *wasted appearance* with asymmetric findings, including larger heads for the size of the body (central nervous system sparing), widened anterior fontanelles, small abdomen, thin arms and legs, decreased subcutaneous fat, dry and redundant skin, decreased muscle mass, and thin (often meconium-stained) umbilical cord. Gestational age is often difficult to assess when based on physical appearance and perceived advanced neurologic maturity. Physical examination should detail the presence of dysmorphic features, abnormal extremities, or gross anomalies that might suggest underlying congenital malformations, chromosomal abnormalities, or exposure to teratogens. Hepatosplenomegaly, jaundice, and skin rashes in addition to ocular disorders, such as chorioretinitis, cataracts, glaucoma, and cloudy cornea, suggest the presence of a congenital infection or inborn error of metabolism. Infants with severe FGR or SGA, particularly in conjunction with fetal distress, may have problems at birth that include metabolic acidosis, asphyxia, hypoxemia, hypotension, hypoglycemia, polycythemia, meconium aspiration syndrome, and persistent pulmonary hypertension of the newborn.

Management of FGR and SGA infants is usually symptomatic and supportive. The diagnostic evaluation at birth should be directed at identifying the cause of the FGR and SGA, if possible. The consequences of FGR and SGA depend on the etiology, severity, and duration of growth restriction. The mortality rates of infants who are severely affected are 5–20 times those of infants who are appropriate for gestational age. Postnatal growth and development depend in part on the etiology, the postnatal nutritional intake, and the care environment. Infants who have FGR and SGA secondary to congenital infection, chromosomal abnormalities, or congenital anomaly syndromes can remain small throughout life. Infants who have growth inhibited late in gestation because of uterine constraints, placental insufficiency, or poor maternal nutrition have "catch-up" growth (rapid growth following the period of reduced growth), and, under optimal environmental conditions, approach their inherited growth and development potential.

HYDROPS FETALIS

Hydrops fetalis is caused by immune and nonimmune conditions. Hydrops fetalis is a fetal clinical condition of excessive

TABLE 59.1 Etiologies for Fetal Growth Restriction and Small for Gestational Age at Birth

BIRTH PARENT FACTORS
Age (young and advanced) Cigarette smoking Genetics (short stature, weight) Illnesses/conditions during pregnancy (preeclampsia, severe diabetes, chronic hypertension, connective tissue disease) Infections (intrauterine) Inadequate/poor prenatal care Oligohydramnios Poor nutrition
FETAL FACTORS
Chromosomal abnormality and nonchromosomal syndromes Congenital infections Inborn errors of metabolism Multiple gestations Insulin resistance or reduced insulin or insulinlike growth factor-1 production
BIRTH PARENT MEDICATIONS
Antimetabolites (methotrexate) Heavy metals (mercury, lead) Hydantoin Narcotics (morphine, methadone) Steroids (prednisone) Substance use (alcohol, cocaine) Warfarin
PLACENTAL AND UTERINE ABNORMALITIES
Abruptio placentae Abnormal implantation Abnormal placental vessels Chorioangioma Circumvallate placenta Fetal vessel thrombosis Ischemic villus necrosis Multiple gestations True knots in umbilical cord Villitis (congenital infection)

fluid accumulation in the skin plus one or more other body compartments, including the pleural space, peritoneal cavity, pericardium, or placenta with resultant high morbidity and mortality. There is often polyhydramnios. Hydrops initially was described in association with Rhesus blood group isoimmunization. The use of Rho (D) immune globulin has reduced the incidence of isoimmune fetal hydrops. Concurrently, the proportion of **nonimmune hydrops** has increased as a cause of this severe clinical condition.

Fetal hydrops results from an imbalance of interstitial fluid accumulation and decreased removal of fluid by the capillaries and lymphatic system. Fluid accumulation can be secondary to congestive heart failure, obstructed lymphatic flow, or decreased plasma oncotic pressure (hypoproteinemic states). Edema formation is the final common pathway for many disease processes that affect the fetus, including fetal cardiac (congenital anomaly, arrhythmia, tumor), genetic, hematologic, lymphatic, metabolic, infection, or malformation syndromes.

The diagnostic work-up of the hydropic fetus should focus on discovering the underlying cause. Maternal findings may include hypertension, anemia, multiple gestation, thickened placenta, polyhydramnios, and edema, whereas fetal findings may include tachycardia, ascites, scalp and body wall edema, and pleural and pericardial effusion. Invasive fetal testing may be indicated. Amniocentesis provides amniotic fluid samples for karyotype, culture, α-fetoprotein, and metabolic and enzyme analysis. Percutaneous umbilical cord blood sampling can provide fetal blood for chromosomal analysis and hematologic and metabolic testing and provide a source for intervention (e.g., fetal transfusion for profound anemia).

Management depends on the underlying cause and the gestational age of the fetus. Resuscitative efforts at delivery are often required. Profound anemia necessitates immediate transfusion with packed red blood cells.

PEARLS FOR PRACTITIONERS

See Fetal and Neonatal Medicine: Pearls for Practitioners at the end of this section.

REVIEW QUESTION

Available online.

CHAPTER 60

Respiratory Diseases of the Newborn

Respiratory distress, often manifested by tachypnea, intercostal retractions, reduced air exchange, cyanosis, expiratory grunting, and nasal flaring, is a nonspecific response to serious illness. The differential diagnosis of respiratory distress includes pulmonary, cardiac, hematologic, infectious, anatomic, and metabolic disorders that may involve the lungs directly or indirectly (Fig. 60.1). Surfactant deficiency causes **respiratory distress syndrome (RDS)**, resulting in tachypnea; **infection**, specifically pneumonia, may require imaging to demonstrate interstitial or lobar infiltrates; **meconium aspiration** results in a chemical pneumonitis with hypoxia and pulmonary hypertension; **hydrops fetalis** causes anemia and hypoalbuminemia with high-output heart failure and pulmonary edema; and congenital or acquired **pulmonary hypoplasia** causes pulmonary hypertension and pulmonary insufficiency. It also is clinically useful to differentiate the common causes of respiratory distress according to gestational age (Table 60.1).

In addition to the specific therapy for the individual disorder, supportive care and evaluation of the infant with respiratory distress can be applied to all the problems mentioned earlier. Continuous pulse oximetry together with blood gas monitoring and interpretation are key components of general respiratory care (Table 60.2).

Treatment of hypoxemia requires knowledge of normal values. In term infants, the arterial Pa_{O_2} level is 55–60 mm Hg at 30 minutes of life, 75 mm Hg at 4 hours, and 90 mm Hg at 24 hours. Preterm infants may have lower values. Pa_{CO_2} levels should be 35–40 mm Hg, and the pH should be 7.35–7.40. It is imperative that blood gas analysis be performed in all infants with *significant* respiratory distress whether or not cyanosis is perceived. Cyanosis becomes evident when there is ~5 g of unsaturated hemoglobin; anemia, jaundice, or melanin concentration may interfere with the perception of cyanosis. Capillary blood gas determinations are useful in determining blood pH and the Pa_{CO_2} level but result in falsely low blood Pa_{O_2} readings. Serial blood gas levels may be monitored by an indwelling arterial catheter placed in the radial artery or through the umbilical artery. Another method for monitoring blood gas levels is to combine capillary blood gas techniques with noninvasive methods used to monitor oxygen (pulse oximetry).

Metabolic acidosis, defined as a reduced pH (<7.25) and bicarbonate concentration (<18 mEq/L) accompanied by a normal or low Pa_{CO_2} level, may be caused by hypoxia or by insufficient tissue perfusion. The origin of the disorder may be pulmonary, cardiac, infectious, renal, hematologic, nutritional, metabolic, or iatrogenic. The initial approach to metabolic acidosis is to determine the cause and treat the pathophysiologic problem. This approach may include, as in the sequence of therapy for hypoxia, increasing the inspired oxygen concentration, applying continuous positive airway pressure (CPAP) nasally, or initiating mechanical ventilation using positive end-expiratory pressure. Patients with hypotension produced by hypovolemia require fluids and may need inotropic or vasoactive drug support.

Respiratory acidosis, defined as an elevated P_{CO_2} level and reduced pH without a reduction in the bicarbonate concentration, may be caused by pulmonary insufficiency or central hypoventilation. Many disorders producing respiratory distress can lead to hypercapnia. Treatment involves assisted ventilation but not sodium bicarbonate.

RESPIRATORY DISTRESS SYNDROME

RDS occurs after the onset of breathing and is associated with an insufficiency of pulmonary surfactant.

Lung Development

The lining of the alveolus consists of 90% type I cells and 10% type II cells. After 20 weeks of gestation, the type II cells contain

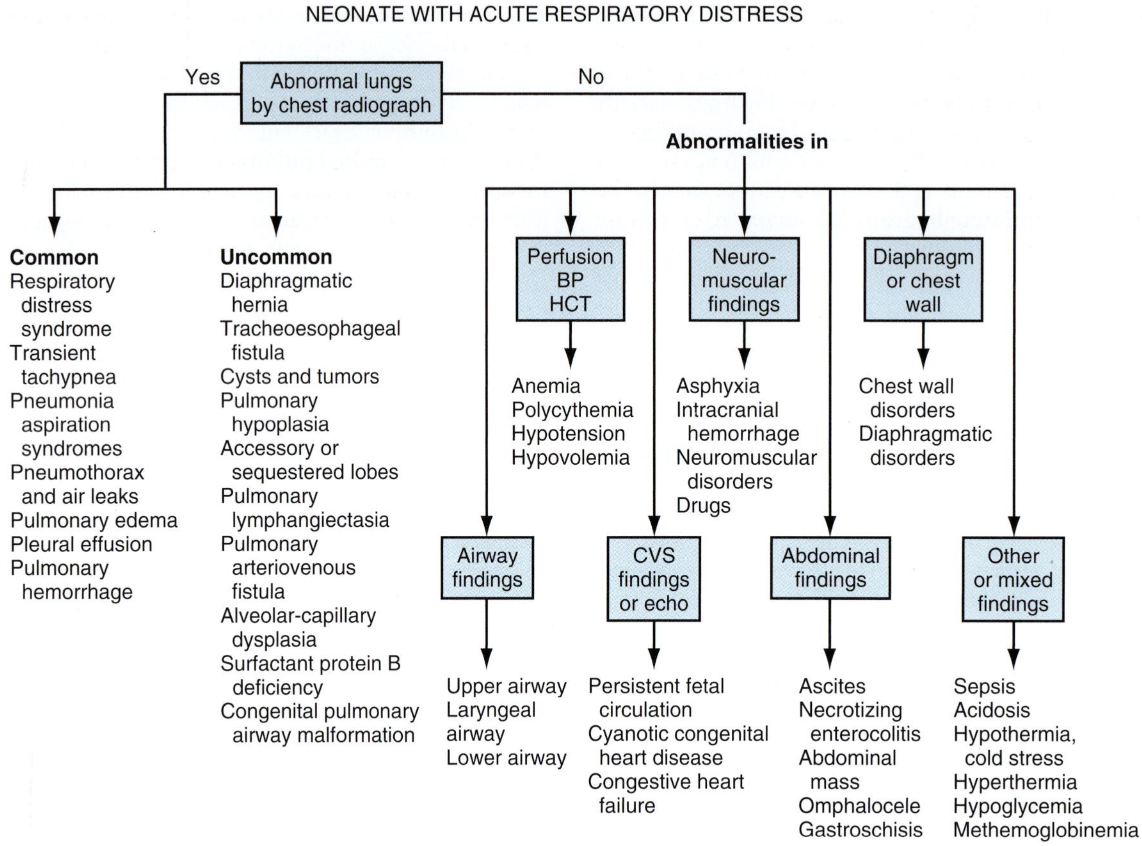

FIGURE 60.1 Diagram of causes of respiratory distress in neonates. *BP,* Blood pressure; *CVS,* cardiovascular system; *echo,* echocardiogram; *HCT,* hematocrit. (Modified from Fanaroff AA, Fanaroff JM. *Klaus & Fanaroff's Care of the High-Risk Neonate.* 7th ed. Philadelphia: Elsevier; 2020: Fig. 10.1.)

TABLE 60.1 Etiology of Respiratory Distress

PRETERM INFANT
Respiratory distress syndrome Erythroblastosis fetalis Nonimmune hydrops Pulmonary hemorrhage
FULL-TERM INFANT
Persistent pulmonary hypertension of the neonate Meconium aspiration pneumonia Polycythemia Amniotic fluid aspiration
PRETERM AND FULL-TERM INFANT
Bacterial sepsis (GBS) Transient tachypnea Spontaneous pneumothorax Congenital anomalies (e.g., congenital lobar emphysema, cystic adenomatoid malformation, diaphragmatic hernia) Congenital heart disease Pulmonary hypoplasia Viral infection (e.g., herpes simplex, CMV) Inborn metabolic errors

CMV, Cytomegalovirus; *GBS,* group B streptococcus.

TABLE 60.2 Initial Evaluation of Respiratory Distress

TEST	RATIONALE
Chest radiograph	To determine reticular granular pattern of RDS; to determine presence of pneumothorax, cardiomegaly, life-threatening congenital anomalies
Blood gas	To determine severity of respiratory compromise, hypoxemia, and hypercapnia and type of acidosis; severity determines treatment strategy
Complete blood count	Hemoglobin/hematocrit to determine anemia and polycythemia; white blood cell count to determine neutropenia/sepsis; platelet count and smear to determine DIC
Blood culture	To recover potential pathogen
Blood glucose	To determine presence of hypoglycemia, which may produce or occur simultaneously with respiratory distress; to determine stress hyperglycemia
Echocardiogram (ECG)	In the presence of a murmur, cardiomegaly, or refractory hypoxia; to determine structural heart disease or PPHN

DIC, Disseminated intravascular coagulation; *ECG,* electrocardiogram; *PPHN,* persistent pulmonary hypertension of the newborn; *RDS,* respiratory distress syndrome.

vacuolated, osmophilic, lamellar inclusion bodies, which are packages of surface-active material (Fig. 60.2). This lipoprotein surfactant is 90% lipid and is composed predominantly of saturated phosphatidylcholine (lecithin) but also contains phosphatidylglycerol, other phospholipids, and neutral lipids. The surfactant proteins, SP-A, SP-B, SP-C, and SP-D, are packaged into the lamellar body and contribute to surface-active properties and recycling of surfactant. Surfactant prevents atelectasis by reducing surface tension at low lung volumes when it is concentrated at end expiration as the alveolar radius decreases; surfactant contributes to lung recoil by increasing surface tension at larger lung volumes when it is diluted during inspiration as the alveolar radius increases. Without surfactant, surface tension forces are not reduced, and atelectasis develops during end expiration as the alveolus collapses.

The timing of surfactant production in quantities sufficient to prevent atelectasis depends on an increase in fetal cortisol levels that begins between 32–34 weeks of gestation. By 34–36 weeks, sufficient surface-active material is produced by the type II cells in the lung, is secreted into the alveolar lumen, and is excreted into the amniotic fluid. Lecithin concentration increases with increasing gestational age, beginning at 32–34 weeks, and indicates fetal pulmonary maturity.

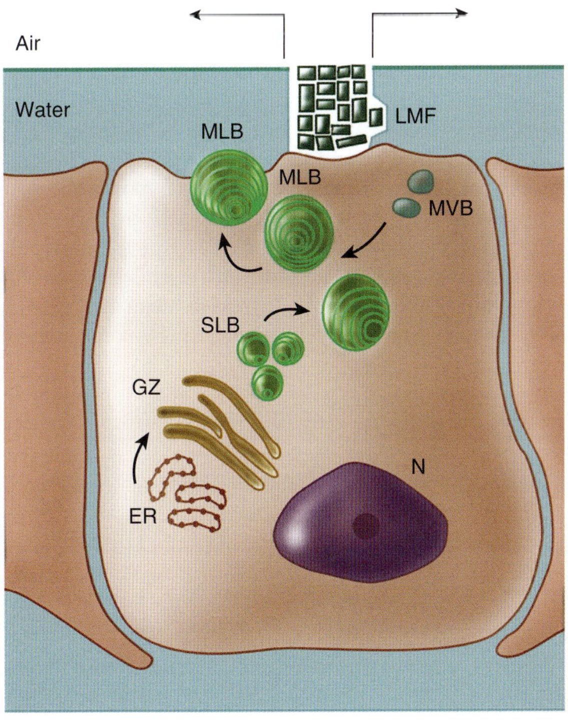

FIGURE 60.2 Proposed pathway of synthesis, transport, secretion, and reuptake of surfactant in the type II alveolar cell. Phospholipids are synthesized in the smooth ER. The glucose/glycerol precursor may be derived from lung glycogen or circulating glucose. Phospholipids and surfactant proteins are packaged in the GZ, emerge as SLB, coalesce to MLB, migrate to the apical membrane, and are released by exocytosis into the liquid hypophase below the air-liquid interface. The tightly coiled lamellar body unravels to form the LMF, the immediate precursor to the phospholipid monolayer at the alveolar surface. Reuptake by endocytosis forms MVB that recycle surfactant. The enzymes, receptors, transporters, and surfactant proteins are controlled by regulatory processes at the transcriptional level in the N. Corticosteroid and thyroid hormones are regulatory ligands that may accelerate surfactant synthesis. *ER*, Endoplasmic reticulum; *GZ*, Golgi apparatus; *LMF*, lattice (tubular) myelin figure; *MLB*, mature lamellar bodies; *MVB*, multivesicular bodies; *N*, nucleus; *SLB*, small lamellar bodies. (From Hansen T, Corbet A. Lung development and function. In: Taeusch HW, Ballard R, Avery ME, eds. *Diseases of the Newborn*. 6th ed. Philadelphia: Saunders; 1991:465.)

Clinical Manifestations

A deficiency of pulmonary surfactant (most often due to prematurity) results in atelectasis, decreased functional residual capacity, arterial hypoxemia, and respiratory distress. Surfactant synthesis may also be reduced because of hypovolemia, hypothermia, acidosis, hypoxemia, and rare genetic disorders of surfactant synthesis. These factors also produce pulmonary artery vasospasm, which may contribute to RDS in larger premature infants who have developed sufficient pulmonary arteriole smooth muscle to produce vasoconstriction. Surfactant deficiency–induced atelectasis causes alveoli to be perfused but not ventilated, which results in a pulmonary shunt and hypoxemia. As atelectasis increases, the lungs become increasingly difficult to expand, and lung compliance decreases (Fig. 60.3). Because the chest wall of the premature infant is very compliant, the infant attempts to overcome decreased lung compliance with increasing inspiratory pressures, resulting in retractions of the chest wall. The sequence of decreased lung compliance and chest wall retractions leads to poor air exchange, an increased physiologic dead space, alveolar hypoventilation, and hypercapnia. A cycle of hypoxia, hypercapnia, and acidosis acts on type II cells to reduce surfactant synthesis and, in some infants, on the pulmonary arterioles to produce pulmonary hypertension.

Premature infants are at greatest risk for RDS. The incidence of RDS increases with decreasing gestational age. RDS occurs in 70–80% of infants with less than 28 weeks of gestation. Other risk factors include delivery of a previous preterm infant with RDS, maternal diabetes, hypothermia, fetal distress, asphyxia, male sex, and delivery by cesarean section without labor.

RDS may develop immediately in the delivery room in extremely immature infants at less than 30 weeks of gestation. Some more mature infants (34 weeks of gestation) may not show signs of RDS until 3–4 hours after birth, correlating with the initial release of stored surfactant at the onset of breathing accompanied by the ongoing inability to replace the surfactant owing to inadequate stores. Clinical manifestations of RDS can

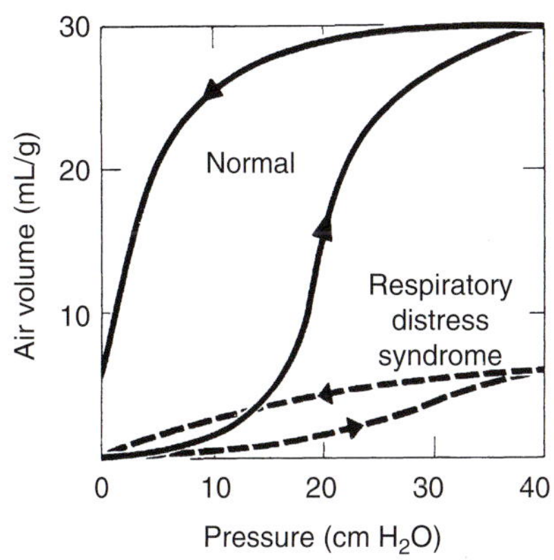

FIGURE 60.3 Air pressure volume curves of normal and abnormal lung. Volume is expressed as milliliters of air per gram of lung. Lung of infant with RDS accepts smaller volume of air at all pressures. Note that deflation pressure volume curve closely follows inflation curve for the RDS lung. *RDS*, Respiratory distress syndrome. (From Fanaroff AA, Fanaroff JM. *Klaus & Fanaroff's Care of the High-Risk Neonate*. 8th ed. Philadelphia: Elsevier; 2026: Fig. 12.3.)

include hypoxia, tachypnea, nasal flaring, intercostal and sternal retractions, and grunting. Grunting is caused by closure of the glottis during expiration, the effect of which is to maintain lung volume (decreasing atelectasis) and gas exchange during exhalation. Atelectasis is well documented by radiographic examination of the chest, which shows a ground-glass haze in the lung surrounding air-filled bronchi (the air bronchogram) (Fig. 60.4). Severe RDS may show an airless lung field *(whiteout)* on a radiograph, even obliterating the distinction between the atelectatic lungs and the heart.

During the first 72 hours, infants with untreated RDS have increasing distress and hypoxemia. In infants with severe RDS, the development of edema, apnea, and respiratory failure necessitates assisted ventilation. Thereafter, uncomplicated cases show a spontaneous improvement that often is heralded by diuresis and a marked resolution of edema. Complications include the development of a pneumothorax, a patent ductus arteriosus (PDA), and bronchopulmonary dysplasia (BPD). The differential diagnosis of RDS includes diseases associated with cyanosis and respiratory distress (see Fig. 60.1 and Table 57.8).

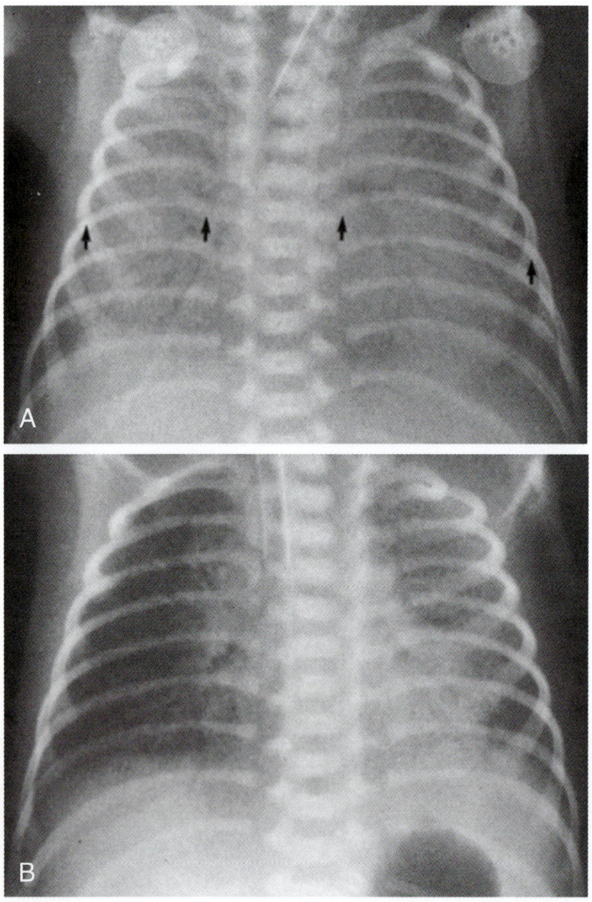

FIGURE 60.4 Respiratory distress syndrome. The infant is intubated, and the lungs show a dense reticulonodular pattern with air bronchograms **(A)**. To evaluate rotation on the frontal chest, the lengths of the posterior ribs are compared from left to right *(arrows)*. Because the infant is supine, the side of the longer ribs indicates to which side the thorax is rotated. In this case, the left ribs are longer, and this radiograph is a left posterior oblique view. Surfactant was administered, resulting in significant improvement in the density of the lung **(B)**. The right lung is slightly better aerated than the left. Uneven distribution of clearing is common. (From Hilton S, Edwards D. *Practical Pediatric Radiology*. 2nd ed. Philadelphia: Saunders; 1994.)

Prevention and Treatment

Strategies to prevent preterm birth include maternal cervical cerclage, treatment of infections, and administration of tocolytic medications. In addition, prevention of neonatal cold stress, birth asphyxia, and hypovolemia reduces the risk of RDS. If premature delivery is unavoidable, the antenatal administration of corticosteroids (usually in the form of betamethasone) to the pregnant person stimulates fetal lung production of surfactant; this approach requires multiple doses for at least 48 hours.

After birth, RDS may be treated or its severity reduced by intratracheal administration of exogenous surfactant immediately after birth in the delivery room or within a few hours of birth. Exogenous surfactant can be administered repeatedly during the course of RDS in patients receiving endotracheal intubation, mechanical ventilation, and oxygen therapy. There are also less-invasive methods to administer surfactant that are becoming standard of care. Early application of nasal CPAP also reduces the severity of RDS (Fig. 60.5).

The Pao_2 level should be maintained between 60 and 70 mm Hg (oxygen saturation 90%), and the pH should be maintained above 7.25. An increased concentration of warm and humidified inspired oxygen administered by CPAP or a nasal cannula may be all that is needed. If respiratory failure ensues ($Pco_2 > 60$ mm Hg, pH < 7.20, and $Pao_2 < 50$ mm Hg with 100% oxygen), assisted ventilation using a ventilator is indicated.

In response to persistent hypercapnia, alveolar ventilation ([tidal volume − dead space] × rate) must be increased. Ventilation can be increased by an increase in the ventilator's rate or an increase in the tidal volume. In response to hypoxia, the inspired oxygen content may be increased. Alternatively, the degree of oxygenation depends on the mean airway pressure. Mean airway pressure is directly related to positive end-expiratory pressure, flow, and inspiratory time. Increased mean airway pressure may improve oxygenation by improving lung volume, enhancing

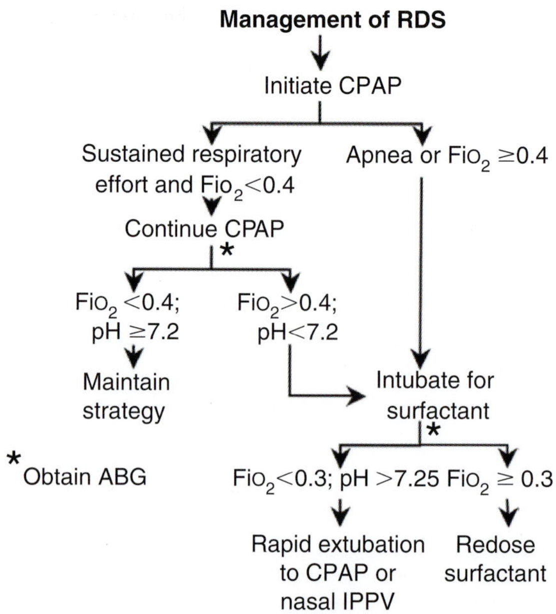

FIGURE 60.5 Algorithm suggesting management strategy of RDS. *ABG*, Arterial blood gas; *CPAP*, continuous positive airway pressure; *FiO2*, fraction of inspired oxygen; *IPPV*, intermittent positive-pressure ventilation; *RDS*, respiratory distress syndrome. (From Fanaroff AA, Fanaroff JM. *Klaus & Fanaroff's Care of the High-Risk Neonate*. 7th ed. Philadelphia: Elsevier; 2020: Fig. 9.5.)

ventilation-perfusion matching. Because of the difficulty in distinguishing sepsis and pneumonia from severe RDS, broad-spectrum parenteral antibiotics (ampicillin and gentamicin) may be administered for 36–48 hours, pending the recovery of an organism from a previously obtained blood culture.

COMPLICATIONS OF RESPIRATORY DISTRESS SYNDROME

Patent Ductus Arteriosus

PDA is a common complication that occurs in many low birth-weight infants who have RDS. The incidence of PDA is inversely related to the gestational age of the infant. In term newborns, the ductus functionally closes within 24–48 hours after birth. However, in preterm newborns, especially those with RDS, the ductus frequently fails to close, requiring medical or surgical closure. The ductus arteriosus in a preterm infant is less responsive to vasoconstrictive stimuli, which, when complicated with hypoxemia during RDS, may lead to a persistent PDA that creates a shunt between the pulmonary and systemic circulations.

During the acute phase of RDS, hypoxia, hypercapnia, and acidosis lead to pulmonary arterial vasoconstriction. The pulmonary and systemic pressures may be equal, and flow through the ductus may be small or bidirectional. When RDS improves and pulmonary vascular resistance declines, flow through the ductus arteriosus increases in a left-to-right direction. Significant systemic-to-pulmonary shunting may lead to heart failure and pulmonary edema. Excessive intravenous fluid administration may increase the incidence of symptomatic PDA. The infant's respiratory status deteriorates because of increased lung fluid, hypercapnia, and hypoxemia.

Clinical manifestations of a PDA usually become apparent on day 2–4 of life. Because the left-to-right shunt directs flow to a low-pressure circulation from one of high pressure, the pulse pressure widens; a previously inactive precordium shows an extremely active precordial impulse, and peripheral pulses become easily palpable and bounding. The murmur of a PDA may be continuous in systole and diastole, but usually only the systolic component is auscultated. Heart failure and pulmonary edema result in rales and hepatomegaly. A chest radiograph shows cardiomegaly and pulmonary edema, a two-dimensional echocardiogram shows ductal patency, and Doppler studies show markedly increased left-to-right flow through the ductus.

Treatment of a PDA during RDS involves initial fluid restriction and diuretic administration. If there is no improvement after 24–48 hours, a prostaglandin synthetase inhibitor, ibuprofen, indomethacin, or acetaminophen is administered. Contraindications to using indomethacin include thrombocytopenia (platelets < 50,000/mm^3), bleeding, serum creatinine measuring more than 1.8 mg/dL, and oliguria. Because 20–30% of infants do not respond initially to medical therapy and because the PDA reopens in 10–20% of infants, a repeat course of medications, surgical ligation, or catheter-based occlusion may be required.

Pulmonary Air Leaks

Assisted ventilation with high peak inspiratory pressures and positive end-expiratory pressures may cause overdistention of alveoli in localized areas of the lung. Rupture of the alveolar epithelial lining may produce pulmonary interstitial emphysema as gas dissects along the interstitial space and the peribronchial lymphatics. Extravasation of gas into the parenchyma reduces lung compliance and worsens respiratory failure. Gas dissection into the mediastinal space produces a pneumomediastinum, occasionally dissecting into the subcutaneous tissues around the neck, causing subcutaneous emphysema.

Alveolar rupture adjacent to the pleural space produces a **pneumothorax** (Fig. 60.6). If the gas is under tension, the pneumothorax shifts the mediastinum to the opposite side of the chest, producing hypotension, hypoxia, and hypercapnia. The diagnosis of a pneumothorax may be based on unequal transillumination of the chest and may be confirmed by chest radiograph. Treatment of a symptomatic pneumothorax requires insertion of a pleural chest tube connected to negative pressure or to an underwater drain. Prophylactic or therapeutic use of exogenous surfactant has reduced the incidence of pulmonary air leaks.

Pneumothorax also is observed after vigorous resuscitation, meconium aspiration pneumonia, pulmonary hypoplasia, and diaphragmatic hernia. Spontaneous pneumothorax may also occur but is seen in fewer than 1% of deliveries.

Bronchopulmonary Dysplasia (Chronic Lung Disease)

BPD is a clinical diagnosis defined by respiratory support at 36 weeks of postconceptual age and accompanied by characteristic clinical and radiographic findings that correspond to anatomic abnormalities (Table 60.3). High airway pressures and inspired oxygen concentrations increase the risk of development of BPD in extremely premature infants. Oxygen-mediated lung injury results from the generation of superoxides, hydrogen peroxide, and oxygen free radicals, which disrupt membrane lipids. Assisted ventilation with high peak pressures produces barotrauma, compounding the damaging effects of highly inspired oxygen levels. In

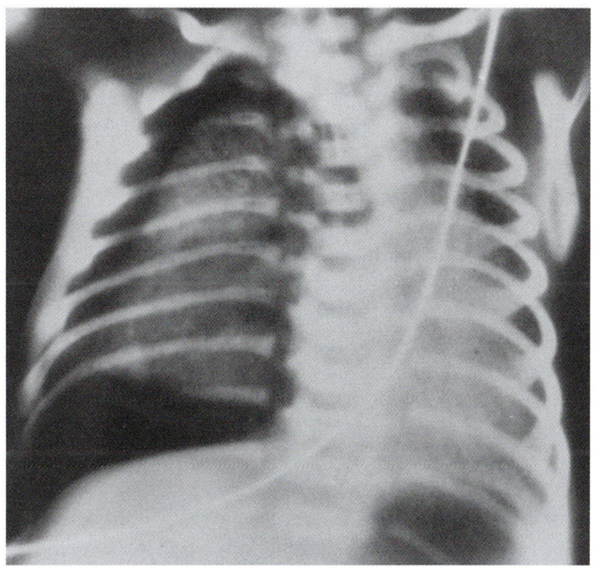

FIGURE 60.6 Pneumothorax. Right-sided hyperlucent pleural air is obvious. The findings of linear interstitial air and the resultant non-compliant but collapsed lung are noted. (From Heller RM, Kirchner SG. *Advanced Exercises in Diagnostic Radiology: The Newborn*. Philadelphia: WB Saunders; 1979.)

TABLE 60.3 Classification of Bronchopulmonary Dysplasia

BPD GRADE	DEFINITION
Mild BPD (Grade 1)	Infant at 36 weeks postmenstrual age requires low flow nasal cannula (<2 liters per minute)
Moderate BPD (Grade 2)	Infant at 36 weeks postmenstrual age requires high flow nasal cannula (>2 liters per minute or noninvasive positive pressure ventilation)
Severe BPD (Grade 3)	Infant at 36 weeks postmenstrual age requires invasive mechanical ventilation

BPD, Bronchopulmonary dysplasia.
Adapted from Jensen EA, Dysart K, Gantz MG, et al. The diagnosis of bronchopulmonary dysplasia in very preterm infants. An evidence-based approach. Am J Respir Crit Care Med. *2019;200(6):751–759.*

most patients, BPD develops after ventilation for RDS that may have been complicated by PDA or pulmonary interstitial emphysema. Inflammation from prolonged assisted ventilation and repeated systemic and pulmonary infections may play a major role. Failure of RDS to improve after 2 weeks, the need for prolonged mechanical ventilation, and oxygen therapy required at 36 weeks of postconceptual age are characteristic of patients with RDS in whom BPD commonly develops. BPD also may develop in infants weighing less than 1,000 g who require mechanical ventilation for poor respiratory drive in the absence of RDS. Fifty percent of infants born at 24–26 weeks gestational age require oxygen at 36 weeks corrected age.

The radiographic appearance of BPD is characterized initially by diffuse haziness eventually progressing to areas of overdistention and atelectasis. The histopathology of BPD reveals interstitial edema, interstitial fibrosis, and smooth muscle hypertrophy with reduced numbers of alveoli.

The clinical manifestations of BPD are oxygen dependence, hypercapnia with a compensatory metabolic alkalosis, pulmonary hypertension, poor growth, and development of right-sided heart failure. These infants also may have increased airway resistance with reactive airway bronchoconstriction. The use of bronchodilating agents may be helpful. Severe chest retractions produce negative interstitial pressure that draws fluid into the interstitial space. Together with cor pulmonale, these chest retractions cause fluid retention, necessitating fluid restriction and the administration of diuretics.

Infants with severe BPD may need treatment with mechanical ventilation for many months. To reduce the risk of subglottic stenosis, a tracheotomy may be indicated. To reduce oxygen toxicity and barotrauma, ventilator settings are reduced to maintain blood gases with slightly lower Pao_2 (50 mm Hg) and higher $Paco_2$ (50–75 mm Hg) levels than for infants during the acute phase of RDS. Dexamethasone therapy may reduce inflammation, improve pulmonary function, and enhance weaning of patients from assisted ventilation. However, steroid therapy in the first week of life may increase the risk of bowel perforation, cerebral palsy, or abnormal neuromotor developmental outcome. Older survivors of BPD may have hyperinflation, reactive airways, and developmental delay. They are at risk for severe respiratory syncytial virus pneumonia and, as infants, should receive prophylaxis against respiratory syncytial virus.

Retinopathy of Prematurity

Retinopathy of prematurity (ROP) is caused by the acute and chronic effects of oxygen toxicity on the developing blood vessels of the premature infant's retina. The completely vascularized retina of the term infant is not susceptible to ROP. ROP is a leading cause of blindness in very low birthweight infants (<1,500 g). Excessive arterial oxygen tensions produce vasoconstriction of immature retinal vasculature in the first stage of this disease. Vaso-obliteration follows if the duration and extent of hyperoxia are prolonged beyond the time when vasoconstriction is reversible. Hypercarbia and hypoxia may contribute to ROP. The subsequent proliferative stages are characterized by extraretinal fibrovascular proliferation, forming a ridge between the vascular and avascular portions of the retina, and by the development of neovascular tufts. In mild cases, vasoproliferation is noted at the periphery of the retina. Severe cases may have neovascularization involving the entire retina, retinal detachment resulting from traction on vessels as they leave the optic disc, fibrous proliferation behind the lens producing leukokoria, and synechiae displacing the lens forward, leading to glaucoma. Both eyes usually are involved, but severity may be asymmetric.

The incidence of ROP may be reduced by careful monitoring of arterial blood gas levels in all patients receiving oxygen. Although there is no absolutely safe Pao_2 level, it is wise to keep the arterial oxygen level between 50–70 mm Hg in premature infants. Infants who weigh less than 1,500 g or who are born before 32 weeks of gestation should be screened when they are 4 weeks of age or starting at 34 weeks of corrected gestational age, whichever comes first. Laser therapy or (less often) cryotherapy may be used for vitreous hemorrhage or for severe, progressive vasoproliferation. Surgery is indicated for retinal detachment. Less severe stages of ROP resolve spontaneously and without visual impairment in most patients.

TRANSIENT TACHYPNEA OF THE NEWBORN

Transient tachypnea of the newborn is a self-limited condition characterized by tachypnea, mild retractions, hypoxia, and occasional grunting, usually without signs of severe respiratory distress. Cyanosis, when present, usually requires treatment with supplemental oxygen in the range of 30–40%. Transient tachypnea of the newborn usually is noted in larger premature infants and in term infants born by precipitous delivery or cesarean section without prior labor. Infants of diabetic mothers and infants with poor respiratory drive as a result of placental passage of analgesic drugs are at risk. Transient tachypnea of the newborn may be caused by retained lung fluid or slow resorption of lung fluid. Chest radiographs show prominent central vascular markings, fluid in the lung fissures, overaeration, and occasionally a small pleural effusion. Air bronchograms and a reticulogranular pattern are not seen; their presence suggests another pulmonary process, such as RDS or pneumonia.

MECONIUM ASPIRATION SYNDROME

Meconium-stained amniotic fluid is seen in 15% of predominantly term and post-term deliveries. Although the passage of meconium into amniotic fluid is common in infants born in the breech presentation, meconium-stained fluid should be considered clinically as a sign of fetal distress in all infants. The presence of meconium in the amniotic fluid suggests in utero distress, which can be accompanied by asphyxia, hypoxia, and acidosis.

Aspiration of amniotic fluid contaminated with particulate meconium may occur in utero in a distressed, gasping fetus; more often, meconium is aspirated into the lung immediately after delivery. Affected infants have areas of lung hyper- and hypoinflation on chest radiographs, showing a high incidence of pneumonia and pneumothoraces.

Meconium aspiration syndrome is characterized by tachypnea, hypoxia, hypercapnia, and small airway obstruction causing a ball-valve effect, leading to air trapping, over-distention, and extra-alveolar air leaks. Complete small-airway obstruction produces atelectasis. Within 24–48 hours, a chemical pneumonitis develops in addition to the mechanical effects of airway obstruction. Abnormal pulmonary function may be caused by the meconium, in part, through inactivation of surfactant. Pulmonary hypertension frequently accompanies meconium aspiration, with right-to-left shunting caused by increased pulmonary vascular resistance. The chest radiograph reveals patchy infiltrates, overdistention, flattening of the diaphragm, increased anteroposterior diameter, and a high incidence of pneumomediastinum and pneumothoraces. Comorbid diseases include those associated with in utero asphyxia that initiated the passage of meconium.

Treatment of meconium aspiration includes general supportive care and assisted ventilation. Newborns with a persistent pulmonary hypertension (PPHN)–like presentation should be treated for PPHN (see next section). If severe hypoxia does not subside with conventional or high-frequency ventilation, surfactant therapy, and inhaled nitric oxide, extracorporeal membrane oxygenation (ECMO) may be beneficial.

Prevention of meconium aspiration syndrome involves careful in utero monitoring to prevent asphyxia. When meconium-stained fluid is observed, the neonatal resuscitation team uses the degree of respiratory distress or failure to guide delivery room intervention; intubation and suctioning below the vocal cords with a meconium aspirator may be utilized if the infant has little to no respiratory effort (see Fig. 57.5).

PERSISTENT PULMONARY HYPERTENSION OF THE NEWBORN

PPHN occurs in post-term, term, or near-term infants. PPHN is characterized by severe hypoxemia, without evidence of parenchymal lung or structural heart disease. PPHN is often seen with asphyxia or meconium-stained fluid. The chest radiograph usually reveals normal lung fields rather than the expected infiltrates and hyperinflation that may accompany meconium aspiration. Additional problems that may lead to PPHN are congenital pneumonia, hyperviscosity-polycythemia, congenital diaphragmatic hernia, pulmonary hypoplasia, congenital cyanotic heart disease, hypoglycemia, and hypothermia. Total anomalous venous return associated with obstruction of blood flow may produce a clinical picture that involves severe hypoxia and that is initially indistinguishable from PPHN; however, a chest radiograph reveals severe pulmonary venous engorgement and a small heart. Echocardiography or cardiac catheterization confirms the diagnosis.

Significant right-to-left shunting through a patent foramen ovale, through a PDA, and through intrapulmonary channels is characteristic of PPHN. The pulmonary vasculature often shows hypertrophied arterial wall smooth muscle, suggesting that the process of or predisposition to PPHN began in utero as a result of previous periods of fetal hypoxia. After birth, hypoxia, hypercapnia, and acidosis exacerbate pulmonary artery vasoconstriction, leading to further hypoxia and acidosis. Some infants with PPHN have extrapulmonary manifestations as a result of asphyxia. Myocardial injuries include heart failure, transient mitral insufficiency, and papillary muscle or myocardial infarction. Thrombocytopenia, right atrial thrombi, and pulmonary embolism also may be noted.

The diagnosis of PPHN is confirmed by echocardiographic examination, which shows elevated pulmonary artery pressures and sites of right-to-left shunting. Echocardiography also rules out structural congenital heart disease and transient myocardial dysfunction.

Treatment of PPHN involves general supportive care; correction of hypotension, anemia, and acidosis; and management of complications associated with asphyxia. If myocardial dysfunction is present, milrinone may be used. The most important therapy for PPHN is assisted ventilation. Reversible mild pulmonary hypertension may respond to conventional assisted ventilation. Patients with severe PPHN do not always respond to conventional therapy. Paralysis with a muscle relaxant may be needed to assist ventilation. Surfactant replacement seems to have no effect when PPHN is the primary diagnosis. If mechanical ventilation and supportive care are unsuccessful in improving oxygenation, inhaled nitric oxide, a selective pulmonary artery vasodilating agent, should be administered. If hypoxia persists, the patient may be a candidate for ECMO. Infants who require extremely high ventilator settings, marked by an alveolar-to-arterial oxygen gradient greater than 620 mm Hg, have a high mortality rate and benefit from ECMO if they do not respond to nitric oxide.

APNEA OF PREMATURITY

Although apnea typically is associated with immaturity of the respiratory control system, it also may be the presenting sign of other diseases or pathophysiologic states that affect preterm infants (Table 60.4). A thorough consideration of possible causes is always warranted, especially with the onset or unexpected increase in the frequency of episodes of apnea (or bradycardia).

Apnea is defined as the cessation of pulmonary airflow for a specific time interval, usually longer than 10–20 seconds. Bradycardia often accompanies prolonged apnea. **Central apnea** refers to a complete cessation of airflow and respiratory efforts with no chest wall movement. **Obstructive apnea** refers to the absence of noticeable airflow but with the continuation of chest wall movements. **Mixed apnea**, a combination of these two events, is the most frequent type. It may begin as a brief episode of obstruction followed by a central apnea. Alternatively, central apnea may produce upper airway closure (passive pharyngeal hypotonia), resulting in mixed apnea.

A careful evaluation to determine the cause of apnea should be performed immediately in any infant with apnea. The incidence of apnea increases as gestational age decreases.

TABLE 60.4 Potential Causes of Neonatal Apnea

Central nervous system	IVH, drugs/medications, seizures, hypoxic injury
Respiratory	Pneumonia, obstructive airway lesions, atelectasis, extreme prematurity (<1,000 grams), laryngeal reflex, phrenic nerve paralysis, severe RDS, pneumothorax
Infectious	Sepsis, necrotizing enterocolitis, meningitis (bacterial, fungal, viral)
Gastrointestinal	Oral feeding, bowel movement, gastroesophageal reflux, esophagitis, intestinal perforation
Metabolic	↓ Glucose, ↓ calcium, ↓ Po_2, ↓↑ sodium, ↑ ammonia, ↑ organic acids, ↑ ambient temperature, hypothermia
Cardiovascular	Hypotension, hypertension, heart failure, anemia, hypovolemia, change in vagal tone
Idiopathic	Immaturity of respiratory center, sleep state, upper airway collapse

IVH, Intraventricular hemorrhage; *RDS*, respiratory distress syndrome.

Apnea of prematurity presents as recurrent apneic events in the absence of any other identifiable disease states during the first week of life and usually resolves by 36–40 weeks of postconceptual age (gestational age at birth + postnatal age). The premature infant's process of regulating respiration is especially vulnerable to apnea. Preterm infants respond paradoxically to hypoxia by developing apnea rather than by increasing respirations as in mature infants. Poor tone of the laryngeal muscles also may lead to collapse of the upper airway, causing obstruction. Isolated obstructive apnea also may occur as a result of flexion or extreme lateral positioning of the premature infant's head, which obstructs the soft trachea.

Treatment of apnea of prematurity involves administration of oxygen to hypoxic infants, transfusion of anemic infants, and physical cutaneous stimulation for infants with mild apnea. Methylxanthines (caffeine or theophylline) are the mainstay of pharmacologic treatment of apnea. Xanthine therapy increases minute ventilation, improves the carbon dioxide sensitivity, decreases hypoxic depression of breathing, enhances diaphragmatic activity, and decreases periodic breathing. Treatment usually is initiated with a loading dose followed by maintenance therapy. High-flow nasal cannula therapy and nasal CPAP of 4–6 cm H_2O also are effective and relatively safe methods of treating obstructive or mixed apneas; they may work by stimulating the infant and splinting the upper airway. CPAP also probably increases functional residual capacity, improving oxygenation.

PEARLS FOR PRACTITIONERS

See Fetal and Neonatal Medicine: Pearls for Practitioners at the end of this section.

REVIEW QUESTIONS

Available online.

CHAPTER 61

Anemia and Hyperbilirubinemia

ANEMIA

Embryonic hematopoiesis begins by the 20th day of gestation and is evidenced by blood islands in the yolk sac. In midgestation, erythropoiesis occurs in the liver and spleen; the bone marrow becomes the predominant site in the last trimester. Hemoglobin concentration increases from 8–10 g/dL at 12 weeks to 16.5–18 g/dL at 40 weeks. Fetal red blood cell (RBC) production is responsive to erythropoietin; the concentration of this hormone increases with fetal hypoxia and anemia. Hemoglobin synthesis in the last two trimesters of pregnancy produces fetal hemoglobin (hemoglobin F), composed of two α chains and two γ chains. Before term, the infant begins to synthesize β-hemoglobin chains; the term infant should have some adult hemoglobin (two α chains and two β chains). Fetal hemoglobin represents 60–90% of hemoglobin at term birth. The levels decline to adult levels of less than 5% by 4 months of age.

For a term infant, blood volume is 75–90 mL/kg, and for a preterm infant, blood volume is 90–100 mL/kg. The placenta and umbilical vessels contain additional blood that can aid in transition of the newborn if fetoplacental circulation continues after birth. This is done by ***delayed cord clamping*** **(DCC)** and umbilical cord milking (UCM). It is recommended to delay umbilical cord clamping for most vigorous term and preterm infants >27 weeks for at least 60 seconds after birth. For 35–42 week infants who remain nonvigorous despite stimulation, ***umbilical cord milking*** **(UCM)**—pushing blood in the umbilical cord towards the infant—may aid resuscitation. DCC and UCM can increase neonatal blood volume and hemoglobin levels transiently for the first 3 days of life. DCC usually has no adverse effects but is not recommended if immediate resuscitation is needed. Umbilical cord milking has been associated with intraventricular hemorrhage in preterm infants and thus is not routinely recommended below 35 weeks gestational age. DCC may increase the risk of polycythemia and jaundice.

After birth, hemoglobin levels increase transiently at 6–12 hours, then decline to 11–12 g/dL at 3–6 months. A premature infant (<32 weeks of gestational age) has a lower hemoglobin concentration and a more rapid postnatal decline of hemoglobin level, which achieves a nadir 1–2 months after birth. Fetal and neonatal RBCs have a shorter life span (70–90 days) and a higher mean corpuscular volume (110–120 fL) than adult cells. The physiologic anemia noted at 2–3 months of age in term infants and at 1–2 months of age in preterm infants is a normal process that does not result in signs of illness and does not require any treatment. It is a physiologic condition believed to be related to several factors, including increased tissue oxygenation experienced at birth, shortened RBC life span, and low erythropoietin levels.

Symptomatic anemia in the newborn period (Fig. 61.1) may be caused by decreased RBC production, increased RBC destruction, or blood loss.

Decreased Red Blood Cell Production

Anemia caused by decreased production of RBCs appears at birth with pallor, a low reticulocyte count, and absence of erythroid precursors in the bone marrow. Potential causes of neonatal

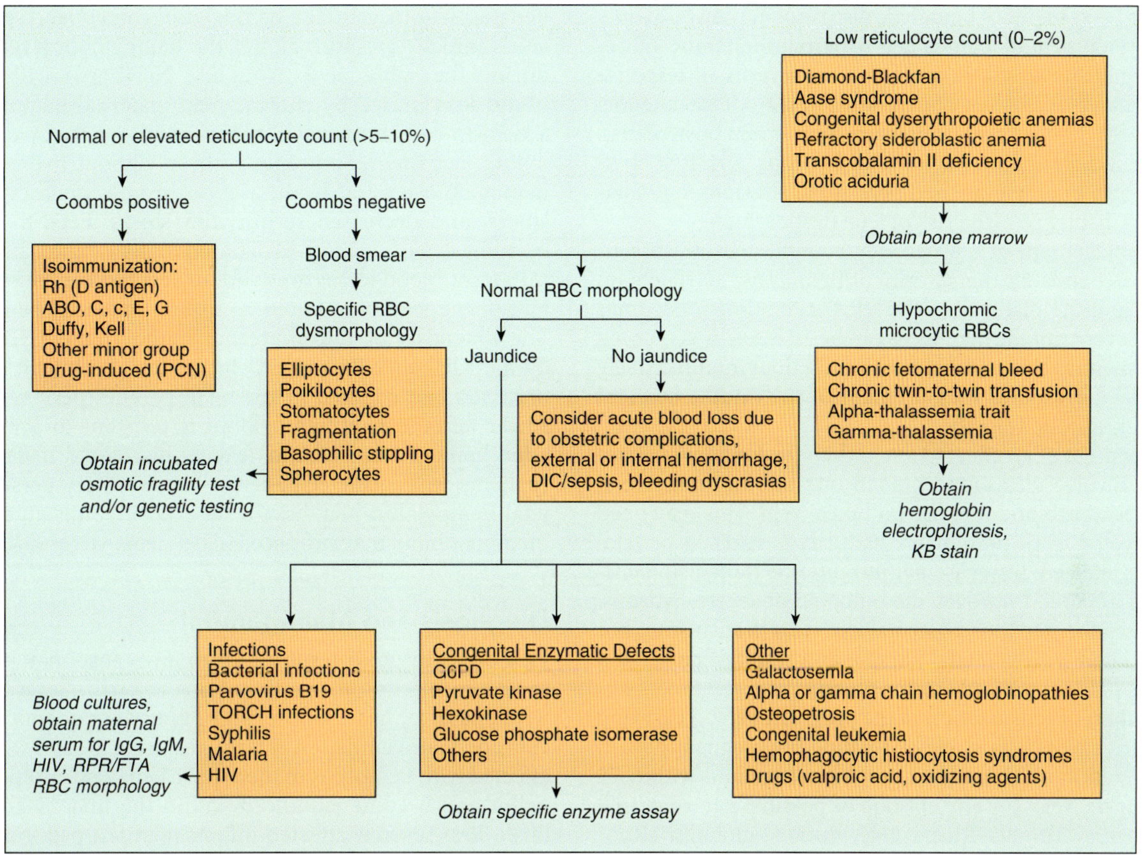

FIGURE 61.1 Differential diagnosis of neonatal anemia. The physician obtains information from the family, maternal and labor and delivery histories, and laboratory tests, including hemoglobin, reticulocyte count, blood type, direct Coombs test, peripheral smear, RBC indices, and bilirubin concentration. *DIC,* Disseminated intravascular coagulation; *FTA,* fluorescent treponemal antibody test; *G6PD,* glucose-6-phosphate dehydrogenase; *KB,* Kleihauer-Betke; *PCN,* penicillin; *RBC,* red blood cell; *RPR,* rapid plasma reagin tests; *TORCH,* toxoplasmosis, other, rubella, cytomegalovirus, herpes simplex. (From Ohls RK. Anemia in the neonate. In: Christensen RD, ed. *Hematologic Problems of the Neonate.* Philadelphia: Saunders; 2000:162.)

decreased RBC production include bone marrow failure syndromes (congenital RBC aplasia [Blackfan-Diamond anemia]), infection (congenital viral infections [parvovirus, rubella], acquired bacterial or viral sepsis), and congenital leukemia.

Increased Red Blood Cell Destruction

Immunologically mediated hemolysis in utero may lead to **erythroblastosis fetalis**, or the fetus may be spared, and **hemolytic disease** may appear in the newborn. Hemolysis of fetal erythrocytes is a result of blood group differences between the sensitized pregnant person and fetus, which causes production of maternal immunoglobulin G (IgG) antibodies directed against an antigen on fetal cells.

ABO blood group incompatibility with neonatal hemolysis develops only if the pregnant person has IgG antibodies from a previous exposure to A or B antigens. These IgG antibodies cross the placenta by active transport and affect the fetus or newborn. Sensitization of the pregnant person to fetal antigens may have occurred by previous transfusions or by conditions of pregnancy that result in transfer of fetal erythrocytes into the maternal circulation, such as first-trimester abortion, ectopic pregnancy, amniocentesis, manual extraction of the placenta, version (external or internal) procedures, or normal pregnancy.

ABO incompatibility may produce **hemolytic disease of the newborn**, which is manifested as significant anemia and hyperbilirubinemia. Because many pregnant people who have blood group O have IgG antibodies to A and B before pregnancy, the firstborn infant of A or B blood type may be affected. In contrast to Rh disease, ABO hemolytic disease does not become more severe with subsequent pregnancies. Hemolysis with ABO incompatibility is less severe than hemolysis in Rh-sensitized pregnancy, either because the anti-A or anti-B antibody may bind to nonerythrocytic cells that contain A or B antigen or because fetal erythrocytes have fewer A or B antigenic determinants than they have Rh sites. With the declining incidence of Rh hemolytic disease, ABO incompatibility has become one of the most common causes of neonatal hyperbilirubinemia requiring therapy. Thus, newborns are often screened after birth with the Coombs test if born to a pregnant person with blood group O.

Erythroblastosis fetalis classically is caused by Rh blood group incompatibility. The Rh antigen system consists of five antigens: C, D, E, c, and e; the D type is most antigenic. In most Rh-sensitized cases, the D antigen of the fetus sensitizes the Rh-negative pregnant person, resulting in IgG antibody production during the first pregnancy. Because most pregnant people are not sensitized to Rh antigens at the start of pregnancy, Rh erythroblastosis fetalis is usually a disease of subsequent pregnancies. The first affected pregnancy results in an antibody response in the pregnant person, which may be detected during antenatal screening with the antibody screen and determined to be anti-D antibody. The first affected newborn may show no serious fetal disease and may manifest hemolytic disease of the newborn only by the development of anemia and hyperbilirubinemia. Subsequent pregnancies result in an increasing severity of response because of an earlier onset of hemolysis in utero. Fetal anemia, heart failure, elevated venous pressure, portal vein obstruction, and hypoalbuminemia result in **fetal hydrops**, which is characterized by ascites, pleural and pericardial effusions, and anasarca (see Chapter 59). The risk of fetal death is high.

The management of a pregnancy complicated by Rh sensitization depends on the severity of hemolysis, its effects on the fetus, and the maturity of the fetus at the time it becomes affected. Severity of the hemolysis can be assessed by screening for fetal anemia; this is most commonly done noninvasively by Doppler ultrasound measurement of the middle cerebral artery peak systolic velocity.

Management of an affected fetus when the lungs are immature may involve ultrasound-guided intrauterine transfusion with O-negative blood into the umbilical vein. This may need to be repeated until pulmonary maturity is reached or fetal distress is detected. Intravascular intrauterine transfusion corrects fetal anemia, improves the outcome of severe hydrops, and reduces the need for postnatal exchange transfusion, but it is associated with neonatal anemia as a result of continued hemolysis plus suppressed erythropoiesis.

Prevention of sensitization of the pregnant person carrying a Rh-positive fetus is possible by treating the pregnant person during gestation at 28 weeks of gestational age and within 72 hours after delivery (or any episode of possible feto-maternal hemorrhage) with anti–Rh-positive immune globulin (RhoGAM). The dose of RhoGAM (300 mcg) is based on the ability of this amount of anti–Rh-positive antibody to bind all the possible fetal Rh-positive erythrocytes entering the maternal circulation during the fetal-to-maternal transfusion at birth (~30 mL). RhoGAM may bind Rh-positive fetal erythrocytes or interfere with maternal anti–Rh-positive antibody production by another, unknown mechanism. RhoGAM is effective only in preventing sensitization to the D antigen. Other blood group antigens that can cause immune hydrops and erythroblastosis include c, E, Kell, and Duffy. Anti-Kell alloimmunity produces lower amniotic bilirubin levels and a lower reticulocyte count because, in addition to hemolysis, it inhibits erythropoiesis.

Nonimmune causes of hemolysis in the newborn include RBC enzyme deficiencies of the Embden-Meyerhof pathway, such as pyruvate kinase or glucose-6-phosphate dehydrogenase deficiency. RBC membrane disorders are another cause of nonimmune hemolysis. Hereditary spherocytosis is inherited as a severe autosomal recessive form or less severe autosomal dominant form and is the result of a deficiency of spectrin, a protein of the RBC membrane. Hemoglobinopathies, such as thalassemia, are another cause of nonimmunologically mediated hemolysis.

Blood Loss

Anemia from blood loss at birth is manifested by two patterns of presentation, depending on the rapidity of blood loss. **Acute blood loss** after fetal-maternal hemorrhage, rupture of the umbilical cord, placenta previa, or internal hemorrhage (hepatic or splenic hematoma; retroperitoneal) is characterized by pallor, diminished peripheral pulses, and shock. There are no signs of extramedullary hematopoiesis and no hepatosplenomegaly. The hemoglobin content and serum iron levels initially are normal, but the hemoglobin levels decline during the subsequent 24 hours. Newborns with **chronic blood loss** caused by chronic fetal-maternal hemorrhage or a twin-to-twin transfusion present with marked pallor, heart failure, hepatosplenomegaly with or without hydrops, a low hemoglobin level at birth, a hypochromic microcytic blood smear, and decreased serum iron stores. Fetal-to-maternal bleeding can occur, with fetal blood losses ranging from 1–150 mL; most blood losses are 1 mL or less but can be more than half of the fetal blood volume in feto-maternal hemorrhage. The diagnosis of **feto-maternal hemorrhage** is confirmed by the Kleihauer-Betke acid elution test. Pink fetal RBCs are observed and counted in the birth parent's peripheral blood smear because fetal hemoglobin is resistant to acid elution; adult hemoglobin is eluted, leaving discolored maternal cells (patients with sickle cell anemia or hereditary persistence of fetal hemoglobin may have a false-positive result, and ABO incompatibility may produce a false-negative result).

Diagnosis and Management

Hemolysis in utero resulting from any cause may produce a spectrum of clinical manifestations at birth. Severe hydrops with anasarca, heart failure, and pulmonary edema may prevent adequate ventilation at birth, resulting in asphyxia. Infants affected with hemolysis in utero have hepatosplenomegaly and pallor and become jaundiced within the first 24 hours after birth. Less severely affected infants manifest pallor and hepatosplenomegaly at birth and can subsequently become rapidly jaundiced. Patients with ABO incompatibility are often asymptomatic and show no physical signs at birth; mild anemia with jaundice develops during the first 24–72 hours of life.

Because hydrops, anemia, or jaundice is secondary to many diverse causes of hemolysis, a laboratory evaluation is needed in all patients with suspected hemolysis. A blood type and antibody screen should be performed on every birth parent. A blood type and screen with direct Coombs test (to determine the presence of antibody-coated RBCs) should be performed in the initial evaluation of all infants with hemolysis. Other laboratory testing that may be useful includes complete blood count, blood smear, and reticulocyte count. An infant's positive Coombs test may be due to **ABO incompatibility** (e.g., maternal blood type O and infant blood type A or B), **Rh incompatibility** (e.g., maternal Rh negative with antibody screen positive for anti-D), **maternal isoimmunization** to a minor antigen (e.g., anti-Kell antibody detected in maternal antibody screen), or transplacental transmission of RhoGAM (passive anti-D antibody given to Rh-negative pregnant people to prevent sensitization). Reduced hemoglobin levels, reticulocytosis, and a blood smear characterized by polychromasia and anisocytosis are expected with isoimmune hemolysis. Spherocytes are commonly observed in ABO incompatibility.

In the absence of a positive Coombs test, maternal isoimmunization, or blood group differences between the birth parent and infant, other causes of nonimmune hemolysis must be considered. RBC enzyme assays, hemoglobin electrophoresis, or RBC membrane tests (osmotic fragility, spectrin assay) should be performed. Internal hemorrhage also may be associated with anemia, reticulocytosis, and jaundice when the hemorrhage reabsorbs; ultrasound evaluation of the brain, liver, spleen, or adrenal gland may be indicated when nonimmune hemolysis is suspected. Shock is more typical in patients with internal hemorrhage, whereas in hemolytic diseases, heart failure may be seen with severe anemia. Evaluation of a possible fetal-maternal hemorrhage should include the Kleihauer-Betke test.

The treatment of *symptomatic* neonatal anemia is transfusion of cross-matched packed RBCs. If immune hemolysis is present, the cells to be transfused must be cross-matched against maternal and neonatal plasma. Acute volume loss may necessitate resuscitation with nonblood products, such as saline if blood is not available; packed RBCs can be given subsequently. To correct anemia and any remaining blood volume deficit, 10–15 mL/kg of packed RBCs should be sufficient. Cytomegalovirus-seronegative blood should be given, and all blood products should be irradiated to reduce the risk of graft-versus-host disease; blood should be screened for HIV, hepatitis B and C, and syphilis. Recombinant erythropoietin may improve the hematocrit in infants with a hyporegenerative anemia after in utero transfusion.

HYPERBILIRUBINEMIA

Hemolytic disease of the newborn is a common cause of neonatal jaundice. Nonetheless, because of the immaturity of the pathways of bilirubin metabolism, many newborn infants without evidence of hemolysis become jaundiced.

Bilirubin is produced by the catabolism of hemoglobin in the reticuloendothelial system. The tetrapyrrole ring of heme is cleaved by heme oxygenase to form equivalent quantities of biliverdin and carbon monoxide. Because no other biologic source of carbon monoxide exists, the excretion of this gas is stoichiometrically identical to the production of bilirubin. Biliverdin is converted to bilirubin by biliverdin reductase. One gram of hemoglobin produces 35 mg of bilirubin. Sources of bilirubin other than circulating hemoglobin represent 20% of bilirubin production; these sources include inefficient (shunt) hemoglobin production and lysis of precursor cells in bone marrow. Compared with adults, newborns have a two- to threefold greater rate of bilirubin production (6–10 mg/kg/24 hours vs. 3 mg/kg/24 hours). This increased production is caused, in part, by an increased RBC mass (higher hematocrit) and a shortened erythrocyte life span of 70–90 days compared with the 120-day erythrocyte life span in adults.

Bilirubin produced after hemoglobin catabolism is lipid soluble and unconjugated and reacts as an indirect reagent in the van den Bergh test. Indirect-reacting, unconjugated bilirubin is toxic to the central nervous system and is insoluble in water, limiting its excretion. Unconjugated bilirubin binds to albumin on specific bilirubin binding sites; 1 g of albumin binds 8.5 mg of bilirubin in a newborn. If the binding sites become saturated or if a competitive compound binds at the site, displacing bound bilirubin, free bilirubin becomes available to enter the central nervous system. Organic acids such as free fatty acids and drugs such as ceftriaxone can displace bilirubin from its binding site on albumin.

Bilirubin dissociates from albumin at the hepatocyte and becomes bound to a cytoplasmic liver protein Y (ligandin). Hepatic conjugation results in the production of bilirubin diglucuronide, which is water soluble and capable of biliary and renal excretion. The enzyme glucuronosyltransferase represents the rate-limiting step of bilirubin conjugation. The concentrations of ligandin and glucuronosyltransferase are lower in newborns, particularly in premature infants, than in older children.

Most conjugated bilirubin is excreted through the bile into the small intestine and eliminated in the stool. Some bilirubin may undergo hydrolysis back to the unconjugated fraction by intestinal glucuronidase, however, and may be reabsorbed **(enterohepatic recirculation)**. In addition, bacteria in the neonatal intestine convert bilirubin to urobilinogen and stercobilinogen, which are excreted in urine and stool and usually limit bilirubin reabsorption. Delayed passage of meconium, which contains bilirubin, also may contribute to the enterohepatic recirculation of bilirubin.

Bilirubin is produced in utero by the normal fetus and by the fetus affected by erythroblastosis fetalis. Indirect, unconjugated, lipid-soluble fetal bilirubin is transferred across the placenta and becomes conjugated by maternal hepatic enzymes. The placenta is impermeable to conjugated water-soluble bilirubin. Fetal bilirubin levels become only mildly elevated in the presence of severe hemolysis but may increase when hemolysis produces fetal hepatic inspissated bile stasis and conjugated hyperbilirubinemia. Maternal indirect (but not direct) hyperbilirubinemia also may increase fetal bilirubin levels.

Etiology of Indirect Unconjugated Hyperbilirubinemia

Physiologic jaundice is a common cause of hyperbilirubinemia among newborns. It is a diagnosis of exclusion, made after careful evaluation has ruled out more serious causes of jaundice, such as hemolysis, infection, and metabolic diseases. Physiologic jaundice is the result of many factors that are normal physiologic characteristics of newborns: increased bilirubin production resulting from an increased RBC mass, shortened RBC life span, and hepatic immaturity of ligandin and glucuronosyltransferase.

The clinical pattern of physiologic jaundice in term infants includes a peak indirect-reacting bilirubin level of around 15 mg/dL typically between 48 and 96 hours after birth. In premature infants, the peak is usually higher and can occur later (days 5–7). The peak level of indirect bilirubin during physiologic jaundice may be higher in breast milk–fed infants than in formula-fed infants. This higher level **(breastfeeding jaundice)** may be partly a result of the variations in fluid intake of breastfeeding infants and is often associated with weight loss and dehydration. Jaundice is nonphysiologic or pathologic if it is clinically evident on the first day of life, if the bilirubin level increases more than 5–7 mg/dL per day, if the direct bilirubin fraction is greater than 1.5 mg/dL, or if hepatosplenomegaly and anemia are present.

Crigler-Najjar syndrome is a serious, rare, autosomal recessive, permanent deficiency of glucuronosyltransferase that results in severe indirect hyperbilirubinemia. Type II responds to enzyme induction by phenobarbital, producing an increase in enzyme activity and a reduction of bilirubin levels. Type I does not respond to phenobarbital and manifests as persistent indirect hyperbilirubinemia, often leading to kernicterus. **Gilbert disease** is caused by a genetic variation of the promoter region of glucuronosyltransferase (*UGT1A1* gene) and results in a mild indirect hyperbilirubinemia, which is indistinguishable from physiologic jaundice in a neonate. In the presence of another icterogenic factor (hemolysis), more severe jaundice may develop.

Breast milk jaundice may be associated with unconjugated hyperbilirubinemia without evidence of hemolysis during the first to second week of life. Interruption of breast-feeding for 1–2 days results in a rapid decline of bilirubin levels, which do not increase significantly after breast-feeding resumes. Breast milk may contain an inhibitor of bilirubin conjugation or may increase enterohepatic recirculation of bilirubin because of breast milk glucuronidase.

Jaundice on the first day of life is always pathologic and may be unconjugated or conjugated; immediate attention is needed to establish the cause. Early onset of predominantly unconjugated hyperbilirubinemia often is a result of hemolysis, internal hemorrhage (subgalealhepatic or splenic hemorrhage), or infection (Table 61.1). Perinatal congenital infections, bacterial sepsis, and neonatal liver failure are also often associated with direct-reacting hyperbilirubinemia (Table 61.2).

TABLE 61.1 Etiology of Unconjugated Hyperbilirubinemia

	HEMOLYSIS PRESENT	HEMOLYSIS ABSENT
Common	*Blood group incompatibility:* ABO, Rh, Kell, Duffy infection	Physiologic jaundice, breast milk jaundice, internal hemorrhage, polycythemia, infant of diabetic mother
Rare	*Red blood cell enzyme defects:* glucose-6-phosphate dehydrogenase, pyruvate kinase *Red blood cell membrane disorders:* spherocytosis, ovalocytosis *Hemoglobinopathy:* thalassemia	Gene variant of glucuronyl transferase enzyme (Crigler-Najjar syndrome, Gilbert disease), pyloric stenosis, hypothyroidism, immune thrombocytopenia

TABLE 61.2 Etiology of Conjugated Hyperbilirubinemia

COMMON
Hyperalimentation cholestasis CMV infection Other perinatal congenital infections (TORCH) Inspissated bile from prolonged hemolysis Neonatal hepatitis Sepsis, urinary tract infection
UNCOMMON
Hepatic infarction Inborn errors of metabolism (galactosemia, tyrosinemia) Cystic fibrosis Biliary atresia Pan-hypopituitarism Choledochal cyst α_1-Antitrypsin deficiency Gestational alloimmune liver disease (neonatal hemochromatosis) Alagille syndrome (arteriohepatic dysplasia) Byler disease, progressive familial intrahepatic cholestasis types 1, 2, 3

CMV, Cytomegalovirus; *TORCH,* toxoplasmosis, other, rubella, cytomegalovirus, herpes simplex.

Therapy of Indirect Hyperbilirubinemia

When jaundice is observed, the laboratory evaluation for hyperbilirubinemia should include a total serum bilirubin measurement to determine the magnitude of hyperbilirubinemia. If treatment of hyperbilirubinemia with phototherapy or exchange transfusion is needed, infants should be evaluated further with measurement of indirect and direct bilirubin levels, blood typing, Coombs test, complete blood count, blood smear, and reticulocyte count.

Phototherapy is an effective and safe method for reducing indirect bilirubin levels, particularly when initiated before serum bilirubin increases to levels associated with kernicterus. Determining when to initiate phototherapy for newborns >35 weeks of gestation is based on gestational age, the hour-specific total serum bilirubin value, and the presence of risk factors for bilirubin neurotoxicity. Factors that increase the risk of neurotoxicity from bilirubin include lower gestational age, an albumin <3.0 g/dL, presence of isoimmune hemolytic disease, G6PD deficiency, or other hemolytic conditions, sepsis, or significant clinical instability in the previous 24 hours. Phototherapy is initiated in premature infants when bilirubin is at lower levels to prevent bilirubin from reaching the high concentrations necessitating exchange transfusion.

Under the effects of phototherapy light in the 460–490 nm wavelength band (ideally at 476 nm), bilirubin is transformed into isomers that are water soluble and easily excreted. For clinical efficacy, phototherapy light sources should have irradiance of at least 30 mW/cm^2/nm, illuminating as much body surface area as possible.

Unconjugated bilirubin (IX) is in the 4Z, 15Z configuration. Phototherapy causes a photochemical reaction producing the reversible, more water-soluble isomer 4Z, 15E bilirubin IX. This isomer can be excreted easily, bypassing the liver's conjugation system. Another photochemical reaction results in the rapid production of lumirubin, a water-soluble isomer which does not spontaneously revert to unconjugated native bilirubin and can be excreted in the urine.

Complications of phototherapy include an increased insensible water loss, which can lead to dehydration. Continued feeding via breast or bottle at regular intervals is important in preventing dehydration during phototherapy and stimulates the infant's physiologic bilirubin excretion. Additional problems are macular-papular red skin rash, lethargy, masking of cyanosis, and potential for retinal damage (infants wear eye protection). Skin bronzing may be noted in infants with direct-reacting hyperbilirubinemia (bronze baby syndrome). Infants with hemolytic disease of the newborn may be managed successfully with phototherapy for hyperbilirubinemia but also may develop anemia later from continued hemolysis.

Exchange transfusion usually is reserved for infants with dangerously high indirect bilirubin levels who are at risk for kernicterus. The exchange transfusion is usually performed through an umbilical venous catheter placed in the inferior vena cava or, if free flow is obtained, at the confluence of the umbilical vein and the portal system. The level of serum bilirubin immediately after the exchange transfusion declines to levels that are about half of those before the exchange; levels rebound 6–8 hours later as a result of continued hemolysis and redistribution of bilirubin from tissue stores.

Complications of exchange transfusion include problems related to the blood (transfusion reaction, metabolic instability, or infection), the catheter (vessel perforation or hemorrhage), or the procedure (hypotension or necrotizing enterocolitis [NEC]). Unusual complications include thrombocytopenia and graft-versus-host disease. Continuation of phototherapy may reduce the necessity for subsequent exchange transfusions.

Etiology of Direct Conjugated Hyperbilirubinemia

Direct-reacting hyperbilirubinemia (defined as a direct bilirubin level >2 mg/dL or >20% of the total bilirubin) is never physiologic and should always be evaluated thoroughly according to the diagnostic categories (Table 61.2). Direct-reacting bilirubin (composed mostly of conjugated bilirubin) is not neurotoxic to the infant but signifies a serious underlying disorder involving cholestasis or hepatocellular injury. The diagnostic evaluation of patients with direct-reacting hyperbilirubinemia involves the determination of the levels of liver enzymes (aspartate aminotransferase, alkaline phosphatase, alanine aminotransferase, and γ-glutamyl transpeptidase) and evaluation of bacterial and viral cultures, metabolic screening tests, liver ultrasound, sweat chloride test, and occasionally liver biopsy. In addition, the presence of dark urine and gray-white (acholic) stools with jaundice after the second week of life strongly suggests biliary atresia. The treatment of disorders manifested by direct bilirubinemia is specific for the diseases that are listed in Table 61.2. These diseases do not respond to phototherapy or exchange transfusion.

Acute Bilirubin Encephalopathy and Kernicterus

Lipid-soluble, unconjugated, indirect bilirubin fraction is toxic to the developing central nervous system, especially when indirect bilirubin concentrations are high and exceed the binding capacity of albumin. Kernicterus results when indirect bilirubin is deposited in brain cells and disrupts neuronal metabolism and function, especially in the basal ganglia. Indirect bilirubin may cross the blood-brain barrier because of its lipid solubility. Other theories propose that a disruption of the blood-brain barrier permits entry of a bilirubin-albumin or free bilirubin–fatty acid complex.

Kernicterus usually is noted when the bilirubin level is excessively high for gestational age or in the presence of other conditions that increase risk, including acidosis, hypoalbuminemia, hemolysis, bilirubin-displacing drugs (sulfa drugs), and prematurity. Other risks for kernicterus in term infants are hemolysis, G6PD deficiency, jaundice noted within 24 hours of birth, and delayed diagnosis of hyperbilirubinemia. Kernicterus has developed in extremely immature infants weighing less than 1,000 g because of a more permeable blood-brain barrier associated with prematurity.

The earliest clinical manifestations of kernicterus are lethargy, hypotonia, irritability, poor Moro response, and poor feeding. A high-pitched cry and emesis also may be present. Later signs include bulging fontanel, opisthotonic posturing, pulmonary hemorrhage, fever, hypertonicity, paralysis of upward gaze, and seizures. Infants with severe cases of kernicterus die in the neonatal period. Spasticity resolves in surviving infants, who may manifest later nerve deafness, choreoathetoid cerebral palsy, enamel dysplasia, and discoloration of teeth as permanent sequelae. Kernicterus may be prevented by avoiding excessively high indirect bilirubin levels and by avoiding conditions or drugs that may displace bilirubin from albumin. Early signs of kernicterus occasionally may be reversed by immediately instituting an exchange transfusion.

Polycythemia (Hyperviscosity Syndrome)

Polycythemia is an excessively high hematocrit (≥65%), which may lead to hyperviscosity that produces symptoms related to vascular stasis, hypoperfusion, and ischemia. As the hematocrit increases from 40–60%, there is a small increase in blood viscosity. When the *central* hematocrit increases to greater than 65%, the blood viscosity begins to increase markedly, and symptoms may appear. Neonatal erythrocytes are less filterable or deformable than adult erythrocytes, which further contributes to hyperviscosity. A central venous hematocrit of 65% or greater is noted in 3–5% of infants. Infants at special risk for polycythemia are term and post-term small for gestational age infants, infants of diabetic mothers, infants with delayed cord clamping, and infants with neonatal hyperthyroidism, adrenogenital syndrome, trisomy 13, trisomy 18, trisomy 21, twin-to-twin transfusion syndrome (recipient), or Beckwith-Wiedemann syndrome. In some infants, polycythemia may reflect a compensation for prolonged periods of fetal hypoxia caused by placental insufficiency; these infants have increased erythropoietin levels at birth.

Polycythemic patients appear plethoric or ruddy and may develop acrocyanosis. Symptoms, if present, are a result of the increased RBC mass and of vascular compromise. Seizures, lethargy, and irritability reflect abnormalities of microcirculation of the brain, whereas hyperbilirubinemia may reflect the poor hepatic circulation or the increased amount of hemoglobin that is being broken down into bilirubin. Additional problems include respiratory distress and persistent pulmonary hypertension of the newborn (PPHN) that result in part from elevated pulmonary vascular resistance. The chest radiograph often reveals cardiomegaly, increased vascular markings, pleural effusions, and interstitial edema. Other problems are NEC, hypoglycemia, thrombocytopenia, priapism, testicular infarction, hemiplegic stroke, and feeding intolerance. Many of these complications also are related to the primary condition associated with polycythemia (small for gestational age infants are at risk for hypoglycemia and PPHN after periods of hypoxia in utero).

Long-term sequelae of neonatal polycythemia relate to neurodevelopmental abnormalities that may be prevented by treatment of symptomatic infants with partial exchange transfusion after birth. A partial exchange transfusion removes whole blood and replaces it with normal saline.

Coagulation Disorders

Disorders of coagulation are common in the neonatal period. Hemorrhage during this time may be a result of trauma, inherited permanent deficiency of coagulation factors, transient deficiencies of vitamin K–dependent factors, disorders of platelets, or disseminated intravascular coagulation (DIC) seen in sick newborns with shock or hypoxia. Thrombosis also is a potential problem in the newborn because of developmentally lower circulating levels of antithrombin III, protein C (a vitamin K–dependent protein that inhibits factors VIII and V), and the fibrinolytic system.

Coagulation factors do not pass through the placenta to the fetus, and newborn infants have relatively low levels of the vitamin K–dependent factors II, VII, IX, and X. Contact factors XI and XII, prekallikrein, and kininogen also are lower in newborns than in adults. Fibrinogen (factor I); plasma levels of factors V, VIII, and XIII; and platelet counts are within the adult normal range.

Because of the transient, relative deficiencies of the contact and vitamin K–dependent factors, the *partial thromboplastin time* (PTT), which is dependent on factors XII, IX, VIII, X, V, II, and I, is prolonged in the newborn period. Preterm infants have the most marked prolongation of the PTT (50–80 seconds) compared with term infants (35–50 seconds) and older, more mature infants (25–35 seconds). The administration of heparin and the presence of DIC, hemophilia, and severe vitamin K deficiency prolong the PTT.

The *prothrombin time* (PT), which is dependent on factors X, VII, V, II, and I, is a more sensitive test for vitamin K deficiency. The PT is only slightly prolonged in term infants (13–20 seconds) compared with preterm infants (13–21 seconds) and more mature patients (12–14 seconds). Abnormal prolongations of the PT occur with vitamin K deficiency, hepatic injury, and DIC. Levels of *fibrinogen* and *fibrin degradation products* are similar in infants and adults. The *bleeding time*, which reflects platelet function and number, is shorter during the newborn period, thought to be due to enhanced platelet/vessel wall interaction (higher hematocrits, higher mean corpuscular volumes, higher concentrations of von Willebrand factor).

Vitamin K is a necessary cofactor for the carboxylation of glutamate on precursor proteins, converting them into the more active coagulation factors II, VII, IX, and X; γ-carboxyglutamic acid binds calcium, which is required for the immediate activation of factors during hemorrhage. There is no congenital deficiency of hepatic synthesis of these precursor proteins, but in the absence of vitamin K, their conversion to the active factor is not possible. Levels of *protein induced by vitamin K absence* increase in vitamin K deficiency and are helpful diagnostic markers; vitamin K administration rapidly corrects the coagulation defects, reducing protein induced by vitamin K absence to undetectable levels.

Although most newborns are born with reduced levels of vitamin K–dependent factors, hemorrhagic complications develop only rarely. Infants at risk for **hemorrhagic disease of the newborn** have the most profound deficiency of vitamin K–dependent factors, and these factors decline further after birth.

Hemorrhage on the first day of life resulting from a deficiency of the vitamin K–dependent factors **(early vitamin K deficiency bleeding)** often is associated with prenatal or intrapartum exposure to medications that affect vitamin K metabolism in the infant. This early pattern of hemorrhage has been seen with maternal warfarin or antibiotic (e.g., isoniazid or rifampin) therapy and in infants of birth parents receiving phenobarbital and phenytoin. **Classic vitamin K deficiency bleeding** occurs in the first week of life. Bleeding usually ensues from the umbilical cord, circumcision site, intestines, scalp, mucosa, and skin, but internal hemorrhage places the infant at risk for fatal complications, such as intracranial bleeding.

Late onset vitamin K deficiency bleeding occurs between 1–6 months after birth, particularly among breast-fed infants because breast milk is a poor source of vitamin K. The most common presentation is with intracranial hemorrhage. Vitamin K deficiency in breast-fed infants also should raise suspicion about the possibility of vitamin K malabsorption resulting from cystic fibrosis, biliary atresia, hepatitis, or antibiotic suppression of the colonic bacteria that produce vitamin K.

Bleeding associated with vitamin K deficiency may be prevented by administration of vitamin K to all infants at birth. Before routine administration of vitamin K, 1–2% of all newborns had hemorrhagic disease of the newborn. One intramuscular dose (1 mg) of vitamin K prevents vitamin K–deficiency bleeding. Treatment of bleeding resulting from vitamin K deficiency involves intravenous administration of 1 mg of vitamin K. If severe, life-threatening hemorrhage is present, fresh frozen plasma also should be given. Higher and/or recurrent doses of vitamin K may be needed for hepatic disease and for maternal warfarin or anticonvulsant therapy.

Clinical Manifestations and Differential Diagnoses of Bleeding Disorders

Bleeding disorders in a newborn may be associated with cutaneous bleeding, such as cephalohematoma, subgaleal hemorrhage, ecchymosis, and petechiae. Facial petechiae are common in infants born by vertex presentation, with or without a nuchal cord, and usually are insignificant. Mucosal bleeding may appear as hematemesis, melena, or epistaxis. Internal hemorrhage results in organ-specific dysfunction, such as seizures associated with intracranial hemorrhage. Bleeding from venipuncture or heel stick sites, circumcision sites, or the umbilical cord also is common with bleeding disorders.

The differential diagnosis depends partly on the clinical circumstances associated with the hemorrhage. In a *sick newborn*, the differential diagnosis should include DIC, hepatic failure, and thrombocytopenia. Thrombocytopenia in an ill neonate may be secondary to consumption by trapping of platelets in a hemangioma **(Kasabach-Merritt syndrome)** or may be associated with perinatal, congenital, or bacterial infections; NEC; thrombotic endocarditis; PPHN; organic acidemia; maternal preeclampsia; or asphyxia. Thrombocytopenia also may be due to peripheral washout of platelets after an exchange transfusion. Treatment of a sick infant with thrombocytopenia should be directed at the underlying disorder, supplemented by infusions of platelets, blood, or both.

The etiology of DIC in a newborn includes hypoxia, hypotension, asphyxia, bacterial or viral sepsis, NEC, death of a twin while in utero, cavernous hemangioma, nonimmune hydrops, neonatal cold injury, neonatal neoplasm, and hepatic disease. The treatment of DIC should be focused primarily on therapy for the initiating or underlying disorder. Supportive management of consumptive coagulopathy involves platelet transfusions and factor replacement with fresh frozen plasma. Heparin and factor C concentrate should be reserved for infants with DIC who also have thrombosis.

Disorders of hemostasis in a *well child* are not associated with systemic disease in a newborn but reflect coagulation factor or platelet deficiency. Hemophilia initially is associated with cutaneous, scalp, or mucosal bleeding and no systemic illness. If bleeding continues, hypovolemic shock may develop.

Bleeding into the brain, liver, or spleen may result in organ-specific signs and shock.

In a well child, thrombocytopenia may be part of a syndrome such as Fanconi anemia syndrome (involving hypoplasia and aplasia of the thumb), radial aplasia-thrombocytopenia syndrome (thumbs present), or Wiskott-Aldrich syndrome. Various maternal drugs also may reduce the neonatal platelet count without producing other adverse effects. These drugs include sulfonamides, quinidine, quinine, and thiazide diuretics.

The most common causes of thrombocytopenia in well newborns are transient isoimmune thrombocytopenia and transient neonatal thrombocytopenia. **Neonatal alloimmune thrombocytopenia** is caused by antiplatelet antibodies produced by the PLA-1–negative birth parent after her sensitization to specific paternal platelet antigen (PA-1a and PA-5b represent 85% and 10% of cases, respectively) expressed on the fetal platelet. This response to maternal-sensitized antibodies that produce alloimmune thrombocytopenia is analogous to the response that produces erythroblastosis fetalis. The maternal antiplatelet antibody does not produce maternal thrombocytopenia, but after crossing the placenta this IgG antibody binds to fetal platelets that are trapped by the reticuloendothelial tissue, resulting in thrombocytopenia. Infants with thrombocytopenia produced in this manner are at risk for development of petechiae, purpura, and intracranial hemorrhage before or after birth. Vaginal delivery may increase the risk of neonatal bleeding; cesarean section may be indicated.

Specific treatment for severe thrombocytopenia (<20,000 platelets/mm^3) or significant bleeding is transfusion of ABO-compatible and RhD-compatible, PA-1a–negative and PA-5b–negative maternal platelets. Because the antibody in isoimmune thrombocytopenia is directed against the fetal rather than the maternal platelet, transfusion of washed and irradiated maternal platelets may be used to treat the affected infant. After one platelet transfusion, the infant's platelet count dramatically increases and usually remains in a safe range. Without treatment, thrombocytopenia resolves during the first month of life as the maternal antibody level declines. Treatment of the birth parent with intravenous immunoglobulin or the thrombocytopenic fetus with intravascular platelet transfusion (cordocentesis) is also effective.

Neonatal thrombocytopenia in infants born to birth parents with idiopathic thrombocytopenic purpura (ITP) also is a result of placental transfer of maternal IgG antibodies. In ITP, these autoantibodies are directed against all platelet antigens; birth parent and newborn may have low platelet counts.

Treatment of an affected infant born to a birth parent with ITP may involve prednisone and intravenous immunoglobulin. In an emergency, random donor platelets may be used and may produce a transient increase in the infant's platelet count. Thrombocytopenia resolves spontaneously during the first month of life as maternal-derived antibody levels decline. Elevated levels of platelet-associated antibodies also have been noted in thrombocytopenic infants with sepsis and thrombocytopenia of unknown cause who were born to birth parents without demonstrable platelet antibodies.

The laboratory evaluation of an infant (well or sick) with bleeding must include a platelet count, blood smear, and evaluation of PTT and PT. Isolated thrombocytopenia in a well infant suggests immune thrombocytopenia. Laboratory evidence of DIC includes a markedly prolonged PTT and PT (minutes rather than seconds), thrombocytopenia, and a blood smear suggesting a microangiopathic hemolytic anemia (burr or fragmented blood cells). Further evaluation reveals low levels of fibrinogen (<100 mg/dL) and elevated levels of fibrin degradation products. Vitamin K deficiency prolongs the PT more than the PTT, whereas hemophilia resulting from factors VIII and IX deficiency prolongs only the PTT. Specific factor levels confirm the diagnosis of hemophilia.

PEARLS FOR PRACTITIONERS

See Fetal and Neonatal Medicine: Pearls for Practitioners at the end of this section.

REVIEW QUESTIONS

Available online.

CHAPTER 62

Necrotizing Enterocolitis

Necrotizing enterocolitis (NEC) is a syndrome of intestinal injury and is the most common intestinal emergency occurring in preterm infants admitted to the neonatal intensive care unit. NEC occurs in 1–3 per 1,000 live births worldwide and accounts for 1–8% of admissions to the neonatal intensive care unit. Prematurity is the most consistent and significant factor associated with neonatal NEC. The disease occurs in 4–13% of infants who weigh less than 1,500 g at birth. NEC is infrequent in term infants (<10% of affected infants).

Most cases of NEC occur in premature infants born before 34 weeks of gestation who have been fed enterally. Prematurity is associated with immaturity of the gastrointestinal tract, including decreased integrity of the intestinal mucosal barrier, depressed mucosal enzymes, suppressed gastrointestinal hormones, suppressed intestinal host defense system, decreased coordination of intestinal motility, and differences in blood flow autoregulation, which is thought to play a significant role in the pathogenesis of NEC. More than 90% of infants diagnosed with NEC have been fed enterally, but NEC has been reported in infants who have never been fed. Feeding with human milk has shown a beneficial role in reducing the incidence of NEC. In addition, probiotics may offer potential benefits for the preterm infant by increasing mucosal barrier function, upregulating the immune system, and reducing mucosal colonization by potential pathogens. It is also theorized that compromised intestinal blood flow contributes to NEC.

Early clinical signs of NEC include abdominal distention, feeding intolerance/increased gastric residuals, emesis, rectal bleeding, and occasional diarrhea. As the disease progresses, patients may develop marked abdominal distention, bilious emesis, ascites, abdominal wall erythema, lethargy, temperature instability, increased episodes of apnea/bradycardia, disseminated intravascular coagulation, and shock. With abdominal perforation, the abdomen may develop a bluish discoloration.

The white blood cell count can be elevated, but often it is depressed. Thrombocytopenia is common. In addition, infants may develop coagulation abnormalities along with metabolic acidosis, electrolyte imbalance, and hypoglycemia and hyperglycemia. No unique infectious agent has been associated with NEC; bacteriologic and fungal cultures may prove helpful but not conclusive.

Radiographic imaging is essential to the diagnosis of NEC. The earliest radiographic finding is intestinal ileus, often associated with thickening of the bowel loops and air-fluid levels. The pathognomonic radiographic finding is **pneumatosis intestinalis** caused by hydrogen gas production from pathogenic bacteria present between the subserosal and muscularis layers of the bowel wall (Fig. 62.1). Radiographic findings also may include a fixed or persistent dilated loop of bowel, intrahepatic venous gas, and *pneumoperitoneum* seen with bowel perforation.

The differential diagnosis of NEC includes sepsis with intestinal ileus or a volvulus. Both conditions can present with systemic signs of sepsis and abdominal distention. The absence of pneumatosis on abdominal radiographs does not rule out the diagnosis of NEC; other causes of abdominal distention and perforation (gastric or ileal perforation) should be considered and investigated. Patients diagnosed with Hirschsprung enterocolitis or severe gastroenteritis may present with pneumatosis intestinalis.

The management of NEC includes the discontinuation of enteral feedings, gastrointestinal decompression with nasogastric suction, fluid and electrolyte replacement, total parenteral nutrition, and systemic broad-spectrum antibiotics. When the diagnosis of NEC is made, consultation with a pediatric surgeon should be obtained. Even with aggressive and appropriate medical management, 25–50% of infants with NEC require surgical intervention. The decision to perform surgery is obvious when the presence of a pneumoperitoneum is observed on abdominal radiograph. Other, not so obvious, indications for surgical intervention include rapid clinical deterioration despite medical therapy, an abdominal mass, and intestinal obstruction. The surgical procedure of choice is laparotomy with removal of the frankly necrotic and nonviable bowel. Many extremely small infants are managed initially with primary peritoneal drainage followed by surgical intervention as needed later, when the infant is stable and a laparotomy can be performed safely. The long-term outcome includes intestinal strictures requiring further surgical intervention, short bowel syndrome with poor absorption of enteral fluids and nutrients, associated cholestasis with resultant cirrhosis and liver failure from prolonged parenteral nutrition, and neurodevelopmental delay from prolonged hospitalization.

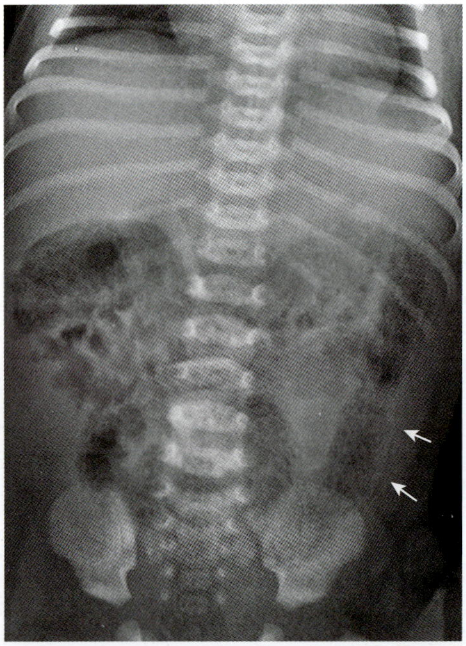

FIGURE 62.1 Necrotizing enterocolitis. Anteroposterior radiograph of the abdomen shows pneumatosis intestinalis with mottled radiolucency over the entire colon and curvilinear radiolucency along the descending colon *(arrows)*. (From Berlin SC, Meyers ML. Neonatal imaging. In: Fanaroff AA, Fanaroff JM, eds. *Klaus and Fanaroff's Care of the High-Risk Neonate*. 7th ed. Philadelphia: Elsevier; 2020: Fig. 18.31.)

PEARLS FOR PRACTITIONERS

See Fetal and Neonatal Medicine: Pearls for Practitioners at the end of this section.

REVIEW QUESTIONS

Available online.

CHAPTER 63

Neurologic Conditions: Seizures, Intracranial Hemorrhage, and Hypoxic-Ischemic Encephalopathy

The human newborn spends more time asleep (predominantly in rapid eye movement or active sleep) than in a wakeful state and is totally dependent on adults. Primitive reflexes, such as the Moro, grasp, stepping, rooting, sucking, and crossed extensor reflexes, are readily elicited and are normal for this age. In addition, the newborn has a wealth of cortical functions that are less easily shown (e.g., the ability to extinguish repetitive or painful stimuli). The newborn also has the capacity for attentive eye fixation and differential responses to the parent's voice. During the perinatal period, many pathophysiologic mechanisms can adversely and permanently affect the developing brain, including prenatal events, such as hypoxia, ischemia, infections, inflammation, malformations, maternal drugs, and coagulation disorders, as well as postnatal events, such as birth trauma, hypoxia-ischemia, inborn errors of metabolism, hypoglycemia, hypothyroidism, hyperthyroidism, polycythemia, hemorrhage, and meningitis.

NEONATAL SEIZURES

Seizures during the neonatal period may be the result of multiple causes, with characteristic historical and clinical manifestations. Seizures caused by **hypoxic-ischemic encephalopathy** (postasphyxial seizures), a common cause of seizures in the full-term infant, usually occur 12–24 hours after a history of birth asphyxia and often are refractory to conventional doses of anticonvulsant medications. Postasphyxial seizures also may be caused by metabolic disorders associated with neonatal asphyxia, such as hypoglycemia and hypocalcemia. **Intraventricular hemorrhage (IVH)** is a common cause of seizures in premature infants and often occurs between 1–3 days of age. Seizures with IVH are associated with a bulging fontanel, hemorrhagic spinal fluid, anemia, lethargy, and coma. Seizures caused by **hypoglycemia** often occur when blood glucose levels decline to the lowest postnatal value (at 1–2 hours of age or after 24–48 hours of poor nutritional intake). Seizures caused by **hypocalcemia** and **hypomagnesemia** develop in high-risk infants and respond well to therapy with calcium, magnesium, or both.

Seizures noted in the delivery room often are caused by direct injection of local anesthetic agents into the fetal scalp (associated with transient bradycardia and fixed dilated pupils), severe anoxia, or congenital brain malformation. Seizures after the first 5 days of life may be the result of infection or parenchymal brain injury. Seizures associated with lethargy, acidosis, and a family history of infant deaths may be the result of an **inborn error of metabolism**. An infant whose parent has a history of a neonatal seizure also is at risk for **benign familial neonatal seizures**; these seizures have onset on days 3–7 ("fifth day fits"), resolve by 1–4 months, and are due to variants in the *KCNQ2* and *KCNQ3* potassium channel genes. In an infant who appears well, a sudden onset on days 1–3 of life of seizures that are of short duration and that do not recur may be the result of a **subarachnoid hemorrhage**. Focal seizures often are the result of local cerebral infarction.

Seizures may be difficult to differentiate from benign jitteriness or from tremulousness in infants of diabetic mothers, in infants with neonatal opioid withdrawal syndrome, and in any infants after an episode of asphyxia. In contrast to seizures, jitteriness and tremors are sensory-dependent, elicited by stimuli, and interrupted by holding the extremity. Seizure activity becomes manifested as coarse, fast and slow clonic activity, whereas jitteriness is characterized by fine, rapid movement. Seizures may be associated with abnormal eye movements, such as tonic deviation to one side. The electroencephalogram often shows seizure activity when the clinical diagnosis is uncertain. Identifying seizures in the newborn period is often difficult because the infant, especially the low birth-weight infant, usually does not show the tonic-clonic major motor activity typical of the older child (Table 63.1). Subtle seizures are a common manifestation in newborns. The subtle signs of seizure activity include apnea, eye deviation, tongue thrusting, eye blinking, fluctuation of vital signs, and staring. Continuous bedside electroencephalographic monitoring can help identify subtle seizures.

The diagnostic evaluation of infants with seizures should involve an immediate determination of capillary blood glucose levels. In addition, blood concentrations of sodium, calcium, glucose, and bilirubin should be determined. When infection is suspected, cerebrospinal fluid and blood specimens should be obtained for culture. After the seizure has stopped, a careful examination should be done to identify signs of increased intracranial pressure, congenital malformations, and systemic illness. If signs of elevated intracranial pressure are absent, a lumbar puncture should be performed. If the diagnosis is not apparent at this point, further evaluation should involve MRI, CT, or cerebral ultrasound and tests to determine the presence of an inborn error of metabolism. Determinations of inborn errors of metabolism are especially important in infants with unexplained lethargy, coma, acidosis, ketonuria, or respiratory alkalosis.

TABLE 63.1 Clinical Characteristics of Neonatal Seizures

DESIGNATION	CHARACTERIZATION
Focal clonic	Repetitive, rhythmic contractions of muscle groups of the limbs, face, or trunk
	May be unilateral or multifocal
	May appear synchronously or asynchronously in various body regions
	Cannot be suppressed by restraint
Focal tonic	Sustained posturing of single limbs
	Sustained asymmetric posturing of the trunk
	Sustained eye deviation
	Cannot be provoked by stimulation or suppressed by restraint
Myoclonic	Arrhythmic contractions of muscle groups of the limbs, face, or trunk
	Typically not repetitive or may recur at a slow rate
	May be generalized, focal, or fragmentary
	May be provoked by stimulation
Generalized tonic	Sustained symmetric posturing of limbs, trunk, and neck
	May be flexor, extensor, or mixed extensor/flexor
	May be provoked by stimulation
	May be suppressed by restraint or repositioning
Ocular signs	Random and roving eye movements or nystagmus
	Distinct from tonic eye deviation
Orobuccolingual movements	Sucking, chewing, tongue protrusions
	May be provoked by stimulation
Progression movements	Rowing or swimming movements of the arms
	Pedaling or bicycling movements of the legs
	May be provoked by stimulation
	May be suppressed by restraint or repositioning

From Mizrahi EM. Neonatal seizures. In: Shinnar S, Branski D, eds. Pediatric and Adolescent Medicine. *Basel: S. Karger; 1995 [vol 6].*

The treatment of neonatal seizures may be specific, such as treatment of meningitis or the correction of hypoglycemia, hypocalcemia, hypomagnesemia, hyponatremia, or vitamin B6 deficiency or dependency. In the absence of an identifiable cause, therapy should involve an anticonvulsant agent, such as phenobarbital, phenytoin, or diazepam. Levetiracetam (Keppra) is an alternative anticonvulsant drug. Treatment of status epilepticus requires repeated doses of phenobarbital and may require diazepam or midazolam, titrated to clinical signs. The long-term outcome for neonatal seizures usually is related to the underlying cause and to the primary pathology, such as hypoxic-ischemic encephalopathy, meningitis, stroke, or hemorrhage.

INTRACRANIAL HEMORRHAGE

Intracranial hemorrhage may be confined to one anatomic area of the brain, such as the subdural, subarachnoid, periventricular, intraventricular, intraparenchymal, or cerebellar region. **Subdural hemorrhages** are seen in association with birth trauma, cephalopelvic disproportion, forceps delivery, large for gestational age infants, skull fractures, and postnatal head trauma. The subdural hematoma does not always cause symptoms immediately after birth; with time, however, the red blood cells undergo hemolysis and water is drawn into the hemorrhage because of the high oncotic pressure of protein, resulting in an expanding symptomatic lesion. Anemia, vomiting, seizures, and macrocephaly may occur in an infant who is 1–2 months of age and has a subdural hematoma. **Nonaccidental trauma** should be considered in this situation and appropriate diagnostic evaluation undertaken to identify other possible signs of skeletal, ocular, or soft tissue injury. Occasionally, a massive subdural hemorrhage in the neonatal period is caused by rupture of the vein of Galen or by an inherited coagulation disorder, such as hemophilia. Infants with these conditions exhibit shock, seizures, and coma. The treatment of all symptomatic subdural hematomas is surgical evacuation.

Subarachnoid hemorrhages may be spontaneous, associated with hypoxia, or caused by bleeding from a cerebral arteriovenous malformation. Seizures are a common presenting manifestation, and the prognosis depends on the underlying injury. Treatment is directed at the seizure and the rare occurrence of posthemorrhagic hydrocephalus.

Periventricular hemorrhage and **IVH** are common in very low birthweight infants; the risk decreases with increasing gestational age. Fifty percent of infants weighing less than 1,500 g have evidence of intracranial bleeding. The pathogenesis for these hemorrhages is unknown (they usually are not caused by coagulation disorders), but the initial site of bleeding may be the weak blood vessels in the periventricular germinal matrix. The vessels in this area have poor structural support. These vessels may rupture and hemorrhage because of passive changes in cerebral blood flow occurring with the variations of blood pressure that sick premature infants often exhibit (failure of autoregulation). In some sick infants, these blood pressure variations are the only identifiable etiologic factors. In others, the disorders that may cause the elevation or depression of blood pressure or that interfere with venous return from the head (venous stasis) increase the risk of IVH; these disorders include asphyxia, pneumothorax, mechanical ventilation, hypercapnia, hypoxemia, prolonged labor, breech delivery, patent ductus arteriosus, heart failure, and therapy with hypertonic solutions such as sodium bicarbonate.

Most periventricular hemorrhages and IVHs occur in the first 3 days of life. It is unusual for IVH to occur after day 5 of life. The clinical manifestations of IVH include seizures, apnea, bradycardia, lethargy, coma, hypotension, metabolic acidosis, anemia not corrected by blood transfusion, bulging fontanel, and cutaneous mottling. Many infants with small hemorrhages (grade 1 or 2) are asymptomatic; infants with larger hemorrhages (grade 4) often have a catastrophic event that rapidly progresses to shock and coma.

The diagnosis of IVH is confirmed and the severity graded by ultrasound through the anterior fontanel or CT examination. Grade 1 IVH is confined to the germinal matrix; grade 2 is an extension of grade 1, with blood noted in the ventricle without ventricular enlargement; grade 3 is an extension of grade 2 with ventricular dilation; and grade 4 has blood in dilated ventricles and in the cerebral cortex, either contiguous with or distant from the ventricle. Grade 4 hemorrhage has a poor prognosis, as does the development of periventricular, small, echolucent cystic lesions, with or without porencephalic cysts and posthemorrhagic hydrocephalus. Periventricular cysts often are noted after the resolution of echodense areas in the periventricular white matter. The cysts may correspond to the development of **periventricular leukomalacia**, which may be a precursor to cerebral palsy. Extensive intraparenchymal echodensities represent hemorrhagic necrosis. They are associated with a high mortality rate and have a poor neurodevelopmental prognosis for survivors.

Treatment of an acute hemorrhage involves standard supportive care, including ventilation for apnea and blood transfusion for hemorrhagic shock. Posthemorrhagic hydrocephalus may be managed with serial daily lumbar punctures, an external ventriculostomy tube, or a permanent ventricular-peritoneal shunt. Implementation of the shunt often is delayed because of the high protein content of the hemorrhagic ventricular fluid. Holding the infant's head in a straight, upright position for the first 96 hours of life and minimizing stimulation may have benefit in the prevention of severe IVH when implemented as part of a comprehensive neuroprotective care bundle.

HYPOXIC-ISCHEMIC ENCEPHALOPATHY

Conditions known to reduce uteroplacental blood flow or to interfere with spontaneous respiration lead to perinatal hypoxia, lactic acidosis, and, if severe enough to reduce cardiac output or cause cardiac arrest, ischemia. The combination of the reduced availability of oxygen for the brain resulting from hypoxia and the diminished or absent blood flow to the brain resulting from ischemia leads to reduced glucose for metabolism and to an accumulation of lactate that produces local tissue acidosis. After reperfusion, hypoxic-ischemic injury also may be complicated by cell necrosis and vascular endothelial edema, reducing blood flow distal to the involved vessel. Typically, hypoxic-ischemic encephalopathy in the term infant is characterized by cerebral edema, cortical necrosis, and involvement of the basal ganglia, whereas in the preterm infant it is characterized by periventricular leukomalacia. Both lesions may result in cortical atrophy, intellectual disability, and spastic quadriplegia or diplegia.

The clinical manifestations and characteristic course of hypoxic-ischemic encephalopathy vary according to the severity of the injury (Table 63.2). Infants with severe stage 3 hypoxic-ischemic encephalopathy are usually hypotonic, although occasionally they initially appear hypertonic and hyperalert at birth. As cerebral edema develops, brain functions are affected in a descending order; cortical depression produces coma, and brainstem depression results in apnea. As cerebral edema progresses, refractory seizures begin 12–24 hours after birth. Concurrently, the infant has no signs of spontaneous respirations, is hypotonic, and has diminished or absent deep tendon reflexes. Hypoxic-ischemic encephalopathy in term infants is often managed with induced hypothermia.

TABLE 63.2 Hypoxic-Ischemic Encephalopathy in Term Infants

SIGNS	STAGE 1	STAGE 2	STAGE 3
Level of consciousness	Hyperalert	Lethargic	Stuporous
Muscle tone	Normal	Hypotonic	Flaccid
Tendon reflexes/clonus	Hyperactive	Hyperactive	Absent
Moro reflex	Strong	Weak	Absent
Pupils	Mydriasis	Miosis	Unequal, poor light reflex
Seizures	None	Common	Decerebration
Electroencephalography	Normal	Low voltage changing to seizure activity	Burst suppression to isoelectric
Duration	>24 hr if progresses, otherwise may remain normal	24 hr to 14 days	Days to weeks

Modified from Sarnat HB, Sarnat MS. Neonatal encephalopathy following fetal distress. Arch Neurol. *1976;33:696.*

Survivors of stage 3 hypoxic-ischemic encephalopathy have a high incidence of seizures and serious neurodevelopmental handicaps. The prognosis of severe asphyxia also depends on other organ system injury (see Table 57.9). Another indicator of poor prognosis is time of onset of spontaneous respiration as estimated by Apgar score. Infants with Apgar scores of 0–3 at 10 minutes have a 20% mortality and a 5% incidence of cerebral palsy; if the score remains this low by 20 minutes, the mortality increases to 60%, and the incidence of cerebral palsy increases to 57%.

PEARLS FOR PRACTITIONERS

See Fetal and Neonatal Medicine: Pearls for Practitioners at the end of this section.

REVIEW QUESTION

Available online.

CHAPTER 64

Sepsis and Meningitis

Systemic and local infections (lung, cutaneous, ocular, umbilical, kidney, bone-joint, and meningeal) are common in the newborn period. Infection may be acquired in utero through the transplacental or transcervical routes and during or after birth. Ascending infection through the cervix, with or without rupture of the amniotic fluid membranes, may result in **intraamniotic infection** ("triple I," also termed *chorioamnionitis*), funisitis (infection of the umbilical cord), congenital pneumonia, and sepsis. The bacteria responsible for ascending infection of the fetus are common bacterial organisms of the maternal genitourinary tract, such as group B streptococci, *Escherichia coli, Haemophilus influenzae,* and *Klebsiella.* Herpes simplex virus (HSV)-1 or HSV-2 also causes ascending infection that at times may be indistinguishable from bacterial sepsis. Syphilis and *Listeria monocytogenes* are acquired by transplacental infection.

Maternal humoral immunity may protect the fetus against some neonatal pathogens, such as group B streptococci and HSV. Nonetheless, various deficiencies of the neonatal antimicrobial defense mechanism probably are more important than maternal immune status as a contributing factor for neonatal infection, especially in the low birthweight infant. The incidence of neonatal sepsis worldwide is approximately 2.2 in 100 live births; incidence and mortality rates are higher in preterm infants in comparison to term infants. The higher rate of sepsis in preterm infants relates to the more immature immunologic systems of preterm infants and to their prolonged periods of hospitalization.

Preterm infants before 32 weeks of gestational age have not received the full complement of maternal antibodies (immunoglobulin G [IgG]), which cross the placenta by active transport predominantly in the latter half of the third trimester. In addition, although low birthweight infants may generate IgM antibodies, their own IgG response to infection is reduced. These infants also have deficiencies of the alternate and, to a smaller degree, the classic complement activation pathways, which results in diminished complement-mediated opsonization. Newborn infants also show a deficit in phagocytic migration to the site of infection (to the lung) and in the bone marrow reserve pool of leukocytes. In addition, in the presence of suboptimal activation of complement, neonatal neutrophils ingest and kill bacteria less effectively than adult neutrophils do. Neutrophils from sick infants seem to have an even greater deficit in bacterial killing capacity compared with phagocytic cells from normal neonates.

Defense mechanisms against viral pathogens also may be deficient in a newborn. Neonatal antibody-dependent, cell-mediated immunity by the natural killer lymphocytes is deficient in the absence of maternal antibodies and in the presence of reduced interferon production; reduced antibody levels occur in premature infants and in infants born during a primary viral infection of the pregnant person, such as with enteroviruses, HSV-2, or cytomegalovirus. In addition, antibody-independent cytotoxicity may be reduced in lymphocytes of newborns.

Bacterial sepsis and meningitis often are linked closely in neonates. Despite this association, the incidence of meningitis relative to neonatal sepsis has been on a steady decline. The causative organisms isolated most frequently are the same as for neonatal sepsis: group B streptococci, *E. coli*, and *L. monocytogenes*. Gram-negative organisms, such as *Klebsiella*, *Salmonella*, and *Serratia marcescens*, are more common in less developed countries, and coagulase-negative staphylococcus needs to be considered in very low birthweight infants. Neonates in the neonatal intensive care unit live in a high-risk environment, with exposure to endotracheal tubes, central arterial and venous catheters, and blood draws, all predisposing to bacteremia and meningitis. Genetic factors have been implicated in the ability of bacteria to cross the blood-brain barrier. This penetration has been noted for group B streptococci, *E. coli*, *Listeria*, *Citrobacter*, and *Streptococcus pneumoniae*.

Neonatal sepsis presents during three periods. **Early-onset sepsis** (defined variably as occurring 0–3 days or 0–7 days of life) often begins in utero and usually is a result of infection caused by the bacteria in the birth parent's genitourinary tract. Organisms related to this sepsis include group B streptococci, *E. coli*, *Klebsiella*, *L. monocytogenes*, and nontypeable *H. influenzae*. Most infected infants are premature and show nonspecific cardiorespiratory signs, such as grunting, tachypnea, and cyanosis at birth. Risk factors for early-onset sepsis include vaginal colonization with group B streptococci, prolonged rupture of the membranes (>18 hours), intraamniotic infection (chorioamnionitis), maternal fever or leukocytosis, fetal tachycardia, low birthweight, and preterm birth.

The incidence of **early-onset sepsis** in the United States is approximately 0.5 in 1,000 live births. It is an overwhelming multiorgan system disease frequently manifested as respiratory failure, shock, meningitis (in 30% of cases), disseminated intravascular coagulation, acute kidney injury, and, less often, symmetric peripheral gangrene. Early manifestations—grunting, poor feeding, pallor, apnea, lethargy, hypothermia, or an abnormal cry—may be nonspecific. Profound neutropenia, hypoxia, and hypotension may be refractory to treatment with broad-spectrum antibiotics, mechanical ventilation, and vasopressors. In the initial stages of early-onset septicemia in a preterm infant, it is often difficult to differentiate sepsis from respiratory distress syndrome. Because of this difficulty, premature infants with respiratory distress syndrome often receive broad-spectrum antibiotics.

Infants with a positive blood culture are diagnosed with early-onset sepsis. Cerebrospinal fluid (CSF) cultures, CSF Gram stain, cell count, protein and glucose levels, in addition to polymerase chain reaction testing, can diagnose associated meningitis. Normal newborns generally have an elevated CSF protein content (100–150 mg/dL) and may have up to 25/mm^3 white blood cells (mean, 6/mm^3), which are 75% lymphocytes in the absence of infection. Some infants with neonatal meningitis caused by group B streptococci do not have an elevated CSF leukocyte count but are seen to have microorganisms in the CSF on Gram stain. In addition to culture, another method of identifying the pathogenic bacteria is the determination of bacterial DNA in samples of CSF. In cases of neonatal meningitis, the ratio of CSF glucose to blood glucose usually is less than 50%. Serial complete blood counts may show neutropenia, an increased number of immature neutrophils (bands), and thrombocytopenia. C-reactive protein levels and procalcitonin are often elevated in neonatal patients with bacterial sepsis; however, elevation may not be specific to infection.

A chest radiograph also should be obtained to determine the presence of pneumonia. In addition to the traditional neonatal pathogens, pneumonia in very low birthweight infants may be the result of acquisition of a maternal genital mycoplasmal agent (e.g., *Ureaplasma urealyticum* or *Mycoplasma hominis*). Arterial blood gases should be monitored to detect hypoxemia and metabolic acidosis that may be caused by hypoxia, shock, or both. Blood pressure, urine output, and peripheral perfusion should be monitored to determine the need to treat septic shock with fluids and vasopressor agents.

The mainstay of treatment for sepsis and meningitis is immediate antibiotic therapy. Antibiotics are used to suppress bacterial growth, allowing the infant's defense mechanisms time to respond. In addition, support measures, such as assisted ventilation and cardiovascular support, are equally important to the management of the infant. A combination of ampicillin and an aminoglycoside (usually gentamicin) for 10–14 days is effective treatment against most organisms responsible for early-onset sepsis. The combination of ampicillin and cefepime also is proposed as an alternative method of treatment. If meningitis is present, the treatment should be extended to 21 days or 14 days after a negative result from a CSF culture. Persistently positive results from CSF cultures are common with neonatal meningitis caused by gram-negative organisms, even with appropriate antibiotic treatment, and may be present for 2–3 days after antibiotic therapy. If gram-negative meningitis is present, some authorities continue to treat with an effective penicillin derivative combined with an aminoglycoside, whereas most change to a third-generation cephalosporin. High-dose penicillin is appropriate for group B streptococcal meningitis. Extracorporeal membrane oxygenation (in term infants) may improve the outcome of sepsis-related pulmonary hypertension or systemic hypotension. Intrapartum penicillin empirical prophylaxis for pregnant people colonized by group B streptococcus or those with risk factors (fever, preterm labor, previous infant with group B streptococci, known colonization, or chorioamnionitis) has reduced the rate of early-onset infection but not late-onset infection.

Late-onset sepsis (8–28 days) most commonly affects preterm infants or infants with chronic medical conditions and prolonged birth hospitalizations. Clinical manifestations may include lethargy, poor feeding, hypotonia, apathy, seizures, bulging fontanel, fever, and direct-reacting hyperbilirubinemia. In addition to bacteremia, hematogenous seeding may result in focal infections, such as meningitis (in 75% of cases), osteomyelitis (group B streptococci, *Staphylococcus aureus*), arthritis (gonococcus, *S. aureus*, *Candida albicans*, gram-negative bacteria), and urinary tract infection (gram-negative bacteria).

The evaluation of infants with late-onset sepsis is similar to that for infants with early-onset sepsis, with special attention given to a careful physical examination of the bones (infants with osteomyelitis may exhibit pseudoparalysis) and to the laboratory examination and culture of urine obtained by sterile suprapubic aspiration or urethral catheterization. Late-onset sepsis may be caused by the same pathogens as early-onset sepsis, but infants exhibiting sepsis late in the neonatal period also may have infections caused by the pathogens usually found in older infants (*H. influenzae*, *S. pneumoniae*, and *Neisseria meningitidis*). In addition, viral agents (HSV, cytomegalovirus, or enteroviruses) may manifest with a late-onset, sepsis-like picture.

Because of the increased rate of resistance of *H. influenzae* and pneumococcus to ampicillin, some centers begin treatment with ampicillin and a third-generation cephalosporin (and vancomycin if meningitis is present) when sepsis occurs in the last week of the first month of life. The treatment of late-onset neonatal sepsis and meningitis is the same as that for early-onset sepsis.

PEARLS FOR PRACTITIONERS

See Fetal and Neonatal Medicine: Pearls for Practitioners at the end of this section.

REVIEW QUESTIONS

Available online.

CHAPTER 65

Congenital Infections

An infection acquired transplacentally during gestation is a congenital infection. Numerous pathogens that produce mild or asymptomatic disease in older infants and children can cause severe disease in neonates who acquire such infections prenatally or perinatally. Sepsis, meningitis, pneumonia, and other infections caused by perinatally acquired pathogens are the cause of significant neonatal morbidity and mortality. Congenital infections include a well-known group of fungal, bacterial, and viral pathogens: toxoplasmosis, rubella, cytomegalovirus (CMV), herpes simplex virus (HSV), varicella-zoster virus, congenital syphilis, parvovirus, HIV, hepatitis B, Zika virus, *Neisseria gonorrhoeae*, *Chlamydia*, and *Mycobacterium tuberculosis*.

Many of the clinical manifestations of congenital infections are similar, including fetal growth restriction, nonimmune hydrops, anemia, thrombocytopenia, jaundice, hepatosplenomegaly, chorioretinitis, and congenital malformations. Some unique manifestations and epidemiologic characteristics of these infections are listed in Table 65.1. Evaluation of patients thought to have a congenital infection can include attempts to isolate the organism by culture (for rubella, CMV, HSV, gonorrhea, and *M. tuberculosis*), to identify the antigen of the pathogen (for hepatitis B and *Chlamydia trachomatis*), to identify the pathogen's genome with polymerase chain reaction ([PCR], useful for CMV, HSV, HIV, gonorrhea, and chlamydia), and to identify specific fetal production of antibodies (immunoglobulin M [IgM] or increasing titer of IgG for *Toxoplasma*, syphilis, parvovirus, HIV, or *Borrelia*).

Treatment is not always available, specific, or effective. Nonetheless, some encouraging results have been reported for preventing the disease and for specifically treating the infant when the correct diagnosis is made (see Table 65.1).

TOXOPLASMOSIS

Vertical transmission of *Toxoplasma gondii* occurs by transplacental transfer of the organism from the birth parent to the fetus after an acute infection during pregnancy. Fetal infection rarely can occur after reactivation of disease in an immunocompromised pregnant person. Transmission from an acutely infected pregnant person to her fetus occurs in about 30–40% of cases, but the rate varies directly with gestational age. Transmission rates and the timing of fetal infection correlate directly with placental blood flow; the risk of infection increases throughout gestation to 90% or greater near term, and the time interval between maternal and fetal infection decreases.

The severity of fetal disease varies inversely with the gestational age at which maternal infection occurs. Most infants have no overt disease at birth; however, specific ophthalmologic and central nervous system (CNS) evaluations may reveal abnormalities. The classic findings of hydrocephalus, chorioretinitis, and intracerebral calcifications suggest the diagnosis of **congenital toxoplasmosis**. Affected infants tend to be small for gestational age, develop early-onset jaundice, have hepatosplenomegaly, and present with a generalized maculopapular rash. Seizures are common, and skull films may reveal diffuse cortical calcifications in contrast to the periventricular pattern observed with CMV. These infants are at increased risk for long-term neurologic and neurodevelopmental complications.

Serologic tests are the primary means of diagnosis. IgG-specific antibodies achieve a peak concentration 1–2 months after infection and remain positive indefinitely. For infants with seroconversion or a fourfold increase in IgG titers, specific IgM antibody determinations should be performed to confirm disease. Especially for congenital infections, measurement of IgA and IgE antibodies can be useful to confirm the disease. Thorough ophthalmologic, auditory, and neurologic evaluations (head CT and cerebrospinal fluid [CSF] examination) are indicated.

For symptomatic and asymptomatic congenital infections, initial therapy should include pyrimethamine (supplemented with folic acid) combined with sulfadiazine. Duration of therapy is often prolonged, even up to 1 year. Optimal dosages of medications and duration of therapy should be determined in consultation with appropriate specialists.

RUBELLA

With the widespread use of vaccination, congenital rubella is rare in developed countries. When acquired in utero during early gestation, rubella can cause severe neonatal consequences. The occurrence of congenital defects approaches 85% if infection is acquired during the first 4 weeks of gestation; close to 40% spontaneously abort or are stillborn. If infection occurs during weeks 13–16, 35% of infants can have abnormalities. Infection after 4 months of gestation does not seem to cause disease.

The most common characteristic abnormalities associated with congenital rubella include ophthalmologic (cataracts, retinopathy, and glaucoma), cardiac (patent ductus arteriosus and peripheral pulmonary artery stenosis), auditory (sensorineural hearing loss), and neurologic (behavioral disorders, meningoencephalitis, and developmental delay) conditions. In addition, infants can present with growth restriction, hepatosplenomegaly, early-onset jaundice, thrombocytopenia, radiolucent bone disease, and purpuric skin lesions ("blueberry muffin" appearance from dermal erythropoiesis).

Detection of rubella-specific IgM antibody usually indicates recent infection. Measurement of rubella-specific IgG over several months can be confirmatory. Rubella virus can be isolated from blood, urine, CSF, and throat swab specimens.

TABLE 65.1 Perinatal Congenital Infections (TORCH)

AGENT	BIRTH PARENT EPIDEMIOLOGY	NEONATAL FEATURES
Toxoplasma gondii	Heterophile-negative mononucleosis	Hydrocephalus, abnormal spinal fluid, intracranial calcifications, chorioretinitis, jaundice, hepatosplenomegaly, fever
	Exposure to cats or raw meat or immunosuppression	Many infants asymptomatic at birth
	High-risk exposure at 10–24 wk of gestation	Treatment: pyrimethamine plus sulfadiazine
Rubella virus*	Unimmunized seronegative birth parent; fever ± rash Detectable defects with infection: by 8 wk, 85%; 9–12 wk, 50%; 13–20 wk, 16%	Fetal growth restriction, microcephaly, microphthalmia, cataracts, glaucoma, "salt and pepper" chorioretinitis, hepatosplenomegaly, jaundice, PDA, deafness, blueberry muffin rash, anemia, thrombocytopenia, leukopenia, metaphyseal lucencies, B-cell and T-cell deficiency
	Virus may be present in infant's throat for 1 yr	Infant may be asymptomatic at birth
	Prevention: vaccinate pregnant person after pregnancy concludes; routine vaccination of toddlers	
CMV	Transmitted by direct contact with infected bodily fluids and often asymptomatic; caregivers of infants and young children are at increased risk	Sepsis, fetal growth restriction, chorioretinitis, microcephaly, periventricular calcifications, blueberry muffin rash, anemia, thrombocytopenia, neutropenia, hepatosplenomegaly, jaundice, sensorineural hearing loss, petechiae, pneumonia
	Heterophile-negative mononucleosis; infant may have viruria for 1–6 yr	90% asymptomatic at birth Prevention: CMV-negative blood products Possible treatment: valganciclovir
Herpes simplex type 2 or 1 virus	Sexually transmitted disease: primary genital infection may be asymptomatic; intrauterine infection rare, acquisition at time of birth more common	Intrauterine infection: chorioretinitis, skin lesions, microcephaly Postnatal: encephalitis, localized or disseminated disease, skin vesicles, keratoconjunctivitis Treatment: acyclovir
Varicella-zoster virus	Intrauterine infection with chickenpox	Microphthalmia, cataracts, chorioretinitis, cutaneous and bony aplasia/hypoplasia/atrophy, cutaneous scars
	Infant develops severe neonatal varicella with maternal illness 5 days before or 2 days after delivery	Zoster as in older child Prevention of neonatal condition with VZIG Treatment of ill neonate: acyclovir
Treponema pallidum (syphilis)*	Sexually transmitted infection	Presentation at birth as nonimmune hydrops, prematurity, anemia, neutropenia, thrombocytopenia, pneumonia, hepatosplenomegaly
	Maternal primary asymptomatic: painless "hidden" chancre	Late neonatal as snuffles (rhinitis), rash, hepatosplenomegaly, condylomata lata, metaphysitis, cerebrospinal fluid pleocytosis, keratitis, periosteal new bone, lymphocytosis, hepatitis
	Penicillin, not erythromycin, prevents fetal infection	Late onset: teeth, eye, bone, skin, central nervous system, ear Treatment: penicillin
Parvovirus	Etiology of fifth disease; fever, rash, arthralgia in adults	Nonimmune hydrops, fetal anemia Treatment: in utero transfusion
HIV*	Progresses to AIDS if not adequately treated	In untreated neonates, mean time to AIDS-defining illness is 5 months (shorter than horizontal transmission cases); growth faltering, recurrent infection, hepatosplenomegaly, neurologic abnormalities Management: trimethoprim/sulfamethoxazole, AZT, other antiretroviral agents Prevention: prenatal, intrapartum, postpartum antiretroviral therapy for the pregnant person; AZT prophylaxis for all exposed neonates In the United States, avoid breastfeeding in cases of uncontrolled maternal disease

(Continued)

TABLE 65.1 Perinatal Congenital Infections (TORCH)—cont'd

AGENT	BIRTH PARENT EPIDEMIOLOGY	NEONATAL FEATURES
Hepatitis B virus*	Most cases are acute; chronic infection may result in cirrhosis, hepatocellular carcinoma	Acute neonatal hepatitis with increased risk of progression to liver failure during childhood
		Prevention: HBIG, vaccine
Neisseria gonorrhoeae	Sexually transmitted infection, infant acquires at birth	Gonococcal ophthalmia, sepsis, meningitis
		Prevention: universal application of erythromycin ocular ointment after birth; ceftriaxone prophylaxis to all exposed infants
	Treatment: cefotaxime, ceftriaxone	Treatment: ceftriaxone
Chlamydia trachomatis	Sexually transmitted infection, infant acquires at birth	Conjunctivitis, pneumonia
		Prevention: no prophylaxis of exposed infants is recommended after birth, but parents should be counseled to watch for symptoms
	Treatment: oral erythromycin	Treatment: oral erythromycin (topical is ineffective)
Mycobacterium tuberculosis	Positive PPD skin test (recent diagnosis), positive chest radiograph, positive family member	Hepatosplenomegaly; congenital pneumonia; acquired primary pulmonary TB
		Prevention: INH, BCG (in certain areas of the world), separation
	Treatment: INH and rifampin ± ethambutol	Treatment: INH, rifampin, pyrazinamide
Trypanosoma cruzi (Chagas disease)	Central South American native, immigrant, travel	Growth faltering, heart failure, achalasia
	Chronic disease in birth parent	Treatment: nifurtimox
Zika virus	Primarily mosquito-borne, infection during 1st and 2nd trimesters of pregnancy carries highest risk of fetal impact	Some infants are asymptomatic; ~5% brain anomalies, microcephaly, feeding difficulties, neurodevelopmental delay, seizures, hypertonia with contracture, hearing loss, blindness

*Indicates that screening for this infection is recommended during each pregnancy.

AZT, Zidovudine (azidothymidine); *BCG,* bacille Calmette-Guerin; *CMV,* cytomegalovirus; *HBIG,* hepatitis B immune globulin; *INH,* isoniazid; *PDA,* patent ductus arteriosus; *PPD,* purified protein derivative; *TB,* tuberculosis; *VZIG,* varicella-zoster immune globulin.

Infants with congenital rubella are chronically and persistently infected and tend to shed live virus in urine, stools, and respiratory secretions for 1 year. Infants should be isolated while in the hospital and kept away from susceptible pregnant people when sent home.

CYTOMEGALOVIRUS

CMV is the most common congenital infection and the leading cause of nonsyndromic sensorineural hearing loss. It is also associated with intellectual disability, retinal disease, and cerebral palsy. Congenital CMV occurs in about 1 in 200 births. When primary infection occurs during a pregnancy, the virus is transmitted to the fetus in approximately 35% of cases, although infection with a different CMV variant or reactivation of a prior infection can also cause congenital CMV. Pregnant people who have direct contact with urine or saliva of young children (i.e., care for young children) are at increased risk of CMV infection. The risk of transmission of CMV to the fetus is independent of gestational age at the time of maternal infection. The earlier in gestation that the primary maternal infection occurs, the more symptomatic the infant may be at birth.

More than 90% of infants who have congenital CMV infection exhibit no clinical evidence of disease at birth. Approximately 10% of infected infants have symptoms at birth. Findings include microcephaly, thrombocytopenia, hepatosplenomegaly, hepatitis, intracranial calcifications, chorioretinitis, and hearing abnormalities. Some infants can present with a blueberry muffin appearance as the result of dermal erythropoiesis. Skull films may reveal periventricular calcifications. Some infected infants present later in infancy or early childhood when they are found to have sensorineural hearing loss and developmental delays. Mortality is 5–10% in symptomatic newborns. Perinatal CMV infection acquired during birth or from breast milk is not associated with newborn illness or CNS sequelae in term infants; in preterm infants, it may present with sepsis-like symptoms.

Congenital CMV infection is diagnosed by detection of virus in bodily fluids in the first 3 weeks after birth. PCR can be used to detect small amounts of CMV DNA in the urine or saliva.

Valganciclovir may mitigate the severity of hearing loss if initiated in the first 3 months of life for symptomatic newborns.

HERPES SIMPLEX VIRUS

HSV-2 accounts for 90% of primary genital herpes. About 70–85% of neonatal herpes simplex infections are caused by HSV-2. Most commonly, neonatal infections are acquired from the birth parent shortly before (ascending infection) or during passage through the birth canal at delivery. Globally, the incidence of neonatal HSV is estimated to range from 1 in 3,000–20,000 live births. Infants with HSV infections are more likely to be born prematurely (40% of affected infants are <36 weeks of gestation). The risk of infection at delivery in an infant born vaginally to a birth parent with primary genital herpes is about 33–50%. The risk to an infant born to a person with a reactivated infection is less than 5%. More than 75% of infants who acquire HSV infection are born to birth parents who have no previous history or clinical findings consistent with HSV infection.

Most infants are normal at birth, and symptoms of infection develop at 5–10 days of life. Symptoms of neonatal HSV infection include disseminated disease involving multiple organ systems, most notably the liver and lungs; localized infection to the CNS; or localized infection to the skin, eyes, and mouth. Symptoms may overlap, and in many cases of disseminated disease, skin lesions are a late finding. Disseminated infection should be considered in any infant with symptoms of sepsis, liver dysfunction, and negative bacteriologic cultures. HSV infection also should be suspected in any neonate who presents with fever, irritability, abnormal CSF findings, and seizures. Initial symptoms can occur anytime between birth and 4 weeks of age, although disseminated disease usually occurs during the first week of life. HSV infections are often severe, and a delay in treatment can result in significant morbidity and mortality.

For the diagnosis of neonatal HSV infection, specimens for culture should be obtained from any skin vesicle, nasopharynx, eyes, urine, blood, CSF, stool, or rectum. Positive cultures obtained from these sites more than 48 hours after birth indicate intrapartum exposure. PCR is a sensitive method for detecting HSV DNA in blood, skin lesions, and CSF.

Parenteral acyclovir is the treatment of choice for neonatal HSV infections. Acyclovir should be administered to all infants suspected to have infection or those diagnosed with HSV. The most benign outcome with regard to morbidity and mortality is observed in infants with disease limited to the skin, eyes, and mouth.

CONGENITAL SYPHILIS

Congenital syphilis most commonly results from transplacental infection of the fetus, although the fetus can acquire infection by contact with a chancre at birth. In addition, hematogenous infection can occur throughout pregnancy.

Syphilis cases in the United States are notably rising. Intrauterine infection can result in stillbirth, hydrops fetalis, or prematurity. Clinical symptoms vary but include hepatosplenomegaly, snuffles, lymphadenopathy, mucocutaneous lesions, osteochondritis, rash, hemolytic anemia, and thrombocytopenia. Untreated infants, regardless of whether they manifest symptoms at birth, may develop late symptoms, which usually appear after 2 years of age and involve the CNS, bones, joints, teeth, eyes, and skin. Some manifestations of disease may not become apparent until many years after birth, such as interstitial keratitis, eighth cranial nerve deafness, Hutchinson teeth, bowing of the shins, frontal bossing, mulberry molars, saddle nose, rhagades, and Clutton joints. The combination of interstitial keratitis, eighth cranial nerve deafness, and Hutchinson teeth is commonly referred to as the *Hutchinson triad.*

Many infants are asymptomatic at birth. If untreated, most infants develop symptoms within the first 5 weeks of life. The most striking lesions affect the mucocutaneous tissues and bones. Early signs of infection may be poor feeding and snuffles (syphilitic rhinitis). Snuffles are more severe and persistent than the common cold and are often bloody. A maculopapular desquamative rash develops over the palms and soles and around the mouth and anus. The rash may progress to become vesicular with bullae. Severely ill infants may be born with hydrops and have profound anemia. Severe consolidated pneumonia may be present at birth, and there may be laboratory findings consistent with a glomerulonephritis. CSF evaluation may reveal a pleocytosis and elevated protein. More than 90% of symptomatic infants exhibit radiographic abnormalities of the long bones consistent with osteochondritis and perichondritis.

All pregnant people should be screened for syphilis during the pregnancy and/or at time of delivery. No newborn should be discharged from the hospital without knowledge or determination of the pregnant person's serologic status for syphilis. All infants born to seropositive birth parents require a careful examination and further evaluation. Diagnosis may be by treponemal or nontreponemal tests. The nontreponemal reaginic antibody assays—the Venereal Disease Research Laboratory (VDRL) and the rapid plasma reagin (RPR)—are indicators of disease activity, used to screen for the disease during pregnancy and trend response to treatment. Comparison of RPR from the parent and infant at birth helps identify active disease in the infant. Treponemal-specific testing ("reverse screening algorithm") may also be used to screen for the disease during pregnancy, but it is not helpful for distinguishing active disease in the infant, as these antibodies remain positive after disease treatment and pass transplacentally to the infant regardless of disease activity during the pregnancy. An infant should be evaluated further if the maternal titer has increased fourfold, if the infant's titer is fourfold greater than the birth parent's titer, if the infant is symptomatic, or if the birth parent has inadequately treated syphilis. A pregnant person infected later in pregnancy may deliver an infant who is incubating active disease. The pregnant person and infant may have negative serologic testing at birth. At-risk infants who had a negative RPR at birth should have repeat RPR at 3 months of age.

When clinical or serologic tests suggest congenital syphilis, CSF should be examined microscopically, and a CSF VDRL test should be performed. An increased CSF white blood cell count and protein concentration suggest neurosyphilis; a positive CSF VDRL is consistent with neurosyphilis but not present in all cases.

Parenteral penicillin is the preferred drug of choice for treatment of syphilis. Penicillin G for 10–14 days is the only documented effective therapy for infants who have congenital syphilis and neurosyphilis. Infants should have nontreponemal antibody titers repeated every 2–3 months until it becomes nonreactive. Infants with persistent titers at 6 to 12 months of age should be reevaluated. See Chapter 117.

HUMAN IMMUNODEFICIENCY VIRUS

See Chapter 126.

HEPATITIS B

See Chapter 114.

NEISSERIA GONORRHOEAE

N. gonorrhoeae infection in a newborn usually involves the eyes (ophthalmia neonatorum). Other sites of infection include scalp abscesses (often associated with fetal monitoring with scalp electrodes), vaginitis, and disseminated disease with bacteremia, arthritis, or meningitis. Transmission to the infant usually occurs during passage through the birth canal when mucous membranes come in contact with infected secretions.

Infection usually is present within the first 5 days of life and is characterized initially by a clear, watery discharge, which rapidly becomes purulent. There is marked conjunctival hyperemia and chemosis. Infection tends to be bilateral; however, one eye may be clinically worse than the other. Untreated infections can spread to the cornea (keratitis) and anterior chamber of the eye. This extension can result in corneal perforation and blindness.

Recommended prophylaxis for exposed infants and treatment for infants with isolated infection, such as ophthalmia neonatorum, is one intramuscular dose of ceftriaxone. Infants with gonococcal ophthalmia should receive eye irrigations with saline solution at frequent intervals. Topical antibiotic therapy alone is inadequate and is unnecessary when recommended systemic antimicrobial therapy is given. Infants with gonococcal ophthalmia should be hospitalized and evaluated for disseminated disease (sepsis, arthritis, meningitis). Disseminated disease should be treated with antimicrobial therapy (ceftriaxone) for 7 days. Cefepime can be used in infants with hyperbilirubinemia. If documented, infants with meningitis should be treated for 10–14 days.

Tests for concomitant infection with *C. trachomatis*, congenital syphilis, and HIV should be performed. Results of the maternal test for hepatitis B surface antigen should be confirmed. Topical prophylaxis with silver nitrate, erythromycin, or tetracycline is recommended for all newborns for the prevention of gonococcal ophthalmia.

CHLAMYDIA

C. trachomatis is the most commonly reported sexually transmitted infection, with a high rate of infection among sexually active adolescents and young adults. Prevalence of the organism in pregnant women ranges from 2–14% and can be even greater in adolescents. *Chlamydia* can be transmitted from the genital tract of an infected birth parent to the newborn. Acquisition occurs in about 50% of infants born vaginally to infected pregnant people. Transmission also has been reported in some infants delivered by cesarean section with intact membranes. In infected infants, the risk of conjunctivitis is 25–50%, and the risk of pneumonia is 5–20%. The nasopharynx is the most commonly infected anatomic site.

Neonatal chlamydial conjunctivitis is characterized by ocular congestion, edema, and discharge developing 5–14 days to several weeks after birth and lasting 1–2 weeks. Clinical manifestations vary from mild conjunctivitis to intense inflammation and swelling. Both eyes are almost always involved; however, one eye may appear to be more swollen and infected than the other. The cornea is rarely involved, and preauricular adenopathy is rare.

Pneumonia in a young infant can occur between 2–19 weeks of age and is characterized by an afebrile illness with a repetitive staccato cough, tachypnea, and rales. Wheezing is uncommon. Hyperinflation with diffuse infiltrates can be seen on chest radiograph. Nasal stuffiness and otitis media can occur.

Diagnosis can be made by scraping the conjunctiva and culturing the material. Giemsa staining of the conjunctival scrapings revealing the presence of blue-stained intracytoplasmic inclusions within the epithelial cells is diagnostic. PCR is also available. Infants with conjunctivitis and pneumonia are treated with oral azithromycin for 3 days or erythromycin for 14 days. Topical treatment of conjunctivitis is ineffective and unnecessary. The recommended topical prophylaxis with silver nitrate, erythromycin, or tetracycline for all newborns for the prevention of gonococcal ophthalmia does not prevent neonatal chlamydial conjunctivitis.

MYCOBACTERIUM TUBERCULOSIS

See Chapter 125.

ZIKA VIRUS

Zika virus is an arthropod-borne flavivirus carried and transmitted by mosquitoes and is associated with severe congenital anomalies. Zika virus is a neurotropic virus that particularly targets progenitor cells. Zika virus causes a maternal infection leading to a placental infection and injury to the fetus. The infection is transmitted to the fetal brain where it kills neuronal progenitor cells, disrupting neuronal proliferation, migration, and differentiation. In utero infections can be transmitted to the fetus at any time during the pregnancy and result in severe brain abnormalities (i.e., microcephaly, cerebellar hypoplasia, ventriculomegaly, lissencephaly) and craniofacial malformations. Additionally, the virus can result in pulmonary hypoplasia and multiple congenital contractures.

COVID-19

SARS-CoV-2 infection in the neonate is uncommon. Neonatal infection is horizontally acquired and may be mild or asymptomatic. Maternal COVID-19 disease may result in premature birth and result in neonatal respiratory distress syndrome and other problems associated with prematurity. Premature infants and neonates with other conditions may develop severe COVID-19 symptoms. The diagnosis of COVID-19 infection in infants should meet the following criteria: (1) at least one clinical symptom, including unstable body temperature, low activity, poor feeding, diarrhea or other mild gastrointestinal symptom, or respiratory distress; (2) chest radiograph showing abnormalities (opacities or ground-glass appearance); (3) infection diagnosed in the infant's family or caregivers; and (4) close contact with people who may have or have confirmed infection with COVID-19.

The diagnosis of COVID-19 in neonates is made by using reverse transcriptase PCR on nasopharyngeal, nasal, or endotracheal samples to detect the presence of SARS-CoV-2.

PEARLS FOR PRACTITIONERS

See Fetal and Neonatal Medicine: Pearls for Practitioners at the end of this section.

REVIEW QUESTIONS

Available online.

Suggested Readings

Engle WA. Infants Born Late Preterm: Definition, Physiologic and Metabolic Immaturity, and Outcomes. *Neoreviews*. 2009;10(6):e280–e286.
Frankovich J, Sandborg C, Barnes P, Hintz S, Chakravarty E. Neonatal Lupus and Related Autoimmune Disorders of Infants. *Neoreviews*. 2008;9(5):e206–e217.
HAPO Study Cooperative Research Group, Metzger BE, Lowe LP, et al. Hyperglycemia and adverse pregnancy outcomes. *N Engl J Med*. 2008;358(19):1991–2002.
Hong H, Wang Y, Chung HT, Chen CJ. Clinical characteristics of novel coronavirus disease 2019 (COVID-19) in newborns, infants and children. *Pediatr Neonatol*. 2020;61(2):131–132.
Jesse N, Neu J. Necrotizing Enterocolitis: Relationship to Innate Immunity, Clinical Features, and Strategies for Prevention. *Neoreviews*. 2006;7(3):e143–e150.
Kates EH, Kates JS. Anemia and polycythemia in the newborn. *Pediatr Rev*. 2007;28(1):33–34.
National Institutes of Health. Extremely Preterm Birth Outcomes Tool. US Department of Health and Human Services. https://www.nichd.nih.gov/research/supported/EPBO. Updated 3/2/2020. Accessed 9/12/2024.
Silva RA, Moshfeghi DM. Interventions in Retinopathy of Prematurity. *Neoreviews*. 2012;13(8):e476–e485.
Steinhorn RH, Farrow KN. Pulmonary Hypertension in the Neonate. *Neoreviews*. 2007;8(1):e14–e21.
Wong RJ, Stevenson DK, Ahlfors CE, Vreman HJ. Neonatal Jaundice: Bilirubin Physiology and Clinical Chemistry. *Neoreviews*. 2007;8(2):e58–e67.

PEARLS FOR PRACTITIONERS

CHAPTER 57

Assessment of the Birth Parent, Fetus, and Newborn

- High-risk pregnancies include those with fetal growth restriction (FGR), maternal hypertension, diabetes, autoimmune diseases (systemic lupus erythematosus), and those with prior intrauterine fetal demise or neonatal deaths. Additional high-risk pregnancies include those with oligo- or polyhydramnios, multiple gestation, or macrosomic fetuses.
- The biophysical profile, which includes fetal movement, fetal breathing, fetal tone, amniotic fluid volume, and fetal heart rate reactivity, is often used to assess fetal well-being. A score of less than 6 of 10 indicates possible fetal compromise and may necessitate delivery of the infant.
- Low birthweight is defined by birthweight less than 2,500 g.
- The Apgar examination performed at 1 and 5 minutes assesses fetal to neonatal transition and identifies infants in need of resuscitation.
- About 10% of neonates will require some form of intervention and/or resuscitation in the delivery room.
- A single intramuscular injection of vitamin K should be administered to all newborns to prevent hemorrhagic disease of the newborn.
- Shock in the delivery room is often due to blood loss such as fetal-maternal hemorrhage or internal bleeding (liver, spleen, subgaleal hemorrhage).
- Erb-Duchenne palsy involves the fifth and sixth cervical nerves.
- Early neonatal hypocalcemia may be due to maternal hyperparathyroidism or neonatal DiGeorge syndrome; it is also seen in infants of diabetic mothers, preterm infants, or following birth asphyxia.
- Erythromycin eye ointment is administered to all infants following delivery to reduce risk of vertically transmitted gonococcal infection. Topical erythromycin ointment is not effective prophylaxis or treatment for chlamydial conjunctivitis.
- Pulse oximetry screening (preductal and postductal) should be performed on all infants before discharge from the hospital. A difference of greater than 3% is suggestive of cyanotic heart disease.
- Each infant should be screened for hearing loss via otoacoustic emissions or auditory brainstem response prior to being discharged from the hospital.
- Failure of a term infant to pass urine in the first 24 hours or meconium in the first 48 hours of life warrants further evaluation, including assessment of feeding efficacy.

CHAPTER 58

Birth Parent Diseases Affecting the Newborn

- Maternal diabetes mellitus represents a high risk for teratogenic changes in the fetus (i.e., congenital heart disease, caudal regression).
- For the fetus, insulin is the primary growth hormone; in situations where fetal insulin levels are increased, the fetus can be overgrown (macrosomic, large for gestational age).
- Infants of diabetic mothers are at risk for birth trauma, hypoglycemia, hypocalcemia, hyperbilirubinemia (increased red cell mass), cardiac disease, and caudal regression.
- The following should be assessed every pregnancy: HIV, syphilis status, hepatitis B surface antigen, rubella immunity, blood type and antibody screen, and group B streptococcus cultures (obtained within 5 weeks of birth).

- Autoimmune diseases of the birth parent may affect the fetus by placental transfer of IgG autoantibodies such as seen in maternal immune thrombocytopenia, systemic lupus erythematosus (SLE), hyperthyroidism, and myasthenia gravis.

CHAPTER 59
Diseases of the Fetus

- Causes of fetal growth restriction (FGR) include poor maternal nutrition, maternal hypertension, fetal anomalies or infection, and twin-twin transfusion syndrome.
- Hepatosplenomegaly, jaundice, dermatitis, chorioretinitis, and micro- or hydrocephaly in an infant with FGR suggests an intrauterine (TORCH) infection.
- Organ anomalies such as congenital heart disease, oral clefts, and limb anomalies suggest a congenital malformation syndrome.
- Hydrops fetalis is often due to fetal anemia secondary to immune hemolysis or decreased red cell production.
- Nonimmune hydrops has many etiologies including infection, malignancy, autoinflammatory diseases, and complex congenital anomalies.

CHAPTER 60
Respiratory Diseases of the Newborn

- Respiratory distress may manifest by cyanosis, sternal and intercostal retractions, nasal flaring, and expiratory grunting.
- Common causes of respiratory distress include infection, respiratory distress syndrome (RDS), and congenital anomalies of the airway, lung, or diaphragm.
- Maternal betamethasone therapy reduces the risk of RDS in at-risk premature infants.
- A patent ductus arteriosus may present with a widened pulse pressure, worsening hypoxia and hypercarbia, and signs of heart failure with a new cardiac murmur.
- Bronchopulmonary dysplasia may develop in infants with severe ventilator-treated RDS and manifests as persistent ventilator and oxygen requirements and chronic changes on chest x-ray.
- Persistent pulmonary hypertension of the newborn (PPHN) often accompanies birth asphyxia, meconium aspiration syndrome, pulmonary hypoplasia, and a congenital diaphragmatic hernia.
- PPHN is managed by oxygen and ventilation therapy; if these are unsuccessful, patients may be treated with inhaled nitric oxide and extracorporeal membrane oxygenation (ECMO).

CHAPTER 61
Anemia and Hyperbilirubinemia

- Neonatal anemia is often due to immune-mediated hemolysis, red cell membrane defects, or red cell enzyme deficiencies. Rarely, it is due to decreased production as seen in Blackfan-Diamond syndrome.
- Prevention of hemolytic disease of the newborn due to Rh factor incompatibility is possible by administering RhoGAM to the Rh-negative birth parent during gestation and within 3 days after the delivery of the Rh-positive infant.
- Fetal-maternal hemorrhage may produce fetal anemia and may be detected by the Kleihauer-Betke test.
- Physiologic jaundice is an indirect hyperbilirubinemia peaking on day 3 of life in term babies; the peak may be later in premature infants.
- Breast milk jaundice is an indirect hyperbilirubinemia that occurs 1–2 weeks after birth; its cause is unknown.
- Rapidly rising indirect bilirubin levels and any direct hyperbilirubinemia are due to potentially serious pathologic processes and require immediate evaluation.

CHAPTER 62
Necrotizing Enterocolitis

- Necrotizing enterocolitis (NEC) manifests with a sepsis-like presentation and with abdominal distention and tenderness.
- Abdominal x-rays in NEC demonstrate pneumatosis intestinalis, portal-hepatic gas, pneumoperitoneum, or intestinal distention.
- Significant bilious emesis is considered a neonatal emergency and deserves further evaluation with an upper gastrointestinal tract series to rule out malrotation and midgut volvulus.

CHAPTER 63
Neurologic Conditions: Seizures, Intracranial Hemorrhage, and Hypoxic-Ischemic Encephalopathy

- Seizures in a neonate within the first 24 hours of birth are most likely secondary to birth asphyxia or hypoxia during labor and delivery.
- Therapeutic hypothermia has been shown to reduce the risk of neurodevelopmental disability following moderate-to-severe in utero hypoxia or ischemia; the outcome is best if hypothermia can be started before 6 hours of age.

CHAPTER 64

Sepsis and Meningitis

- Maternal intraamniotic infection (chorioamnionitis) puts the fetus at increased risk for early-onset sepsis.
- The most common organisms causing early-onset neonatal sepsis include group B streptococcus and *Escherichia coli*; a synergistic combination of ampicillin and an aminoglycoside (usually gentamicin) is appropriate initial therapy for early-onset sepsis.

CHAPTER 65

Congenital Infections

- "Blueberry muffin" appearance is most commonly seen in neonates with congenital rubella or cytomegalovirus infection. A biopsy of a blueberry muffin lesion will reveal dermal hematopoiesis. The "skin" is the first organ system to produce red cells.
- CMV is the most common congenital infection.

SECTION 12

ADOLESCENT MEDICINE

Kim Blake | Nancy Van Eyk

CHAPTER 66

Overview and Assessment of Adolescents

Adolescents have distinct health concerns that differ from those of children and adults, many of which revolve around puberty, psychosocial development, and behavior-driven risks. The leading causes of morbidity (Table 66.1) and mortality in U.S. adolescents are behavior mediated, with over 75% of deaths attributable to motor vehicle accidents, injuries, and risky behaviors. Unhealthy dietary habits and insufficient physical activity contribute to adolescent obesity, leading to complications such as diabetes and hypertension.

Table 66.2 describes key chronic health conditions in adolescents. It is crucial for providers caring for adolescents to assess both risk-taking behaviors and protective or resilience factors at every visit, regardless of the presenting complaint, while ensuring confidentiality to foster open and honest communication. Because physical symptoms in adolescence may often be linked to psychosocial issues, a structured approach is essential. The HEADDSSS mnemonic (Home, Education, Activities, Drugs, Diet, Sex, Suicide, and Safety) can be adapted in various ways depending on the context (Table 66.3). For example, an additional "S" might represent "Self," "A" could be changed to "Alcohol" (especially relevant for young adolescents, for whom alcohol is a common gateway substance), and "E" might stand for both "Education" and "Exercise." These modifications allow the mnemonic to better address individual needs, age, and specific risk factors. The Structured Communication Adolescent Guide (SCAG) is a validated tool for a comprehensive adolescent evaluation and provides an example of how the HEADDSSS mnemonic can be applied effectively. The SCAG (Fig. 66.1) encourages clinicians not only to identify areas of risk-taking but also to explore the positive actions adolescents are taking to support their well-being.

TABLE 66.1 Leading Causes of Death in Adolescents (15–19 Years Old) in the United States From 2018 to 2023

RANK	CAUSE	RATE (PER 100,000)
1	Unintentional injuries	22.0
2	Assault (homicide)	12.9
3	Suicide	10.0
4	Malignant neoplasms (cancer)	2.9
5	Diseases of the heart	1.3
6	Congenital malfunctions	1.0
7	COVID-19	0.7
8	Diabetes	0.3

From the Centers for Disease Control and Prevention, National Center for Health Statistics. National Vital Statistics. *Atlanta, GA: CDC; 2024.*

MENTAL HEALTH CRISIS IN ADOLESCENTS

The mental health crisis among adolescents has been exacerbated by social media; anxiety and depression have been linked to excessive screen time. Adolescent females may experience heightened anxiety due to social media while males are increasingly exposed to violent content online. The COVID-19 pandemic worsened these issues by increasing isolation and academic pressure, often at the expense of physical activity and healthy relationships. Balancing discussions of these risk factors with attention to activities that foster well-being—such as positive relationships, healthy coping mechanisms, physical activity, and hobbies—can be central to supporting adolescents' overall health.

LEGAL RIGHTS OF MINORS

The law confers certain rights on adolescents, depending on their health condition and personal characteristics; this allows them to receive health services without parental permission (Table 66.4). Adolescents can seek health care without parental consent for reproductive, mental, and emergency health services. Emancipated adolescents and *mature minors* may be treated without parental consent; this status should be documented in the medical record. The key characteristics of mature minors are their competence and capacity to understand, not their chronological age. There must be a reasonable judgment that the health intervention is in the best interest of the minor.

OPEN ELECTRONIC HEALTH RECORD AND ADOLESCENT CONFIDENTIALITY

A key issue with electronic health records (EHRs) and adolescent care is maintaining confidentiality for sensitive health information (e.g., sexual or mental health). Federal laws such as HIPAA (Health Insurance Portability and Accountability

TABLE 66.2 Description of the Key Chronic Health Conditions in Adolescents

CAUSE	DESCRIPTION	KEY STATISTICS
Mental health disorders	Anxiety, depression, and mood disorders are leading cause of illness in teens.	About 1 in 5 U.S. teens has a diagnosable mental health condition.
Unintentional injuries	Motor vehicle accidents, falls, firearms, and sports injuries are major health risks.	Leading cause of death in teens; around 45% of teen deaths are due to unintentional injuries.
Substance use	Alcohol, tobacco (including vaping), and drug use are significant concerns.	Approximately 20% of high school students report using tobacco or marijuana.
Obesity	Poor diet and sedentary lifestyles lead to obesity, increasing risk for diabetes.	1 in 5 U.S. adolescents are obese.
Sexually transmitted infections	Infections like chlamydia, gonorrhea, and human papillomavirus (HPV) are common among sexually active teens.	Adolescents account for nearly half of all new STI cases each year.
Chronic diseases	Asthma, type 1 and type 2 diabetes, and autoimmune diseases are prevalent.	Asthma affects about 10% of teens.
Eating disorders	Anorexia, bulimia, binge-eating disorders, and avoidant restrictive food intake disorder are prevalent, particularly in females.	Estimated 2–3% of U.S. teens struggle with an eating disorder.
Suicide	Suicide is a leading cause of death among adolescents.	Suicide rates have increased, particularly among young males.

STI, Sexually transmitted infection.

TABLE 66.3 Interviewing the Adolescent Alone: Discussion of HEADDSSS Topics*

HOME/ FRIENDS	Family, relationships, and activities. "What do you do for fun?" "What social media do you use?" "How much screen time in a day?"
EDUCATION	How school is going. "What do you like best at school?" "Any bullying?"
ALCOHOL*	Assessment of alcohol use. "Are any of your friends drinking?" "Are you drinking?"
DRUGS	Cigarettes, vaping, marijuana, street drugs. "Have you ever smoked or tried e-cigarettes?" "Many adolescents experiment with different drugs and substances. Have you tried anything?"
DIET*	Weight, diet/eating habits. "Many adolescents worry about their weight and try dieting. Have you ever done this?"
SEX	Sexual activity, contraception. "Are you going out with anybody?" "Have you dated in the past?" "Are you sexually active with males, females, or both?"
SUICIDE/ DEPRESSION	Mood swings, depression, suicide attempts or thoughts, self-image. "Feeling down or depressed is common for everyone. Have you ever felt so bad that you wanted to harm yourself?"

**The acronym HEADDSSS can represent other terms; that is, A, Activities; D, Depression.*

Act) and state minor consent laws provide guidelines, but they vary by state, making it challenging to balance transparency and privacy. Understanding each state's laws around confidentiality and communicating these laws clearly with both the adolescent and their guardians is crucial for protecting patient trust and well-being.

PHYSICAL GROWTH AND DEVELOPMENT OF ADOLESCENTS

Females

Adrenarche, the increased production of androgens by the adrenal glands, is the first physiologic change associated with puberty. Breast development **(thelarche)** is typically the first visible sign in females, occurring at around 8.8 years of age in Black females and 9.6 years in White females. The growth of pubic hair **(pubarche)** usually follows approximately 6 months after thelarche, but breast development and pubic hair growth may happen at the same time for some females.

Obesity is associated with earlier onset of puberty. Progression through puberty is denoted by Tanner staging (Fig. 66.2) for each of breast and pubic hair growth, stages 1 (no growth/prepubertal) through 5 (complete development). Not all females achieve Tanner 5 pubic hair.

An increase in height velocity occurs at the onset of puberty. The peak height velocity or "growth spurt" usually occurs approximately 1 year after thelarche, at Tanner stage 3 breast development. Females only grow an additional 2–5 cm in height after menarche.

Onset of menstruation **(menarche)** occurs at stage 4 breast development. The mean ages of menarche are 11.6 and 12.1 years for Black and White females, respectively. Important predictors for menarche are when the female's mother had menarche and body mass index (BMI). Higher BMI in childhood is associated with early menarche. The interval from the initiation of thelarche to the onset of menses (menarche) is 2.3 years plus or minus 1 year.

Males

Testicular enlargement (≥2.5 cm) corresponds to Tanner stages 1 to 2 for males (Fig. 66.3). Testicular enlargement is followed by pubic hair development at the base of the penis (**adrenarche**) and then axillary hair within the year. The growth spurt is a relatively late event; it can occur from 10.5 to 16 years of age. Deepening of the voice, the appearance of facial hair, and acne indicate the early stages of puberty. See Chapter 175 for discussion of disorders of puberty.

Changes Associated With Physical Maturation

Tanner stages mark biologic maturation, which can be related to specific changes in laboratory values and certain physical conditions. The higher hematocrit values in adolescent males than in females are the result of greater androgenic stimulation of the bone marrow and not loss through menstruation.

Structured Communication Adolescent Guide (SCAG)

Instructions for scoring this form

After your check-up, please score your doctor (or medical student) using this form.

Examples:

0 = Did Not	1 = Did	2 = Did Well
Dr. didn't ask at all.	Dr. asked as if reading a list. Dr. asked as if embarrassed. I felt judged. I felt a bit uncomfortable.	Dr. established a relationship. Dr. comfortable with questions. Dr. did not judge. I felt comfortable.

General Rating: Give a general impression of each section.
A = Excellent, B = Good, C = Average, D = Poor, F = Fail

	Did Not 0	Did 1	Did Well 2	Give examples of things that stood out in your interview, one positive and one negative.
A. GETTING STARTED				*Example: I liked that you talked to me and not just my mom.*
1. Greeted me.	0	1	2	
2. Introduced self.	0	1	2	
3. Discussed confidentiality.	0	1	2	
GENERAL RATING A B C D F				

	Did Not 0	Did 1	Did Well 2	Give examples of things that stood out in your interview, one positive and one negative.
B. GATHERING INFORMATION				*Example: I felt bad when you asked about smoking with my mom in the room.*
4. Good body language.	0	1	2	
5. Encouraged me to speak by asking questions other than ones with a yes/no answer.	0	1	2	
6. Encouraged parent to speak *(leave out if no parent present).*	0	1	2	
7. Listened and did not judge me.	0	1	2	
8. Established relationship with me by appropriate choice of words.	0	1	2	
GENERAL RATING A B C D F				

FIGURE 66.1 The Structured Communication Adolescent Guide (SCAG). The SCAG is an interviewing and feedback tool developed for learners to use with real or standardized adolescent patients. The SCAG incorporates the three major interview components: confidentiality, separation of the adolescent from the adult, and psychosocial data gathering (using the HEADDSSS mnemonic). The SCAG is at a grade 5 reading level and has demonstrated reliability and validity. A printable version (2020) is available at www.drkimblake.com.

Continued

	Did Not 0	Did 1	Did Well 2	Give examples of things that stood out in your interview, one positive and one negative.
C. TEEN ALONE				*Example: I was glad you talked about confidentiality. I need lots of reassurance that you won't tell my mom.*
9. Separated me and parent. *(Leave out if no parent present.)*	0	1	2	
10. Discussed confidentiality.	0	1	2	
11. Gave me a chance to talk about things other than what I came in to discuss.	0	1	2	
12. Reflected on my feelings or concerns (example: You seem...).	0	1	2	
LIFESTYLES: Physician asks or talks about the following:				
13. **Home:** Family	0	1	2	
14. **Education:** School	0	1	2	
15. Friends/	0	1	2	
16. **Activities** social media	0	1	2	
17. **Alcohol:** Beer and hard liquor	0	1	2	
18. **Drugs:** Cigarettes	0	1	2	
19. Marijuana	0	1	2	
20. Street drugs	0	1	2	
21. **Diet:** Weight/diet/eating habits	0	1	2	
22. **Sex:** Boyfriend/girlfriend	0	1	2	
23. Sexual activity	0	1	2	
24. Safe sex/ contraception	0	1	2	
25. **Self:** Body image, self-esteem	0	1	2	*Example: You weren't embarrassed to talk about sex. OR You seemed embarrassed to talk about sex.*
26. Moods/depression/ suicide	0	1	2	
GENERAL RATING A B C D F				

	Did Not 0	Did 1	Did Well 2	Comments: Please give examples of things that stood out in your interview.
D. WRAP UP				*Example: I wasn't sure what the next step would be.*
27. Summary, recapped issues	0	1	2	
28. Kept the confidentiality	0	1	2	
29. Asked if there were any questions	0	1	2	
30. Talked about what to do next (plan and follow-up)	0	1	2	
GENERAL RATING A B C D F				

FIGURE 66.1, cont'd

TABLE 66.4 Legal Rights of Minors

Age of majority (≥18 yr of age in most states)
Exceptions in which health care services can be provided to a minor*
Emergency care (e.g., life-threatening condition or condition in which a delay in treatment would increase significantly the likelihood of morbidity)
Diagnosis and treatment of sexuality-related health care
Diagnosis and treatment of drug-related health care
Emancipated minors (physically and financially independent of family; Armed Forces, married, childbirth)
Mature minors (able to comprehend the risks and benefits of evaluation and treatment)
All exceptions should be documented clearly in the patient's health record.

**Determined by individual state laws.*

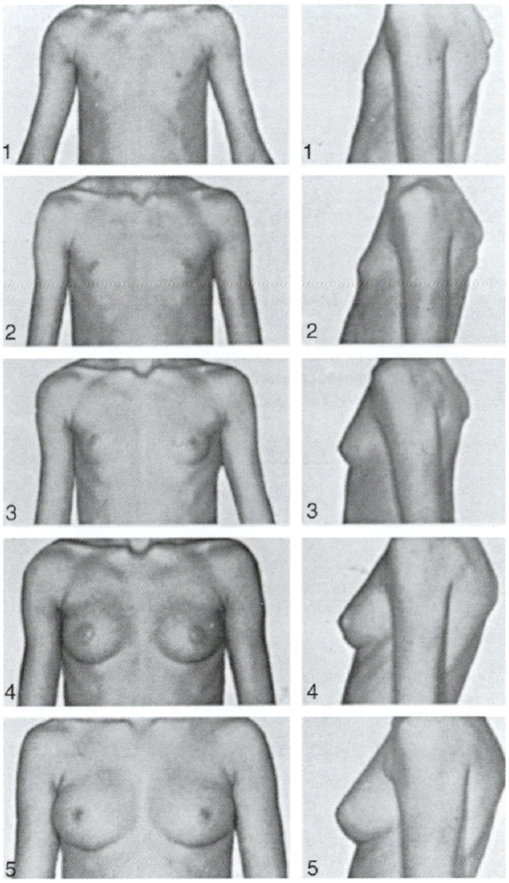

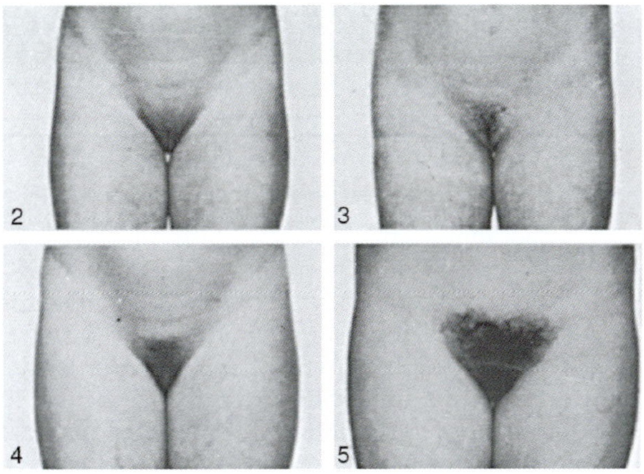

FIGURE 66.2 Typical progression of female pubertal development, Stages 1–5. **(A)** Pubertal development in the size of female breasts. **(B)** Pubertal development of female pubic hair. Note that at stage 1 (not shown) there is no pubic hair. (Courtesy JM Tanner. Institute of Child Health, Department of Growth and Development. London, England: University of London.)

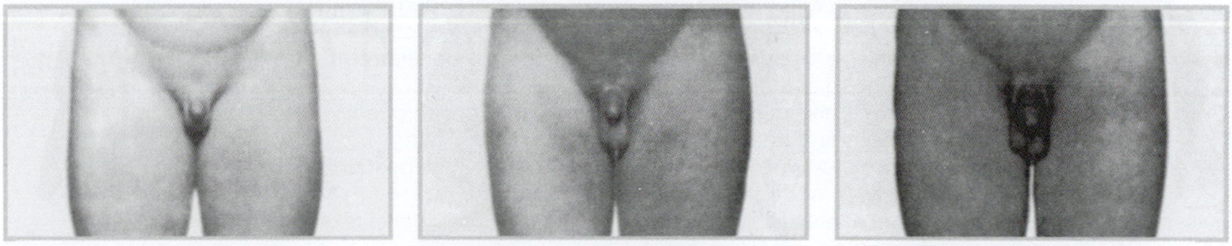

Stage 1 The penis, testes, and scrotum are of childhood size.

Stage 2 There is enlargement of the scrotum and testes, but the penis usually does not enlarge. The scrotal skin reddens.

Stage 3 There is further growth of the testes and scrotum and enlargement of the penis, mainly in length.

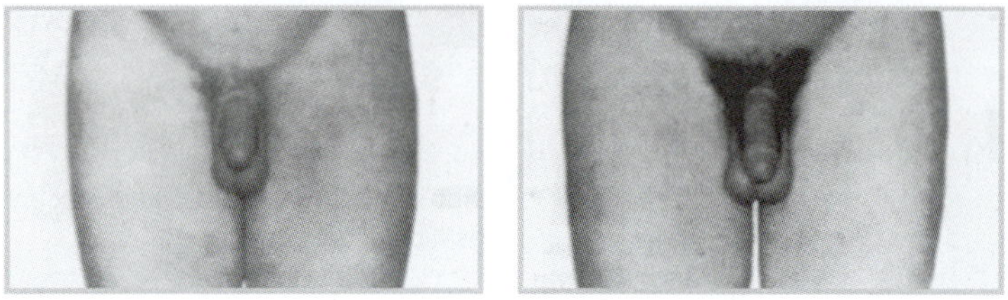

Stage 4 There is still further growth of the testes and scrotum and increased size of the penis, especially in breadth.

Stage 5 The genitalia are adult in size and shape.

A

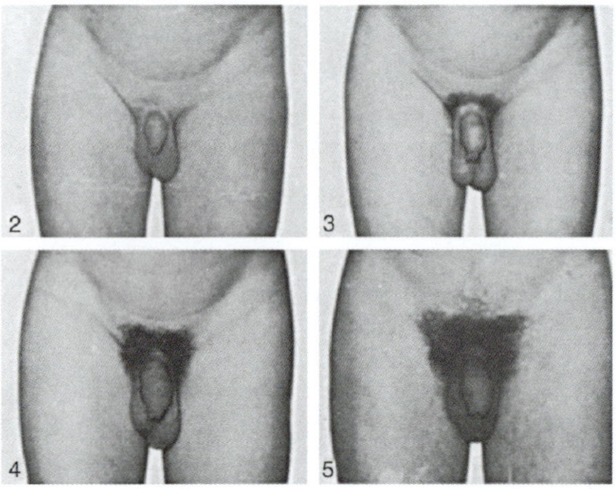

Stage 2 There is sparse growth of long, slightly pigmented, downy hair, straight or only slightly curled, primarily at the base of the penis.

Stage 3 The hair is considerably darker, coarser, and more curled. The hair spreads sparsely over the junction of the pubes.

Stage 4 The hair, now adult in type, covers a smaller area than in the adult and does not extend onto the thighs.

Stage 5 The hair is adult in quantity and type, with extension onto the thighs.

B

FIGURE 66.3 Typical progression of male pubertal development. **(A)** Pubertal development in the size of male genitalia. **(B)** Pubertal development of male pubic hair. Note that at stage 1 there is no pubic hair. (Courtesy JM Tanner. Institute of Child Health, Department of Growth and Development. London, England: University of London.)

Alkaline phosphatase levels in males and females increase during puberty because of rapid bone turnover, especially during the growth spurt. Worsening of mild scoliosis can occur in adolescents during the growth spurt.

PSYCHOLOGIC GROWTH AND DEVELOPMENT OF ADOLESCENTS

See Chapters 7 and 9.

PEARLS FOR PRACTITIONERS

See Adolescent Medicine: Pearls for Practitioners at the end of this section.

REVIEW QUESTION

Available online.

CHAPTER 67

Adolescent Well Care

INTERVIEWING ADOLESCENTS

The adolescent interview shifts the focus of information gathering from the parent to the adolescent. Interviewing the adolescent alone and ensuring confidentiality are crucial for obtaining an accurate history, assessing risk-taking behaviors (see Table 66.3), providing anticipatory guidance, and identifying resilience/protective factors. It is important to confirm the adolescent's preferred name and pronouns during the interview. The nature of the questions should consider the developmental age of the adolescent. Conversations about sports, friends, videogames, and activities outside of school can be useful for all ages and help build rapport.

Confidentiality is a key element in interviewing an adolescent (Table 67.1). An open discussion about risk-taking and activities that foster well-being is more likely to happen when the adolescent is alone. Certain issues cannot be kept confidential, such as suicidal intent, serious harm to self and others, and disclosure of sexual or physical abuse. This needs to be explained to the parent/guardian and adolescent before the discussion alone with the adolescent. In caring for an adolescent, the health care provider should encourage them to have open discussions with a parent, guardian, or other trusted adult.

When interviewing adolescents, providers should use a nonjudgmental approach and find some common ground to engage the adolescents to talk about themselves. Adolescents who experiment in one area of risk-taking often have contemplated or tried multiple other risk-taking behaviors. When all the protective factors and risk-taking information has been gathered, choose one or two health care issues to discuss, making it clear that the information is confidential and that you are there in partnership to help the adolescent. Although the focus in adolescent care is on psychosocial issues, a general examination must also be performed (Table 67.2). The physical examination of an adolescent should prioritize good communication, consent, and comfort.

General pediatric issues, such as immunizations (see Chapter 95) and health screening, should be included (see Table 9.5).

Adolescent psychological development can be divided into three broad timelines (early, middle, and late teens) (Fig. 67.1).

EARLY ADOLESCENCE (AGES 10–13 YEARS)

Rapid changes in physical appearance and behavior are the major characteristics of early adolescence, leading to a great deal of self-consciousness and need for privacy. The history focuses on the early adolescent's physical and psychosocial health.

MIDDLE ADOLESCENCE (AGES 14–17 YEARS)

Autonomy and a global sense of identity are the major characteristics of middle adolescence. The history focuses on the middle adolescent's interactions with family, school, and peers. High-risk behaviors because of experimentation are common.

TABLE 67.1 Guidelines for Confidentiality

Prepare the preadolescent and parent for confidentiality and being interviewed alone at future adolescent visits.
Discuss confidentiality at the start of the interview.
Conversations with parents/guardians/adolescent are confidential (with exceptions*).
Reaffirm confidentiality when you are alone with your adolescent patient.

**Exceptions to confidentiality include major or impending harm to any person (i.e., abuse, suicide, homicide).*

LATE ADOLESCENCE (AGES 18–21 YEARS)

Individuality and planning for the future are the major characteristics of late adolescence. Greater emphasis is placed on late adolescents' responsibility for their own health care.

GYNECOLOGICAL EXAMINATION

Prior to any gynecologic exam, the patient should be informed about the importance of the assessment and exactly what will occur, including any potential discomfort. The patient should be encouraged to ask questions and know that they can request to stop at any time. A chaperone should be offered if a caregiver is not present. The examiner should maintain eye contact during the exam and explain what is happening during each step. A padded examination table with the patient in a frog-leg position improves comfort during a gynecologic examination. The examination room, lubricants, and instruments should be warm. The examination should be unhurried but efficient.

TABLE 67.2 How to Foster Trust and Cooperation in the Adolescent's Examination

Build rapport	Start by establishing a connection with the adolescent. Introduce yourself and explain the purpose of the exam in clear, age-appropriate language.
Provide clear explanations	As you proceed with the exam, explain each step so the adolescent understands what you are doing and why. This helps reduce anxiety and makes them feel more in control.
Seek consent	Always ask for permission before beginning the exam or touching the patient. This reinforces the adolescent's autonomy and comfort.
Offer a chaperone	Ensure that the adolescent knows they have the option to have a chaperone present. This can increase their sense of security and trust.
Respect privacy and comfort	Regularly check in with the adolescent about their comfort level throughout the exam. Be observant of nonverbal cues that may indicate discomfort or anxiety.
Use draping	When performing the exam, use draping to maintain the adolescent's privacy and modesty. If possible, work around the regular clothes they are wearing rather than asking them to change into a gown.
Focus on comfort and consent	Remember that the adolescent's comfort and consent are paramount. If at any point the adolescent feels uncomfortable, be prepared to adjust your approach.

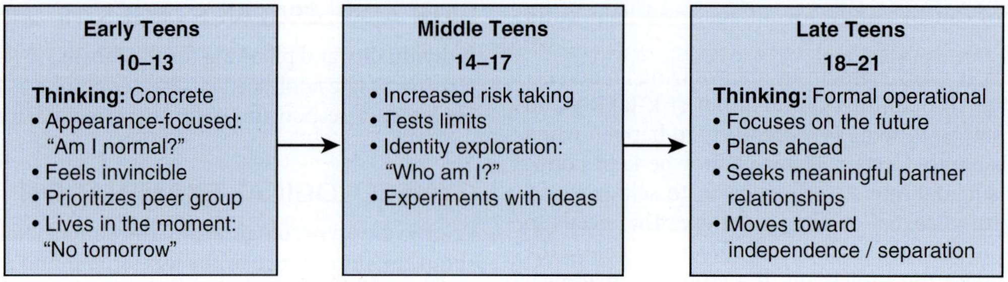

FIGURE 67.1 Adolescent psychologic development.

A pelvic exam is rarely required in an adolescent female who has never been sexually active unless there are specific gynecologic concerns. Routine Papanicolaou (Pap) smears are not required for normal-risk adolescents. Current American College of Obstetrics and Gynecology (ACOG) screening guidelines recommend initiating Pap smears at age 21, regardless of whether the patient is sexually active or not. Screening for sexually transmitted infections (STIs) should be performed at least annually in all sexually active adolescents <25 years old; testing should also be performed anytime new exposure risk or symptoms are present. STI screening can be performed by the patient doing a vaginal self-swab or a urine specimen.

Inspection of the external genitalia includes evaluation of the pubic hair, labia majora and minora, clitoris, urethra, and hymenal ring. A knee-chest position can be used to better assess abnormalities of the hymen. Stirrups should be used when a speculum exam is required. The speculum allows visualization of the vagina, assessing for any discharge or signs of infection, and the cervix if a Pap smear is required. In the rare circumstance that a speculum examination is necessary in a female who has not previously had vaginal intercourse, a Huffman (pediatric) or small Pederson (narrow) speculum should be used. Bimanual exam allows palpation of the internal genitalia and should be performed after any vaginal swabs are taken, because lubricants can interfere with the evaluation of microscopic and microbiologic samples.

BREAST CHANGES IN FEMALES AND MALES

Breast Asymmetry and Masses in Females

The breast bud is a pea-sized mass below the nipple that is often tender. One breast may begin to grow before the other or grow more rapidly, with resulting asymmetry. Reassurance should be provided that after full maturation, the asymmetry will be less obvious and that all women have some degree of asymmetry. Occasionally adolescents present with a breast mass; usually these are benign fibroadenomas or cysts (Table 67.3). An ultrasound is superior to mammography in this population.

Gynecomastia in Males

Breast enlargement (gynecomastia) in males is common (50–60%) and usually benign and self-limited. Gynecomastia may be noted in various conditions including morbid obesity (Table 67.4).

Typical findings include the appearance of a round (1–3 cm) freely mobile, often tender, and firm mass immediately beneath the areola during sexual maturity rating stage 3. Large, hard, or fixed enlargement and masses associated with any nipple discharge warrant further investigation. Reassurance is usually the only treatment required for benign gynecomastia. If the condition worsens and is associated with psychologic morbidity, it may be treated with surgery or medication.

TABLE 67.3 Etiology of Breast Masses in Adolescents
Classic or juvenile fibroadenoma (most common)
Fibrocystic disease
Breast cyst
Abscess/mastitis
Intraductal papilloma
Fat necrosis/lipoma
Cystosarcoma phyllodes (low-grade malignancy)
Adenomatous hyperplasia
Hemangioma, lymphangioma, lymphoma (rare)
Carcinoma (<1%)

TABLE 67.4 Etiology of Gynecomastia
Idiopathic
Hypogonadism (primary or secondary)
Liver disease
Kidney disease
Hyperthyroidism
Neoplasms
Adrenal
Ectopic human chorionic gonadotropin secretion
Testicular
Medications
Antiandrogens
Antibiotics (isoniazid, ketoconazole, metronidazole)
Antacids (H_2 blockers)
Cancer chemotherapy (especially alkylating agents)
Cardiovascular drugs
Psychoactive agents (diazepam, phenothiazines, tricyclics)
Drugs of abuse
Alcohol
Amphetamines
Heroin
Marijuana
Hormone imbalance
Anabolic steroid use

PEARLS FOR PRACTITIONERS

See Adolescent Medicine: Pearls for Practitioners at the end of this section.

REVIEW QUESTIONS

Available online.

CHAPTER 68
Adolescent Gynecology

VAGINAL DISCHARGE

Physiologic leukorrhea is due to estrogen's effects on the vagina and cervix following puberty and may be increased mid-cycle at the time of ovulation. Physiologic leukorrhea is clear or white. Yeast is a thick, white, clumpy discharge and is associated with pruritus. Bacterial vaginosis may have a stereotypical "fishy" odor. STIs may be asymptomatic. A focused history should be obtained, particularly inquiring whether the patient is sexually active. Swabs can be obtained for STIs, yeast, and bacterial vaginosis. Adolescents can be instructed to do their own vaginal swab, so a speculum exam is not required. If sexually active, this opportunity also allows the discussion of condom use for STI protection and contraceptive options. Up-to-date treatment options for vaginal infections and STIs are available on the Centers for Disease Control and Prevention website (cdc.gov).

MENSTRUAL DISORDERS

Amenorrhea

Primary amenorrhea is defined as the absence of menstruation by 15 years of age in the *presence* of secondary sexual characteristics, 13 years of age in the *absence* of secondary sexual characteristics, or no onset of menses within 3–4 years of thelarche. Features that should prompt earlier evaluation include signs of hirsutism, a history of excessive exercise or an eating disorder, or absence of menses at any age with symptoms suggestive of an outflow tract obstruction (e.g., cyclic abdominal pain).

Primary amenorrhea may be a result of functional or anatomic abnormalities of the hypothalamus, pituitary gland, ovaries, uterus, cervix, or vagina. The most common etiologies are ovarian failure (e.g., primary ovarian insufficiency, Turner syndrome) and Müllerian agenesis. The history and physical examination should guide further evaluation.

An outflow tract obstruction should be suspected in adolescents with primary amenorrhea, cyclic abdominal pain, and normal secondary sexual characteristics. The most common cause is an **imperforate hymen**, which is easily evident on exam, with a characteristic blue, bulging membrane. Higher outflow tract anomalies require imaging to confirm the diagnosis and should be strongly suspected with a history of kidney anomalies. A single-digit vaginal/bimanual examination or rectoabdominal exam may allow palpation of a hematocolpos or hematometra (blood accumulated in the vagina or uterus).

An endocrine evaluation is indicated for females with primary amenorrhea without secondary sexual characteristics (see Chapter 175). An elevated follicle-stimulating hormone (FSH) over 25 IU/L on two occasions 4 weeks apart indicates hypergonadotropic hypogonadism, which may reflect ovarian dysgenesis/agenesis and warrants a karyotype looking for **Turner syndrome.** Other etiologies include autoimmune diseases and fragile X pathogenic variant carriers. Low levels of FSH indicate hypogonadotropic hypogonadism, which may be due to constitutional delay (more common in males than females), isolated gonadotropin deficiency (e.g., Kallmann syndrome or CHARGE syndrome), a central nervous system (CNS) lesion, or hypothalamic dysfunction (chronic illness, low body weight/disordered eating, stress). Additional hormone evaluation may include thyroid-stimulating hormone (TSH) and prolactin. Hypothyroidism is a common cause of menstrual dysfunction. If prolactin is elevated, imaging to evaluate for a prolactinoma should be performed.

Secondary amenorrhea refers to the cessation of menses for more than 3 consecutive months in females who previously had regular menses or greater than 6 months in females who had irregular menses. The most common causes of secondary amenorrhea are pregnancy, anorexia/stress (low luteinizing hormone [LH], FSH, and estradiol), and **polycystic ovary syndrome (PCOS)**. With PCOS there may be symptoms of androgen excess, such as acne and hirsutism, weight gain, and, with insulin resistance, acanthosis. If hirsutism or virilization is present, free (or bioavailable) and total testosterone, androstenedione, and dehydroepiandrosterone sulfate (DHEAS) should be measured to evaluate for ovarian or adrenal tumors. A normal 17-hydroxyprogesterone level rules out late-onset **congenital adrenal hyperplasia.** The diagnosis of PCOS may be difficult in adolescence because there is considerable overlap between normal pubertal development and PCOS. After excluding other etiologies of irregular menses and hyperandrogenism, PCOS may be diagnosed with infrequent menstrual bleeding (or amenorrhea) that has persisted for more than 2 years after menarche in conjunction with clinical or biochemical evidence of hyperandrogenism. Hyperandrogenism in adolescents is defined as moderate or severe hirsutism, persistent acne that is poorly responsive to treatment, or persistent elevation of total and/or free testosterone. There are no compelling criteria for polycystic ovarian morphology on imaging in adolescents; ovarian ultrasound imaging can be deferred during the evaluation of PCOS in this age group. Patients may have impaired glucose tolerance or hypercholesterolemia even in adolescence.

Treatment for amenorrhea should be directed at the underlying cause. Anovulation can be managed with either cyclic progesterone withdrawal or combined hormonal contraceptives (CHCs). For ovarian failure, therapy is directed at replacing estrogen and progesterone, either with a combined hormone replacement regimen or a CHC. With reversible etiologies of hypothalamic amenorrhea, therapy is directed at modifying the contributing factors (e.g., stress, exercise, or dietary changes). For PCOS, conservative measures include weight loss and exercise, which may restore ovulatory cycles. Some individuals will require cyclic progesterone or CHC. If there is evidence of androgen excess, CHCs reduce androgen production from the ovaries and increase sex hormone–binding globulin to reduce the amount of bioavailable testosterone. The need for contraception can make a CHC a good choice. Other options include spironolactone, which improves hirsutism, or metformin, which can restore ovulatory cycles.

Abnormal Uterine Bleeding

The International Federation of Gynecology and Obstetrics (FIGO) nomenclature and classification of **abnormal uterine bleeding (AUB)** define menstrual disorders (Table 68.1).

Normal menses occur at intervals of 21–35 days. The average duration of flow is 3–7 days. More than 8 well-soaked pads or 12 tampons per day may be considered heavy menstrual bleeding (HMB). Charting on a menstrual calendar and use of a pictorial bleeding assessment chart (PBAC) can more accurately quantify the volume of blood loss (Fig. 68.1). A PBAC score above 100 is consistent with greater than 80 mL of menstrual loss and HMB.

The differential diagnosis of AUB uses the PALM COEIN classification system (Table 68.2). The PALM categories include anatomic abnormalities (polyp, adenomyosis, leiomyoma, and malignancy) and are rare causes of AUB in adolescents. Far more common are the categories of AUB-C (coagulopathy) and AUB-O (ovulatory).

Anovulation is the most common etiology of AUB in adolescents, resulting in irregular cycles. Without progesterone (which is produced by the corpus luteum following ovulation), unopposed estrogen causes endometrial thickening and irregular endometrial shedding, which can be prolonged and heavy. Progesterone induces a secretory endometrium ("luteinizes"); when it is withdrawn, the endometrium sheds in a synchronous fashion with myometrial and vascular contractions (causing dysmenorrhea but limiting blood loss). This typically resolves within 2 years postmenarche as the hypothalamic-pituitary-ovarian (HPO) axis matures but can persist up to 4 years, particularly if menarche was late. If concerning symptoms occur at any time (e.g., hirsutism, symptoms of anemia) or if they persist beyond 4 years, investigation is warranted. When irregular bleeding occurs after regular cycles have been established, this usually indicates an organic abnormality. The differential diagnosis of anovulatory bleeding at that time would include thyroid dysfunction, PCOS, and adrenal and pituitary disorders.

Approximately 20% of adolescents with heavy or prolonged menses have a coagulation disorder (even higher if presenting at/soon after menarche) and 10% have other pathology. Clues on history to suspect a coagulopathy are onset of heavy menses with menarche, severity requiring hospital admission or blood transfusion, failure of initial medical therapy, a family

TABLE 68.1 Definition of Menstrual Disorders

CLINICAL DIMENSION	DESCRIPTIVE TERM	DEFINITION
Frequency	Frequent menstrual bleeding	<21 days/cycle
	Infrequent menstrual bleeding	>35 days/cycle
Regularity	Amenorrhea	Absent for ≥6 mo
	Irregular menstrual bleeding	>20-day variation in cycle length
Duration	Prolonged menstrual bleeding	>8 days of flow
	Shortened menstrual bleeding	<2 days of flow
Flow	Heavy menstrual bleeding	>80 mL loss
	Light menstrual bleeding	<5 mL loss
Intermenstrual bleeding		Bleeding between normally timed periods

TABLE 68.2 Differential Diagnosis of Abnormal Uterine Bleeding—PALM COEIN Classification

STRUCTURAL (PALM)	NONSTRUCTURAL (COEIN)
P—Polyps	C—Coagulopathies
A—Adenomyosis	O—Ovulatory disorder
L—Leiomyoma	E—Endometrial
M—Malignancy	I—Iatrogenic
	N—Not otherwise specified

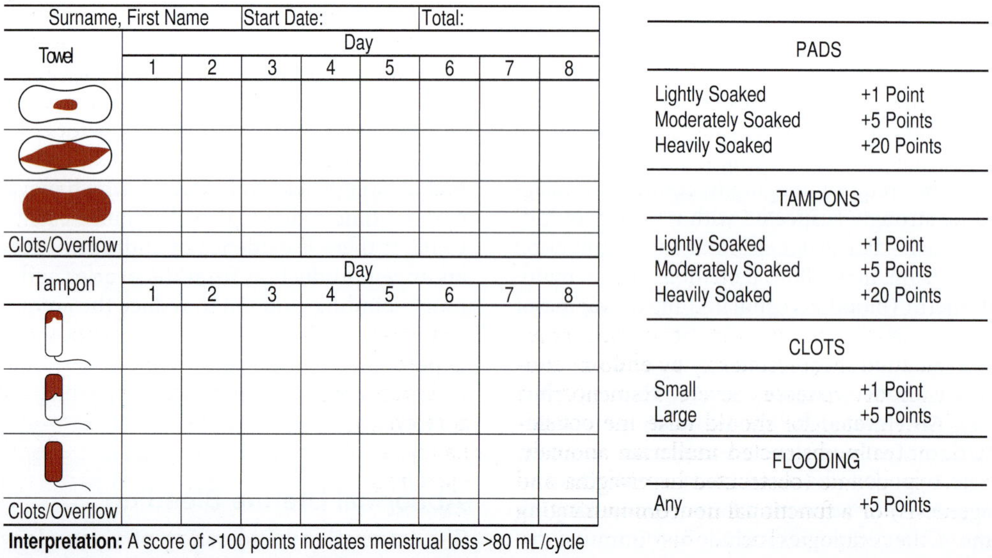

FIGURE 68.1 Pictorial bleeding assessment chart (PBAC). (Modified from Higham JM, O'Brien PM, Shaw RW. Assessment of menstrual blood loss using a pictorial chart. *Br J Obstet Gynaecol.* 1990;97[8]:734–739.)

history of a bleeding disorder, or a personal history of bleeding, easy bruising, or epistaxis. If an underlying pathology is discovered, treatment should be directed at the primary disorder and the secondary menstrual dysfunction. It is important to remember that AUB in sexually active adolescents can be due to pregnancy or STIs or as a side effect of contraception (AUB-I [iatrogenic]).

Physical examination should assess for signs of anemia, bruising, or petechiae and signs of hyperandrogenism or thyroid disease. A pelvic examination should be performed in sexually active adolescents and swabs sent for STIs. A complete blood count, pregnancy test, TSH, and coagulation screen should be performed if appropriate. With a suspicion of PCOS or in the setting of clinical hyperandrogenism, androgens should be included. Due to the infrequency of structural etiologies of AUB at this age, pelvic ultrasound is not recommended as an initial investigation. Unpredictable, heavy, and prolonged menses may impair school attendance and social functioning; iron-deficiency anemia is associated with lower academic scores.

Treatment for AUB should be initiated if there are detrimental effects on health (e.g., anemia) or quality of life. Menstrual irregularity and HMB can be managed with CHCs, which can be prescribed either cyclically or in an extended fashion (e.g., 84 days of active CHC followed by a 5- to 7-day hormone-free interval). Extended use is a good strategy to consider for females with a recognized **bleeding disorder**, such as von Willebrand disease or thrombocytopenia. For acute heavy bleeding, multiple daily doses of CHC may be required until blood loss is controlled and occasionally requires hospitalization for more intensive management. If estrogen is contraindicated, progestin-only methods can be prescribed. The levonorgestrel-releasing intrauterine system has high rates of amenorrhea, provides over 70% reduction in blood loss, and is the most effective contraceptive. Parents may express concern that using contraceptives will encourage their daughter to become sexually active, but literature and experience do not support this. Tranexamic acid is an antifibrinolytic taken only on the heavy days of flow, which can decrease blood loss by up to 50% but does not provide cycle regulation or contraceptive benefits.

Dysmenorrhea

The most common gynecologic complaint of adolescent females is painful menstruation, or dysmenorrhea. **Primary dysmenorrhea** is defined as pelvic pain during menstruation in the absence of pelvic pathology. It develops once ovulation is established. Pain occurs due to prostaglandins and leukotrienes being released from the degenerating endometrium, causing increased uterine tone and contractions.

Secondary dysmenorrhea is menstrual pain associated with pelvic pathology; it accounts for 10% of dysmenorrhea in adolescents and is caused most frequently by **endometriosis** or **pelvic inflammatory disease**. Severe dysmenorrhea within a few months of menarche should raise the consideration of an asymmetrically obstructed mullerian anomaly, such as an OHVIRA syndrome (obstructed hemivagina and ipsilateral renal agenesis) or a functional noncommunicating uterine horn. Secondary dysmenorrhea is often more severe, fails initial medical therapy, and is more commonly associated with atypical features (e.g., pain outside of menstrual cycle, dyschezia, dyspareunia). Ultrasound is the recommended initial evaluation for obstructing genital tract lesions. Magnetic resonance imaging is the gold standard for diagnosing complex reproductive tract anomalies in this age group.

Treatment of primary dysmenorrhea should start with nonsteroidal antiinflammatory drugs (NSAIDs) such as ibuprofen, naproxen, or mefenamic acid. To maximize efficacy, NSAIDs should be taken prior to or immediately at onset of bleeding, closely following the dosing schedule. If NSAIDs fail to provide adequate relief, if contraception is needed, or if features of AUB are also present, then hormonal treatment can be initiated. CHCs (cyclical or extended) or long-acting reversible contraceptives (LARCs), such as the levonorgestrel-releasing intrauterine system, can be used. If dysmenorrhea persists despite an adequate trial of hormonal therapy, an alternative diagnosis should be considered, such as endometriosis. The patient should be referred to gynecology to consider additional investigations, alternative medical treatments for endometriosis (such as dienogest or gonadotropin-releasing hormone agonists), or possible surgical exploration with laparoscopy.

PREGNANCY

In 2023, 32% of American never-married teenagers aged 15–19 years old reported ever having had sexual intercourse. This has gradually declined since 2013 (47%). Risk factors for adolescent pregnancy include lower socioeconomic status, lower educational attainment, low self-esteem, lack of access to contraception, alcohol and drug use, and adverse early life experiences in the home. In 2023 the teen birth rate was 13.1/1,000, which has continued to decline every year from a peak of 61.8 in 1991. The teen birth rate in the United States remains higher than that in other developed countries.

Diagnosis

Pregnancy should be considered in any adolescent female presenting with secondary amenorrhea. Frequently, pregnant adolescents delay seeking a diagnosis until several periods have been missed and initially may not disclose having had intercourse. Young adolescents may present with other symptoms, such as vomiting, vague pain, or deteriorating behavior and may report normal periods. Because of the varied presentations of adolescent pregnancy, a thorough menstrual history should be obtained from all menstruating adolescents. Urine pregnancy tests are sensitive approximately 7–10 days after conception. Sexual assault or coercion should be screened for in all cases of adolescent pregnancy. It is important to recognize that adolescent pregnancies are not all unwanted or unplanned. Sensitivity to that awareness and to culture is important in the approach to the pregnant adolescent.

When pregnancy is confirmed, an ultrasound for dating is recommended. Options to continue or terminate the pregnancy should be discussed. Pregnant adolescents should be encouraged to involve their families in decision making, but if competent, these adolescents should be encouraged to make the decision that is right for them.

Continuation of the Pregnancy

Pregnancy risks are influenced by behavior and socioeconomic status as well as inherent biologic risks, particularly in those younger than age 15 years. Adolescents have an increased incidence of preterm and very preterm births, low birthweight infants, infant neonatal admission, neonatal mortality, child abuse, subsequent maternal unemployment, and poor maternal educational achievement. When compared with their peers, children of adolescent parents are more likely to have lower educational achievement, be involved with drugs and alcohol, and become adolescent parents themselves.

Prenatal care for these adolescents should be multidisciplinary, be easily accessible, and focus on both social support and nutritional counseling, which has been shown to improve pregnancy outcomes. Pregnant adolescents should be screened frequently for mood disorders, alcohol and/or drug use, STIs, and interpersonal violence, because reported rates are higher in this age group than in adults. Pregnancy is the most common cause for young women to drop out of school; special attention should be given to continuing education. Contraceptive planning should be initiated in the antenatal care period with continued focus postpartum. Many teens choose to parent the child themselves, but the option of adoption should also be discussed.

Termination

Abortion laws vary by state. The options for pregnancy termination depend on the gestational age, including medical (mifepristone [RU-486]) if less than 10 weeks or surgical (manual vacuum aspiration or suction curettage). Psychosocial support and subsequent contraceptive counseling should be provided.

CONTRACEPTION

Although the proportion of adolescents using contraception the first time they have sex has increased, 20% still initiate intercourse with no contraception, and only 33% report using an effective hormonal birth control method. The best form of contraception is the one an individual will use; thus counseling adolescents about all methods and supporting their choice is important. A history and physical should be performed to determine whether any contraindications exist to specific methods; the U.S. Medical Eligibility Criteria (U.S. MEC website or app) provides recommendations for using specific contraceptive methods by women who have certain characteristics or medical conditions. Contraceptives can be divided into user-based methods and LARCs. Although LARCs are recommended as first-line options, only the minority of adolescents choose these methods. Focused education around LARCs and removing the barriers of cost and access have been shown to improve uptake. It is important to remind young women that any hormonal method requires concomitant use of condoms for STI protection.

Steroidal Contraception

Long-Acting Reversible Contraceptives

Implants

The subdermal etonogestrel (progestin) implant is a single rod inserted subcutaneously in the upper inner arm. Effective for 3 years, it has the lowest failure rate of any contraceptive method (0.05% of 100 women during the first year of typical use). The primary mechanism of action is suppression of ovulation; there may be additional efficacy from thickening cervical mucus and endometrial atrophy. Quick starts are possible, with insertion on the day of presentation once pregnancy has been excluded. The implant does not need to be inserted at a specific time in the menstrual cycle. Patients should be counseled that the most common side effect is irregular bleeding, particularly in the first 3 months of use. The continuation rate in adolescents is over 80% at 1 year.

Intrauterine Devices

Intrauterine devices (IUDs) are inserted into the uterus, where they release either copper ions or levonorgestrel. Either IUD method is safe for adolescents. A sterile foreign-body reaction in the uterine cavity is a common mechanism of action of both IUD methods. In addition, the copper IUD impairs sperm function and fertilization, whereas the levonorgestrel IUDs induce an atrophic endometrium as well as thickening cervical mucus. The copper IUD has the longest approval for duration of use, up to 10 years; it may increase the amount and duration of bleeding as well as dysmenorrhea. The levonorgestrel-releasing intrauterine systems (L-IUS) contain differing amounts of levonorgestrel, with durations of use of 3 years (for the 13.5 mg IUS), 5 years (for 19.5 mg IUS), and 8 years (for the 52 mg IUS). The 52 mg product decreases menstrual flow by up to 70%, and complete amenorrhea is noted in approximately 20% of users at 1 year. They are prescribed frequently for heavy menstrual bleeding and dysmenorrhea. The two lower dose L-IUSs also decrease menstrual flow but to a lesser extent, less frequently achieving amenorrhea. All IUDs are highly effective (failure rates of 8/1,000 for copper and 2/1,000 for L-IUS) and have high continuation rates (>85% at 1 year). There is a small increased risk of pelvic inflammatory disease for 21 days after insertion; hence adolescents should be screened for STIs prior to or at the time of IUD insertion. Oral analgesia can decrease insertion-related discomfort and a paracervical block can also be considered, particularly for nulliparous people.

Hormonal Injections

Depo-medroxyprogesterone acetate (DMPA) is available in two formulations: intramuscular injection of 150 mg every 12–14 weeks or 104 mg/0.65 mL for subcutaneous use every 12–14 weeks. The primary mechanism of action is suppression of ovulation with a secondary effect on cervical mucus and the endometrium. DMPA is associated with very high rates of amenorrhea (70%); some may experience frequent or irregular menstrual bleeding. The average weight gain on DMPA is 5 lb in the first year; some continue to gain weight following that. A decrease in bone mineral density is reversible after cessation, but adolescents should be counseled about adequate calcium and vitamin D intake and not smoking. Continuation rates of DMPA in adolescents at 1 year are less than with other LARCs.

Combined Hormonal Contraceptives

CHCs are available in oral, transdermal, and vaginal routes of administration. All contain synthetic estrogen and progesterone that suppress gonadotropin secretion and ovulation. CHCs also induce endometrial atrophy (inhospitable for blastocyst implantation) and thicken cervical mucus to inhibit sperm penetration. Absolute (category 4) and relative (category 3) contraindications to CHCs are listed in Table 68.3. CHCs are 99% effective with perfect use and have numerous noncontraceptive benefits including improved acne, dysmenorrhea, and menstrual flow. Any CHC can be used in an extended fashion by limiting hormone-free days to extend intervals between withdrawal bleeds.

Oral contraceptive pills need to be taken at approximately the same time daily. Due to poor compliance, oral CHCs tend to have higher failure rates (~8%/year) and continuation rates at 1 year are low. There are different formulations of oral CHCs available that vary in the type, dose, and duration of estrogen and progestin, as well as variation in the number of placebo pills. The contraceptive patch is a 25-cm^2 pink patch containing ethinyl estradiol and norelgestromin that is applied to the skin of the torso, buttocks, or arm. A new patch is applied each week for 3 weeks, then no patch is worn the fourth week to allow for a withdrawal bleed. It is less efficacious in women weighing more than 90 kg. The contraceptive vaginal ring is a flexible, silastic ring that releases 15 mcg of ethinyl estradiol and 120 mcg of etonogestrel per day. Each ring is placed in the vagina for 3 weeks, and a new ring is inserted 7 days later.

After a history, physical examination (including blood pressure), and confirming the patient is not pregnant, CHCs can be started on the first day of the next menstrual period or as a "quick start." The quick start method refers to starting on any day of the cycle as soon as the teen has the medication available. A backup method should be used for 7 days. The adolescent should be seen again within a few months to reinforce good contraceptive use and safer sex.

Initial **side effects**, such as nausea, breast tenderness, and breakthrough bleeding, are common and usually transient. CHCs do not generally cause weight gain. Usually 3–4 months on one CHC are needed to determine acceptability. If there is breakthrough bleeding, the physician should determine compliance with the method before prescribing something new. Adolescents should be taught the appropriate response to missed doses.

TABLE 68.3 Absolute and Relative Contraindications to Combined Hormonal Contraceptives

ABSOLUTE CONTRAINDICATIONS (CATEGORY 4)	RELATIVE CONTRAINDICATIONS (CATEGORY 3)
Smoker age >35 yr and >15 cigarettes/day	Smoker age >35 yr and <15 cigarettes/day
Hypertension: >160 systolic or >100 diastolic	Hypertension: controlled or 140–159 systolic or 90–99 diastolic
Cardiac: ischemic heart disease, complicated valvular heart disease, atrial fibrillation, peripartum cardiomyopathy <6 mo	Cardiac: multiple risk factors for arterial cardiovascular disease, peripartum cardiomyopathy >6 mo with no/mild impaired function
Vascular: vascular disease, venous thromboembolic (VTE) disease: acute or high recurrence risk (e.g., thrombophilia), systemic lupus with antiphospholipid antibodies, complicated solid organ transplant	Vascular: VTE on treatment or past history and low recurrence risk, diabetes with end-organ damage (nephropathy, retinopathy, neuropathy)
Neurologic: migraines with focal neurologic symptoms, stroke history	Neurologic: migraine without neurologic symptoms and age >35 yr
Breast: current cancer, postpartum <4 wk + breast-feeding (BF), postpartum <3 wk no BF	Breast: cancer disease-free history >5 yr, postpartum 4–6 wk + BF + other VTE risks, postpartum 3–6 wk + no BF + other VTE risks
Gastrointestinal (GI): liver failure, hepatocellular adenoma, malignant hepatoma, severe cirrhosis	GI: acute viral hepatitis (oral contraceptive pill [OCP] only), symptomatic gallbladder disease, history of combined hormonal contraceptive (CHC)–related cholestasis, malabsorptive bariatric procedures (OCP only)
Immobilization (prolonged): major surgery	Immobilization (prolonged): multiple sclerosis
	Drug interactions: certain anticonvulsants, rifampicin, rifabutin, certain antiretroviral therapies

Modified from Centers for Disease Control and Prevention. U.S. Medical Eligibility Criteria for Contraceptive Use. *CDC, Atlanta: GA, 2024. https://www.cdc.gov/mmwr/volumes/73/rr/rr7304a1.htm.*

Progestin-Only Pills

The norethindrone progestin-only pill is an effective form of contraception when used consistently and is safe with very few contraindications. The norethindrone progestin-only pill is supplied in packages of 28 tablets, each containing norethindrone with no hormone-free interval. The primary mechanism of action is by thickening the cervical mucus, thereby inhibiting penetration by sperm, but it also decreases implantation due to endometrial atrophy. Ovulation is inconsistently suppressed with approximately 40% of cycles still being ovulatory. Progestin-only pills are considered for females with contraindications to estrogen but are chosen less often than CHCs due to the stringent compliance needed (must take within 3 hours of the same time every day, due to a short half-life of only 22 hours); they may not be the best first choice for adolescents. In 2024 the norgestrel progestin-only pill was approved for over-the-counter release in the United States and has very similar qualities.

The drospirenone progestin-only pill has a longer half-life than norethindrone, so the compliance window is similar to a CHC and has comparable efficacy. Its main mechanism of action is inhibition of ovulation. A monthly pack has 24 hormonal pills and 4 placebo pills.

Barrier Methods

Condoms

Condoms are readily accessible without a prescription and provide excellent protection against STIs; due to incorrect use and breakage (higher with non-latex), the contraceptive failure rates are quite high (~15%). Condoms may be chosen by individuals who have infrequent intercourse, but a more reliable method of regular contraception should be encouraged for adolescents long term. The female condom is an additional barrier method made of polyurethane that affords females more control, but adolescents usually do not consider it aesthetically pleasing. Any adolescent using barrier methods should be counseled regarding emergency contraceptive (EC) options.

Sponge, Caps, and Diaphragm

The vaginal sponge is a single-use "one size fits all" spermicide-impregnated synthetic sponge. Both the cervical cap and diaphragm come in various sizes so must be fitted by a health care professional and used with a spermicidal gel. Each of these methods can be difficult to source/get fitted, require placement in advance of intercourse, must be left in place for 6 hours following, and have significantly higher failure rates than hormonal methods. For all these reasons, they are a less favorable choice for adolescents.

Emergency Postcoital Contraception

Emergency postcoital contraception (EC) should be discussed at every visit and a prescription given in advance when over-the-counter access is unavailable. EC reduces the risk of pregnancy after unprotected intercourse or in the case of condom breakage. Indications and contraindications are listed in Table 68.4. There are several forms of EC. The copper IUD can be inserted up to 7 days after unprotected intercourse; it is the most effective EC method with an efficacy of greater than 99%, but access can be a barrier.

A single dose of levonorgestrel 1.5 mg (or two 0.75 mg tablets) or ulipristal acetate (UPA) 30 mg can be taken up to 5 days after unprotected intercourse. Effectiveness is higher the earlier the method is used. Both hormonal methods are equally effective if taken within 72 hours; UPA is superior to levonorgestrel if treatment is delayed more than 72 hours and in young women with a body mass index (BMI) greater than 25 kg/m^2. Another hormonal contraceptive can be started immediately after levonorgestrel use; it should be delayed for 5 days after UPA use. Multiple CHC pills may be taken to deliver the equivalent of 100 mcg of ethinyl estradiol and 500 mcg of levonorgestrel 12 hours apart (Yuzpe regimen). This method is associated with significantly more nausea and vomiting (an antiemetic should be given) and is less effective. Following EC use, a pregnancy test should be completed if normal menstrual bleeding does not occur within 21 days. Young women who use EC should be counseled on alternative contraceptive methods.

Coitus Interruptus and Rhythm Method (Periodic Coital Abstinence)

Neither coitus interruptus nor the rhythm method are reliable methods of pregnancy prevention. Withdrawal is ineffective because sperm are released into the vagina before ejaculation, and withdrawal may occur after ejaculation has begun. The rhythm method attempts to avoid intercourse around the time of ovulation, which cannot be accurately predicted with any degree of certainty, particularly in adolescents who are more likely to have irregular cycles.

Oral and Anal Sex

Some adolescents engage in oral or anal sex because they believe that it eliminates the need for contraception; they do not consider this activity as "having sex." Condoms generally are not used during oral or anal sex, but the risk of acquiring an STI is still present. Adolescents should be asked specifically about nonvaginal forms of sexual activity. Adolescents who engage in oral and anal sex require STI (including HIV) counseling and screening.

TABLE 68.4 Emergency Contraception

INDICATIONS
• No method of contraception being used • Condom breaks, slips, or leaks • Diaphragm or cervical cap dislodged/removed <6 hr • Missed hormonal contraceptive • Error in using withdrawal (ejaculation on external genitalia or in vagina) • Sexual assault on no reliable contraceptive
CONTRAINDICATIONS
• Known pregnancy • If strong contraindications to estrogens, use progestin • If uterine anomaly, do not use intrauterine device

SEXUAL VIOLENCE

One in 9 females and 1 in 53 males under the age of 18 experience sexual abuse or assault at the hands of an adult. The perpetrator is known in 93% of cases; 34% are family members. Fifteen percent of all sexual assaults occur in adolescents age 12–17, and the vast majority are female. Although gathering historical and physical evidence for a criminal investigation is important, the physician's primary responsibility is to perform these functions in a supportive, nonjudgmental manner. The history should include details of the sexual assault, time from the assault until presentation, whether the victim cleaned themselves already, date of last menstrual period, and previous sexual activity, if any.

For optimal results, forensic material should be collected within 72 hours of the assault. Clothes, especially undergarments, need to be placed in a paper bag for drying (plastic holds humidity, which allows organisms to grow, destroying forensic evidence). The patient should be inspected for bruising and bites as well as oral, genital, and anal trauma. Photographs are the best record to document injuries. Specimens should be obtained from the fingernails, mouth, genitalia, pubic hair, and anus. The sexual assault evidence kit (SAEK) provides materials to obtain DNA from semen, saliva, blood, fingernail swabs, and pubic hair. A wet mount of vaginal fluids shows the presence or absence of sperm under the microscope. STI testing should occur but is usually negative (unless the patient was previously infected) because 72 hours are needed for the bacterial load to be sufficient for a positive result. Blood should be drawn for baseline HIV and syphilis testing. The full timeline of treatment for sexual assault is outlined in Table 68.5. All materials must be maintained in a "chain of evidence" that cannot be called into question in court.

SEX TRAFFICKING AND EXPLOITATION IN ADOLESCENCE

Sex trafficking and exploitation are critical risks for adolescents that health care providers must be prepared to recognize. Clinicians in any setting may encounter youth who are at risk of, or already experiencing, exploitation. Because few adolescents openly disclose exploitation, providers need a trained eye for risk factors and indicators. A trauma-informed, rights-based, and culturally sensitive approach helps build trust, making it easier for adolescents to feel safe and understood during clinical interactions. Table 68.6 summarizes common risk factors and indicators that clinicians can use as a reference during adolescent visits.

There are validated screening tools shown to be effective in identifying risks of exploitation (Table 68.7). These tools incorporate trauma-informed elements to ensure patient comfort, privacy, and empowerment during the screening process. Screening tools specifically developed for identifying online victimization risks are also available, and when used in conjunction with a trauma-informed approach, can aid in the early identification of at-risk adolescents.

Alongside screening, it is essential to engage families in open, sensitive discussions about the potential for exploitation, ensuring that they understand the risk factors that may affect their child. This awareness can empower caregivers to support their child's safety. A trauma-informed, culturally

TABLE 68.5 Treatment for Sexual Assault

- Empiric treatment for chlamydia, gonorrhea, and trichomonas for females and for chlamydia and gonorrhea for males
  - Females: Ceftriaxone 500 mg intramuscular (IM) in a single dose PLUS doxycycline 100 mg orally 2 times per day for 7 days PLUS metronidazole 500 mg orally 2 times per day for 7 days
  - Males: Ceftriaxone 500 mg IM in a single dose PLUS doxycycline 100 mg orally 2 times per day for 7 days
- Emergency contraception should be considered when the assault could result in pregnancy.
- Human immunodeficiency virus (HIV) postexposure prophylaxis recommended based on risk assessment if assault survivor presents within 3 days of assault.
- Hepatitis B postexposure vaccination if hepatitis status of the assailant is unknown and survivor not previously or incompletely vaccinated; if assailant is known to be HBsAg positive, hepatitis B immune globulin (HBIG) should also be given. Human papillomavirus (HPV) vaccination for survivors who are unvaccinated or incompletely vaccinated.
- At 1–3 weeks, repeat sexually transmitted infection (STI) and pregnancy testing.
- At 4–6 weeks and 12 weeks, serology for syphilis, hepatitis, and HIV.
- Immediate and ongoing psychological support.

Adapted from the Centers for Disease Control and Prevention. Sexually Transmitted Infections Treatment Guidelines, 2021: Sexual Assault and Abuse and STIs—Adolescents and Adults. *CDC. Atlanta, GA. https://www.cdc.gov/std/treatment-guidelines/sexual-assault-adults.htm. Accessed May 17, 2025.*

TABLE 68.6 Common Risk Factors and Indicators for Adolescent Sex Trafficking

RISK FACTOR	INDICATOR DESCRIPTION
Homelessness or runaway youth	Adolescents lacking stable housing are at heightened risk due to vulnerability and limited support systems.
Previous history of abuse	Past experiences of physical, emotional, or sexual abuse increase susceptibility to further exploitation.
Family dysfunction or instability	Unstable or disruptive family environments can lead to increased risk behaviors or seeking support elsewhere.
Poverty and socioeconomic challenges	Economic hardship may push youth toward exploitative situations as a means of survival.
Involvement in child protection services	Youth involved in child protection often lack consistent support networks, heightening vulnerability.
Involvement in the juvenile justice system	Justice system involvement may indicate prior risky behaviors or lack of stable, positive influences.
Marginalization due to LGBTQ+ status	LGBTQ+ adolescents may face social exclusion or discrimination, increasing isolation and vulnerability.
Recent migration or refugee status	Migration or refugee status can create social isolation and economic vulnerability, raising exploitation risks.
Exposure to community or family violence	Living in or experiencing violent settings can normalize risky or exploitative relationships.
Cultural isolation or barriers	Cultural isolation can limit access to support and increase vulnerability due to lack of resources.

TABLE 68.7 Screening Tools for Sex Trafficking

TOOL NAME	PURPOSE	KEY FEATURES	TRAUMA-INFORMED ELEMENTS
Human Trafficking Screening Tool (HTST)	Identifies trafficking risks in clinical and social service settings	Includes questions on housing, work, relationships, and exploitation history	Uses nonjudgmental language and emphasizes confidentiality
Commercial Sexual Exploitation-Identification Tool (CSE-IT)	Assesses risk of sexual exploitation in children and adolescents	Validated tool designed for use by child welfare and juvenile justice professionals	Culturally sensitive approach; avoids retraumatization through neutral phrasing
Child Sex Trafficking Victim Identification Tool (CST-VIT)	Helps identify youth at risk of or experiencing sex trafficking	Focuses on red flags such as inconsistent stories, branding, or controlling relationships	Encourages rapport-building to reduce stress during screening
Quick Youth Indicators for Trafficking (QYIT)	Provides a brief, targeted screening for trafficking indicators	Short, trauma-informed format for quick assessment in busy clinical settings	Focuses on patient comfort, privacy, and empowerment during the process

TABLE 68.8 Common Types of Online Victimization, Risk Factors, and Indicators That Clinicians Can Reference During Adolescent Visits to Screen for Exploitation

TYPE OF ONLINE VICTIMIZATION	RISK FACTORS	INDICATORS
Cyberbullying	High social media use, low self-esteem, lack of parental supervision	Sudden withdrawal from social interactions, anxiety about using devices
Sexual solicitation	History of abuse, social isolation, unsupervised online access	Secretive behavior online, reluctance to discuss online interactions
Exposure to harmful content	Frequent internet access, lack of digital literacy, mental health challenges	Emotional distress, exposure to age-inappropriate material, mood swings
Privacy invasion	Sharing personal information online, insufficient privacy settings, peer pressure	Identity theft concerns, anxiety over personal data misuse
Online grooming	Frequent online gaming or chat use, low self-confidence, lack of trusted adult support	Meeting strangers online, inappropriate messages, secretive about online friends

sensitive approach is essential when working with at-risk or trafficked youth. This care model emphasizes respect, awareness of cultural context, and the need to establish comfort and trust with each patient, fostering an environment where adolescents are more likely to disclose risks or concerns.

ONLINE VICTIMIZATION

With the widespread use of digital platforms, online victimization is now a significant concern for adolescents. Health care providers need to be aware of the various forms of online victimization, such as cyberbullying, sexual solicitation, and exposure to harmful content (see Table 68.8). Adolescents may not readily disclose these experiences, making it essential for clinicians to recognize indicators of online victimization. By using trauma-informed, culturally sensitive approaches and validated screening tools, providers can create a safe environment that encourages adolescents to share their online experiences. Educating caregivers about online risks and encouraging open family discussions on safe internet practices can further support adolescent well-being.

PEARLS FOR PRACTITIONERS

See Adolescent Medicine: Pearls for Practitioners at the end of this section.

REVIEW QUESTIONS

Available online.

CHAPTER 69
Eating Disorders

Eating disorders are common chronic diseases in adolescents, especially in females. The *Diagnostic and Statistical Manual of Mental Disorders*, Fifth Edition–Text Revision (DSM-5-TR) classifies these as psychiatric illnesses. The diagnosis in young adolescents (pregrowth spurt, premenstrual) may not follow the typical diagnostic criteria for anorexia nervosa (Table 69.1). Avoidant/restrictive food intake disorder (ARFID) is showing a rise in prevalence and can be seen associated with numerous other primary diagnoses.

ANOREXIA NERVOSA

The prevalence of anorexia nervosa is 1.5% in teenage females. The female:male ratio is approximately 20:1, and the condition shows a familial pattern. The cause of anorexia nervosa is unknown but involves a complex interaction between social, environmental, psychologic, and biologic events (Fig. 69.1).

Clinical Manifestations and Diagnosis

Screening for eating disorders is important and is best done as part of the larger psychosocial screen for risk-taking behaviors (see Fig. 66.1). Although it is recommended to interview the teen alone, the adolescent may minimize the problem; thus it is also important to interview the caregivers alone as well. The first event usually described by an affected patient is a behavioral change in eating or exercise (i.e., food obsession, food-related ruminations, overexercise, and/or mood changes). The patient may have an unrealistic body image and feels overweight or even obese, despite appearing excessively thin. The caregivers' response to this situation can be anger, self-blame, focusing attention on the adolescent, ignoring and minimizing the disorder, or even approving the behavior.

The provider should be nonjudgmental, collect information, and assess the differential diagnosis. The **differential diagnosis** of weight loss includes gastroesophageal reflux, peptic ulcer, malignancy, chronic diarrhea, malabsorption, inflammatory bowel disease, increased energy demands, hypothalamic lesions, hyperthyroidism, diabetes mellitus, and Addison disease. Psychiatric disorders (primary or comorbid) must also be considered (e.g., substance use disorder, depression, obsessive-compulsive disorder).

The **clinical features** of anorexia can include wearing oversized, layered clothing to hide appearance or, conversely, tight-fitting clothing to exaggerate appearance. Other signs include fine hair on the face and trunk (lanugo-like hair), rough and scaly skin, bradycardia, hypothermia, decreased body mass index, erosion of tooth enamel (due to acid from emesis), and acrocyanosis of the hands and feet. Signs of hyperthyroidism should not be present (see Chapter 176). The diagnostic criteria for anorexia nervosa are listed in Table 69.1.

Treatment and Prognosis

Treatment requires a multidisciplinary approach with family-based therapy. Feeding is accomplished through voluntary intake of regular foods, nutritional formula orally, or use of nasogastric tube. When vital signs are stable, discussion and negotiation of a detailed treatment contract with the patient and the parents or guardians is essential. The first step is to restore body weight.

TABLE 69.1 Diagnostic Criteria for Anorexia Nervosa

A. Restriction of energy intake relative to requirements, leading to a significantly low body weight in the context of age, sex, developmental trajectory, and physical health. *Significantly low weight* is defined as a weight that is less than minimally normal or, for children and adolescents, less than that minimally expected. B. Intense fear of gaining weight or of becoming fat, or persistent behavior that interferes with weight gain, even though at a significantly low weight. C. Disturbance in the way in which one's body weight or shape is experienced, undue influence of body weight or shape on self-evaluation, or persistent lack of recognition of the seriousness of the current low body weight.
Specify whether: **Restricting type:** During the last 3 months, the individual has not engaged in recurrent episodes of binge-eating or purging behavior (i.e., self-induced vomiting or the misuse of laxatives, diuretics, or enemas). This subtype describes presentations in which weight loss is accomplished primarily through dieting, fasting, and/or excessive exercise. **Binge-eating/purging type:** During the last 3 months, the individual has engaged in recurrent episodes of binge-eating or purging behavior (i.e., self-induced vomiting or the misuse of laxatives, diuretics, or enemas).
Specify if: **In partial remission:** After full criteria for anorexia nervosa were previously met, criterion A (low body weight) has not been met for a sustained period, but either criterion B (intense fear of gaining weight or becoming fat or behavior that interferes with weight gain) or criterion C (disturbances in self-perception of weight and shape) is still met. **In full remission:** After full criteria for anorexia nervosa were previously met, none of the criteria have been met for a sustained period of time.
Specify current severity: The minimum level of severity is based, for adults, on current BMI (see below) or, for children and adolescents, on BMI percentile. The ranges below are derived from World Health Organization categories for thinness in adults; for children and adolescents, corresponding BMI percentiles should be used. The level of severity may be increased to reflect clinical symptoms, the degree of functional disability, and the need for supervision. **Mild:** BMI $\geq$ 17 kg/m^2 **Moderate:** BMI 16–16.99 kg/m^2 **Severe:** BMI 15–15.99 kg/m^2 **Extreme:** BMI < 15 kg/m^2

Reprinted with permission from the Diagnostic and Statistical Manual of Mental Disorders, *Fifth Edition, Text Revision (Copyright © 2022). American Psychiatric Association. All Rights Reserved.*

Hospitalization may be necessary (Table 69.2), and a multidisciplinary approach should be taken for the acute management of patients hospitalized with an eating disorder (Table 69.3).

When 80% of normal weight is achieved, the patient is permitted to gain weight at a personal pace. The prognosis includes a 3–5% mortality rate (suicide, malnutrition), the development of bulimic symptoms (30% of individuals), and persistent anorexia nervosa symptoms (20% of individuals).

BULIMIA NERVOSA

The prevalence of bulimia nervosa is 5% in female college students. The female:male ratio is 10:1. Binge-eating episodes consist of large quantities of what the adolescent perceives as forbidden foods or leftovers, consumed rapidly, followed by vomiting. Metabolic abnormalities can result from the excessive vomiting or laxative and diuretic intake. Binge-eating episodes and the loss of control over eating often occur in young women who are overweight with a history of dieting.

Nutritional, educational, and self-monitoring techniques are used to increase awareness of the maladaptive behavior, following which efforts are made to change the eating behavior. Patients with bulimia nervosa may respond to antidepressant therapy, which may help impulse control and/or depression. Be aware that attention deficit/hyperactivity disorder (ADHD) in females is often missed at this age and should be considered. There may be a family history of affective disorders. Patients often feel embarrassed, guilty, and ashamed of their actions. Attempted suicide and completed suicide (5%) are important concerns.

AVOIDANT RESTRICTIVE FOOD INTAKE DISORDER (ARFID)

Avoidant/restrictive food intake disorder (ARFID) is characterized by an extreme avoidance of certain foods or severely restricted food intake that is not driven by body image concerns (Table 69.4). ARFID can present at any age and may be associated with other mental and physical illnesses. Individuals with ARFID may avoid foods due to sensory issues (e.g., texture, color), fear of aversive consequences (e.g., choking or

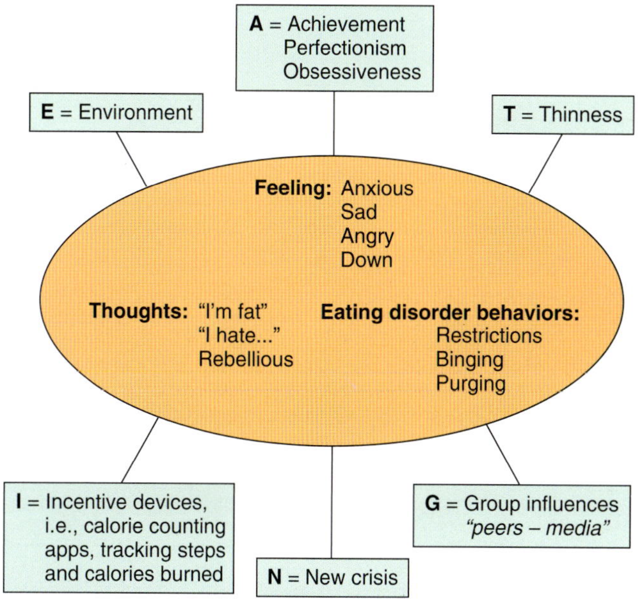

FIGURE 69.1 The "EATING" disorder cycle.

TABLE 69.2 When to Hospitalize a Patient With Eating Disorders

Extremely low body weight (weight <75th percentile ideal body weight)
Acute food refusal
Risk of suicide
Physiologic instability: bradycardia, hypothermia, hypotension, orthostatic changes in heart rate or blood pressure
Dehydration or electrolyte disturbances (hypokalemia, hypophosphatemia)
Dysrhythmias
Failure of outpatient treatment

TABLE 69.3 Acute Management of Patients Admitted With Eating Disorders

- Feed slowly with dietitian advice.
- Monitor electrolytes as refeeding can cause hypophosphatemia,* hypokalemia, and hypomagnesemia.
- Monitor glucose, liver function, calcium, complete blood count, kidney function.
- In prolonged malnutrition, thiamine supplementation to prevent Wernicke encephalopathy.
- Monitor vital signs carefully including orthostatic changes in heart rate and blood pressure.
- Observe individual at risk of self-harm.
- Observe individual at risk of increasing exercise even if in bed.
- Involve psychology team early in admission to start individual- and family-based therapy.

**Hypophosphatemia is a hallmark of refeeding syndrome and requires very close monitoring.*

TABLE 69.4 Diagnostic Criteria for Avoidant/Restrictive Food Intake Disorder

A. An eating or feeding disturbance (e.g., apparent lack of interest in eating or food; avoidance based on the sensory characteristics of food; concern about aversive consequences of eating) associated with one (or more) of the following:
   1. Significant weight loss (or failure to achieve expected weight gain or faltering growth in children)
   2. Significant nutritional deficiency
   3. Dependence on enteral feeding or oral nutritional supplements
   4. Marked interference with psychosocial functioning

B. The disturbance is not better explained by lack of available food or by an associated culturally sanctioned practice.

C. The eating disturbance does not occur exclusively during the course of anorexia nervosa or bulimia nervosa, and there is no evidence of a disturbance in the way in which one's body weight or shape is experienced.

D. The eating disturbance is not attributable to a concurrent medical condition or not better explained by another mental disorder. When the eating disturbance occurs in the context of another condition or disorder, the severity of the eating disturbance exceeds that routinely associated with the condition or disorder and warrants additional clinical attention.

Specify if:

In remission: After full criteria for avoidant/restrictive food intake disorder were previously met, the criteria have not been met for a sustained period of time.

Reprinted with permission from the Diagnostic and Statistical Manual of Mental Disorders, *Fifth Edition, Text Revision (Copyright © 2022). American Psychiatric Association. All Rights Reserved.*

vomiting), or a general lack of interest in eating. This can lead to significant nutritional deficiencies, weight loss, dependence on nutritional supplements, and interference with daily functioning. There is a growing recognition of ARFID, particularly among children and adolescents (including those with comorbid conditions such as anxiety, autism spectrum disorder, and sensory processing issues). With ARFID, early identification and multidisciplinary treatment approaches are important, including medical, psychological, and dietary interventions. Cognitive-behavioral therapy (CBT) and exposure therapy are often used to help individuals gradually increase their food variety and manage anxiety around eating.

PEARLS FOR PRACTITIONERS

See Adolescent Medicine: Pearls for Practitioners at the end of this section.

REVIEW QUESTIONS

Available online.

CHAPTER 70 Substance Use

Substance use among adolescents is common, with vaping and marijuana use increasing, particularly among early teens. The rise in the use of vapes and cannabis edibles, both of which often contain high concentrations of nicotine or tetrahydrocannabinol (THC), introduces unpredictable effects that heighten their dangers. Cocaine use remains prevalent, as does misuse of prescribed amphetamines (i.e., Adderall use during exam periods). The older adolescent population has also seen continued use of nitrous oxide and MDMA (ecstasy), particularly in festival and club settings. Although heroin use has decreased, a far more concerning trend is the rise in fentanyl and fentanyl-laced heroin, both of which have been responsible for overdoses among young people. These shifts highlight the growing complexity and dangers of substance use in the adolescent population.

A history of substance use should be taken in a nonjudgmental and supportive manner and should include the types of substances as well as the frequency, timing, circumstances, and outcomes of substance use. Table 70.1 is a helpful screening tool. There are few physical findings on exam, even with chronic adolescent substance use, outside of acute intoxication. Risk factors for substance use should be explored, as well as protective factors and prevention strategies (Table 70.2).

There are numerous illicit substances available to adolescents, each with their own unique profile and associated symptoms. An adolescent may present in an overdose or in an intoxicated state or in a psychosis triggered by a hallucinogen (Table 70.3). Some drugs used in party settings can have direct (coma and seizures) and indirect (sexual assault and dehydration) adverse effects. Anabolic steroids also have direct (gynecomastia and testicular atrophy) and indirect (mood swings and violence) adverse effects.

The vaping epidemic among adolescents has led to e-cigarettes being the most used tobacco product in this age group. Flavored products and targeted marketing have contributed to increased use, with concerns for nicotine addiction and potential long-term health impacts. Adolescents may also perceive vaping as less harmful than smoking, despite growing evidence of serious risks. Addressing this epidemic requires education, regulation, and preventive measures in schools and health care settings.

The opioid crisis has become increasingly deadly for adolescents. Fentanyl, a potent synthetic opioid, is often mixed with other drugs without the user's knowledge, increasing the risk of overdose. Adolescents may accidentally access fentanyl through household prescriptions or illicit sources, sometimes even within school environments. Its easy availability and the rise of counterfeit pills have made education, awareness, and proper storage crucial in preventing adolescent exposure and overdose. Overdose deaths among adolescents aged 10–19 significantly increased from 2020 to 2022 (following the COVID-19 pandemic), with fentanyl being a key factor. Many deaths involved counterfeit pills, and a large percentage of decedents had mental health conditions. Despite the presence of bystanders, most failed to intervene in overdose situations. Public health responses should focus on educating teens about the risks of fentanyl, reducing access to counterfeit pills, and improving access to mental health and substance use treatment to prevent future deaths.

ACUTE OVERDOSE

Some drugs (most commonly alcohol, amphetamines, opioids, and cocaine) can result in a toxicologic emergency (Table 70.3). Initial management should be directed at appropriate supportive medical treatment, with follow-up counseling after the toxic effects have diminished.

ACUTE AND CHRONIC EFFECTS

Heavy alcohol use can cause acute gastritis and acute pancreatitis. Intravenous drug use can result in hepatitis B, bacterial endocarditis, osteomyelitis, septic pulmonary embolism, infection, and HIV. Chronic marijuana or tobacco use is associated with bronchoconstriction and bronchitis. Compulsive drug or alcohol use results in an adolescent being unable to navigate out of the psychosocial sequelae that attend such habituation (e.g., stealing, prostitution, drug dealing, unemployment, school failure, and social isolation).

TREATMENT

Treatment should be targeted at the specific effects of substances: paranoia (haloperidol), seizures (diazepam), hyperthermia (slow cooling), hypertension (β blockers), and opiate

TABLE 70.1 CRAFFT: A Screening Tool for Adolescent Substance Use

C	Car	Driving under the influence of drugs
R	Relax	Using drugs to relax, fit in, feel better
A	Alone	Drugs/alcohol consumption while alone
F	Forgetting	Forgetting things as a result of drugs/alcohol
F	Family/friends	Family and friends tell teen to stop/cut down
T	Trouble	Getting into trouble because of drugs/alcohol

TABLE 70.2 Risk and Protective Factors for Substance Use

RISK FACTORS	PROTECTIVE FACTORS
• Family history of substance use • Favorable parental attitudes toward the behavior • Poor parental monitoring • Parental substance use • Family rejection of sexual orientation or gender identity • Association with delinquent or substance using peers • Lack of school connectedness • Low academic achievement • Childhood sexual abuse • Mental health issues	• Family support • Parental disapproval of substance use • Parental monitoring • School connectedness • Sports/activity connectedness

TABLE 70.3 Substances Used by Adolescents

SUBSTANCE (STREET/ ALTERNATIVE NAME)	EFFECTS	ROUTE OF ADMINISTRATION (TIME OF ACTION)	DETECTION
Alcohol/liquor	Disinhibition, ataxia, slurred speech, respiratory and CNS depression	Oral (depends on amount and tolerance)	Urine and blood
Nicotine	Relaxation, CNS dependence, ↑ blood pressure, ↑ heart rate, ↓ temperature	Inhaled (minutes); snuffed, dipped, chewed Vape, pens, electronic cigarettes (e-cigs)	Urine
Marijuana (cannabis, weed, joints, pot) Synthetic cannabinoids (K2/ Spice, Scooby Snax)	Euphoria, relaxation, ↑ appetite, ↓ reaction time	Inhaled (minutes); may be smoked (joints, blunts, pipes, bongs) or vaped (often with THC oils) Oral (30 min+) (edibles)	Urine (for up to 1 month after use)

(Continued)

TABLE 70.3 Substances Used by Adolescents—cont'd

SUBSTANCE (STREET/ ALTERNATIVE NAME)	EFFECTS	ROUTE OF ADMINISTRATION (TIME OF ACTION)	DETECTION
STIMULANTS			
Cocaine (coke, crack, blow, snow, powder, rock)	Alertness, euphoria Insomnia, ↓ appetite, irritability, paranoia	Injected (dissolved into water), inhaled (crack cocaine), and snorted (powder) (quick high); oral (longer effect)	Urine (up to 2 days)
Amphetamines (bennies, black beauties, ice) Amphetamines/Adderall (Addy's, study drug, speed, uppers)	Insomnia, ↓ appetite, irregular heartbeat, hypertension	Inhaled, oral, injection Crushed, swallowed, or snorted	Urine (test associated with false positives)
HALLUCINOGENS			
Mescaline (buttons, cactus, mesc)	Psychosis, dilated pupils	Injected, sniffed, ingested (onset: 20–90 min; duration 6–12 hr)	Immunoassay
Psilocybin (magic mushrooms, shrooms)	Dysphoria	Ingested (dry, raw mushrooms, tea) (onset: 20–90 min; duration 6–12 hr)	Immunoassay
Nitrous oxide (whippets, NOS, nitro, buzz bombs)	Hallucinations, dissociation, euphoria	Inhaled via balloons or directly from canisters	Timely screen not available.
LSD (acid)	"Artistic high" "Lucy in the sky with diamonds"	Oral: tablets, liquid, absorbed through mouth using drug-soaked paper (onset: 20–90 min; duration 6–12 hr)	Timely screen not available
Phencyclidine (PCP, angel dust)	Microdots in many colors Can induce suicide attempts	Ingested, inhaled, injected (onset: 20–90 min; duration 6–12 hr)	Urine immunoassay
MDMA (ecstasy, molly, X, E, rolls, beans)*	Euphoria, drowsiness, memory impairment	Oral: tablet or liquid, powder (snorted) (duration: 3–6 hr)	Not detected by routine urine screen MDMA popular at musical festivals and clubs often mixed with other substances
Codeine and morphine	Euphoria, ataxia, miosis, slurred speech	Oral, IV, smoked, snorted, and sniffed	Urine or blood
Heroin (H, horse, smack, junk, black tar)	Euphoria, alternating wakefulness, and drowsiness	Injected, smoked, snorted	Urine or blood
Fentanyl (China white, Apache, jackpot)	Euphoria It is potent and often fatal in small doses, especially the illicitly manufactured fentanyl	Pills, powder (snorted, injected, or absorbed in skin through patches) Often mixed with other drugs such as heroin	Urine
Opium and heroin (free base)	A common adolescent mix	Injected, smoked	Urine
Oxycodone (cotton, hillbilly)	Pain relief, sedation	Oral, IV, inhaled	Urine
TRANQUILIZERS			
Flunitrazepam (Rohypnol, roofies, date rape drugs)		Often mixed in alcohol	Urine (1–24 hr)
Sedatives (barbs, downers)	Sedation	Oral	Urine or blood
Inhalants (solvents, gasoline)	Like alcohol	Inhaled	
Amyl nitrite or butyl nitrite (Poppers, Rush, Snappers, Liquid gold)	Short and intense high and muscle relaxing effects	Inhaled directly from the bottle; sniffing or huffing	
Anabolic steroids	To enhance athletic performance	Oral	Urine

Both a stimulant and hallucinogen.
CNS, Central nervous system; *IV*, intravenous; *LSD*, lysergic acid diethylamide; *MDMA*, 3,4-ethylenedioxy-N-methylamphetamine; *PCP*, phencyclidine.

overdose (naloxone). Long-term management of substance use by adolescents depends on individual patient factors.

Due to the highly addictive (physical and psychologic) nature of substances, intensive counseling and, if necessary, residential drug treatment facilities are suggested, especially for younger adolescents.

PEARLS FOR PRACTITIONERS

See Adolescent Medicine: Pearls for Practitioners at the end of this section.

REVIEW QUESTIONS

Available online.

CHAPTER 71

Sexuality and Gender Identity

The development of sexuality occurs throughout a child's life. Sexuality includes the interplay of gender roles, gender identity, sexual orientation, and sexual behaviors. Sexuality is influenced by biologic and social factors, as well as individual experience. Transgender and gender-diverse (TGD) individuals are those whose gender identity differs from their sex assigned at birth (Table 71.1). Among youth ages 13–17 years in the United States, 1.4% identify as transgender; it is important for all providers to be comfortable providing medical care for these adolescents. The World Professional Association for Transgender Health (WPATH) has established Standards of Care for all health care professionals to assist TGD people in accessing safe and effective pathways to achieving lasting personal comfort with their gendered selves (https://wpath.org/publications/soc8/).

DEVELOPMENT OF SEXUALITY

Sexual development begins early on in childhood. A male infant may have erections, or a toddler may touch their genitals during diaper changes or bathing. During the preschool period, masturbation occurs in both sexes. Reassurance is critical because these behaviors are part of typical child development and represent normal exploration of the body. It is important for preschool age children to learn the proper anatomic names for their body parts and that genitals and sexual behaviors are private. Although it is common for pre-elementary–age children to touch their genitals in public, show their genitals to others, or "play doctor," it would be highly unusual for a child at that age to imitate intercourse or other adult sexual behaviors. If this behavior is occurring, the child should be evaluated for exposure to inappropriate sexual material and possible sexual abuse (see Chapter 21).

Children in elementary school are often intrigued by the topics of pregnancy, birth, and gender roles; often they will begin to preferentially play with children of the same gender. Their curiosity and inquiries should be met with accurate information and limited judgment so that future questions will be directed to reliable resources and not answered by peers or social media.

The biologic, social, and cognitive changes that occur during adolescence place a focus on sexuality. Puberty can be both scary and exciting. One of the principal developmental tasks of this period is to become comfortable with one's own sexuality, and this is often achieved through questioning and experimentation. Some teenagers may try out different sexual practices, including those with members of the same sex, as they explore their own emerging sexuality. The nature of these experiences does not necessarily predict sexual orientation; stereotypical masculine and feminine traits do not predict sexual orientation either.

SEXUAL ORIENTATION

Sexual orientation, the pattern of physical and emotional arousal toward another person, is not always the same as sexual behavior. An individual's sexual orientation emerges before or early in adolescence. Although many adolescents have sexual experiences with a same-sex partner (10–25%, more often reported by males than females), fewer will affirm LGBTQ (lesbian, gay, bisexual, transgender, queer or questioning) orientation by late adolescence. By 18 years of age, most individuals endorse certainty around their sexual orientation.

There is no reliable way to predict an individual's sexual orientation. Identical twins (even twins raised in separate families) show a higher concordance rate for sexual orientation than would be expected by chance alone but nowhere near 100%, as would be expected if genetics were the sole determinant. Attempts to correlate brain imaging or levels of androgens and estrogens with sexual orientation are inconsistent. Although it is well established that parents tend to treat males and females differently, there is no evidence that parental behavior alters the developmental trajectory toward sexual orientation.

Classic definitions of heterosexuality, homosexuality, and bisexuality do not account for the complex interplay of sexual identity, behaviors, and attraction. It is important that providers use patient preferred pronouns to promote an environment of inclusivity and to appropriately counsel based on sexual behaviors and not solely on sexual orientation. TGD children and adolescents may face stigmatization derived from homophobia and heterosexism, ostracism, and family rejection. A persistent negative societal attitude toward TGD individuals is reflected in higher rates of social isolation, verbal harassment, and physical assault experienced by sexual minority youth. Educational and unbiased information is often not available in school and community settings where homophobic jokes, teasing, and violence are common. Not surprisingly, sexual minority youth are at high risk for having negative self-esteem, mental health issues, substance use, and sexual risk-taking behaviors. Sexual minority youth are more than twice as likely to report considering suicide than their heterosexual peers, and rates of legal and illegal substance use are significantly higher.

There are significant health disparities for sexual minority youth related to sexual health outcomes. Although sexual behaviors, not sexual orientation, determine risk of STIs, sexual minority youth are more likely to have intercourse at a younger age, are less likely to use contraception, and report a greater number of sexual partners compared to heterosexual peers. Rates of STIs in the minority group of men who have sex with men (MSM) have not declined along with the

TABLE 71.1 Definition of Terms

Biological sex, biological male or female: These terms refer to physical aspects of maleness and femaleness. As these may not be in line with each other (e.g., a person with XY chromosomes may have female-appearing genitalia), the terms biological sex and biological male or female are imprecise and should be avoided.
Cisgender: This means not transgender. An alternative way to describe individuals who are not transgender is "non-transgender people."
Gender dysphoria: This is the distress and unease experienced if gender identity and designated gender are not completely congruent. In 2013 the American Psychiatric Association released the fifth edition of the DSM-5, which replaced "gender identity disorder" with "gender dysphoria" and changed the criteria for diagnosis.
Gender expression: This refers to external manifestations of gender, expressed through one's name, pronouns, clothing, haircut, behavior, voice, or body characteristics. Typically, transgender people seek to make their gender expression align with their gender identity, rather than their designated gender.
Gender identity/experienced gender: This refers to one's internal, deeply held sense of gender. For transgender people, their gender identity does not match their sex designated at birth. Most people have a gender identity of male or female. For some people, their gender identity does not fit neatly into one of those two choices. Unlike gender expression (see below), gender identity is not visible to others.
Gender identity disorder: This is the term used for gender dysphoria/ gender incongruence in previous versions of DSM (see "gender dysphoria"). The *International Classification of Diseases,* 11th revision (ICD-11) now uses "gender incongruence of childhood."
Gender incongruence: This is an umbrella term used when the gender identity and/or gender expression differs from what is typically associated with the designated gender. Gender incongruence is the term used for gender identity–related diagnoses in ICD-11. Not all individuals with gender incongruence have gender dysphoria or seek treatment.
Gender reassignment: This refers to the treatment procedure for those who want to adapt their bodies to the experienced gender by means of hormones and/or surgery. This is also called gender-confirming or gender-affirming treatment.
Gender role: This refers to behaviors, attitudes, and personality traits that a society (in a given culture and historical period) designates as masculine or feminine and/or that society associates with or considers typical of the social role of men or women.
Sex designated at birth: This refers to sex assigned at birth, usually based on genital anatomy.
Sex: This refers to attributes that characterize biological maleness or femaleness. The best known attributes include the sex-determining genes, the sex chromosomes, the H-Y antigen, the gonads, sex hormones, internal and external genitalia, and secondary sex characteristics.
Sexual orientation: This term describes an individual's enduring physical and emotional attraction to another person. Gender identity and sexual orientation are not the same. Irrespective of their gender identity, transgender people may be attracted to women (gynephilic), attracted to men (androphilic), bisexual, asexual, or queer.
Transgender: This is an umbrella term for people whose gender identity and/or gender expression differs from what is typically associated with their sex designated at birth. Not all transgender individuals seek treatment.
Transgender male (also: trans man, female-to-male, transgender male): This refers to individuals assigned female at birth but who identify and live as men.
Transgender woman (also: trans woman, male-to-female, transgender female): This refers to individuals assigned male at birth but who identify and live as women.
Transition: This refers to the process during which transgender persons change their physical, social, and/or legal characteristics consistent with the affirmed gender identity. Prepubertal children may choose to transition socially.
Transsexual: This is an older term that originated in the medical and psychological communities to refer to individuals who have permanently transitioned through medical interventions or desired to do so.

Modified from Hembree WC, Cohen-Kettenis PT, Gooren L, et al. Endocrine treatment of gender-dysphoric/gender-incongruent persons: an Endocrine Society clinical practice guideline. J Clin Endocrinol Metab. *2017;102:3869–3903, table 1.*

downward trend of STIs in adolescents overall, including rates of HIV. Although education about safe sexual practices should be part of all adolescent well-child visits, the Centers for Disease Control and Prevention (CDC) guidelines recommend asking about the gender of all sex partners as part of STI risk assessment. Health care providers should be aware of specific STI screening recommendations for MSM related to anal intercourse (see Chapter 117). Some adolescents who identify as women who have sex with women (WSW) have also had sex with men and require cervical cancer screening per guidelines. Immunization for human papillomavirus per CDC guidelines is recommended for adolescents regardless of gender or sexual behavior. Discussions around highly effective birth control methods are prudent with both heterosexual and sexual minority youth.

Acknowledging that one is LGBTQ and disclosing it to one's parents or caregivers is often extremely stressful. Although many families are supportive of their child's sexual orientation, some may respond very negatively and ostracize their child. Adolescents should be counseled that even parents whose initial reaction is one of shock, fear, or grief can come to accept their child's sexuality. TGD youth are at a high risk for homelessness following parental rejection. Interventions designed to change sexual orientation are strongly opposed and are not only unsuccessful but can be detrimental to the mental health of the child or adolescent. Health care providers should provide reassurance to parents who feel guilt or shame by affirming that sexual minority youth are normal and sexual orientation is not related to parenting practices. Evidence supports improved health outcomes for sexual minority youth who experience family connectedness and receive encouragement and positive support from their parents. For medical and psychosocial reasons, health care providers need to provide an environment in which adolescents feel comfortable discussing their sexual orientation and families can find the support and resources they need (Table 71.2).

DEVELOPMENT OF GENDER IDENTITY

Developing an awareness and appreciation for one's gender identity is an important milestone in psychosocial development. A child can identify oneself as a male or a female by 3 years of age and begins to demonstrate initial expressions of gender identity. Gender atypical behavior is common in young children and may be part of typical development. Gender constancy, the understanding that one is always a male or always a female, is achieved by age 6 years.

Most elementary school–age children show a strong and consistent **gender identity**, and their behaviors **(gender roles)** reflect this. If a child this age is engaging in cross-gender role behaviors or playing with toys that are stereotypically associated with the opposite gender, parents may be concerned about teasing/bullying or about the child's eventual sexual orientation. In assessing parental concerns, the type of behavior exhibited and its consistency and persistence over time should be considered. Gender nonconformity may be seen temporarily, in response to a stressor, such as the birth of an infant of the opposite sex or divorce of the parents. Stating the desire to be of the opposite gender or to be called a name classically used for the opposite gender is more suggestive of persistent gender discordance.

TABLE 71.2 Providing Supportive Health Care Environments for Sexual Minority Youth

Offices should be welcoming to all, regardless of sexual orientation and behavior.
Ensure that office staff and information-gathering forms do not presume heterosexuality of patients or parents (i.e., use gender-neutral language).
All adolescents should have a confidential adolescent psychosocial history including screening and referral for depression, suicidality, other mood disorders, substance use, and eating disorders.
Adolescents should have sexual behaviors and risks assessed, with particular attention to sexually transmitted infection testing guidelines affecting sexual minority youths. This should include contraceptive counseling.
Target behavioral interventions to maximize the individual's strengths and resources and minimize risk-taking behaviors.
Be available to answer questions, correct misinformation, and reinforce that minority sexual orientations are normal.
Support and affirm transgender youth and refer as appropriate.
Support parents in working through adjustment issues related to having a child with a minority sexual orientation and encouraging the commitment to a loving and supportive family environment.
Support gay–straight alliances at schools and zero-tolerance policies for bullying and violence.
Provide information about support groups and resources for sexual minority youth and their families.
If a health care provider does not feel competent to provide appropriate care for sexual minority youth, this person has the responsibility to evaluate and refer families for medically appropriate care.

Data from Levine DA; Committee on Adolescence. Office-based care for lesbian, gay, bisexual, transgender, and questioning youth. Pediatrics. *2013;132(1):198–203.*

TABLE 71.3 Diagnostic Criteria for Gender Dysphoria in Children

A. A marked incongruence between one's experienced/expressed gender and assigned gender, of at least 6 months' duration, as manifested by at least six of the following (one of which must be criterion A1):
1. A strong desire to be of the other gender or an insistence that one is the other gender (or some alternative gender different from one's assigned gender)
2. In boys (assigned gender), a strong preference for cross-dressing or simulating female attire or, in girls (assigned gender), a strong preference for wearing only typical masculine clothing and a strong resistance to the wearing of typical feminine clothing
3. A strong preference for cross-gender roles in make-believe play or fantasy play
4. A strong preference for the toys, games, or activities stereotypically used or engaged in by the other gender
5. A strong preference for playmates of the other gender
6. In boys (assigned gender), a strong rejection of typically masculine toys, games, and activities and a strong avoidance of rough-and-tumble play or, in girls (assigned gender), a strong rejection of typically feminine toys, games, and activities
7. A strong dislike of one's sexual anatomy
8. A strong desire for the primary and/or secondary sex characteristics that match one's experienced gender

B. The condition is associated with clinically significant distress or impairment in social, school, or other important areas of functioning.

Specify if:
With a disorder/difference of sex development (e.g., a congenital adrenogenital disorder such as E25.0 congenital adrenal hyperplasia or E34.50 androgen insensitivity syndrome).

Reprinted with permission from the Diagnostic and Statistical Manual of Mental Disorders, *Fifth Edition, Text Revision (Copyright © 2022). American Psychiatric Association. All Rights Reserved.*

GENDER DYSPHORIA

Gender dysphoria (GD) is defined as marked distress related to the inconsistency between the way an individual may feel and think of oneself (experienced/expressed gender) and the individual's physical or assigned gender. The diagnostic criteria for gender dysphoria differs between children and adolescents/adults (see Table 71.3). GD is 2–4.5 times more common among children assigned male at birth (AMAB) than assigned female at birth (AFAB). By adolescence, the male:female ratio is closer to even. There are some associations between gender atypical behavior in young children and the ultimate development of same-sex attraction; many children with GD grow up to be adults who identify as LGBTQ.

In contrast, the term **transgender** refers to an individual who does not conform to the culturally derived gender role for the sex assigned at birth. A person can have gender dysphoria, a medical diagnosis, without being considered transgender. Most children with GD will not identify as transgender during adolescence and adulthood. Children with GD who demonstrate more insistence in affirming their gender identity, use more declarative language, and are more significantly distressed by their body may be more likely to identify as transgender in adolescence or adulthood.

Transgender youth are often faced with rejection from their community and family, leading to rates of depression, anxiety, and suicidality that greatly exceed those in the general population. Allowing social transitions for prepubescent transgender children may be linked to improved mental health outcomes. This involves family acceptance and allows the child to present in all aspects as the gender role that aligns with the child's gender identity and not the gender assigned at birth. In 2018 the American Academy of Pediatrics confirmed a commitment to gender-affirmative care comprising developmentally appropriate support for the child's gender experience.

GENDER-AFFIRMING CARE

There are multidisciplinary specialty centers across the country to address the needs of transgender children and their families. The Endocrine Society 2017 guideline supports treatment of gender dysphoric/gender-incongruent adolescents who have entered puberty using puberty blockers, following a comprehensive evaluation to confirm the diagnosis and capacity for informed consent. Pubertal onset (Tanner stage 2) corresponds to development of breast buds for AFAB and testicular volume of 4 cc for AMAB individuals. Puberty blockers are GnRH analogues, such as depot leuprolide acetate or the histrelin implant. These GnRH analogues prevent further development of secondary sexual characteristics and help minimize gender dysphoria. The suppression effects are reversible, so with cessation, pubertal development would again continue. During treatment with GnRH analogues, height, weight, Tanner staging, and hormone levels should

TABLE 71.4 World Professional Association for Transgender Health Readiness Standards for Gender-Affirming Surgery

Diagnosis of gender incongruence by a qualified clinician
Marked sustained gender incongruence
Capacity to consent (assent in case of a minor)
Understanding the effects of the specific surgery on reproductive health
Management of mental health and physical comorbidities that can affect the outcomes of the surgery
A minimum of 6 months on hormone therapy (12 months for adolescents) unless it is medically contraindicated or not desired

be monitored every 3 months, as well as annual bone mineral density (BMD) testing.

The initiation of gender-affirming hormones (estrogen or testosterone) is supported by the Endocrine Society for age 16 and over. Timing of gender-affirming surgery is more controversial and rarely performed before the age of majority/18 years old. Access to these surgeries is more limited as well by state and expertise (Table 71.4). It is important to note that access to all forms of gender-affirming care varies state by state.

PEARLS FOR PRACTITIONERS

See Adolescent Medicine: Pearls for Practitioners at the end of this section.

REVIEW QUESTIONS

Available online.

Suggested Readings

Archibald T, Bryant-Waugh R. Current evidence for avoidant restrictive food intake disorder: Implications for clinical practice and future directions. *JCPP Adv*. 2023;3(2):e12160. Published 2023 Apr 3.

Centers for Disease Control and Prevention Centers for Disease Control and Prevention. Emergency contraception. https://www.cdc.gov/reproductivehealth/contraception/mmwr/spr/emergency.html.

Committee on Practice Bulletins-Gynecology, Long-Acting Reversible Contraception Work Group. Practice Bulletin No. 186: Long-Acting Reversible Contraception: Implants and Intrauterine Devices. *Obstet Gynecol*. 2017;130(5):e251–e269.

Das JK, Salam RA, Arshad A, Finkelstein Y, Bhutta ZA. Interventions for Adolescent Substance Abuse: An Overview of Systematic Reviews. *J Adolesc Health*. 2016;59(4S):S61–S75.

Fleming N, O'Driscoll T, Becker G, Spitzer RF; CANPAGO COMMITTEE. Adolescent Pregnancy Guidelines. *J Obstet Gynaecol Can*. 2015;37(8):740–756.

Graham RA, Davis JA, Corrales-Medina FF. The Adolescent with Menorrhagia: Diagnostic Approach to a Suspected Bleeding Disorder. *Pediatr Rev*. 2018;39(12):588–600.

Hay P. Current approach to eating disorders: a clinical update. *Intern Med J*. 2020;50(1):24–29.

Jones K, Salzman GA. The Vaping Epidemic in Adolescents. *Mo Med*. 2020;117(1):56–58.

Klein D, Goldenring J, Adelman W. HEEADSSS 3.0 the psychosocial interview for adolescents updated for a new century fueled by media. *Contemp Pediatr*. 2014;31:16–1628.

Norris ML, Spettigue WJ, Katzman DK. Update on eating disorders: current perspectives on avoidant/restrictive food intake disorder in children and youth. *Neuropsychiatr Dis Treat*. 2016;12:213–218.

Rape, Abuse & Incest National Network. Children and teens: Statistics. https://www.rainn.org/statistics/children-and-teens.

PEARLS FOR PRACTITIONERS

CHAPTER 66

Overview and Assessment of Adolescents

General Adolescent

- Leading causes of adolescent deaths in the United States include unintentional injuries, suicide, and homicide.
- Physical symptoms in an adolescent are often related to psychosocial problems.
- A psychosocial history, including protective and risk-taking behaviors, is important.
- Mental health concerns and substance use are important issues, often intertwined with other problems like stress, peer pressure, and social medical influences.

Laboratory and Physical Changes

- High hematocrit values (males > females) occur because of androgenic stimulation of the bone marrow.
- Alkaline phosphatase levels increase during puberty because of rapid bone turnover.
- Worsening of mild scoliosis can occur during growth spurt.
- Female puberty: thelarche (breast budding) typically starts at around 9 years and is followed by pubarche (pubic hair) approximately 1 year later. Growth spurt occurs 1 year after thelarche at Tanner stage 3 breast development. The mean age of menarche in the United States is 11.9 years.
- Male puberty: (9–14 years) deepening of voice, facial hair, and acne are good indicators of the early stages of male puberty. Testicular enlargement (Tanner stages 1–2) followed by pubic hair at the penis (adrenarche) precedes the axillary hair and growth spurt, which is often much later. Penile enlargement occurs before the growth spurt.

Key Elements for Interviewing an Adolescent Alone

- Discussing confidentiality.
- Separating the caregiver and adolescent.
- Being nonjudgmental—build rapport by discussing activities, hobbies, and interests.
- Use HEADDSSS approach (**h**ome, **e**ducation [friends/bullies], **a**ctivities/**a**lcohol, **d**rugs [including e-cigarettes], **d**iet/**d**epression, **s**ex, **s**uicide/**s**afety, **s**elf).
- Explain which issues cannot be kept confidential: suicidal intent, serious harm to someone else, or experiencing physical or sexual abuse/neglect.

Mature Minor

- Has competence and capacity to understand (is not age specific).
- Can be treated without parental consent.
- Any intervention should be in the best interest of the minor (and documented).

CHAPTER 67
Adolescent Well Care

Interview and Examination of the Adolescent

- The interview shifts from the parent to the adolescent.
- Check pronouns with the adolescent alone.
- Confidentiality is key.
- Examination: explain what you're doing, use simple language, seek consent and offer chaperone, work around regular clothes, and use draping.
- Adolescent psychological development can be divided into early, middle, and late teens.
  - Early (10–13 years): focused on appearance and fitting in with peers
  - Middle (14–17 years): risk-taking behaviors
  - Late (18–21 years): future planning

Gynecological Exam

- A chaperone should be offered.
- A pelvic exam is rarely indicated unless there is a specific gynecologic concern.
- Routine Pap smears are not required in the adolescent.
- STI testing can be performed by the adolescent doing their own vaginal swab or providing a urine specimen.

Breast Changes

- Breast asymmetry in females is common. Most breast masses in adolescents are benign.
- Gynecomastia in males is common and is often self-limiting.

CHAPTER 68
Adolescent Gynecology

- Evaluation for primary amenorrhea should be initiated by age 15 with secondary sexual characteristics, age 13 without secondary sexual characteristics, or earlier in the presence of cyclic pelvic pain, suspicion of an eating disorder, or hyperandrogenism.
- Pregnancy should be excluded in any adolescent presenting with amenorrhea.
- Treatment in reversible causes of hypothalamic amenorrhea (disordered eating, stress) are directed at changing the underlying state to allow resumption of menses.
- Physiologic anovulation is the most common etiology of abnormal uterine bleeding (AUB) in adolescents; treatment may be required if the associated symptoms affect health status or quality of life.
- A coagulopathy should be considered in adolescents with heavy menstrual bleeding that begins at menarche, especially with anemia or a family/personal history of bleeding; anatomical causes are rare.
- Polycystic ovary syndrome (PCOS) is difficult to diagnose in adolescence because it overlaps with physiologic changes in puberty; the diagnosis should be considered with the persistence of both infrequent menstrual bleeding and clinical or biochemical hyperandrogenism.
- First-line therapies for primary dysmenorrhea should consider the need for contraception for an adolescent and include combined hormonal contraceptives, progestin-only contraception, and levonorgestrel intrauterine device (IUD).
- Failure of nonsteroidal antiinflammatory drugs (NSAIDs) and hormonal contraceptives for dysmenorrhea should prompt investigation for secondary etiologies such as endometriosis, pelvic inflammatory disease (PID), or Müllerian anomalies.
- Multidisciplinary adolescent-specific antenatal care can decrease risks associated with teen pregnancy, such as preterm birth, low birthweight infants, and neonatal admissions to intensive care settings.
- Long-acting reversible contraceptives (LARCs) are an acceptable method of contraception for adolescents with high continuation rates and should be offered as first-line methods.
- There are multiple progestin-only methods of contraception for adolescents with contraindications or side effects related to estrogen.
- All sexually active teens should be counseled on emergency contraception (EC), particularly those using only condoms.
- Be aware that there are trauma-informed screening tools available to identify risks of sex trafficking.
- Common types of online victimization are cyberbullying, sexual solicitation, exposure to harmful content, privacy invasion, and online grooming.

CHAPTER 69
Eating Disorders

- Anorexia nervosa occurs in 1–2% of teenage females. There is a female:male ratio of 20:1. Initial signs are behavioral changes in eating, exercise, and mood. Physical signs include oversized clothing, fine hair on face and trunk (lanugo-like hair), bradycardia, hypothermia, decreased body mass index, and erosion of tooth enamel. Diagnostic criteria may be difficult to meet in a younger adolescent.

- Bulimia occurs in 5% of females (with a female:male ratio of 10:1). Patients with bulimia demonstrate binge or excessive eating within a set period of time. There is a sense of lack of control, and patients exhibit behavior to prevent gaining weight (i.e., vomiting, laxatives, diuretics, exercise).
- Avoidant/restrictive food intake disorder (ARFID) is characterized by an extreme avoidance of certain foods or severely restricted food intake that is not driven by body image concerns. Individuals with ARFID may avoid foods due to sensory issues (e.g., texture, color), fear of aversive consequences (e.g., choking or vomiting), or a general lack of interest in eating.
- Patients with an eating disorder should be hospitalized when weight loss exceeds 25% of ideal body weight (less weight loss accepted in young adolescent), with a risk of suicide, or when outpatient treatment fails. Physiologic signs include bradycardia, hypothermia, dehydration, hypokalemia, and dysrhythmias.

CHAPTER 70

Substance Use

- There are specific screening tools such as the CRAFFT (**c**ar, **r**elax, **a**lone, **f**orgetting, **f**amily/friends, **t**rouble) to screen for substance use in adolescents.
- Numerous substances are used by adolescents, often with several different names and routes. Substances may include depressants, barbiturates, tranquilizers, opioids, stimulants, hallucinogens, psilocybin, marijuana, ecstasy, and anabolic steroids.
- Common side effects (with suggested treatment) of substance use are paranoia (haloperidol), seizures (diazepam), hyperthermia (slow cooling), hypertension (β blockers), and opiate overdose (naloxone).
- Substances vary in their popularity, but marijuana and vaping (both nicotine and THC) remain the most used drugs among teens. Being aware of the evolving street names and forms of these drugs is critical for understanding usage trends.
- Fentanyl and illicitly manufactured fentanyl (IMF), which can be 50–100 times more potent than morphine, are the most common drugs in overdoses that cause death. Fentanyl and IMF are often mixed with other drugs without people being aware of this, making them highly dangerous.

CHAPTER 71

Sexuality and Gender Identity

- There is no reliable way to predict an individual's sexual orientation and no evidence that parental behavior alters the developmental trajectory toward a particular sexual orientation.
- Providers should discuss and use language, terminology, and pronouns preferred by transgender and gender-diverse (TGD) youth.
- There are significant health disparities for sexual minority youth related to sexual health outcomes. Education about safe sexual practices should be part of all adolescent well visits, including asking about the gender of all sex partners as part of STI risk assessment.
- TGD youth have higher rates of depression, anxiety, self-destructive choices, and suicide. Connecting with a specialty center with a multidisciplinary team to address the needs of TGD children and their families is vital.

IMMUNOLOGY

James W. Verbsky

CHAPTER 72

Immunologic Assessment

The major components of host defense include anatomic barriers and the innate and adaptive immune systems (Fig. 72.1). Integrity of the **anatomic** and **mucociliary barrier** (i.e., skin and mucous membranes) is essential for protection against infection (Table 72.1). The **innate immune system** acts as the first line of defense against pathogens, responding rapidly but nonspecifically before development of the more versatile **adaptive immune system**. The innate immune system includes soluble factors, including acute-phase proteins, cytokines, chemokines, and complement, as well as cellular components, including neutrophils, monocytes/macrophages, innate lymphoid cells, and natural killer (NK) cells. The adaptive immune system consists of T and B lymphocytes and their effector molecules (Table 72.2).

Recognition of pathogens by the innate immune system is facilitated by receptors on macrophages, NK cells, and neutrophils that recognize conserved pathogen motifs called **pathogen-associated molecular patterns (PAMPs)** such as lipopolysaccharide of gram-negative bacteria, lipoteichoic acid of gram-positive bacteria, mannans of yeast, and specific nucleotide sequences of bacterial and viral DNA. Recognition of PAMPs by the innate immune system leads to the production of cytokines that initiate inflammation and induce an acute phase response (e.g., C-reactive protein, mannose-binding lectin, complement) and chemokines that recruit inflammatory cells. This also activates antigen-presenting cells, stimulating the adaptive immune system. Complement protein activation on pathogens facilitates their uptake by phagocytic cells or results in lysis of pathogens. Polymorphonuclear neutrophils ingest pyogenic bacteria and some fungi. Macrophages are effective in killing facultative intracellular organisms such as *Mycobacterium, Toxoplasma, Salmonella,* and *Legionella.* NK lymphocytes mediate cytotoxic activity against virus-infected cells and cancer cells.

The key features of the **adaptive immune system** are antigen specificity and the development of immunologic memory, produced by expansion and maturation of antigen-specific

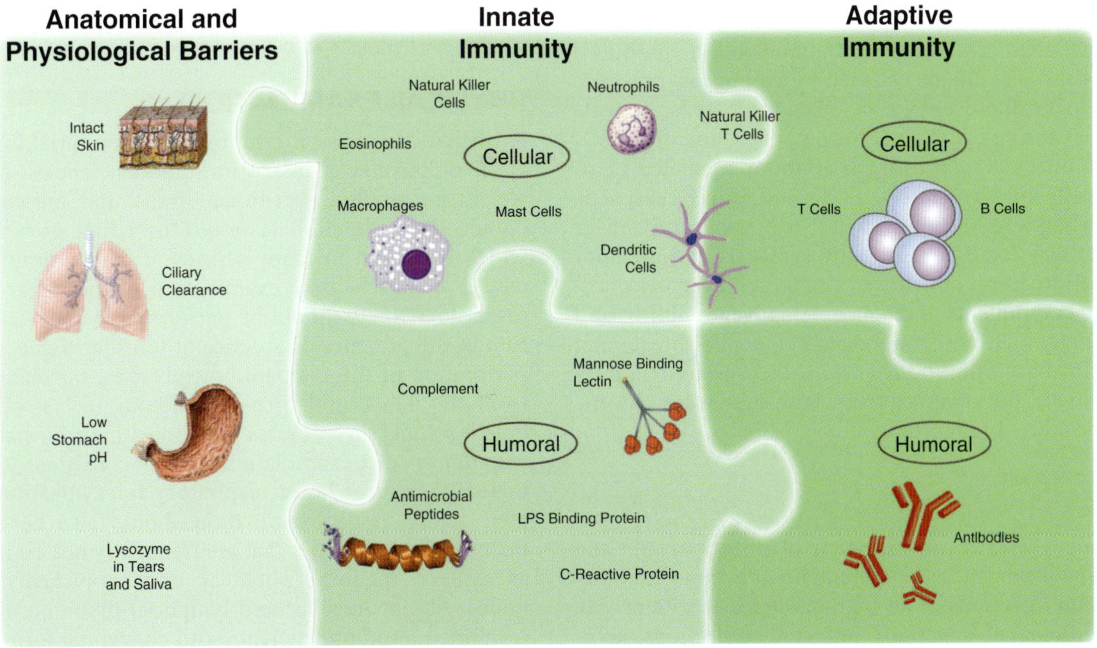

FIGURE 72.1 Integrated human immune system. The human microbial defense system can be simplistically viewed as consisting of three levels: (1) anatomic and physiologic barriers, (2) innate immunity, and (3) adaptive immunity. In common with many classification systems, some elements are difficult to categorize. For example, natural killer T cells and dendritic cells could be classified as being on the cusp of innate and adaptive immunity rather than being firmly in one camp. (From Turvey SE, Broide DH. Innate immunity. *J Allergy Clin Immunol.* 2010;125:S24–S32, Fig. 1.)

TABLE 72.1 Anatomic and Mucociliary Defects That Result in Recurrent or Opportunistic Infections

ANATOMIC DEFECTS IN UPPER AIRWAYS
Aspiration syndromes (gastroesophageal reflux, ineffective cough, foreign body) Cleft palate, choanal atresia, eustachian tube dysfunction Adenoidal hypertrophy Nasal polyps Obstruction of paranasal sinus drainage (osteomeatal complex disease), encephaloceles Posttraumatic or congenital sinus tracts (CSF rhinorrhea)
ANATOMIC DEFECTS IN THE TRACHEOBRONCHIAL TREE
Tracheoesophageal fistula, bronchobiliary fistula, CPAM Pulmonary sequestration, bronchogenic cysts Vascular ring Tumor, foreign body, or enlarged lymph nodes
PHYSIOLOGIC DEFECTS IN UPPER AND LOWER AIRWAYS
Primary ciliary dyskinesia syndromes Cystic fibrosis Bronchopulmonary dysplasia Bronchiectasis Allergic disease (allergic rhinitis, asthma) Chronic cigarette smoke exposure
OTHER DEFECTS
Burns Exfoliative cutaneous lesions* Chronic atopic dermatitis Ureteral obstruction, vesicoureteral reflux IV drug use Central venous line, artificial heart value, CSF shunt, peritoneal dialysis catheter, urinary catheter Dermal sinus tract

**Toxic epidermal necrolysis, Stevens-Johnson syndrome, epidermolysis bullosa.*
CPAM, Congenital pulmonary airway malformation; *CSF,* cerebrospinal fluid; *IV,* intravenous.

T cells and B cells. Antibodies (immunoglobulin) produced by **B cells** neutralize toxins released by pathogens, opsonize pathogens to facilitate uptake by phagocytic cells, activate complement causing cytolysis of the pathogen, and direct NK cells to kill infected cells through antibody-mediated cytotoxicity. **T cells** kill virus-infected cells and cancer cells, activate macrophages to kill intracellular pathogens, and deliver signals necessary for B-cell antibody synthesis and memory B-cell formation. Immunodeficiency can result from defects in one or more components of innate or adaptive immunity, and lead to recurrent, chronic, opportunistic, or life-threatening infections. Primary immunodeficiency diseases are relatively rare individually, but together they cause significant chronic disease, morbidity, and mortality (Table 72.3).

HISTORY

The frequency, severity, and location of infections and the pathogens involved can help differentiate infections in a normal host from infections in an immunodeficient patient (see Table 72.3). Frequent infections, intractable infections, invasive or deep-seated infections, infections that require multiple courses of oral or intravenous antibiotics, or infections with opportunistic pathogens suggest a primary immunodeficiency. Recurrent sinopulmonary infections with encapsulated bacteria suggest a defect in antibody-mediated immunity. Growth faltering, diarrhea, malabsorption, and infections with opportunistic pathogens (i.e., fungi, *Candida* sp., *Pneumocystis jirovecii*) suggest T-cell immunodeficiency. Recurrent viral infections can result from T-cell or NK-cell deficiency. Deep-seated abscesses and infections with *Staphylococcus aureus, Serratia marcescens,* and *Aspergillus* suggest a disorder of neutrophil function, such as chronic granulomatous disease (CGD). **Delayed separation of the umbilical cord**, especially in the presence of omphalitis, severe periodontal disease, and poorly formed abscesses, suggests leukocyte adhesion deficiency (LAD). Invasive infections with *Neisseria* or early-onset autoimmunity may suggest a complement defect.

Age of onset of symptoms can be helpful in defining an immune deficiency, although significant variability occurs. Neutrophil defects (e.g., congenital neutropenia, LAD, CGD) typically present in the first several months of life. Antibody defects (e.g., congenital agammaglobulinemia) and severe T-cell defects (e.g., severe combined immunodeficiency [SCID]) typically present after 3 months of life when maternal antibody levels have waned. Presentation with symptoms of an antibody deficiency later in life (adolescence or adulthood) suggests common variable immunodeficiency (CVID) rather than congenital agammaglobulinemia, although milder phenotypes of primary immunodeficiency disease may not present until later in life. The presence of associated problems, such as congenital heart disease and hypocalcemia (DiGeorge syndrome), abnormal gait and telangiectasia (ataxia-telangiectasia), atopic dermatitis (hyper-IgE syndrome, Omenn syndrome), and easy bruising or bleeding (Wiskott-Aldrich syndrome), can be informative in guiding the workup. Early-onset autoimmunity, such as autoimmune cytopenias, and early-onset inflammatory bowel disease are important potential manifestations of primary immunodeficiencies. A **family history** of a primary immune deficiency or death of a young child due to infections should prompt an immune evaluation, particularly in the setting of recurrent infections.

PHYSICAL EXAMINATION

A meticulous physical examination is essential in the evaluation of possible primary immunodeficiencies. Height and weight percentiles, nutritional status, and presence of subcutaneous fat should be assessed to exclude growth faltering, which is present in many serious primary immunodeficiencies. A comprehensive examination of the upper and lower respiratory tracts should be performed, paying careful attention to the presence or absence of tonsillar tissue, scarring or perforation of the tympanic membranes, purulent discharge from the nares, oral thrush, aphthous ulcers, or abnormal breath sounds such as rales and rhonchi. Abnormalities in the respiratory tract examination may be consistent with past or ongoing upper or lower respiratory tract infections. A complete lymph node examination should also be performed, including lymph nodes that are frequently not examined such as axillary, inguinal, popliteal, and supraclavicular lymph nodes. Absent tonsillar and lymphoid tissue occur in severe combined immunodeficiency and congenital forms of agammaglobulinemia, whereas lymphadenopathy and splenomegaly are found in CVID and autoimmune lymphoproliferative syndrome (ALPS). The presence or absence of skin abnormalities such as petechiae, scarring from recurrent skin infections,

TABLE 72.2 Cytokines and Chemotactic Cytokines and Their Functions

FACTOR	SOURCE	FUNCTION
IL-1	Macrophages	Costimulatory effect on T cells, enhances antigen presentation, acute phase response, fever
IL-2	T cells	Primary T-cell growth factor; B-cell and NK-cell growth factors; required for T-regulatory cell function and survival
IL-3	T cells	Mast cell growth factor; multicolony-stimulating factor
IL-4	T cells	T-cell growth factor; enhances IgE synthesis; enhances B-cell differentiation; mast cell growth
IL-5	T cells	Enhances eosinophil differentiation; enhances immunoglobulin synthesis; enhances IgA synthesis
IL-6	T cells, macrophages, fibroblasts, endothelium	Enhances immunoglobulin synthesis, antiviral activity; induces acute phase response, fever, hematopoietic effects
IL-7	Stromal cells	Enhances growth of pre-T cells
IL-8	T cells, macrophages, epithelium	Neutrophil-activating protein; T-lymphocyte and neutrophil chemotactic factor
IL-9	T cells	Acts in synergy with IL-4 to induce IgE production, mast cell growth
IL-10	T cells, including regulatory T cells, macrophages	Cytokine synthesis inhibitory factor; suppresses macrophage function; enhances B-cell growth; inhibits IL-12 production; suppresses inflammation at mucosal surfaces
IL-12	Macrophages, neutrophils	NK-cell stimulatory factor; cytotoxic lymphocyte maturation factor; enhances IFN-γ synthesis; inhibits IL-4 synthesis
IL-13	T cells	Enhances IgE synthesis; enhances B-cell growth; inhibits macrophage activation; causes airway hyperreactivity
IL-17	T cells	Induces IL-1β and IL-6 synthesis, important in fungal infections
IL-18	Macrophages	Enhances IFN-γ synthesis
IFN-γ	T cells	Macrophage activation; inhibits IgE synthesis; antiviral activity
TNF-α	Macrophage/monocytes, T cells, B cells	Induces endothelial cell adhesion and immune cell recruitment to promote inflammation, role in apoptosis, cachexia, cytokine and chemokine production, activates numerous cell types
TGF-β	T cells, including regulatory T cells, many other cells	Inhibits T-cell and B-cell proliferation and activation, induces T-regulatory cells
RANTES	T cells, endothelium	Chemokine for monocytes, T cells, eosinophils
MIP-1α	Mononuclear cells, endothelium	Chemokine for T cells; enhances differentiation of $CD4^+$ T cells
Eotaxin 1, 2, and 3	Epithelium, endothelium, eosinophils, fibroblasts, macrophages	Chemokine for eosinophils, basophils, and Th2 cells
IP-10	Monocytes, macrophages, endothelium	Chemokine for activated T cells, monocytes, and NK cells

IFN, Interferon; *Ig*, immunoglobulin; *IL*, interleukin; *IP-10*, interferon gamma induced protein 10Kda; *NK*, natural killer; *RANTES*, regulated on activation, normal T-cell expressed and secreted; *TGF-β*, transforming growth factor β; *Th2*, T-helper 2; *TNF-α*, tumor necrosis factor alpha.

severe eczema, telangiectasias, or chronic infections (e.g., molluscum contagiosum, candida) may help lead to the diagnosis of a variety of primary immunodeficiencies such as hyper-IgE syndrome, ataxia-telangiectasia, Wiskott-Aldrich syndrome, or mucocutaneous candidiasis.

DIFFERENTIAL DIAGNOSIS

There are many secondary causes of immunodeficiency that should be considered, particularly if the immunologic testing is nonrevealing (Table 72.4). In patients with primary immunodeficiencies, infections develop at multiple sites (e.g., ears, sinuses, lungs, skin); individuals with anatomic problems (e.g., sequestered pulmonary lobe, ureteral reflux) experience infections confined to a single anatomic site. Asplenia is associated with recurrent and severe infections, even in the presence of protective antibody titers. Infection with HIV should be considered at any age in any patient presenting with a history of opportunistic infections.

DIAGNOSTIC EVALUATION

The diagnosis of patients with primary immunodeficiency diseases depends on early recognition of signs and symptoms (Table 72.3) followed by laboratory tests to evaluate immune function (Fig. 72.2).

TABLE 72.3 Clinical Characteristics of Primary Immunodeficiencies

B-CELL DEFECTS
Recurrent pyogenic infections with extracellular encapsulated organisms (such as *Streptococcus pneumoniae, Haemophilus influenzae* type b, and group A streptococcus), *Mycoplasma* sp., and *Ureaplasma* sp., as well as *Giardia* and enteroviruses
Otitis, sinusitis, recurrent pneumonia, bronchiectasis, and conjunctivitis
Few problems with fungal or viral infections (except enterovirus and poliomyelitis)
Diarrhea common, especially secondary to infection with *Giardia lamblia* and due to enteropathy
Minimal growth retardation
Long-term survival expected with early diagnosis and treatment except in cases with severe autoimmunity-immune dysregulation
COMPLEMENT DEFECTS
Recurrent bacterial infections with extracellular encapsulated organisms, such as *S. pneumoniae* and *H. influenzae*
Susceptibility to recurrent infections with *Neisseria meningitidis*
Increased incidence of autoimmune disease
Severe or recurrent skin and respiratory tract infection
T-CELL DEFECTS
Recurrent infections with common pathogens as well as less virulent pathogens or opportunistic organisms, such as fungi, *Candida* sp., atypical mycobacteria, *Pneumocystis jirovecii*, viruses, and protozoa as well as bacteria
Growth retardation, malabsorption, diarrhea, and growth faltering common
Anergy
Susceptible to graft versus host disease from nonirradiated blood or from maternal engraftment
Fatal reactions may occur from live virus or bacille Calmette-Guérin vaccination
Increased incidence of malignancy
Poor survival beyond infancy or early childhood in the absence of stem cell transplantation
NEUTROPHIL DEFECTS
Recurrent dermatologic infections with bacteria such as *Staphylococcus, Pseudomonas,* and *Escherichia coli, Nocardia,* and fungi such as *Aspergillus*
Subcutaneous, lymph node, lung, and liver abscesses
Pulmonary infections common, including abscess and pneumatocele formation, contributing to chronic disease
Bone and joint infections common
Delayed separation of umbilical cord
Absence of pus at site(s) of infection
Poor wound healing
TOLL-LIKE RECEPTOR DEFECTS
Recurrent bacteremia, meningitis; pneumococcus, *Staphylococcus aureus, Pseudomonas,* meningococcus; herpes simplex
Lack of fever
Early-onset infections with *S. aureus* or *Streptococcus pyogenes* with a normal immune workup

TABLE 72.4 Causes of Secondary Immunodeficiency

VIRAL INFECTIONS
HIV (destroys CD4 T cells)
Measles
Rubella
Influenza
METABOLIC DISORDERS
Diabetes mellitus
Malnutrition
Advanced renal or liver disease
Sickle cell disease
Zinc and vitamin deficiency
Multiple carboxylase deficiency
Burns (via hypermetabolism)
PROTEIN-LOSING STATES
Nephrotic syndrome
Protein losing enteropathy
OTHER CAUSES
Prematurity
Immunosuppressive agents (e.g., corticosteroids, radiation, and antimetabolites)
Malignancy (leukemia, Hodgkin lymphoma, nonlymphoid cancer)
Acquired asplenia
Acquired neutropenia (autoimmune, viral, or drug induced)
Stem cell transplantation/graft versus host disease
Systemic lupus erythematosus and other autoimmune diseases
Sarcoidosis

Laboratory Tests

A diagnosis of primary immunodeficiency disease cannot be established without the use of laboratory tests guided by the clinical history (Table 72.5). A **complete blood count with differential** should always be obtained to identify neutropenia or lymphopenia (SCID) as well as the presence of eosinophils (allergic disease) and anemia (chronic disease). **Serum immunoglobulin levels (serum IgG, IgA, IgM, and IgE)** are essential. Antibody levels vary with age, with normal adult values of immunoglobulin G (IgG) at full-term birth from transplacental transfer of maternal IgG, a physiologic nadir occurring between 3 and 6 months of age, and a gradual increase to adult values over several years. IgA and IgM are low at birth and increase gradually over several years; IgA takes the longest to reach normal adult values. Low albumin levels with low immunoglobulin levels suggest low synthetic rates for all proteins or increased loss of proteins, as in protein-losing enteropathy. Elevated immunoglobulin levels suggest intact B-cell immunity and can be found in diseases with recurrent infections, such as CGD, primary ciliary dyskinesia, cystic fibrosis, HIV infection, and autoimmune diseases. Elevated IgE levels occur in a number of immune deficiencies such as hyper-IgE syndrome as well as in atopic diseases, allergic bronchopulmonary aspergillosis, and tissue invasive parasites. Undiagnosed atopic disease such as asthma, where viral respiratory tract infections can lead to chronic cough, frequently masquerade as a primary immunodeficiency.

Specific antibody titers after childhood vaccination (tetanus, diphtheria, *Haemophilus influenzae* type b, or *Streptococcus pneumoniae* vaccines) reflect the capacity of the immune system to synthesize specific antibodies and to develop memory B cells. If titers are low, immunization with a specific vaccine and titers obtained 4–6 weeks later can confirm response to the immunization. Poor response to bacterial polysaccharide antigens is normal before 24 months of age but is also associated with specific antibody deficiency. The development of protein-conjugate polysaccharide vaccines prevents infections with encapsulated organisms in early childhood. Antibody responses to the *S. pneumoniae* serotypes found in the 23-valent polysaccharide vaccine, but not in the conjugate vaccine, can

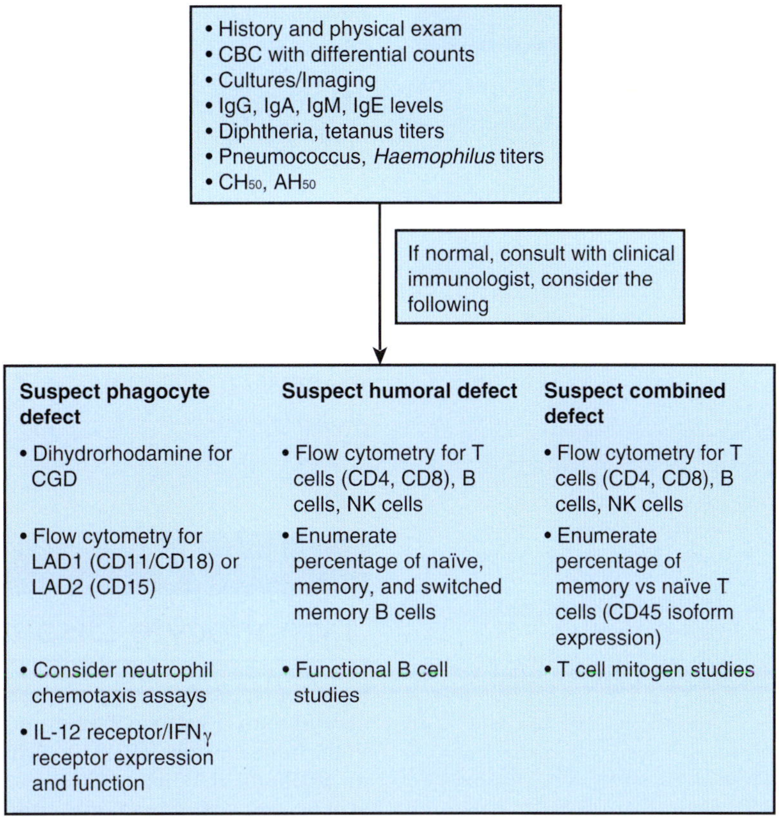

FIGURE 72.2 Algorithm showing initial workup and follow-up studies of patients with suspected immune deficiency. Consultation with a clinical immunologist is recommended to guide advanced testing and interpret results. *CBC*, Complete blood count; *CGD*, chronic granulomatous disease; *IFN*, interferon; *Ig*, immunoglobulin; *IL*, interleukin; *LAD*, leukocyte adhesion defect; *NK*, natural killer cell. (From Kliegman RM, Toth H, Bordini BJ, Basel D, eds. *Nelson Pediatric Symptom-Based Diagnosis*. Philadelphia: Elsevier; 2023, fig. 54.9.)

be used to test antibody responses to polysaccharide antigens. With the development of conjugated vaccines covering more of these specific serotypes, the assessment of pure polysaccharide responses is becoming more difficult. Other polysaccharide responses, such as *Salmonella* Typhi, can be performed.

Delayed-type hypersensitivity skin tests to protein antigens such as tetanus, diphtheria, *Candida,* or mumps are used as a measurement of T-cell function and specifically demonstrate the presence of antigen-specific T cells and functional antigen-presenting cells. Due to the drawbacks of delayed-type hypersensitivity skin testing (need to be read 72 hours after subcutaneous injection of antigen; occasional exaggerated, painful delayed skin reactions; or anergic responses of control antigens), T-cell proliferation assays (see later) are often substituted for delayed-type hypersensitivity skin testing to assess T-cell function.

Lymphocyte phenotyping by flow cytometry enumerates the percentage and absolute numbers of T-cell, B-cell, and NK-cell subsets. Flow cytometry can also test for the presence of proteins that are necessary for normal immunity, such as major histocompatibility complex molecules or adhesion molecules, as well as intracellular analysis of signaling proteins and cytokines. **T-cell proliferation** assays to mitogens (phytohemagglutinin, concanavalin A, pokeweed mitogen, or CD3) or antigens (tetanus toxoid or *Candida*) are in vitro assays that assess the capacity of T cells to proliferate in response to a nonspecific stimulus (mitogens) or the presence of antigen-specific memory T cells (antigens). **Tests for cytokine synthesis, intracellular signaling pathways, or expression of activation markers** may be performed in specialized laboratories.

Complement assays include the CH_{50} test, which measures the presence of proteins in the classic pathway of complement (C1, C2, C3, C4), and the AH_{50} test, which tests the proteins of the alternative pathway of complement (C3, factor B, properdin). If both the CH_{50} and AH_{50} levels are abnormal, a defect in the common pathway is likely (C5–C9). Specialized laboratories measure the presence or function of specific complement proteins. Tests for C1-inhibitor antigen levels and function are used to diagnose hereditary or acquired angioedema.

Tests for neutrophil function include the nitroblue tetrazolium (NBT) or the more commonly used dihydrorhodamine 123 (DHR) assay. Both the DHR and NBT tests assess the ability of neutrophils to generate a respiratory burst generated by the enzyme complex NADPH oxidase, which is abnormal in CGD. In the DHR test, neutrophils are treated with dihydrorhodamine and then activated, which normally leads to the production of superoxide. Superoxide subsequently leads to the production of H_2O_2, which oxidizes the dihydrorhodamine to rhodamine-1,2,3 emitting a robust fluorescent signal, which is quantitated by flow cytometry. Neutrophils from patients with CGD produce low or no superoxide (markedly reduced fluorescence). Other in vitro tests for neutrophils include phagocytosis, chemotaxis, and bacterial killing, which are available in specialized clinical immunology laboratories. Tests for the expression of adhesion molecules such as CD18 (leukocyte function–associated antigen type 1 [LFA-1]) and CD15 (LFA-2) can also be performed by flow cytometry.

TABLE 72.5 Tests for Suspected Immune Deficiency

GENERAL
Complete blood count, including hemoglobin, white blood cell count with differential and morphology, and platelet count including MPV
Radiographs to document infection in chest, sinus, mastoids, and long bones, if indicated by clinical history
Cultures, if appropriate
ANTIBODY-MEDIATED IMMUNITY
Quantitative immunoglobulin levels: IgG, IgA, IgM, IgE, isohemagglutinin titers (anti-A, anti-B, measures IgM function)
Specific antibody levels:
Protein antigens: diphtheria, tetanus
Protein-conjugated antigens: *Haemophilus influenzae, Streptococcus pneumoniae* (conjugate vaccine)
Polysaccharide antigens: *S. pneumoniae* (nonconjugated vaccine); *Salmonella* Typhi Vi vaccine
B-cell numbers and subsets by flow cytometry
CELL-MEDIATED IMMUNITY
Lymphocyte count and morphology
Delayed hypersensitivity skin tests (*Candida*, tetanus toxoid, mumps): measure T-cell and macrophage function
T-cell and NK-cell numbers and subsets by flow cytometry
T-lymphocyte functional analyses (mitogen responses, cytokine production)
NK-cell cytotoxicity assays
PHAGOCYTE FUNCTION
Neutrophil cell count and morphology
Dihydrorhodamine 123 using flow cytometry/nitroblue tetrazolium dye test
Staphylococcal killing, chemotaxis assay
Myeloperoxidase stain
COMPLEMENT
Total hemolytic complement CH_{50}: measures classic and common pathway activity
AH_{50}: measures alternative and common pathway activity
Levels of individual complement components
C1-inhibitor level and function

Ig, Immunoglobulin; *MPV*, mean platelet volume; *NK*, natural killer.

Genetic testing to confirm the diagnosis of a primary immunodeficiency is often needed. Defining a genetic cause facilitates the optimal course of treatment, determining the natural history and prognosis of the disease, and aids in genetic counseling and prenatal diagnosis. Genetic panels, which include genes known to be implicated in specific types of immunodeficiencies, are frequently performed. More extensive genetic testing, such as whole exome sequencing, may be used in particularly complicated cases or when individual genetic panels fail to yield a diagnosis. Fluorescent in situ hybridization or chromosomal microarray studies (preferred) detect specific deletions or duplications that occur in syndromes associated with immunodeficiency (e.g., DiGeorge syndrome).

Diagnostic Imaging

Radiographic studies may screen for commonly found abnormalities associated with the specific immunodeficiency. A CT scan of the chest can reveal bronchiectasis in patients with serious antibody deficiencies such as common variable immunodeficiency. Chest radiographs may detect the presence or absence of a thymus. Abnormalities in the cerebellum are found by MRI in patients with ataxia telangiectasia. CT or MRI studies may detect the presence of widespread lymphadenopathy or splenomegaly in some immunodeficiencies such as CVID.

PEARLS FOR PRACTITIONERS

See Immunology: Pearls for Practitioners at the end of this section.

REVIEW QUESTIONS

Available online.

CHAPTER 73

Lymphocyte Disorders

Hematopoietic stem cells give rise to lymphoid precursors that develop into T lymphocytes in the thymus or B lymphocytes in the bone marrow (Fig. 73.1). Isolated B-cell disorders result in **antibody deficiency diseases**, whereas T-cell disorders usually cause **combined immunodeficiency** because they are necessary for cell-mediated immunity to clear intracellular pathogens and for antibody synthesis by B cells. Natural killer (NK) cells are an important component of the **innate immune response**, develop from lymphoid precursors, and can kill virus-infected cells and tumor cells. Antibodies can enhance NK-cell function by antibody-mediated cellular cytotoxicity.

ETIOLOGY AND CLINICAL MANIFESTATIONS

Antibody Deficiency Diseases

Disorders of B cells result in an increased susceptibility to infections by encapsulated bacteria, mycoplasma, and certain viruses. **Agammaglobulinemia** results from the absence or defective function of B cells with subsequent severe decrease in immunoglobulin (Ig) levels and an absence of specific antibody. **X-linked agammaglobulinemia** (XLA), which accounts for approximately 80% of all congenital agammaglobulinemias, is characterized by a profound deficiency of B cells, severe panhypogammaglobulinemia, and absence of lymphoid tissue (Table 73.1; see Fig. 73.1). The defect is caused by pathogenic variants in the gene *BTK* encoding the Bruton's tyrosine kinase protein. *BTK* is necessary for downstream signaling of the pre–B-cell receptor and the B-cell antigen receptor, which is necessary for normal differentiation of B cells. **Autosomal recessive agammaglobulinemia** presents similar to XLA, is due to defects in components of the pre–B-cell and B-cell antigen receptor complexes, and includes pathogenic variants in the μ heavy-chain gene, λ5, Igα, Igβ, and BLNK.

Patients with agammaglobulinemia usually present during the first 6–12 months of life as maternally derived antibodies wane; however, patients can present years later. These patients develop infections with *Streptococcus pneumoniae, Haemophilus influenzae* type b, *Staphylococcus aureus, Mycoplasma,* and *Pseudomonas,* organisms for which antibody is an important

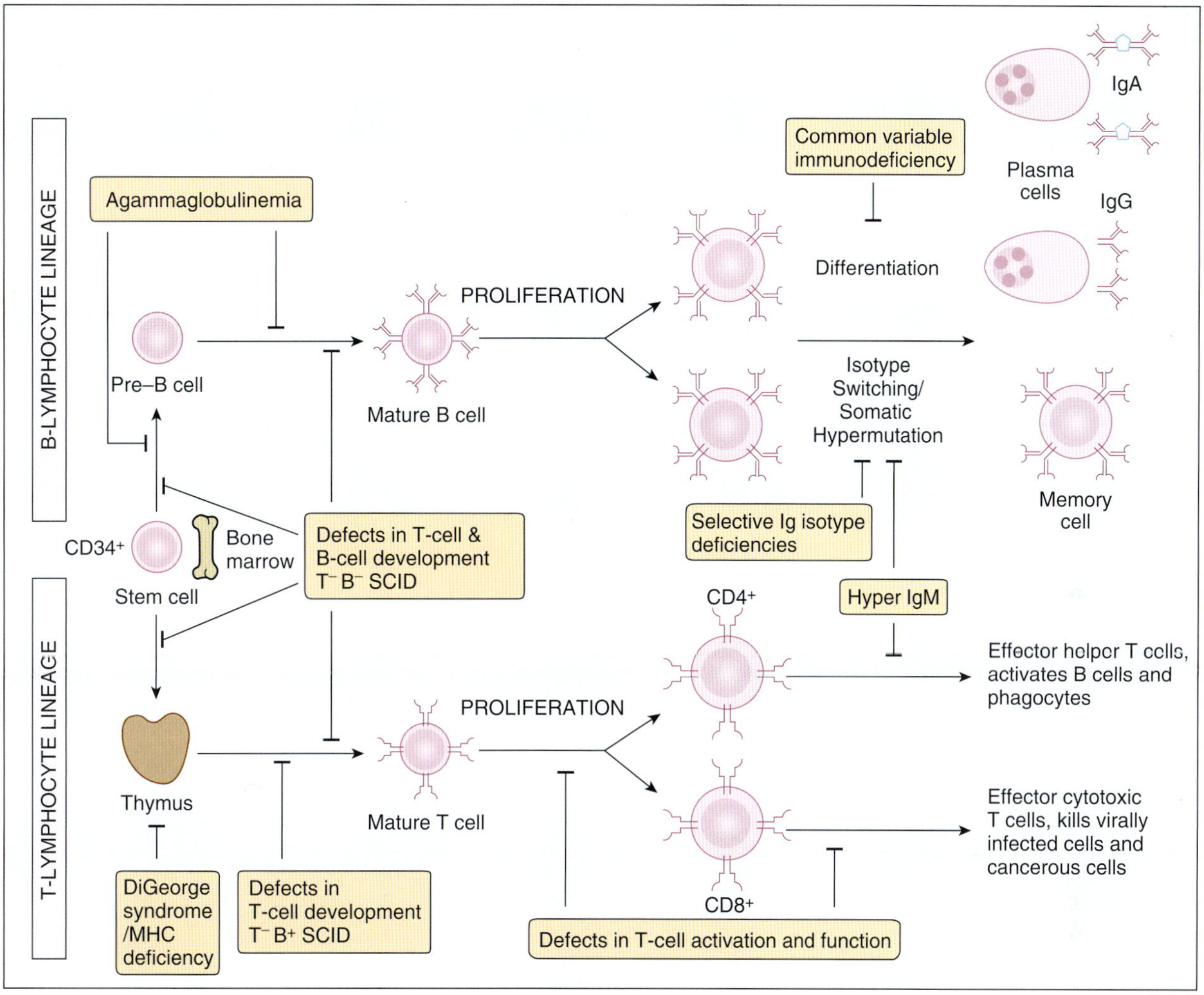

FIGURE 73.1 Sites of cellular abnormalities in congenital immunodeficiencies. In primary immunodeficiency diseases, the maturation or activation of B or T lymphocytes may be blocked at different stages. *B*, B lymphocyte; *Ig*, immunoglobulin; *MHC*, major histocompatibility complex; *SCID*, severe combined immunodeficiency; *T*, T lymphocyte. (Modified from Abbas AK, Lichtman AH, Pober JS. *Cellular and Molecular Immunology*. 3rd ed. Philadelphia: Saunders; 1997.)

opsonin. They also have increased susceptibility to giardiasis and enteroviral infections and vaccine-associated poliomyelitis (if immunized with oral live attenuated poliovirus vaccine).

Common variable immunodeficiency (CVID) is a heterogeneous disorder characterized by hypogammaglobulinemia developing after an initial period of normal immune function, most commonly in the second and third decades of life (see Table 73.1). Serum IgG levels are <500 mg/dL (usually <300 mg/dL) with IgA levels <10 mg/dL and/or low IgM levels. Secondary causes of hypogammaglobulinemia (e.g., corticosteroids, rituximab, protein-losing enteropathy) can present with a preferential reduction in IgG but can have normal IgA or IgM levels. Antibody titers to polysaccharide antigens, such as pneumococcus, are nearly always absent. Reduced specific antibody responses to protein antigens, such as tetanus and diphtheria, are frequently abnormal. T-cell numbers and function are highly variable. Although B-cell numbers are variable, they are typically present, which helps distinguish CVID from congenital agammaglobulinemia. Patients exhibit normal-sized or enlarged tonsils and lymph nodes and may have splenomegaly. They are susceptible to frequent respiratory tract infections due to *S. pneumoniae, H. influenzae* type b, and *Mycoplasma*. Gastrointestinal infections with *Giardia, Campylobacter, Salmonella, Helicobacter,* and enteroviruses are common. Noninfectious complications due to autoimmune disease (e.g., autoimmune cytopenias), malignancies (e.g., B-cell lymphomas), and immune dysregulation (e.g., multisystemic granulomatous disease, interstitial lung disease, nodular regenerative hyperplasia of the liver, enteropathy, seronegative arthritis) occur in a substantial proportion of subjects and are the major causes of morbidity and mortality.

Genetic defects causing CVID occur in approximately 20% of patients, but in most cases a single gene defect is not present. Increasing use of DNA sequencing reveals monogenic disorders as the cause of some CVID or CVID-like immunodeficiencies, especially with early-onset CVID or CVID complicated by autoimmunity or disorders of immune regulation. In patients with early-onset CVID, it is important to exclude congenital agammaglobulinemia and other monogenic disorders that can present with CVID-like immunodeficiencies (e.g., *CLTA4, LRBA, PIK3CD*). Some patients have defects in inducible costimulator (ICOS), transmembrane activator and calcium-modulating cyclophilin ligand interactor (TACI), CD19, CD21, CD81, or BAFF-R. Before making the diagnosis

TABLE 73.1 Antibody Deficiency Diseases

DISORDER	GENETICS	ONSET	MANIFESTATIONS	PATHOGENESIS	ASSOCIATED FEATURES
Agammaglobulinemia	X-linked, AR	Infancy (6–9 mo)	Recurrent infections, sinusitis, pneumonia, meningitis (encapsulated bacteria, enteroviruses, atypical bacteria)	Arrest in B-cell differentiation (pre-B level); pathogenic variants in: *BTK* gene (X-linked); μ-chain, BLNK, Igα, Igβ, λ5, BLNK (AR)	Lymphoid hypoplasia
Common variable immunodeficiency	AR; AD; sporadic	Second to third decade	Sinusitis, bronchitis, bronchiectasis pneumonia, interstitial lung disease, chronic diarrhea, autoimmune cytopenias, lymphomas	Arrest in plasma cell differentiation, genetic defects in ICOS, TACI, CD19, CD81, CD20, CD21, CTLA4, NFKB1, and other genetic causes leading to CVID-like disorders	Autoimmune disease, RA, SLE, Graves disease, ITP, malignancy, multisystemic granulomatous disease
Transient hypogammaglobulinemia of infancy		Infancy (3–7 mo)	Recurrent viral and pyogenic infections	Unknown; delayed plasma cell maturation	Frequently in families with other immunodeficiencies
IgA deficiency	Variable	Variable	Most normal, sinopulmonary infections	Failure of IgA expression	IgG subclass deficiency common, autoimmune diseases
IgG subclass deficiency	Variable	Variable	Most normal, sinopulmonary infections	Defect in IgG isotype production	IgA deficiency, ataxia telangiectasia, polysaccharide antibody deficiency
Specific antibody deficiency	Variable	After 2 yr of age	Sinopulmonary infections	Unknown	IgG subclass deficiency
Hyper-IgM syndrome	AR	Variable	Sinopulmonary infections	Defect in AID, UNG	Autoimmunity

AD, Autosomal dominant; *AID*, activation-induced cytidine deaminase; *AR*, autosomal recessive; *Ig*, immunoglobulin; *ITP*, idiopathic thrombocytopenic purpura; *RA*, rheumatoid arthritis; *SLE*, systemic lupus erythematosus; *UNG*, uracil-DNA glycosylase.

of CVID, X-linked agammaglobulinemia, X-linked lymphoproliferative disease, or hyper-IgM syndrome as well as other causes of hypogammaglobulinemias (e.g., protein losing enteropathy, medications) should be excluded.

Selective **IgA deficiency** is defined as serum IgA levels <10 mg/dL with normal levels of the other Ig isotypes. The diagnosis cannot be confirmed until the patient is at least 4 years of age when IgA levels usually reach adult levels. Selective IgA deficiency occurs in approximately 1 in 500 individuals. Most patients with selective IgA deficiency are asymptomatic. A small percentage of patients present with recurrent sinopulmonary infections, which may be associated with specific antibody deficiency and/or IgG_2 subclass deficiency. In selected cases, patients may require antibiotic prophylaxis and, rarely, antibody replacement therapy. Patients with IgA deficiency are at increased risk to develop atopic diseases, selected autoimmune diseases, and celiac disease. Some cases of IgA deficiency occur in families, suggesting autosomal inheritance.

IgG subclass deficiency occurs when the level of antibodies in one or more of the four IgG subclasses is selectively decreased while total IgG levels are normal. Normal individuals can express low levels or absence of one or more subclasses, so a history of significant and recurrent infections is important. An inability to synthesize specific antibody titers to protein or polysaccharide antigens is the best marker of clinically significant IgG subclass deficiency that leads to recurrent infections.

Transient hypogammaglobulinemia of infancy is a temporary condition characterized by a prolongation of the physiologic hypogammaglobulinemia of infancy. The immunoglobulin nadir at 6 months of age is accentuated, with IgG levels less than 200 mg/dL. Ig levels remain diminished throughout the first year of life and usually increase to normal, age-appropriate levels by 2–4 years of age. The incidence of sinopulmonary infection is increased in some patients. The diagnosis is supported by normal levels of both B and T cells and by normal antibody responses to protein antigens such as diphtheria and tetanus toxoids. The transient nature of this disorder cannot be confirmed, however, until Ig levels return to normal ranges.

Specific antibody deficiency syndrome is characterized by recurrent infections with normal Ig levels and normal lymphocyte numbers and subsets but an inability to synthesize specific antibody to polysaccharide antigens, such as to the 23-valent pneumococcal vaccine. The pathogenesis of this disorder is unknown. In selected, rare patients, specific antibody deficiency may be responsible for increased sinopulmonary infections and require either antibiotic prophylaxis or immunoglobulin replacement therapy.

Combined Immunodeficiency Diseases

Combined immunodeficiencies are defined by defects in antibody production and cell mediated immunity. The most severe form is **severe combined immunodeficiency (SCID)**, which is characterized by a profound lack of T-cell numbers or function and B-cell dysfunction resulting from the absence of B cells from the gene defect itself or secondary to lack of T-cell function (Table 73.2). T cells develop from bone marrow–derived precursors in the thymus (Fig. 73.1), where they undergo several stages of development characterized by DNA recombination of the variable region of T-cell antigen receptor genes to generate a diverse T-cell receptor repertoire. A process of positive selection occurs in the thymus to select thymocytes with antigen receptors that can interact with major histocompatibility complex (MHC) molecules to ensure their survival (Fig. 73.1). Thymocytes differentiate into CD4 or CD8 T cells if they interact with MHC class II or class I molecules, respectively. Some of the positively selected thymocytes, however, have antigen receptors that recognize self-antigens presented by MHC molecules in the thymus. These cells are deleted in the thymus by a process of negative selection, or they become regulatory T cells. Positive selection and negative selection in the thymus ensure that the mature T cells that leave the thymus can function with the individual's MHC molecules and recognize a multitude of foreign antigens without mounting autoimmune responses. SCID can result from any specific pathogenic variant that interferes with T-cell development in the thymus or T-cell function in the periphery.

Clinical manifestations of SCID include growth faltering, severe bacterial infections, chronic candidiasis and other fungal infections, chronic viral infections, infection with *Pneumocystis jirovecii* and other opportunistic organisms, and intractable diarrhea. Patients may have skin disease similar to eczema, possibly related to **graft versus host disease (GVHD)** from engraftment of maternal lymphocytes or by selecting for self-reactive clones of T cells (Omenn syndrome). Patients with SCID are extremely susceptible to fatal GVHD from lymphocytes in blood transfusions and can be infected by cytomegalovirus-positive blood products. *Patients with T-cell disorders should always receive irradiated, leukocyte-depleted, cytomegalovirus (CMV)–negative blood products.*

X-linked SCID, the most common cause of SCID, is caused by pathogenic variants in the gene coding the common γ-chain of the interleukin (IL)-2, IL-4, IL-7, IL-9, IL-15, and IL-21 receptors. Affected patients have no T cells or NK cells in the peripheral blood but have normal numbers of B cells. Ig levels are low or undetectable because there are no CD4 T cells to stimulate B cells. Defects in IL-2 and IL-7 signaling lead to impaired T-cell proliferation and T-cell development, whereas IL-15 is required for NK-cell development. There are many causes of **autosomal recessive SCID**. Defects in Janus kinase 3 (Jak3), which binds to the common γ-chain, result in a similar phenotype as X-linked SCID. Defects in the IL-7 receptor, ZAP-70, and subunits of the CD3 molecule result in a deficiency of T cells with normal B-cell and NK-cell numbers. In addition, there are a variety of defects that affect DNA recombination in T and B cells; these include two genes called *recombinase activating gene (RAG)1* and *RAG2* as well as genes important in DNA excision and repair (e.g., DNA cross-link repair 1C gene *[DCLRE1C]*, encoding Artemis). Defects in any of the genes that abolish DNA recombination or DNA repair result in autosomal recessive SCID with no T or B cells present. Variants in *RAG1, RAG2,* or *Artemis* that do not completely abrogate enzymatic activity may result in **Omenn syndrome**, a variant form of SCID that is characterized by exfoliative erythroderma, lymphadenopathy, hepatosplenomegaly, marked eosinophilia, elevated serum IgE, and impaired T-cell function. Patients with Omenn syndrome have T cells in the periphery, but these T cells have a limited T-cell receptor repertoire which is self-reactive.

Deficiencies in **adenosine deaminase (ADA)** and **purine nucleoside phosphorylase**, two enzymes involved in the purine salvage pathway, also result in SCID. Accumulation of nucleoside substrates or their metabolic products in the plasma is toxic to lymphocytes, including T, B, and NK cells. Most patients exhibit severe infection early in life, although the diagnosis in patients with partial enzyme function may not be established until after 5 years of age or, occasionally, in adulthood. Patients with late-onset diagnosis are generally lymphopenic; they may have B cells and normal total Ig levels but little functional antibody.

Other disorders that affect T-cell development or function that are less severe than SCID are referred to as **combined immunodeficiencies (CIDs)**. **X-linked hyper-IgM syndrome** is a combined immunodeficiency with deficient T-cell function due to defects in CD40 ligand. Defects in CD40 cause **autosomal recessive hyper-IgM syndrome** and present similarly to X-linked hyper-IgM syndrome (Fig. 73.2; Table 73.2). Hyper-IgM syndrome is characterized by a failure of Ig isotype switching from IgM and IgD to IgG, IgA, or IgE and lack of memory responses. Affected patients have normal or elevated serum levels of IgM with low or absent levels of IgG, IgA, and IgE. Ig isotype switching allows a B cell to maintain antigen specificity while altering Ig function and is directed by cytokines and interaction between CD40 ligand on CD4 T cells and CD40 on B cells (Fig. 73.2). Signal transduction via CD40 activates several signaling molecules and transcription factors, including nuclear factor kappa B (NF-κB) and two enzymes, activation-induced cytidine deaminase (AID) and uracil-DNA glycosylase (UNG), which are required for class switching. Autosomal recessive forms of hyper IgM deficiency due to pathogenic variants in *AID* or *UNG* also lead to the same abnormal pattern in serum immunoglobulins but without T-cell function abnormality. Thus patients with these forms of hyper-IgM clinically present in a manner similar to antibody deficiencies but do not exhibit susceptibility to opportunistic infections (see Table 73.1).

All patients with hyper-IgM syndrome have increased susceptibility to sinopulmonary infections due to defective antibody production; patients with defects in CD40 ligand or CD40 are susceptible to opportunistic infections, such as *P. jirovecii* and *Cryptosporidium parvum*. Antiviral immunity is generally preserved. Signaling via CD40 on B cells, macrophages, and other antigen-presenting cells leads to upregulation of costimulatory molecules important for promoting T-cell differentiation and for activating cell-mediated immune responses. The hyper-IgM phenotype is also found in an X-linked disorder associated with ectodermal dysplasia, resulting from defects in the gene encoding the NF-κB essential modulator (NEMO). Patients with defects in NEMO are susceptible to a wider spectrum of infectious organisms, especially meningitis and infection with atypical mycobacteria, because NF-κB signaling is important for the function of both innate and adaptive immune systems.

TABLE 73.2 Combined Immunodeficiency Diseases

DISORDER	GENETICS	ONSET	MANIFESTATIONS	PATHOGENESIS	ASSOCIATED FEATURES
Hyper-IgM syndrome (see Table 73.1)	X-linked, AR	First year	Sinopulmonary infections, opportunistic infections, Pneumocystis jirovecii	Defect in CD40 ligand (X-linked) or CD40 (AR)	Neutropenia, liver disease, cancer
DiGeorge anomaly	22q11.2 (or 10p) deletion	Newborn, early infancy	Hypocalcemic tetany, pyogenic infections, partial or complete T-cell deficiency	Hypoplasia of third and fourth pharyngeal pouch	Congenital heart disease (aortic arch anomalies), hypoparathyroidism, micrognathia, hypertelorism
Severe combined immunodeficiency ($T^- B^+$ SCID)	X-linked; AR	1–3 mo	Candidiasis, all types of infections, growth faltering, chronic diarrhea	Pathogenic variants in IL-2Rγ chain, Jak3 kinase, ZAP-70, IL-7Ra, CD3 subunits	GVHD from maternal-fetal transfusions, severe GVHD from nonirradiated blood transfusion
Severe combined immunodeficiency ($T^- B^-$ SCID)	AR	1–3 mo	Same as $T^- B^+$ SCID	Pathogenic variants in RAG1/2, Artemis, ADA/PNP deficiency	Same as $T^- B^+$ SCID ADA deficiency: chondro-osseous dysplasia PNP deficiency: neurologic disorders
Omenn syndrome	AR	1–3 mo	Same as $T^- B^-$ SCID, exfoliative erythroderma, lymphadenopathy, hepatosplenomegaly	Hypomorphic variants in SCID-causing genes (RAG1/2, Artemis, others)	Restricted T-cell receptor heterogeneity, eosinophilia, elevated IgE
Reticular dysgenesis ($T^- B^-$ SCID)	AR	1–3 mo	Same as $T^- B^-$ SCID	Defective maturation of common stem cells due to AK2 pathogenic variants	Agammaglobulinemia, alymphocytosis, agranulocytosis
Bare lymphocyte syndrome (MHC class I deficiency)	AR	First decade	Sinopulmonary infections	Pathogenic variants in TAP1 or TAP2 (transporter associated with antigen processing)	Decreased CD8 T cells, chronic lung inflammation
Bare lymphocyte syndrome (MHC class II deficiency)	AR	Early infancy	Respiratory tract infections, chronic diarrhea, viral infections	Pathogenic variants in CIITA, RFX5, RFXAP, and RFX-B (DNA binding factors)	Decreased CD4 T cells, autoimmune disease

ADA, Adenosine deaminase; *AR,* autosomal recessive; *GVHD,* graft versus host disease; *IL,* interleukin; *IL-2Rγ,* interleukin-2 receptor γ-chain; *MHC,* major histocompatibility complex; *PNP,* purine nucleoside phosphorylase; *SCID,* severe combined immunodeficiency; $T^- B^+$, T cells absent and B cells present; $T^- B^-$, T cells absent and B cells absent.

Bare lymphocyte syndrome results from defects in transcription factors (i.e., CIITA, RFX5, RFXAP, and RFXANK) that regulate expression of MHC class II molecules, which leads to the absence of MHC class II molecules. Lymphoid tissue and B cells may be present in normal amounts, but CD4 T cells are decreased or absent. Defects in genes that affect processing and transport of intracellular peptides (i.e., TAP1, TAP2, tapasin) leads to MHC class I deficiency with decreased or absent CD8 cells. Some patients may have normal numbers of CD4 or CD8 T cells, but none of the T cells are functional because peptide antigens cannot be presented to T cells.

DiGeorge syndrome, also known as **velocardiofacial syndrome** or **CATCH 22 syndrome** (**c**ardiac anomalies, **a**bnormal facies, **t**hymic hypoplasia, **c**left palate, and **h**ypocalcemia), is the result of dysmorphogenesis of the third and fourth pharyngeal pouches, resulting in hypoplasia of the thymus required for T-cell maturation. Most, but not all, patients with DiGeorge syndrome have a deletion on chromosome 22q11.2. DiGeorge syndrome is classically characterized by hypocalcemic (hypoparathyroidism) tetany, conotruncal and aortic arch anomalies, and increased infections. The diagnosis is established by fluorescence in situ hybridization, chromosomal microarray studies, or a polymerase chain reaction with a DNA probe to detect the chromosomal deletion. Most affected patients have partial DiGeorge syndrome, with a less severe immunodeficiency with low T-cell numbers and function that generally improve with age. In complete DiGeorge syndrome, the thymus is absent and patients present similarly to SCID due to a complete lack of T cells. Importantly, complete DiGeorge syndrome and bare lymphocyte syndrome

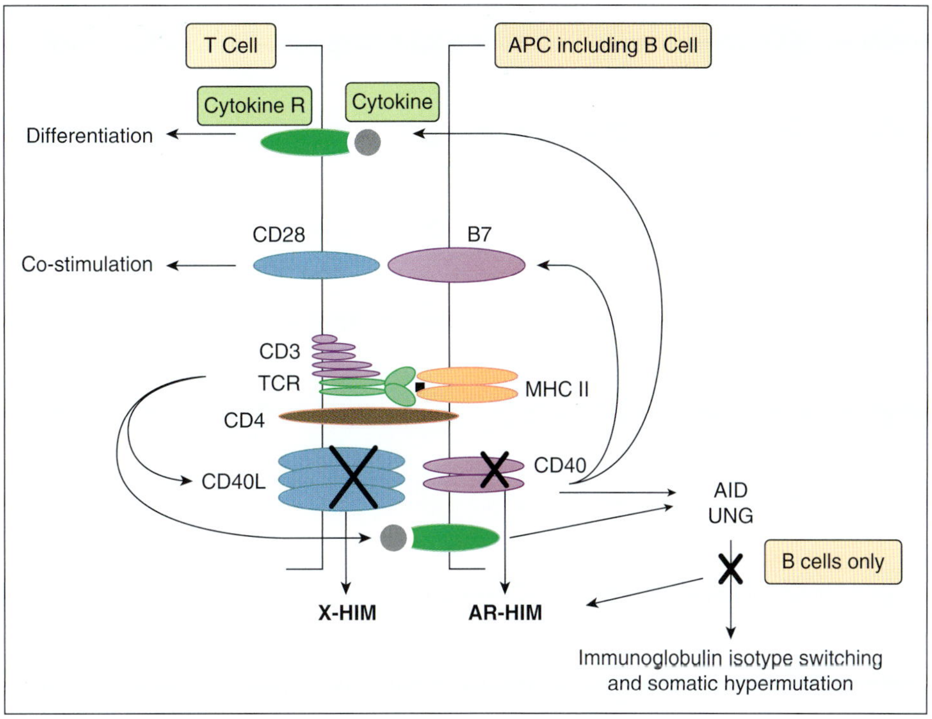

FIGURE 73.2 Schematic representation of the interaction between a CD4 T cell and a B cell. T-cell activation follows T-cell receptor *(TCR)* recognition of peptide antigen presented via major histocompatibility complex *(MHC)* class II molecules resulting in CD40 ligand (CD40L) expression and cytokine synthesis. CD40L stimulates the B cell via CD40, resulting in expression of costimulatory molecules *(B7)* that are important in T-cell priming and cytokine synthesis that drives T-cell differentiation. CD40 and cytokine signaling in B cells activate activation-induced cytidine deaminase *(AID)* and uracil-DNA glycosylase *(UNG)* to promote Ig isotype switching and somatic hypermutation. Defects in CD40L cause X-linked hyper-IgM *(X-HIM)*, and defects in CD40, AID, or UNG cause autosomal recessive hyper-IgM *(AR-HIM)*. Defects in either CD40L or CD40 affect T-cell costimulation and priming, leading to T-cell defects and susceptibility to opportunistic infections, whereas defects in AID and UNG maintain normal T-cell costimulation and function.

(both with an intrinsic thymic defect) do not respond as well to bone marrow transplantation as do other forms of SCID. Transfer of mature donor T cells in such patients may confer some immune function. Thymic transplants have been utilized in cases of severe T-cell lymphopenia in DiGeorge syndrome.

Wiskott-Aldrich syndrome is an X-linked disorder characterized by thrombocytopenia, eczema, defects in cell-mediated and humoral immunity, and a predisposition to lymphoproliferative disease (Table 73.3). Wiskott-Aldrich syndrome is caused by pathogenic variants of the *WAS* gene coding for the Wiskott-Aldrich syndrome protein (WASP), which is expressed in lymphocytes, platelets, and monocytes. Deficiency of this protein results in elevated levels of IgE and IgA, decreased IgM, poor responses to polysaccharide antigens, waning T-cell function, and profound thrombocytopenia. Opportunistic infections and autoimmune cytopenias become problematic in older children. **Isolated X-linked thrombocytopenia** also results from *WAS* variants. One-third of patients with Wiskott-Aldrich syndrome die as a result of hemorrhage, and two-thirds die as a result of recurrent infection caused by bacteria, cytomegalovirus, *P. jirovecii,* or herpes simplex virus. Hematopoietic stem cell transplantation is the treatment of choice for severe forms of Wiskott-Aldrich syndrome and corrects the immunologic and hematologic problems in these patients.

Ataxia telangiectasia is a syndrome caused by pathogenic variants in the ataxia telangiectasia *(ATM)* gene on chromosome 11q22.3 (Table 73.3). Patients have cutaneous and conjunctival telangiectasias and progressive cerebellar ataxia with degeneration of Purkinje cells. IgA deficiency, IgG_2 subclass deficiency of variable severity, low IgE levels, and variably depressed T-cell function may be seen. The normal function of the *ATM* gene appears to be involved in detecting DNA damage and blocking cell division until the damage is repaired. Ataxia telangiectasia cells are exquisitely sensitive to irradiation. Malignancies including leukemia or lymphoma can occur. Diabetes also may be present, and sexual maturation is delayed. There is no uniformly effective therapy, but antimicrobial therapy and intravenous immunoglobulin (IVIG) replacement therapy may be helpful.

Chronic mucocutaneous candidiasis (autoimmune-polyendocrinopathy-candidiasis-ectodermal dystrophy [APECED]) is characterized by chronic or recurrent candidal infections of the mucous membranes, skin, and nails (Table 73.3). There is normal antibody production but significantly decreased or absent lymphocyte proliferation and delayed skin reactivity to *Candida*. Patients usually do not respond to topical antifungal therapy and must be treated with oral antifungal agents. In most patients, an autoimmune endocrine disorder develops by early adulthood, such as hypoparathyroidism and Addison disease. Other autoimmune disorders have been reported. The insidious onset requires the need for frequent evaluation for autoimmune endocrine disorders. This disease results from a defect in the gene for the transcription factor autoimmune regulator *(AIRE),* which is necessary for expression of peripheral tissue antigens in the thymus. In the absence of these tissue antigens in the thymus, defects in negative selection occur, and autoreactive T cells to specific organs (e.g., adrenal glands, parathyroid glands) lead to specific endocrinopathies.

Hyper-IgE syndrome is characterized by markedly elevated serum IgE levels, a rash that resembles atopic dermatitis,

TABLE 73.3 Other Immunodeficiency Diseases

DISORDER	GENETICS	ONSET	MANIFESTATIONS	PATHOGENESIS	ASSOCIATED FEATURES
Wiskott-Aldrich syndrome	X-linked (Xp11.22)	Early infancy	Thrombocytopenia and bleeding, atopic dermatitis, recurrent infections	53-kDa protein (WASP) defect	Polysaccharide antibody deficiency, small platelets, decreased cell-mediated immunity, lymphoproliferation
Ataxia telangiectasia	AR (11q22.3)	2–5 yr	Recurrent otitis media, pneumonia, meningitis with encapsulated organisms	*ATM* gene pathogenic variant; disorder of DNA double-strand break repair	Neurologic and endocrine dysfunction, malignancy, telangiectasis; sensitivity to radiation
Nijmegen breakage syndrome	AR (8q21)	Infancy	Sinopulmonary infections, bronchiectasis, urinary tract infections	Defect in chromosomal repair mechanisms; hypomorphic variant in NBS1 (Nibrin)	Sensitivity to ionizing radiation; microcephaly with mild neurologic impairment; malignancy
Cartilage-hair hypoplasia (short-limbed dwarf)	AR (9p13–21)	Birth	Variable susceptibility to infections	Pathogenic variant in *RMRP*	Metaphyseal dysplasia, short extremities
Chronic mucocutaneous candidiasis (APECED)	AR	3–5 yr	Candidal infections of mucous membranes, skin, and nails	Pathogenic variants in *AIRE* gene	Autoimmune endocrinopathies
Hyper-IgE syndrome	AD, AR	Variable	Skin and pulmonary abscesses, fungal infections, eczema, elevated IgE	Pathogenic variants in STAT3 (AD), TYK2 (AR), and DOCK8 (AR)	Coarse facial features, failure to shed primary teeth, frequent fractures (STAT3), viral and other infections (TYK2 and DOCK8)
Interferon-γ receptor deficiency 1,2	AR, AD	Variable	Recurrent nontuberculous *Mycobacterium* and *Salmonella* infections	Pathogenic variants in IFN-γR1, IFN-γR2	Absent interferon signaling
Interleukin 12 receptor β1 deficiency	AR	Variable	Recurrent nontuberculous *Mycobacterium* and *Salmonella* infections	IL-12β1	Absent IL-12 signaling
Interleukin 12p40 deficiency	AR	Variable	Recurrent nontuberculous *Mycobacterium* and *Salmonella* infections	IL-12p40	Lack of IL-12 with resulting low IFN-γ

AD, Autosomal dominant; *APECED*, autoimmune-polyendocrinopathy-candidiasis-ectodermal dystrophy; *AR*, autosomal recessive; *IFN*, interferon.

eosinophilia, and staphylococcal abscesses of the skin, lungs, joints, and viscera (Table 73.3). Variants in the *STAT3* gene cause autosomal dominant hyper-IgE syndrome, which is the most common form of hyper-IgE syndrome. Infections with *H. influenzae* type b, *Candida*, and *Aspergillus* also may occur. These patients have coarse facial features, joint laxity, and osteopenia with fractures and may have giant pneumatoceles in the lungs after staphylococcal pneumonias. Although serum IgG, IgA, and IgM levels are normal, humoral immune responses to specific antigens are reduced, as is cell-mediated immunity. Long-term treatment with antistaphylococcal medications is indicated, and Ig replacement therapy may be helpful. Some patients with a hyper-IgE phenotype have autosomal recessive inheritance due to variants in the *TYK2* and *DOCK8* genes.

Since the implementation of next-generation sequencing, the number of combined immunodeficiencies has increased exponentially, and currently there are greater than 50 genetic defects that cause a combined immune deficiency. These include defects in proximal T-cell receptor signaling molecules (CD3γ, ZAP70, LCK, MALT1/CARD11/BCL10 complex, ITK), defects in NF-κB activation (IKBKB, IKBKA, relB), defects in T- and B-cell interacting molecules similar to CD40/CD40L (OX40, IL21, IL21R), and defects in transcription factors (NFATC1, Helios). These can also involve genetic syndromes (Table 73.3). These conditions can have variable numbers of T cells; highly variable infectious susceptibility with bacterial, fungi, and opportunistic organisms; and variable associated features such as autoimmunity. There is not good testing to rule out most of these defects, and thus genetic sequencing panels are useful to screen for many diseases at once.

TREATMENT

The approach to therapy of lymphocyte disorders depends on the diagnosis, clinical findings, and laboratory findings (Table 73.4). When immunodeficiency is suspected and while the evaluation is in process, all blood products need to be irradiated and negative for cytomegalovirus. Lymphocytes present in blood products can cause fatal GVHD in patients with SCID. Cytomegalovirus infection can be fatal in an immunodeficient patient undergoing stem cell transplantation. Live virus vaccines should be withheld from patients *and* household members until a diagnosis is established.

Infections should be treated with appropriate antibiotics; **antibiotic prophylaxis** can be used to prevent recurrent infections, provide a better quality of life, and decrease possible consequences. Patients with severe T-cell deficiencies should receive prophylaxis against *Pneumocystis,* fungi, and herpesviruses, as well as immunoglobulin replacement therapy until treatment with stem cell transplantation. Patients with milder forms may benefit from **vaccination** with protein-conjugate vaccines to *H. influenzae* type b and *S. pneumonia.*

Ig replacement therapy, intravenously or subcutaneously, is a lifesaving therapy for patients with severe antibody deficiency diseases and SCID. Intravenous or subcutaneous gammaglobulin contains polyclonal IgG antibodies isolated from at least 1,000 healthy donors, and its use provides passive immunity against common microorganisms and reduces the frequency and severity of infection in most patients. Ig replacement therapy is usually administered at a total monthly dose of 400–600 mg/kg of body weight administered intravenously every 3–4 weeks or subcutaneously by infusion pump every 1–2 weeks. IVIG therapy should be monitored by regularly measuring trough Ig levels and, more important, the patient's clinical course. Patients who continue to have recurrent infections, especially in the last week before the administration of IVIG, may require higher doses or more frequent administration. A combination of prophylactic antibiotics and Ig replacement therapy may be indicated in patients who continue to have recurrent infections. **Complications of IVIG** therapy include transfusion reactions with chills, fever, and myalgias. Pretreatment with an antihistamine, an antipyretic, and a slower rate of infusion usually prevents these reactions in subsequent infusions. Headache from aseptic meningitis can develop after IVIG therapy, usually in the first 24 hours. It most often responds to treatment with ibuprofen. Hemolysis can also occur. Allergic reactions to IVIG may rarely occur in patients with absent IgA. Subcutaneous administration of Ig has fewer adverse effects but may be complicated by local reactions at the site(s) of infusion. In rare cases, Ig replacement therapy has been linked to the development of pulmonary emboli, stroke, myocardial infarction, or kidney failure, particularly in subjects with underlying medical issues. The risk of transmission of infectious agents, despite preparation from large numbers of selected donors, is extremely low.

Therapy for severe T-cell disorders is stem cell transplantation, preferably from a human leukocyte antigen–matched sibling (see Chapter 76). Some patients continue to have poor B-cell function after stem cell transplantation and require lifelong Ig replacement therapy. GVHD, in which the transplanted cells initiate an immune response against the host tissues, is the main complication of stem cell transplantation. Patients with the ADA deficiency form of SCID who lack matched sibling donors can receive repeated intramuscular replacement doses of ADA, stabilized by coupling to polyethylene glycol. Gene therapy has been performed in patients with common γ-chain deficiency and ADA deficiency by transfer of a normal gene into bone marrow stem cells, which are infused into the patient. Gene therapy for common γ-chain deficiency (X-SCID) and ADA deficiency results in immune reconstitution in most patients. However, in X-SCID, but not ADA-SCID, initial gene therapy trials were complicated by the development of leukemia in most patients. Newer viral vectors have been developed that appear not to cause leukemia, making it a likely option in the future for some forms of SCID. Gene therapy for ADA-SCID has been approved by the European Medicines Agency (equivalent of the U.S. Food and Drug Administration) and is currently a therapeutic option in European countries.

TABLE 73.4 General Management of Patients With Immunodeficiency

Avoid transfusions with blood products unless they are irradiated and cytomegalovirus negative.
Avoid live virus vaccines, especially in patients with severe T-cell deficiencies or agammaglobulinemia, and in household members.
Use prophylaxis to *Pneumocystis jirovecii* in T-cell immunodeficiency including X-linked hyper-IgM and CD40 deficient AR hyper-IgM; consider antifungal prophylaxis in T-cell immunodeficiency.
Consider using prophylactic antibacterials (essential in severe immunodeficiencies and in patients with severe bronchiectasis).
Follow pulmonary function in patients with recurrent pneumonia.
Use chest physiotherapy and postural drainage in patients with recurrent pneumonia.
Examine diarrheal stools for *Giardia lamblia* and *Clostridium difficile*.
Avoid unnecessary exposure to individuals with infection.
Boil water for T-cell defects and hyper-IgM syndrome (*Cryptosporidium* risk).
Use Ig for severe antibody deficiency states (400–600 mg/kg IV monthly or SC every 1–2 weeks).

AR, Autosomal recessive; *Ig*, immunoglobulin; *IV*, intravenous; *SC*, subcutaneous.

PREVENTION AND NEWBORN SCREENING

Population-based screening programs to detect SCID in newborns are routine in the United States, parts of Europe, South America, and Asia. The T-cell receptor excision circle (TREC) assay is the newborn screening test for SCID. The TREC assay enumerates the numbers of a specific TREC isolated from newborn blood spot cards, which serves as a biomarker for normal, newly formed, naïve T cells. Absent or severely low TREC assays indicate low or absent numbers of naïve T cells and identify infants with SCID. Newborn screening for SCID is highly sensitive in identifying infants prior to the development of infectious complications and substantially decreases mortality following stem cell transplantation. Newborn screening for SCID has also led to the identification of additional genetic causes of SCID, but it does not pick up all forms of SCID or all severe forms of combined immunodeficiencies such as CD40L deficiency or MHC class II deficiency.

PEARLS FOR PRACTITIONERS

See Immunology: Pearls for Practitioners at the end of this section.

REVIEW QUESTIONS

Available online.

CHAPTER 74

Neutrophil Disorders

Neutrophils play important roles in immunity and wound healing; their primary function is ingesting and killing pathogens. Neutrophil disorders can result from deficient cell numbers or defective function (Table 74.1). Patients with neutrophil disorders are susceptible to a variety of bacterial infections and certain fungi. Suggestive signs include mucous membrane infections (gingivitis), abscesses in the skin and viscera, lymphadenitis, poor wound healing, delayed umbilical cord separation, or absence of pus. Neutrophils develop in the bone marrow from hematopoietic stem cells by the action of several colony-stimulating factors (CSFs), including stem cell factor, granulocyte-monocyte CSF, granulocyte CSF (G-CSF), and interleukin (IL)-3. On leaving the bone marrow, mature neutrophils are found in the circulation or reside in the marginating pool. Adhesion molecules are necessary for neutrophils to roll and adhere to vascular endothelium and extravasate from the blood into sites of infection, where they phagocytose and kill pathogens, especially those coated by complement or antibodies. Chemotactic factors, including the complement fragment C5a, IL-8, and bacterial formulated peptides, mobilize neutrophils to enter tissues and sites of infections. Neutrophils kill ingested pathogens using enzymes contained in their granules and by the production of superoxide by nicotinamide adenine dinucleotide phosphate (NADPH) oxidase. Immunodeficiencies may result from abnormalities in the production, turnover, adherence and/or extravasation, or killing mechanisms by neutrophils.

ETIOLOGY AND CLINICAL MANIFESTATIONS

Disorders of Neutrophil Numbers

The normal neutrophil count varies with age. **Neutropenia** is defined as an absolute neutrophil count (ANC) less than 1,500/mm^3 for White children 1 year of age or older. Black children of African heritage normally have lower total white blood cell and neutrophil counts. The effect of neutropenia depends on its severity. The susceptibility to infection is minimally increased until the ANC is less than 1,000/mm^3. Most patients do well with an ANC greater than 500/mm^3. At these levels, localized infections are more common than generalized bacteremia. Serious bacterial infections are more common with an ANC less than 200/mm^3. The major types of infections associated with neutropenia are cellulitis, pharyngitis, gingivitis, lymphadenitis, abscesses (cutaneous or perianal), enteritis (typhlitis), and pneumonia. The sites of the infection are usually colonized heavily with normal bacterial flora that becomes invasive in the presence of neutropenia. Neutropenia may be congenital or acquired (Table 74.2) and may be associated with specific diseases, especially infections (Table 74.3), or result from drug reactions (Table 74.4).

There are several forms of congenital neutropenia. **Severe congenital neutropenia (Kostmann syndrome)** is an autosomal recessive disorder in which myeloid cells fail to mature beyond the early stages of the promyelocyte due to pathogenic variants in the *HAX-1* gene (Table 74.1). The peripheral blood may show an impressive monocytosis. Exogenous G-CSF is commonly used to treat this disorder by increasing the production of neutrophils. Acute myeloid leukemia has developed in a few patients who have survived to adolescence. Stem cell transplantation may be curative. Defects in *G6PC3, GFI1,* and other genes have also been shown to cause severe congenital neutropenia (Table 74.1). **Cyclic neutropenia** is a stem cell disorder in which all marrow elements cycle resulting in transient neutropenia. It may be transmitted as an autosomal dominant, recessive, or sporadic disorder. Because of the short half-life of neutrophils in the blood (6–7 hours) compared to platelets (10 days) and red blood cells (120 days), neutropenia is the only clinically significant abnormality. The usual cycle is 21 days, with neutropenia lasting 4–6 days, accompanied by monocytosis and often by eosinophilia. Severe, debilitating bone pain is common when the neutrophil count is low. G-CSF results in increasing neutrophil numbers and a shorter duration of neutropenia. Defects in *ELANE,* the gene encoding for neutrophil elastase, have been found in patients with cyclic neutropenia. Further analysis has demonstrated *ELANE* variants in some cases of severe congenital neutropenia.

Severe congenital neutropenia that may be either persistent or cyclic also is a component of **Shwachman-Diamond syndrome**, an autosomal recessive syndrome of pancreatic insufficiency accompanying bone marrow dysfunction (Table 74.1). This is a panmyeloid disorder in which neutropenia is the most prominent manifestation. Metaphyseal dysostosis and dwarfism may occur. Patients usually respond to G-CSF. A gain of function variant in the Wiskott-Aldrich syndrome protein has also been associated with an X-linked form of severe congenital neutropenia. **Benign congenital neutropenia** is a condition in which significant neutropenia develops but in whom major infectious complications do not occur. Many patients whose ANC ranges from 100 to 500/mm^3 have an increased frequency of infections, particularly respiratory infections, but the major problem is the slow resolution of infections that develop. Severe congenital neutropenia may be associated with severe combined immunodeficiency in **reticular dysgenesis**, a disorder of hematopoietic stem cells affecting all bone marrow lineages due to variants of the *AK2* gene.

Isoimmune neutropenia occurs in neonates as the result of transplacental transfer of maternal antibodies to fetal neutrophil antigens. The mother is sensitized to specific neutrophil antigens on fetal leukocytes that are inherited from the father and are not present on maternal cells. Isoimmune neonatal neutropenia, similar to isoimmune anemia and thrombocytopenia, is a transient process (see Chapter 61). Cutaneous infections are common, and sepsis is rare. Early treatment of infection while the infant is neutropenic is the major goal of

TABLE 74.1 Phagocytic Disorders

NAME	GENETICS	DEFECT	COMMENT
Congenital neutropenia, cyclic neutropenia	AR (*HAX1, GFI1*, others) AD (*GFI1, ELANE*)	Severe neutropenia	Cellulitis, pharyngitis, gingivitis, lymphadenitis, abscesses, typhlitis, and pneumonia
Chronic granulomatous disease	X-linked (gp91^{phox}), AR (p22^{phox}, p47^{phox}, and p67^{phox})	Bactericidal, fungicidal	X-linked recessive (66%), autosomal recessive (33%); eczema, osteomyelitis, granulomas, abscesses caused by *Staphylococcus aureus, Burkholderia cepacia, Aspergillus fumigatus*, colitis
Chédiak-Higashi syndrome (1q42l-44)	AR (*LYST*)	Bactericidal plus chemotaxis; poor natural killer function	Autosomal recessive; oculocutaneous albinism, neuropathy, giant neutrophilic cytoplasmic inclusions; malignancy, neutropenia
Myeloperoxidase deficiency	AR (*MPO*)	Bactericidal, fungicidal but low risk of infections	Reduced chemiluminescence; autosomal recessive (1:4,000); persistent candidiasis in patients with diabetes
Glucose-6-phosphate dehydrogenase deficiency	X-linked (*G6PD*)	Bactericidal, fungicidal	Phenotypically similar to chronic granulomatous disease
Leukocyte adhesion deficiency type 1, 2, and 3	AR (*ITGB2, FUCT1, FERMT3*, respectively)	Adherence, chemotaxis, phagocytosis; reduced lymphocyte cytotoxicity	Type 1: Delayed separation or infection of umbilical cord; lethal bacterial infections without pus; neutrophilia Type 2: Also short stature Type 3: Also bleeding disorder
Shwachman-Diamond syndrome	AR (*SBDS*)	Chemotaxis, neutropenia	Pancreatic insufficiency, metaphyseal chondrodysplasia; autosomal recessive
WHIM	AD (*CXCR4*)	Impaired chemokine receptor	Low IgG, warts, myelokathexis
Mono MAC	AD (*GATA2*)	Monocytopenia, macrophage dysfunction	Mycobacterial, viral, fungal, bacterial opportunistic infections, warts, pulmonary alveolar proteinosis, lupus

AD, Autosomal dominant; *AR*, autosomal recessive; *Mono MAC*, monocytopenia, B- and NK-cell lymphopenia, opportunistic infections, virus-induced cancers, myelodysplasia; *WHIM*, warts, hypogammaglobulinemia, infections, myelokathexis.

therapy. Intravenous immune globulin may decrease the duration of neutropenia.

Autoimmune neutropenia usually develops in children 5–24 months of age and often persists for prolonged periods. Neutrophil autoantibodies may be IgG, IgM, IgA, or a combination of these. Usually the condition resolves in 6 months to 4 years. Although intravenous immune globulin and corticosteroids have been used, most patients respond to G-CSF. Autoimmune neutropenia may rarely be an early manifestation of systemic lupus erythematosus, rheumatoid arthritis, or autoimmune lymphoproliferative disease.

Disorders of Neutrophil Migration

Neutrophils normally adhere to endothelium and migrate to areas of inflammation by the interaction of membrane proteins, called *integrins* and *selectins*, with endothelial cell adhesion molecules. A hallmark of defects in neutrophil migration is the absence of pus at sites of infection. In **leukocyte adhesion deficiency type I (LAD-I)**, infants lacking the β_2 integrin CD18 exhibit the condition early with failure of separation of the umbilical cord (often 2 months after birth) with attendant omphalitis and sepsis (Table 74.1). The neutrophil count usually is greater than 20,000/mm^3 because of failure of the neutrophils to adhere normally to vascular endothelium and to migrate out of blood to the tissues (Fig. 74.1). Cutaneous, respiratory, and mucosal infections occur. Children with this condition often have severe gingivitis. Sepsis can lead to death in early childhood. This disorder is transmitted as an autosomal recessive trait. Stem cell transplantation can be lifesaving.

LAD-II results from impairment of neutrophil rolling along the vascular wall, which is the first step in neutrophil migration into tissues and at sites of infection. Rolling is mediated by sialylated and fucosylated tetrasaccharides related to the sialylated Lewis X (S-LeX) blood group found on the surface of neutrophils, monocytes, and activated lymphocytes binding to selectin molecules on vascular endothelium (Fig. 74.1). LAD-II results from a defect in the FUCT1 protein resulting in abnormal fucose metabolism leading to the absence of S-LeX blood group on the surface of neutrophils and other leukocytes. Patients with LAD-II can be dysmorphic, have short stature, and experience severe developmental delay (Table 74.1). LAD-III is a rare disorder caused by defects in the KINDLIN-3 protein resulting in defective neutrophil adhesion as well as platelet defects. Defective migration of neutrophils has also been described in **hyper-IgE syndrome** and with pathogenic variants in the *RAC2* gene (see Chapter 73).

TABLE 74.2 Mechanisms of Neutropenia

ABNORMAL BONE MARROW
Marrow Injury
Medications: idiosyncratic, cytotoxic (myelosuppressive) Radiation Chemicals: DDT, benzene Immune mediated: T and B cells and immunoglobulin Infections (viruses, rickettsia) Infiltrative processes: tumor, storage disease Myelodysplasia Aplastic anemia
Maturation Defects
Folic acid deficiency Vitamin B_{12} Copper
Congenital Disorders
Severe congenital neutropenia (HAX-1, G6PC3, ELANE, GFI-1) Cyclic neutropenia (ELANE) Cartilage-hair hypoplasia Shwachman-Diamond syndrome Diamond-Blackfan syndrome Griscelli syndrome, type 2 Chédiak-Higashi syndrome WHIM syndrome (warts, hypogammaglobulinemia, infections, myelokathexis) Glycogen storage disease type Ib Methylmalonic acidemia
PERIPHERAL CIRCULATION
Pseudoneutropenia: Shift to Bone Marrow/Spleen
Splenomegaly Severe infection
Intravascular
Destruction: neonatal isoimmune, autoimmune, hypersplenism Autoimmune diseases (systemic lupus erythematosus, rheumatoid arthritis, Sjögren syndrome)

DDT, Dichloro-diphenyl-trichloroethane; *ELANE*, elastase, neutrophil expressed; *G6PC3*, glucose-6-phosphatase catalytic subunit 3; *GFI-1*, growth factor independent 1; *HAX-1*, HS1-associated protein X-1.

TABLE 74.3 Infection-Associated Neutropenia

Viral	Cytomegalovirus, dengue, Epstein-Barr virus, hepatitis viruses, HIV, influenza, measles, parvovirus B19, rubella, varicella, HHV-6, SARS-CoV-2
Bacterial	Brucellosis, paratyphoid, pertussis, tuberculosis (disseminated), tularemia, psittacosis, Shigella, typhoid, congenital syphilis; any form of sepsis, including neonatal sepsis
Fungal	Histoplasmosis (disseminated)
Protozoan	Malaria, leishmaniasis (kala-azar)
Rickettsial	*Anaplasma* (formerly *Ehrlichia*) *phagocytophilum*, Rocky Mountain spotted fever, typhus, rickettsialpox

HHV-6, Human herpesvirus-6.
Adapted from Michniacki TF. Walkovich KJ. Leukopenia. In: Kliegman RM, St. Geme J, eds. Nelson Textbook of Pediatrics. *22nd ed. Philadelphia: Elsevier; 2025, table 171.4.*

TABLE 74.4 Drug-Associated Neutropenia

CYTOTOXIC
Myelosuppressive, chemotherapeutic agents Immunosuppressive agents
IDIOSYNCRATIC
Indomethacin Para-aminophenol derivatives Pyrazolone derivatives (aminopyrine, dipyrone, oxyphenbutazone) Chloramphenicol Sulfonamides Antithyroid drugs (propylthiouracil, methimazole, carbimazole) Phenothiazines (chlorpromazine, phenothiazines) Penicillins, semisynthetic penicillins, and cephalosporins

Modified from Dale DC. Neutropenia. In: Lichtman MA, Kipps TJ, Seligsohn U, et al., eds. Williams Hematology. *8th ed. New York: McGraw-Hill; 2010.*

Disorders of Neutrophil Function

Defects in neutrophil function are relatively rare inherited disorders and tend to be associated with a marked susceptibility to bacterial and fungal infections. **Chronic granulomatous disease (CGD)** is a disorder of white blood cells that results from defective intracellular killing of bacteria and pathogens by neutrophils and macrophages because of an inability to activate the "respiratory burst," the catalytic conversion of molecular oxygen to superoxide (O_2^-). NADPH oxidase is the enzyme that catalyzes the respiratory burst and consists of five essential subunits: gp91^{phox}, p22^{phox}, p47^{phox}, p67^{phox}, and p40^{phox}. Additionally, cytochrome B-245 (Eros) is necessary for gp91^{phox}-p22^{phox} heterodimer formation, which is essential for NADPH oxidase function. Defects in any of these enzymes lead to CGD and an inability to kill catalase-positive pathogens such as *Staphylococcus aureus*, gram-negative bacteria *(Burkholderia, Nocardia, Serratia)*, and fungi *(Aspergillus fumigatus, Candida albicans)*. The gp91^{phox} gene, located on chromosome Xp21.1, is responsible for the most common form of the disease. The other gene variants are inherited in an autosomal recessive manner. Glucose-6-phosphate dehydrogenase is also involved in the production of superoxide, and severe forms of glucose-6-phosphate dehydrogenase deficiency also result in CGD. Patients with CGD characteristically have lymphadenopathy, hypergammaglobulinemia, hepatosplenomegaly, dermatitis, growth faltering, anemia, chronic diarrhea, and abscesses. Infections occur in the lungs, middle ear, gastrointestinal tract, skin, urinary tract, lymph nodes, liver, and bones. Granulomas are prominent and may obstruct the pylorus or ureters.

Chédiak-Higashi syndrome, an abnormality of secondary granules, is an autosomal recessive disorder caused by a pathogenic variant in a cytoplasmic protein (LYST) thought to be involved in organellar protein trafficking, resulting in a fusion of the primary and secondary granules in neutrophils. Giant granules are present in many cells, including lymphocytes, platelets, and melanocytes. Patients usually have partial oculocutaneous albinism. The defect in Chédiak-Higashi syndrome results in defective neutrophil and natural killer–cell function, leading to recurrent and sometimes fatal infections with streptococci and staphylococci. Most patients progress to an accelerated phase associated with Epstein-Barr virus infection and characterized by a **lymphoproliferative syndrome** with generalized lymphohistiocytic infiltrates, fever, jaundice, hepatomegaly,

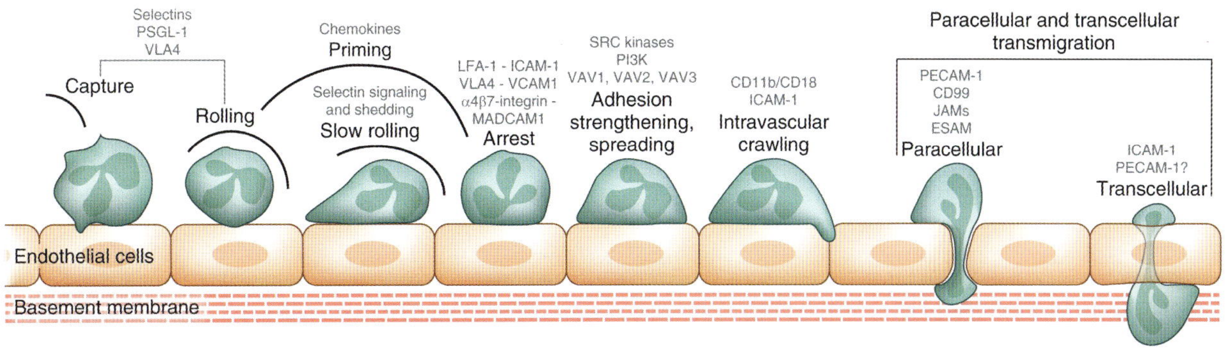

FIGURE 74.1 Steps in the emigration of neutrophils from the vascular space. Neutrophils are depicted entering the marginating pool in a postcapillary venule, and the effector molecules participating in each event are indicated in *gray* text. Initial capture is mediated by interactions between neutrophil/leukocyte (L)–selectin and endothelial cell (E, P)–selectins and their respective carbohydrate ligands on the opposing cell surface (e.g., P-selectin glycoprotein ligand-1 *[PSGL-1]*), whereas integrins (e.g., very late antigen 4 *[VLA4]*) are responsible for firm adherence. Selectin-mediated signaling slows the rolling or tumbling neutrophils, partially countering the shear forces resulting from blood flow. Chemokines diffusing into the bloodstream from sites of microbial invasion in the tissues bind to specific receptors and activate the neutrophil, which is then arrested by integrin-dependent interactions. The activated neutrophil flattens against the endothelium and crawls along the luminal surface of the vessel wall. Platelet–endothelial cell adhesion molecule-1 *(PECAM-1)*, junctional adhesion molecules *(JAMs)*, and endothelial cell–selective adhesion molecule *(ESAM)* localized to interendothelial cell junctions interact with PECAM-1 and CD99 on the neutrophil surface to permit neutrophil migration between and through endothelial cells. Once in the tissues, the polarized neutrophils move up the mediator concentration gradient to reach the site of microbial invasion. *ICAM-1*, Intercellular adhesion molecule; *LFA-1*, leukocyte function–associated antigen; *MADCAM1*, mucosal addressing cell adhesion molecule 1; *PI(3)K*, phosphatidylinositol-3-phosphate kinase; *SRC*, sarcoma; *VAV1*, vav1 guanine nucleotide exchange factor; *VCAM1*, vascular cell adhesion molecule 1. (From DeLeo FR, Nauseef WM. Granulocytic phagocytes. In Bennett JE, Dolin R, Blaser MJ, eds. *Mandell, Douglas, and Bennett's Principles and Practice of Infectious Diseases*. 9th ed. Philadelphia: Elsevier; 2020, fig. 8.3.)

lymphadenopathy, and pancytopenia. The condition resembles hemophagocytic lymphohistiocytosis (see Chapter 77).

LABORATORY DIAGNOSIS

The evaluation of a neutropenic child depends on clinical signs of infection, family and medication history, age of the patient, cyclic or persistent nature of the condition, signs of bone marrow infiltration (malignancy or storage disease), and evidence of involvement of other cell lines. Neutropenia is confirmed by a complete blood count and differential. A bone marrow aspirate and biopsy may be necessary to determine whether the neutropenia is due to a failure of production in the bone marrow, infiltration of the bone marrow, or loss of neutrophils in the periphery. Antineutrophil antibodies can be useful in the diagnosis of autoimmune neutropenia, although their interpretation can be difficult.

Neutrophil chemotactic defects can be excluded by the presence of neutrophils at the site of infection. The **Rebuck skin window** is a 4-hour in vivo test for neutrophil chemotaxis that is not performed routinely by most laboratories. In vitro studies of neutrophil chemotaxis and migration are available in specialized laboratories. Flow cytometry for the presence of adhesion molecules, such as CD18 or CD15, can help diagnose leukocyte adhesion defects. Point variants that affect the function of the adhesion molecule but do not alter antibody binding are missed using flow cytometry. CGD can be diagnosed by the flow cytometry–based test using **dihydrorhodamine 123** or the nitroblue tetrazolium test (see Chapter 72). Light microscopy of neutrophils for the presence of giant granules can help diagnose Chédiak-Higashi syndrome.

TREATMENT

Therapy for neutropenia depends on the underlying cause. Patients with severe bacterial infections require broad-spectrum antibiotics; the resolution of neutropenia is the most important prognostic factor. Most patients with severe congenital neutropenia or autoimmune neutropenia respond to therapy with G-CSF. Granulocyte transfusion should be reserved for life-threatening infection. Chronic mild neutropenia not associated with immunosuppression can be managed expectantly with prompt antimicrobial treatment of soft tissue infections, which usually are caused by *S. aureus* or group A streptococcus.

In the past, CGD has been treated by antimicrobial prophylaxis with trimethoprim-sulfamethoxazole, itraconazole, and interferon-γ. Stem cell transplantation has become the preferred treatment if an acceptable human leukocyte antigen–matched donor can be identified. Prompt diagnosis and treatment of infections are required in CGD. Because *A. fumigatus* can cause serious infection in patients with CGD, moldy hay, decomposing compost, and other nests of fungi must be avoided.

PROGNOSIS AND PREVENTION

The prognosis depends on the particular defect. Milder and transient defects in neutrophil numbers have a better prognosis. Prolonged absence of neutrophils or their function has a poor prognosis, especially with the risk of bacterial and fungal sepsis. Stem cell transplantation has improved the prognosis of CGD and is also the treatment of choice for other severe neutrophil defects that cannot be managed with G-CSF. Prenatal diagnosis and genetic counseling are possible for known gene variants.

PEARLS FOR PRACTITIONERS

See Immunology: Pearls for Practitioners at the end of this section.

REVIEW QUESTIONS

Available online.

CHAPTER 75

Complement System

The **complement system** consists of plasma and membrane proteins that function in the innate immune response as well as in facilitating adaptive immunity. **Complement proteins** can kill pathogens with or without antibodies, opsonize pathogens to facilitate their uptake by phagocytes, or mediate inflammation. The complement system can be activated through three pathways—classic, alternative, or lectin—that involve a cascade-like sequential activation of complement factors resulting in an amplified response (Fig. 75.1). Disorders of the complement system predispose to recurrent infection, autoimmunity, and angioedema (Table 75.1).

ETIOLOGY

The three pathways for complement activation are initiated by different mechanisms. The classic pathway is initiated by antigen-antibody complexes or by C-reactive protein and activated by C1q and two proteases, C1R and C1S. The alternative pathway may be activated by C3b generated through the classical pathway or by spontaneous hydrolysis of C3 on microbial surfaces, which is then amplified when C3b binds to factor B, which is cleaved by factor D to form the C3 convertase, C3bBb. The alternative pathway is an amplification mechanism of complement activation. The lectin pathway is initiated by the interaction of mannose-binding lectin with microbial carbohydrate, and then mannose-binding protein-associated proteases (MASP) cleave C4 and C2. Figure 75.1 depicts the steps in each of these pathways that converge with the generation of C3b and result in the formation of a membrane attack complex (MAC). The MAC is a complex of C5b, C6, C7, C8, and C9 molecules that is common to all three pathways. The MAC generates pores in the cell membrane, leading to lysis of the cells. C3a and C5a, produced by cleavage of C3 and C5, respectively, can release histamine from mast cells and basophils, leading to increased vascular permeability and smooth muscle contraction. C5a attracts phagocytes to the site of complement activation and can cause degranulation of phagocytic cells. C3b acts as an opsonin when attached to the surface of a pathogen by binding to phagocytes via complement receptor 1 (CR1). Its degradation product, iC3b, can bind to the complement receptor CR3 on the surface of phagocytes, leading to the ingestion of the C3b-coated or iC3b-coated pathogen. iC3b and its breakdown product C3dg can bind complement receptor 2 (CR2) on B cells, leading to activation and differentiation.

The complement system is under tight regulation because it has potent inflammatory activity and the potential to cause significant damage to host cells. The complement cascade is inherently regulated by the short half-life of C4b and C3b and by instability of the C3 convertases, C4b2b, and C3bBb. C1-inhibitor regulates the cascade by blocking active sites on C1r, C1s, and MASP. Factor I destabilizes C3 convertase complexes and degrades the active fragments. Other inhibitors include membrane proteins, such as decay accelerating factor, CR1, membrane cofactor protein (MCP), and plasma proteins such as C4b-binding protein, factor H, and factor I. Formation of the MAC can be blocked by cell surface CD59, protein S, and other plasma proteins. Deficiency of any of these regulatory proteins can result in an inflammatory response, tissue damage, or excessive complement consumption.

Disorders of complement proteins can result from inherited deficiency or can be secondary to increased consumption. The consequences of decreased complement depend on the affected factor (see Table 75.1). **Deficiencies of early components** of the classic pathway (C1, C2, or C4) may present with recurrent infections with encapsulated bacteria, such as pneumococcus. Patients with C1, C2, or C4 deficiency are susceptible to autoimmune diseases, especially systemic lupus erythematosus. The exact mechanism of this susceptibility is not known but is thought to arise from the role of these early components in clearing immune complexes.

Deficiency of properdin, C3, or the terminal components predisposes patients to severe recurrent infections. Deficiency of C3, the major opsonin, due to a genetic defect or secondary to excessive consumption, predisposes patients to infections, especially with encapsulated organisms. Deficiency of one of the terminal components that compose the MAC

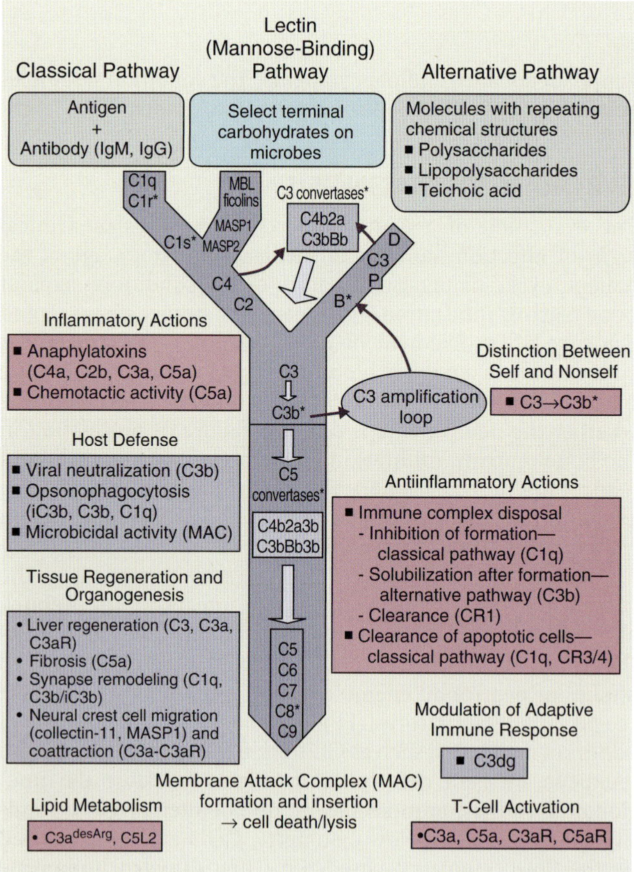

FIGURE 75.1 The complement cascade. Within each pathway, the components are arranged in order of their activation and aligned opposite their functional and structural analogues in the other pathways. Rounded boxes relate to activation of the pathways; squared boxes reflect complement functions; asterisks indicate sites of downregulation of complement activity. *B*, Factor B; *C*, complement; *CR1*, complement receptor 1; *D*, factor D; *Ig*, immunoglobulin; *MAC*, membrane attack complex; *MASP*, MBL-associated serine protease; *MBL*, mannose-binding lectin; *P*, properdin. (From Ram S. Complement and deficiencies. In: Bennett JE, Dolin R, Blaser MJ, eds. *Mandell, Douglas, and Bennett's Principles and Practice of Infectious Diseases.* 9th ed. Philadelphia: Elsevier; 2020, fig. 9.1.)

TABLE 75.1 Deficiency of Complement and Associated Disease

DEFICIENT PROTEIN	ASSOCIATED DISEASE
C1q, C1r	SLE, glomerulonephritis; encapsulated bacterial infections
C2	SLE, glomerulonephritis; encapsulated bacterial infections
C3	Recurrent bacterial infections, rare glomerulonephritis, or SLE
C4	SLE, glomerulonephritis; encapsulated bacterial infections
C5	Recurrent meningococcal infections
C6	Recurrent meningococcal infections
C7	Recurrent meningococcal infections
C8	Recurrent meningococcal infections
C9	Occasional meningococcal infection
Properdin	Recurrent infections, severe meningococcal infection
MBL	Mildly increased susceptibility to infections
Factor H	Glomerulonephritis, atypical HUS
Factor I	Recurrent infections, glomerulonephritis
MCP	Glomerulonephritis, atypical HUS
C1 inhibitor	Hereditary angioedema

HUS, Hemolytic uremic syndrome; *MBL,* mannose-binding lectin; *MCP,* membrane cofactor protein; *SLE,* systemic lupus erythematosus.

predisposes patients to infection with *Neisseria meningitidis.* Complement deficiency may be found in 40% of patients presenting with recurrent neisserial infections. Deficiency of mannose-binding lectin may be associated with an increased frequency of bacterial infections, but the clinical significance of mannose-binding lectin deficiency is controversial.

Congenital deficiency of C1-inhibitor results in **hereditary angioedema**, characterized by recurrent episodes of nonpruritic angioedema lasting 48–72 hours that occur spontaneously or after minor trauma, stress, or anxiety (see Chapter 82). Intestinal edema can cause acute abdominal pain; edema of the upper airway can be life-threatening and may necessitate emergency tracheostomy. Importantly, the angioedema in this disorder is not responsive to corticosteroids, and this feature is useful in distinguishing from more common forms of idiopathic angioedema. Hereditary angioedema is inherited as an autosomal dominant disease and results from a heterozygous deficiency of C1-inhibitor, leading to serum levels <30% of normal values. Some pathogenic variants (type II hereditary angioedema) result in normal levels of C1-inhibitor with defective function. Hereditary angioedema with normal C1-inhibitor (formally known as hereditary edema type 3) may occur due to variants in factor XII, but the etiology in most cases is unknown. An acquired form of angioedema results from autoantibodies to C1-inhibitor in lymphoid malignancies or autoimmune disorders but is uncommon in childhood. C1-inhibitor is a regulator of Hageman factor (clotting factor XIIa), clotting factor XIa, plasma kallikrein, and plasmin in addition to C1r and C1s. Lack of inhibition of the contact system, Hageman factor, and plasma kallikrein leading to the overproduction of bradykinin is responsible for the development of angioedema. Deficiencies in the complement regulatory proteins factor H, factor I, and MCP result in **atypical hemolytic uremic syndrome** or **membranoproliferative glomerulonephritis type II** and have been linked to **age-related macular degeneration**.

LABORATORY STUDIES

The **CH_{50} test** tests the classic complement pathway function, based on an antibody-dependent hemolytic assay, which measures the serum dilution that results in lysis of 50% of sheep red blood cells. The CH_{50} test depends on the function of all nine complement proteins, C1 through C9. The **AH_{50} test**, which measures complement activation using red blood cells from different species (e.g., rabbit) that can activate the alternative pathway without antibody, is less widely available than the CH_{50} test and requires the alternative pathway components and C5–C9. Abnormal results of both tests indicate a deficiency in a terminal component common to both pathways (C5–C9), whereas an abnormal result of CH_{50} or AH_{50} indicates a deficiency of an early component (C1q, C2, C4, or C3) or of the alternative pathway (factor B, properdin), respectively. If the CH_{50} or AH_{50} levels are abnormal, individual components can be analyzed in specialized laboratories.

Low C1-inhibitor levels or function results in chronically decreased C4 levels; therefore C4 levels are commonly used as a screening test for hereditary angioedema type 1 and type 2, but definitive diagnosis requires determination of C1-inhibitor levels and function. Low C1 levels are found in acquired C1-inhibitor deficiency, which distinguishes it from hereditary angioedema since the C1 esterase blocks cleavage of C4 and C3 but does not affect C1 levels. Tests for autoantibodies to C1-inhibitor can be performed by enzyme-linked immunosorbent assay.

TREATMENT

Specific treatment of complement deficiencies with component replacement is not available. Long, frequent courses of antibiotics constitute the primary therapy. Immunization of patients and close contacts with pneumococcal and meningococcal vaccines may be useful, but infections may still occur in immunized complement-deficient patients. Replacement of complement proteins by plasma transfusion has been used in some patients with C2 deficiency, factor H deficiency, or factor I deficiency; however, these are short-lived proteins made in the liver and required frequent transfusions, making this less than optimal therapy. Eculizumab, which binds to C5 and inhibits activation of the complement system, has been used. MCP deficiency is treated with kidney transplantation because it is a membrane protein.

There are several therapeutic options available for **C1-inhibitor deficiency**. Acute attacks of angioedema in this disorder should be treated as promptly as possible with plasma-derived or recombinant C1-inhibitor, icatibant (a bradykinin B2-receptor antagonist), or ecallantide (a kallikrein inhibitor). Importantly, the angioedema in these disorders is not responsive to epinephrine, antihistamines, or corticosteroids. In the case of acute airway obstruction nonresponsive to medications, an emergency tracheostomy may be required.

Long-term prophylaxis of hereditary angioedema can be treated by several medications. The prophylactic use of an oral attenuated androgen (**stanozolol** or **danazol**), which increases serum concentrations of C1-inhibitor, can be used; adverse effects, including masculinization in females, growth arrest, and hepatitis, limit their use. Chronic administration of recombinant or plasma derived C1-inhibitor or lanadelumab (a human monoclonal antibody to kallikrein) is increasingly used in the disorder. Alternatively, prompt breakthrough treatment with icatibant or ecallantide is also used. Angiotensin-converting enzyme inhibitors, such as captopril, should be avoided in patients with C1-inhibitor deficiency because these medications can precipitate episodes of angioedema by inhibiting degradation of kinins that mediate angioedema formation.

PEARLS FOR PRACTITIONERS

See Immunology: Pearls for Practitioners at the end of this section.

REVIEW QUESTIONS

Available online.

TABLE 76.1 Immunodeficiency Diseases Curable by Stem Cell Transplantation

Severe combined immunodeficiency (SCID)
X-linked SCID (γ_c deficiency)
Jak3 kinase deficiency
ZAP-70 deficiency and other T-cell activation defects
RAG1/RAG2 deficiency and other T^- B^- SCID
Omenn syndrome
Adenosine deaminase deficiency
Purine nucleoside phosphorylase deficiency
Reticular dysgenesis
Bare lymphocyte syndrome
Wiskott-Aldrich syndrome
X-linked hyper-IgM
X-linked lymphoproliferative syndromes
Chronic granulomatous disease
Autoimmune lymphoproliferative syndrome (Fas defect)
Severe congenital neutropenia
Shwachman-Diamond syndrome
Immune dysregulation, polyendocrinopathy, enteropathy, X-linked (IPEX)
Cyclic neutropenia
Chédiak-Higashi syndrome
Leukocyte adhesion deficiency type I
Familial hemophagocytic lymphohistiocytosis

CHAPTER 76

Hematopoietic Stem Cell Transplantation

Hematopoietic stem cell transplantation (HSCT) can cure some patients with primary immunodeficiency disease (Table 76.1). Use of HSCT is primarily limited to immunodeficiency diseases, some metabolic storage diseases (see Chapter 55), malignancies (see Chapter 155), aplastic anemia (see Chapter 151), and hemoglobinopathies (see Chapter 151).

The principle of HSCT is to replace a patient's defective bone marrow stem cells with normal stem cells. Hematopoietic stem cells reside in the bone marrow but can also be obtained from peripheral blood or cord blood. Peripheral blood does not contain a significant proportion of stem cells unless the donor's bone marrow is actively stimulated to generate stem cells. Cord blood is a good source of stem cells and is used for sibling and unrelated HSCT.

Major histocompatibility complex (MHC) compatibility is crucial in the choice of a stem cell donor to avoid rejection of the donor cells by the host immune system and to prevent **graft versus host disease (GVHD)** caused by contaminating mature T cells. The donor stem cells give rise to T cells that develop in the host thymus and need to interact with donor and host antigen-presenting cells. In cases with MHC mismatched donors, mature T cells need to be removed from the donor to reduce the risk of GVHD; this complication outweighs the disadvantage of a prolonged time of 90–120 days before T-cell development. Patients are at risk for developing **B-cell lymphoproliferative disease**, usually associated with Epstein-Barr virus, when T-cell depletion techniques are used, likely due to the delay in T-cell engraftment.

The most important factor affecting outcomes in HSCT is the similarity of the donor MHC. The best outcomes are obtained using MHC-identical siblings (25% chance of a matched sibling) as donors, followed by matched unrelated donors. Unlike transplantation for other disorders, MHC haploidentical bone marrow from a parent (preferred) or a sibling can be used to treat severe combined immunodeficiency (SCID), likely the result of these patients lacking functioning T cells. Stem cells from a partially mismatched donor, such as a parent, can give rise to a functioning immune system because the patient shares at least half of the MHC molecules with the donor stem cells.

MHC molecules are highly polymorphic, and typing is currently performed on DNA rather than by serology. Bone marrow and cord blood registries are available worldwide. Searching and identifying a donor can be a lengthy process, especially for some underrepresented ethnic backgrounds. Finding a suitable cord blood donor is faster because the cord blood already has been obtained and stored, whereas bone marrow donors have to be identified, located, and tested.

Patients with SCID require definitive treatment as survival is unlikely beyond 1–2 years of age. Stem cell transplantation is the main option for treatment of SCID, with some gene therapies available. The development of transplantation using T-cell–depleted, haploidentical bone marrow from a parent for SCID has provided almost every patient with SCID a potential donor. The mother is the preferred source for haploidentical bone marrow, if she is able to donate, because some transfer of maternal T cells can occur during pregnancy, and these maternal T cells can reject cells obtained from the father. The need for conditioning prior to stem cell transplantation for SCID is controversial and an area of ongoing research. In nations that use newborn screening for SCID, the long-term survival rate after stem cell transplantation is over 90%, reflecting the improvement in outcomes that occur with transplantation prior to infection.

DNA sequencing is often needed to obtain a genetic diagnosis to ascertain the cause of a primary immunodeficiency. Consequently, information about the natural history of these disorders is increasingly available and a better, more informed decision on the need for stem cell transplantation can be made. In those cases where a genetic diagnosis is not obtained, several factors are taken into consideration when considering stem cell transplantation such as age, severity of the immunodeficiency, functional status of the patient, and availability of a human leukocyte antigen (HLA)–matched donor. Disorders of B cells have not been treated with HSCT because in many cases these disorders respond well to antibody replacement therapy. Furthermore, normal immunoglobulin production does not necessarily occur following stem cell transplantation in a substantial percentage of patients, despite normal donor B-cell engraftment. Regardless, stem cell transplantation is commonly used to treat a number of combined immunodeficiencies (see Table 76.1).

COMPLICATIONS

Rejection of the grafted stem cells is the first potential complication of HSCT and depends on the immunocompetence of the patient, the degree of MHC incompatibility, and the number of stem cells administered. Preconditioning with cytotoxic drugs such as busulfan and cyclophosphamide can prevent graft rejection but may be complicated by pulmonary toxicity and by veno-occlusive disease of the liver, which results from damage to the hepatic vascular endothelium and can be fatal. Conditioning prior to stem cell transplantation results in anemia, leukopenia, and thrombocytopenia, making patients susceptible to infection and bleeding disorders. Neutropenic precautions should be maintained, and patients supported with red blood cell and platelet transfusions until the red blood cell, platelet, and neutrophil lineages engraft. Reduced intensity preconditioning is increasingly used to prevent graft rejection and decrease the adverse effects of more intensive forms of conditioning. **B-cell lymphoproliferative disorders** due to Epstein-Barr virus infection can develop after T-cell–depleted bone marrow transplantation. GVHD can arise from an MHC-mismatched transplantation or from mismatch in minor histocompatibility antigens that are not tested before transplantation. T-cell depletion of haploidentical bone marrow reduces the risk of GVHD. Patients with SCID transplanted with T-cell–depleted haploidentical bone marrow do not usually develop severe GVHD. **Acute GVHD** begins 6 or more days after transplantation due to transfer of mature lymphocytes or can result from transfusion of nonirradiated blood products in patients with no T-cell function. Acute GVHD presents with fever, skin rash, and severe diarrhea. Patients develop a high, unrelenting fever; a morbilliform maculopapular erythematous rash that is painful and pruritic; hepatosplenomegaly and abnormal liver function tests; and nausea, vomiting, abdominal pain, and watery diarrhea. Acute GVHD is staged from grades 1 to 4, depending on the degree of skin, fever, gastrointestinal, and liver involvement. **Chronic GVHD** typically occurs after acute GVHD, is diagnosed after 100 days, and can develop without acute GVHD or after acute GVHD has resolved. Chronic GVHD is characterized by skin lesions (hyperkeratosis, reticular hyperpigmentation, fibrosis, and atrophy with ulceration), limitation of joint movement, interstitial pneumonitis, and immune dysregulation with autoantibody and immune complex formation.

PEARLS FOR PRACTITIONERS

See Immunology: Pearls for Practitioners at the end of this section.

REVIEW QUESTIONS

Available online.

CHAPTER 77

Hemophagocytic Lymphohistiocytosis

James W. Verbsky | Julie-An M. Talano

Hemophagocytic lymphohistiocytosis (HLH) and **macrophage activation syndrome (MAS)** are a spectrum of disorders characterized by an excessive inflammatory response resulting in life threatening complications. These can be primary genetic disorders or secondary to severe infections (e.g., viruses, fungus, parasites), autoimmunity, or malignancy. Primary HLH occurs due to defects in the granule exocytosis pathway of cytotoxic lymphocytes, and MAS occurs secondary to autoimmune disorders such as systemic juvenile idiopathic arthritis. Regardless of the cause of HLH/MAS, excessive inflammation results in the activation of macrophages resulting in end organ damage most notably of the liver, bone marrow, and brain. Cytokines such as interferon-gamma, interleukin (IL)-1, and IL-18 appear important in the pathophysiology of these diseases. Rapid recognition and treatment are essential to prevent morbidity and mortality.

PATHOPHYSIOLOGY OF HLH

HLH is the common clinicopathologic outcome of an excessive inflammatory response to infection, malignancy, or autoimmune diseases. In primary HLH, the failure to kill virally infected cells leads to high levels of virus and persistent T-cell activation. T cells produce cytokines, such as interferon-γ (IFN-γ) and TNF-α, that activate macrophages resulting in further cytokine production by these cells. Many inflammatory cytokines are elevated in HLH, including IFN-γ, IL-1, IL-6, IL-12, IL-18, and TNF-α. IFN-γ appears to be central in the pathophysiology of HLH as it is a potent activator of macrophages. In *NLRC4*-associated MAS, IL-18 appears to be a key cytokine as it induces IFN-γ. Similar findings of high IL-18 levels are seen in systemic-onset juvenile idiopathic arthritis (JIA) or Still's disease. However, IFN-γ is not absolutely required for HLH as shown in cases of HLH associated with IFN-γ receptor defects in response to mycobacterial infections. This highlights the observation that multiple cytokines likely contribute to the pathophysiology of HLH.

The cytokine storm causes excessive inflammation and organ dysfunction such as fever, hyperferritinemia, and hyperlipidemia, in addition to macrophage activation. The activated macrophages infiltrate the bone marrow, liver, and other organs and phagocytize cells, resulting in the pathologic finding of hemophagocytosis. Activated macrophages also activate clotting pathways resulting in fibrinogen consumption and bleeding. The reasons for the excessive inflammation and its effects can vary. Uncontrolled viral, bacterial, or fungal infection results in persistent inflammation, continued T cell activation, and resulting HLH. Poorly controlled inflammation in systemic-onset JIA or other autoimmune disease can give the same result. Malignancy-associated HLH may occur due to excessive cytokine production by malignant cells or due to infections associated with these diseases or their treatment.

Spectrum of Disease

HLH and MAS are characterized by similar pathologic and clinical findings and are thus considered a spectrum of disorders, which can be **primary** (genetic) or **secondary** to other illnesses/infections (Table 77.1).

Primary HLH

Perforin is a critical component of the granule exocytosis pathway and the pathophysiology of HLH. Perforin is mainly expressed in the cytotoxic granules of human natural killer (NK) cells and activated $CD8^+$ T lymphocytes together with granzymes. Cytotoxic lymphocytes kill target cells by binding the infected cells and forming a synapse, followed by movement of cytotoxic granules containing perforin, granzymes, and other cytotoxic molecules to the synapse, which then fuses with the cellular membrane and releases the granule contents into the extracellular space. Perforin then facilitates movement of granzyme into the target cells, which activates apoptotic pathways. Several proteins are required for granule formation, movement toward the target cells, and fusion with the cellular membrane: lysosomal trafficking regulator (LYST) is required for granule formation, RAB27A is a guanosine triphosphate (GTP)-binding protein required for granule movement, and syntaxin 11 (STX11), syntaxin-binding protein 2 (STXBP2), and UNC13D are involved in fusion of the cytotoxic granules to the plasma membrane.

Perforin deficiency accounts for approximately 25% of cases of HLH and typically presents very early in life, although there are rare reports of teenage- and adult-onset disease. Pathogenic variants in UNC13D and STXBP2 each make up about 20% of primary HLH patient cohorts (see Table 77.1). STX11, RAB27A, and LYST make up less than 10% of cases of HLH. All of these disorders have autosomal recessive inheritance. RAB27A deficiency results in Griscelli syndrome, characterized by albinism, neurological deficits, and variable degrees of cellular immunodeficiency including HLH. LYST deficiency causes Chédiak-Higashi syndrome (CHS), characterized by albinism, bleeding tendency, neurological symptoms, and frequent pyogenic infections as well as HLH. CHS exhibits large granules in multiple cell types, which can indicate the diagnosis.

In addition to the defects of the granule exocytosis pathway, several other X-linked disorders can cause HLH. X-linked lymphoproliferative (XLP) disease affects males, is usually triggered by Epstein-Barr virus (EBV), and has two genetic variants. XLP-1 is caused by a deficiency in SAP (SLAM-associated protein), an adaptor protein that is critical for signaling transduction in lymphocytes. These patients also develop hypogammaglobulinemia and lymphoma. XLP-2 is caused by deficiency of X-linked inhibitor of apoptosis (XIAP). In addition, XLP-2 is associated with colitis, likely due to its role in signaling of NOD1 and NOD2 proteins (NOD2 variants are a risk factor for inflammatory bowel disease). XLP-2 does not appear to be associated with lymphoma. Pathogenic variants in a number of genes that result in EBV susceptibility and may result in HLH have been reported, including *CD27, CD70, CORO1A, CTPS1, ITK, RASGRP1, TNFSFR9,* and *MAGT1*. Most of these have autosomal recessive inheritance except for *MAGT1*, which is X-linked.

All of the above genetic causes of HLH typically have an infectious trigger, which is most commonly viral, but other disorders can exhibit a similar outcome. For example, genetic defects in the *NLRC4* gene, involved in inflammasome activation, cause MAS with early onset enterocolitis. Other infections, including fungal infections or mycobacterial infections, can also trigger HLH. Primary immune deficiencies that affect control of infections can also present with HLH. For example, genetic defects in IL-12 and interferon-gamma (IFN-γ) signaling result in susceptibility to intracellular infections (e.g., mycobacteria, salmonella), and case reports have demonstrated HLH in these patients. Finally, a variety of inborn errors of metabolism, including lysinuric protein intolerance, Gaucher disease, and Wolman disease, can also exhibit HLH.

Secondary HLH

Secondary HLH refers to conditions that meet criteria for HLH but are not associated with a genetic pathogenic variant. Secondary HLH is subdivided into infection-related HLH, malignancy-related HLH, and autoimmunity-related HLH, or MAS (see Table 77.1). Secondary HLH is more common in older children and adults than primary HLH. Infection-related HLH can occur due to viruses, including CMV, EBV, other herpetic viruses, HIV, influenza, parvovirus, and others. HLH has also been reported in severe fungal infections, parasitic infections, and bacterial infections. Primary

TABLE **77.1** Diseases Characterized by Hemophagocytosis

PRIMARY HLH (GENETIC CAUSE)
Familial hemophagocytic lymphohistiocytosis *(PRF1, STX11, STXBP2, UNC13D)*
Chédiak-Higashi syndrome *(LYST)*
Griscelli syndrome *(RAB27A)*
X-linked lymphoproliferative disease *(SH2D1A, XIAP)*
SECONDARY HLH
Infection-associated HLH
Viral: Herpes virus infection (EBV, CMV, HHV-6, others), HIV, influenza, parvovirus, others
Bacterial: *Staphylococcus aureus, Streptococcus pneumoniae*, enteric gram-negative rods, *Mycobacterium tuberculosis*
Fungal: *Candida, Cryptococcus, Histoplasma*
Malignancy-associated HLH
T, B, or NK cell lymphoma or leukemia
Myeloid malignancies
Others
Macrophage activation syndrome (MAS) associated with autoimmune disease
Systemic-onset juvenile rheumatoid arthritis (SOJRA)
Adult-onset Still disease
Others (systemic lupus erythematosus, vasculitis)

CMV, Cytomegalovirus; *EBV,* Ebstein-Barr virus; *HHV,* human herpesvirus; *HLH,* hemophagocytic histiocytosis.

immune deficiencies should also be considered in these cases. Malignancy-associated HLH also occurs and has a high mortality rate; T- and B-cell lymphomas and leukemias, NK lymphomas, and myeloid malignancies have all been implicated. In addition, treatment of malignancies with chemotherapy can result in HLH, which can be due to infectious susceptibility. Finally, autoimmune diseases, in particular systemic-onset JIA and adult-onset Still disease, can cause MAS. Other autoimmune diseases can also be a trigger including systemic onset lupus erythematosus and vasculitis.

Clinical Presentation

HLH/MAS is a potentially fatal disease that largely affects children. Typical clinical features include high-grade fever, lymphoproliferation manifesting as hepatosplenomegaly and lymphadenopathy, edema, hypotension and shock, bleeding, and central nervous system symptoms. Laboratory abnormalities include cytopenias affecting at least two cell lines, liver dysfunction (e.g., transaminitis, hypertriglyceridemia, hyperbilirubinemia), coagulopathy (hypofibrinogenemia, elevated prothrombin time [PT], elevated partial thromboplastin time [PTT], and elevated thrombin time), hyperferritinemia, cerebral spinal fluid (CSF) pleocytosis, hyponatremia, and hypoproteinemia. Histopathology of affected organs (liver, bone marrow, lymph node, CSF) may demonstrate histiocytosis with evidence of hemophagocytic activity (i.e., engulfed platelets, red blood cells, and neutrophils). However, the lack of biopsy-confirmed hemophagocytosis does not rule out the diagnosis.

Guidelines for the diagnosis of HLH require either molecular diagnosis or five of eight clinical and laboratory criteria to establish the diagnosis (Table 77.2). Accuracy of NK killing assays may be compromised in clinically ill patients, and false positives are common in patients without a genetic variant. More specific tests of NK function, such as perforin staining and degranulation of NK cells by analyzing CD107 testing, have become more common. Importantly, patients may not have sufficient criteria to diagnose HLH, and treatment should not be withheld if there is a strong clinical suspicion in the setting of clinical deterioration. Genetic confirmation is sufficient for the diagnosis as well.

TABLE 77.2 Diagnostic Guidelines for Hemophagocytic Histiocytosis

The diagnosis of HLH is established if criterion 1 or 2 is fulfilled:

1. A molecular diagnosis consistent with HLH (e.g., pathogenic variants of *PRF1, UNC13D, STXBP2, Rab27a, STX11, SH2D1A*, or XIAP)

OR

2. Having 5 out of 8 of the following clinical and laboratory findings:
   a. Fever
   b. Splenomegaly
   c. Cytopenias affecting ≥2 cell lineages (Hgb <9 g/dL [or <10 g/dL for infants <4 weeks of age], platelets <100 × 10^3/mL, neutrophils <1 × 10^3/mL)
   d. Hypertriglyceridemia (≥265 mg/dL) and/or hypofibrinogenemia (≤150 mg/dL)
   e. Hemophagocytosis in the bone marrow, spleen, or lymph nodes without evidence of malignancy
   f. Low or absent NK-cell cytotoxicity
   g. Hyperferritinemia (≥500 mcg/L)
   h. Elevated soluble CD25 (IL-2Rα chain; ≥2,400 U/mL)

Adapted from Jordan MB, Allen CE, Greenberg J, et al. Challenges in the diagnosis of hemophagocytic lymphohistiocytosis: recommendations from the North American Consortium (NACHO). Pediatr Blood Cancer. 2019;66(11)e27929, table 1.

THERAPEUTIC MANAGEMENT OF HLH

Survival rates for children with primary HLH have improved with immunosuppressive treatment regimens. The HLH-94 protocol includes dexamethasone, cyclosporin A (CSA), etoposide, and intrathecal methotrexate and hydrocortisone. This, together with hematopoietic stem cell transplantation (HSCT), improved the 3-year overall survival rate to ~50–70%. Establishing a genetic diagnosis is also essential because this not only confirms the diagnosis of HLH but also affects prognosis and the need for stem cell transplantation.

The treatment of secondary HLH uses similar immunosuppressive therapies but with some modifications. In secondary HLH, it is critical to treat the underlying condition while also treating the inflammation that is driving the HLH. Corticosteroids are often given to treat the inflammatory complications. In infection-associated HLH, aggressive treatment of the infection needs to be incorporated with the immunosuppression. Malignancy-associated HLH is treated with appropriate chemotherapies, which often include corticosteroids. In MAS associated with autoimmunity, specific treatments for the autoimmune disorder may treat MAS, and steroids are often used. For example, in MAS associated with systemic onset JIA, IL-1 and IL-6 neutralizing therapies are effective. If HLH symptoms persist, other agents may be added. Etoposide can be given in severe cases, or newer agents can be tried.

With more understanding of the pathophysiology of these disorders, directed therapies are available. Because IFN-γ is a critical effector molecule in primary HLH, IFN-γ neutralizing antibody can be given in severe cases or refractory HLH, although this increases the infectious risk. Anti-IL-1, anti-IL-6, and anti-TNF-α therapies have been tried in refractory primary HLH. Because many of these cytokines utilize the Janus kinase/signal transducers and activators of transcription (JAK/STAT) signaling pathway, JAK inhibitors have been used in primary or secondary forms of HLH. Additionally, IL-18 has been implicated in MAS associated with systemic-onset JIA or *NLRC-4* MAS, so clinical trials with IL-18–blocking agents are underway.

PEARLS FOR PRACTITIONERS

See Immunology: Pearls for Practitioners at the end of this section.

REVIEW QUESTIONS

Available online.

Suggested Readings

Bousfiha A, Moundir A, Tangye SG, et al. The 2022 Update of IUIS Phenotypical Classification for Human Inborn Errors of Immunity. *J Clin Immunol.* 2022;42(7):1508–1520.

Frank MM. Complement disorders and hereditary angioedema. *J Allergy Clin Immunol.* 2010;125(2 Suppl 2):S262–S271.

Ricklin D, Hajishengallis G, Yang K, Lambris JD. Complement: a key system for immune surveillance and homeostasis. *Nat Immunol.* 2010;11(9):785–797.

Szabolcs P, Cavazzana-Calvo M, Fischer A, Veys P. Bone marrow transplantation for primary immunodeficiency diseases. *Pediatr Clin North Am.* 2010;57(1):207–237.

Turvey SE, Broide DH. Innate immunity. *J Allergy Clin Immunol.* 2010;125(2 Suppl 2):S24–S32.

PEARLS FOR PRACTITIONERS

CHAPTER 72

Immunologic Assessment

- Primary immune deficiency disorders (PIDDs) result in severe, recurrent, or unusual (opportunistic) infections.
- Secondary causes of immune deficiency (e.g., protein-losing enteropathy, drug effects, impaired barrier function such as eczema or burns, anatomic defects, malignancies) should be excluded in the evaluation of primary immunodeficiencies.
- PIDDs typically present in childhood but can occur at any age, and the age of onset can give clues to the diagnosis.
  - Congenital neutropenia and other phagocyte defects typically present with infections in the first several months of life.
  - Severe combined immunodeficiency (SCID) and other serious combined immunodeficiencies present within the first year of life.
  - Antibody deficiencies typically present after 6 months of age but can present after several years of life.
  - Common variable immunodeficiency (CVID) typically presents in young adulthood.
- The type and location of infections can help to narrow the diagnosis.
  - Gingivitis, poor wound healing, omphalitis, granulomas, or abscesses without pus point to a neutrophil/phagocyte defect.
  - Recurrent sinopulmonary infections suggest a humoral or B-cell defect.
  - Infection with opportunistic infections or severe viral infections suggests a T-cell or combined immunodeficiency.
  - *Neisseria* infections or early-onset autoimmunity may represent a complement defect.
- The initial workup of a suspected PIDD is guided by the type and locations of the infections as noted earlier. However, a complete blood count (CBC) with differential should be obtained in all patients with a suspected PIDD.
  - Suspected neutrophil/phagocyte defects: CBC with differential, examination of peripheral smear and dihydrorhodamine 123 (DHR) or nitroblue tetrazolium (NBT) test, which examines the integrity of the nicotinamide adenine dinucleotide phosphate (NADPH) oxidase pathway. Bone marrow biopsy is performed when more than one blood lineage is affected or there is a poor response to therapy.
  - Suspected humoral or B-cell disorder: immunoglobulin G (IgG), IgA, IgM levels; specific titers to diphtheria, tetanus, and pneumococcus
  - Suspected T-cell or combined defect: IgG, IgA, IgM levels; specific titers to diphtheria, tetanus, and pneumococcus; flow cytometry for lymphocyte subsets
  - Suspected complement defects: CH_{50}, AH_{50}
- Genetic testing is increasingly used to obtain a definitive diagnosis and has implications as to treatment and long-term monitoring. In addition, expanded genetic sequencing panels allow for the rapid and economical diagnosis of many PIDDs.
- Treatment of PIDDs is tailored to the diagnosis.
  - Humoral/B-cell defects are treated with immunoglobulin replacement.
  - Neutrophil/phagocyte defects are treated with granulocyte colony-stimulating factor (G-CSF) or hematopoietic stem cell transplant (HSCT).
  - T-cell/combined defects are treated with antibody replacement therapy and antimicrobial (bacterial, viral fungal) prophylaxis until HSCT can be performed.
  - Complement defects are treated with frequent vaccinations and in some cases antibiotic prophylaxis.
- Practical aspects of patients with PIDDs
  - No live-virus vaccines. If patient has SCID, family members should not receive live viral vaccines.
  - Clean water sources, which may involve boiling water. Bottled water is not acceptable.
  - All blood products given to patients with PIDDs should be cytomegalovirus (CMV) negative and irradiated.
  - Limit sick contacts.

CHAPTER 73

Lymphocyte Disorders

- Agammaglobulinemia may be inherited as either an X-linked or autosomal recessive disorder.
- Patients with agammaglobulinemia have an increased risk of infection with encapsulated bacteria as well as enteroviruses and giardia.
- Congenital agammaglobulinemia and common variable immunodeficiency (CVID) have low IgG levels with low IgA or IgM levels.
- Patients with CVID are at risk for infection, autoimmunity, immune dysregulation, and B-cell lymphomas.
- Hyper-IgM syndrome is most commonly X-linked due to CD40L deficiency and is a combined immunodeficiency.
- Severe combined immunodeficiency (SCID) diseases present with growth faltering, severe bacterial or virus infections, diarrhea, eczema-like skin rash, and graft versus host disease from transfused lymphocytes and require early stem cell transplantation.

- DiGeorge syndrome is characterized by hypocalcemia, congenital heart disease, T-cell immunodeficiency, and deletions on chromosome 22q11.2.

CHAPTER 74

Neutrophil Disorders

- Neutrophil disorders may manifest with abscesses, lymphadenitis, gingivitis, poor wound healing, delayed separation of the umbilical cord, or poor pus formation.
- Neutropenia is defined as an absolute neutrophil count of less than 1,500/mm^3 in White children over 1 year of age. It is somewhat lower in children of Black African heritage.
- Cyclic neutropenia has ~21-day cycles of low neutrophil counts that then recover.
- Autoimmune neutropenia develops in children between 5 and 24 months of age and may persist; it responds to G-CSF.
- Chronic granulomatous disease results from defective intracellular neutrophil killing of bacteria that produce catalase.

CHAPTER 75

Complement System

- Deficiencies of early components of the classic complement pathway are associated with encapsulated bacteria, and deficiencies of the late components of the complement cascade are associated with neisserial infections.
- Patients with C1, C2, or C4 deficiency are at risk for autoimmune diseases (especially systemic lupus erythematosus).
- Deficiency of C1-inhibitor produces hereditary angioedema.

CHAPTER 76

Hematopoietic Stem Cell Transplantation

- Hematopoietic stem cell transplantation (HSCT) has been used to treat malignancies, some metabolic disorders, aplastic anemia, immunodeficiency or immune dysregulation syndromes, and hemoglobinopathies.

CHAPTER 77

Hemophagocytic Lymphohistiocytosis

- Hemophagocytic lymphohistiocytosis (HLH) and macrophage activation syndrome (MAS) are a spectrum of severe disease characterized by life-threatening excessive inflammatory response.
- MAS is a complication of severe autoimmune disorders such as systemic-onset juvenile idiopathic arthritis or systemic lupus erythematosus.
- Primary HLH is caused by genetic pathogenic variants.
- Secondary HLH describes when excessive inflammatory response occurs in the absence of a genetic pathogenic variant. Secondary HLH can be associated with infections, malignancies, and autoimmune disorders (MAS).
- Survival improves with broad immunosuppressive therapy. Management of secondary HLH requires aggressive treatment of the underlying illness.

SECTION 14

ALLERGY

Barry J. Pelz | Matthew T. Tallar | Asriani M. Chiu

CHAPTER 78

Allergy Assessment

Atopy is a result of complex interactions between multiple genes and environmental factors. It implies specific immunoglobulin (Ig)E–mediated diseases, including allergic rhinitis, asthma, and food allergy. An **allergen** is an antigen that triggers an IgE response in genetically predisposed individuals.

Hypersensitivity disorders of the immune system are classified into four groups, based on the mechanism of tissue inflammation (Table 78.1). **Type I (immediate hypersensitivity) reactions** result from the binding of antigen to cell surface–bound IgE on high-affinity IgE receptors on tissue mast cells, circulating basophils, or both, causing the release of preformed chemical mediators, such as histamine and tryptase, and newly generated mediators, such as leukotrienes, prostaglandins, and platelet-activating factor. These mediators contribute to the development of allergic symptoms, with anaphylaxis as the most profound syndrome. Several hours after the initial response, a **late-phase reaction** may develop with an influx of other inflammatory cells such as basophils, eosinophils, monocytes, lymphocytes, and neutrophils, and their inflammatory mediators. Recruitment of these cells leads to more persistent and chronic symptoms.

Type II (cytotoxic antibody) reactions involve IgM, IgG, or IgA antibodies binding to cell surface antigens and activating the entire complement pathway, resulting in lysis of the cell or release of **anaphylatoxins**, such as C3a, C4a, and C5a (see Chapter 75). These anaphylatoxins trigger mast cell degranulation, resulting in inflammatory mediator release. The target can be cell surface membrane antigens, such as red blood cells causing hemolytic anemia, platelet cell surface molecules, glomerular basement membrane molecules, acetylcholine receptor α chain at the neuromuscular junction, and thyroid-stimulating hormone receptor on thyroid cells causing Graves disease.

Type III (immune complex) reactions involve the formation of antigen-antibody or immune complexes that enter into the circulation and are deposited in tissues such as blood vessels and filtering organs (i.e., liver, spleen, and kidney). These complexes initiate tissue injury by activating the complement cascade and recruiting neutrophils that release their toxic mediators. Local reactions caused by the injection of antigen into tissue are called ***Arthus reactions***. The administration of large amounts of antigen leads to **serum sickness**. Other type III reactions include hypersensitivity pneumonitis and some vasculitic syndromes.

TABLE **78.1** Gell and Coombs Classification of Hypersensitivity Disorders

TYPE	INTERVAL BETWEEN EXPOSURE AND REACTION	EFFECTOR MOLECULE	TARGET OR ANTIGEN	EXAMPLES OF MEDIATORS	EXAMPLES
I Immediate Late phase	<30 min 2–12 hr	IgE	Pollens, food, venom, drugs	Histamine, tryptase, leukotrienes, prostaglandins, platelet-activating factor	Anaphylaxis, urticaria, allergic rhinitis, allergic asthma
II Cytotoxic antibody	Variable (min–hr)	IgM, IgG, IgA	Red blood cells, platelets	Complement	Hemolytic anemia, thrombocytopenia, Goodpasture syndrome
III Immune complex	1–3 wk after drug exposure	Antigen-antibody complexes	Blood vessels, liver, spleen, kidney, lung	Complement, anaphylatoxin	Serum sickness, hypersensitivity pneumonitis
IV Delayed type	2–7 days after drug exposure	Lymphocytes	*Mycobacterium tuberculosis*, chemicals	Cytokines (IFN-γ, TNFα, GM-CSF)	TB skin test reactions, contact dermatitis, graft-vs-host disease

GM-CSF, Granulocyte-macrophage colony-stimulating factor; *IFN-γ*, interferon-γ; *Ig*, immunoglobulin; *TB*, tuberculosis; *TNFα*, tumor necrosis factor-α.

Type IV (cellular immune–mediated or delayed-hypersensitivity) reactions involve recognition of antigen by sensitized T cells. Antigen-presenting cells present peptides on the cell surface in association with major histocompatibility complex class II (MHC-II) molecules. Memory T cells recognize the peptide/MHC-II complex, resulting in cytokine release (e.g., interferon-γ, tumor necrosis factor-α, and granulocyte-macrophage colony-stimulating factor), which activates and attracts tissue macrophages. **Contact allergies** (e.g., nickel dermatitis and poison ivy) and immunity to tuberculosis are examples of type IV reactions.

HISTORY

The history may reveal allergic symptoms after exposure to a potential trigger that usually has occurred upon previous exposures.

A family history of allergic disease is often present in affected patients. If one parent has allergies, the risk that a child will develop an allergic disease is 25%. If both parents have allergies, the risk increases to 50–70%. Other atopic diseases tend to occur in families.

PHYSICAL EXAMINATION

Allergic disease may involve the skin, nose, eyes, lungs, or gastrointestinal tract alone or in combination. Many patients have more than one organ system involved.

Children with allergic rhinitis exhibit frequent nasal itching and rubbing of the nose with the palm of the hand, called the **allergic salute**, which leads to a transverse nasal crease across the nose. Pale nasal mucosa and edematous turbinates are common examination findings. **Allergic shiners**, blue-gray to purple discoloration below the lower eyelids attributed to venous congestion, along with swollen eyelids or conjunctival injection, are often present in children. Dermatologic findings of atopy include pruritic, erythematous plaques of atopic dermatitis, prominent creases under the lower eyelids (**Dennie-Morgan folds** or **Dennie lines**), urticaria, and **keratosis pilaris** (see Chapter 81). Wheezing may be noted on auscultation of the lower respiratory tract.

INITIAL DIAGNOSTIC EVALUATION

Screening Tests

Atopy is characterized by elevated levels of IgE (Table 78.2) and **eosinophilia** (3–10% of white blood cells or an absolute eosinophil count of >250 eosinophils/mm^3) with a predominance of T helper 2 cytokines, including interleukin (IL)-4, IL-5, and IL-13. Extreme eosinophilia suggests a nonallergic disorder such as infection, hypereosinophilic syndrome, drug reaction, or malignancy (Table 78.3).

TABLE 78.2 Select Disorders Associated With Elevated Serum Immunoglobulin E

Allergic disease
Atopic dermatitis (eczema)
Tissue-invasive helminthic infections
Hyperimmunoglobulin E syndromes
Allergic bronchopulmonary aspergillosis
Systemic candidiasis
HIV
Wiskott-Aldrich syndrome
Bone marrow transplantation
Hodgkin disease
Bullous pemphigoid
Idiopathic nephrotic syndrome
Cystic fibrosis
Kawasaki disease

TABLE 78.3 Disorders Associated With Eosinophilia

ALLERGIC DISEASE
Allergic rhinitis
Atopic dermatitis
Asthma
GASTROINTESTINAL
Eosinophilic esophagitis and gastroenteritis
Allergic colitis
Inflammatory bowel disease
INFECTIOUS
Tissue-invasive helminthic infections
Fungal infections
NEOPLASTIC
Eosinophilic leukemia
Hodgkin disease
RESPIRATORY
Eosinophilic pneumonia
Allergic bronchopulmonary aspergillosis
SYSTEMIC
Idiopathic hypereosinophilic syndrome
Adrenal insufficiency
Mastocytosis
IATROGENIC
Medication induced

There are two methods for identifying allergen-specific IgE: in vivo skin testing and in vitro serum testing (Table 78.4). **In vivo skin testing** introduces allergen into the skin via a prick/puncture or intradermal injection. The allergen diffuses through the skin to interact with IgE that is bound to mast cells. Cross-linking of IgE causes mast cell degranulation, which results in histamine release and the development of a **central wheal** and **erythematous flare**. The wheal and flare are measured 15–20 minutes after the allergen has been applied. Properly performed skin tests are the most sensitive method for detecting the presence of allergen-specific IgE.

In vitro serum testing, such as immunoassays like the enzyme-linked immunosorbent assay **(ELISA)**, measures levels of antigen-specific IgE. Many allergists and laboratories regard the ImmunoCAP System (ThermoFisher Scientific, Waltham, MA) as the method of choice. This method uses a solid phase and shows higher sensitivity, specificity, and reproducibility. The assay uses a quantitative fluorescent immunoassay that is more sensitive than other methods. Serum-based tests are indicated for patients who have dermatographism or extensive dermatitis, who cannot discontinue medications such as antihistamines that interfere with skin test results, or who are noncompliant for skin testing. The presence of specific IgE antibodies suggests sensitization *but is not sufficient* for the diagnosis of allergic

TABLE 78.4 Determination of Allergen-Specific IgE by Skin Testing vs In Vitro Testing

VARIABLE	SKIN TEST*	sIgE ASSAY
Risk of allergic reaction	Yes (especially ID)	No
Relative sensitivity	High	High
Affected by antihistamines	Yes	No
Affected by corticosteroids	Usually not	No
Affected by extensive dermatitis or dermographism	Yes	No
Broad selection of antigens	Fewer	Yes
Immediate results	Yes	No
Expensive	No	Yes
Lability of allergens	Yes	No
Results evident to patient	Yes	No

Skin testing may be the prick test or ID injection.
ID, Intradermal; *Ig*, immunoglobulin; *sIgE*, allergen-specific IgE.
From Bunyavanich S, Kattan J, Sicherer SH. Diagnosis of allergic disease. In: Kliegman RM, St. Geme J, eds. Nelson Textbook of Pediatrics. *22nd ed. Philadelphia: Elsevier; 2025. [table 183.3].*

disease. Diagnosis must be based on the physician's assessment of the entire clinical picture, including the history and physical examination, the presence of specific IgE antibodies, and the correlation with IgE-mediated symptoms.

DIAGNOSTIC IMAGING

Diagnostic imaging has a limited role in the evaluation of allergic disease. Chest radiography may be helpful with the differential diagnosis of asthma. Sinus radiography and computed tomography may be useful, but when these images are abnormal, they do not distinguish allergic disease from nonallergic disease.

PEARLS FOR PRACTITIONERS

See Allergy: Pearls for Practitioners at the end of this section.

REVIEW QUESTIONS

Available online.

CHAPTER 79
Asthma

ETIOLOGY

Inflammatory cells (mast cells, eosinophils, T lymphocytes, neutrophils), chemical mediators (histamine, leukotrienes, platelet-activating factor, bradykinin), and chemotactic factors (cytokines, eotaxin) mediate the underlying inflammation found in asthmatic airways. Inflammation contributes to **airway hyperresponsiveness** (airways constricting in response to allergens, irritants, viral infections, and exercise). It also results in edema, increased mucus production in the lungs, influx of inflammatory cells into the airway tissue, and epithelial cell denudation. Chronic inflammation can lead to **airway remodeling**, which results from a proliferation of extracellular matrix proteins and vascular hyperplasia and may lead to irreversible structural changes and progressive loss of pulmonary function.

EPIDEMIOLOGY

Asthma is the most common chronic disease of childhood in industrialized countries, affecting over 6 million children younger than 18 years of age in the United States (6.5% of children). In adults, females are more likely than males to have asthma, but in children the reverse is true. Mortality from asthma occurs; in the United States, approximately 181 pediatric deaths per year are attributed to asthma. Morbidity and mortality rates from asthma vary widely across contexts, suggesting the impact of environmental factors, differential access to medical care, and social determinants of health.

CLINICAL MANIFESTATIONS

Children with asthma have symptoms of coughing, wheezing, shortness of breath, exercise intolerance, and chest tightness. The history should elicit the frequency, severity, and precipitating factors as well as a family history of asthma and allergy. Common exacerbating factors include respiratory viral infections, exposure to allergens and irritants (e.g., smoke, air pollution, strong odors, fumes), exercise, emotions, and change in weather/humidity. Nocturnal symptoms are common. Rhinosinusitis, gastroesophageal reflux, and aspirin can aggravate asthma. Treatment of these conditions may lessen the frequency and severity of asthma exacerbations.

During acute episodes, tachypnea, tachycardia, cough, wheezing, and a prolonged expiratory phase may be present. Physical findings may be subtle. Wheezing may not be prominent if there is poor aeration from airway obstruction. As the attack progresses, cyanosis, diminished air movement, retractions, agitation, inability to speak, tripod sitting position, diaphoresis, and pulsus paradoxus (decrease in blood pressure of >15 mm Hg with inspiration) may be observed. Physical examination may show evidence of other atopic diseases such as eczema or allergic rhinitis.

LABORATORY AND IMAGING STUDIES

While no single test or study can confirm the diagnosis of asthma, many elements contribute to establishing the diagnosis.

Objective measurements of pulmonary function aid in the diagnosis and direct the treatment of asthma. **Spirometry** is used to monitor response to treatment, assess degree of reversibility with therapeutic intervention, and measure the severity of an asthma exacerbation. Children older than 5 years of age can usually perform spirometry maneuvers. **Peak expiratory flow** offers a simple, inexpensive way to measure asthma control at home; variability in predicted peak flow reference values make spirometry preferred over peak flow measures in the diagnosis of asthma. For younger children who cannot perform spirometry maneuvers or peak flow, a therapeutic trial of controller medications aids in the diagnosis of asthma.

Measurement of a biomarker, **exhaled nitric oxide**, reflects eosinophilic airway inflammation and provides information on those patients who may better respond to corticosteroid treatment, aids in monitoring response to therapy and dose optimization, and detects nonadherence to corticosteroid therapy.

Allergy skin testing should be included in the evaluation of all children with persistent asthma but not during an exacerbation of symptoms. Positive skin test results, identifying sensitization to **aeroallergens** (e.g., pollens, mold, dust mite, pet dander), correlate strongly with bronchial allergen provocative challenges. In vitro serum tests, such as enzyme-linked immunosorbent assay, are generally less sensitive in defining clinically pertinent allergens, are more expensive, and require several days for results, compared to several minutes for skin testing (see Table 78.4).

A **chest x-ray** may be useful at the time of the first episode of asthma or with recurrent episodes of undiagnosed cough or wheeze to exclude anatomic abnormalities. Repeat chest x-rays are not needed with new episodes unless there is fever (suggesting pneumonia) or localized findings on physical examination.

DIFFERENTIAL DIAGNOSIS

Many childhood conditions can cause wheezing and coughing like asthma (Table 79.1), but not all cough and wheeze is asthma. Misdiagnosis delays correcting the underlying cause and exposes children to inappropriate therapy (Table 79.2).

Allergic bronchopulmonary aspergillosis is a hypersensitivity reaction to antigens of the mold *Aspergillus fumigatus*. It occurs primarily in patients with steroid-dependent asthma and in patients with cystic fibrosis.

TREATMENT

Optimal medical treatment of asthma includes several key components: environmental control, pharmacologic therapy, and patient education, including attainment of self-management skills. Children with asthma who develop symptoms in response to indoor allergens may benefit from specific allergen-mitigation interventions (Table 79.3). For all children with asthma, influenza immunization is indicated; exposure to tobacco and wood smoke should be avoided. Asthma medications can be divided into long-term control medications and quick-relief medications.

Long-Term Control Medications

Inhaled Corticosteroids

Inhaled corticosteroids (ICS) are the most effective antiinflammatory medications for the treatment of chronic, persistent asthma and are the preferred therapy when initiating long-term control therapy. Early intervention with ICS reduces morbidity but does not alter the natural history of asthma. Regular use reduces airway hyperreactivity, the need for rescue bronchodilator therapy, risk of hospitalization, and risk of death from asthma. ICS are available as inhalation aerosols, dry powder inhalers, and nebulizer solution.

The potential risks of ICS are favorably balanced with their benefits. A reduction in growth velocity may occur with poorly controlled asthma or ICS use. Low-to-medium dose ICS may decrease growth velocity, although these effects are small (approximately 1 cm in the first year of treatment). Height measurements should be monitored. ICS do not have clinically significant adverse effects on hypothalamic-pituitary-adrenal axis function, glucose metabolism, subcapsular cataracts, or glaucoma when used at low-to-medium doses in children. Rinsing the mouth after inhalation and using large volume spacers help lessen the local adverse effects of dysphonia and candidiasis and decrease systemic absorption from the gastrointestinal tract. ICS should be titrated to the lowest dose needed to maintain control of a child's asthma. For children with severe asthma, high-dose ICS may be needed

TABLE 79.2 Mnemonic of Causes of Cough in the First Months of Life

C—Cystic fibrosis
R—Respiratory tract infections
A—Aspiration (swallowing dysfunction, gastroesophageal reflux, tracheoesophageal fistula, foreign body)
D—Dyskinetic cilia
L—Lung and airway malformations (laryngeal webs, laryngotracheomalacia, tracheal stenosis, vascular rings and slings)
E—Edema (heart failure, congenital heart disease)

From Schidlow DV. Cough. In: Schidlow DV, Smith DS, eds. *A Practical Guide to Pediatric Disease.* Philadelphia: Hanley & Belfus; 1994.

TABLE 79.1 Differential Diagnoses of Cough and Wheeze in Infants and Children

UPPER AIRWAY DISEASES	OBSTRUCTION INVOLVING LARGE AIRWAYS	OBSTRUCTION INVOLVING SMALL AIRWAYS	OTHER
Allergic rhinitis Sinusitis	Tracheal or bronchial foreign body Paradoxical vocal fold motion Vascular rings or laryngeal webs Enlarged lymph nodes or tumor	Viral bronchiolitis or obliterative bronchiolitis Cystic fibrosis Bronchopulmonary dysplasia (chronic lung disease of prematurity)	Recurrent cough not caused by asthma (infection, habit cough, postnasal drip) Aspiration from swallowing mechanism dysfunction or gastroesophageal reflux disease Heart failure, pulmonary edema

From Guilbert TW, Lemanske RF, Jackson DJ. Diagnosis of asthma in infants and children. In: Adkinson Jr NF, Bochner BS, Burks AW, et al., eds. *Middleton's Allergy: Principles and Practice.* 8th ed. Philadelphia: Saunders; 2014:870.

TABLE 79.3 Controlling Factors Contributing to Asthma Severity

INDOOR TRIGGERS FOR ASTHMA	SUGGESTIONS FOR REDUCING EXPOSURE IF CHILD HAS DEMONSTRATED SENSITIVITY
Viral upper respiratory tract infection (e.g., RSV, rhinovirus, influenza virus)	Limit exposure to viral infections
	Annual influenza immunization
Tobacco smoke, wood smoke	No smoking around the child or in child's home
	Help parents and caregivers quit smoking
	Eliminate use of wood stoves and fireplaces
Dust mites	Encase pillow, mattress, and box spring in allergen-impermeable encasements
	Wash bedding in hot water weekly
	Avoid sleeping or lying on upholstered furniture
	Minimize number of stuffed toys in child's bedroom
	Reduce indoor humidity to <50%
	If possible, remove carpets from bedroom and play areas; if not possible, vacuum weekly
Animal dander	Remove the pet from the home or keep outdoors (if removal is not acceptable)
	Keep pet out of bedroom/no sleeping with pet
	Use a filter on air ducts in child's room
	Wash pet weekly (the evidence to support this has not been firmly established)
Cockroach allergens	Do not leave food or garbage exposed
	Pesticides
	Sealing cracks and holes
Indoor mold	Avoid vaporizers
	Reduce indoor humidity to <50%
	Use of mold-inhibiting cleaner
	Use of dehumidifier
	Fix leaky faucets, pipes

RSV, Respiratory syncytial virus.
Adapted from American Academy of Allergy Asthma & Immunology. Pediatric Asthma: Promoting Best Practice. *Milwaukee, WI: American Academy of Allergy Asthma & Immunology; 1999:50.*

to minimize oral corticosteroid use, but other complementary therapy should be considered (see the following sections).

Leukotriene Modifiers

Leukotrienes, synthesized via the arachidonic acid metabolism cascade, are potent mediators of inflammation and smooth muscle bronchoconstriction. Leukotriene modifiers are oral, daily-use medications that inhibit these biologic effects in the airway. Two classes of leukotriene modifiers include cysteinyl leukotriene receptor antagonists (zafirlukast and montelukast) and leukotriene synthesis inhibitors (zileuton). The leukotriene receptor antagonists have much wider appeal than zileuton. Zafirlukast is approved for children older than 5 years of age and is given twice daily. Montelukast is dosed once daily at night as 4-mg granules or chewable tablets (for children 6 months to 5 years of age), 5-mg chewable tablets (6–14 years of age), and 10-mg tablets (≥15 years of age). Pediatric studies show the usefulness of leukotriene modifiers in mild asthma and the attenuation of exercise-induced bronchoconstriction. These agents may be helpful as steroid-sparing agents in patients with asthma that is more difficult to control.

Long-Acting β_2 Agonists

Long-acting β_2 agonists (LABAs) relax airway smooth muscle for 12–24 hours but do not have any significant antiinflammatory effects. LABAs are not intended for use as monotherapy, but adding a LABA to ICS therapy is more beneficial than doubling the dose of inhaled corticosteroids. Multiple formulations are available. Formoterol is approved for use in children older than 5 years of age for maintenance asthma therapy and for prevention of exercise-induced asthma. It has a rapid onset of action similar to albuterol (15 min) and is dosed twice daily. Salmeterol is approved for children 4 years of age or older, has an onset of 30 min, and is given twice daily. Vilanterol, an ultralong-acting β_2 agonist, is approved in patients aged 5 years and older and has the advantage of once-daily dosing. Combination ICS/LABA products are available. Because combination inhalers administer two medications simultaneously, compliance is generally improved.

Theophylline

Theophylline was more widely used previously, but because current management is aimed at inflammatory control, its use has declined. It is mildly to moderately effective as a bronchodilator and is considered an alternative add-on treatment to low- and medium-dose inhaled corticosteroids. Its therapeutic window is narrow, necessitating monitoring of blood levels.

Biologics

Biologic agents are genetically engineered proteins that target specific antibodies, inflammatory molecules, and receptors; several biologics are U.S. Food and Drug Administration approved for the treatment of asthma in children (Table 79.4). Omalizumab is a humanized anti-immunoglobulin (Ig)E monoclonal antibody that prevents binding of free IgE to high-affinity receptors on basophils and mast cells. It is delivered by subcutaneous injection every 2–4 weeks, depending on body weight and pretreatment serum IgE level.

Mepolizumab is an add-on maintenance therapy for severe asthma with an eosinophilic phenotype. It decreases the production and survival of eosinophils, a major inflammatory cell involved in asthma pathogenesis.

Dupilumab binds to the interleukin (IL)-4 receptor, which blocks intracellular signaling of IL-4 and IL-13. This medication can be administered at home.

Benralizumab binds the IL-5 receptor, inhibiting IL-5 activity, and induces eosinophil apoptosis. Reslizumab also

TABLE 79.4 List of U.S. Food and Drug Administration–Approved Biologic Medications for the Treatment of Asthma in Children and Their Characteristics

NAME	INDICATION	MECHANISM OF ACTION	DOSE	MOST COMMON SIDE EFFECTS	ADMINISTRATION CONSIDERATIONS	OTHER
Benralizumab (Fasenra)	• Add-on controller therapy for severe eosinophilic asthma ≥12 yr of age	• IL-5 receptor blocker (at the α-subunit) • Induces apoptosis of eosinophils through ADCC	• 30-mg SC every 4 wk × 3 • Then every 8 wk	• Injection site reactions • Headache • Pharyngitis	• Treat preexisting helminth infections • 30-min observation from first dose	• Improved efficacy if AEC >150 cells/µL
Dupilumab (Dupixent)	• Add-on controller therapy for moderate-to-severe persistent asthma of eosinophilic phenotype or oral corticosteroid dependent ≥12 yr of age	• IL-4 receptor blocker (at α subunit) preventing IL-4 and IL-13 signaling	• 400-mg SC once then 200-mg SC every 2 wk OR • 600-mg SC once then 300 mg every 2 wk • With concomitant moderate-to-severe atopic dermatitis, 600 mg once then 300 mg every 2 wk	• Injection site reactions • Eosinophilia • Oropharyngeal pain	• Avoid live vaccines • Treat preexisting helminth infections • Option for self-administration	• Improved efficacy if AEC >150 cells/µL
Mepolizumab (Nucala)	• Add-on controller therapy for severe persistent asthma of eosinophilic phenotype ≥6 yr of age	• IL-5 antagonist; binds to circulating IL-5 to prevent its binding to IL-5 receptors on eosinophils	• Patients >12 yr of age: 100-mg SC every 4 wk • Patients 6–11 yr of age 40 mg SC every 4 wk	• Injection site reactions • Herpes zoster • Headache • Back pain • Fatigue	• Zoster vaccination • Treat preexisting helminth infections • 30-min observation from first dose	• AEC >150 in last 6 wk OR • AEC 300 in last 12 months required
Omalizumab (Xolair)	• Moderate-to-severe persistent asthma ≥6 yr of age with sensitivity to perennial aeroallergens	• Binds free IgE preventing IgE binding to high-affinity IgE receptors on mast cells and basophils minimizing release of chemical mediators involved in allergic inflammatory cascade	• Dependent on age, weight, and total IgE level • Administered SC every 2–4 wk	• Anaphylaxis • Injection site reactions • Arthralgia	• Patients should have autoinjectable epinephrine available at time of injection • 90-min wait after first 3 injections, then 30-min wait with subsequent doses • Equipment available to treat anaphylaxis	• Total IgE >30 ku/L AND • Positive skin prick test or serum-specific IgE to perennial aeroallergen
Tezepelumab (Tezspire)	• Severe persistent asthma ≥12 yr of age	• Binds TSLP preventing it from binding to the TSLP receptor	• 210 mg SC every 4 wk	• Pharyngitis • Arthralgia • Back pain	• Avoid live vaccines • Treat preexisting helminth infections	

ADCC, Antibody-dependent cell-mediated cytotoxicity; *AEC*, absolute blood eosinophil count; *Ig*, immunoglobulin; *IL*, interleukin; *SC*, subcutaneous; *TSLP*, thymic stromal lymphopoietin.

binds to IL-5, preventing its binding to the IL-5 receptor, but it is only approved for patients over 18 years of age.

Tezepelumab binds thymic stromal lymphopoietin (TSLP), preventing binding to the TSLP receptor. It is approved for patients 12 years of age and older for severe persistent asthma.

Quick-Relief Medications

Short-Acting β_2 Agonists

Short-acting β_2 agonists (SABAs) such as albuterol and levalbuterol are effective bronchodilators that relax bronchial smooth muscle within 5–10 minutes of administration. These effects last 4–6 hours. Generally, a SABA is prescribed for acute symptoms and as prophylaxis before allergen exposure and exercise. The inhaled route is preferred because adverse effects—tremor, prolonged tachycardia, and irritability—are fewer. Overuse of SABAs implies inadequate control, and a change in medications may be warranted. The definition of *bronchodilator overuse* depends on the severity of the child's asthma; use of more than one metered-dose inhaler canister per month or daily use suggests poor control.

Albuterol-budesonide (AirSupra) is a combination SABA/ICS indicated in those 18 and older. It is indicated for as-needed treatment rather than a maintenance controller. It has the dual benefit of treating bronchospasm in addition to inflammation associated with the onset of exacerbations. There are limits to the number of puffs that can be used within a 24-hour period.

Anticholinergic Agents

Ipratropium bromide is a short-acting anticholinergic bronchodilator that relieves bronchoconstriction, decreases mucus hypersecretion, and counteracts cough-receptor irritability by binding acetylcholine at the muscarinic receptors found in bronchial smooth muscle. It seems to have an additive effect with SABAs when used for acute asthma exacerbations.

A long-acting anticholinergic agent (tiotropium) is approved for use in moderate-to-severe persistent asthma in children 6 years or older. It inhibits muscarinic receptors on bronchial smooth muscle to induce bronchodilation.

Oral Corticosteroids

Short bursts of oral corticosteroids (1–10 days) are administered to children with acute exacerbations. The usual dose is 1–2 mg/kg/day of prednisone for 5 days or 0.6 mg/kg/day of dexamethasone for 1–2 days. Oral corticosteroids are available in liquid or tablet formulations. Prolonged use of oral corticosteroids can result in systemic adverse effects such as hypothalamic-pituitary-adrenal suppression, cushingoid features, weight gain, hypertension, diabetes, cataracts, glaucoma, impaired immunity, osteoporosis, and growth suppression. Children with severe asthma may require oral corticosteroids over extended periods. The dose should be tapered as soon as

AGES 0–4 YEARS Stepwise Approach for Management of Asthma

	Intermittent Asthma	Management of Persistent Asthma in Individuals Ages 0–4 Years				
Treatment	**STEP 1**	**STEP 2**	**STEP 3**	**STEP 4**	**STEP 5**	**STEP 6**
Preferred	PRN SABA and At the start of RTI: Add short course daily ICS	Daily low-dose ICS and PRN SABA	Daily medium-dose ICS and PRN SABA	Daily medium-dose ICS-LABA and PRN SABA	Daily high-dose ICS-LABA and PRN SABA	Daily high-dose ICS-LABA + oral systemic corticosteroid and PRN SABA
Alternative		Daily montelukast* or Cromolyn,** and PRN SABA		Daily medium-dose ICS + montelukast* and PRN SABA	Daily high-dose ICS + montelukast* and PRN SABA	Daily high-dose ICS + montelukast* + oral systemic corticosteroid and PRN SABA
			For children age 4 years only, see Step 3 and Step 4 on Management of Persistent Asthma in Individuals Ages 5–11 Years diagram.			

Assess Control

- First check adherence, inhaler technique, environmental factors, and comorbid conditions.
- **Step up** if needed; reassess in 4–6 weeks
- **Step down** if possible (if asthma is well controlled for at least 3 consecutive months)

Consult with asthma specialist if Step 3 or higher is required. Consider consultation at Step 2.

Control assessment is a key element of asthma care. This involves both impairment and risk. Use of objective measures, self-reported control, and health care utilization are complementary and should be employed on an ongoing basis, depending on the individual's clinical situation.

* Montelukast had a Boxed Warning issued by the FDA in March 2020 noting a risk of serious neuropsychiatric events.
** Cromolyn inhalation solution historically with limited availability in the United States.

FIGURE 79.1 Stepwise long-term approach for managing asthma in children, 0–4 years of age. *ICS*, Inhaled corticosteroid; *LABA*, long-acting β_2-agonist; *PRN*, as needed; *RTI*, respiratory tract infection; *SABA*, inhaled short-acting β_2-agonist. (Adapted from 2020 Focused Updates to the Asthma Management Guidelines: A Report from the National Asthma Education and Prevention Program Coordinating Committee Expert Panel Working Group. National Heart Lung Blood Institute. NIH Publication No. 20-HL-8142. Bethesda, MD: U.S. Department of Health and Human Services; 2021. nhlbi.nih.gov/asthmaguidelines.)

possible to the minimum effective dose, preferably administered on alternate days (for prednisone).

Administration of one or two doses of dexamethasone for the treatment of *acute asthma* exacerbations is used for intermittent, mild persistent, or moderate persistent asthma. This long-acting oral corticosteroid has properties that may increase compliance with therapy, decrease missed school days, and decrease readmission rates.

Approach to Therapy

Therapy is based on the concept that chronic airway inflammation is a fundamental feature of asthma, which can vary in intensity over time, requiring treatment to be adjusted accordingly. Classification of asthma severity is emphasized for initiation of therapy in patients not currently receiving controller medications. A child with **intermittent asthma** has asthma symptoms less than two times per week. To determine whether a child is having more **persistent asthma**, using the *Rules of Two* is helpful: daytime symptoms occurring two or more times per week or nocturnal awakenings two or more times per month implies a need for daily antiinflammatory medication.

Assessing control is emphasized for monitoring and adjusting therapy. A stepwise approach is used for management of infants and young children 0–4 years of age (Fig. 79.1), children 5–11 years of age (Fig. 79.2), and youths 12 years or older (Fig. 79.3). Medication type, dose, and dosing intervals are determined by the level of asthma severity or asthma control. Therapy is then increased **(stepped up)** as necessary and decreased **(stepped down)** when possible. A short-acting bronchodilator should be available for all children with asthma.

Inhaled corticosteroids are the preferred initial long-term control therapy for children of all ages. For children with a

AGES 5–11 YEARS Stepwise Approach for Management of Asthma

	Intermittent Asthma	Management of Persistent Asthma in Individuals Ages 5–11 Years				
Treatment	**STEP 1**	**STEP 2**	**STEP 3**	**STEP 4**	**STEP 5**	**STEP 6**
Preferred	PRN SABA	Daily low-dose ICS and PRN SABA	Daily and PRN combination low-dose ICS-formoterol	Daily and PRN combination medium-dose ICS-formoterol	Daily high-dose ICS-LABA and PRN SABA	Daily high-dose ICS-LABA + oral systemic corticosteroid and PRN SABA
Alternative		Daily LTRA,* or Cromolyn,* or Nedocromil,* or Theophylline,* and PRN SABA	Daily medium-dose ICS and PRN SABA or Daily low-dose ICS-LABA, or daily low-dose ICS + LTRA,* or daily low-dose ICS +Theophylline,* and PRN SABA	Daily medium-dose ICS-LABA and PRN SABA or Daily medium-dose ICS + LTRA* or daily medium-dose ICS + Theophylline,* and PRN SABA	Daily high-dose ICS + LTRA* or daily high-dose ICS + Theophylline,* and PRN SABA	Daily high-dose ICS + LTRA* + oral systemic corticosteroid or daily high-dose ICS + Theophylline* + oral systemic corticosteroid, and PRN SABA
		Steps 2–4: Conditionally recommend the use of subcutaneous immunotherapy as an adjunct treatment to standard pharmacotherapy in individuals ≥ 5 years of age whose asthma is controlled at the initiation, build up, and maintenance phases of immunotherapy			Consider Omalizumab**	

Assess Control

- First check adherence, inhaler technique, environmental factors, and comorbid conditions.
- **Step up** if needed; reassess in 2–6 weeks
- **Step down** if possible (if asthma is well controlled for at least 3 consecutive months)

Consult with asthma specialist if Step 4 or higher is required. Consider consultation at Step 3.

Control assessment is a key element of asthma care. This involves both impairment and risk. Use of objective measures, self-reported control, and health care utilization are complementary and should be employed on an ongoing basis, depending on the individual's clinical situation.

* Cromolyn, Nedocromil, LTRAs including montelukast, and Theophylline have limited availability for use in the United States, and/or have an increased risk of adverse consequences and need for monitoring that make their use less desirable. The FDA issued a Boxed Warning for montelukast in March 2020.

** Omalizumab is the only asthma biologic FDA-approved for this age range.

FIGURE 79.2 Stepwise long-term approach for managing asthma in children, 5–11 years of age. *ICS*, Inhaled corticosteroid; *LABA*, long-acting β_2-agonist; *LTRA*, leukotriene receptor antagonist; *SABA*, inhaled short-acting β_2-agonist. (Adapted from 2020 Focused Updates to the Asthma Management Guidelines: A Report from the National Asthma Education and Prevention Program Coordinating Committee Expert Panel Working Group. National Heart Lung Blood Institute. NIH Publication No. 20-HL-8142. Bethesda, MD: U.S. Department of Health and Human Services; 2021. nhlbi.nih.gov/asthmaguidelines.)

history of wheezing with respiratory tract infections, a short 7–10 day course of daily ICS with SABA therapy starting at the onset of a respiratory tract infection may reduce the need for systemic steroids.

For children over 5 years of age with moderate persistent asthma, combining long-acting bronchodilators with low-to-medium doses of inhaled corticosteroids improves lung function and reduces rescue medication use. For children with severe persistent asthma, a high-dose inhaled corticosteroid combined with a long-acting bronchodilator is the preferred therapy. Treatment should be re-evaluated within 4–6 weeks of initiating therapy. Once asthma is under control, control should be assessed on an ongoing basis every 1–6 months. Asthma should be well controlled for at least 3 months before stepping down therapy.

Single maintenance and reliever therapy (SMART) describes using a combined ICS (budesonide) and LABA

AGES 12+ YEARS Stepwise Approach for Management of Asthma

	Intermittent Asthma	Management of Persistent Asthma in Individuals Ages 12+ Years				
Treatment	STEP 1	STEP 2	STEP 3	STEP 4	STEP 5	STEP 6 ■
Preferred	PRN SABA	Daily low-dose ICS and PRN SABA or PRN concomitant ICS and SABA	Daily and PRN combination low-dose ICS-formoterol	Daily and PRN combination medium-dose ICS-formoterol	Daily medium-high dose ICS-LABA + LAMA and PRN SABA	Daily high-dose ICS-LABA + oral systemic corticosteroids + PRN SABA
Alternative		Daily LTRA* and PRN SABA or Cromolyn,* or Nedocromil,* or Zileuton,* or Theophylline,* and PRN SABA	Daily medium-dose ICS and PRN SABA or Daily low-dose ICS-LABA, or daily low-dose ICS + LAMA, or daily low-dose ICS + LTRA,* and PRN SABA or Daily low-dose ICS + Theophylline* or Zileuton,* and PRN SABA	Daily medium-dose ICS-LABA or daily medium-dose ICS + LAMA, and PRN SABA or Daily medium-dose ICS + LTRA,* or daily medium-dose ICS + Theophylline,* or daily medium-dose ICS + Zileuton,* and PRN SABA	Daily medium-high dose ICS-LABA or daily high-dose ICS + LTRA,* and PRN SABA	
		Steps 2–4: Conditionally recommend the use of subcutaneous immunotherapy as an adjunct treatment to standard pharmacotherapy in individuals ≥ 5 years of age whose asthma is controlled at the initiation, build up, and maintenance phases of immunotherapy			Consider adding Asthma Biologics (e.g., anti-IgE, anti-IL5, anti-IL5R, anti-IL4/IL13)**	

Assess Control

- First check adherence, inhaler technique, environmental factors, and comorbid conditions.
- **Step up** if needed; reassess in 2–6 weeks
- **Step down** if possible (if asthma is well controlled for at least 3 consecutive months)

Consult with asthma specialist if Step 4 or higher is required. Consider consultation at Step 3.

Control assessment is a key element of asthma care. This involves both impairment and risk. Use of objective measures, self-reported control, and health care utilization are complementary and should be employed on an ongoing basis, depending on the individual's clinical situation.

* Cromolyn, Nedocromil, LTRAs including Zileuton and montelukast, and Theophylline have limited availability for use in the United States, and/or have an increased risk of adverse consequences and need for monitoring that make their use less desirable. The FDA issued a Boxed Warning for montelukast in March 2020.

** Specific recommendations for the use of biologics in asthma are not provided in 2020 NHLBI guidelines.

■ Data on the use of LAMA therapy in individuals with severe persistent asthma (Step 6) were not included in the AHRQ systematic review and thus no recommendation is made.

FIGURE 79.3 Stepwise approach for managing asthma in youths, 12 years of age or older. *ICS*, Inhaled corticosteroid; *LABA*, long-acting β_2-agonist; *LAMA*, long-acting muscarinic antagonist; *LTRA*, leukotriene receptor antagonist; *SABA*, inhaled short-acting β_2-agonist. (Adapted from 2020 Focused Updates to the Asthma Management Guidelines: A Report from the National Asthma Education and Prevention Program Coordinating Committee Expert Panel Working Group. National Heart Lung Blood Institute. NIH Publication No. 20-HL-8142. Bethesda, MD: U.S. Department of Health and Human Services; 2021. nhlbi.nih.gov/asthmaguidelines.)

(formoterol) for both rescue and maintenance therapy and is recommended in children aged 4 years and older with moderate persistent asthma that is not responsive to ICS alone. Mometasone-formoterol may also be used in children 5 years and older. Formoterol has been shown to have similar and as rapid onset of action as albuterol. Salmeterol is a slower onset LABA and is not indicated in SMART therapy. SMART therapy may reduce total corticosteroid exposure and thus minimize potential growth side effects. However, there are limitations, including the number of puffs a patient can use per day, high cost of the inhaler, and insurance reimbursement constraints. There are no specific exclusionary criteria for this therapy.

COMPLICATIONS

Most asthma exacerbations can be successfully managed at home. **Status asthmaticus** is an acute exacerbation of asthma that does not respond adequately to therapeutic measures and may require hospitalization. Exacerbations may progress over several days or occur suddenly and can range in severity from mild to life threatening. Significant respiratory distress, dyspnea, wheezing, cough, and a decrease in spirometry or peak expiratory flow rate (PEFR) characterize deterioration in asthma control. During a severe episode, pulse oximetry is helpful in monitoring oxygenation. In status asthmaticus, arterial blood gases may be necessary for measurement of ventilation. As airway obstruction worsens and chest compliance decreases, carbon dioxide retention can occur. In the context of persistent tachypnea, a *normal* P_{CO_2} (35–45 mm Hg) indicates impending respiratory arrest.

First-line management of asthma exacerbations includes supplemental oxygen if needed and repetitive or continuous administration of SABAs. Early administration of oral or intravenous corticosteroids (Fig. 79.4) is important in treating the underlying inflammation. Administration of anticholinergic agents (ipratropium) with bronchodilators decreases rates of hospitalization and duration of time in the emergency department. Intravenous **magnesium sulfate** may be administered in the emergency department if there is clinical deterioration despite treatment with β_2 agonists, ipratropium, and systemic corticosteroids. The typical dose of magnesium sulfate is 25–75 mg/kg (maximum 2 g) intravenously administered over 20 minutes. Intramuscular epinephrine or subcutaneous terbutaline is rarely used except when severe asthma is associated with anaphylaxis or is unresponsive to continuous administration of SABAs.

PROGNOSIS

For some children, symptoms of wheezing with respiratory infections subside in the preschool years, whereas others have more persistent asthma symptoms. Prognostic indicators for children younger than 3 years of age who are at risk for persistent asthma are known as the *Modified Asthma Predictive Index for Children* (Table 79.5). Atopy is the strongest predictor for wheezing continuing into persistent asthma (Table 79.6).

TABLE 79.5 Modified Asthma Predictive Index for Children

At least four wheezing episodes *plus:*	
ONE MAJOR CRITERION	**OR TWO MINOR CRITERIA**
Parental asthma	Allergic rhinitis
Eczema	Wheezing apart from colds
Inhalant allergen sensitization	Eosinophils ≥4%
	Food allergen sensitization

From Liu AH, Martinez FD. Natural history of allergic diseases and asthma. In: Leung DYM, Akdis CA, Bacharier LB, et al., eds. Pediatric Allergy: Principles and Practice. *4th ed. Philadelphia: Elsevier; 2021: Fig. 2.4.*

TABLE 79.6 Risk Factors for Persistent Asthma

ALLERGY
• Atopic dermatitis • Allergic rhinitis • Elevated total serum IgE levels (first year of life) • Peripheral blood eosinophilia >4% (2–3 yr of age) • Inhalant and food allergen sensitization
LOWER RESPIRATORY TRACT INFECTIONS
• Rhinovirus, respiratory syncytial virus • Severe bronchiolitis (i.e., requiring hospitalization) • Pneumonia
PARENTAL ASTHMA
ENVIRONMENTAL TOBACCO SMOKE EXPOSURE (INCLUDING PRENATAL)
GENDER
Males
• Transient wheezing • Persistent allergy-associated asthma
Females
• Asthma associated with obesity and early-onset puberty • "Triad" asthma (adulthood)*

**Triad asthma—nasal polyps, aspirin sensitivity, asthma.*
Ig, Immunoglobulin.
From Liu AH, Martinez FD. Natural history of allergic diseases and asthma. In: Leung DYM, Akdis CA, Bacharier LB, et al., eds. Pediatric Allergy: Principles and Practice. *4th ed. Philadelphia: Elsevier; 2021: Box 2.2.*

PREVENTION

Education plays an important role in helping patients and their families adhere to the prescribed therapy and needs to begin at the time of diagnosis. Successful education involves teaching basic asthma facts, explaining the role of medications, teaching environmental control measures, and improving patient skills in the use of spacer devices for metered-dose inhalers and peak flow monitoring. Families should have an asthma management plan (Fig. 79.5) for daily care and for exacerbations.

Peak flow monitoring is a self-assessment tool that may be helpful for children over 5 years of age with asthma who are poor perceivers of airway obstruction, have moderate-to-severe asthma, or have a history of severe exacerbations. Peak flow monitoring also can be useful in children who are still learning to recognize asthma symptoms. It must be emphasized that peak flow monitoring is not for the diagnosis of asthma but for monitoring.

A child's personal best PEFR is the highest value achieved over a 2-week period when asthma is controlled. Percentages

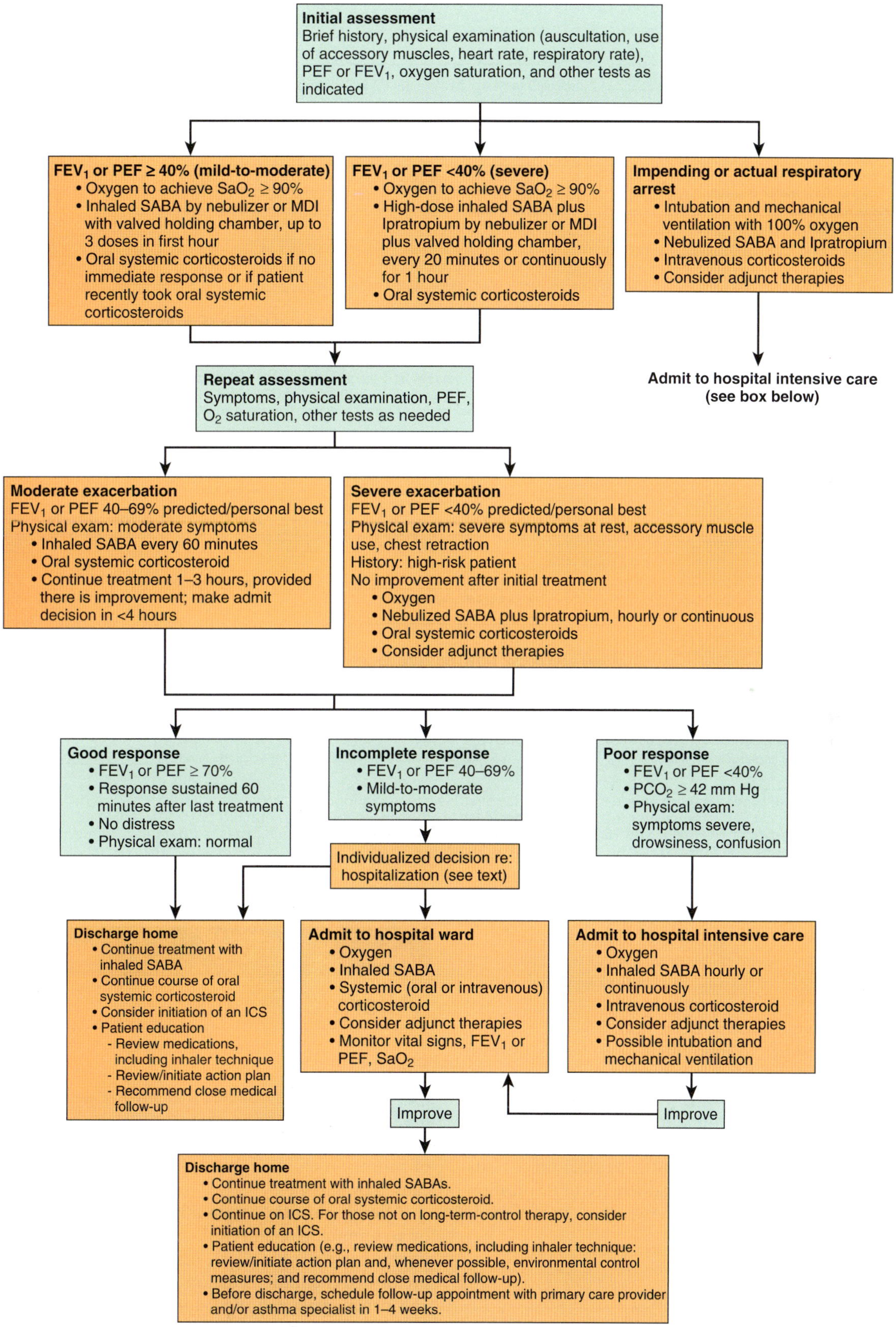

Key: *FEV_1*, Forced expiratory volume in 1 second; *ICS*, inhaled corticosteroid; *MDI*, metered-dose inhaler; *PCO_2*, partial pressure carbon dioxide; *PEF*, peak expiratory flow; *SABA*, short-acting beta$_2$-agonist; *SaO_2*, oxygen saturation

FIGURE 79.4 Management of asthma exacerbations: emergency department and hospital-based care. (From National Heart Lung Blood Institute, National Asthma Education and Prevention Program. Expert Panel Report 3: Guidelines for the Diagnosis and Management of Asthma. Summary Report 2007, NIH Publication No. 08-5846. Bethesda, MD: U.S. Department of Health and Human Services; 2007:55. https://www.nhlbi.nih.gov/sites/default/files/media/docs/asthsumm.pdf.)

Asthma Action Plan

For: ______ Doctor: ______ Date: ______

Doctor's Phone Number ______ Hospital/Emergency Department Phone Number ______

GREEN ZONE

Doing Well

- No cough, wheeze, chest tightness, or shortness of breath during the day or night
- Can do usual activities

And, if a peak flow meter is used,

Peak flow: more than ______ (80 percent or more of my best peak flow)

My best peak flow is: ______

Take these long-term-control medicines each day (include an anti-inflammatory).

Medicine	How much to take	When to take it

Identify and avoid and control the things that make your asthma worse, like (list here):

______ ______ ______

Before exercise, if prescribed, take: ☐ 2 or ☐ 4 puffs ______ 5 to 60 minutes before exercise

YELLOW ZONE

Asthma Is Getting Worse

- Cough, wheeze, chest tightness, or shortness of breath, or
- Waking at night due to asthma, or
- Can do some, but not all, usual activities

-Or-

Peak flow: ______ to ______ (50 to 79 percent of my best peak flow)

First → **Add: quick-relief medicine–and keep taking your GREEN ZONE medicine.**

______ (short-acting $beta_2$-agonist) ☐ 2 or ☐ 4 puffs, every 20 minutes for up to 1 hour ☐ Nebulizer, once

If applicable, remove yourself from the thing that made your asthma worse.

Second → If your symptoms (and peak flow, if used) return to GREEN ZONE after 1 hour of above treatment:

☐ Continue monitoring to be sure you stay in the green zone.

-Or-

If your symptoms (and peak flow, if used) do not return to GREEN ZONE after 1 hour of above treatment:

☐ Take: ______ (short-acting $beta_2$-agonist) ☐ 2 or ☐ 4 puffs or ☐ Nebulizer

☐ Add: ______ (oral corticosteroid) mg per day. For ______ (3–10) days

☐ Call the doctor ______ (phone) ☐ before/ ☐ within ______ hours after taking the oral corticosteroid.

RED ZONE

Medical Alert!

- Very short of breath, or
- Quick-relief medicines have not helped, or
- Cannot do usual activities, or
- Symptoms are same or get worse after 24 hours in Yellow Zone.

-Or-

Peak flow: less than ______ (50 percent of my best peak flow)

Take this medicine:

☐ ______ (short-acting $beta_2$-agonist) ☐ 4 or ☐ 6 puffs or ☐ Nebulizer

☐ ______ (oral corticosteroid) mg

Then call your doctor NOW. Go to the hospital or call an ambulance if

- You are still in the red zone after 15 minutes AND
- You have not reached your doctor.

DANGER SIGNS

- Trouble walking and talking due to shortness of breath
- Lips or fingernails are blue

→

- Take ☐ 4 or ☐ 6 puffs of your quick-relief medicine **AND**
- Go to the hospital or call for an ambulance ______ (phone) **NOW!**

FIGURE 79.5 Asthma self-management guideline. (From National Heart Lung Blood Institute, National Asthma Education and Prevention Program. Expert Panel Report 3: Guidelines for the Diagnosis and Management of Asthma. Summary Report 2007, NIH Publication No. 05-5251. Bethesda, MD: U.S. Department of Health and Human Services; 2007:119. https://www.nhlbi.nih.gov/sites/default/files/media/docs/asthsumm.pdf.)

based on the best PEFR reading may then be incorporated into a written asthma management plan as a means of providing an objective indication of airway obstruction to guide home-based asthma care. Limitations exist, however, to PEFR: they are effort- and technique-dependent, peak flow meters may lose accuracy with time, and appropriate range meters (low vs. high) must be provided.

Utilizing PEFR and written asthma management plans simultaneously may impact asthma monitoring and management. Children with asthma should be seen not only when they are ill but also when they are healthy. Regular office visits allow the health care team to review adherence to medication and control measures and to determine whether doses of medications need adjustment.

PEARLS FOR PRACTITIONERS

See Allergy: Pearls for Practitioners at the end of this section.

REVIEW QUESTIONS

Available online.

CHAPTER 80

Allergic Rhinitis

ETIOLOGY

Rhinitis describes diseases that involve inflammation of the nasal epithelium and is characterized by sneezing, pruritus, rhinorrhea, and congestion. There are many different causes of rhinitis in children, but approximately half of all cases are caused by allergies.

Allergic rhinitis, commonly known as ***hay fever***, is caused by an immunoglobulin (Ig)E-mediated allergic response. During the early allergic phase, mast cells degranulate and release preformed chemical mediators, such as histamine and tryptase, and newly generated mediators such as leukotrienes, prostaglandins, and platelet-activating factor. After a quiescent phase in which other cells are recruited, a late phase occurs approximately 4–8 hours later. Eosinophils, basophils, CD4 T cells, monocytes, and neutrophils release their chemical mediators, which leads to the development of chronic nasal inflammation.

Allergic rhinitis can be seasonal, perennial, or episodic depending on the specific causative allergen and exposure. Some children experience perennial symptoms with seasonal exacerbations. **Seasonal allergic rhinitis** is caused by airborne pollens, which have seasonal patterns. Typically, trees pollinate in the spring, grasses in late spring to summer, and weeds in the summer and fall. The pollen, microscopic in size, can travel airborne for hundreds of miles and be inhaled easily into the respiratory tract. **Perennial allergic rhinitis** is primarily caused by indoor allergens, such as house dust mites, animal dander, mold, and cockroaches. **Episodic rhinitis** occurs with intermittent exposure to allergens, such as visiting a friend's home where a pet lives.

EPIDEMIOLOGY

Chronic rhinitis is one of the most common disorders encountered in infants and children. Overall, allergic rhinitis is observed in 10–25% of the general population, with children and adolescents more commonly affected than adults. The prevalence of physician-diagnosed allergic rhinitis has been estimated as high as 40%.

CLINICAL MANIFESTATIONS

The hallmark symptoms of allergic rhinitis are clear, thin rhinorrhea, nasal congestion, sneezing paroxysms, and pruritus of the eyes, nose, ears, and palate. Postnasal drip may result in frequent attempts to clear the throat, nocturnal cough, and hoarseness. It is important to correlate the onset, duration, and severity of symptoms with seasonal or perennial exposures, changes in the home or school environment, and exposure to nonspecific irritants such as tobacco smoke.

The physical examination includes a thorough nasal examination and an evaluation of the eyes, ears, throat, chest, and skin. Physical findings may be subtle. Classic physical findings include pale or bluish, boggy and edematous nasal turbinates with clear, watery secretions. Frequent nasal itching and rubbing of the nose superiorly with the palm of the hand, the **allergic salute**, can lead to a transverse nasal crease found across the nose. Children may produce clucking sounds by rubbing the soft palate with their tongue. Oropharyngeal examination may reveal lymphoid hyperplasia of the posterior oropharynx, visible mucus, or both. Orthodontic abnormalities may be seen in children with chronic mouth breathing. **Allergic shiners**, dark, edematous infraorbital areas caused by venous congestion, along with eyelid edema or conjunctival injection, are often present in children. Retracted tympanic membranes from eustachian tube dysfunction or serous otitis media also may be seen. Evidence of other atopic diseases, such as asthma or eczema, may be present, which helps lead the clinician to the correct diagnosis.

LABORATORY AND IMAGING STUDIES

Allergy testing can be performed by in vivo skin tests or by in vitro serum tests (enzyme-linked immunosorbent assay) to pertinent allergens found in the patient's environment (see Table 78.4). Skin tests (prick/puncture) provide immediate and accurate results. Positive tests correlate strongly with nasal and bronchial allergen provocative challenges. In vitro serum tests are useful for patients with diffuse dermatitis, dermatographism, poor tolerance to skin testing, or for those taking medications that interfere with skin testing. Disadvantages of serum tests include increased cost, inability to obtain immediate results, and reduced sensitivity compared with skin tests. Testing should include relevant allergens in the home and regional flora. Broad screening testing without regard to symptoms is not recommended. Measurement of total serum IgE or blood eosinophils generally is not helpful. The presence of eosinophils on the nasal smear suggests a diagnosis of allergy, but eosinophils also can be found in patients with **nonallergic rhinitis with eosinophilia**. Nasal smear eosinophilia is often predictive of a good clinical response to nasal corticosteroid sprays but is not commonly performed in clinical practice.

DIFFERENTIAL DIAGNOSIS

Rhinitis can be divided into allergic and nonallergic rhinitis (Table 80.1). Nonallergic rhinitis describes a group of nasal diseases in which there is no evidence of allergic etiology. It can be divided further into nonanatomic and anatomic etiologies. The most common form of nonallergic rhinitis in children is infectious rhinitis, which may be acute or chronic. Acute infectious rhinitis **(the common cold)** is caused by viruses, including rhinoviruses and coronaviruses, and typically resolves within 7–10 days (see Chapter 103). An average child has three to six common colds per year, with the most affected being younger children and children attending day care. Infection is suggested by the presence of sore throat, fever, and poor appetite, especially with a history of exposure

TABLE 80.1 Classification of the Etiology of Rhinitis in Children

ALLERGIC	NONALLERGIC	
	NONANATOMIC	ANATOMIC
Seasonal Perennial Episodic	Nonallergic, noninfectious (vasomotor) rhinitis Infectious rhinosinusitis Nonallergic rhinitis with eosinophilia Rhinitis medicamentosa	Adenoidal hypertrophy CSF rhinorrhea Choanal atresia Congenital anomalies Foreign body Nasal polyps Septal deviation Tumors Turbinate hypertrophy

CSF, Cerebrospinal fluid.

to others with colds. Chronic infectious **rhinosinusitis**, or sinusitis, should be suspected if there is mucopurulent nasal discharge with symptoms that persist beyond 10 days (see Chapter 105). Classic signs of acute sinusitis in older children include facial tenderness, tooth pain, headache, and fever. Classic signs are usually not present in young children who may present with postnasal drainage with cough, throat clearing, halitosis, and rhinorrhea. The character of the nasal secretions with infectious rhinitis varies from purulent to minimal or absent. Coexistence of middle ear disease, such as otitis media or eustachian tube dysfunction, may be additional clues of infection.

Nonallergic, noninfectious rhinitis (formerly known as *vasomotor rhinitis*) can manifest as rhinorrhea and sneezing in children with profuse clear nasal discharge. Exposure to irritants, such as cigarette smoke and dust, and strong fumes and odors, such as perfumes and chlorine in swimming pools, can trigger these nasal symptoms. **Nonallergic rhinitis with eosinophilia syndrome** is associated with clear nasal discharge and eosinophils on nasal smear and is seen infrequently in children. Cold air **(skier's nose)**, hot/spicy food ingestion **(gustatory rhinitis)**, and exposure to bright light **(reflex rhinitis)** are examples of nonallergic, noninfectious rhinitis. Treatment with topical ipratropium before exposure may be helpful.

Rhinitis medicamentosa is due primarily to overuse of topical nasal decongestants, such as oxymetazoline or phenylephrine, resulting in rebound nasal congestion. This condition is not common in younger children. Adolescents or young adults may become dependent on these over-the-counter medications. Treatment requires discontinuation of the offending decongestant spray, topical corticosteroids, and, frequently, a short course of oral corticosteroids.

The most common anatomic problem seen in young children is obstruction secondary to **adenoidal hypertrophy**, which can be suspected from symptoms such as mouth breathing, snoring, hyponasal speech, sleep disordered breathing, and persistent rhinitis with or without chronic otitis media (see Chapter 136). Infection of the nasopharynx may be secondary to infected hypertrophied adenoid tissue.

Nasal polyps typically appear as bilateral, gray, glistening tissue originating from the sinus ostia and may be associated with anosmia, nasal obstruction, and clear or purulent nasal discharge. Nasal polyps are rare in children younger than 10 years of age, but if present they warrant evaluation for an underlying disease process such as cystic fibrosis or primary ciliary dyskinesia. **Aspirin-exacerbated respiratory disease** consists of asthma, aspirin sensitivity, and nasal polyps with chronic or recurrent sinusitis.

Foreign bodies are seen more commonly in young children who place food, small toys, stones, or other objects in their nose. The index of suspicion should be raised by a history of unilateral, purulent nasal discharge or foul odor. The foreign body can often be seen on anterior nasal examination.

TREATMENT

Management of allergic rhinitis is based on disease severity, impact of the disease on the patient, and the ability of the patient to comply with recommendations. Treatment modalities include allergen avoidance, pharmacologic therapy, and immunotherapy. Environmental control and steps to minimize allergen exposure, similar to preventive steps for asthma, should be implemented whenever possible (see Table 79.3).

Pharmacotherapy

Intranasal corticosteroids are the most effective pharmacologic therapy for treatment of allergic and nonallergic rhinitis. These include beclomethasone, budesonide, ciclesonide, flunisolide, fluticasone, mometasone, and triamcinolone. These topical agents work to reduce inflammation, edema, and mucus production. They are effective for symptoms of nasal congestion, rhinorrhea, pruritus, and sneezing but less helpful for ocular symptoms. Daily administration is necessary for maximum effectiveness. Nasal corticosteroid sprays have been used safely in long-term therapy. Deleterious effects on adrenal function or nasal membranes have not been reported when these agents are used appropriately. The most common adverse effects include local irritation, burning, and sneezing, which occur in 10% of patients. Nasal bleeding from improper technique (spraying the nasal septum) can occur. Rare cases of nasal septal perforation have been reported.

Antihistamines are the medications used most frequently to treat allergic rhinitis. They are useful in treating rhinorrhea, sneezing, nasal itching, and ocular itching but are less helpful in treating nasal congestion. **First-generation antihistamines**, such as diphenhydramine and hydroxyzine, easily cross the blood-brain barrier, with sedation as the most common reported adverse effect. Use of first-generation antihistamines in children has an adverse effect on cognitive and academic function. In very young children, a paradoxical stimulatory central nervous system effect resulting in irritability and restlessness has been noted. Other adverse effects of first-generation antihistamines include anticholinergic effects, such as blurred vision, urinary retention, dry mouth, tachycardia, and constipation. **Second-generation antihistamines**, such as cetirizine, desloratadine, fexofenadine, levocetirizine, and loratadine, are less likely to cross the blood-brain barrier, resulting in less sedation. Cetirizine, fexofenadine, levocetirizine, and loratadine are available without prescription. Azelastine and olopatadine, topical nasal antihistamine sprays, are approved for children older than 5 years and 6 years, respectively. Azelastine is available without a prescription.

Decongestants, taken orally or intranasally, may be used to relieve nasal congestion. Oral medications, such as pseudoephedrine and phenylephrine, are available either alone or in combination with antihistamines. Adverse effects of oral decongestants include insomnia, nervousness, irritability, tachycardia, tremors, and palpitations; oral decongestants are not recommended for children less than 4 years old. For older children participating in sports, oral decongestant use may be restricted. Topical nasal decongestant sprays are effective for immediate relief of nasal obstruction but should not be used more than 3 consecutive days to prevent rhinitis medicamentosa.

Topical ipratropium bromide, an anticholinergic nasal spray, is used primarily for nonallergic rhinitis and rhinitis associated with viral upper respiratory infection. Leukotriene modifiers have been studied in the treatment of allergic rhinitis. Montelukast is approved for use in seasonal allergic rhinitis.

Allergen Immunotherapy

If environmental control measures and medication intervention are only partially effective or produce unacceptable adverse effects, immunotherapy may be recommended. The mechanism of action for allergen immunotherapy is complex but includes increased production of an IgG_4-blocking antibody, decreased production of allergen-specific IgE, induction of allergen-specific T-regulatory cells, and alteration of cytokine expression produced in response to an allergen challenge. Immunotherapy is effective for desensitization to pollens, dust mites, and cat and dog proteins. Use in young children may be limited by the need for frequent injections. *Subcutaneous immunotherapy* (injections or **"allergy shots"**) must be administered in a physician's office with 30 minutes of observation after the allergen injection. Anaphylaxis may occur, and the physician must be experienced in the treatment of these severe adverse allergic reactions. *Sublingual immunotherapy* (tablets placed under the tongue) is only indicated for ragweed pollen, some grass pollens, and dust mite allergy. It can be used in children 5 years or older. The first dose must be given in a physician's office, but subsequent doses can be administered at home.

COMPLICATIONS

Approximately 60% of children with allergic rhinitis have symptoms of bronchial hyperresponsiveness (see Chapter 79). Chronic allergic inflammation leads to chronic cough from postnasal drip, eustachian tube dysfunction, otitis media, sinusitis, and tonsillar and adenoid hypertrophy, which may lead to obstructive sleep apnea. Children with allergic rhinitis may experience sleep disturbances, limitations of activity, irritability, and mood and cognitive disorders that adversely affect their performance at school and their sense of well-being.

PROGNOSIS AND PREVENTION

Seasonal allergic rhinitis is a common and prominent condition that may not improve as children grow older. Patients become more adept at self-management. Perennial allergic rhinitis improves with allergen control of indoor allergens.

Removal or avoidance of the offending allergen is advised. The only effective measure for minimizing pet allergen exposure is removal of the pet from the home. Avoidance of pollen and outdoor molds can be accomplished by staying indoors in a controlled environment. Air conditioning and keeping windows and doors closed lower exposure to pollen. High-efficiency particle air filters reduce exposure to allergens (e.g., pet dander). Sealing the mattress and pillow in allergen-proof encasings is the most effective strategy for reduction of dust mite allergen. Bedding should be washed in hot water (>130°F) every week.

PEARLS FOR PRACTITIONERS

See Allergy: Pearls for Practitioners at the end of this section.

REVIEW QUESTIONS

Available online.

CHAPTER 81

Atopic Dermatitis

ETIOLOGY

Atopic dermatitis is a chronic, pruritic, relapsing inflammatory skin condition. The pathogenesis is multifactorial and involves a complex interplay of genetics, immunologic abnormalities, impaired skin barrier function, environmental interactions, and infectious triggers. A diverse set of genes encoding epidermal structural proteins (filaggrin) and elements of the immune system play a major role in atopic dermatitis.

Several immunoregulatory abnormalities have been described in patients with atopic dermatitis. There is an exaggerated cutaneous inflammatory response to environmental triggers, including irritants and allergens. Activated Langerhans cells in the dermis expressing surface-bound immunoglobulin E (IgE) stimulate T cells. In acute lesions, activated Th2 lymphocytes infiltrate the dermis. They initiate and maintain local tissue inflammation primarily through interleukin (IL)-4, IL-13, and IL-5, promoting IgE production (IL-4, IL-13) and eosinophil differentiation (IL-5). As the disease progresses from an acute to chronic phase, the Th2 response switches to Th1/Th0 response. Chronic lesions are characterized by increased IL-12 and IL-18.

Patients with atopic dermatitis have **hyperirritable skin**; many factors can cause the disease to worsen or relapse. Known triggers include anxiety and stress, climate (extremes of temperature and humidity), irritants, allergens, and infections. Approximately 30% of infants and young children with severe atopic dermatitis have coexisting food allergies. The more severe the atopic dermatitis and the younger the patient, the more likely a food allergy will be identified as a contributing factor. Egg allergy is the most common cause of food-induced eczematous reactions.

EPIDEMIOLOGY

The prevalence of atopic dermatitis has increased two- to threefold over the past 30 years. Approximately 15–20% of children and 2–10% of adults are affected. Atopic dermatitis often starts in early infancy. Approximately 50% of affected children show symptoms in the first year of life, and 80% experience disease onset before 5 years of age. Atopic dermatitis is often the first manifestation of the **atopic march**. Approximately 80% of children with atopic dermatitis develop other allergic diseases, such as asthma or allergic rhinitis. Symptoms of dermatitis may and often do disappear before the later onset of respiratory allergies.

CLINICAL MANIFESTATIONS

The clinical manifestations of atopic dermatitis vary with age. In infants, atopic dermatitis involves the face, scalp, cheeks, and extensor surfaces of the extremities (Fig. 81.1). The diaper area is spared. In older children, the rash localizes to the antecubital and popliteal fossae, head, and neck. In adolescents and adults, **lichenified plaques** are seen in flexural areas (Fig. 81.2) and head and neck regions. Pruritus has a significant impact on the child and family's quality of life because it is

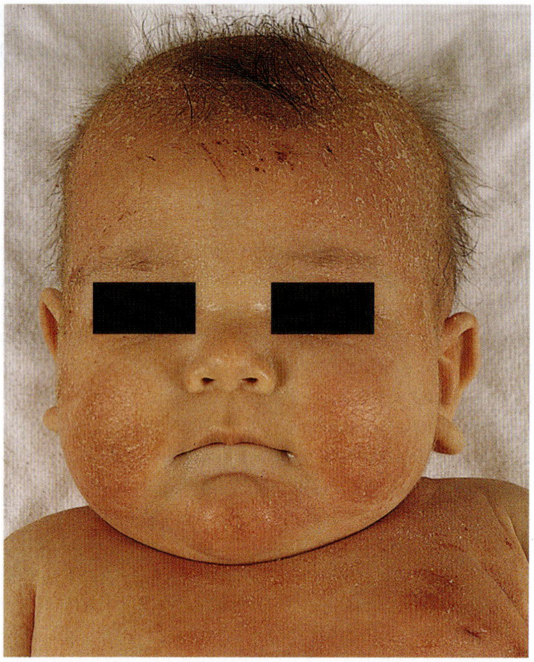

FIGURE 81.1 Atopic dermatitis typical cheek involvement. (From Eichenfield LF, Frieden IJ, Esterly NB. *Textbook of Neonatal Dermatology*. Philadelphia: Saunders; 2001:242.)

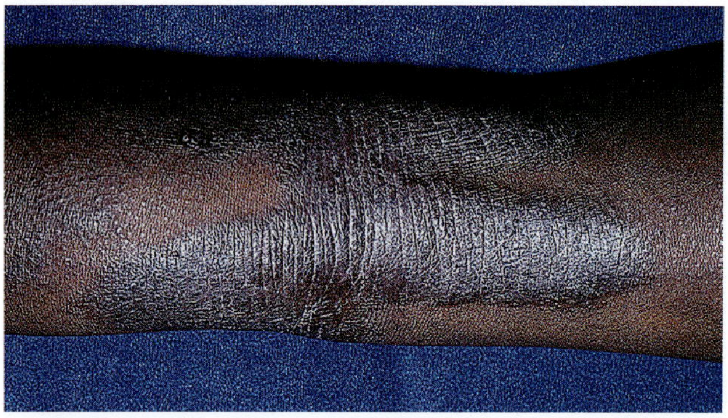

FIGURE 81.2 Adolescent with lichenification of the popliteal fossa from chronic atopic dermatitis. (From Weston WL, Morelli JG, Lane A [eds]. Color Textbook of Pediatric Dermatology, 4th ed. St. Louis: Mosby, 2007.)

often worse at night, disturbing sleep. Physical examination may also show hyperlinearity of the palms and soles, dermatographism, pityriasis alba, creases under the lower eyelids (**Dennie-Morgan folds** or **Dennie lines**), and **keratosis pilaris** (asymptomatic horny follicular papules on the extensor surfaces of the arms).

LABORATORY AND IMAGING STUDIES

The diagnosis of atopic dermatitis is based on clinical features rather than laboratory tests (Table 81.1). Skin biopsy is of little value but may be performed to exclude other skin diseases that mimic atopic dermatitis. Skin testing or serum-specific IgE testing may be helpful in assessing the contribution of food or environmental allergies to disease expression if history is suggestive.

TABLE 81.1 Clinical Features of Atopic Dermatitis

ESSENTIAL FEATURES
• Pruritus • Facial, neck, and extensor eczema in infants and children • Flexural eczema that spares the groin • Chronic or relapsing dermatitis
FREQUENTLY ASSOCIATED FEATURES
• Personal or family history of atopic disease • Xerosis • Lichenification • Elevated serum IgE levels • Positive immediate-type allergy skin tests • Early age of onset
OTHER FEATURES
• Ichthyosis, palmar hyperlinearity, keratosis pilaris • Dermatographism and delayed blanch response • Dennie-Morgan infraorbital folds, orbital darkening • Facial erythema or pallor • Periorbital changes • Regional involvement (perioral, periauricular) • Perifollicular accentuation

Ig, Immunoglobulin.
Adapted from Boguniewicz M, Leung DYM. Evaluation and management of atopic dermatitis. In: Leung DYM, Akdis CA, Bacharier LB, et al., eds. Pediatric Allergy: Principles and Practice. *4th ed. Philadelphia: Elsevier; 2021:Table 38.1.*

DIFFERENTIAL DIAGNOSIS

Many conditions share signs and symptoms of atopic dermatitis (Table 81.2). Infants presenting in the first year of life with growth faltering, recurrent skin or systemic infections, and scaling, erythematous rash should be evaluated for immunodeficiency disorders. Wiskott-Aldrich syndrome is an X-linked recessive syndrome characterized by atopic dermatitis, thrombocytopenia, small-sized platelets, and recurrent infections. Langerhans cell histiocytosis is characterized by hemorrhagic or petechial lesions. **Scabies** is an intensely pruritic skin condition caused by the human scabies mite. The presence of burrows in interdigital spaces and flexor surfaces of the wrists, elbows, axilla, or genitals is pathognomonic. Burrows may be few or absent, however.

TREATMENT

The goals of eczema therapy are to reduce the number and severity of flares and to increase duration of disease-free periods. Successful management involves skin hydration with emollients, pharmacologic therapy to reduce pruritus and inflammation, and identification and avoidance of triggers. Patients with atopic dermatitis have impaired skin barrier function and enhanced transepidermal water loss. Daily, lukewarm baths for 15–20 minutes followed immediately by the application of fragrance-free emollients to retain moisture are major components of therapy. Prevention of xerosis is important for pruritus control and for maintaining the integrity of the epithelial barrier. Emollients should be ointments or creams. Lotions are not as effective because they contain water or alcohol and may have a drying effect owing to evaporation. A mild nonsoap cleanser also is recommended.

Topical antiinflammatory agents, including corticosteroids and immunomodulators, are the cornerstone of therapy for acute flares and prevention of relapses. Topical corticosteroids

TABLE 81.2 Differential Diagnoses of Atopic Dermatitis

CONGENITAL DISORDERS
Netherton syndrome Familial keratosis pilaris
CHRONIC DERMATOSES
Seborrheic dermatitis Contact dermatitis (allergic or irritant) Nummular eczema Psoriasis Ichthyoses
INFECTIONS AND INFESTATIONS
Scabies HIV-associated dermatitis Dermatophytosis
MALIGNANCIES
Cutaneous T-cell lymphoma (mycosis fungoides/Sezary syndrome) Langerhans cell histiocytosis Letterer-Siwe disease
AUTOIMMUNE DISORDERS
Dermatitis herpetiformis Pemphigus foliaceus Graft-vs.-host disease Dermatomyositis
IMMUNODEFICIENCIES
Wiskott-Aldrich syndrome (*WAS* gene) Severe combined immunodeficiency Autosomal dominant hyper-IgE syndrome (*STAT3* gene) DOCK8-associated immunodeficiency X-linked immune dysregulation, polyendocrinopathy, enteropathy syndrome (IPEX; *FOXP3* gene)
METABOLIC DISORDERS
Zinc deficiency Pyridoxine (vitamin B_6) and niacin deficiency Multiple carboxylase deficiency Phenylketonuria

DOCK 8, Dedicator of cytokinesis 8; *Ig*, immunoglobulin.
Modified from Boguniewicz M, Leung DYM. Evaluation and management of atopic dermatitis. In: Leung DYM, Akdis CA, Bacharier LB, et al., eds. Pediatric Allergy: Principles and Practice. *4th ed. Philadelphia: Elsevier; 2021:Table 38.2.*

are used for reducing inflammation and pruritus. They are effective for the acute and chronic phases of the disease. Ointments generally are preferred over creams and lotions because of enhanced potency due to easier skin penetration. Corticosteroids are ranked by potency into seven classes. The least potent corticosteroid that is effective should be used. Higher potency corticosteroids may be necessary to diminish the dermatitis flare but should be used for limited periods. Low-potency nonfluorinated corticosteroids should be used on the face, intertriginous areas (groin, axilla), and large areas to reduce the risk of adverse effects. Reduced efficacy of topical corticosteroids may be related to disease severity rather than glucocorticoid resistance. Local adverse effects (skin atrophy and striae) and systemic adverse effects (hypothalamic-pituitary-adrenal axis suppression and hyperglycemia) are related to the potency, length of use, and applied surface area. In infants and younger children, the possibility of corticosteroid-induced adverse effects may be greater. When control of inflammatory lesions is achieved, most patients can be managed with emollients and low-potency topical corticosteroids.

The topical calcineurin inhibitors tacrolimus and pimecrolimus are second-line agents for short-term and intermittent treatment of atopic dermatitis in patients (≥2 years) unresponsive to or intolerant of other therapies. These agents may be used on all body locations and are especially useful on delicate skin sites, such as the face, neck, and axilla, without the adverse effect of cutaneous atrophy seen with topical corticosteroids. Crisaborole, a topical phosphodiesterase 4 (PDE-4) inhibitor, is approved for treatment of mild-to-moderate atopic dermatitis in patients ages 2 and older and offers an alternative to topical corticosteroids or calcineurin inhibitors. The most common adverse effect of both calcineurin and PDE-4 inhibitors is local skin irritation.

In cases of severe, refractory atopic dermatitis, systemic medications may be considered, including systemic corticosteroids, cyclosporine, dupilumab, and, rarely, antimetabolites such as mycophenolate mofetil or methotrexate. Janus kinase inhibitors like topical ruxolitinib and oral upadacitinib have been approved by the Food and Drug Administration in the treatment of moderate-to-severe atopic dermatitis for adults and children over age 12. Phototherapy is also considered for patients who have failed standard treatments.

COMPLICATIONS

Defective cell-mediated immunity leads to increased susceptibility to many bacterial, viral, and fungal infections of the skin. More than 90% of patients with atopic dermatitis have colonization of lesional skin with *Staphylococcus aureus (S. aureus)*, and more than 75% of patients have colonization of uninvolved skin. Colonization and infection by *S. aureus* are associated with disease severity. *S. aureus* secretes exotoxins that act as superantigens, stimulating T cells and increasing IgE production. Secondarily infected atopic dermatitis often presents as impetiginous, pustular lesions with crusting and honey-colored exudate. Topical antibiotics, such as mupirocin or retapamulin, can be used to treat local areas of infection. Oral antibiotics such as cephalexin, dicloxacillin, or amoxicillin-clavulanate can be used for multifocal disease or for infection around the eyes and mouth that is difficult to treat topically. Bacterial cultures may be helpful in patients who do not respond to oral antibiotics or who have infection after multiple antibiotic courses given the possibility of community-acquired methicillin-resistant *S. aureus*.

Herpes simplex superinfection of affected skin, or **Kaposi varicelliform eruption** or **eczema herpeticum**, results in vesiculopustular lesions that appear in clusters and can become hemorrhagic. Herpes simplex virus infection can be misdiagnosed as bacterial infection and should be considered if skin lesions fail to respond to antibiotics. Coxsackieviruses may produce similar lesions.

Widespread infections with human papillomavirus (warts) and molluscum contagiosum are also common in children with atopic dermatitis.

PROGNOSIS

Atopic dermatitis is a chronic, relapsing skin disorder that tends to be more severe and prominent in young children. Symptoms become less severe in two-thirds of children, with complete remission for approximately 20%. More widespread early onset disease that is concomitant with asthma and allergic rhinitis, family history of atopic dermatitis, and elevated serum IgE levels may predict a more persistent course. Patients and families should be taught that a single cause and cure for atopic dermatitis is unlikely, but that good control is possible for the majority of affected patients.

PREVENTION

An important step in the management of atopic dermatitis is to identify and avoid allergens and irritants including soaps, detergents, fragrances, chemicals, smoke, and extremes of temperature and humidity. Because wool and synthetic fabrics can be irritating to the skin, 100% cotton fabric is preferred. Sweating is a recognized trigger. Fingernails should be trimmed frequently to minimize excoriations from scratching.

In infants and younger children who do not respond to the usual therapies, identifying and removing a food allergen from the diet may lead to clinical improvement. Food allergy is not a common trigger for older patients. Other environmental exposures, such as dust mites, can also contribute to the disease state; using allergen-proof encasings on pillows and bedding can be helpful.

PEARLS FOR PRACTITIONERS

See Allergy: Pearls for Practitioners at the end of this section.

REVIEW QUESTIONS

Available online.

CHAPTER 82
Urticaria, Angioedema, and Anaphylaxis

ETIOLOGY

Urticaria, commonly referred to as ***hives***, is swelling of the dermis and one of the most common skin conditions seen in clinical practice. **Angioedema** results from a process similar to urticaria, but the reaction extends below the dermis. Urticaria and angioedema occur in response to the release of inflammatory mediators, including histamine, leukotrienes, platelet-activating factor, prostaglandins, and cytokines, from mast cells residing in the skin. A variety of stimuli can trigger mast cells to release their chemical mediators. Typically, mast cells degranulate when antigen cross-links cell surface immunoglobulin E (IgE). Release of mediators results in vasodilation, increased vascular leak, and pruritus. In addition, basophils from the peripheral blood can localize to tissue and release mediators. Patients with urticaria have elevated histamine content in the skin that is more easily released.

Anaphylaxis is mediated by IgE, whereas **anaphylactoid reactions** result from mechanisms that are due to nonimmunologic mechanisms. Both reactions are acute, severe, and can be life threatening due to massive release of inflammatory mediators.

Not all mast cell activation is IgE mediated. Immunologic, nonimmunologic, physical, and chemical stimuli can produce degranulation of mast cells and basophils. **Anaphylatoxins**, C3a and C5a, can cause histamine release in a non–IgE-mediated reaction. Anaphylatoxins are generated in serum sickness (see Chapter 83) and in infectious, neoplastic, and rheumatic diseases. In addition, mast cell degranulation can occur from direct pharmacologic effect or physical or mechanical activation, such as urticaria after exposure to opiate medications or dermatographism (see later).

Urticaria and angioedema can be classified into three subcategories: acute, chronic, and physical. **Acute urticaria** and **angioedema** are hives and diffuse swelling that last less than 6 weeks. Often, the history is quite helpful in eliciting the cause of the acute reaction (Table 82.1). An IgE mechanism is more commonly found in acute urticaria than in chronic urticaria. In the pediatric population, viral illnesses are responsible for the majority of acute urticaria.

Chronic urticaria and **angioedema** are characterized by persistence of symptoms beyond 6 weeks (see Table 82.1). Some have daily symptoms of hives and swelling, whereas others have intermittent or recurrent episodes. Chronic urticaria can be idiopathic with unknown causal factors. Thirty-five percent to 40% of chronic urticaria cases have an autoimmune process due to IgG autoantibodies binding directly to IgE or the high-affinity IgE receptor. **Physical urticaria** and **angioedema** are characterized by known eliciting external factors that may include pressure, cold, heat, exercise, vibration, and exposure to sun.

The most common physical urticaria is dermatographism, affecting 2–5% of persons. **Dermatographism** means "writing on the skin" and is easily diagnosed by firmly scratching the skin with a blunt point, such as the wooden tip of a cotton swab or tongue depressor. It is characterized by an urticarial reaction localized to the site of skin trauma. It has been suggested that trauma induces an IgE-mediated reaction, causing histamine to be released from the mast cells.

Cholinergic urticaria, characterized by the appearance of 1- to 3-mm wheals surrounded by large erythematous flares after an increase in core body temperature, occurs commonly in young adults. Lesions may develop during strenuous exercise, after a hot bath, or with emotional stress. The lack of airway symptoms differentiates it from exercise-induced anaphylaxis.

Cold urticaria occurs with exposure to cold and may develop within minutes on areas directly exposed to cold or on rewarming of the affected areas. Ingestion of cold drinks may precipitate lip swelling. Cold urticaria syndromes can be categorized into acquired and familial disorders. Severe reactions resulting in death can occur with swimming or diving into cold water. Patients must never swim alone, should avoid total body exposure to cold, and should have autoinjectable epinephrine available.

TABLE 82.1 Etiologies of Acute and Chronic Urticaria

ACUTE URTICARIA	CHRONIC URTICARIA
Food	Physical
Medication	Chronic spontaneous (formerly *idiopathic*)
Insect sting or bite	Autoantibody associated
Infection	Neoplastic
Contact allergy	Idiopathic
Transfusion reaction	Autoinflammatory diseases
Idiopathic	

Hereditary angioedema (HAE) is an autosomal dominant disease due to a deficiency of C1-esterase inhibitor. The genetic defect may be caused by a spontaneous pathogenic variant because approximately 25% of cases occur in patients without any family history. The disease is estimated to affect approximately 10,000 persons in the United States. It is characterized by unpredictable, recurrent attacks of episodic swelling that involves the face, peripheral extremities, genitalia, abdomen, oropharynx, and pharynx. Episodes are often triggered by trauma. Asphyxiation from laryngeal attacks is a significant cause of mortality. Patients with HAE rarely have urticaria associated with angioedema, and the swelling is not relieved with antihistamines or oral corticosteroids. Most patients (85%) have **type I** disease, which is due to decreased production of C1-esterase inhibitor. A minority of patients (15%) have **type II** disease, which is due to production of dysfunctional C1-esterase inhibitor. A low C4 level serves as an initial screening test. Patients with reduced C4 should have quantitative and functional levels of C1-esterase inhibitor measured. C2 levels are low during an acute attack. Patients with **HAE with normal C1 inhibitor** have normal laboratory evaluation of C1-esterase inhibitor; the disease is more common in females. Treatment for HAE is divided into on-demand treatment for acute attacks and prophylaxis. Prophylactic C1 inhibitor concentrate has advantage over other prophylactic therapies in terms of availability, effectiveness, and side effects. Bradykinin is an important mediator in the pathophysiology of HAE, and newer treatments are aimed at blocking this mediator.

Anaphylactic reactions are type I IgE-mediated reactions and result from many causes (Table 82.2). Cross linking of cell surface IgE by allergen leads to high-affinity IgE receptor activation on the mast cells and basophils, resulting in release of mediators, including histamine, tryptase, tumor necrosis factor, platelet-activating factor, leukotrienes, prostaglandins, and cytokines. Other cell types involved in the reactions include monocytes, macrophages, eosinophils, neutrophils, and platelets. The mediator release results in the clinical picture of anaphylaxis.

Anaphylactoid reactions are due to nonimmunologic mechanisms. Mast cells and basophils can be activated by direct, nonspecific stimulation, although the exact underlying mechanism is unknown. Reactions to opiates and radiocontrast material are classic examples. Complement system activation also can result in mast cell and basophil activation. **Anaphylatoxins**, C3a and C5a, are named because of their ability to trigger mediator release and are generated in serum sickness. There are other causes of anaphylactoid reactions for which the mechanism has not been clarified.

TABLE **82.2** Common Causes of Anaphylaxis in Children

IgE-MEDIATED ANAPHYLAXIS	DIRECT MAST CELL ACTIVATORS
Food/food additives	Exercise
Medications	Heat or cold
Insect sting or bite	Sunlight/ultraviolet radiation
Natural rubber latex	Medications (opioids)
Allergen immunotherapy and challenge tests	
Biologic agent	
Blood products	

Ig, Immunoglobulin.

Modified from Wang J. Anaphylaxis: assessment and management. In: Leung DYM, Akdis CA, Bacharier LB, et al., eds. Pediatric Allergy: Principles and Practice. *4th ed. Philadelphia: Elsevier; 2021:Table 44.2.*

EPIDEMIOLOGY

Urticaria and angioedema are common skin conditions affecting 15–25% of individuals at some point in their lives. Most cases of urticaria are self-limited, but for some patients they are chronic. In approximately 50% of patients, urticaria and angioedema occur together. In the remaining 50%, 40% have urticaria alone and 10% have angioedema alone. The worldwide incidence of anaphylaxis in children is unknown.

CLINICAL MANIFESTATIONS

Raised, erythematous lesions with pale centers that are intensely pruritic characterize **urticaria** (Fig. 82.1). The lesions vary in size and can occur anywhere on the body. Typically, urticaria arise suddenly and may resolve within 1–2 hours or may persist for up to 24 hours. **Angioedema** is a similar process that involves the deeper dermis or subcutaneous tissue, with swelling as the principal symptom. Generally, angioedema is not pruritic, may be mildly painful, and persists for longer than 24 hours. In rare cases, it may become life threatening if swelling affects the upper airway.

The clinical manifestations of **anaphylaxis** and **anaphylactoid reactions** are the same for children and adults. The signs and symptoms vary and can range from mild skin findings to a fatal reaction. Ninety percent of patients present with cutaneous symptoms, including urticaria, angioedema, flushing, and warmth, but the absence of dermal symptoms does not exclude the diagnosis of anaphylaxis. Other affected organ systems include the respiratory tract (rhinorrhea, oropharyngeal edema, laryngeal edema, hoarseness, stridor, wheezing, dyspnea, and asphyxiation), cardiovascular system (tachycardia, hypotension, shock, syncope, and arrhythmias), gastrointestinal tract (nausea, abdominal pain, diarrhea, and vomiting), and neurologic system (syncope, seizure, dizziness, and a sense of impending doom). The severity of an anaphylactic reaction is often proportionate to the speed of symptom onset. *A clinical diagnosis of anaphylaxis can be made when there is acute onset of symptoms with involvement of the skin and/or mucosal tissue along with one of the following: respiratory compromise, reduced blood pressure, or end-organ dysfunction (total of two affected organ systems)* (Fig. 82.2). Similarly, if a patient has a known exposure to a personal allergen, anaphylaxis should be diagnosed with skin symptoms (hives, swollen lips/tongue), respiratory compromise, or persistent gastrointestinal symptoms or if the patient has reduced blood pressure following the known exposure.

LABORATORY AND IMAGING STUDIES

The laboratory evaluation of patients with urticaria and angioedema must be tailored to the clinical situation. Acute urticaria and angioedema do not require specific laboratory evaluation except to document the suspected cause. For patients with chronic urticaria and angioedema, current recommendations advise against routine lab testing unless history suggests a potential etiology. Patients with recurrent angioedema *without* urticaria should be evaluated for HAE (Table 82.3).

Measurement of the mast cell mediators, histamine and tryptase, may be helpful when the diagnosis of anaphylaxis is in question. A tryptase level is a more useful test because histamine is released quickly, has a very short half-life, and is often difficult to detect in the serum. Serum tryptase levels peak 1–1.5

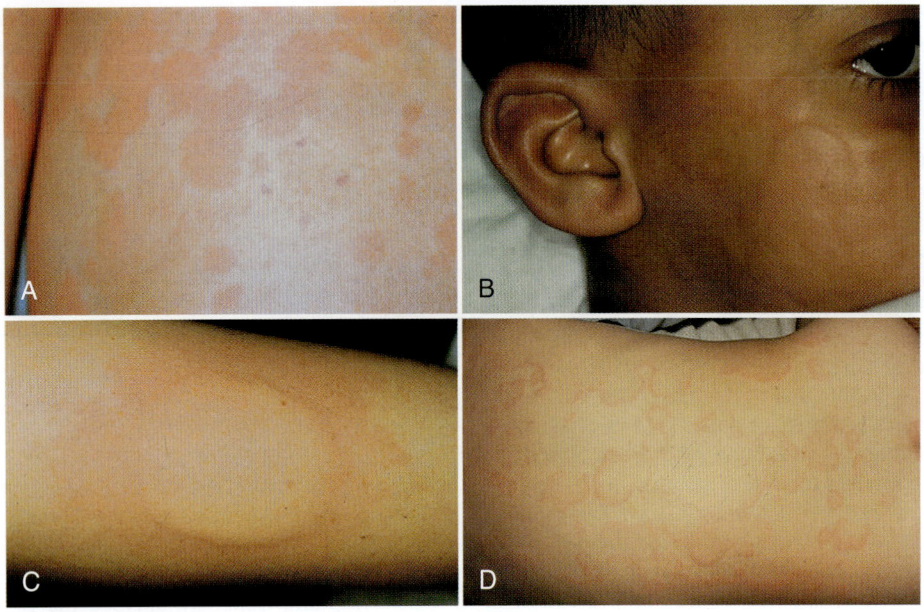

FIGURE 82.1 Examples of urticaria. (From Zitelli BJ, Davis HW, eds. *Pediatric Physical Diagnosis Electronic Atlas.* Philadelphia: Mosby; 2018.)

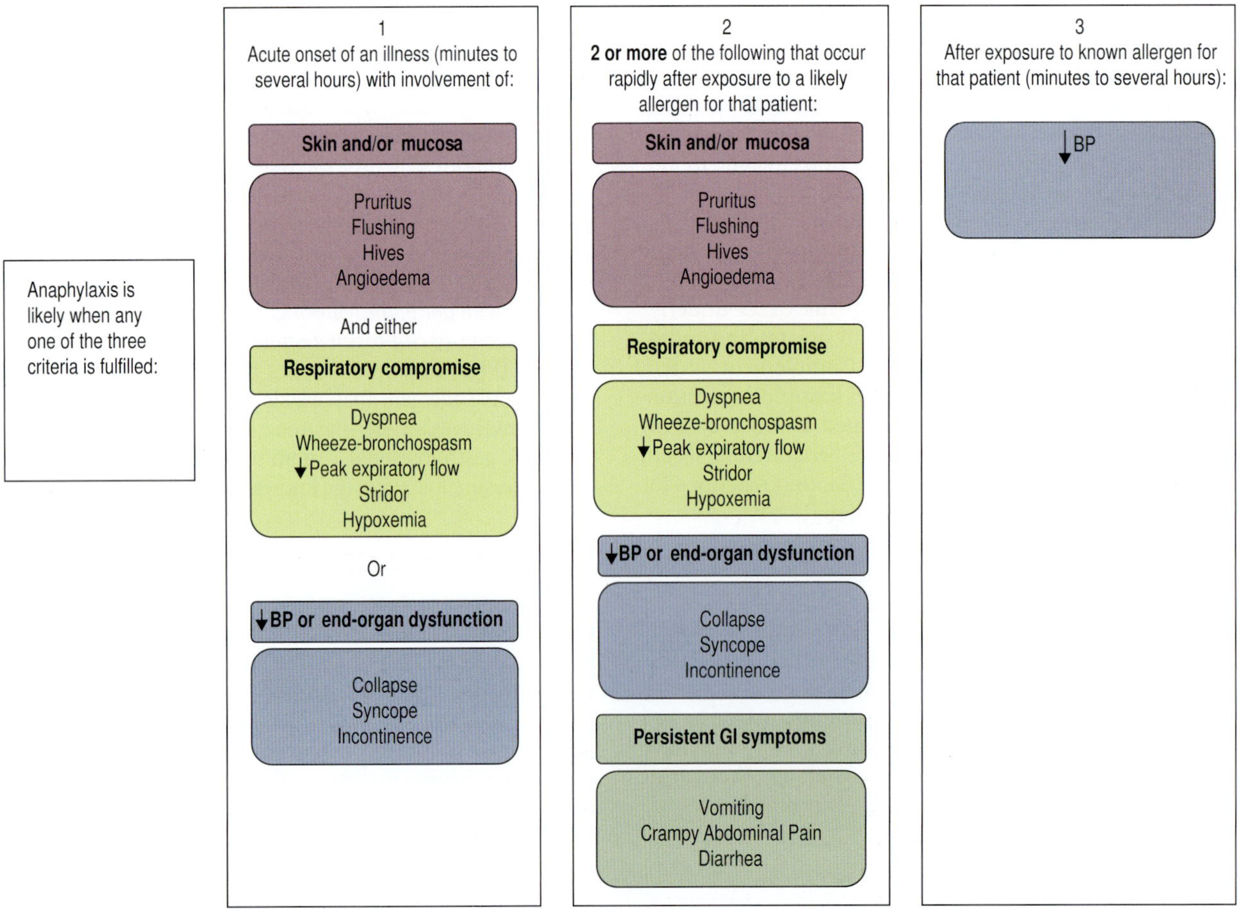

FIGURE 82.2 Visual representation of anaphylaxis diagnostic criteria. (From Campbell RL, Li JTC, Nicklas RA, et al. Emergency department diagnosis and treatment of anaphylaxis: a practice parameter. *Ann Allergy Asthma Immunol.* 2014;113:599–608 [Fig. 1:601].)

TABLE 82.3 Complement Evaluation of Patients With Recurrent Angioedema

ASSAY	IDIOPATHIC ANGIOEDEMA	TYPE I HEREDITARY ANGIOEDEMA	TYPE II HEREDITARY ANGIOEDEMA	HEREDITARY ANGIOEDEMA WITH NORMAL C1 INHIBITOR	ACQUIRED C1-ESTERASE INHIBITOR DEFICIENCY	VASCULITIS
C4	Normal	Low	Low	Normal	Low	Low or normal
C1-esterase inhibitor level	Normal	Low	Normal	Normal	Low	Normal
C1-esterase inhibitor function	Normal	Low	Low	Normal	Low	Normal
C1q	Normal	Normal	Normal	Normal	Low	Low or normal

Modified from Joshi SR, Khan DA. Urticaria and angioedema. In: Leung DYM, Akdis CA, Bacharier LB, et al., eds. Pediatric Allergy: Principles and Practice. *4th ed. Philadelphia: Elsevier; 2021:Table 39.3.*

hours after anaphylaxis. Elevated levels may be helpful in establishing the diagnosis, but normal tryptase levels do not rule out the diagnosis. It is best to measure a serum tryptase level 1–2 hours after the onset of symptoms. It also can be measured retrospectively on stored serum that is less than 2 days old.

DIFFERENTIAL DIAGNOSIS

The diagnosis of urticaria and angioedema is straightforward; finding the etiology may be more difficult. Other dermatologic conditions can mimic urticaria. **Erythema multiforme** has target-shaped, erythematous, macular, or papular lesions that may look similar to urticaria, but the lesions are fixed and last for several days. Other dermatologic diseases such as dermatitis herpetiformis and bullous pemphigoid are quite pruritic, and early on, the lesions may resemble urticaria. Mastocytosis is characterized by mast cell infiltration of various organs, including the skin. Some patients have skin lesions similar in appearance to urticaria rather than the classic urticaria pigmentosa. Urticaria pigmentosa appears as hyperpigmented, red-brown macules that may coalesce. When these lesions are stroked, they urticate, which is called the ***Darier sign***. A rare disorder that should be included in the differential diagnosis of urticaria is **Muckle-Wells syndrome**. It is an autosomal dominant autoinflammatory disorder (variant in the *NLRP3* gene) characterized by episodic urticaria presenting in infancy with sensorineural deafness, amyloidosis, arthralgias, and skeletal abnormalities. Also rare, **Schnitzler syndrome** is an acquired/late onset autoinflammatory disease characterized by chronic urticaria, macroglobulinemia, bone pain, anemia, fever, fatigue, and weight loss. **Urticarial vasculitis** is a small vessel vasculitis with histologic features of a leukocytoclastic response. The main distinguishing feature is that the lesions last longer than 24 hours, may be tender, and leave behind skin pigmentation. Skin biopsy is required for definitive diagnosis.

The diagnosis of anaphylaxis is usually apparent from the acute and often dramatic onset of multisystem involvement of the skin, respiratory tract, and cardiovascular system. Sudden cardiovascular collapse in the absence of cutaneous symptoms suggests vasovagal collapse, seizure disorder, aspiration, pulmonary embolism, or myocardial infarction. Laryngeal edema, especially with abdominal pain, suggests HAE. Many patients with anaphylaxis are initially thought to have septic shock (see Chapter 39).

TREATMENT

Avoidance of triggering agents is important in the management of acute urticaria and angioedema. Most cases resolve spontaneously. However, use of antihistamines will provide symptom relief. If acute urticaria and angioedema do not respond to this therapy, a short course of oral steroids may be considered.

Chronic urticaria treatment employs H_1 antihistamines. Second-generation H_1 antihistamines, such as cetirizine, desloratadine, fexofenadine, levocetirizine, and loratadine, are preferred because they have fewer adverse effects. If second-generation H_1 antihistamine monotherapy does not provide adequate relief, increasing the dose of antihistamines is indicated as is the addition of a sedating H_1 antihistamine at bedtime or H_2 antihistamines, such as cimetidine or famotidine. While results on the effectiveness of antileukotriene medications as mono- or add-on therapy are mixed, a trial of this medication can be considered. Omalizumab, a monoclonal anti-IgE antibody, has proven to be effective for chronic urticaria. Other immunomodulating agents, such as cyclosporine, hydroxychloroquine, methotrexate, cyclophosphamide, and intravenous immunoglobulin, have also been used. However, data supporting their use are limited, and they require laboratory monitoring due to potential adverse effects. Corticosteroids are effective in treating chronic urticaria, although adverse effects from long-term use mandate using the lowest effective dose for a brief time.

Anaphylaxis is a medical emergency. Prompt recognition and immediate treatment are crucial (Fig. 82.3). Early administration of intramuscular epinephrine is the mainstay of therapy and should be given at the same time basic measures of cardiopulmonary resuscitation are being performed. If the child is not in a medical setting, emergency medical services should be activated. Supplemental oxygen and intravenous fluid should be administered with the child lying in Trendelenburg position. An airway must be secured as intubation or tracheotomy may be required. Additional pharmacologic therapies, such as corticosteroids, antihistamines, H_2-receptor antagonists, and bronchodilators, may be given to improve symptoms. Up to 15% of people with anaphylaxis have biphasic or protracted anaphylaxis. The **biphasic reaction** is a recurrence of anaphylactic symptoms after an initial remission, typically occurring within 4–6 hours after the initial reaction. A person with **protracted anaphylaxis** has signs and symptoms that persist for hours or even days despite treatment, although this is rare.

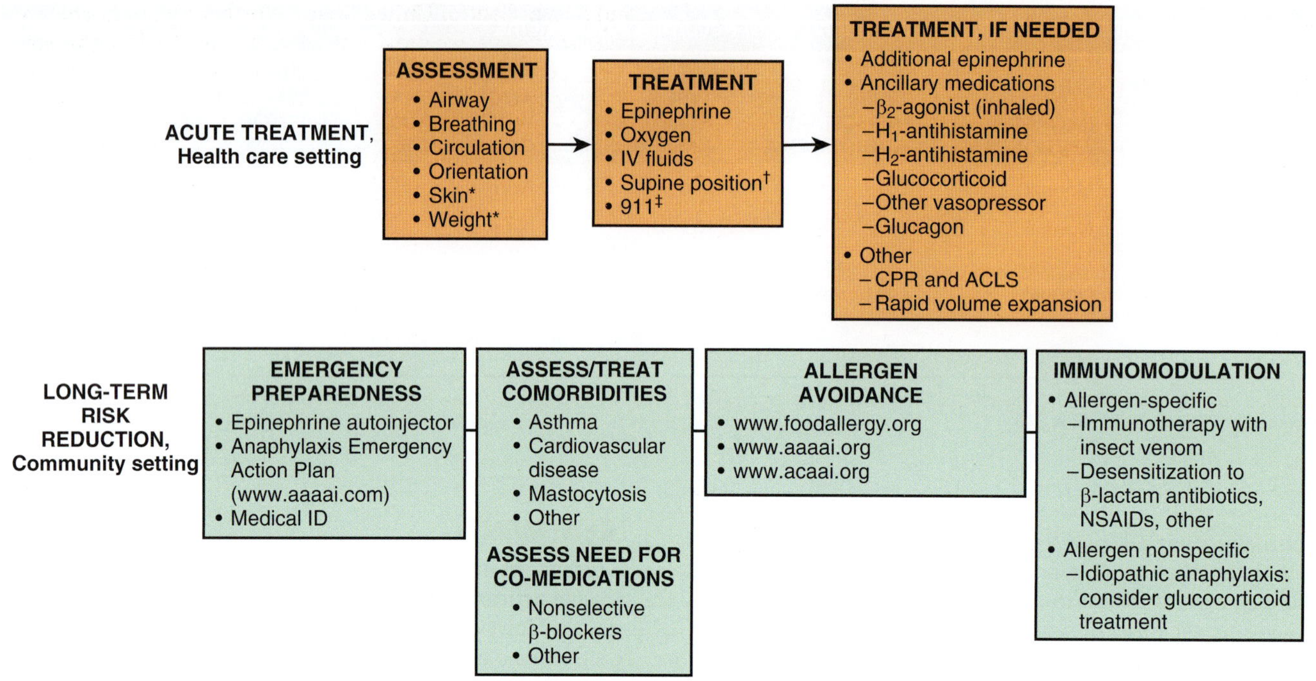

FIGURE 82.3 Summary of anaphylaxis management. Acute treatment is the same regardless of the mechanism or trigger involved in anaphylaxis. In contrast, for long-term risk reduction, avoidance measures and immunomodulation are trigger specific; currently, immunomodulation is available only for a minority of individuals with anaphylaxis. All at-risk individuals need to have comorbidities and current medications assessed, be taught the importance of emergency preparedness, and be instructed in the use of autoinjectable epinephrine. *The skin should be inspected, and weight estimation is important, especially in infants and children, and also in overweight and obese teens and adults, to calculate an optimal dose of epinephrine and other medications needed in treatment and resuscitation. †Supine position, as tolerated, to prevent empty ventricle syndrome. ‡Call 911/emergency medical services for anaphylaxis occurring in community health care facilities such as medical, dental, or infusion clinics, where optimal backup might not be available for resuscitation. *ACLS,* Advanced cardiac life support; *CPR,* cardiopulmonary resuscitation; *CVS,* cardiovascular; *GI,* gastrointestinal; *ID,* identification (e.g., bracelet, wallet card); *IV,* intravenous; *NSAIDs,* nonsteroidal antiinflammatory drugs. (From Simon FER. Anaphylaxis. *J Allergy Clin Immunol.* 2008;121:S405.)

PREVENTION

Prevention of urticaria, angioedema, and anaphylaxis focuses on avoidance of known triggers. A referral to an allergy specialist for a thorough history, diagnostic testing if indicated, and recommendations for avoidance of triggers is suggested for patients following severe reactions or anaphylaxis. Skin testing and serum IgE-specific testing are available for foods, inhalants, insect venoms, medications (penicillin), vaccines, and latex. Educating the patient and family members about the signs and symptoms of anaphylaxis and using autoinjectable epinephrine early results in better outcomes. Fatal anaphylaxis has occurred despite timely and appropriate treatment. Medical alert jewelry with appropriate information should be worn. Medications such as β blockers, angiotensin-converting enzyme inhibitors, and monoamine oxidase inhibitors should be discontinued if there are alternatives, because they may exacerbate anaphylaxis or interfere with its treatment.

PEARLS FOR PRACTITIONERS

See Allergy: Pearls for Practitioners at the end of this section.

REVIEW QUESTIONS

Available online.

CHAPTER **83**

Serum Sickness

ETIOLOGY

Serum sickness is a type III hypersensitivity reaction (see Table 78.1). The patient's immune system recognizes the proteins in a drug or antiserum as foreign and produces antibodies against them. The newly formed antibodies bind with the foreign protein to form antigen-antibody or immune complexes, which may enter the circulation and be deposited in blood vessels and filtering organs. These complexes cause tissue injury by activating the complement cascade and recruiting neutrophils, resulting in increased capillary permeability, toxic mediator release, and tissue damage.

EPIDEMIOLOGY

Common inciting agents include blood products and foreign proteins, such as antithymocyte globulin and antivenoms. Medications frequently implicated include penicillin, sulfonamides, minocycline, cefaclor, hydantoins, and thiazides. The availability of *human-derived* biologics, bioengineered antibodies, and alternative pharmacotherapies has greatly reduced the incidence of serum sickness.

CLINICAL MANIFESTATIONS

The symptoms of serum sickness typically occur 7–21 days after the administration of medications, foreign proteins, or infections. Symptom onset may be more rapid (within 1–4 days) in previously sensitized individuals. The classic clinical manifestations consist of fever, polyarticular arthralgias, lymphadenopathy, and cutaneous symptoms. Cutaneous lesions vary and may include urticaria, angioedema, erythema multiforme, morbilliform rash, and palpable purpura or serpiginous rash at the interface of the dorsal and palmar or plantar aspects of the hands and feet. Carditis, glomerulonephritis, Guillain-Barré syndrome, encephalomyelitis, and peripheral neuritis are rare complications.

LABORATORY AND IMAGING STUDIES

Laboratory tests may show an elevated erythrocyte sedimentation rate, thrombocytopenia, and depressed complement (C3 and C4) levels. Skin biopsy specimens show immune deposits of immunoglobulin (Ig)M, IgA, IgE, or C3. Hematuria, proteinuria, or both may be present. The diagnosis is established by history of exposure to an inciting cause, characteristic clinical manifestations, and laboratory testing showing circulating immune complexes and depressed complement levels.

TREATMENT AND PREVENTION

Serum sickness is self-limited and resolves within 1–2 weeks. Treatment is symptomatic relief. Antihistamines may be administered to relieve pruritus. Nonsteroidal antiinflammatory drugs reduce fever and joint pain, and in severe cases, systemic glucocorticoids may be considered. Allergy skin testing does not predict the likelihood of serum sickness development and is not indicated. The primary means of prevention is to avoid exposure to the implicated cause.

PEARLS FOR PRACTITIONERS

See Allergy: Pearls for Practitioners at the end of this section.

REVIEW QUESTIONS

Available online.

CHAPTER **84**

Insect Allergies

ETIOLOGY

Systemic allergic reactions usually result from stinging insects of the order **Hymenoptera**, which include **apids** (honeybee and bumblebee), **vespids** (yellow jacket, wasp, yellow-face and white-face hornets, northern giant hornets), and **formicids** (fire and harvester ants). Honeybees have a barbed stinger that remains embedded after a sting. Yellow jackets are responsible for most allergic reactions in most parts of the United States, whereas wasps are the most frequent cause of sting reactions in Texas. Fire ants are found in Southeastern and South-Central United States. Northern giant hornets are an invasive species previously detected in Washington state; they are currently thought to have been eradicated from North America.

Biting insects rarely cause anaphylaxis. Anaphylaxis has been described, however, after the bites from the kissing bug *Triatoma*, bed bugs, blackflies, and deerflies. Large local reactions from biting insects, such as mosquitoes, fleas, and flies, are a more common occurrence; large local reactions to mosquito bites are known as ***skeeter syndrome***. The reaction appears urticarial, is caused by the salivary secretions deposited by the biting insect, and does not represent an allergic response.

EPIDEMIOLOGY

Insect sting allergy may develop at any age and typically manifests after several uneventful stings. Although children are stung more frequently than adults, systemic allergic reactions occur in only about 1% of children and 3% of adults. Reactions in adults are generally more severe than in children and can result in death. Large local reactions to insect stings are more common in children, with an estimated incidence of 20% for children and 10% for adults.

CLINICAL MANIFESTATIONS

The diagnosis of insect sting allergy is dependent on the history of the reaction and the presence of venom-specific immunoglobulin (Ig)E. Normal reactions to insect stings, observed in 90% of children, include localized pain, swelling, and erythema at the sting site that usually subside within 24 hours. Large local reactions are usually late-phase, IgE-mediated reactions, with large swelling contiguous to the sting site that develops over 24–48 hours and resolves within 2–7 days. Virtually all individuals with large local reactions have similar reactions with subsequent stings. Systemic reactions are IgE-mediated. They can be mild and nonlife threatening with cutaneous symptoms only or life threatening with respiratory, cardiovascular, or neurologic symptoms of anaphylaxis (see Chapter 82). Toxic reactions may result if a person receives a large number of simultaneous stings (50–100). Symptoms include malaise, nausea, and emesis resulting from the toxic effects of the venom. Unusual reactions, such as vasculitis, nephrosis, neuritis, serum sickness, and encephalitis, may occur as delayed reactions (Table 84.1).

LABORATORY AND IMAGING STUDIES

A positive skin test to Hymenoptera venom extract demonstrates the presence of venom-specific IgE and in the context of a positive sting reaction history helps identify specific insects to which an individual is allergic. Venom-specific IgE antibodies also may be measured by in vitro serum tests. Both testing methods should be considered complementary because neither test alone detects all patients with insect sting allergy. Future reactions correlate more with past individual patterns than the level of sensitivity of venom skin testing or serum-specific IgE testing.

Patients presenting with history of anaphylaxis to stinging insect venoms require evaluation of a baseline tryptase level to screen for an underlying mast cell disorder in addition to assessment of specific IgE. Patients with mast cell disorders are

TABLE 84.1 Classification of Insect Sting Reactions

REACTION TYPE	CHARACTERISTICS
Normal	<2 in. in diameter
	Transient pain and erythema
	Duration <24 hr
Large local reaction	>2 in. in diameter
	Swelling contiguous to the site
	Duration 2–7 days
SYSTEMIC	
Nonlife threatening	Immediate generalized reaction confined to the skin (erythema, urticaria, angioedema)
Life threatening	Immediate generalized reaction not confined to the skin with respiratory (laryngeal edema, bronchospasm) or cardiovascular (hypotension, shock) symptoms
Toxic	Follows multiple simultaneous stings, produced by exogenous vasoactive amines in venom
Unusual	Serum sickness, vasculitis, nephrosis, neuritis, encephalitis
	Symptoms start several days to weeks after the insect sting

at higher risk for severe reactions to stings. Likewise, they are more likely to have no skin manifestations during their reaction, systemic reactions to vespid stings, hypotensive anaphylaxis, and negative evaluation of specific IgE despite a highly suggestive history. Mast cell disorders have further implications for venom immunotherapy. During immunotherapy, these patients have higher risk of side effects, higher risk of systemic sting reactions, and higher risk of relapse after discontinuing therapy. They should receive venom immunotherapy indefinitely.

DIFFERENTIAL DIAGNOSIS

A history of an immediate systemic reaction is necessary before venom testing and consideration of immunotherapy. Testing for venom-specific IgE without a history of a systemic reaction to a sting is not recommended. Identification of the offending insect is often unreliable. Honeybee stings may be identified by the stinger that remains in place. Vespid stings are usually unprovoked and occur at summer's end when the insects are more aggressive.

TREATMENT

Local reactions should be treated by cleaning the site, applying cold compresses, and administering oral antihistamines and analgesics. Stingers should be removed promptly. Occasionally, large local reactions may be mistaken for cellulitis. Infection is unlikely if the reaction occurs within 24–48 hours after a sting. Treatment is with oral antihistamines and corticosteroids for 4–5 days rather than oral antibiotics.

Treatment of systemic reactions is guided by the severity of the reaction, but epinephrine is the cornerstone of therapy and should be administered without delay for all anaphylactic reactions. Antihistamines may be administered concurrently with epinephrine. Corticosteroids should be given to prevent prolonged symptoms. For severe reactions, intravenous fluids and epinephrine, oxygen, and respiratory support in an intensive care unit may be needed. After acute care of a systemic sting reaction, patients should be provided an epinephrine autoinjector, referral to an allergist, and instructions on prevention of insect stings.

COMPLICATIONS

At least 50–100 fatalities per year in the United States are attributed to insect sting reactions. Most deaths (80%) occur in adults older than 40 years of age; only 2% occur in individuals younger than 20 years of age. Approximately half of deaths occur in persons without a previous history of a sting reaction.

PROGNOSIS

Successfully avoiding the stinging insect is the most important prognostic factor. More than 85% of adults who complete 5 years of immunotherapy tolerate sting challenges without systemic reactions for 5–10 years after completion.

PREVENTION

Measures to reduce the chance of accidental sting include exterminating infested areas, avoiding eating or drinking outdoors, wearing long pants and shoes, and avoiding brightly colored clothing, fragrances, or hairspray when outdoors. Common insect repellents are not effective against Hymenoptera.

Current recommendations are to administer **venom immunotherapy** to individuals who have had a systemic life-threatening reaction from an insect sting and have positive venom skin tests or elevated venom-specific IgE. All persons with a history of systemic reactions to stinging insects should be instructed in the use of an epinephrine autoinjector and encouraged to wear medical information jewelry. Children and adults who have had only a cutaneous reaction generally do not require immunotherapy because their risk of life-threatening reaction is low.

PEARLS FOR PRACTITIONERS

See Allergy: Pearls for Practitioners at the end of this section.

REVIEW QUESTIONS

Available online.

CHAPTER 85

Adverse Reactions to Foods

ETIOLOGY AND EPIDEMIOLOGY

An **adverse reaction to food** is a generic description of any untoward reaction after food ingestion, including toxic reactions such as food poisoning and nontoxic reactions, which can be subdivided further into nonimmune and immune reactions. **Food intolerances** such as lactose intolerance represent a nonimmune reaction. **Food allergy** or hypersensitivity reactions encompass immune reactions to food and can be divided further into immunoglobulin (Ig)E–mediated reactions, which are typically rapid in onset, and non–IgE-mediated reactions.

Oral tolerance is the suppression of the immune response to the array of dietary elements ingested daily. **Food allergy** or **hypersensitivity reactions** are the result of immune reactions to glycoproteins and develop in genetically predisposed individuals. In children, cow's milk, eggs, peanuts, soybean, wheat, tree nuts, fish, shellfish, and sesame seed cause 90% of IgE-mediated reactions. In older children and adults, peanuts, tree nuts, fish, and shellfish account for most reactions. Exposure to the allergenic food protein results in cross linking of cell surface–specific IgE molecules found on mast cells and basophils, resulting in activation and degranulation. Numerous potent mediators and cytokines are released within minutes to hours of ingestion. Non–IgE-mediated reactions typically occur hours to days after the ingestion and manifest as gastrointestinal symptoms. A cell-mediated immune mechanism may be responsible.

Approximately 6–8% of children are affected with food allergy. In adults, estimates vary from 2–10%.

CLINICAL MANIFESTATIONS

Symptoms of hypersensitivity reactions vary from single-system involvement of the skin, gastrointestinal tract, or respiratory tract to multisystem involvement in anaphylaxis. Non–IgE-mediated food allergy typically presents during infancy as proctitis/proctocolitis, enteropathy, or enterocolitis (Table 85.1).

LABORATORY AND IMAGING STUDIES

In suspected IgE-mediated food reactions, skin prick allergy testing and serum-specific IgE testing to foods help confirm the suspected food allergy. Despite the availability of two methods to evaluate food allergy, neither test can predict the severity of the reaction or the quantity of food ingested to elicit symptoms. Positive skin tests or serum-specific tests to foods in the context of a positive history can only indicate risk of an allergic reaction when exposed to that allergen.

TABLE 85.1 Adverse Food Reactions

DISORDER	AGE GROUP	CHARACTERISTICS	DIAGNOSIS	PROGNOSIS/COURSE
IgE-MEDIATED				
Food allergy	Any	Symptom onset: min–2 hr of urticaria, angioedema, cough, wheeze, dyspnea, rhinitis, conjunctivitis, nausea, abdominal pain, emesis, diarrhea, altered mental status, loss of consciousness, death	History, positive SPT, and/or serum food IgE Confirmatory OFC	Variable, food dependent Milk, soy, egg, and wheat typically outgrown Peanut, tree nuts, seeds, and shellfish typically persist
Pollen-food allergy syndrome (oral allergy syndrome)	Any, most common in young adults (50% of birch pollen allergic adults)	Immediate symptoms on contact of raw fruit or vegetables with oral mucosa Pruritus, tingling, erythema, or angioedema of the lips, tongue, oropharynx, throat pruritus/tightness	History, positive SPT with raw fruits or vegetables, OFC positive with raw fruit, negative with cooked	Severity of symptoms may vary with pollen season Symptoms may improve with pollen immunotherapy in subset of patients
IgE- AND/OR NON–IgE-MEDIATED				
Allergic eosinophilic esophagitis	Any, but especially infants, children, adolescents	Children: chronic/intermittent symptoms of gastroesophageal reflux, emesis, dysphagia, abdominal pain, irritability Adults: abdominal pain, dysphagia, food impaction	History, positive SPT, and/or food IgE in 50%, but poor correlation with clinical symptoms Elimination diet and OFC Endoscopy, biopsy provide conclusive diagnosis and response to treatment information	Variable, not well established, improvement with elimination diet within 6–8 wk Elemental diet may be required Often responds to swallowed topical steroids
Allergic eosinophilic gastroenteritis	Any	Chronic/intermittent abdominal pain, emesis, irritability, poor appetite, growth faltering, weight loss, anemia, protein-losing gastroenteropathy	History, positive SPT, and/or food IgE in 50% but poor correlation with clinical symptoms, elimination diet, and OFC Endoscopy, biopsy provide conclusive diagnosis and response to treatment information	Variable, not well established, improvement with elimination diet within 6–8 wk Elemental diet or systemic steroids may be required

(Continued)

TABLE **85.1** Adverse Food Reactions—cont'd

DISORDER	AGE GROUP	CHARACTERISTICS	DIAGNOSIS	PROGNOSIS/COURSE
Atopic dermatitis	Infant and child; 90% start <5 yr	Relapsing pruritic vesiculopapular rash; generalized in infants, localized to flexor areas in older children; food allergy in about 35% of children with severe atopic dermatitis	History, SPT, and/or serum food IgE level; elimination diet and OFC	60–80% improve significantly or allergy resolves by adolescence
Asthma	Any	Chronic cough, wheezing, dyspnea; food allergy is risk factor for intubation in children who have asthma	History, SPT, and/or serum food IgE level; OFC	Varies
NON–IgE-MEDIATED				
Food protein-induced allergic proctocolitis	Young infants (<6 mo), frequently breast-fed	Blood-streaked or heme-positive stools, otherwise healthy appearing	History, prompt response (resolution of gross blood in 48 hr) to allergen elimination Biopsy conclusive but not necessary in vast majority	Majority able to tolerate milk or soy by 1–2 yr of age
Food protein-induced enterocolitis syndrome	Young infants	Chronic: emesis, diarrhea, growth faltering on chronic exposure Subacute: repetitive emesis, dehydration (15% shock), diarrhea on repeat exposure after elimination period Breast-feeding protective	History, response to dietary restriction; OFC; SPT is negative	Most resolve in 1–3 yr; rarely persists into late teenage years
Food protein-induced enteropathy	Young infants; incidence has decreased	Protracted diarrhea, (steatorrhea), emesis, growth faltering, anemia in 40%	History, endoscopy, and biopsy Response to dietary restriction	Most resolve in 1–2 yr
Celiac disease (gluten-sensitive enteropathy)	Any	Chronic diarrhea, malabsorption, abdominal distention, flatulence, growth faltering, or weight loss May be associated with oral ulcers and/or dermatitis herpetiformis	Biopsy diagnostic: villous atrophy Screening with serum IgA antitissue transglutaminase and antigliadin Resolution of symptoms with gluten elimination and relapse on oral challenge	Lifelong
Contact dermatitis	Any; more common in adults	Relapsing, pruritic eczematous rash, often on hands or face; often occurs in occupational contact with food stuff	History, patch testing	Varies
Dermatitis herpetiformis	Any	Intensely pruritic vesicular rash on extensor surfaces and buttocks	Biopsy diagnostic, shows IgA granule deposits at the dermal-epidermal junction; resolves with dietary gluten avoidance	Lifelong
Pulmonary hemosiderosis (Heiner syndrome)	Infants, children (rare)	Chronic cough, hemoptysis, lung infiltrates, wheezing, anemia; described in cow's milk- and buckwheat-allergic infants	History, SPT and serum food IgE negative but milk and buckwheat IgG precipitins positive; lung biopsy with deposits of IgG and IgA	

Ig, Immunoglobulin; *OFC*, oral food challenge; *SPT*, skin prick test.
Modified from Nowak-Wegrzyn A, Burks AW, Sampson HA. Reactions to foods. In: Adkinson Jr NF, Bochner BS, Burks AW, et al., eds. Middleton's Allergy: Principles and Practice. *9th ed. Philadelphia: Elsevier; 2020:1294–1325e.1, Table 79.7.*

DIAGNOSIS

A careful history focuses on symptoms, the time interval from ingestion to onset of symptoms, the quantity of food necessary to evoke the reaction, the most recent reaction, patterns and reproducibility of reactivity, and associated factors such as exercise and medication use. Skin prick testing can be performed to confirm suspected IgE-mediated food allergies. The history dictates what food allergens should be evaluated. Testing to a wide variety of food allergens as a screening tool has little clinical value and is strongly discouraged. A negative skin test virtually excludes an IgE-mediated mechanism. A positive skin test indicates sensitization but does not prove clinical reactivity and must be interpreted in the context of the history.

An in vitro serum-specific IgE assay can be used to help confirm clinical allergy. Many allergists and laboratories regard the ImmunoCAP system as the method of choice. These tests provide supplementary information to skin tests. Food-specific IgE levels exceeding the diagnostic values help predict which patients are highly likely to experience clinical reactions (Table 85.2). Patients with allergen-specific IgE levels greater than 95% of the predictive value will likely be symptomatic upon ingestion, so an oral food challenge is not necessary. Monitoring the allergen-specific IgE level and/or wheal size on skin prick testing may be helpful in predicting whether a child has outgrown the food allergy. *Oral food challenges remain the gold standard of diagnosis* and can be performed to determine whether a child has developed oral tolerance to the food allergen.

Component resolved diagnostics (CRD) is a food allergy testing method that employs allergens purified from natural sources or recombinant DNA technology. Thus, an individual allergen is being evaluated versus whole allergens in hopes of improved information about risk, tolerance, and prognosis. CRD is helpful in peanut, cow's milk, egg, cashew, walnut, and hazelnut allergy but not for soy allergies.

TABLE **85.2** Interpretation of Serum IgE Antibody Concentrations

FOOD		FOOD-SPECIFIC IgE ANTIBODY CONCENTRATIONS AT OR ABOVE WHICH CLINICAL REACTIONS ARE HIGHLY LIKELY (KUa/L)	POSITIVE PREDICTIVE VALUE (%)
Egg	>2 yr of age	7	98
	≤2 yr of age	0.35	95
Milk	>2 yr of age	15	95
	≤1 yr of age	5	95
Peanut		14	99
Fish		20	99
Soybean		30	73
Wheat		26	74
Tree nuts		15	95

Ig, Immunoglobulin.
Modified from Nowak-Wegrzyn A, Burks AW, Sampson HA. Reactions to foods. In: Adkinson Jr NF, Bochner BS, Burks AW, et al., eds. Middleton's Allergy: Principles and Practice. 9th ed. Philadelphia: Elsevier; 2020:1294–1325.e1, Table 79.11.

TREATMENT

Currently, the main treatment modality of IgE-mediated food allergy is avoidance of the allergen and use of rescue medications in the event of a reaction. This requires the education of the patient and family on how to avoid ingestion of the responsible allergen and when to initiate therapy if ingestion occurs. If the food allergen is ingested and severe symptoms of an IgE-mediated reaction ensue, autoinjectable epinephrine should be immediately administered intramuscularly. In most cases, it is recommended that epinephrine administration be followed by emergent evaluation by medical personnel. In cases of mild allergic reactions, antihistamines can be given, but patients need to be monitored as the reaction can evolve. The severity of the reaction is unpredictable. There are approximately 100 deaths per year due to food allergies, and most cases are secondary to a delay in or lack of administration of epinephrine.

Oral immunotherapy entails ingesting *increasing* amounts of the food allergen to achieve desensitization. Pharmaceutical-grade peanut protein containing relevant peanut allergens *(Arachis hypogaea)* is U.S. Food and Drug Administration approved for oral immunotherapy in children with peanut allergy aged 1–17 years of age. This treatment modality is not a cure but mitigates the allergic reaction should peanut be accidentally ingested. The monoclonal antibody omalizumab (Xolair) also can reduce allergic reactions, including anaphylaxis, that may occur with accidental exposure to one or more foods that trigger IgE-mediated food allergies. Omalizumab is approved for children 1 year of age and older and is intended to be used in conjunction with food allergen avoidance.

Other therapies for IgE-mediated food allergy aim to either desensitize patients to food allergens or induce tolerance. Sublingual immunotherapy requires placing increasing doses of food allergen under the tongue. This treatment is effective for desensitization, but compliance is poor. In epicutaneous therapy, food allergens are embedded in a patch that is applied to the skin.

COMPLICATIONS

Anaphylaxis is the most serious complication of allergic food reactions and can result in death (see Chapter 82). Patients need to be monitored for alterations in growth and potential nutritional deficiencies from food avoidance. This is especially important for children avoiding multiple foods or if one of their food allergens is cow's milk.

PROGNOSIS AND PREVENTION

The natural history of food allergies or "is my child going to outgrow this?" is a common concern of parents. For cow's milk–allergic patients who have multiple food allergies, asthma, and allergic rhinitis, 21% of patients have persistent milk allergy at age 16 years; 85% of children who do not have additional atopic disease develop cow's milk *tolerance* by 3 years of age. Similarly, 66% of children with egg allergy but no other atopic disease develop tolerance by 5 years of age; 32% of those with additional atopic disease will still be sensitive to egg by age 16 years. The natural histories of soy and wheat allergy are similar: oral tolerance in 25–29% by age 4 years, 45–56% by age 6 or 8 years, and 65–69% by age 10 or 12 years. Twenty percent of children with peanut allergy outgrow their allergy. Between 9–15% of tree nut allergic patients will develop oral tolerance. Food allergies to seafood are most often a lifelong affliction.

Avoidance of the suspect food is crucial. Careful reading of food labels is a priority. Medical identification jewelry with appropriate information may be worn or utilized. The Food Allergy Research & Education organization (www.foodallergy.org) is a useful educational resource for families and physicians.

Recommendations for prevention of allergic diseases aimed at the *high-risk* newborn who has not manifested atopic disease include exclusive breast-feeding for the first 4–6 months. Other approaches, such as hydrolyzed formulas, maternal avoidance diets during pregnancy and during lactation, or avoidance of allergenic foods for infants beyond 6 months of age, have not shown preventative effects.

Early introduction of peanuts in high-risk infants, defined as those infants with severe atopic dermatitis and/or the presence of IgE-mediated allergy to egg, significantly decreases the development of peanut allergy; this effect is durable. It is thought that the potential protection against peanut allergy by early introduction may be generalizable to nonhigh-risk infants; however, some infants develop food allergy even with attempts at early introduction.

PEARLS FOR PRACTITIONERS

See Allergy: Pearls for Practitioners at the end of this section.

REVIEW QUESTIONS

Available online.

CHAPTER 86

Adverse Reactions to Drugs

ETIOLOGY

An **adverse drug reaction** is defined as an unwanted, negative consequence associated with the use of a medication (drug) or biologic agent. Drug reactions can be classified as immunologic or nonimmunologic reactions (Table 86.1). Nearly 75–80% of adverse drug reactions are caused by a predictable, nonimmunologic mechanism; between 5–10% of all drug reactions are explained by an immune-mediated mechanism (see Table 78.1). The remaining drug reactions are caused by an unpredictable mechanism, which may or may not be immune mediated. Many drug reactions cannot be classified because the exact immune mechanism has not been defined. Most drugs cannot elicit an immune response because of their small size; rather, the drug or a metabolite acts as a hapten and binds to larger molecules, such as tissue or serum proteins, a process called ***haptenation***. The multivalent hapten-protein complex forms a new immunogenic epitope that stimulates T- and B-lymphocyte responses.

EPIDEMIOLOGY

Reactions to penicillins and cephalosporins are the most common allergic drug reactions encountered in the pediatric population. Approximately 6–10% of children are labeled as *penicillin allergic*; however, less than 1% of people have a true immunoglobulin (Ig)E–mediated reaction. Risk factors for drug reactions include previous drug exposure, increasing age (>20 years of age), parenteral or topical administration, higher dose, intermittent repeated exposure, and a genetic predisposition of slow drug metabolism. An atopic background does not predispose an individual to the development of drug reactions but may indicate a greater risk of serious reaction.

CLINICAL MANIFESTATIONS

Allergic reactions can be classified as **immediate (anaphylactic) reactions**, which occur within 60 minutes of drug administration; **accelerated reactions**, which begin 1–72 hours after drug administration; and **late reactions**, which occur after 72 hours. The most common form of adverse drug reaction is cutaneous. Accelerated reactions are usually dermatologic. Late reactions include desquamating dermatitis, Stevens-Johnson syndrome, toxic epidermal necrolysis, and serum sickness.

LABORATORY AND IMAGING STUDIES

Skin prick testing protocols are standardized for penicillin and are well described for other agents, such as local anesthetics, muscle relaxants, vaccines, and insulin. Positive skin testing to such reagents confirms the presence of antigen-specific IgE and supports the diagnosis of a type I hypersensitivity reaction in the appropriate clinical setting. Patch testing is the most reliable way to test for allergy to topically applied drugs.

DIFFERENTIAL DIAGNOSIS

The broadest experience with managing adverse drug reactions is with penicillin. Penicillin allergy should be evaluated when the individual is well and not in acute need of treatment. Penicillin skin testing is helpful for IgE-mediated reactions because of its negative predictive value; only 1–3% of patients with negative skin tests have a reaction, which is mild, when re-exposed to penicillin. Skin testing for penicillin should be performed using the major determinant, penicilloyl polylysine (available as Pre-Pen [ALK-Abelló, Inc, Hørsholm, Denmark]), and minor determinants, which include penicillin G, penicilloate, and penilloate. Skin testing to penicillin does not predict non–IgE-mediated reactions. For patients with a history consistent with serum sickness or desquamative-type reactions, skin testing should not be performed, and penicillin should be avoided indefinitely. To promote antibiotic stewardship, increased attention has been paid to delabelling those with penicillin allergy if safe to do so. A thorough history can be used to triage a patient into low risk or high risk of having a penicillin allergy, and low-risk patients may be offered an oral drug challenge directly in lieu of penicillin skin testing that is followed by oral drug exposure.

The risk of having an allergic reaction to a cephalosporin in a child who has reacted positively to penicillin skin testing is less than 2%. It is believed that the first-generation cephalosporins are more likely than second- or third-generation cephalosporins to be cross reactive. This is due to the chemical similarity of side chains of the β-lactam ring between penicillin and first-generation cephalosporins.

TABLE 86.1 Classification of Adverse Drug Reactions

TYPE	EXAMPLE
IMMUNOLOGIC	
Type I reaction (IgE mediated)	Anaphylaxis from β-lactam antibiotic
Type II reaction (cytotoxic)	Hemolytic anemia from cephalosporins
Type III reaction (immune complex)	Serum sickness from antithymocyte globulin
Type IV reaction (delayed, cell mediated)	Contact dermatitis from topical antihistamine
Specific T-cell activation	Morbilliform rash from sulfonamides
Fas/Fas ligand-induced apoptosis	Stevens-Johnson syndrome; toxic epidermal necrolysis
Other	Drug-induced lupuslike syndrome; anticonvulsant hypersensitivity syndrome
NONIMMUNOLOGIC	
Predictable	
Pharmacologic adverse effect	Dry mouth from antihistamines; tremor from albuterol
Secondary pharmacologic adverse effect	Thrush while taking antibiotics; *Clostridium difficile*–associated colitis (pseudomembranous colitis) from clindamycin (and other antibiotics)
Drug toxicity	Hepatotoxicity from methotrexate
Drug-drug interactions	Increased carbamazepine levels with clarithromycin
Drug overdose	Hepatic necrosis from acetaminophen
Unpredictable	
Pseudoallergic	Anaphylactoid reaction after radiocontrast media
Idiosyncratic	Hemolytic anemia in a patient with G6PD deficiency after primaquine therapy
Intolerance	Tinnitus after a single, small dose of aspirin

G6PD, Glucose-6-phosphate dehydrogenase; *Ig*, immunoglobulin.
Modified from Riedl MA, Casillas AM. Adverse drug reactions: types and treatment options. Am Fam Physician. *2003;68(9):1781–1790.*

TREATMENT

If penicillin skin testing is positive, penicillin should be avoided, and an alternative antibiotic should be used. If there is a definite need for penicillin, **desensitization** can be accomplished by administration of increasing amounts of drug over a short time in a hospital setting. The exact mechanism of desensitization is unclear; however, it is thought to render mast cells unresponsive to the drug. Depending on the half-life, the drug must be given at least twice daily to maintain desensitization. If the drug is stopped for longer than 48 hours, the patient is no longer *desensitized* and the same protocol must be repeated before continuing antibiotic use.

For other antibiotics, the relevant allergenic determinants produced by metabolism or degradation are not well defined. Skin testing to the native antibiotic in nonirritating concentrations can be performed. However, a negative response does not exclude allergy while a positive response suggests the presence of IgE-mediated allergy. In the case of a negative skin test response, a graded challenge or test dose may be administered, depending on the clinical history of the reaction. Patients who have experienced Stevens-Johnson syndrome, toxic epidermal necrolysis, or serum sickness should not be challenged. There are emerging data to suggest that children who have been diagnosed with a serum sickness–like reaction are likely to tolerate re-exposure to the inciting agent after a period of time; a consultation with an allergist should be arranged in this scenario.

Management of nonpharmacologic drug reactions varies; some reactions may be managed symptomatically while others require avoidance or reduced dose of the offending agent.

COMPLICATIONS

Anaphylaxis is the most serious complication of IgE-mediated drug reactions and can result in death (see Chapter 82).

PROGNOSIS

Most drug reactions do not seem to be allergic in nature. Repeated, intermittent exposure during childhood or early adulthood contributes to an increased incidence of adverse drug reactions in adults.

PREVENTION

Avoidance of the suspect drug is paramount. Medical identification jewelry with appropriate information should be worn. In the medical community, responsible antibiotic use has been emphasized to improve patient outcomes, decrease selection for resistant organisms, and minimize spread of multidrug-resistant organisms. Ideally, sensitive and specific testing to any drug for allergy evaluation is highly desirable. However, standardized testing reagents do not exist for antibiotics other than penicillin. The penicillin family of antimicrobials is very effective to treat a multitude of pediatric infections; limiting their use due to suspected drug allergy may result in undesirable outcomes. In addition to skin testing, oral penicillin challenge may be a useful tool to safely delabel patients with a history of low-risk reactions.

One of the most common concerns in regard to allergic drug reactions is cross reactivity between penicillin and cephalosporins. In children with a history of penicillin allergy, it is important to determine whether they are truly allergic by skin testing to penicillin using the major and minor determinants. If penicillin skin testing is negative, there is a very low risk of an allergic reaction to cephalosporins. A positive penicillin skin test leads to use of an alternate noncross-reacting antibiotic, a graded challenge to the required cephalosporin under appropriate monitoring, or desensitization to the required cephalosporin.

For children with a history of a cephalosporin allergy who require another cephalosporin, clinicians should consider using a graded challenge with a cephalosporin with a different side chain.

PEARLS FOR PRACTITIONERS

See Allergy: Pearls for Practitioners at the end of this section.

REVIEW QUESTIONS

Available online.

Suggested Readings

Cosme-Blanco W, Arroyo-Flores E, Ale H. Food Allergies. *Pediatr Rev.* 2020;41(8):403–415.

Du Toit G, Roberts G, Sayre PH, et al. Randomized trial of peanut consumption in infants at risk for peanut allergy [published correction appears in N Engl J Med. 2016 Jul 28;375(4):398.]. *N Engl J Med.* 2015;372(9):803–813.

Du Toit G, Sayre PH, Roberts G, et al. Effect of Avoidance on Peanut Allergy after Early Peanut Consumption. *N Engl J Med.* 2016;374(15):1435–1443.

Keeney GE, Gray MP, Morrison AK, et al. Dexamethasone for acute asthma exacerbations in children: a meta-analysis. *Pediatrics.* 2014;133(3):493–499.

Leung D, Akdis C, Bacharier L, et al. *Pediatric Allergy: Principles and Practice.* 4th ed. Oxford: Elsevier; 2020.

2020 Focused Updates to the Asthma Management Guidelines. A Report from the National Asthma Education and Prevention Program Coordinating Committee Expert Panel Working Group. National Heart Lung Blood Institute. NIH Publication No. 20-HL-8142. Bethesda, MD: U.S. Department of Health and Human Services; 2021. nhlbi.nih.gov/asthmaguidelines.

PEARLS FOR PRACTITIONERS

CHAPTER 78

Allergy Assessment

- Type I immediate hypersensitivity reactions involve immunoglobulin E (IgE) antibodies bound to mast cell and basophil cell surfaces. Upon binding of antigen to these antibodies, chemical mediators such as histamine, tryptase, leukotrienes, and prostaglandins are released, resulting in allergic symptoms, the most serious syndrome being anaphylaxis.
- Type II cytotoxic antibody reactions, such as hemolytic anemia and Goodpasture syndrome, occur when antibodies (IgM, IgG, or IgA) bind to cell surface antigens causing complement activation and, ultimately, cell lysis or release of anaphylatoxins.
- Type III immune complex reactions result when antigen-antibody complexes are formed, causing injury to vasculature and organs such as liver, spleen, and kidney. The classic type III reaction is serum sickness.
- Type IV delayed type hypersensitivity reactions result when T cells recognize antigens in the context of major histocompatibility complex class II, which activates cytokine release. Contact dermatitis to poison ivy represents an example of type IV delayed hypersensitivity reactions.
- The history, family history, and physical examination may indicate existing atopic disease in patients.
- Allergic rhinitis, allergic asthma, and food allergies are examples of atopic disease involving IgE antibodies.
- Of the two methods for assessing antigen-specific IgE antibodies, in vivo skin testing (via prick or intradermal testing) is the most sensitive. Serum-based testing with quantitative fluorescent immunoassay is useful in those patients unable to have skin testing performed.
- The presence of specific IgE antibodies does not equate to diagnosis of allergic disease; positive results must be correlated with the history. Therefore, obtaining screening tests of multiple allergens is not recommended.

CHAPTER 79

Asthma

- Asthma involves many different cells, chemical mediators, and chemotactic factors, resulting in airway inflammation and airway hyperresponsiveness. Typical symptoms include cough, wheeze, shortness of breath, and chest tightness.
- Evaluation of patients with asthma should include history, response to treatment, spirometry (>5 years of age), and allergy testing.
- Treatment of asthma involves numerous interventions: patient and caregiver education, reduction of exposure to nonspecific irritants such as secondhand tobacco smoke or sensitized indoor allergens such as dust mites, pharmacologic therapy, possible immunologic therapy, and yearly influenza vaccination.
- To relieve smooth muscle airway bronchoconstriction, short-acting β_2 agonists (SABAs) should be employed on an as-needed basis and/or prior to physical activity.
- The most effective antiinflammatory pharmacologic therapy for persistent asthma is inhaled corticosteroids (ICS). Due to steroid side effects, it is important to find the minimum dose that is able to achieve control and minimize risk and impairment from the disease.
- All metered-dose inhalers need to be administered with the use of an aerochamber to maximize lung deposition of the medication.
- For some patients with more severe asthma, additional therapies may be required to achieve treatment goals: combination therapy with long-acting β_2 agonists, leukotriene modifiers, theophylline, biologic agents, anticholinergic agents, allergen immunotherapy, and oral corticosteroids.
- Use of peak flow monitoring and written asthma action plans may assist patients and their parents with at-home monitoring and adherence to medical therapy.

- Asthma exacerbations may be treated with frequent administration of short-acting bronchodilators and a course of systemic corticosteroids. Despite these interventions, status asthmaticus may ensue, requiring supplemental oxygen, continuous bronchodilation, intravenous corticosteroids, blood gas monitoring, magnesium sulfate, and/or hospitalization.

CHAPTER 80
Allergic Rhinitis

- Allergic rhinitis and conjunctivitis are IgE-mediated atopic diseases in response to relevant aeroallergens in a perennial and/or seasonal fashion. Common symptoms include nasal pruritus, sneezing, clear rhinorrhea, nasal obstruction, lacrimation, ocular pruritus, and conjunctival injection.
- Like asthma, treatment for allergic rhinitis and conjunctivitis employs numerous modalities: education, avoidance of triggers, pharmacologic therapy, and immunotherapy.
- The most effective pharmacologic class of medications for the treatment of allergic rhinitis is intranasal corticosteroids. Other treatments include oral and nasal antihistamines, oral decongestants, and leukotriene modifiers.

CHAPTER 81
Atopic Dermatitis

- Atopic dermatitis is a chronic relapsing skin condition characterized by pruritus and skin inflammation. The pathogenesis is complex and multifactorial.
- Restoring the skin barrier is an important treatment modality as is control of pruritus, reduction of inflammation, and minimizing exposure to known triggers.
- In severe atopic dermatitis, 30% of pediatric patients may have a food allergy trigger; for moderate eczema, 15%; for mild, less than 10%.

CHAPTER 82
Urticaria, Angioedema, and Anaphylaxis

- The pathophysiology of urticaria involves swelling of the dermis due to inflammatory mediators released from skin mast cells.
- Angioedema is swelling below the dermis.
- Acute urticaria refers to urticaria occurring less than 6 weeks of duration; chronic urticaria occurs for 6 weeks or more. A causal agent is more likely to be found in acute urticaria such as a food, medication, insect sting, infection, blood transfusion, or contact agent. With chronic urticaria, an etiology is less likely to be found, and most cases are idiopathic.
- Physical urticaria refers to lesions due to physical stimuli such as dermatographia, cold, heat, and/or exercise and pressure.
- There are two types of hereditary angioedema, and both are inherited in an autosomal-dominant fashion. Type I accounts for the majority of cases and is due to decreased production of C1-esterase inhibitor. Patients with type II have normal levels of C1-esterase inhibitor, but function is reduced.
- Patients with hereditary angioedema with normal C1 inhibitor experience angioedema like type I and II hereditary angioedema but have normal levels and function of C1-esterase inhibitor.
- Anaphylaxis refers to a severe allergic reaction (usually involving two or more organ systems) due to type I immediate hypersensitivity. Causative agents are numerous.
- Anaphylactoid reactions result from direct, nonspecific mast cell and basophil activation but are not immune-mediated. Examples include reactions to radiocontrast media and opioids.

CHAPTER 83
Serum Sickness

- Serum sickness is the prototypical type III reaction where antibody binds to antigen, forming immune complexes that can cause vascular injury or end-organ damage. Symptoms classically are fever, arthralgias, lymphadenopathy, and rash.

CHAPTER 84
Insect Allergies

- Stinging insect hypersensitivity refers to allergic reactions to Hymenoptera, which include bees, yellow jackets, wasps, hornets, and fire ants. Biting insects such as the kissing bug, bed bugs, blackflies, and deerflies have also caused anaphylaxis.
- Patients of any age who suffer from anaphylaxis due to Hymenoptera stings with positive specific IgE testing benefit from immunotherapy and should have an autoinjector of epinephrine. However, pediatric and adult patients who experience only cutaneous symptoms do not require testing, immunotherapy, or epinephrine because their risk of life-threatening reaction is low.

CHAPTER 85
Adverse Reactions to Foods

- Cow's milk, egg, soy, wheat, peanut, tree nut, finned fish, shellfish, and sesame account for 90% of IgE-mediated food allergies in children.

- Positive food skin-specific and/or serum-specific IgE testing alone does not equate to clinical reactivity and must be interpreted in the context of the history.
- The clinical history should dictate what food allergens should be tested; testing too many different foods as a screening tool has very little clinical value and is strongly discouraged.
- Neither skin nor serum testing for food allergies can predict severity of allergy or the amount required to elicit a reaction. Only risk for an allergic reaction can be inferred from a positive allergy test to a food.
- The mainstay of treatment of food allergies is avoidance and the use of autoinjectable epinephrine in the case of accidental ingestion resulting in symptoms. Oral immunotherapy with pharmaceutical-grade peanut protein containing relevant allergens is available. Omalizumab, a monoclonal antibody against IgE, has been approved for the mitigation of allergic reactions in conjunction with ongoing food avoidance.
- Studies indicate that even for high-risk infants, early introduction of peanut into the diet decreased the development of peanut allergy.

CHAPTER 86

Adverse Reactions to Drugs

- Predictable adverse drug reactions are classified as either immunologic or nonimmunologic, with the former being less common.
- Standardized allergy skin testing for reactions due to IgE is available for penicillin determinants but unavailable for most other medications. Drug challenges and drug desensitization may be an appropriate approach in this setting.

SECTION 15

RHEUMATIC DISEASES OF CHILDHOOD

Grant D. Syverson | Leanne M. Mansfield

CHAPTER 87

Rheumatic Assessment

The **rheumatic diseases** (**collagen vascular** or **connective tissue diseases**) **of childhood** are characterized by autoimmunity and inflammation, which may be localized or generalized. The classic rheumatic diseases of children include **juvenile idiopathic arthritis (JIA)**, **systemic lupus erythematosus (SLE)**, and **juvenile dermatomyositis (JDM)**. *Vasculitis* may be a component of rheumatic diseases. **Musculoskeletal pain syndromes** are a set of overlapping conditions characterized by poorly localized, diffuse pain. Scleroderma (systemic sclerosis), Behçet syndrome, and Sjögren syndrome are rare in childhood. The differential diagnosis of rheumatologic disorders includes infections, postinfectious processes, and malignancies (Table 87.1).

HISTORY

The patient history is one of the most important tools in diagnosing rheumatic diseases. History can identify symptoms that reflect the source of the inflammation, including whether it is localized or systemic. Symptoms of systemic inflammation can be nonspecific. *Fever*, caused by cytokine release, can take different patterns. A hectic fever, without periodicity or pattern, is commonly found in vasculitides such as Kawasaki disease but can also occur in children with underlying acute infectious process. Certain illnesses, such as systemic JIA, produce a *patterned fever* with regular temperature spikes once or twice a day. Other rheumatic illnesses may cause low-grade fevers. Monitoring the child's fever pattern, particularly in the absence of antipyretics, is useful. Rashes occur in several varied forms, from evanescent to fixed and scarring (see Table 87.1). Other systemic symptoms (malaise, anorexia, weight loss, and fatigue) can vary from mild to debilitating.

Symptoms of localized inflammation vary depending on the involved site. **Arthritis**, or inflammation of the synovium (synovitis), leads to joint pain, swelling, decreased range of motion, and functional limitations. Stiffness (gelling) is commonly described in the morning or after periods of inactivity and improves with movement. Children may refrain from or alter activities or sports participation. **Enthesitis** is inflammation at the insertion of a ligament to a bone. **Serositis**, inflammation of serosal lining such as pleuritis, pericarditis, or peritonitis, gives rise to chest pain, shortness of breath, and/or abdominal pain. **Myositis**, inflammation of the muscle, may lead to symptoms of muscle pain, weakness, and difficulty performing tasks of daily living. **Vasculitis**, inflammation of the blood vessels, leads to nonspecific symptoms of rash (petechiae, purpura) and edema when small vessels deep in the papillary dermis are involved; involvement of medium-sized vessels results in a circumscribed tender nodule, and large vessel disease can lead to claudication and hypertension.

PHYSICAL EXAMINATION

A physical examination added to a thorough history is frequently sufficient to narrow the differential diagnosis and elicit the diagnosis. The child's overall appearance and evidence of growth faltering may point to a significant underlying inflammatory disorder. The head and neck examination may show evidence of mucosal ulceration seen in diseases such as SLE. The eye examination may show pupillary irregularity and synechiae from uveitis or the nonpurulent conjunctivitis of Kawasaki disease. Diffuse lymphadenopathy may be found and is nonspecific. The respiratory and cardiac examinations may show pericardial or pleural friction rubs, indicating serositis. Splenomegaly or hepatomegaly raises suspicion of activation of the reticuloendothelial system that occurs in systemic JIA or SLE.

The joint examination is crucial for the diagnosis of arthritis and may identify evidence of inflammation, such as joint swelling, effusion, tenderness, and warmth from increased blood flow. Joint contractures may be seen if the process is chronic. The joint lining, or synovium, may be thickened from chronic inflammation. Activation of epiphyseal growth plates in an area of arthritis can lead to localized bony proliferation and limb length discrepancies. Conversely, inflammation at sites of immature growth centers may lead to maldevelopment of bones, such as the carpals or tarsals (resulting in crowding) or the temporomandibular joints (resulting in micrognathia). A rash or evidence of underlying skin disorders, such as skin thickening from scleroderma or sclerodactyly, may be noted. Chronic Raynaud phenomenon may result in nail fold capillary changes, ulceration, or digital tuft wasting.

COMMON MANIFESTATIONS

Rheumatic diseases of childhood encompass a heterogeneous group of diseases with a shared underlying pathogenesis: chronic inflammation from a disordered immune response. This leads to inflammation directed against native proteins, with secondary increases in numbers of activated lymphocytes, inflammatory cytokines, and circulating antibodies. This antibody production can be nonspecific, or it can be targeted against specific native proteins, leading to subsequent

TABLE 87.1 Differential Diagnoses of Pediatric Arthritis Syndromes

CHARACTERISTIC	SYSTEMIC LUPUS ERYTHEMATOSUS	JUVENILE IDIOPATHIC ARTHRITIS	RHEUMATIC FEVER	LYME DISEASE	LEUKEMIA	GONOCOCCEMIA	KAWASAKI DISEASE
Gender	F > M	Type-dependent	M = F	M = F	M = F	F > M	M > F
Age	10–20 yr	1–16 yr	5–15 yr	5–20 yr	2–10 yr	>12 yr	<5 yr
Arthralgia	Yes	Yes	Yes	Yes	Yes	Yes	Yes
Morning stiffness	Yes	Yes	No	No	No	No	No
Rash	Butterfly; discoid	Salmon-pink macules (sJIA)	Erythema marginatum	Erythema migrans	No, petechiae	Palms/soles, papulopustular	Diffuse maculopapular, desquamation
Oligoarticular (up to four joints)	Yes	Yes (30%)	No	Yes (often monoarticular)	Yes	Yes	—
Polyarticular	Yes	Yes (70%)	Yes	No	Yes	No	Yes
Small joints	Yes	Yes	No	Rare	Yes	No	Yes
Temporomandibular joint	No	Yes	No	Rare	No	No	No
Eye disease	Uveitis, retinitis	Uveitis, iridocyclitis (rare sJIA)	No	Conjunctivitis, keratitis	No	No	Conjunctivitis, uveitis
Total WBC count	Decreased	Increased (decreased in MAS)	Normal to increased	Normal	Increased or neutropenia ± blasts	Increased	Increased
ANA positive*	>99% positive	~50%	Nondiagnostic	Nondiagnostic	Nondiagnostic	Nondiagnostic	Nondiagnostic
RF*	Positive or negative	Positive (10%) (polyarticular)	Nondiagnostic	Nondiagnostic	Nondiagnostic	Nondiagnostic	Nondiagnostic
Other laboratory results	↓ Complement, ↑ antibodies to double-stranded DNA	Anti-CCP antibody + in adult-type RA	↑ ASO, anti-DNase B	↑ Cryoglobulin, ↑ immune complexes	+ Bone marrow blasts	+ Culture for *Neisseria gonorrhoeae*	Thrombocytosis, ↑ immune complexes
Erosive arthritis	Rare	Yes	Rare	Rare	No	Yes	No
Other clinical manifestations	Proteinuria, serositis	Fever, serositis (sJIA)	Carditis, nodules, chorea	Carditis, neuropathy, meningitis , facial nerve palsy	Thrombocytopenia	History of sexual activity	Fever, lymphadenopathy, swollen hands/feet, oral lesions
Pathogenesis	Autoimmune	Autoimmune	Group A streptococcus	*Borrelia burgdorferi*	Acute lymphoblastic leukemia	*N. gonorrhoeae*	Unknown
Treatment	NSAIDs, corticosteroids, hydroxychloroquine, immunosuppressive agents, biologic agents	NSAIDs, methotrexate, sulfasalazine, biologic agents	Penicillin prophylaxis, aspirin, corticosteroids	Doxycycline, amoxicillin, ceftriaxone	Corticosteroids, chemotherapy	Ceftriaxone	Intravenous immunoglobulin, aspirin

**Up to 20% of normal children will have a false-positive ANA or RF, most likely due to infection.*

ANA, Antinuclear antibody; *ASO*, antistreptolysin-O titer; *CCP*, cyclic citrullinated protein; *MAS*, macrophage activation syndrome; *NSAID*, nonsteroidal antiinflammatory drug; *RA*, rheumatoid arthritis; *RF*, rheumatoid factor; *sJIA*, systemic juvenile idiopathic arthritis; *WBC*, white blood cell.

disease manifestations (Table 87.2). Although immune system hyperactivity may be self-limited, the hallmark of most rheumatic diseases of childhood is chronicity or the perpetuation of the inflammatory process, which may lead to long-term disability.

INITIAL DIAGNOSTIC EVALUATION

Rheumatic diseases can initially present with nonspecific symptoms; over time, a characteristic set of symptoms and physical findings can be elicited. In conjunction with carefully chosen testing, an appropriate differential diagnosis is made, and eventually the correct diagnosis is made and a treatment plan is developed.

Most rheumatologic diagnoses are established by clinical findings and fulfillment of classification criteria. Laboratory testing should be judicious and based on a differential diagnosis rather than random screening in search of a diagnosis. Laboratory tests confirm clinical diagnoses rather than developing them.

LABORATORY TESTING

Evidence of an underlying systemic inflammation may be indicated by *elevated acute phase reactants*, especially the erythrocyte sedimentation rate (ESR), but also the white blood cell (WBC) count and C-reactive protein (CRP). The complete blood count (CBC) may demonstrate a normochromic, normocytic anemia of chronic disease. These laboratory findings are nonspecific for any rheumatologic diagnosis. Certain laboratory tests may help confirm a diagnosis, such as autoantibody production in SLE or muscle enzyme elevation in JDM, or identify increased risk for complications, such as uveitis in a patient with JIA with a positive antinuclear antibody.

TABLE 87.2 Manifestations of Autoantibodies

Coombs-positive hemolytic anemia
Immune neutropenia
Immune thrombocytopenia
Immune lymphopenia
Thrombosis (anticardiolipin, antiphospholipid, lupus anticoagulant)
Antimitochondrial (primary biliary cirrhosis, SLE)
Antimicrosomal (chronic active hepatitis, SLE)
Antithyroid (thyroiditis, SLE)
ANCA-cytoplasmic (granulomatosis with polyangiitis)
ANCA-perinuclear (microscopic polyangiitis or other vasculitides)
Anti-CCP (rheumatoid-positive JIA)
ANTINUCLEAR ANTIBODIES TO SPECIFIC NUCLEAR ANTIGENS AND ASSOCIATED MANIFESTATIONS
Single-stranded DNA (nonspecific, indicates inflammation)
Double-stranded DNA (SLE, kidney disease)
DNA-histone (drug-induced SLE)
Sm (SLE, kidney, CNS)
RNP (SLE, Sjögren syndrome, scleroderma, polymyositis, MCTD)
Ro (SSA) (SLE, neonatal lupus-congenital heart block, Sjögren syndrome)
La (SSB) (SLE, neonatal lupus-congenital heart block, Sjögren syndrome)
Jo-1 (polymyositis, dermatomyositis)
Scl-70 (systemic sclerosis)
Centromere (CREST; limited scleroderma)
PM-Scl (scleroderma, UCTD)

ANCA, Antineutrophil cytoplasmic antibody; *CCP*, cyclic citrullinated protein; *CNS*, central nervous system; *CREST syndrome*, calcinosis, Raynaud phenomenon, esophageal dysfunction, sclerodactyly, telangiectasia; *JIA*, juvenile idiopathic arthritis; *La*, Lane; *MCTD*, mixed connective tissue disease; *PM-Scl*, polymyositis-scleroderma; *RNP*, ribonucleoprotein; *Ro*, Robert; *SLE*, systemic lupus erythematosus; *Sm*, Smith; *SSA*, Sjögren syndrome antigen A; *SSB*, Sjögren syndrome antigen B; *UCTD*, undifferentiated connective tissue disease.

Modified from Condemi J. The autoimmune disease. JAMA. *1992;268:2882–2892.*

DIAGNOSTIC IMAGING

Radiologic studies should focus on areas of concern identified by history or physical examination. Radiography of joints in patients with arthritis on examination may be beneficial, but radiographic abnormalities lag behind the clinical examination. Tests with greater sensitivity, such as MRI, may be useful when trying to differentiate between synovitis and traumatic soft tissue injury. MRI may also be useful to identify evidence of central nervous system involvement with SLE or evidence of myositis with JDM.

PEARLS FOR PRACTITIONERS

See Rheumatic Diseases of Childhood: Pearls for Practitioners at the end of this section.

REVIEW QUESTIONS

Available online.

CHAPTER 88

Immunoglobulin A Vasculitis

ETIOLOGY

Immunoglobulin (Ig) A vasculitis (IgAV) (formerly known as *Henoch-Schönein purpura*) is a vasculitis of unknown etiology characterized by inflammation of small blood vessels with IgA immune complex deposition, leukocytic infiltration of tissue, hemorrhage, and ischemia.

EPIDEMIOLOGY

IgAV is the most common systemic vasculitis of childhood and a cause of *nonthrombocytopenic purpura*, with an incidence of 3–27 per 100,000 children. IgAV presents primarily in children 3–15 years of age and is more common in males than females. IgAV occurs more frequently in the autumn and winter months.

CLINICAL MANIFESTATIONS

IgAV is characterized by rash, arthritis or arthralgias, and, less frequently, gastrointestinal and kidney involvement. The hallmark of IgAV is *palpable purpura*, caused by small vessel inflammation in the skin, leading to extravasation of blood into the surrounding tissues, frequently with IgA deposition. The rash is classically found in dependent areas such as the buttocks and lower extremities (Fig. 88.1). The rash of IgAV can begin as small macules, papules, or urticarial lesions and

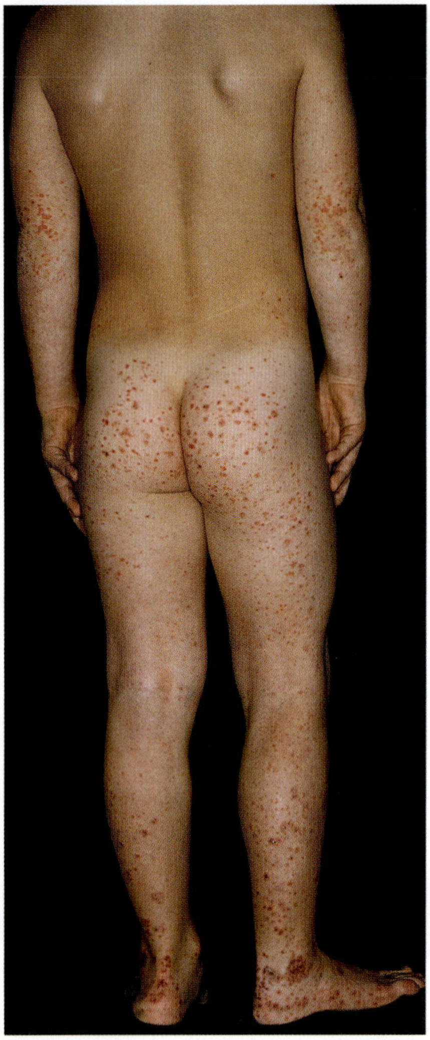

FIGURE 88.1 Distribution of immunoglobulin A vasculitis. Palpable purpuric lesions are most common on the lower extremities and buttocks but can appear on the arms, face, and ears; the trunk is usually spared. (From Dinulos JGH, ed. *Habif's Clinical Dermatology: A Color Guide to Diagnosis and Therapy*. 7th ed. Philadelphia: Elsevier; 2021:738, Fig. 18.18.)

progress to petechiae, ecchymoses, purpura, or hemorrhagic bullae. The rash also can be accompanied by edema, particularly of the dorsum of the feet and hands, scalp, and scrotum. Although uncommon, IgAV can be associated with encephalopathy, pancreatitis, and orchitis.

Arthritis or arthralgia occurs in 80% of patients with IgAV and is most common in the lower extremities, particularly the ankles and knees. The arthritis is acute, edematous, painful, and limits range of motion.

Gastrointestinal involvement occurs in about one half of individuals with IgAV. Gastrointestinal symptoms commonly present as mild-to-moderate crampy abdominal pain (due to edema and/or ischemia caused by small vessel involvement); there can be significant abdominal distention, bloody diarrhea, intussusception, and/or abdominal perforation, which require emergent intervention. Arthritis and gastrointestinal symptoms may precede the onset of rash.

Approximately 30% of children with IgAV develop kidney involvement, which can be acute or chronic. Kidney involvement is mild in most cases; glomerulonephritis manifested by proteinuria, hematuria, hypertension, or kidney failure can occur. Most cases of glomerulonephritis occur within the first few months of presentation, but rarely, patients develop late kidney disease, which ultimately can lead to chronic kidney disease including kidney failure.

LABORATORY AND IMAGING STUDIES

Assessment of the platelet count is crucial because IgAV is characterized by *nonthrombocytopenic purpura* with a normal or elevated platelet count, differentiating IgAV from other causes of purpura that are associated with thrombocytopenia (autoimmune thrombocytopenia, systemic lupus erythematosus, or leukemia). Serum IgA may only be elevated in 30% of patients. Erythrocyte sedimentation rate (ESR), C-reactive protein (CRP), and white blood cell (WBC) count are often elevated in patients with IgAV. A urinalysis screens for evidence of hematuria as well as proteinuria; a urine protein:urine creatinine ratio should be evaluated. A serum blood urea nitrogen and creatinine should be obtained to evaluate kidney function. A complete blood count (CBC) demonstrating anemia and testing the stool for blood may identify evidence of gastrointestinal involvement. Any question of severe gastrointestinal pain requires urgent imaging; an ultrasound can quickly evaluate for intussusception. If performed, skin biopsy will show leukocytoclastic vasculitis (LCV) with predominant IgA deposition differentiating it from other forms of LCV.

DIFFERENTIAL DIAGNOSIS

The diagnosis of IgAV is based on the presence of purpura (mandatory) with a classic lower limb distribution and at least one of the following: abdominal pain, arthritis or arthralgia, kidney involvement, and/or consistent histopathology (Table 88.1), which provides 100% sensitivity and 87% specificity for the disease. The differential diagnosis for IgAV includes other systemic vasculitides (Table 88.2) and diseases associated with thrombocytopenic purpura, such as idiopathic thrombocytopenic purpura or leukemia.

TREATMENT

Treatment for IgAV is supportive. A short-term course of **nonsteroidal antiinflammatory drugs** can be administered for arthritis or painful manifestations if there are no kidney involvement concerns. **Systemic corticosteroids** are usually reserved for children with significant pain from gastrointestinal disease or orchitis. A typical dosing regimen is prednisone (1–2 mg/kg/day, maximum 60 mg/day) with a gradual taper plan over several weeks. When IgAV nephritis is present, it is treated with corticosteroids but may require the addition of more aggressive immunosuppressive therapy.

COMPLICATIONS

Most cases of IgAV are monophasic, last 3–4 weeks, and resolve completely. The arthritis of IgAV does not result in any permanent joint damage. The most significant complications acutely are gastrointestinal, such as intussusception, infarction, and bowel perforation; the chronic concern is development of kidney disease leading to kidney failure. Kidney function should be monitored for months following a diagnosis of IgAV.

TABLE 88.1 Criteria for Diagnosis of IgA Vasculitis*

CRITERIA	DEFINITION
Purpura (mandatory)	Purpura (typically palpable) or petechiae with classic lower limb distribution in the absence of thrombocytopenia
Abdominal pain	Acute, diffuse, colicky abdominal pain, which may include gastrointestinal bleeding or intussusception
Arthritis or arthralgia	Arthritis: acute joint pain or swelling with limited range of motion Arthralgia: acute joint pain without swelling or limited range of motion
Kidney involvement	Proteinuria and/or hematuria
Histopathology	Leukocytoclastic vasculitis or proliferative glomerulonephritis with IgA deposits Biopsy to be obtained if purpura has an atypical distribution

*The diagnosis of IgA vasculitis is based on the presence of purpura and then at least one of the additional four criteria.
Ig, Immunoglobulin.
Adapted from Ozen S, Pistorio A, Iusan SM, et al. EULAR/PRINTO/PRES criteria for Henoch-Schönlein purpura, childhood polyarteritis nodosa, childhood Wegener granulomatosis and childhood Takayasu arteritis: Ankara 2008. Part II: final classification criteria. Ann Rheum Dis. 2010;69(5):798–806.

TABLE 88.2 Classification of Pediatric Vasculitides

LARGE VESSEL
Takayasu arteritis
MEDIUM-SIZED VESSEL
Childhood polyarteritis nodosa Cutaneous polyarteritis nodosa Kawasaki disease
GRANULOMATOUS SMALL VESSEL
Eosinophilic granulomatosis with polyangiitis Granulomatosis with polyangiitis
NONGRANULOMATOUS SMALL VESSEL
Immunoglobulin A vasculitis Hypocomplementemic urticarial vasculitis Other leukocytoclastic vasculitides Microscopic polyangiitis
OTHER VASCULITIDES
Vasculitis associated with infections, drugs, malignancies, or other rheumatic diseases Behçet syndrome Central nervous system vasculitis

PROGNOSIS

The prognosis of IgAV is excellent. Most children have complete resolution of the illness without any significant sequelae, though recurrence is possible. Patients with kidney disease from IgAV are at highest risk for long-term complications, particularly if the initial course was marked by significant kidney involvement. There is a long-term risk of progression to end-stage kidney disease in less than 5% of children with IgAV; they may require kidney transplantation.

PEARLS FOR PRACTITIONERS

See Rheumatic Diseases of Childhood: Pearls for Practitioners at the end of this section.

REVIEW QUESTIONS

Available online.

CHAPTER 89

Kawasaki Disease

ETIOLOGY

Kawasaki disease (KD) is a vasculitis of unknown etiology that is characterized by multisystem involvement and inflammation of predominately medium-sized arteries with risk of aneurysm formation.

EPIDEMIOLOGY

KD is the second most common vasculitis of childhood. It has been described with variable frequency in all parts of the world, with the highest incidence in Japan. KD occurs more often in males and in children younger than 5 years of age. The disease occurs throughout the year, but a seasonal variability has been described with a peak in the winter and spring months. In the United States, KD is the leading cause of acquired heart disease in children.

CLINICAL MANIFESTATIONS

The clinical course of KD can be divided into three phases (acute, subacute, convalescent), each with unique manifestations. Abnormalities of the coronary arteries are the most concerning manifestation of KD.

Acute Phase

The acute phase of KD, which lasts 1–2 weeks, is marked by sudden onset of a high fever without an infectious or alternative explanation. The onset of fever is often followed by conjunctivitis, mucosal changes, rash, edema and/or erythema of the hands and feet, and cervical lymphadenopathy (Fig. 89.1). Conjunctivitis is bilateral, bulbar, and nonexudative with perilimbal sparing. Mucosal changes may include dry, cracked lips and a *strawberry tongue*. A rash, which can vary in appearance, occurs in >80% of children with KD and may be particularly accentuated on the chest and perineal region. Cervical lymphadenopathy is most often unilateral and, for the purposes of diagnosis, greater than 1.5 cm in diameter. Extreme irritability is prominent, especially in infants. Diarrhea, abdominal pain, and hydrops of the gallbladder may occur. Tachycardia, particularly while febrile, and carditis may be present. Some patients present with **KD shock syndrome**, which is marked by sustained systolic hypotension or clinical signs of poor perfusion. Monitoring for coronary artery abnormalities, including aneurysms, begins in the acute phase and continues throughout the course of the disease.

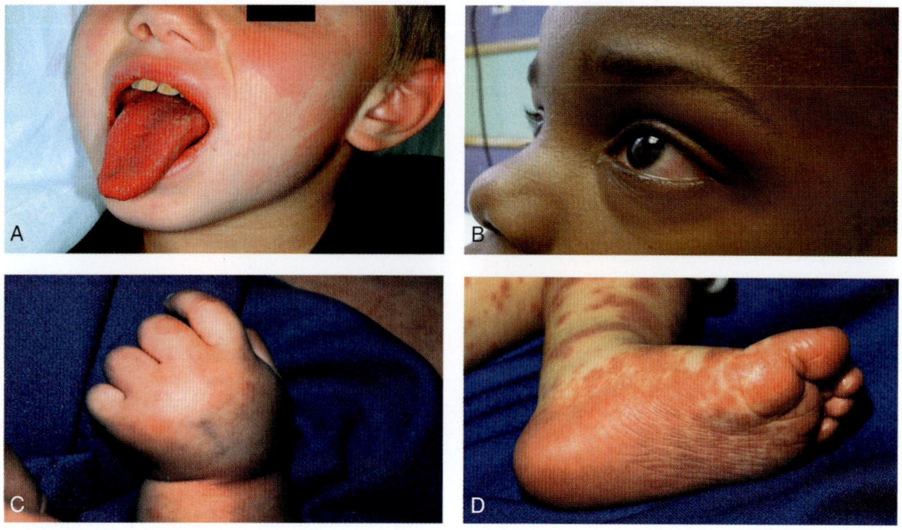

FIGURE 89.1 **(A)** Kawasaki disease. Hyperemia of the tongue with prominent lingual papillae ("red strawberry tongue"). **(B)** The conjunctivitis in this patient demonstrates the notable perilimbal sparing (halo of noninvolvement adjacent to the iris). **(C)** Nonpitting edema of the hand in a young male with Kawasaki disease. **(D)** Confluent, erythematous patches and plaques of the sole in a young male with Kawasaki disease. (From Paller AS, Mancini AJ. *Hurwitz Clinical Pediatric Dermatology*. 6th ed. Philadelphia, PA: Elsevier; 2022:Figs. 21-21, 21-24, 21-25, 21-27.)

Subacute Phase

The subacute phase is characterized by continued systemic inflammation but has resolution of fever and improvement in other clinical symptoms. *Periungual desquamation* of the fingers and toes may appear during this phase. Arthritis occurs most often during the subacute phase but can occur throughout the course and resolves without long-term sequelae.

Convalescent Phase

The convalescent phase begins with the disappearance of all clinical symptoms and continues until the inflammatory markers (C-reactive protein [CRP] and platelets) return to normal. Linear nail creases known as *Beau lines* of the nails may appear during this phase.

TABLE 89.1 Criteria for Diagnosis of Kawasaki Disease
Fever of >5-day duration associated with at least four* of the following five changes:
Bilateral nonsuppurative conjunctivitis
One or more changes of the oropharyngeal mucous membranes, including pharyngeal injection, dry fissured lips, injected lips, and "strawberry" tongue
One or more changes of the peripheral extremities, including edema and/or erythema of the hands and feet or periungual desquamation
Polymorphous rash, primarily truncal
Cervical lymphadenopathy >1.5 cm in diameter and most commonly unilateral
Disease cannot be explained by some other known disease process

**A diagnosis of Kawasaki disease can be made if fever and fewer than four criteria are met if coronary artery disease is demonstrated by two-dimensional echocardiography or coronary angiography.*

LABORATORY AND IMAGING STUDIES

With KD, it is particularly important to exclude other causes of fever; appropriate infectious evaluation (i.e., blood and urine cultures, chest x-ray, viral testing) should occur. In the acute phase, inflammatory parameters are elevated, including white blood cell (WBC), CRP, and erythrocyte sedimentation rate (ESR). Platelet counts may be inappropriately low or normal until a week after fever onset when thrombocytosis occurs. Sterile pyuria may be present. A lumbar puncture, if performed to exclude meningitis, may reveal pleocytosis with normal protein and glucose. Tests of hepatobiliary function may be abnormal. Echocardiograms need to be completed at baseline, 2 weeks after onset (or more frequently if there are concerns), and then through the completion of disease follow-up to monitor for development of coronary artery abnormalities.

DIFFERENTIAL DIAGNOSIS

The diagnosis of KD is based on the presence of fever for more than 5 days without an identifiable source and the presence of four of five other clinical criteria (Table 89.1).

The diagnosis of **incomplete KD**, which occurs more commonly in infants, is made when fever is present for at least 5 days, with two or three clinical criteria, elevated ESR and/or CRP, and three or more supplemental laboratory findings with particular definitions (anemia, elevated alanine aminotransferase, hypoalbuminemia, sterile pyuria, thrombocytosis, leukocytosis) or the presence of coronary artery abnormalities on echocardiogram (Fig. 89.2). The diagnosis of KD should be considered in infants younger than 6 months of age with fever for at least 7 days even if no other criteria are present, and an echocardiogram should be obtained. Manifestations of KD are found in other illnesses; a broad differential must be considered and excluded before the diagnosis of KD can be established (Table 89.2). The differential diagnosis of KD should include **multisystem inflammatory syndrome in children (MIS-C)**, which is a complication of COVID-19 characterized by fever, multiorgan involvement, and inflammation. MIS-C can be difficult to distinguish from KD if rash, peripheral extremity changes, oropharyngeal changes, cervical lymphadenopathy, and conjunctival injection are present. Patients with MIS-C are typically older and tend to have more

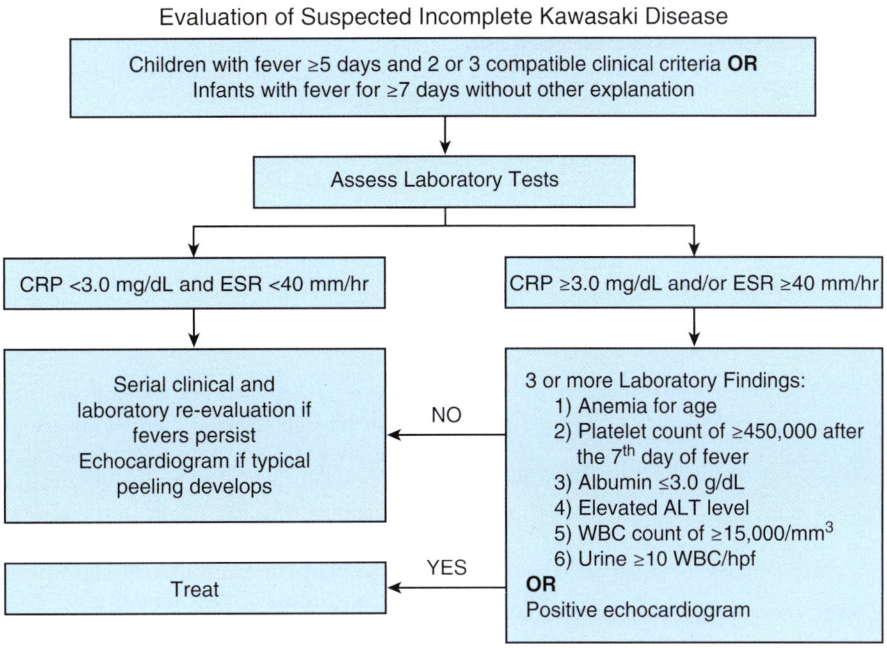

FIGURE 89.2 Algorithm for the evaluation of suspected incomplete Kawasaki disease. *ALT*, Alanine aminotransferase; *CRP*, C-reactive protein; *ESR*, erythrocyte sedimentation rate; *WBC*, white blood cell. (From McCrindle BW, Rowley AH, Newburger JW, et al. Diagnosis, treatment, and long-term management of Kawasaki disease: a scientific statement for health professionals from the American Heart Association. *Circulation*. 2017;135[17]:e927–e999. Published correction appears in *Circulation*. 2019;140[5]:e181–e184.)

TABLE 89.2 Differential Diagnoses of Kawasaki Disease

INFECTIOUS
Scarlet fever
Epstein-Barr virus
Adenovirus
Meningococcemia
Measles
Rubella
Roseola infantum
Staphylococcal toxic shock syndrome
Scalded skin syndrome
Toxoplasmosis
Leptospirosis
Rocky Mountain spotted fever
Multisystem inflammatory syndrome in children (SARS-CoV-2)
INFLAMMATORY
Systemic juvenile idiopathic arthritis
Polyarteritis nodosa
Behçet syndrome
HYPERSENSITIVITY
Drug reaction
Stevens-Johnson syndrome

neurologic and gastrointestinal symptoms, cardiac dysfunction rather than coronary artery aneurysms (though they can occur), higher CRP, thrombocytopenia, and lower absolute lymphocyte counts.

TREATMENT

Intravenous immunoglobulin (IVIG) is the mainstay of therapy for KD, although the mechanism of action is unknown. A single dose of IVIG (2 g/kg over 8–12 hours) usually results in rapid defervescence and improvement of clinical symptoms in most patients and, most importantly, reduces the incidence of coronary artery aneurysms. **Aspirin** is initially given at higher dosing (30–50 mg/kg/day divided every 6 hours) in the acute phase. Once the fever resolves, aspirin is reduced to lower dosing (3–5 mg/kg/day as a single dose) and given until 6 weeks after illness onset and when follow-up echocardiography documents the absence of coronary artery aneurysms.

Up to 20% of children with KD may have IVIG resistance, which is defined as persistent or recurrent fevers >36 hours after completion of the IVIG infusion. Patients considered high risk at diagnosis (age <6 months or coronary artery z-score ≥2.5) or with IVIG resistance may be treated with adjunctive or alternative therapies such as retreatment with IVIG, corticosteroids, or infliximab. Of note, IVIG impacts laboratory results; ESR should not be used following IVIG to monitor disease response to therapy.

COMPLICATIONS

Most cases of KD resolve without sequelae, though 5% of treated patients develop coronary artery aneurysms. The most common cause of morbidity and mortality for patients with KD is large/giant aneurysms with coronary thrombosis leading to ischemia, infarct, or death. Children who are <6 months old are considered high risk for aneurysms. Patients who present with thrombocytopenia, severe anemia, and unexpectedly normal or low ESR should be further evaluated for macrophage activation syndrome in the setting of KD, which is an inflammatory cytokine storm that may be life-threatening. Other complications are listed in Table 89.3.

TABLE 89.3 Complications of Kawasaki Disease
Coronary artery thrombosis
Peripheral artery aneurysm
Coronary artery aneurysm
Myocardial infarction
Myopericarditis
Heart failure
Kawasaki shock syndrome
Hydrops of gallbladder
Aseptic meningitis
Irritability
Arthritis
Sterile pyuria (urethritis)
Thrombocytosis (late)
Diarrhea
Pancreatitis
Peripheral gangrene
Macrophage activation syndrome

PROGNOSIS

Most patients with KD who receive treatment have an excellent prognosis. Timely treatment reduces the risk of coronary artery aneurysms from 20–25% to less than 5%.

PEARLS FOR PRACTITIONERS

See Rheumatic Diseases of Childhood: Pearls for Practitioners at the end of this section.

REVIEW QUESTIONS

Available online.

CHAPTER 90

Juvenile Idiopathic Arthritis

ETIOLOGY

The chronic arthritides of childhood include several types, the most common of which is **juvenile idiopathic arthritis (JIA)**. The classification of JIA includes different types of juvenile arthritis, such as enthesitis-related arthritis, spondyloarthropathies, and psoriatic arthritis. The etiology of this autoimmune disease is unknown; the common underlying manifestation is the presence of chronic **synovitis**, or inflammation of the synovial lining of the joint. The synovium becomes thickened and hypervascular with infiltration by lymphocytes, which also can be found in the synovial fluid along with inflammatory cytokines. The inflammation leads to production and release of tissue proteases and collagenases. If left untreated, the inflammation can lead to tissue destruction, particularly of the articular cartilage and, eventually, the underlying bony structures.

EPIDEMIOLOGY

JIA is the most common chronic rheumatologic disease of childhood, with a prevalence of 1:1,000 children. The disease has two peaks, one at 1–3 years and one at 8–12 years, but it can occur at any age. Females are affected more commonly than males, particularly with the oligoarticular form of the illness.

CLINICAL PRESENTATION

JIA can be divided into several subtypes, depending on the number of joints involved (<5 vs. ≥5), the presence of sacroiliac or axial involvement, and the presence of systemic features, each with unique disease characteristics (Table 90.1). Although the onset of the arthritis is slow, the actual joint swelling is often noticed acutely by the child or parent, such as after an accident or fall, and can be confused with trauma (even though traumatic effusions are rare in children). Children often develop pain and stiffness in the joint that limit use, but refusing to walk or severe pain is rare. *Morning stiffness* and gelling also can occur in the joint and, if present, can be followed in response to therapy.

On physical examination, signs of inflammation are present, including joint tenderness, erythema, and effusion (Fig. 90.1). Joint range of motion may be limited because of pain, swelling, or contractures from lack of use. In children, due to the presence of an active growth plate, it may be possible to find bony abnormalities of the surrounding bone, causing bony proliferation and localized growth disturbance. In a lower extremity joint, a leg length discrepancy may be appreciable if the arthritis is asymmetric.

All children with chronic arthritis are at risk for chronic **iridocyclitis** or **uveitis**. There is an association between human leukocyte antigens (HLAs; HLA-DR5, HLA-DR6, and HLA-DR8) and uveitis. The presence of a positive **antinuclear antibody (ANA)** identifies children with arthritis who are at higher risk for chronic uveitis. Although all children with JIA are at increased risk, the subgroup of children, particularly young females, with oligoarticular (less than five affected joints) JIA and a positive ANA are at highest risk, with an incidence of uveitis of 80%. The uveitis associated with JIA can be asymptomatic until the point of visual loss, making it the primary treatable cause of blindness in children. It is crucial for children with JIA to undergo regular ophthalmologic screening with a slit-lamp examination to identify anterior chamber inflammation and to initiate prompt treatment of any active disease.

Oligoarticular Juvenile Idiopathic Arthritis

Oligoarticular JIA is defined as the presence of arthritis in fewer than five joints within 6 months of diagnosis. This is the most common form of JIA, accounting for approximately 50% of cases.

Oligoarticular JIA presents in young children, with a peak at 1–3 years. The arthritis is found in medium-sized to large joints; the knee is the most common joint involved, followed by the ankle and the wrist. It is unusual for small joints, such as the fingers or toes, to be involved, although this may occur. Neck and hip involvement are uncommon; temporomandibular joint involvement occurs in more than 75% of patients. Children with oligoarticular JIA may be otherwise well without any evidence of systemic inflammation (fever, weight loss, or growth faltering) or any laboratory evidence of systemic inflammation (elevated white blood cell [WBC] count

TABLE 90.1 Features of Juvenile Idiopathic Arthritis Subgroups

FEATURE	OLIGOARTICULAR	POLYARTICULAR	SYSTEMIC	ENTHESITIS RELATED
Number of joints	<5	≥5	Varies, usually ≥5	Varies
Types of joints	Medium to large (also small in extended oligoarthritis)	Small to medium	Small to medium	Medium to large, including sacroiliac joints
Gender predominance	F > M (especially in younger children)	F > M	F = M	M > F
Systemic features	None	Some constitutional	Prominent	Some constitutional
Eye disease	+++ (uveitis)	++ (uveitis)	+ (uveitis)	++ (iritis)
Extraarticular manifestations	None	None	Systemic features, MAS, lung disease	Enthesopathy, psoriasis, bowel disease
ANA positivity	++	+	—	—
RF or anti-CCP positivity	—	+ (in older children with early-onset RA)	—	N/A
Outcomes	Excellent, >90% complete remission	Excellent with proper diagnosis and treatment; some risk of disability	Significantly improved with newer therapies	Variable

ANA, Antinuclear antibody; *CCP*, cyclic citrullinated peptide; *MAS*, macrophage activation syndrome; *RA*, rheumatoid arthritis; *RF*, rheumatoid factor.

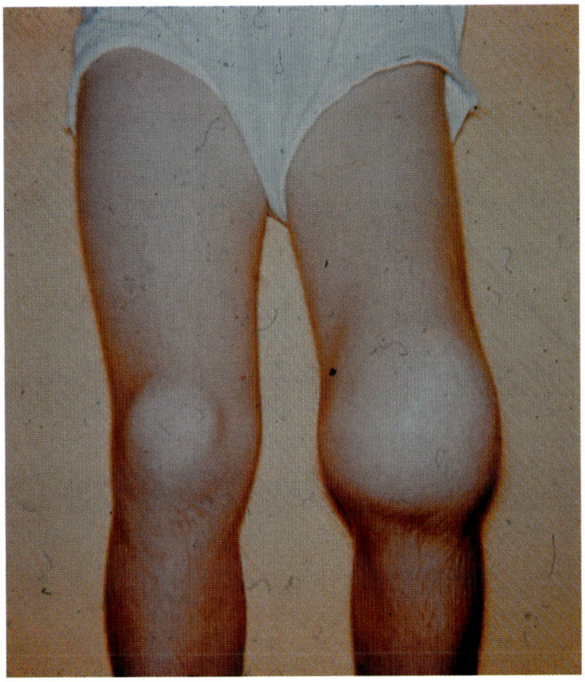

FIGURE 90.1 An affected knee in a patient with oligoarticular juvenile idiopathic arthritis. Note sizable effusion, bony proliferation, and flexion contracture.

or erythrocyte sedimentation rate [ESR]). A subset of these children later develop polyarticular disease (called *extended oligoarthritis*).

Polyarticular Juvenile Idiopathic Arthritis

Polyarticular JIA describes children with arthritis in five or more joints within the first 6 months of diagnosis and accounts for 20–30% of cases. Children with polyarticular JIA tend to have symmetric arthritis, which can affect any joint but most commonly involves the small joints of the hands, feet, ankles, wrists, and knees. The cervical spine can be involved, leading to fusion of the spine over time. In contrast to oligoarticular JIA, children with polyarticular disease can present with evidence of systemic inflammation, including malaise, low-grade fever, growth faltering, anemia of chronic disease, and elevated markers of inflammation. Polyarticular JIA can present at any age, although there is a peak in early childhood. There is a second peak in adolescence, but these children differ by the presence of a positive **rheumatoid factor** or **anticyclic citrullinated protein (anti-CCP) antibody** and most likely represent a subgroup with true adult rheumatoid arthritis; the clinical course and prognosis are similar to the adult entity.

Systemic Juvenile Idiopathic Arthritis

A small subgroup of patients (approximately 10%) with juvenile arthritis does not present with onset of arthritis but rather with preceding systemic inflammation. **Systemic JIA**, thought to be an autoinflammatory (rather than autoimmune) disease, manifests with a typical recurring, spiking fever, usually once or twice per day (also known as *quotidian fever*), which can occur for several weeks to months. This is accompanied by a rash that is morbilliform, salmon colored, and may be *evanescent* (occurs at times of high fever only). Rarely, the rash can be urticarial in nature. Internal organ involvement also occurs. Serositis, such as pleuritis and pericarditis, occurs in 50% of children. Pericardial tamponade may rarely occur. Hepatosplenomegaly occurs in 70% of children. Children with systemic JIA appear sick; they have significant constitutional symptoms, including malaise and growth faltering. Laboratory findings show inflammation, with elevated ESR, C-reactive protein (CRP), WBC, and platelet counts and anemia. The arthritis can follow the systemic inflammation by 6 weeks to 6 months. The arthritis is polyarticular in nature and can be extensive and resistant to treatment, placing these children at highest risk for long-term disability.

Enthesitis-Related Arthritis

Enthesitis-related arthritis describes a group of arthritides that includes inflammation of the axial skeleton, sacroiliac joints, peripheral large joints, and entheses (inflammation of tendinous insertions); these were previously referred to as *spondyloarthropathies.* These include juvenile ankylosing spondylitis, psoriatic arthritis, reactive arthritis, arthritis of inflammatory bowel disease, and undifferentiated juvenile arthritis. This group of diseases can also present with peripheral arthritis and can be initially classified in other subgroups. It is only later, when the patient develops evidence of sacroiliac arthritis, psoriasis, or gastrointestinal disease, that the diagnosis becomes clear (Table 90.2). Other important features of this group include the frequent presence of **HLA-B27** and the need for earlier treatment with tumor necrosis factor (TNF) blockers as axial disease can have a poor response to conventional disease-modifying antirheumatic drugs like methotrexate.

LABORATORY AND IMAGING STUDIES

History and physical exam are the most important diagnostic tools for juvenile arthritis. Most children with oligoarticular JIA have no laboratory abnormalities. Children with polyarticular and systemic disease commonly show elevated acute phase reactants and anemia of chronic disease. In all pediatric patients with joint or bone pain, a complete blood count should be performed to exclude leukemia, which also can present with limb pain (see Chapter 156). Oligoarticular and polyarticular patients with JIA should have an ANA test to help identify those at higher risk for uveitis. Older children and adolescents with polyarticular disease should also have a rheumatoid factor and anti-CCP antibody performed to identify children with early-onset adult rheumatoid arthritis.

Diagnostic arthrocentesis may be necessary to exclude suppurative arthritis in children who present with acute onset of monoarticular symptoms or patients with severe pain. The synovial fluid WBC count is less than 50,000–100,000/mm^3 and should be predominantly lymphocytes, rather than neutrophils as seen with suppurative arthritis. Gram stain, polymerase chain reaction, and culture should be negative.

The most common radiologic finding in the early stages of JIA is a normal bone x-ray. Over time, periarticular osteopenia, resulting from decreased mineralization, is the most common finding. Growth centers may be slow to develop; there may be accelerated maturation of growth plates or evidence of bony proliferation. Erosions of bony articular surfaces may be a late finding. If the cervical spine is involved, fusion of C1–4 and atlantoaxial subluxation may occur.

DIFFERENTIAL DIAGNOSIS

The diagnosis of JIA is established by the presence of arthritis, the duration of the disease for at least 6 weeks, and exclusion of other possible diagnoses. Although a presumptive diagnosis of systemic JIA can be established for a child during the systemic phase, a definitive diagnosis is not possible until arthritis develops. Children must be younger than 16 years of age at the time of onset of the disease; the diagnosis of JIA does not change when the child becomes an adult. As there are a myriad of other causes of arthritis, these disorders need to be excluded before providing a definitive diagnosis of JIA (Table 90.3). The acute arthritides can affect the same joints as JIA but have a shorter time course.

TREATMENT

The treatment of JIA focuses on suppressing inflammation, preserving and maximizing function, preventing deformity, and preventing blindness. **Nonsteroidal antiinflammatory drugs** are often the first choice in the treatment of JIA. Naproxen, sulindac, ibuprofen, indomethacin, and others have been used successfully. Systemic corticosteroid medications, such as prednisone and prednisolone, should be avoided in all but the most extreme circumstances, such as for severe systemic JIA with internal organ involvement or for significant

TABLE **90.2** Comparison of Juvenile Idiopathic Arthritis and Enthesitis-Related Arthritis

CLINICAL MANIFESTATIONS	JIA	JAS	PSA	IBD
Gender predominance	F > M	M > F	Equal	Equal
Peripheral arthritis	+++	+	++	+
Back symptoms	–	+++	+	++
Family history	–	++	++	+
ANA positivity	++	–	–	–
HLA-B27 positivity	–	++	–	+
RF or anti-CCP antibody positivity	+ (in late-onset JIA)	–	–	–
Extraarticular manifestations	Systemic symptoms (systemic JIA)	Enthesopathy	Psoriasis, nail changes	Bowel symptoms
Eye disease	Anterior uveitis, iritis	Iritis	Posterior uveitis	Anterior uveitis

ANA, Antinuclear antibody; *CCP,* cyclic citrullinated peptide; *HLA,* human leukocyte antigen; *IBD,* inflammatory bowel disease; *JAS,* juvenile ankylosing spondylitis; *JIA,* juvenile idiopathic arthritis; *PSA,* psoriatic arthritis; *RF,* rheumatoid factor.

TABLE 90.3 Differential Diagnoses of Juvenile Arthritis

CONNECTIVE TISSUE DISEASES
Juvenile idiopathic arthritis Systemic lupus erythematosus Juvenile dermatomyositis Scleroderma with arthritis
INFECTIOUS ARTHRITIS
Bacterial arthritis Viral arthritis Fungal arthritis Lyme disease
REACTIVE ARTHRITIS
Poststreptococcal arthritis Rheumatic fever Toxic synovitis Immunoglobulin A (IgA) vasculitis Postinfectious arthritis
ORTHOPEDIC DISORDERS
Traumatic arthritis Legg-Calve-Perthes disease Slipped capital femoral epiphysis Osteochondritis dissecans Chondromalacia patellae
MUSCULOSKELETAL PAIN SYNDROMES
Growing pains Hypermobility syndromes Myofascial pain syndromes/fibromyalgia Complex regional pain syndrome
HEMATOLOGIC/ONCOLOGIC DISORDERS
Leukemia Lymphoma Sickle cell disease Thalassemia Malignant and benign tumors of bone, cartilage, or synovium Metastatic bone disease Hemophilia
MISCELLANEOUS
Rickets/metabolic bone disease Lysosomal storage diseases Heritable disorders of collagen

active arthritis leading to functional disability. In this circumstance, the corticosteroids are used as *bridging therapy* until other medications take effect. For patients with isolated inflamed joints, intraarticular corticosteroids may be helpful at any point in the treatment course.

Methotrexate, preferably given subcutaneously, has become the drug of choice for polyarticular JIA (which may not respond to baseline agents alone) and for oligoarticular patients who do not respond to standard therapy and have high disease activity with risk factors for poor prognosis. Methotrexate can cause bone marrow suppression and hepatotoxicity; regular monitoring can minimize these risks. Leflunomide, with a similar adverse effect profile to methotrexate, has also been used. *Biologic agents* that inhibit TNFα and block the inflammatory cascade, including **etanercept**, **infliximab**, **adalimumab** and **golimumab**, are effective in the treatment of JIA and are superior to methotrexate in the spondyloarthropathy group. **Abatacept** blocks co-stimulation of T cells and is approved for polyarticular juvenile arthritis. **Tofacitinib**, a Janus kinase inhibitor, is an oral therapy approved for polyarticular juvenile arthritis. **Anakinra**, an interleukin 1 (IL-1) receptor antagonist, **canakinumab**, an IL-1β monoclonal antibody, and **tocilizumab** and **sarilumab**, monoclonal antibodies to the IL-6 receptor, are very beneficial and are recommended as the initial treatment for systemic JIA.

COMPLICATIONS

Complications with JIA result primarily from the loss of function of an involved joint secondary to contractures, bony fusion, or loss of joint space. Physical and occupational therapies, professionally and through home programs, are crucial to preserve and maximize function. More serious complications arise from associated uveitis; if left untreated, it can lead to blindness.

A very serious complication of systemic JIA, **macrophage activation syndrome** (MAS), has received increasing recognition. Occurring in 10–30% of systemic JIA patients, MAS can be seen in the context of overwhelming inflammation, which leads to activation of proliferation of T lymphocytes and macrophages, resulting in overwhelming release of proinflammatory cytokines. The patient develops high fevers, hepatosplenomegaly, lymphadenopathy, and a bleeding diathesis. Laboratory studies reveal pancytopenia, elevated ferritin, transaminases, and triglycerides, as well as elevated soluble CD25. There is evidence of disseminated intravascular coagulation with low fibrinogen, increased D-dimer, and abnormal blood smear. Bone marrow sampling may identify mature macrophages displaying *hemophagocytic activity*. MAS can lead to multisystem organ failure. Even with early detection and aggressive treatment, mortality rates for MAS approximate 8–20%.

PROGNOSIS

The prognosis of JIA can be excellent if diagnosed early and treated appropriately. Remission rates vary depending on the subtype. Children with oligoarticular JIA uniformly tend to do well; children with polyarticular disease and systemic disease constitute most children with functional disability. Systemic disease, a positive rheumatoid factor or anti-CCP antibody, poor response to therapy, and the presence of bony erosions on x-ray all connote a poorer prognosis. The importance of physical and occupational therapy cannot be overstated; when the disease remits, the physical limitations remain with the patient into adulthood.

PEARLS FOR PRACTITIONERS

See Rheumatic Diseases of Childhood: Pearls for Practitioners at the end of this section.

REVIEW QUESTIONS

Available online.

CHAPTER 91

Childhood-Onset Systemic Lupus Erythematosus

ETIOLOGY

Systemic lupus erythematosus (SLE) is a multisystem disorder of unknown etiology characterized by a production of large amounts of *circulating autoantibodies.* This antibody production may be due to loss of T-lymphocyte control on B-lymphocyte activity, leading to hyperactivity of B lymphocytes, which leads to nonspecific and specific antibody and autoantibody production. The antibodies form immune complexes that become trapped in the microvasculature, leading to inflammation and ischemia. Monogenic defects in complement (C1q, C2, C4) or genes in the interferon production pathway *(IFIH1, IRF5, STAT4)* are responsible for only a small percentage of patients with SLE; the majority of SLE is polygenic, with both genetic and environmental influence.

EPIDEMIOLOGY

SLE affects primarily females, with 65% having disease onset between the ages of 16–55 and 10–20% before the age of 16. SLE is rare in children younger than 5 years of age. Although there is a female predominance of this disease in adolescence and adulthood, there is an equal gender distribution in children <5 years of age. The overall prevalence of SLE in the pediatric population ranges from 1.89 to 25.7 per 100,000 children and is highest among non-Whites.

CLINICAL MANIFESTATIONS

Patients with SLE can present either in an abrupt fashion with fulminant disease or in an indolent manner (Tables 91.1 and 91.2). Nonspecific symptoms can be quite profound; significant fatigue and malaise, low-grade fever, and weight loss are common.

Skin disease may be a prominent finding, occurring in up to 90% of patients. **Acute cutaneous lupus** can present as a raised, erythematous rash on the cheeks, called a *malar butterfly rash,* and is a common clinical manifestation (Fig. 91.1). The rash can also occur across the bridge of the nose, on the forehead, and on the chin but spares the nasolabial folds. **Photosensitivity** can be problematic, particularly during summer months. Both rashes improve with appropriate therapy. **Chronic cutaneous lupus** presents as **discoid lupus**, an inflammatory process that disrupts the dermal-epidermal junction, resulting in permanent scarring and loss of pigmentation in the affected area. Discoid lupus is less common in children. If discoid lupus occurs in the scalp, permanent alopecia ensues because of loss of hair follicles. **Alopecia** and **Raynaud phenomenon** may occur, although these are not specific for SLE. **Livedo reticularis** also can occur.

Mouth and nasal sores from mucosal ulceration are a common complaint and can lead to ulceration and perforation of the nasal septum. Due to reticuloendothelial system stimulation, lymphadenopathy and splenomegaly are common findings. Axillary lymphadenopathy can be a sensitive indicator of SLE activity. Serositis can present with chest pain, pleural or pericardial friction rubs, or frank effusion.

Kidney involvement is one of the most serious manifestations of SLE and is common in pediatric SLE, occurring in 20–80% of children. Kidney disease may range from microscopic proteinuria or hematuria to gross hematuria, nephrotic syndrome, and kidney failure. Hypertension or the presence of edema suggests lupus nephritis.

Arthralgias and arthritis are common. The arthritis is rarely deforming and involves the small joints of the hands; any joint may be involved. Myalgias or frank myositis, with muscle weakness and muscle fatigability, may occur. SLE can affect the central nervous system (CNS), leading to a myriad of symptoms ranging from poor school performance and difficulty concentrating to seizures, psychosis, and stroke.

LABORATORY AND IMAGING STUDIES

Testing for SLE is performed to establish the diagnosis, determine prognosis, and monitor response to therapy. Although nonspecific, a positive **antinuclear antibody** is found in more than 99% of patients with SLE, usually at high titers. Because of its high sensitivity, a negative antinuclear antibody has a high negative predictive value for SLE. The presence of **antibodies**

TABLE 91.1 SLICC Criteria for Diagnosis of SLE*

PHYSICAL SIGNS
Acute cutaneous lupus Chronic cutaneous lupus Nonscarring alopecia Oral or nasopharyngeal ulcers Joint disease (two or more joints with effusion and tenderness or tenderness in two or more joints with 30 minutes of morning stiffness) Pleuritis, ascites, or pericarditis (serositis) Seizures or psychosis in absence of metabolic toxins or drugs
LABORATORY DATA
Kidney Disease (Nephritis)
Proteinuria (>500 mg/24 hr) or cellular casts (RBC, granular, or tubular)
Hematologic Disease
Hemolytic (autoimmune) anemia with reticulocytosis Leukopenia (<4,000/mm^3 at least once) or lymphopenia (<1,000/mm^3 at least once) Thrombocytopenia (<100,000/mm^3)
SEROLOGIC DATA
Positive anti-dsDNA Positive anti-Sm Antiphospholipid antibodies (positive lupus anticoagulant; medium- or high-titer IgA, IgG, or IgM anticardiolipin antibodies; or positive anti-beta 2 glycoprotein I [IgA, IgG, or IgM]) Direct Coombs in the absence of hemolytic anemia Low complement (low C3, low C4, OR low CH50) Positive ANA above laboratory reference range

These are the 2012 SLICC criteria for diagnosing SLE. A patient must have 4 of the 17 criteria, including 1 clinical criterion and 1 immunologic criterion, or biopsy-proven lupus nephritis, to establish the diagnosis of SLE. Criteria are cumulative and need not be present concurrently. Additional, less specific diagnostic manifestations are noted in Table 91.2.

ANA, Antinuclear antibody; *dsDNA,* double-stranded DNA; *Ig,* immunoglobulin; *RBC,* red blood cell; *SLE,* systemic lupus erythematosus; *SLICC,* Systemic Lupus International Collaborating Clinics; *Sm,* Smith.

TABLE 91.2 Additional Manifestations of Systemic Lupus Erythematosus

SYSTEMIC
Fever Malaise Weight loss Fatigue
MUSCULOSKELETAL
Myositis, myalgia Arthralgia
CUTANEOUS
Raynaud phenomenon Urticaria-angioedema Panniculitis Livedo reticularis
NEUROPSYCHIATRIC
Personality disorders Stroke Peripheral neuropathy Chorea Transverse myelitis Migraine headaches Depression
CARDIOPULMONARY
Endocarditis (noninfectious) Myocarditis Pneumonitis
OCULAR
Episcleritis Sicca syndrome Retinal cytoid bodies
GASTROINTESTINAL
Pancreatitis Mesenteric arteritis Serositis Hepatomegaly Hepatitis (chronic lupoid) Splenomegaly
KIDNEY
Nephritis Nephrosis Uremia Hypertension
REPRODUCTIVE
Repeat spontaneous abortions Neonatal lupus erythematosus Congenital heart block in fetus

to double-stranded DNA (dsDNA) should raise suspicion for SLE; these antibodies are present in most patients with SLE and are found almost exclusively in the disease. Titers of dsDNA antibodies are quantifiable and can vary with disease activity. Antibodies directed against Sm (Smith) are specific to SLE but are found in only approximately 30% of persons with SLE. Antibodies to Ro (SSA) and La (SSB) can also be found in patients with SLE but also occur in patients with Sjögren syndrome.

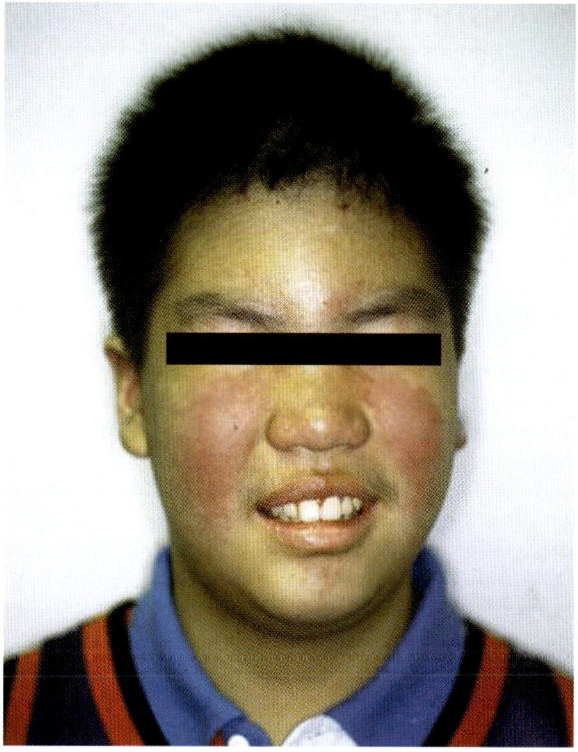

FIGURE 91.1 Malar butterfly rash on teenage male with systemic lupus erythematosus. Note erythema on cheeks and chin, sparing the nasolabial folds.

Patients with SLE may have antibodies directed against phospholipids, which also can be seen in other rheumatologic diseases and in primary antiphospholipid syndrome. These antibodies lead to an increased risk of arterial and venous thrombosis and can be detected by the presence of anticardiolipin antibodies, lupus anticoagulant, and/or beta-2 glycoprotein antibodies.

Hematologic abnormalities also are prevalent with SLE. Leukopenia, and specifically lymphopenia, is common. Thrombocytopenia and anemia of chronic disease may be found. Patients with SLE can develop a Coombs-positive autoimmune hemolytic anemia. Excessive antibody production can lead to polyclonal hypergammopathy, with an elevated globulin fraction in the serum. Excessive circulating antibodies and immune complexes also lead to the consumption of complement proteins, with low levels of C3 and C4 and decreased complement function as measured by CH50. Effective therapy returns the low complement levels to normal. This is one way to monitor therapy, except in patients with familial deficiency in complement components, which itself predisposes to SLE.

Urinalysis may show hematuria and proteinuria, identifying patients with lupus nephritis. Serum blood urea nitrogen and creatinine evaluate kidney function. Hypoalbuminemia and hypoproteinemia may be present due to leakage at the glomerular level. Elevation of muscle enzymes may be a clue for the presence of myositis. Elevated cerebrospinal fluid (CSF) protein and an elevated immunoglobulin (Ig)G-to-albumin ratio when comparing CSF with serum (IgG index) can indicate antibody production in the CSF and help diagnose SLE affecting the CNS. CNS lupus has a specific pattern on gadolinium-enhanced MRI.

DIFFERENTIAL DIAGNOSIS

As SLE is a multisystem disease, it can be difficult to diagnose early in the disease course. Suspicion must be high in patients who present with diffuse symptoms, particularly adolescent females. Clinical manifestations of SLE are found in other inflammatory or infectious diseases. Criteria have been developed for the diagnosis of SLE (see Table 91.1). The presence of 4 of 17 of these criteria has 94% sensitivity and 92% specificity for SLE.

TREATMENT

Corticosteroids have been the mainstay of treatment for SLE for decades. Initial use of pulse methylprednisolone and high-dose oral prednisone (up to 2 mg/kg) frequently is required, followed by cautious tapering to minimize recurrence of symptoms. **Nonsteroidal antiinflammatory drugs** have been used to treat the arthralgias and arthritis associated with SLE. **Hydroxychloroquine** is used not only for the treatment of lupus skin disease, such as discoid lupus, but as maintenance therapy. Hydroxychloroquine treatment results in longer periods of remission, reduces vascular complications, and improves dyslipidemia.

Corticosteroids and hydroxychloroquine frequently are not sufficient therapies for lupus nephritis or cerebritis. Both **mycophenolate mofetil** and **cyclophosphamide** are effective for the most severe forms of lupus nephritis, with significant improvements in outcome and decreased rates of progression to kidney failure. **Azathioprine** also has a role in the treatment of lupus nephritis due to the improved side effect profile compared to cyclophosphamide. CNS lupus responds to cyclophosphamide. For patients who are not able to tolerate the tapering of corticosteroids, the use of steroid-sparing agents, such as azathioprine, methotrexate, or mycophenolate mofetil, may be indicated. Biologic therapies such as **belimumab** have been approved for children >5 years of age with SLE to treat musculoskeletal, cutaneous, cardiac, and renal manifestations. **Rituximab** and **intravenous immunoglobulin (IVIG)** can be used to treat hematologic manifestations.

Patients with SLE should be counseled to wear sun block and avoid sun exposure because exposure to the sun precipitates flares of the disease. Because of this prohibition, patients benefit from calcium and vitamin D supplementation to reduce the risk of osteoporosis that may result from prolonged corticosteroid use. Early treatment of hyperlipidemia to decrease long-term cardiovascular complications is also indicated.

COMPLICATIONS

Long-term complications include avascular bone necrosis secondary to corticosteroid use, infections, and myocardial infarction. Patients with SLE develop accelerated atherosclerosis, not only from prolonged corticosteroid use but also due to the underlying chronic inflammation. All patients with SLE should be counseled regarding their weight and maintaining an active lifestyle to reduce other cardiac risk factors.

PROGNOSIS

Outcomes for SLE have improved significantly over the past several decades and depend largely on the organ systems that are involved. Worse prognoses are seen in patients with severe lupus nephritis or cerebritis, with risk of chronic disability or progression to kidney failure. Due to advances in therapy for the disease and the success of kidney transplantation, most patients live well into adulthood.

PEARLS FOR PRACTITIONERS

See Rheumatic Diseases of Childhood: Pearls for Practitioners at the end of this section.

REVIEW QUESTIONS

Available online.

CHAPTER 92

Juvenile Dermatomyositis

ETIOLOGY

Juvenile dermatomyositis (JDM) is an idiopathic inflammatory myopathy of unknown etiology. It is thought to involve type I interferon pathway dysregulation, including activation of T and B lymphocytes, production of autoantibodies, vasculopathy affecting small vessels, and subsequent inflammation, particularly of the muscle and skin. Environmental factors such as infections or sun exposure in genetically susceptible children may contribute to JDM.

EPIDEMIOLOGY

JDM is a rare disease, with an incidence of approximately 3.2 per million children. JDM can occur in all age groups with a peak incidence of approximately 7 years of age. The disease is more common in females than males.

CLINICAL MANIFESTATIONS

JDM presentation is variable and may be insidious or acute. Patients may have constitutional symptoms including fatigue, malaise, and fevers.

The muscle disease of JDM primarily affects the proximal muscles, particularly the limb girdles, core, and neck muscles. Children have difficulty raising their arms, climbing steps, getting out of chairs, and getting off the floor. The patient may have a positive **Gower sign**. In severe cases, the patient is not able to sit up from a supine position or even lift the head off the examination table. If muscles of the upper airway and pharynx are involved, the patient may have a nasal voice, difficulty swallowing, and respiratory symptoms.

JDM is characterized by several classic rashes. A **malar** or erythematous rash can occur on the face and across the cheeks; the erythematous **shawl sign** can be found on the posterior neck, shoulders, and back; and the erythematous V sign can be found on the anterior neck and upper chest. Patients may have a violaceous **heliotrope rash** (Fig. 92.1) of the eyelids. Scaly, erythematous **Gottron papules** (Fig. 92.2) (may also be patches or plaques) are classically found across the knuckles but can be found on the extensor surfaces of other joints.

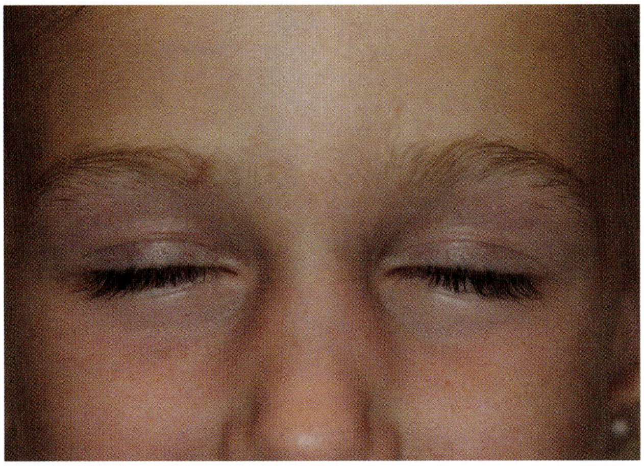

FIGURE 92.1 Heliotrope rash. (From Pilkington CA, Feldman BM, Sontichai W. Juvenile dermatomyositis and other inflammatory muscle diseases. In: Petty RE, Laxer RM, Lindsley CB, et al., eds. *Textbook of Pediatric Rheumatology.* 8th ed. Philadelphia: Elsevier; 2021:Fig. 26.2.)

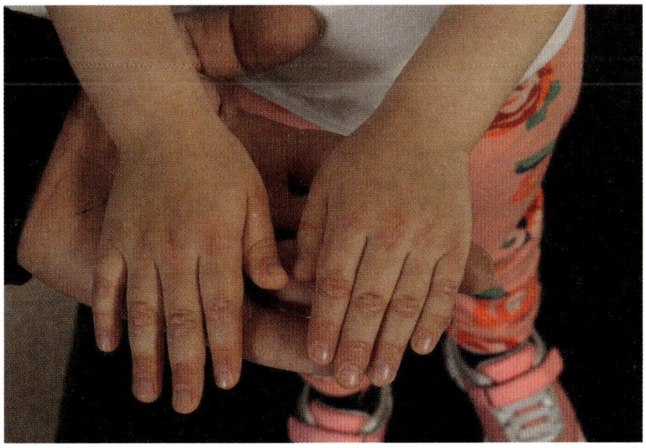

FIGURE 92.2 Gottron papules over metacarpophalangeal and interphalangeal joints. (From Pilkington CA, Feldman BM, Sontichai W. Juvenile dermatomyositis and other inflammatory muscle diseases. In: Petty RE, Laxer RM, Lindsley CB, et al., eds. *Textbook of Pediatric Rheumatology.* 8th ed. Philadelphia: Elsevier; 2021:Fig. 26.3.)

Patients may have periungual erythema and swelling with **abnormal nailfold capillaries** (Fig. 92.3). Less commonly, patients develop cutaneous vasculitis, with inflammation, erythema, and skin breakdown.

Patients with JDM can also develop arthritis, Raynaud phenomenon, and cardiac, pulmonary, and gastrointestinal involvement.

LABORATORY AND IMAGING STUDIES

Patients with active JDM may have no evidence of systemic inflammation (normal blood counts, erythrocyte sedimentation rate [ESR], and C-reactive protein [CRP]). Evidence of myositis can be identified in most children with active JDM by elevated serum muscle enzymes, including aspartate aminotransferase, alanine aminotransferase, creatine kinase, aldolase, and lactate dehydrogenase. Myositis-specific antibodies can identify subsets of JDM patients with shared clinical features to possibly predict phenotypes and outcomes. Evidence of inflammatory myositis can also be found on electromyography and muscle biopsy, which are both invasive procedures. Noncontrast MRI (pelvic and thigh) is a noninvasive means of demonstrating muscle inflammation.

DIFFERENTIAL DIAGNOSIS

Diagnosis of JDM is based on the presence of documented muscle inflammation in the setting of classic rash (Table 92.1). If the patient has muscle disease without skin manifestations, a muscle biopsy should be obtained to exclude other causes of muscle weakness such as muscular dystrophy (particularly in males) or polymyositis. The differential diagnoses include other idiopathic inflammatory myopathies, overlap myositis with other connective tissue diseases, infectious or postinfectious myositis, noninflammatory myopathies (see Chapter 183), and malignancy-associated myositis.

TREATMENT

Methotrexate, supplemented by **systemic corticosteroids**, is the cornerstone of treatment for JDM. Initial steroid therapy is high dose oral prednisone or pulse intravenous methylprednisolone followed by several months of tapering oral prednisone. Early initiation of methotrexate as a steroid-sparing agent significantly decreases the duration of corticosteroid use and its associated toxicities. **Intravenous immunoglobulin** can provide significant benefit as an adjunctive therapy. In severe or refractory cases, it may be necessary to use cyclosporine, mycophenolate mofetil, azathioprine, tacrolimus, cyclophosphamide, or biologic agents. **Hydroxychloroquine** has been used for the skin manifestations without significant muscle disease. Exposure to the sun worsens the cutaneous manifestations and exacerbates the muscle disease. Patients should be advised to wear sunblock and refrain from prolonged sun exposure to avoid disease flares. Supplementation with calcium and active forms of vitamin D is also indicated, particularly with steroid treatment. Physical and occupational therapies are encouraged.

COMPLICATIONS

Rare but serious complications of JDM that can lead to mortality include gastrointestinal vasculopathy and interstitial lung disease. Another serious complication of JDM is the development of **calcinosis**. Dystrophic calcification can occur in the skin, muscles, and soft tissues and ranges from mild to extensive (calcinosis universalis). Calcinosis can lead to ulceration, joint contractures, and pain. Although it is difficult to predict who will develop calcinosis, it occurs more commonly in children with prolonged disease activity or delays in diagnosis and onset of therapy. JDM has been associated with lipodystrophy with metabolic abnormalities such as hyperlipidemia, insulin resistance, and diabetes.

PROGNOSIS

The outcome of JDM depends greatly on the extent of muscle disease and the time between disease onset and initiation of therapy. JDM follows one of three clinical courses: a monophasic course, in which patients are treated and improve without significant sequelae; a chronic recurrent course; or a chronic progressive course marked by poor response to therapy and resulting loss of function. Patients who ultimately develop

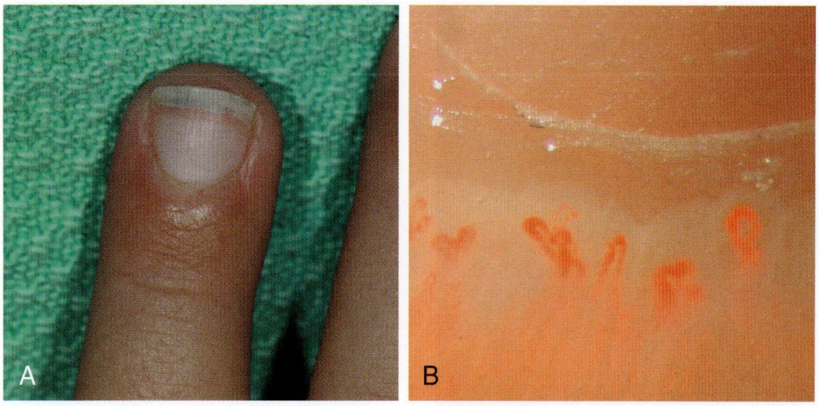

FIGURE 92.3 **(A)** Abnormal nailfold capillary pattern with the classic changes of dermatomyositis. **(B)** Capillary dropout, enlargement, and tortuosity. (From Pilkington CA, Feldman BM, Sontichai W. Juvenile dermatomyositis and other inflammatory muscle diseases. In: Petty RE, Laxer RM, Lindsley CB, et al., eds. *Textbook of Pediatric Rheumatology.* 8th ed. Philadelphia: Elsevier; 2021:Fig. 26.7.)

TABLE **92.1** Criteria for Diagnosis of Juvenile Dermatomyositis*

Cutaneous findings typical of dermatomyositis (Gottron signs, heliotrope rash)
Symmetric proximal muscle weakness
Elevated serum muscle enzymes (ALT, AST, LDH, CK, and aldolase)
EMG abnormalities typical of inflammatory myositis
Muscle biopsy typical of inflammatory myositis

**To make a definitive diagnosis of dermatomyositis, the patient must have typical cutaneous findings and three of the additional criteria.*
ALT, Alanine aminotransferase; *AST,* aspartate aminotransferase; *CK,* creatine kinase; *EMG,* electromyography; *LDH,* lactate dehydrogenase.

calcinosis are at risk for chronic loss of mobility, depending on the extent of calcium deposition. The association of dermatomyositis with malignancy is uncommon with childhood disease.

PEARLS FOR PRACTITIONERS

See Rheumatic Diseases of Childhood: Pearls for Practitioners at the end of this section.

REVIEW QUESTIONS

Available online.

CHAPTER 93
Musculoskeletal Pain Syndromes

GROWING PAINS

Growing pains, or benign musculoskeletal pains of childhood, occur in up to 37% of school-age children. The peak age range is 3–12 years, and it is more common in males than females. There is no known etiology, although there appears to be a familial predisposition.

Children with growing pains complain of deep, crampy pain in the legs that is not centered in the joints. The pain occurs in the evening or as nocturnal pain that occasionally can awaken the child from sleep. Growing pains tend to be more common in children who are extremely active; bouts are exacerbated by increased physical activity. The physical examination is unremarkable, with no evidence of arthritis, muscular tenderness, or weakness. Laboratory studies or x-rays, if performed, are normal.

The diagnosis of growing pains is based on a typical history and a normal physical examination. It is important to consider leukemia as a cause of nocturnal leg pain in children of this age group, and a complete blood count should be considered.

The treatment of growing pains consists of reassurance and a regular bedtime ritual of stretching and relaxation. The pain can be relieved by massage. Some patients may benefit from a nighttime dose of acetaminophen or an analgesic dose of a nonsteroidal antiinflammatory drug (NSAID). Occasionally, nocturnal awakening is of long duration, leading to disruptive behavior patterns. In these cases, intervention must be aimed at decreasing the secondary gain associated with nighttime parental attention and should focus on sleep hygiene. Other than the negative behavioral patterns that can occur, there are no significant complications. Growing pains are not associated with other illnesses and resolve over time.

BENIGN HYPERMOBILITY

Hypermobility syndromes are disorders that cause musculoskeletal pain secondary to excessive mobility of joints. These disorders most commonly present in children 3–10 years of age. Females are more commonly affected than males and there is a familial predisposition to some hypermobility syndromes. Specific diseases causing hypermobility include Marfan syndrome, homocystinuria, Stickler syndrome, Ehlers-Danlos syndromes, osteogenesis imperfecta, Williams syndrome, and trisomy 21. Most children with hypermobility do not have an identifiable associated syndrome or disease.

Hypermobility can be isolated to a specific joint group or can present as a generalized disorder. Symptoms vary depending on the joints involved. The most consistent symptom is pain, which may occur during the day or night. The discomfort increases after exertion and can interfere with physical activity. Children with hypermobility of the ankles or feet may complain of chronic leg or back pain.

Joint hypermobility may be quite marked. Range of motion may be exaggerated, with excessive flexion or extension at the metacarpophalangeal joints, wrists, elbows, or knees *(genu recurvatum)* (Fig. 93.1). There may be excessive pronation of the ankles. Hypermobility of the foot (flat foot; *pes planus*) is shown by the presence of a longitudinal arch of the foot that disappears with weight bearing and may be associated with a shortened Achilles tendon. These findings are rarely associated with tenderness on examination. No laboratory test abnormalities are apparent, and radiographs of affected joints are normal.

The diagnosis of isolated hypermobility is made through physical examination with demonstration of exaggerated mobility of a joint. Generalized hypermobility is diagnosed by the presence of sufficient criteria (Table 93.1) and the absence of evidence of other underlying disorders. Excessive skin elasticity, easy bruisability, or mitral valve prolapse suggests **Ehlers-Danlos syndrome** or **Marfan syndrome** rather than benign hypermobility.

The treatment of hypermobility consists of reassurance and regular stretching. NSAIDs can be administered as needed but do not need to be prescribed on a regular basis. Arch supports can be helpful in children with symptomatic pes planus but are not indicated in the absence of symptoms. Patients benefit from formal physical therapy and conditioning exercises. Benign hypermobility tends to improve with increasing age and is not associated with long-term complications.

TABLE 93.1 Criteria for Hypermobility

MODIFIED CRITERIA OF CARTER AND WILKINSON
Three of Five Are Required to Establish a Diagnosis of Hypermobility
• Touch thumb to volar forearm • Hyperextend metacarpophalangeal joints so fingers parallel forearm • >10-degree angle hyperextension of elbows • >10-degree angle hyperextension of knees • Touch palms to floor with knees straight
BEIGHTON SCALE

• ≥6 points defines hypermobility:
  • Touch thumb to volar forearm (one point each for right and left)
  • Extend fifth metacarpophalangeal joint to 90-degree angle (one point each for right and left)
  • >10-degree angle hyperextension of elbow (one point each for right and left)
  • >10-degree angle hyperextension of knee (one point each for right and left)
  • Touch palms to floor with knees straight (one point)

Other Noncriteria Features of Many Children With Hypermobility
• Put heel behind head • Excessive internal rotation to hip • Excessive ankle dorsiflexion • Excessive eversion of the foot • Passively touch elbows behind the back

Data from Carter C, Wilkins J. Persistent joint laxity and congenital dislocation of the hip. J Bone Joint Surg Br. *1964;46:40–45.*

MYOFASCIAL PAIN SYNDROMES AND FIBROMYALGIA

The myofascial pain syndromes are a group of noninflammatory disorders characterized by diffuse musculoskeletal pain, the presence of multiple *tender points*, fatigue, malaise, and poor sleep patterns. The etiology of these disorders is unknown, although there seems to be a familial predisposition. Although these disorders sometimes follow viral infection or trauma, there is no definitive causal relationship. Myofascial pain syndromes are uncommon in children <12 years of age and are seen more frequently in females than in males. The prevalence of fibromyalgia in children is 1–6%.

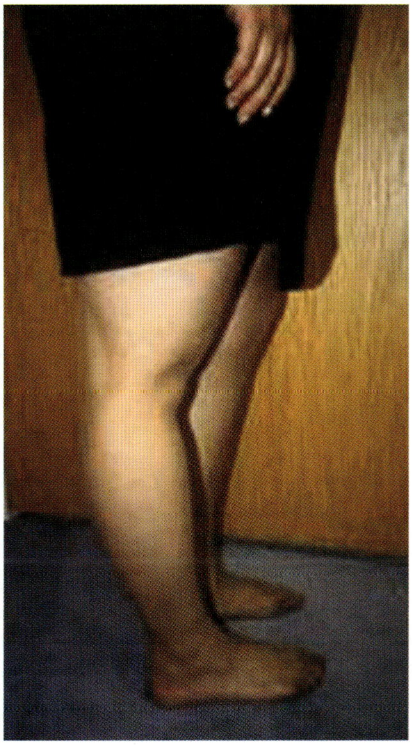

FIGURE 93.1 Hyperextension of the knees—an example of hypermobility.

Patients with myofascial pain syndromes complain of longstanding diffuse pain in muscles and in the soft tissues around joints that can occur at any time of day, awaken the patient from sleep, and interfere with regular activities. There is frequently a high degree of school absenteeism, despite maintaining adequate school performance. A significant percentage of patients with myofascial pain syndromes exhibit symptoms consistent with anxiety and depression. Stressful life events, family dysfunction, and emotional, physical, or sexual abuse may precede these conditions.

Physical examination is unremarkable except for the presence of specific points that are painful—not just tender—to digital palpation. Pain is often out of proportion with the exam, and patients will report significant pain without other physical clues. There is no evidence of arthritis or muscular weakness. Some patients experience postural autonomic dysfunction and others report disordered thinking or "brain fog."

Patients with myofascial pain syndromes frequently undergo extensive medical testing due to concern for underlying inflammatory disease. These tests are normal other than a clinically insignificant positive antinuclear antibody, which is found in up to 20% of the normal pediatric population.

The diagnosis of myofascial pain syndrome is based on the presence of multiple tender points in the absence of other illness. To fulfill strict criteria for a diagnosis of fibromyalgia, the patient must have a history of diffuse pain for at least 3 months, the presence of multiple pain sites, and an elevated symptom profile as measured by formal instruments. It is important to exclude underlying inflammatory diseases, such as systemic lupus erythematosus, or the postinfectious fatigue that characteristically follows Epstein-Barr virus and influenza virus infection. Mood and somatic symptom related disorders also should be considered.

Treatment consists of pain control and restoration of function. Physical therapy, psychologic therapy, development of coping mechanisms, and education about sleep hygiene and the concept of the pain response system are all highly valuable interventions. Patients may require medications, such as amitriptyline to regulate sleep or gabapentin to reduce pain sensitivity. Due to the disability associated with myofascial pain syndromes, patients and parents frequently believe that the child has a serious underlying condition that makes education and reassurance crucial. It should be emphasized that there is no simple cure, and time and perseverance are required.

The long-term outcomes in the myofascial pain syndromes vary. Patients and families who focus on therapy and are positive in their approach tend to have better outcomes. Patients who pursue prolonged evaluations, especially from multiple health care providers, may do more poorly.

PEARLS FOR PRACTITIONERS

See Rheumatic Diseases of Childhood: Pearls for Practitioners at the end of this section.

REVIEW QUESTIONS

Available online.

Suggested Readings

Barut K, Sahin S, Kasapcopur O. Pediatric vasculitis. *Curr Opin Rheumatol.* 2016;28(1):29–38.

Cattalini M, Khubchandani R, Cimaz R. When flexibility is not necessarily a virtue: a review of hypermobility syndromes and chronic or recurrent musculoskeletal pain in children. *Pediatr Rheumatol Online J.* 2015;13(1):40.

Couture J, Silverman ED. Update on the pathogenesis and treatment of childhood-onset systemic lupus erythematosus. *Curr Opin Rheumatol.* 2016;28(5):488–496.

Giancane G, Consolaro A, Lanni S, Davì S, Schiappapietra B, Ravelli A. Juvenile Idiopathic Arthritis: Diagnosis and Treatment. *Rheumatol Ther.* 2016;3(2):187–207.

Henderson LA, Canna SW, Friedman KG, et al. American College of Rheumatology Clinical Guidance for Multisystem Inflammatory Syndrome in Children Associated With SARS-CoV-2 and Hyperinflammation in Pediatric COVID-19: Version 3. *Arthritis Rheumatol.* 2022;74(4):e1–e20.

Jone PN, Tremoulet A, Choueiter N, et al.; American Heart Association Rheumatic Fever, Endocarditis, and Kawasaki Disease Committee of the Council on Lifelong Congenital Heart Disease and Heart Health in the Young; Council on Cardiovascular and Stroke Nursing; Council on Cardiovascular Radiology and Intervention; and Council on Clinical Cardiology. Update on Diagnosis and Management of Kawasaki Disease: A Scientific Statement From the American Heart Association. *Circulation.* 2024;150(23):e481–e500. Erratum in: *Circulation.* 2025;151(8):e677–e679. Erratum in: *Circulation.* 2025;151(13):e863.

Lundberg IE, Tjärnlund A, Bottai M, et al. 2017 European League Against Rheumatism/American College of Rheumatology classification criteria for adult and juvenile idiopathic inflammatory myopathies and their major subgroups. *Ann Rheum Dis.* 2017;76(12):1955–1964. [published correction appears in Ann Rheum Dis. 2018;77(9):e64].

McCrindle BW, Rowley AH, Newburger JW, et al. Diagnosis, Treatment, and Long-Term Management of Kawasaki Disease: A Scientific Statement for Health Professionals From the American Heart Association. *Circulation.* 2017;135(17):e927–e999 [published correction appears in Circulation. 2019;140(5):e181–e184].

Rider LG, Nistala K. The juvenile idiopathic inflammatory myopathies: pathogenesis, clinical and autoantibody phenotypes, and outcomes. *J Intern Med.* 2016;280(1):24–38.

Thakral A, Klein-Gitelman MS. An Update on Treatment and Management of Pediatric Systemic Lupus Erythematosus. *Rheumatol Ther.* 2016;3(2):209–219.

Zhu FH, Ang JY. The Clinical Diagnosis and Management of Kawasaki Disease: a Review and Update. *Curr Infect Dis Rep.* 2016;18(10):32.

PEARLS FOR PRACTITIONERS

CHAPTER 87

Rheumatic Assessment

- The hallmarks of rheumatic diseases of childhood are inflammation (localized or generalized) and autoimmunity.
- The differential diagnoses of rheumatologic disease include infections, postinfectious processes, and malignancy.
- The diagnosis of most rheumatologic diseases can be made from the history and physical exam in conjunction with carefully chosen confirmatory laboratory or radiologic tests.
- Enthesitis is inflammation at the insertion of a ligament to a bone such as at the heel.
- Vasculitis often results in a petechial or purpuric rash.
- Morning stiffness may be seen in rheumatologic disorders and is suggestive of inflammatory joint disease.
- Certain laboratory tests will reveal generalized inflammation, such as an elevated white blood cell or platelet count or an elevated ESR or CRP; they may also reveal anemia of chronic disease. Other laboratory tests, such as those that measure autoantibodies, are used to detect only specific disorders.

CHAPTER 88

Immunoglobulin A Vasculitis

- Immunoglobulin A vasculitis (IgAV) is a small vessel vasculitis with nonthrombocytopenic palpable purpura, which predominantly occur on the buttocks and lower extremities. Other features may include joint, gastrointestinal, and kidney involvement.
- Immunoglobulin A deposits are often present in skin and renal lesion biopsies with IgAV.
- The differential diagnoses of IgAV include other vasculitis syndromes, leukemia, and immune thrombocytopenic purpura.
- Treatment of IgAV is largely supportive; nonsteroidal anti-inflammatory drugs are used for arthritis in the absence of kidney involvement. In rare cases, such as gastrointestinal or kidney involvement, steroids are used with a prolonged taper.
- The prognosis of IgAV is excellent. Most cases of IgAV are monophasic and resolve within 3–4 weeks, but symptoms can recur. In rare cases, patients can develop severe, chronic kidney disease.

CHAPTER 89

Kawasaki Disease

- Kawasaki disease (KD) is a medium vessel vasculitis that most commonly affects children under the age of 5 years.
- KD has a triphasic course: acute, subacute, and convalescent.
  - The acute phase is characterized by at least 5 days of fever, followed by clinical symptoms including bilateral nonsuppurative conjunctivitis, mucosal changes, polymorphous rash, cervical lymphadenopathy >1.5 cm, swelling and/or edema of the hands and feet, and elevated inflammatory markers.
  - The subacute phase is noted by resolution of the fevers and periungual desquamation and has continued elevation of inflammatory markers including thrombocytosis.
  - The convalescent phase is characterized by the resolution of all clinical symptoms and development of dystrophic nails (Beau lines) and ends with normalization of laboratory studies.
- The most serious complication of KD is coronary artery aneurysms.
- The main treatment of KD is intravenous immunoglobulin (which reduces the incidence of coronary artery aneurysms from 20–25% to less than 5%) and aspirin.

CHAPTER 90

Juvenile Idiopathic Arthritis

- Juvenile idiopathic arthritis (JIA) is the most common rheumatologic disease of childhood and is classified into subtypes, including oligoarticular, polyarticular, systemic, juvenile psoriatic arthritis, and enthesitis-related arthritis (spondyloarthropathies).
- Chronic arthritis is characterized by gradual onset, morning stiffness and joint pain, swelling, and limitation of range of motion, either from pain or contracture. Due to the presence of active growth plates, patients also develop localized growth disturbance, which causes the ends of the surrounding bones to be longer and wider.
- Systemic JIA differs from the other subtypes of arthritis, as the presence of arthritis is preceded by a systemic inflammatory process characterized by high diurnal fever, rash, hepatosplenomegaly, and elevated inflammatory parameters.
- The goal of JIA treatment is to control inflammation and preserve joint function. Nonsteroidal antiinflammatory medications are often the first line of therapy, followed by methotrexate and biologic agents. Steroids are used sparingly as bridge therapy and should not be used for maintenance therapy.
- Long-term prognosis of JIA can be excellent if diagnosed early and treated appropriately. Higher rates of remission are seen in the oligoarticular group and are lowest in the systemic and polyarticular groups.
- The most common complication of JIA is uveitis. The uveitis is frequently asymptomatic until the point of visual loss and therefore the patient requires regular screening with a slit-lamp exam. All children with JIA are at increased risk for uveitis, but those with a positive antinuclear antibody are at even higher risk and need to be screened more often.
- The most severe complication of systemic JIA is macrophage activation syndrome (MAS), caused by massive release of cytokines with overwhelming inflammation, leading to pancytopenia, liver dysfunction, disseminated intravascular coagulation, and multiorgan failure. Even with appropriate treatment, mortality rates from MAS are approximately 8–20%.

CHAPTER 91

Childhood-Onset Systemic Lupus Erythematosus

- Systemic lupus erythematosus (SLE) is a multisystem disease characterized by large amounts of circulating autoantibodies that form immune complexes that become trapped in the microvasculature, leading to inflammation and ischemia.
- The most serious features of SLE are nephritis and central nervous system (CNS) involvement, which can lead to long-term morbidity. Other features include malar rash, discoid rash, photosensitivity, mucosal ulceration, arthritis, myositis, and hemolytic anemia.
- Diagnosis of SLE is made based on specific criteria, including screening with sensitive autoantibodies (antinuclear

antibody) and confirming diagnosis with specific autoantibodies (anti–double-stranded DNA antibody, anti-Smith antibody).

- Corticosteroids have been the mainstay of treatment for SLE. For more aggressive disease, including kidney or CNS disease, medications like cyclophosphamide, azathioprine, and mycophenolate mofetil may be used. In patients for whom steroids cannot be reduced, use of steroid-sparing agents such as methotrexate, mycophenolate mofetil, or azathioprine may be indicated.
- Long-term outcomes in SLE are determined primarily by the presence or absence of nephritis or neurologic involvement, with most patients living well into adulthood.

CHAPTER 92

Juvenile Dermatomyositis

- Juvenile dermatomyositis (JDM) is a rare disease characterized by inflammation of muscles and skin. Patients have muscle weakness, particularly in proximal muscle groups, which can develop slowly or in a fulminant fashion. Involvement of muscles of the upper airway can lead to difficulty phonating or swallowing. The skin disease is characterized by classic rashes including a facial malar rash, heliotrope discoloration of the eyelids, and scaly red papules on extensor surfaces (Gottron papules).
- Diagnosis of JDM is made by the presence of classic rash and evidence of myositis with three of the following four criteria: symmetric proximal muscle weakness, elevated serum muscle enzymes, muscle biopsy, and electromyography. MRI without contrast of the pelvis or thighs demonstrating muscle inflammation is also supportive of the diagnosis and is noninvasive.
- Treatment of JDM consists of an initial course of high-dose corticosteroids and a longer course of a steroid-sparing agent, most commonly methotrexate.
- Prognosis in JDM depends greatly on the extent of muscle disease and the time between disease onset and initiation of therapy. Patients may have a monophasic course, a chronic recurrent course, or a chronic progressive course.
- A complication of JDM is calcinosis. Dystrophic calcification can occur in the skin, muscles, and soft tissues and can range from mild to extensive. Treatment for calcinosis is challenging, and therapies are not consistently effective.

CHAPTER 93

Musculoskeletal Pain Syndromes

- Growing pains are common in pediatric patients, affecting up to 37% of school-age children. Children report deep aching pain in their legs, particularly at night, but have no evidence of underlying disease. Treatment is symptomatic, but other causes of nocturnal leg pain, particularly leukemia, should be excluded.
- Hypermobility syndromes can be either generalized (benign hypermobility, Ehlers-Danlos syndrome) or localized (pes planus). Beighton criteria are used to diagnose generalized hypermobility. Treatment is symptomatic and focused on stretching, joint protection, arch supports when appropriate, and nonsteroidal antiinflammatory drug therapy as needed.
- Myofascial pain syndromes, such as fibromyalgia, are characterized by diffuse musculoskeletal pain, tender points, and generalized malaise, fatigue, and poor sleep patterns. These syndromes are noninflammatory, and an underlying cause for the pain cannot be found. Comorbid anxiety and depression are common.
- The treatment of myofascial pain syndrome consists of pain control and restoration of function. Physical therapy, psychologic therapy, development of coping mechanisms and education about sleep hygiene and the concept of the pain response system are valuable interventions.

SECTION 16

INFECTIOUS DISEASES

Matthew P. Kronman | Yasaman Fatemi | Victoria J.L. Konold | Caitlin L. McGrath | Surabhi B. Vora

CHAPTER 94

Infectious Disease Assessment

Overlapping clinical symptoms caused by infectious and noninfectious illnesses make the diagnosis of some diseases difficult. Clinicians may be concerned that, untreated or inappropriately treated, a minor infection may progress to a life-threatening illness. Conversely, unnecessary treatment with antimicrobial agents may lead to emergence of antimicrobial-resistant organisms, antibiotic-associated diarrhea, or allergic reactions. Therefore accurate diagnosis of infection is critical to ensure the provision of specific treatment only as indicated and thereby reduce the unnecessary use of antibiotics.

A thorough patient assessment, including a detailed history, complete physical examination, and appropriate diagnostic testing, is the cornerstone of optimal care.

INITIAL DIAGNOSTIC EVALUATION

The ability to accurately diagnose specific infections begins with an understanding of the epidemiology: risk factors, including exposures to sick contacts or environmental risks (e.g., travel to endemic areas, zoonoses), and infection susceptibility related either to age (reflecting the maturity of the immune system) or to primary or secondary immunodeficiencies. Obtaining a thorough history and physical examination identifies most of these elements (Tables 94.1 and 94.2) and guides the appropriate use of other diagnostic tests.

Unique questions that help identify whether an infection is causing the patient's symptoms include a detailed environmental history (including sick contacts, travel, food, water, and animal exposure) (see Table 94.1). Certain infections are more common in specific geographic areas. For instance, many parasitic infections are more common in tropical climates. Certain fungal infections have specific geographic distribution (coccidioidomycosis in the Southwestern United States, blastomycosis in the Upper Midwest, and histoplasmosis in the Central United States). In other areas, fungal pneumonias are rare except in immunocompromised persons.

An immunization history is critical for determining susceptibility to vaccine-preventable diseases. Family history, especially unexpected deaths of infants, may suggest familial immunodeficiency (see Chapters 72 through 77). Localization of symptoms to a specific body site may narrow diagnostic possibilities (see Table 94.2).

A complete physical examination is essential to identify signs of infection, which may be systemic (e.g., fever and shock) or focal (e.g., swelling, erythema, tenderness, pain, and limitation of function). Many infectious diseases are associated with characteristic cutaneous signs (see Table 98.1). Accurate otolaryngologic examination is critical for diagnosing upper respiratory tract infections and otitis media, the most common childhood infectious diseases in the United States.

DIFFERENTIAL DIAGNOSIS

Fever does not always represent infection. Rheumatologic diseases, inflammatory bowel disease, Kawasaki disease, poisoning, periodic fever syndromes, and malignancy also may present with fever. *Children with overwhelming infection may be afebrile or hypothermic.* Common symptoms, such as bone pain or lymphadenopathy that suggest infection, may also be due to leukemia, lymphoma, juvenile idiopathic arthritis, or Kawasaki disease (see Chapters 89, 90, and 154). Acute mental status changes or focal neurologic impairment could be manifestations of infections (encephalitis, meningitis, or brain abscess) or noninfectious causes (trauma, brain or spinal

TABLE 94.1 Clues From the History for Risk of Infection
Season of year
Age
General health
Weight change
Fever—presence, duration, and pattern
Previous similar symptoms
Previous infections and other illnesses
Previous surgeries, dental procedures
Preceding trauma
Presence of outbreaks or epidemics in the community
Exposures to infected individuals
Exposures to farm or feral animals and pets
Exposures to ticks and mosquitoes
Sexual history, including possibility of sexual abuse
Illicit drug use
Transfusion of blood or blood products
Travel history
Daycare or school attendance
Sources of water and food (e.g., undercooked meat, unpasteurized dairy products)
Home sanitary facilities and hygiene
Pica
Exposure to soil-borne and water-borne organisms (e.g., swimming in brackish water)
Presence of foreign bodies (e.g., indwelling catheters, shunt, grafts)
Immunization history
Immunodeficiency (chemotherapy, acquired, congenital)
Current medications

TABLE 94.2 Localizing Manifestations of Infection

SITE	LOCALIZING SYMPTOMS	LOCALIZING SIGNS*
Eye	Eye pain, double vision, photophobia, conjunctival discharge	Periorbital erythema, periorbital edema, drainage, chemosis, limitation of extraocular movements
Ear	Ear pain, drainage	Red, bulging tympanic membrane, drainage from ear canal
Upper respiratory tract	Rhinorrhea, sore throat, cough, drooling, stridor, trismus, sinus pain, tooth pain, hoarse voice	Nasal congestion, pharyngeal erythema, enlarged tonsils with exudate, swollen red epiglottis, regional lymphadenopathy
Lower respiratory tract	Cough, chest pain, dyspnea, sputum production, cyanosis	Tachypnea, crackles, wheezing, localized diminished breath sounds, intercostal retractions
Gastrointestinal tract	Nausea, vomiting, diarrhea, abdominal pain (focal or diffuse), anorexia, weight loss	Hypoactive or hyperactive bowel sounds, abdominal tenderness (focal or generalized), hematochezia
Liver	Anorexia, vomiting, dark urine, light stools	Jaundice, hepatomegaly, hepatic tenderness, bleeding diatheses, coma
Genitourinary tract	Dysuria, frequency, urgency, flank or suprapubic pain, vaginal or urethral discharge	Costovertebral angle or suprapubic tenderness, cervical motion and adnexal tenderness, scrotal swelling and pain
Central nervous system	Lethargy, irritability, headache, neck stiffness, seizures	Nuchal rigidity, Kernig sign, Brudzinski sign, bulging fontanelle, focal neurologic deficits, altered mental status, coma
Cardiovascular	Dyspnea, palpitations, fatigue, exercise intolerance, chest pain	Tachycardia, hypotension, cardiomegaly, hepatomegaly, splenomegaly, crackles, petechiae, Osler nodes, Janeway lesions, Roth spots, new or change in murmur, distended neck veins, pericardial friction rub, muffled heart sounds
Musculoskeletal	Limp, bone pain, limited function (pseudoparalysis)	Local swelling, erythema, warmth, limited range of motion, point bone tenderness, joint line tenderness

**Fever usually accompanies infection as a systemic manifestation.*

tumors, inflammatory conditions, postinfectious sequelae, or impairment from toxic ingestions or inhalants). Many manifestations of mucosal allergy (rhinitis, diarrhea) may mimic common infectious diseases (see Chapter 78).

Some infections are prone to recurrence, especially if treatment is suboptimal (wrong antimicrobial or insufficient duration). Recurrent, severe, or unusual (opportunistic) infections suggest the possibility of immunodeficiency (see Chapters 72 and 126).

SCREENING TESTS

Laboratory diagnosis of infection includes determining the presence of a pathogen using Gram stain, various culture techniques, molecular microbiologic methods (e.g., polymerase chain reaction [PCR] or matrix-assisted laser desorption/ionization time of flight [MALDI-TOF]), and assessment of the immune response with antibody titers or skin testing. The **acute phase response** is a nonspecific metabolic and inflammatory response to infection, trauma, autoimmune disease, and some malignancies. **Acute phase reactants**, such as erythrocyte sedimentation rate, C-reactive protein, and procalcitonin, are commonly elevated during a bacterial infection but are not specific for infection and do not identify any specific infection. These tests can be used to monitor response to therapy.

A **complete blood count** is frequently obtained for evidence of infection. The initial response to infection, especially in children, is usually **leukocytosis** (increased number of circulating leukocytes) with an initial neutrophilic response to both bacterial and viral infections. With most viral infections, this response is transient and is followed quickly by a characteristic mononuclear response. In general, bacterial infections are associated with greater neutrophil counts than viral infections (Table 94.3). A **left shift** is an increase in the numbers of circulating immature cells of the neutrophil series, including band forms, metamyelocytes, and myelocytes. It indicates the rapid release of cells from the bone marrow and is characteristic of both the early stages of infection and, if sustained, bacterial infections. Transient lymphopenia at the beginning of illness and lasting 24–48 hours has been described with many viral infections. **Atypical lymphocytes** are mature T lymphocytes with larger, eccentrically placed, and indented nuclei classically seen with infectious mononucleosis caused by Epstein-Barr virus. Other infections associated with atypical lymphocytosis include cytomegalovirus infection, toxoplasmosis, viral hepatitis, rubella, roseola, mumps, and some drug reactions. **Eosinophilia** is characteristic of allergic diseases but may be seen with tissue-invasive multicellular parasites, such as the migration of the larval stages of parasites through skin, lung, connective tissue, and viscera. High-grade eosinophilia (>30% eosinophils, or a total eosinophil count >3,000/μL) frequently occurs during the muscle invasion phase of trichinellosis, the pulmonary phases of ascariasis, hookworm infection (eosinophilic pneumonia), and the hepatic and central nervous system phases of visceral larva migrans.

Other common screening tests include **urinalysis** for urinary tract infections, transaminases for liver inflammation,

TABLE 94.3 Differentiating Viral From Bacterial Infections

VARIABLE	VIRAL	BACTERIAL
Petechiae	Present	Present
Purpura	Rare	If severe
Leukocytosis	Uncommon*	Common
Left-shift (↑ bands)	Uncommon	Common
Neutropenia	Possible	Suggests overwhelming infection
↑ CRP	Common	Common
↑ TNF, IL-1, PAF	Uncommon	Common
↑ Procalcitonin	Unusual	Common
Meningitis (pleocytosis)	Lymphocytic†	Neutrophilic
Meningeal signs positive‡	Present	Present

**Some viruses such as adenovirus and herpes simplex may cause leukocytosis.*
†Early viral (enterovirus, arbovirus) meningitis initially may have a neutrophilic pleocytosis.
‡Nuchal rigidity, bulging fontanelle, Kernig sign, Brudzinski sign.
CRP, C-reactive protein; *IL,* interleukin; *PAF,* platelet-activating factor; *TNF,* tumor necrosis factor.

and **lumbar puncture** for evaluation of the cerebrospinal fluid if there is concern for meningitis or encephalitis (see Chapters 101 and 102). Various tests may help distinguish viral versus bacterial infection, but definitive diagnosis requires identifying the agent by culture or molecular means.

Cultures are the mainstay of diagnosis of many infections. **Blood cultures** are sensitive with sufficient volume and specific for bacteremia (when disregarding common contaminants), which may be primary or secondary to a focal infection (osteomyelitis, pyelonephritis, and endocarditis). Urine cultures are important to confirm urinary tract infection, which may be occult in young infants. Cultures can be obtained with lumbar puncture, aspiration, or biopsy of other fluid collections or abscesses. Specific types of cultures (bacterial, fungal, viral, or mycobacterial) are guided by the clinical presentation and history.

Antibiotics often are begun before a definitive diagnosis is established, complicating the ability to rely on subsequent cultures for microbiologic diagnosis (see Chapter 96). Although persistent or progressive symptoms, despite antibiotic treatment, may indicate the need to change the regimen, more frequently this indicates the need to stop all antibiotics to facilitate definitive diagnosis by obtaining appropriate cultures. Antibiotics should not be given before obtaining appropriate cultures unless there is a life-threatening situation (e.g., septic shock or increased intracranial pressure).

Rapid tests, such as antigen tests, are useful for preliminary diagnosis and are available for numerous bacterial, viral, fungal, and parasitic infections. **Serologic tests**, using enzyme-linked immunosorbent assay or Western blotting, showing an immunoglobulin M (IgM) response, high IgG titer, or seroconversion between acute and convalescent sera, also can be used for diagnosis. **Molecular tests**, such as **polymerase chain reaction** (PCR: nucleic acid amplification tests) for DNA or RNA, offer the specificity of culture, high sensitivity, and rapid results. PCR is the standard method of testing for viral and some bacterial infections; its limitation is the inability to do antibiotic sensitivity testing. Microbial cell free DNA, a form of metagenomic sequencing, is a culture-free method of detecting pathogens from blood. In addition, detection of bacterial (16S ribosomal RNA) or fungal (18S ribosomal RNA) pathogens can be performed on tissue.

DIAGNOSTIC IMAGING

The choice of diagnostic imaging modality should be based on the location of the findings and the differential diagnosis. **Plain x-rays** are useful initial tests for respiratory tract infections. **Ultrasonography** is a noninvasive, nonirradiating technique well suited to infants and children for imaging solid organs. It also is useful to identify soft tissue abscesses with lymphadenitis and to diagnose suppurative arthritis of the hip or other joints. **Computed tomography (CT)** and **magnetic resonance imaging (MRI)** allow characterization of lesions and precise anatomic localization and are the modalities of choice for the brain. CT shows greater bone detail, and MRI shows greater soft tissue detail. MRI is especially useful for diagnosis of osteomyelitis, myositis, and necrotizing fasciitis. High-resolution CT is useful for complicated chest infections. Judicious use of CT scans is important because of the long-term effects of radiation on children's health. CT or MRI is preferred for evaluation of intraabdominal infections. A voiding cystourethrogram may be used to evaluate for vesicoureteral reflux, a predisposing factor for upper urinary tract infections.

PEARLS FOR PRACTITIONERS

See Infectious Diseases: Pearls for Practitioners at the end of this section.

REVIEW QUESTIONS

Available online.

CHAPTER 95 Immunization and Prophylaxis

IMMUNIZATION

Childhood immunization has markedly reduced the impact of major infectious diseases. **Active immunization** induces immunity through the administration of all or part of a microorganism or a modified product of a microorganism (e.g., toxoid). **Passive immunization** involves administration of protective antibodies and includes transplacental transfer of maternal antibodies and the administration of preformed antibody, either as immunoglobulin or as monoclonal antibody.

Vaccinations may be with live-attenuated viruses (measles, mumps, rubella [MMR], varicella, nasal influenza, oral polio, rotavirus), inactivated or killed viruses (intramuscular polio, hepatitis A, intramuscular influenza), recombinant products (hepatitis B, human papillomavirus, respiratory syncytial virus), messenger RNA or mRNA-based (SARS-CoV-2) or immunogenic components of bacteria (pertussis, *Haemophilus influenzae* type b, *Neisseria meningitidis,* and *Streptococcus pneumoniae*), including toxoids (diphtheria, tetanus). Many purified polysaccharides are T-cell–independent antigens that initiate B-cell proliferation without involvement of CD4 T lymphocytes and are poor immunogens in children younger than 2 years of age. Conjugation of a polysaccharide to a **protein carrier** induces a T-cell–dependent response in infants and creates immunogenic vaccines for *H. influenzae* type b, *S. pneumoniae,* and *N. meningitidis.*

Childhood immunization standards and recommendations in the United States (Figs. 95.1, 95.2, and 95.3) are formulated by the Advisory Committee on Immunization Practices of the Centers for Disease Control and Prevention (ACIP), the American Academy of Pediatrics (AAP), and the American Academy of Family Physicians. In the United States, due to state laws requiring immunization for school entry, approximately 93% of children entering kindergarten are vaccinated for the common infectious diseases. The COVID-19 pandemic contributed to decline in routine childhood vaccine rates in the United States, with school-aged children declining from 95% coverage (2019–2020 school year) to 93% coverage (2023–2024 school year). The AAP recommends that children in the United States routinely receive vaccines and monoclonal antibodies against 18 diseases (see Fig. 95.1). Infants and children who are at increased risk for meningococcal infections should receive the two- or four-dose meningococcal series depending on age. Children who are behind in immunization should receive catch-up immunizations as rapidly as feasible. Infants born prematurely, regardless of birthweight, should be vaccinated at the same chronological age and according to the same schedule as full-term infants and children (see Fig. 95.2). The single exception to this practice is providing hepatitis B vaccine at 1 month of age instead of at birth for infants weighing less than 2,000 g if the mother is hepatitis B virus surface antigen (HB_sAg) negative. Vaccines for older children and adolescents include human papillomavirus (HPV), meningococcal, and tetanus/diphtheria/pertussis (Tdap) (see Fig. 95.1).

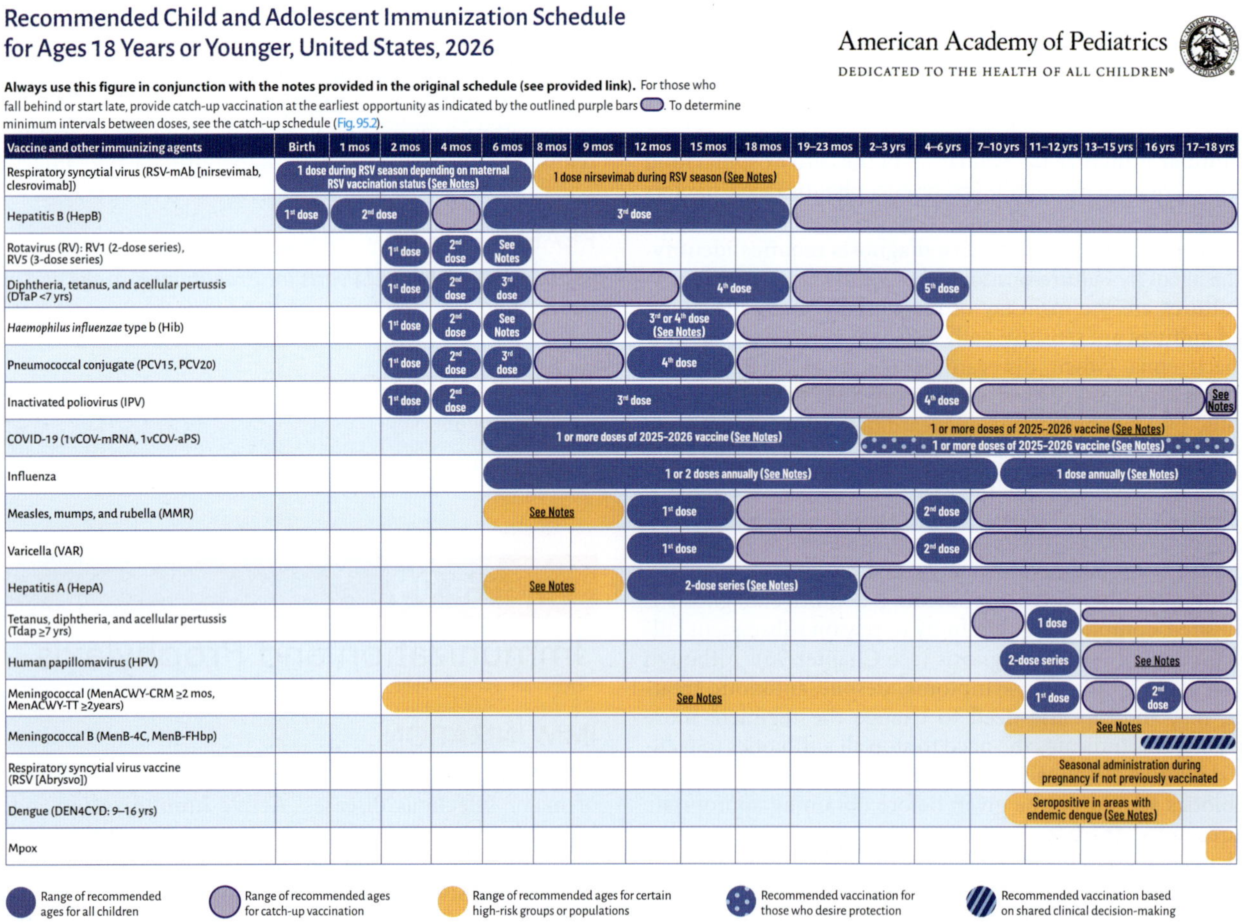

FIGURE 95.1 Recommended child and adolescent immunization schedule for ages 18 years or younger, United States, 2026. **These recommendations must be read with the notes provided in the original schedule (see provided link).** For those who fall behind or start late, provide catch-up vaccination at the earliest opportunity as indicated by the outlined purple bars. To determine minimum intervals between doses, see the catch-up schedule (Fig. 95.2). (Reproduced with permission from the American Academy of Pediatrics, Recommended Child and Adolescent Immunization Schedule 2026, AAP.org/Immunization Schedule, Updated January 26, 2026. Accessed [27-Jan-26].)

The **National Childhood Vaccine Injury Act** requires that all health care providers provide parents or patients with copies of **Vaccine Information Statements** prepared by the Centers for Disease Control and Prevention (http://www.cdc.gov/vaccines/hcp/vis/index.html) before administering each vaccine dose.

Most vaccines are administered by intramuscular or subcutaneous injection. The preferred sites for administration are the anterolateral aspect of the thigh in infants and the deltoid region in children and adults. Multiple vaccines can be administered simultaneously at anatomically separate sites (different limbs or separated by >1 in) without diminishing the immune response. MMR and varicella vaccines should be administered simultaneously or more than 28 days apart. The conjugate and polysaccharide pneumococcal vaccines should be spaced at least 8 weeks apart when both are indicated, and the conjugate vaccine should be administered first, if possible. Tuberculosis testing, either with a skin test or gamma interferon release blood test, can be performed at the time of vaccination. If tuberculosis testing is not performed at the same visit as MMR vaccination, then testing should be delayed for 4 weeks because MMR vaccination can temporarily suppress response to tuberculin antigens. Administration of blood products and immunoglobulin can diminish response to live-virus vaccines administered before the recommended interval.

General contraindications to vaccination include serious allergic reaction (anaphylaxis) after a previous vaccine dose or to a vaccine component, certain immunocompromised states, or pregnancy (live-virus vaccines) and moderate or severe acute illness with or without fever. History of *anaphylactic-like* reactions to eggs has historically been a contraindication to influenza and yellow fever vaccines, which are produced in embryonated chicken eggs; however, in 2016 the ACIP recommended that even persons with severe egg allergy receive any licensed influenza vaccine. Current preparations of measles and mumps vaccines, which are produced in chick embryo

Recommended Catch-up Immunization Schedule for Children and Adolescents Who Start Late or Who Are More than 1 Month Behind United States 2026,

American Academy of Pediatrics
DEDICATED TO THE HEALTH OF ALL CHILDREN®

The table below provides catch-up schedules and minimum intervals between doses for children whose vaccinations have been delayed. A vaccine series does not need to be restarted, regardless of the time that has elapsed between doses. Use the section appropriate for the child's age. **Always use this figure in conjunction with Fig. 95.1 and the notes provided in the original schedule (see provided link).**

Children age 4 months through 6 years					
Vaccine	Minimum Age for Dose 1	Minimum Interval Between Doses			
		Dose 1 to Dose 2	Dose 2 to Dose 3	Dose 3 to Dose 4	Dose 4 to Dose 5
Hepatitis B	Birth	**4 weeks**	**8 weeks *and* at least 16 weeks after first dose:** minimum age for the final dose is 24 weeks		
Rotavirus	6 weeks: Maximum age for first dose is 14 weeks, 6 days.	**4 weeks**	**4 weeks:** maximum age for final dose is 8 months, 0 days		
Diphtheria, tetanus, and acellular pertussis	6 weeks	**4 weeks**	**4 weeks**	**6 months**	**6 months:** A fifth dose is not necessary if the fourth dose was administered at age 4 years or older ***and*** at least 6 months after dose 3
Haemophilus influenzae type b	6 weeks	**No further doses needed** if first dose was administered at age 15 months or older **4 weeks** if first dose was administered before the 1st birthday **8 weeks (as final dose)** if first dose was administered at age 12 through 14 months	**No further doses needed** if previous dose was administered at age 15 months or older **4 weeks** if current age is younger than 12 months and first dose was administered at younger than age 7 months ***and*** at least 1 previous dose was PRP-T (ActHib, Pentacel, Hiberix), Vaxelis, or unknown **8 weeks and age 12 through 59 months (as final dose)** if current age is younger than 12 months ***and*** first dose was administered at age 7 through 11 months; **OR** if current age is 12 through 59 months ***and*** first dose was administered before the 1st birthday ***and*** second dose was administered at younger than 15 months; **OR** if both doses were PedvaxHIB and were administered before the 1st birthday	**8 weeks (as final dose):** This dose only necessary for children age 12 through 59 months who received 3 doses before the 1st birthday	
Pneumococcal conjugate	6 weeks	**No further doses needed** for healthy children if first dose was administered at age 24 months or older **4 weeks** if first dose was administered before the 1st birthday **8 weeks (as final dose for healthy children)** if first dose was administered at the 1st birthday or after	**No further doses needed** for healthy children if previous dose was administered at age 24 months or older **4 weeks:**if current age is younger than 12 months ***and*** previous dose was administered at <7 months old **8 weeks (as final dose for healthy children)** if previous dose was administered between 7–11 months (wait until at least 12 months old); **OR** if current age is 12 months or older ***and*** at least 1 dose was administered before age 12 months	**8 weeks (as final dose):** This dose is only necessary for children age 12 through 59 months regardless of risk, or age 60 through 71 months with any risk, who received 3 doses before age 12 months	
Inactivated poliovirus	6 weeks	**4 weeks**	**4 weeks** if current age is <4 years **6 months (as final dose)** if current age is 4 years or older	**6 months (minimum age 4 years for final dose)**	
Measles, mumps, and rubella	12 months	**4 weeks**			
Varicella	12 months	**3 months**			
Hepatitis A	12 months	**6 months**			
Meningococcal ACWY	2 months MenACWY-CRM 2 years MenACWY-TT	**8 weeks**	See Notes	See Notes	
Children and adolescents age 7 through 18 years					
Meningococcal ACWY	Not applicable (N/A)	**8 weeks**			
Tetanus, diphtheria; tetanus, diphtheria, and acellular pertussis	7 years	**4 weeks**	**4 weeks:** if first dose of DTaP/DT was administered before the 1st birthday **6 months (as final dose):** if first dose of DTaP/DT or Tdap/Td was administered at or after the 1st birthday	**6 months:** if first dose of DTaP/DT was administered before the 1st birthday	
Human papillomavirus	9 years	**Routine dosing intervals are recommended**			
Hepatitis A	N/A	**6 months**			
Hepatitis B	N/A	**4 weeks**	**8 weeks *and* at least 16 weeks after first dose**		
Inactivated poliovirus	N/A	**4 weeks**	**6 months:** A fourth dose is not necessary if the third dose was administered at age 4 years or older ***and*** at least 6 months after the previous dose	A fourth dose of IPV is indicated if all previous doses were administered at <4 years **OR** if the third dose was administered <6 months after the second dose	
Measles, mumps, and rubella	N/A	**4 weeks**			
Varicella	N/A	**3 months** if younger than age 13 years **4 weeks** if age 13 years or older			
Dengue	9 years	**6 months**	6 months		

FIGURE 95.2 Recommended catch-up immunization schedule for children and adolescents who start late or who are more than 1 month behind, United States, 2026. The table below provides catch-up schedules and minimum intervals between doses for children whose vaccinations have been delayed. A vaccine series does not need to be restarted, regardless of the time that has elapsed between doses. Use the section appropriate for the child's age. **Always use this table in conjunction with Fig. 95.1 and the notes provided in the original schedule (see provided link).** (Reproduced with permission from the American Academy of Pediatrics, Recommended Child and Adolescent Immunization Schedule 2026, AAP.org/Immunization Schedule, Updated January 26, 2026. Accessed [27-Jan-26].)

fibroblast tissue culture, do not contain significant amounts of egg proteins and may be administered without testing children with history of egg allergy. Mild acute illness with or without fever, convalescent phase of illness, recent exposure to infectious diseases, current antimicrobial therapy, breast-feeding, mild to moderate local reaction or low-grade to moderate fever after previous vaccination, and a history of penicillin or other nonvaccine allergy or receiving allergen extract immunotherapy are **not contraindications** to immunization.

Severe immunosuppression resulting from congenital immunodeficiency, HIV infection, leukemia, lymphoma, cancer therapy, or a prolonged course of high-dose corticosteroids (≥2 mg/kg/day for >2 weeks) predisposes to complications and is a contraindication for live-virus vaccines (Fig. 95.3). For children with HIV who do not have evidence of severe immunosuppression, MMR vaccination is recommended as per the regular schedule. Varicella vaccine is contraindicated for persons with cellular immunodeficiency but is recommended for persons with impaired humoral immunity (hypogammaglobulinemia or dysgammaglobulinemia) and at 12 months of age for children with HIV without evidence of severe immunosuppression, given as two doses 3 months apart. Rotavirus vaccine should not be given to children with a history of intussusception or severe combined immunodeficiency syndromes.

The National Childhood Vaccine Injury Act requires that clinically significant adverse events after vaccination be reported to the **Vaccine Adverse Event Reporting System (VAERS)** (http://www.vaers.hhs.gov or 800-822-7967). Suspected cases of vaccine-preventable diseases should be reported to state or local health departments. The act also established the **National Vaccine Injury Compensation Program**, a no-fault system in which persons thought to have suffered an injury or death as a result of administration of a covered vaccine can seek compensation.

PROPHYLAXIS

Prophylaxis may include antibiotics, immunoglobulin or monoclonal antibody, and vaccine, alone or in combination. They may be used pre-exposure, for perinatal exposure, and

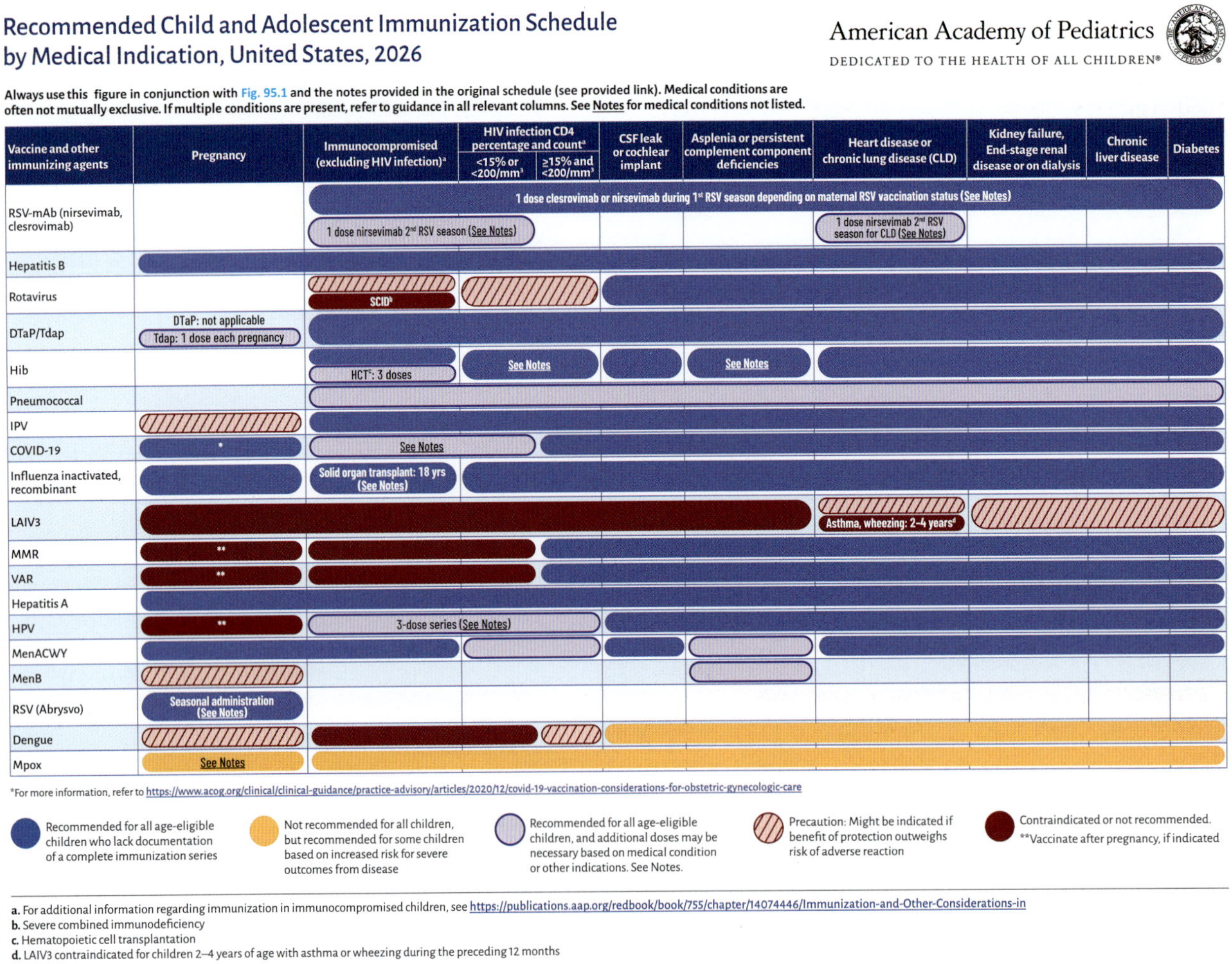

FIGURE 95.3 Recommended child and adolescent immunization schedule by medical indication, United States, 2026. **Always use this figure in conjunction with Fig. 95.1 and the notes provided in the original schedule (see provided link).** Medical conditions are often not mutually exclusive. If multiple conditions are present, refer to guidance in all relevant columns. See notes for medical conditions not listed. (Reproduced with permission from the American Academy of Pediatrics, Recommended Child and Adolescent Immunization Schedule 2026, AAP.org/Immunization Schedule, Updated January 26, 2026. Accessed [27-Jan-26].)

postexposure for persons at increased risk for infection. **Primary prophylaxis** is used to prevent infection before a first occurrence. **Secondary prophylaxis** is used to prevent recurrence after a first episode.

Meningococcus

Primary prophylaxis to all close contacts of index cases of *N. meningitidis* infection should be administered as soon as possible (see Chapter 101). Prophylaxis is recommended for all household contacts, especially young children; child-care or preschool contacts in the 7 days before illness onset; contacts with direct exposure to the index patient's secretions through kissing or sharing of toothbrushes or eating utensils in the 7 days before illness onset; and for mouth-to-mouth resuscitation or unprotected contact during endotracheal intubation within 7 days before illness onset. Prophylaxis is also recommended for contacts who frequently sleep or eat in the same dwelling as the index patient or passengers seated directly next to the index case during airline flights lasting longer than 8 hours. Chemoprophylaxis is not recommended for casual contacts with no history of direct exposure to the patient's oral secretions (school or work), indirect contact with the index patient, or medical personnel without direct exposure to the patient's oral secretions. Rifampin twice daily for 2 days, ceftriaxone once, and ciprofloxacin once are the recommended regimens. Clinicians should be aware that cases of ciprofloxacin-resistant strains of *Neisseria meningitidis* have risen since 2019. Azithromycin may be used in the case of resistant organisms.

Respiratory Syncytial Virus

Primary prophylaxis with one dose of nirsevimab should be given to all infants age 0–8 months whose birthing parent was not given the respiratory syncytial virus (RSV) vaccine during pregnancy. Infants with certain medical complexity, including but not limited to chronic lung disease or in certain populations, may require an additional dose of nirsevimab prior to their second RSV season (Table 95.1).

Tetanus

All postexposure wound treatment begins with immediate, thorough cleansing using soap and water; removal of foreign bodies; and debridement of devitalized tissue. Tetanus prophylaxis after wounds and injuries for persons with incomplete immunization includes vaccination for all wounds as well as tetanus immunoglobulin for contaminated wounds (soil, feces, saliva), puncture wounds, avulsions, and wounds resulting from missiles, crushing, burns, and frostbite (Table 95.2).

Rabies

Rabies immune globulin (RIG) and rabies vaccine are extremely effective for prophylaxis after exposure to rabies but are of no known benefit after symptoms appear. Because rabies is one of the deadliest infections, recognition of potential exposure and prophylaxis are crucial. Any healthy-appearing domestic animal (dog, cat) responsible for an apparently unprovoked bite should be observed for 10 days for signs of rabies without immediate

TABLE 95.1 Infants and Children Aged 8–19 Months With Increased Risk for Severe Disease Who Are Recommended to Receive Nirsevimab When Entering Their Second Respiratory Syncytial Virus Season

- Children with chronic lung disease of prematurity who required medical support (chronic corticosteroid therapy, diuretic therapy, or supplemental oxygen) any time during the 6-month period before the start of the second RSV season
- Children with severe immunocompromise
- Children with cystic fibrosis who have either (1) manifestations of severe lung disease (previous hospitalization for pulmonary exacerbation in the first year of life or abnormalities on chest imaging that persist when stable) or (2) weight-for-length <10th percentile
- American Indian or Alaska Native children

RSV, Respiratory syncytial virus.
From Jones JJ, Fleming-Dutra KE, Prill MM, et al. Use of nirsevimab for the prevention of respiratory syncytial virus disease among infants and young children: recommendations of the advisory committee on immunization practices—United States, 2023. MMWR. *2023;73(34):920–925.*

TABLE 95.2 Guide to Tetanus Prophylaxis in Routine Wound Management

HISTORY OF ADSORBED TETANUS TOXOID (DOSES)	CLEAN, MINOR WOUNDS		ALL OTHER WOUNDS*	
	DTaP, TdaP, OR Td†	TIG‡	DTaP, Tdap, OR Td†	TIG‡
Fewer than 3 or unknown	Yes	No	Yes	Yes
3 or more	No if <10 yr since last tetanus-containing vaccine dose	No	No if <5 yr since last tetanus-containing vaccine dose	No
	Yes if ≥10 yr since the last tetanus toxoid-containing vaccine dose	No	Yes if ≥5 yr since the last tetanus toxoid-containing vaccine dose	No

Such as, but not limited to, wounds contaminated with dirt, feces, soil, or saliva; puncture wounds; avulsions; and wounds resulting from flying or crushing objects, animal bites, burns, and frostbite.
†*Tdap is preferred for children ≥10 years of age who have never received Tdap; Td is preferred for children 7 through 9 years.*
‡*Immune globulin intravenous should be used if TIG is not available.*
DTap, Diphtheria and tetanus toxoids, acellular pertussis vaccine; *Td,* tetanus-diphtheria toxoid; *Tdap,* tetanus and diphtheria toxoids, acellular pertussis vaccine; *TIG,* tetanus immunoglobulin.
From American Academy of Pediatrics. Tetanus (Lockjaw). In: Kimberlin DW, Banerjee R, Barnett ED, et al., eds. Red Book: 2024–2027 Report of the Committee on Infectious Diseases. *Itasca, IL: American Academy of Pediatrics; 2024;fig 3.19.*

treatment of the victim. Prophylaxis should be administered if the animal is rabid or suspected to be rabid or if the animal develops signs of rabies while under observation. A captured wild animal should be euthanized (by animal control officials) without a period of observation and its brain examined for evidence of rabies. If the biting animal is not captured, particularly if it is a wild animal of a species known to harbor the virus in the region, rabies should be presumed and prophylaxis administered to the victim. Bats, raccoons, skunks, foxes, coyotes, and bobcats are the most important wild animal potential sources of rabies infection. Prophylaxis also should be provided following exposure to a bat for persons who might be unaware or unable to relate that a bite or direct contact has occurred, such as a sleeping child or an unattended infant. Local public health departments are important resources for determining rabies risk based on local epidemiology.

All rabies postexposure management begins with immediate thorough cleansing of the bite using soap and water. RIG at a dose of 20 IU/kg should be administered, with the full dose of RIG infiltrated subcutaneously into the area around the wound, if possible. Any remaining RIG that cannot be infiltrated into the wound should be administered as an intramuscular injection. Inactivated rabies vaccine should be administered simultaneously as soon as possible, at a site away from where RIG was administered, with additional vaccine doses at 3, 7, and 14 days.

PEARLS FOR PRACTITIONERS

See Infectious Diseases: Pearls for Practitioners at the end of this section.

REVIEW QUESTIONS

Available online.

CHAPTER 96

Antimicrobial Therapy

The selection of antimicrobial therapy depends on a number of factors: the site of infection and clinical syndrome, host immunity, probable causative agents, the pathogen's susceptibility to antimicrobial agents or the local epidemiology of resistance, the pharmacokinetics of the selected agents, and their pharmacodynamics in specific patient populations.

Empirical or presumptive antimicrobial therapy is based on a clinical diagnosis combined with published evidence and experience of the probable causative pathogens. **Definitive therapy** relies on microbiologic diagnosis by isolation or other direct evidence of a pathogen. Microbiologic diagnosis through culture permits characterization of the pathogen's antimicrobial drug **susceptibilities** and delivery of the appropriate antimicrobial agent to the site of infection in concentrations sufficient to kill or alter the pathogen and facilitate an effective immune response. Antiviral therapy must include consideration of the intracellular nature of viral replication and, to avoid toxicity to host cells, must be targeted to viral-specific proteins, such as the thymidine kinase of herpesviruses or the reverse transcriptase of HIV.

Empirical antimicrobial therapy is best initiated *after* obtaining appropriate cultures or molecular testing of fluids or tissues. In high-risk circumstances, such as neonatal sepsis or bacteremia in immunocompromised persons, empirical therapy includes broad-spectrum antimicrobials (see Chapters 97 and 121). Empirical antimicrobial therapy may be tailored to specific pathogens based on the clinical diagnosis (e.g., streptococcal pharyngitis) or defined risks (e.g., close exposure to tuberculosis). Definitive therapy can additionally minimize drug toxicity, development of resistant microorganisms, and cost.

Antimicrobial agents are an adjunct to the normal host immune response. Infections associated with foreign bodies, such as an intravascular catheter, are difficult to eradicate with antimicrobials alone because of organism-produced biofilms that impair phagocytosis. Similarly, it is difficult for phagocytic cells to eradicate bacteria amid vegetations of fibrin and platelets on infected heart valves. Prolonged bactericidal therapy may be required with these types of infections, and foreign body devices may have to be removed if sterilization does not occur promptly on antimicrobial therapy. Infections in closed spaces with limited perfusion (e.g., abscesses or chronic osteomyelitis with poorly perfused bone) are difficult to cure without surgical drainage, debridement of the infected tissue, and re-establishment of a good vascular supply.

Optimal antimicrobial therapy requires an understanding of both the **pharmacokinetics** (e.g., absorption, distribution, metabolism, excretion) of the administered drugs and their **pharmacodynamics** (e.g., mechanism of action, dose-response relationship, efficacy-potency, outcomes/effects) in specific patient populations. The bioavailability of orally administered antibiotics varies depending on the acid stability of the drug, degree of gastric acidity, and whether it is taken with food, antacids, H_2 blockers, or other medications. An ileus, underlying intestinal disease or substantial resection, or profuse diarrhea may alter intestinal transit time and result in unpredictable absorption.

The **site and nature** of the infection may affect the choice of antimicrobials. Aminoglycosides, active against aerobic organisms only, have significantly reduced activity in abscesses with low pH and oxygen tension. Infections of the central nervous system or the eye necessitate treatment with antimicrobials that penetrate and achieve therapeutic levels in these sites.

Limited kidney function (as in premature infants or those with kidney failure) requires lengthening dosing intervals to allow time for excretion of certain drugs. The larger volume of distribution of certain hydrophilic antimicrobials and increased renal clearance in some populations (e.g., in cystic fibrosis) requires higher doses to achieve therapeutic levels. Weight-based dosage regimens may result in overdoses in obese children due to significantly smaller volumes of distribution for hydrophilic drugs. Determining serum drug levels for antibiotics with narrow safety margins (e.g., aminoglycosides and vancomycin) minimizes adverse effects of treatment.

Drug-drug interactions must be considered when multiple antimicrobial agents are used to treat infection or for patients on other medications (e.g., chemotherapy or immunosuppressants). Use of two or more antimicrobial agents may be justified before organism identification or for the benefit of different mechanisms of action. Several antimicrobials are administered routinely in combination (e.g., trimethoprim-sulfamethoxazole or amoxicillin-clavulanate) because of **synergism** (significantly greater bacterial killing or spectrum of activity than when either is used alone). The use of a bacteriostatic drug, such as a tetracycline, along with a β-lactam agent, effective against growing organisms only, may result in antibiotic **antagonism**, or less bacterial killing in the presence of both drugs, than if either is used alone.

PEARLS FOR PRACTITIONERS

See Infectious Diseases: Pearls for Practitioners at the end of this section.

REVIEW QUESTIONS

Available online.

CHAPTER 97

Fever Without a Focus

Core body temperature is normally maintained within 1–1.5°C in a range of 37–38°C. Normal body temperature is generally considered to be 37°C (98.6°F; range, 97–99.6°F). Normal diurnal variation exists, with maximum temperature in the late afternoon. Sustained rectal temperatures higher than 38.3–38.5°C (>100.9–101.3°F) generally are considered abnormal, especially if associated with other symptoms.

Normal body temperature is maintained by a complex regulatory system in the anterior hypothalamus. The development of fever begins with the release of endogenous pyrogens into the circulation as the result of infection, inflammatory processes, or malignancy. Microbes and microbial toxins act as **exogenous pyrogens** by stimulating release of **endogenous pyrogens**, including cytokines such as interleukin 1 (IL-1), IL-6, tumor necrosis factor, and interferons. These cytokines reach the anterior hypothalamus, liberating arachidonic acid, which is metabolized to prostaglandin E_2. Elevation of the hypothalamic thermostat occurs via a complex interaction of complement and prostaglandin E_2 production. Antipyretics (acetaminophen, ibuprofen, aspirin) inhibit hypothalamic cyclooxygenase, decreasing production of prostaglandin E_2. Aspirin is associated with Reye syndrome in children and is not recommended as an antipyretic. The response to antipyretics does not distinguish bacterial from viral infections.

The **pattern of fever** in children may vary, depending on age and the nature of the illness. Neonates may not have a febrile response and may instead be hypothermic despite significant infection, whereas older infants and children younger than 5 years of age may have an exaggerated febrile response with temperatures of up to 105°F (40.6°C) or beyond in response to either a serious bacterial infection or an otherwise benign viral infection. Fever to this degree is unusual in older children and adolescents and suggests a serious process. The fever pattern does not reliably distinguish fever caused by infectious microorganisms from that resulting from malignancy, autoimmune diseases, or drugs.

Children with fever without a focus present a diagnostic challenge that includes identifying bacteremia and sepsis. **Bacteremia**, the presence of bacteria in the bloodstream, may be primary or secondary to a focal infection. **Sepsis** is the systemic response to infection that is manifested by hyperthermia or hypothermia, tachycardia, tachypnea, shock, and organ dysfunction (see Chapter 39). Children with septicemia and signs of CNS dysfunction (irritability, lethargy), cardiovascular impairment (cyanosis, poor perfusion), or disseminated intravascular coagulation (petechiae, ecchymosis) are readily recognized as **toxic appearing** or **septic**. Most febrile illnesses in children may be categorized as follows:

- **Fever of short duration** accompanied by localizing signs and symptoms, in which a diagnosis can often be established by clinical history and physical examination
- **Fever without localizing signs (fever without a focus)**, frequently occurring in children younger than 3 years of age, in which a history and physical examination fail to establish a cause
- **Fever of unknown origin (FUO)**, defined as daily fever for more than 14 days without an identified etiology despite history, physical examination, and routine laboratory tests or after 1 week of intense evaluation

FEVER IN INFANTS YOUNGER THAN 2 MONTHS OF AGE

Fever or **temperature instability** in infants younger than 2 months of age is associated with a higher risk of **serious bacterial infections** than in older infants. These younger infants usually exhibit only fever and poor feeding, without localizing signs of infection. Most febrile illnesses in this age group are caused by common viral pathogens, but serious infections include **bacteremia** (most commonly caused by group B streptococcus [GBS], *Escherichia coli,* and *Listeria monocytogenes* in neonates and *Streptococcus pneumoniae, Haemophilus influenzae* type b [Hib], nontyphoidal *Salmonella,* and *Neisseria meningitidis* in 1- to 3-month-old infants), **urinary tract infection (UTI)** *(E. coli),* **pneumonia** (*S. pneumoniae,* GBS, or *Staphylococcus aureus*), **meningitis** (GBS, *E. coli, L. monocytogenes, S. pneumoniae, N. meningitidis,* Hib), herpes simplex virus (HSV), enteroviruses, **bacterial diarrhea** *(Salmonella, Shigella, E. coli),* and **osteomyelitis** or **septic arthritis** (*S. aureus* or GBS).

Differentiating between viral and bacterial infections in young infants is difficult, but emerging studies demonstrate that doing so may be possible with the examination of inflammatory markers and gene expression profiles. Febrile infants younger than 60 days of age who appear ill, especially if follow-up is uncertain, and all febrile infants younger than 21 days of age should be admitted to the hospital for empirical antibiotics pending culture results. After blood, urine, and cerebrospinal fluid cultures are obtained, broad-spectrum parenteral antibiotics (typically ampicillin with either ceftazidime or gentamicin for infants under 21 days or ceftriaxone for infants over 21 days) are administered. The choice of antibiotic depends on the pathogens suggested by localizing findings. The possibility of neonatal HSV should also be considered in febrile children younger than 4 weeks and empirical acyclovir begun in those in whom neonatal HSV is a concern. Well-appearing febrile infants 4 weeks of age and older without an identifiable focus and with certainty of follow-up are at a low risk of developing a serious bacterial infection (0.8% develop bacteremia, and 2% develop a serious localized bacterial infection). Specific criteria identifying these low-risk infants include age older than 21 days, well appearing without a focus of infection, no history of prematurity or prior antimicrobial therapy, a white blood cell (WBC) count of 5,000–15,000/µL, normal urinalysis, procalcitonin below 1.7 ng/mL, and spinal fluid, if obtained, with less than 20 WBC/µL. Fecal leukocyte testing and chest radiograph can be considered in infants with diarrhea or respiratory signs. Low-risk infants may be followed as outpatients without empirical antibiotic treatment or, alternatively, may be treated with intramuscular ceftriaxone. Regardless of antibiotic treatment, close follow-up for at least 72 hours, including re-evaluation in 24 hours or immediately with any clinical change, is essential (Table 97.1).

FEVER IN CHILDREN 2 MONTHS TO 3 YEARS OF AGE

A common problem is the evaluation of a febrile but well-appearing child 2 months to 3 years of age without localizing signs of infection. Although most of these children have self-limited viral infections, some have **occult bacteremia** (bacteremia without identifiable focus) or UTIs, and a few have severe and potentially life-threatening illnesses. It is difficult, even for experienced clinicians, to differentiate patients with occult bacteremia from those with benign illnesses.

Observational assessment is a key part of the evaluation. Descriptions of normal appearance and **alertness** include *child looking at the observer* and *looking around the room,* with eyes that are *shiny* or *bright.* Descriptions that indicate severe impairment include *glassy eyes* and *stares vacantly into space.* Observations such as *sitting, moving arms and legs on table or lap,* and *sits without support* reflect normal motor ability, whereas *no movement in caregiver's arms* and *lies limply on table* indicate severe impairment. Normal behaviors, such as *vocalizing spontaneously, playing with objects, reaching for objects, smiling,* and *crying with noxious stimuli,* reflect **playfulness**; abnormal behaviors reflect **irritability** or central nervous system infection. Normally, crying children are **consolable** and *stop crying when held by the caregiver,* whereas severe impairment is indicated by *continual cry despite being held and comforted.*

Children between 2 months and 3 years of age are at increased risk for infection with organisms with polysaccharide capsules, including *S. pneumoniae,* Hib, *N. meningitidis,* and nontyphoidal *Salmonella.* Effective phagocytosis of these organisms requires opsonic antibody. Transplacentally acquired maternal immunoglobulin G (IgG) initially provides immunity to these organisms, but as the maternal IgG gradually dissipates, the risk of infection increases. In the United States, use of conjugate Hib and *S. pneumoniae* vaccines has dramatically reduced the incidence of these infections, and determining the child's immunization status is essential to evaluate the risk of these infections. An approach to evaluating these children is outlined in Table 97.1.

Most episodes of fever in children younger than 3 years of age have a demonstrable source of infection elicited by history, physical examination, or a simple laboratory test. In this age group, the most commonly identified serious bacterial infection is a UTI. A blood culture to evaluate for occult bacteremia and urinalysis and urine culture to evaluate for a UTI should be considered for all children younger than 3 years of age with ongoing fever without localizing signs. Stool culture or molecular testing should be obtained in those with diarrhea marked by blood or mucus. Ill-appearing children should be admitted to the hospital and treated with empirical antibiotics after obtaining appropriate diagnostic samples.

Approximately 0.2% of well-appearing febrile children 3–36 months of age vaccinated against *S. pneumoniae* and Hib and without localizing signs have occult bacteremia. Signs associated with occult bacteremia include temperature of 102.2°F (39°C) or greater, WBC count of 15,000/mm^3 or more, and elevated absolute neutrophil count, band count, erythrocyte sedimentation rate (ESR), or C-reactive protein (CRP). No combination of demographic factors (socioeconomic status, ethnicity, gender, and age), clinical parameters, or laboratory tests in these children reliably predicts occult bacteremia. Occult bacteremia due to pneumococcus in otherwise healthy children is usually transient and self-limited but may progress to serious localizing infections. Well-appearing children usually are followed as outpatients without empirical antibiotic treatment. Regardless of antibiotic treatment, close follow-up for at least 72 hours, including re-evaluation in 24 hours or immediately with any clinical change, is essential. Children with a positive blood culture require immediate re-evaluation, repeat blood culture, consideration for lumbar puncture, and empirical antibiotic treatment.

Children with **sickle cell disease** have both impaired splenic function and properdin-dependent opsonization that places them at increased risk for bacteremia due to encapsulated organisms, especially during the first 5 years of life. Children with sickle cell disease and fever who appear seriously ill, have a temperature of 104°F (40°C) or above or WBC count less than 5,000/mm^3 or more than 30,000/mm^3 should be hospitalized and treated empirically with antibiotics. Other children with sickle cell disease and fever should have blood culture, empirical treatment with ceftriaxone, and close outpatient follow-up. Osteomyelitis resulting from *Salmonella* or *S. aureus* is more common in children with sickle cell disease; blood culture is not always positive in the presence of osteomyelitis.

FEVER OF UNKNOWN ORIGIN

FUO is defined as a daily temperature greater than 100.4°F (38°C) lasting for more than 14 days without an obvious cause or a fever documented by a health care provider for which the cause could not be identified after at least 8 days of work-up despite a complete history, physical examination, and routine screening laboratory evaluation. It is important to distinguish persistent fever from recurrent fevers, which often represent serial acute illnesses.

The initial FUO evaluation requires a thorough history and physical examination supplemented with a few screening laboratory tests (Fig. 97.1). Additional laboratory and imaging tests are guided by abnormalities on initial evaluation. Important historical elements include the impact the fever has on the child's health and activity; weight loss; the use of drugs, medications, or immunosuppressive therapy; a history of unusual, severe, or chronic infection suggesting immunodeficiency (see Chapter 72); immunizations; exposure to unpasteurized or raw foods; a history of pica or exposure to soil-borne or water-borne organisms; exposure to industrial or hobby-related chemicals; blood transfusions; domestic or foreign travel;

TABLE 97.1 Management of Fever Without Source in Infants 0–36 Months Old

GROUP	MANAGEMENT
Any toxic-appearing child 0–36 mo and temperature ≥38°C (100.4°F)	Hospitalize, cultures (blood, urine, CSF) plus other tests,* parenteral antibiotics
WELL-APPEARING CHILD	
Child <22 days and temperature ≥38°C (100.4°F)	Hospitalize, cultures (blood, urine, CSF) plus other tests,* parenteral antibiotics
Child 22–60 days and temperature ≥38°C (100.4°F)	**Three-Step Process** 1. Determine risk based on history, physical examination, and laboratory studies. Low risk: • Uncomplicated medical history • Well-appearing physical examination • Normal laboratory studies • Urine: negative leukocyte esterase and nitrite, ≤5 WBC/hpf centrifuged and <10 WBC/hpf uncentrifuged • Inflammatory markers: temperature ≤38.5°C, procalcitonin ≤0.5 ng/mL, CRP ≤20 mg/L, absolute neutrophil count ≤4,000–5,200/mm³ • Stool studies if diarrhea (no RBC and <5 WBC/hpf) 2. If child *fulfills all low-risk criteria*, use age to determine need for LP, parenteral antimicrobials, and hospital observation. • **Age 22–28 days:** Obtain UA, blood culture, inflammatory markers. May perform LP. May administer parenteral antimicrobials. Observe in hospital. • **Age 29–60 days old:** Obtain UA, blood culture, inflammatory markers. Need not perform LP. Need not administer antimicrobials. Observe closely at home with follow-up within 24–36 hr. 3. If child does not fulfill all low-risk criteria, use age and lab results to determine need for LP, antimicrobials, and hospital observation. • **Age 22–28 days** with abnormal UA and normal inflammatory markers: May perform LP. Administer parenteral antimicrobials. Observe in hospital. • **Age 22–28 days** with abnormal inflammatory markers: Perform LP. If CSF pleocytosis, CSF uninterpretable, or abnormal UA, administer parenteral antimicrobials and observe in hospital. If CSF and UA are normal, may observe at home after parenteral antimicrobials or observe in the hospital with or without parenteral antimicrobials. • **Age 29–60 days** with abnormal UA and normal inflammatory markers: Administer oral antimicrobials. May observe closely at home with follow-up in 12–24 hr. • **Age 29–60 days** with abnormal inflammatory markers: May perform LP. If CSF pleocytosis, administer parenteral antimicrobials and observe in hospital. If CSF is normal, may administer parenteral or oral antimicrobials and may observe closely in hospital or at home. If CSF is not available or uninterpretable, administer parenteral antimicrobials and may observe closely in hospital or at home.
Child 2–36 mo and temperature 38–39°C (100.4–102.2°F)	Reassurance that diagnosis is likely self-limited viral infection, but advise return with persistence of fever, temperatures >39°C (102.2°F), and/or new signs and symptoms.
Child 2–36 mo and temperature >39°C (102.2°F)	**Two-Step Process** 1. Determine immunization status. 2. If received conjugate pneumococcal and *Haemophilus influenzae* type b vaccines, obtain urine studies (urine WBC, leukocyte esterase, nitrite, and culture) for all females, all males <6 mo old, all uncircumcised males <2 yr, and all children with recurrent urinary tract infections. If did not receive conjugate pneumococcal and *H. influenzae* type b vaccines, manage according to the 1993 Guidelines (see Baraff et al. *Ann Emerg Med.* 1993;22:1198–1210).

*Other tests may include chest radiograph, stool studies, herpes simplex and other virus polymerase chain reaction.

CSF, Cerebrospinal fluid; *hpf,* high-powered field; *LP,* lumbar puncture; *RBC,* red blood cell; *UA,* urinalysis; *WBC,* white blood cell.

Adapted from Nield LS, Kamat D. Fever without a focus. In: Kliegman RM, Stanton BF, St. Geme JW III, et al., eds. Nelson Textbook of Pediatrics. *20th ed. Philadelphia: Elsevier; 2016: Table 177.3; with data from Pantell RH, Roberts KB, Adams WG, et al.* Evaluation and Management of Well Appearing Febrile Infants 8 to 60 Days Old. Pediatrics. *2021;148(2).*

exposure to animals; exposure to ticks or mosquitoes; ethnic background and family history; recent surgical procedures or dental work; tattooing and body piercing; and sexual activity.

The etiology of most occult infections causing FUO is an unusual presentation of a common disease. Sinusitis, endocarditis, intraabdominal abscesses (perinephric, intrahepatic, subdiaphragmatic), and CNS lesions (tuberculoma, cysticercosis, abscess, toxoplasmosis) may be relatively asymptomatic. **Infections** are the most common identified cause of FUO in children, accounting for approximately 40–50% of FUO episodes, followed by **inflammatory diseases** (about 20% of all episodes), **malignancy** (about 10% of all episodes), and other etiologies (Table 97.2). Approximately 15% of children with FUO have no diagnosis. Fever eventually resolves in many of these cases, usually without sequelae, although some may develop definable signs of rheumatic disease over time. Common infections causing FUO in patients with known or newly diagnosed **immunodeficiency** include viral hepatitis, Epstein-Barr virus, cytomegalovirus, *Bartonella henselae,* ehrlichiosis, *Salmonella,* and tuberculosis.

Factitious fever or fever produced or feigned intentionally by the patient **(factitious disorder imposed on self/Munchausen syndrome)** or the parent/guardian of a child **(factitious disorder imposed on another/Munchausen syndrome by**

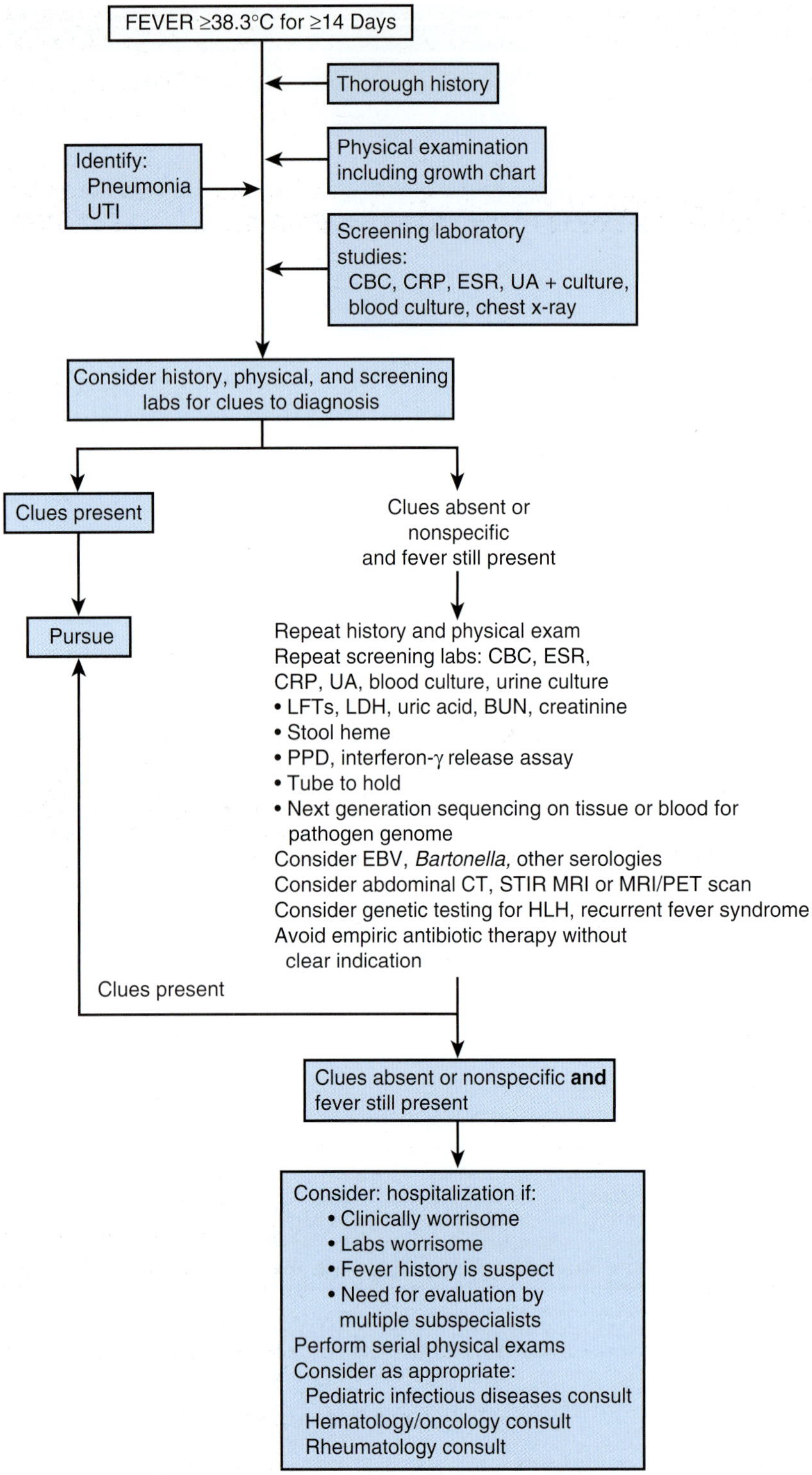

FIGURE 97.1 Algorithmic approach to the evaluation of fever of unknown origin (FUO). *EBV,* Epstein-Barr virus; *HLH,* hemophagocytic lymphohistiocytosis; *LDH,* lactate dehydrogenase; *LFT,* liver function test; *PPD,* purified protein derivative; *STIR,* short tau inversion recovery MRI; *UTI,* urinary tract infection. (Modified from Huppler AR. Fever. In: Kliegman RM, Toth H, Bordini BJ, Basel D, eds. *Nelson Pediatric Symptom-Based Diagnosis.* 2nd ed. Philadelphia: Elsevier; 2023:fig. 52.2.)

proxy) is an important consideration, particularly if family members are familiar with health care practices (see Chapter 21). Fever should be recorded in the hospital by a reliable individual who remains with the patient when the temperature is taken. Continuous observation over a long period and repetitive evaluation are essential.

Screening tests for FUO include complete blood count with WBC and differential, CRP, ESR, procalcitonin, basic metabolic panel, hepatic transaminase levels, urinalysis, and cultures of urine and blood. Chest radiograph should be included for patients with pulmonary symptoms. Additional tests for FUO may include throat culture, stool culture or molecular testing, tuberculin skin test or interferon-γ release assay, HIV, Epstein-Barr virus, cytomegalovirus, and *B. henselae* antibodies (Fig. 97.1). Consultation with infectious disease, immunology, rheumatology, or oncology specialists should be considered. Further tests may include lumbar puncture for cerebrospinal fluid analysis and culture; evaluation

TABLE **97.2** Causes of Fever of Unknown Origin

INFECTIOUS		
Abscesses	**Bacterial Diseases**	**Rickettsiae**
Abdominal	Actinomycosis	African tick-bite fever
Brain	*Bartonella henselae* (cat-scratch)	Anaplasmosis
Dental	Brucellosis	*Ehrlichia canis*
Hepatic	*Campylobacter*	Ehrlichiosis *(E. chaffeensis, E. ewingii)*
Paraspinal	Chlamydia	Q fever *(Coxiella burnetii)*
Pelvic	*Francisella tularensis* (tularemia)	Rocky Mountain spotted fever
Perinephric	*Listeria monocytogenes* (listeriosis)	Tick-borne typhus
Rectal	Meningococcemia (chronic)	**Spirochetes**
Retroperitoneal	*Mycobacterium* (nontuberculosis)	*Borrelia burgdorferi* (Lyme disease)
Subphrenic	*Mycoplasma pneumoniae*	Relapsing fever *(Borrelia recurrentis)*
Psoas	*Neisseria* meningitis (chronic)	Leptospirosis
Infected urachal cyst	Rat-bite fever *(Streptobacillus moniliformis)*	Rat-bite fever *(Spirillum minus)*
Vertebral	*Salmonella*	Syphilis
Viruses	Tuberculosis	**Parasitic Diseases**
Adenovirus	Whipple disease	Amebiasis
Arborviruses	Yersiniosis	Babesiosis
Cytomegalovirus	Localized Infections	Giardiasis
Epstein-Barr virus	Cholangitis	Leishmania
Hanta virus	Infective endocarditis	Malaria
Hepatitis viruses	Lymphogranuloma venereum	Toxoplasmosis
HIV	Mastoiditis	Trichinosis
Human picornavirus	Osteomyelitis	Trypanosomiasis
Fungal Diseases	Pneumonia	Visceral larva migrans *(Toxocara canis/cati)*
Blastomycosis (extrapulmonary)	Pyelonephritis	
Coccidioidomycosis (disseminated)	Psittacosis	
Histoplasmosis (disseminated)	Sinusitis	
NONINFECTIOUS IMMUNE-MEDIATED DISEASES		
Rheumatologic Diseases	**Miscellaneous Inflammatory**	**Granulomatous Diseases**
Autoimmune cholangitis	Hemophagocytic syndromes	Granulomatosis with polyangiitis
Aortitis	Kawasaki disease	Crohn disease
Behçet disease	Kikuchi-Fujimoto disease	Granulomatous colitis
Juvenile dermatomyositis	Immunoblastic lymphadenopathy	Granulomatous hepatitis
Juvenile idiopathic arthritis	Löfgren syndrome	Granulomatous peritonitis
Rheumatic fever	Periodic fever syndromes	Sarcoidosis
Sjögren syndrome	Schnitzler syndrome	Other vasculitis syndromes
Systemic lupus erythematosus	Subacute necrotizing lymphadenitis	
Polyarteritis nodosa		
NEOPLASMS		
Hodgkin lymphoma	Hepatocellular carcinoma	Cholesterol granuloma
Non-Hodgkin's Lymphoma	Neuroblastoma	Inflammatory pseudotumor
Leukemia	Other solid tumor malignancies	Pheochromocytoma
Wilms tumor		Lymphomatoid granulomatosis
		Myeloproliferative neoplasms
OTHER		
Hypersensitivity Diseases	**Miscellaneous**	**Miscellaneous (continued)**
Drug fever	Addison disease	Paroxysmal hemoglobinurias
Hypereosinophilic syndrome	Cardiac myxomas	Pericarditis
Hypersensitivity pneumonitis	Castleman disease	Poisoning
Serum sickness	Chronic active hepatitis	Postpericardiotomy syndrome
Weber-Christian disease	Cyclic neutropenia	Pulmonary embolism
Familial and Hereditary Diseases	Diabetes insipidus (central and nephrogenic)	Resorbing hematoma
Anhidrotic ectodermal dysplasia	Drug fever	Retroperitoneal fibrosis
Autonomic neuropathies	Factitious fever	Rosai-Dorfman disease
Fabry disease	Hemoglobinopathies	Spinal cord/brain injury
Familial dysautonomia	Hemolytic anemias	Thrombophlebitis
Familial Hibernian fever	Hypothalamic-central fever	Thyrotoxicosis, thyroiditis
Familial Mediterranean fever	Infantile cortical hyperostosis	Thrombotic thrombocytopenic purpura
Hypertriglyceridemia	Metal fume fever	Ulcerative colitis
Ichthyosis	Pancreatitis	Veno-occlusive disease
Other autoinflammatory diseases	Parathyroid apoplexy	Vitamin B_{12} deficiency
Sickle cell crisis		

Adapted from Steenhoff, A., Fever of Unknown Origin, in Nelson textbook of pediatrics, *R. Kliegman, and colleagues, Editors. 2016, Elsevier: Philadelphia, Pennsylvania. p. 1397 to 1402.; with permission.*

for rheumatic disease with antinuclear antibody, rheumatoid factor, ferritin, and serum complement (C3, C4, CH_{50}); uric acid and lactate dehydrogenase; computed tomography or magnetic resonance (often with positron emission tomography [PET] scan) imaging of the chest, abdomen, and head; and bone marrow biopsy for cytology and culture.

PEARLS FOR PRACTITIONERS

See Infectious Diseases: Pearls for Practitioners at the end of this section.

REVIEW QUESTIONS

Available online.

CHAPTER 98
Infections Characterized by Fever and Rash

Rashes are a common manifestation of many infections; this chapter describes five common childhood viral exanthems characterized by fever and rash. Rash distribution and appearance provide important clues to the differential diagnosis, including other infectious agents (Table 98.1).

MEASLES (RUBEOLA)

Etiology

Measles (rubeola) is highly contagious and is caused by a single-stranded RNA paramyxovirus with one antigenic type. Humans are the only natural hosts. The measles virus infects the upper respiratory tract and regional lymph nodes and is spread systemically during a brief, low-titer primary viremia. Secondary viremia occurs within 5–7 days as virus-infected monocytes spread the virus to the respiratory tract, skin, and other organs. The virus is present in respiratory secretions, blood, and the urine of infected individuals. It is transmitted by droplets or via the airborne route and is extremely contagious. Infected persons are contagious from 1–2 days before onset of symptoms and from about 5 days before to 4 days after the appearance of rash; immunocompromised persons can have prolonged excretion of contagious virus.

Epidemiology

Measles remains endemic in regions of the world where vaccination is not readily available and is responsible for about 11 million infections and 95,000 deaths annually (based on 2024 data). There have typically been fewer than 100 cases of measles reported annually in the United States; however, outbreaks have occurred resulting from imported virus after international travel and declines in vaccine coverage. In 2025 there were over 2,000 measles cases in the United States, the highest number since 1992. Infections of children without travel history may occur during outbreaks among those too young to be vaccinated or in communities with low immunization rates.

TABLE 98.1 Differential Diagnosis of Fever and Rash

LESION	PATHOGEN OR DISEASE
MACULAR OR MACULOPAPULAR RASH	
Viruses	Adenovirus
	Measles
	Rubella
	Roseola (HHV-6 or HHV-7)
	Erythema infectiosum (fifth disease, parvovirus B19)
	Epstein-Barr virus
	Enteroviruses
	Parechoviruses
	HBV (papular acrodermatitis or Gianotti-Crosti syndrome)
	HIV
Bacteria	Erythema marginatum (rheumatic fever)
	Scarlet fever (group A streptococcus)
	Erysipelas (group A streptococcus)
	Arcanobacterium haemolyticum
	Secondary syphilis
	Leptospirosis
	Pseudomonas aeruginosa (folliculitis or early ecthyma gangrenosum)
	Meningococcal infection (early)
	Salmonella typhi (typhoid fever, "rose spots")
	Lyme disease (erythema migrans)
	Mycoplasma pneumonia
Rickettsiae	Rocky Mountain spotted fever (early)
	Typhus (scrub, endemic)
	Ehrlichiosis
Other	Kawasaki disease
	Juvenile idiopathic arthritis
	Drug reaction
DIFFUSE ERYTHRODERMA	
Bacteria	Scarlet fever (group A streptococcus)
	Staphylococcal scalded skin syndrome
	Toxic shock syndrome (*Staphylococcus aureus*, group A streptococcus)
Fungi	*Candida albicans*
Other	Kawasaki disease
URTICARIAL RASH	
Viruses	Epstein-Barr virus
	HBV
	HIV
Bacteria	*M. pneumonia*
	Group A streptococcus
Other	Drug reaction
	Serum sickness
VESICULAR, BULLOUS, PUSTULAR	
Viruses	Herpes simplex viruses
	Varicella-zoster virus
	Coxsackievirus
	Mpox

(Continued)

TABLE 98.1 Differential Diagnosis of Fever and Rash—cont'd

LESION	PATHOGEN OR DISEASE
VESICULAR, BULLOUS, PUSTULAR (cont'd)	
Bacteria	Staphylococcal scalded skin syndrome
	Staphylococcal bullous impetigo
	Group A streptococcal crusted impetigo
Rickettsiae	Rickettsialpox
Other	Toxic epidermal necrolysis
	Erythema multiforme
	Stevens-Johnson syndrome
PETECHIAL-PURPURIC	
Viruses	Adenovirus
	Atypical measles
	Congenital rubella
	Congenital cytomegalovirus
	Enterovirus
	Papular-purpuric gloves and socks (parvovirus B19)
	HIV
	Hemorrhagic fever viruses
	SARS-CoV-2
Bacteria	Sepsis (meningococcal, gonococcal, pneumococcal, *Haemophilus influenzae* type b)
	Infective endocarditis
	Ecthyma gangrenosum *(P. aeruginosa)*
	Vibrio vulnificus
Rickettsiae	Rocky Mountain spotted fever
	Epidemic typhus
	Ehrlichiosis
Other	Vasculitis
	IgA vasculitis (Henoch-Schönlein purpura)
	Acute hemorrhagic edema of infancy
	Malaria
NECROTIC ESCHAR	
Bacteria	*Bacillus anthracis*
	Francisella tularensis
	Rickettsiae rickettsialpox
Fungi	*Aspergillus, Mucor*
ERYTHEMA NODOSUM	
Viruses	Epstein-Barr virus
	HBV
Bacteria	Group A streptococcus
	Mycobacterium tuberculosis
	Yersinia
	Cat-scratch disease *(Bartonella henselae)*
Fungi	Coccidioidomycosis
	Histoplasmosis
Other	Sarcoidosis
	Inflammatory bowel disease
	Estrogen-containing oral contraceptives
	Systemic lupus erythematosus
	Behçet disease

HBV, Hepatitis B virus; *HHV,* human herpesvirus.

Clinical Manifestations

Measles infection is divided into four phases: incubation, prodromal (catarrhal), exanthematous (rash), and recovery. The incubation period is 8–12 days from exposure to symptom onset and a mean of 14 days (range of 7–21) from exposure to rash onset. The manifestations of the 3-day prodromal period are cough, coryza, conjunctivitis, and the pathognomonic **Koplik spots** (gray-white, sand grain–sized dots on the buccal mucosa opposite the lower molars) that last 12–24 hours. The conjunctiva may reveal a characteristic transverse line of inflammation along the eyelid margin (**Stimson line**). Cough, coryza, and conjunctivitis continue to occur during the secondary viremia of the exanthematous phase, which often is accompanied by high fever (40–40.5°C [104–105°F]). The macular rash begins on the head (often above the hairline) and spreads over most of the body in a cephalad-to-caudal pattern over 24 hours. Areas of the rash are often confluent. The rash fades in the same pattern, and illness severity is related to the extent of the rash. It may be petechial or hemorrhagic (**black measles**). As the rash fades, it undergoes brownish discoloration and desquamation. Generalized lymphadenopathy may be noted with the rash, with cervical nodes being most prominent. Mesenteric lymphadenopathy with abdominal pain may be noted with the rash. Otitis media, pneumonia, and diarrhea are more common in infants. Liver involvement is more common in adults.

The term **modified measles** describes mild cases of measles occurring in persons with partial protection against measles. Modified measles occurs in persons vaccinated before 12 months of age, in infants with disease modified by transplacentally acquired antibody, or in persons receiving immunoglobulin.

Laboratory and Imaging Studies

Routine laboratory findings are nonspecific and do not aid in diagnosis. Leukopenia is characteristic. In patients with acute encephalitis, the cerebrospinal fluid reveals an increased protein, lymphocytic pleocytosis, and normal glucose levels. Measles virus culture is not generally available, though identification of measles RNA via reverse transcriptase-polymerase chain reaction (PCR) may be available through state public health departments or the Centers for Disease Control and Prevention (CDC). Serologic testing for immunoglobulin M (IgM) antibodies that appear within 1–2 days of the rash and persist for 1–2 months in unimmunized persons confirms the clinical diagnosis, though IgM antibodies may be present only transiently in immunized people. Suspected cases should be **reported immediately** to the local or state health department.

Differential Diagnosis

The constellation of fever, rash, cough, and conjunctivitis is highly suggestive of measles. Measles must be differentiated from rubella, roseola, enteroviral or adenoviral infection, infectious mononucleosis, toxoplasmosis, meningococcemia, scarlet fever, rickettsial disease, Kawasaki disease, serum sickness, and drug rash.

Treatment

Routine supportive care includes maintaining adequate hydration and antipyretics. High-dose vitamin A supplementation improves the outcome of infants with measles in low- and middle-income countries. The World Health Organization recommends routine administration of vitamin A for 2 days to children with acute measles, regardless of country of residence.

Complications and Prognosis

Otitis media is the most common complication of measles infection. Interstitial (measles) pneumonia can occur, or pneumonia may result from secondary bacterial infection with *Streptococcus pneumoniae, Staphylococcus aureus,* or group A streptococcus. Persons with impaired cell-mediated immunity may develop **giant cell pneumonia**, which is usually fatal. Myocarditis and mesenteric lymphadenitis are infrequent complications.

Encephalomyelitis occurs in 1–3 per 1,000 cases and usually occurs 2–5 days after the onset of the rash. Early encephalitis probably is caused by direct viral infection of brain tissue, whereas later onset encephalitis is a demyelinating, and probably an immunopathologic, phenomenon. **Subacute sclerosing panencephalitis (SSPE)** is a late neurologic complication of slow measles infection that is characterized by progressive behavioral and intellectual deterioration and eventual death. It occurs in approximately 1 in every million cases of measles, an average of 8–10 years after measles. There is no effective treatment.

Deaths most frequently result from bronchopneumonia or encephalitis, with much higher risk in persons with malignancy, severe malnutrition, age under 5 years, or immunocompromise (such as HIV infection). Late deaths in adolescents and adults usually result from SSPE. Other forms of measles encephalitis in immunocompetent persons are associated with a mortality rate of approximately 15%, with 20–30% of survivors having serious neurologic sequelae.

Prevention

Live measles vaccine prevents infection and is recommended as measles, mumps, and rubella (MMR) for children at 12–15 months and 4–6 years of age. MMR can be given as early as 6 months for children traveling internationally or for infants who live in or are traveling to an area experiencing a measles outbreak. If the first dose of MMR is given prior to 12 months of age, the child should still receive doses at 12–15 months and 4–6 years. The MMRV (MMR combined with varicella vaccine) is an alternative vaccine for children 12 months to 12 years of age, provided there are no contraindications, but is associated with a higher rate of febrile seizures following administration. The second dose of MMR significantly reduces the primary vaccine failure rate, from less than 5% to less than 1%. Contraindications to measles vaccine include immunocompromised states or an immunosuppressive course of corticosteroids (>2 mg/kg/day or >20 mg/day for those weighing >10 kg, for >14 days), pregnancy, or recent administration of immunoglobulin (within 3–11 months, depending on the type and dose). MMR vaccination *is recommended* for all persons with HIV without evidence of severe immunosuppression (low age-specific CD4 T lymphocytes), children with cancer in remission who have not received chemotherapy in the previous 3 months, and children who have not received immunosuppressive corticosteroids in the previous month. Susceptible household contacts (6–11 months old or unimmunized) should receive **postexposure prophylaxis** with measles vaccine within 72 hours of measles exposure if immunocompromised or immunoglobulin within 6 days of exposure.

RUBELLA (GERMAN OR 3-DAY MEASLES)

Etiology

Rubella, also known as **German measles** or **3-day measles**, is caused by a single-stranded RNA virus with a glycolipid envelope and is a member of the togavirus family. Humans are the only natural hosts. Rubella virus invades the respiratory epithelium and disseminates via primary viremia. After replication in the reticuloendothelial system, a secondary viremia ensues, and the virus can be isolated from peripheral blood monocytes, cerebrospinal fluid, and urine. Rubella virus is most contagious through direct or droplet contact with nasopharyngeal secretions from 2 days before until 5–7 days after rash onset, although the virus may be present in nasopharyngeal secretions from 7 days before until 14 days after the rash.

Infection **in utero** results in significant morbidity from **congenital rubella syndrome (CRS)** with associated ophthalmologic, cardiac, and neurologic manifestations (see Chapter 65). Maternal infection during the first trimester results in fetal infection with generalized tissue damage or vasculitis in more than 90% of cases. Infants with CRS may shed the virus in nasopharyngeal secretions and urine for more than 12 months after birth and transmit it to susceptible contacts.

Epidemiology

In unvaccinated populations, rubella usually occurs in the spring, with epidemics occurring in cycles of every 6–9 years. Approximately 25–50% of cases are subclinical. Fewer than 20 cases of rubella occur annually in the United States. Outbreaks occasionally occur in nonvaccinated groups from internationally imported cases. Transplacentally acquired antibody is protective during the first 6 months of life.

Clinical Manifestations

The incubation period for postnatal rubella is typically 16–18 days (range of 14–21 days). The mild catarrhal symptoms of the prodromal phase of rubella may go unnoticed. The characteristic signs of rubella are posterior auricular, posterior cervical, and posterior occipital lymphadenopathy accompanied by an erythematous, maculopapular, discrete rash. The rash begins on the face and spreads to the body, lasting for 3 days, and is less prominent than that of measles. Rose-colored spots on the soft palate, known as **Forchheimer spots**, develop in 20% of patients and may appear before the rash. Other manifestations of rubella include mild pharyngitis, conjunctivitis, anorexia, headache, malaise, and low-grade fever. Polyarthritis, usually of the hands, may occur, especially among adult females, but usually resolves without sequelae. Paresthesias and tendinitis may occur.

Laboratory and Imaging Studies

Routine laboratory findings are nonspecific and generally do not aid in diagnosis. The white blood cell count usually is normal or low, and thrombocytopenia rarely occurs. Diagnosis is confirmed by serologic testing for IgM antibodies (typically positive 5 days after symptom onset) or by a fourfold or greater increase in specific IgG antibodies in paired acute and convalescent sera. CRS cases can have detectable IgM until 3 months of age and stable or rising IgG titers over the first 7–11 months of age. False-positive IgM results can occur. Cases of suspected CRS and postnatal rubella infection should be reported to the local and state health departments.

Differential Diagnosis

The rash must be differentiated from measles, roseola, enteroviral or adenoviral infection, infectious mononucleosis, toxoplasmosis, scarlet fever, rickettsial disease, Kawasaki disease, serum sickness, and drug rash.

Treatment

There is no specific therapy for rubella, and treatment is supportive.

Complications and Prognosis

Other than CRS (see Chapter 65) arising from fetal rubella infection during pregnancy, complications are rare. Death rarely occurs with rubella encephalitis.

Prevention

Live rubella vaccine prevents infection and is recommended as MMR for children at 12–15 months and at 4–6 years of age. After vaccination, vaccine-rubella virus is shed from the nasopharynx for several weeks, but it is not communicable. In children, rubella vaccine rarely is associated with adverse effects, but in postpubertal females it causes arthralgias in 25% of vaccinated individuals and acute arthritis-like symptoms in 10% of vaccinated individuals. These symptoms typically develop 1–3 weeks after vaccination and last 1–3 days.

Contraindications to rubella vaccine include immunocompromised states or an immunosuppressive course of corticosteroids (>2 mg/kg/day or >20 mg/day for those weighing >10 kg, for >14 days), pregnancy, or recent administration of immunoglobulin (within 3–11 months, depending on the type and dose). Vaccine virus has been recovered from fetal tissues, although no cases of CRS have been identified among infants born to women inadvertently vaccinated against rubella during pregnancy. Nevertheless, women are cautioned to avoid pregnancy for 28 days after receiving the rubella-containing vaccine. All pregnant women should have prenatal serologic testing to determine their immune status to rubella, and susceptible mothers should be vaccinated after delivery and before hospital discharge.

Susceptible, nonpregnant persons exposed to rubella should receive rubella vaccination. Immunoglobulin is not recommended for postexposure prophylaxis of susceptible, pregnant women exposed to rubella.

ROSEOLA INFANTUM (EXANTHEM SUBITUM)

Etiology

Roseola infantum (exanthem subitum, sixth disease) is caused primarily by human herpesvirus type 6 (HHV-6) in most cases and by HHV-7 in 10–30% of cases. HHV-6 and HHV-7 are large, enveloped double-stranded DNA viruses that are members of the herpesvirus family. Two species of HHV-6 (HHV-6A and HHV-6B) exist, with almost all postnatal infections caused by HHV-6B. These viruses infect mature mononuclear cells and cause a relatively prolonged (3–5 days) viremia during primary infection. They can be detected in the saliva of healthy adults, which suggests, as with other herpesviruses, the development of lifelong latent infection and intermittent viral shedding.

Epidemiology

Transplacentally acquired antibody protects most infants until 6 months of age. The incidence of infection increases as maternally derived antibody levels decline. By 12 months of age, approximately 60–90% of children have antibodies to HHV-6, and essentially all children are seropositive by 2–3 years of age. The virus is likely acquired from asymptomatic adults who periodically shed these viruses. HHV-6 is a major cause of acute febrile illnesses in infants and may be responsible for up to 20% of visits to the emergency department for children 6–18 months of age.

Clinical Manifestations

Roseola is characterized by high fever (often >40°C) with an abrupt onset that lasts 3–5 days. A maculopapular, rose-colored rash erupts coincident with defervescence, although it may be present earlier. The rash usually lasts 1–3 days but may fade rapidly; rash *is not* present in all infants with HHV-6 infection. Upper respiratory symptoms, nasal congestion, erythematous tympanic membranes, and cough may occur. Gastrointestinal symptoms are described. Roseola is associated with ~30% of febrile seizures. Roseola cases caused by HHV-6 and HHV-7 are clinically indistinguishable, although HHV-6–associated roseola typically occurs in younger infants. Reactivation of HHV-6 following bone marrow transplantation may result in bone marrow suppression, hepatitis, rash, and encephalitis.

Laboratory and Imaging Studies

Routine laboratory findings are nonspecific and do not aid in diagnosis. Encephalitis with roseola is characterized by pleocytosis (30–200 cells/mm^3) with mononuclear cell predominance, elevated protein concentration, and normal glucose concentration. Serologic testing showing a fourfold rise in acute and convalescent sera or documentation of HHV-6 DNA by PCR in the cerebrospinal fluid is diagnostic. PCR has also been used to detect HHV-6 in blood but may not be able to differentiate latent, reactivation, or primary infection. A rising viral titer is indicative of reactivation or primary infection. HHV-6 may also integrate in human chromosomes, making viral PCR on white blood cells difficult to interpret.

Differential Diagnosis

The pattern of high fever for 3–5 days without significant physical findings followed by onset of rash with subsequent defervescence is characteristic. Many febrile illnesses may be easily confused with roseola during the preeruptive stage. Serious infections must be excluded, although most children with roseola are alert, behave normally, and continue with their usual daily activities.

Treatment

There is no specific therapy for roseola. Routine supportive care includes maintaining adequate hydration and antipyretics. In immunocompromised hosts, use of ganciclovir or foscarnet can be considered.

Complications and Prognosis

The prognosis for roseola is excellent. A few deaths have been attributed to HHV-6, usually in cases complicated by encephalitis or virus-associated **hemophagocytosis syndrome**.

Prevention

No preventative measures are available.

ERYTHEMA INFECTIOSUM (FIFTH DISEASE)

Etiology

Erythema infectiosum (fifth disease) is caused by the human parvovirus B19, a single-stranded DNA virus producing a benign viral exanthem in healthy children. The viral affinity for red blood cell progenitor cells makes it an important cause of aplastic crisis in patients with chronic hemolytic anemias, including sickle cell disease, spherocytosis, and thalassemia. Parvovirus B19 also causes fetal anemia and hydrops fetalis after primary infection during pregnancy. The cell receptor for parvovirus B19 is the **erythrocyte P antigen**, a glycolipid present on erythroid cells. The virus replicates in actively dividing erythroid stem cells, leading to cell death that results in erythroid aplasia and anemia.

Epidemiology

Erythema infectiosum is common. Parvovirus B19 seroprevalence is only 2–9% in children younger than 5 years of age but increases to 15–35% in children 5–18 years and 30–60% in adults. Community epidemics usually occur in the spring. The virus is transmitted by respiratory secretions and by blood product transfusions.

Clinical Manifestations

The incubation period is typically 4–14 days and, rarely, may last 21 days. Parvovirus B19 infections usually begin with a mild, nonspecific illness characterized by fever, malaise, myalgias, and headache. In some cases, the characteristic rash appears 7–10 days later. Erythema infectiosum is manifested by rash, low-grade or no fever, and occasionally pharyngitis and mild conjunctivitis. The rash appears in three stages. The initial stage is typically a **"slapped cheek" rash** with circumoral pallor. An erythematous symmetric, maculopapular, truncal rash appears 1–4 days later and then fades as central clearing takes place, giving a distinctive **lacy, reticulated rash** that lasts 2–40 days (mean of 11 days). This rash may be pruritic, does not desquamate, and may recur with exercise, bathing, rubbing, or stress. Adolescents and adults may experience myalgias, significant arthralgias or arthritis, headache, pharyngitis, coryza, and gastrointestinal upset.

Children with shortened erythrocyte life span (e.g., sickle cell disease) may develop a **transient aplastic crisis**, which is characterized by ineffective erythroid production typically lasting 7–10 days (see Chapter 151). Most children with parvovirus B19–induced transient aplastic crisis have multiple symptoms, including fever, lethargy, malaise, pallor, headache, gastrointestinal symptoms, and respiratory symptoms. The reticulocyte count is extremely low, and the hemoglobin level is lower than usual for the patient. Transient neutropenia and thrombocytopenia also commonly occur. Parvovirus may also cause hepatitis, myocarditis, and the **papular-purpuric gloves and socks syndrome**.

Persistent parvovirus B19 infection may develop in children with immunodeficiency, causing severe anemia resulting from pure red blood cell aplasia. These children do not display the typical manifestations of erythema infectiosum.

Laboratory and Imaging Studies

Hematologic abnormalities occur with parvovirus infection, including reticulocytopenia lasting 7–10 days, mild anemia, thrombocytopenia, lymphopenia, and neutropenia. Parvovirus B19 can be detected by PCR and by electron microscopy of erythroid precursors in the bone marrow. Serologic tests showing specific IgM antibody to parvovirus are diagnostic, demonstrating an infection that probably occurred in the prior 2–4 months. Parvovirus PCR of blood and cerebrospinal fluid is also available, primarily for use in severe illness or immunocompromised patients.

Differential Diagnosis

The diagnosis of erythema infectiosum in children is based on the clinical findings of typical facial rash with absent or mild prodromal symptoms, followed by a reticulated rash over the body that waxes and wanes. The differential diagnosis includes measles, rubella, scarlet fever, enteroviral or adenoviral infection, infectious mononucleosis, Kawasaki disease, systemic lupus erythematosus, serum sickness, and drug reaction.

Treatment

There is no specific therapy other than routine supportive care. Transfusions may be required for transient aplastic crisis. Intrauterine transfusion has been performed for hydrops fetalis associated with fetal parvovirus B19 infection. Intravenous immunoglobulin may be used for immunocompromised persons with severe anemia or chronic infection.

Complications and Prognosis

The prognosis for erythema infectiosum is excellent. Fatalities associated with transient aplastic crisis are rare. Parvovirus B19 is not teratogenic, but in utero infection of fetal erythroid cells may result in fetal heart failure, hydrops fetalis, and fetal death. Of the approximately 50% of women of childbearing age susceptible to parvovirus B19 infection, 30% of exposed women develop infection, with 25% of exposed fetuses becoming infected and 10% of these culminating in fetal death.

Prevention

The greatest risk is to pregnant women. Effective control measures are limited. The exclusion of affected children from school is not recommended because children generally are not infectious by the time the rash is present. Good handwashing and hygiene are practical measures that should help reduce transmission.

VARICELLA-ZOSTER VIRUS INFECTION (CHICKENPOX AND ZOSTER)

Etiology

Chickenpox and zoster are caused by varicella-zoster virus (VZV), an enveloped, icosahedral, double-stranded DNA virus that is a member of the herpesvirus family. Humans are the only natural hosts. **Chickenpox (varicella)** is the manifestation of primary infection. VZV infects susceptible individuals via the conjunctivae or respiratory tract and replicates in the nasopharynx and upper respiratory tract. It disseminates by primary viremia and infects regional lymph nodes, the liver, the spleen, and other organs. Secondary viremia follows, resulting in a cutaneous infection with the typical vesicular rash. After resolution of chickenpox, the virus persists in latent infection in the dorsal root ganglia cells. **Zoster (shingles)** is the manifestation of reactivated latent infection of endogenous VZV. Chickenpox is highly communicable in susceptible individuals, with a secondary attack rate of more than 90%. The period of communicability ranges from 2 days before to 7 days after the onset of the rash, when all lesions are crusted.

Epidemiology

In the postvaccine era, the incidence of varicella has declined in all age groups, with peak incidence during outbreaks in the 5–9 year age group. VZV transmission is by direct person-to-person contact of vesicular fluid or droplets and via inhalation of aerosols from vesicular fluid (either varicella or zoster lesions) or infected respiratory secretions. The incidence and severity of zoster are increased in immunocompromised persons.

Clinical Manifestations

The incubation period of **chickenpox** is generally 14–16 (range of 10–21) days after exposure. Prodromal symptoms of fever, malaise, and anorexia may precede the rash by 1 day. The characteristic rash appears initially as small red papules that rapidly progress to nonumbilicated, oval, teardrop-like vesicles on an erythematous base. The fluid progresses from clear to cloudy, and the vesicles ulcerate, crust, and heal. New crops appear for 3–4 days, usually beginning on the trunk followed by the head, the face, and, less commonly, the extremities. There may be a total of 100–500 lesions, with all forms of lesions present at the same time. Pruritus is universal and marked. Lesions may be present on mucous membranes. Lymphadenopathy may be generalized. The severity of the rash varies, as do systemic signs and fever, which generally abate after 3–4 days.

The preeruption phase of **zoster** includes intense localized and burning pain and tenderness **(acute neuritis)** along a dermatome, accompanied by malaise and fever. In several days, the eruption of papules, which quickly vesiculate, occurs in the dermatome or in two adjacent dermatomes. Groups of lesions occur for 1–7 days and then progress to crusting and healing. Thoracic and lumbar regions are typically involved. Lesions generally are unilateral and are accompanied by regional lymphadenopathy. In one third of patients, a few vesicles occur outside the primary dermatome. Any branch of cranial nerve V may be involved, which also may cause corneal and intraoral lesions. Involvement of cranial nerve VII may result in facial paralysis and ear canal vesicles **(Ramsay Hunt syndrome)**. Ophthalmic zoster may be associated with ipsilateral cerebral angiitis and stroke. Immunocompromised persons may have unusually severe, painful herpes zoster that involves multiple cutaneous regions and, potentially, visceral dissemination (to liver, lungs, and central nervous system). **Postherpetic neuralgia**, defined as pain persisting longer than 1 month, is uncommon in children.

Laboratory and Imaging Studies

Laboratory testing confirmation for diagnosis is usually unnecessary. PCR of vesicular fluid is the current diagnostic method of choice, and genotyping to distinguish vaccine and wild-type strains is available through the CDC.

Differential Diagnosis

The diagnosis of varicella and zoster is based on the distinctive characteristics of the rash. **Eczema herpeticum**, or **Kaposi varicelliform eruption**, is a localized, vesicular eruption caused by herpes simplex virus (HSV) that develops on skin affected by underlying eczema or trauma. The differentiation between zoster and HSV infection may be difficult because HSV may cause an eruption that appears to be in a dermatomal distribution. Coxsackievirus A infection has a vesiculopustular appearance, but lesions are usually localized to the extremities and oropharynx. A previously healthy patient with more than one recurrence probably has HSV infection, which can be confirmed by PCR. Mpox should also be considered in the differential diagnosis.

Treatment

Symptomatic therapy of **chickenpox** includes nonaspirin antipyretics and other supportive care. Routine administration of acyclovir is not recommended in otherwise healthy children with varicella. The decision to use antiviral medications, the route, and the duration of treatment depend on host factors and the risk for severe infection or complications. Early therapy with antivirals (especially within 24 hours of rash onset) in *immunocompromised* persons is effective in preventing severe complications, including pneumonia, encephalitis, and death from varicella. Acyclovir or valacyclovir may be considered in those at risk of severe varicella, such as unvaccinated persons older than 12 years; those with chronic cutaneous or pulmonary disease; or those receiving short-course, intermittent, oral, or aerosolized corticosteroids. The dose of acyclovir used for VZV infections is higher than that for HSV.

Antiviral treatment of **zoster** accelerates cutaneous healing, hastens the resolution of acute neuritis, and reduces the risk of postherpetic neuralgia. Oral valacyclovir and famciclovir have much greater oral bioavailability than acyclovir and are recommended for treatment of zoster in adults. Valacyclovir is approved for use in children 2 years and older, and acyclovir is available for use in all age groups.

Complications and Prognosis

Secondary infection of skin lesions by streptococci or staphylococci is the most common complication of chickenpox. These infections may be mild, resembling impetigo, or life-threatening, with toxic shock syndrome or necrotizing fasciitis. Pneumonia is uncommon in healthy children but occurs in 15–20% of healthy adults and immunocompromised persons. Myocarditis, pericarditis, orchitis, hepatitis, ulcerative gastritis, glomerulonephritis, and arthritis may complicate varicella. Reye syndrome may follow varicella; thus salicylate use is contraindicated during varicella infection.

Neurologic complications frequently include postinfectious encephalitis, cerebellar ataxia, nystagmus, and tremor. Less common neurologic complications include Guillain-Barré syndrome, transverse myelitis, cranial nerve palsies, optic neuritis, and hypothalamic syndrome.

Primary varicella can be fatal in immunocompromised persons due to visceral dissemination, encephalitis, hepatitis, and pneumonitis. The mortality rate approaches 15% in children with leukemia who do not receive prophylaxis or therapy (see Chapter 156).

A severe form of neonatal varicella may develop in newborns of mothers with primary varicella (but not shingles) occurring 5 days before to 2 days after delivery. The fetus is exposed to a large inoculum of virus but is born before the maternal antibody response develops and can cross the placenta. These infants should be treated as soon as possible with varicella-zoster immunoglobulin (VZIG) or intravenous immunoglobulin if VZIG is unavailable, to attempt to prevent or ameliorate the infection.

Zoster is usually self-limited, especially in children. Advanced age and severity of pain at presentation and at 1 month are predictors of prolonged pain. Scarring is more common with zoster because of the involvement of the deeper layers of the skin.

Prevention

Children with chickenpox should not return to school until all vesicles have crusted. A hospitalized child with chickenpox and immunocompromised patients with zoster should be isolated in a negative-pressure room to prevent transmission. Zoster transmission can be minimized by covering the affected area.

A live, two-dose attenuated varicella vaccine is recommended for all children. The first dose should be administered at age 12–15 months and the second dose at 4–6 years. The two-dose varicella vaccine is 98% effective in preventing any disease (92% effective in postlicensure trials) and 100% effective in preventing severe disease. Transmission of vaccine virus from a healthy vaccinated individual is rare but possible.

Passive immunity can be provided by VZIG, which is indicated within 96 hours of exposure for susceptible individuals at increased risk for severe illness, such as immunocompromised children and some hospitalized preterm infants. Administration of VZIG does not eliminate the possibility of disease in recipients and prolongs the incubation period up to 28 days.

PEARLS FOR PRACTITIONERS

See Infectious Diseases: Pearls for Practitioners at the end of this section.

REVIEW QUESTIONS

Available online.

CHAPTER 99

Cutaneous Infections

SUPERFICIAL BACTERIAL INFECTIONS

Impetigo

Nonbullous or crusted impetigo is caused most often by *Staphylococcus aureus* and occasionally by group A streptococcus. It begins as a single erythematous papulovesicle that progresses to one or many **honey-colored, crusted lesions** weeping serous drainage. **Bullous impetigo** accounts for approximately 30% of all impetigo. The skin lesions are thin-walled (0.5–3 cm) bullae with erythematous margins resembling second-degree burns and are associated with *S. aureus*. Impetigo most frequently occurs on the face, around the nares and mouth, and on the extremities. Fever is uncommon. The diagnosis usually is established by the clinical appearance alone.

Recommended treatment for nonbullous impetigo is topical 2% mupirocin or oral antistaphylococcal antibiotics. Extensive or disseminated lesions, bullous impetigo, lesions around the eyes, or lesions otherwise not amenable to topical therapy are best treated with oral antibiotics. Streptococcal impetigo is associated with increased risk of postinfectious glomerulonephritis but not acute rheumatic fever (see Chapter 164). Antibiotic treatment does not decrease the risk of postinfectious glomerulonephritis, but it does decrease the possible spread of nephritogenic strains to close contacts. Children with impetigo should remain out of school or day care until 24 hours of antibiotic therapy have been completed.

Cellulitis

Cellulitis is infection involving the subcutaneous tissues and the dermis and is usually caused by *S. aureus* or group A streptococci. Cellulitis typically presents with indurated, warm, and erythematous macules with indistinct borders that can expand. Additional manifestations commonly include fever, lymphangitis, and regional lymphadenitis. **Erysipelas** is a superficial variant of cellulitis usually caused by group A streptococcus that involves the dermis only. The rapidly advancing lesions are tender, bright red in appearance, and have sharp margins. The patients may appear toxic. Blood cultures are recommended for erysipelas. Empirical antibiotic treatment for cellulitis is recommended with a first-generation cephalosporin unless the local *S. aureus* methicillin-resistance rate is high, in which case alternatives include clindamycin or trimethoprim-sulfamethoxazole. Many patients may be managed with oral antibiotics and close follow-up; hospitalization and intravenous antibiotics are recommended for erysipelas and cellulitis of the face, hands, feet, or perineum; those with lymphangitis; and those not responding to outpatient therapy.

Ecthyma usually is caused by group A streptococcus and may complicate impetigo. Initially, it is characterized by a lesion with a rim of erythematous induration surrounding an eschar, which if removed reveals a shallow ulcer. **Ecthyma gangrenosum** is a serious skin infection occurring in immunocompromised persons due to hematogenous spread of septic emboli to the skin, classically caused by *Pseudomonas aeruginosa,* other gram-negative organisms, or occasionally *Aspergillus.* The lesions begin as purple macules that undergo central necrosis to become exquisitely tender, deep, punched-out ulcers 2–3 cm in diameter with a dark necrotic base, raised red edges, and sometimes a yellowish-green exudate. Fever usually is present.

Necrotizing fasciitis is the most extensive form of cellulitis and involves deeper subcutaneous tissues and fascial planes. It may progress to **myonecrosis** of the underlying muscle. Common causes include *S. aureus* and group A streptococcus alone or in combination with anaerobic organisms, such as *Clostridium perfringens.* Risk factors include underlying immunodeficiency, recent surgery or trauma, and varicella infection. Lesions progress rapidly with raised or sharply demarcated margins, although disease typically extends on a deeper plane beyond superficially evident lesions. A **compartment syndrome** may be a complication. Warning signs of necrotizing fasciitis include pain out of proportion to evident skin lesions, shock or toxic appearance, or crepitus due to subcutaneous gas formation by anaerobes. Necrotizing fasciitis is a surgical emergency, and early consultation with an experienced surgeon is recommended. Adjunctive tests such as magnetic resonance imaging can confirm the presence of gas in tissues, but obtaining imaging should not delay surgical consultation. Treatment includes rapid surgical debridement of all necrotic tissues and broad-spectrum intravenous antibiotics, such as clindamycin, linezolid, or vancomycin plus ceftriaxone or piperacillin-tazobactam.

Folliculitis

Folliculitis refers to small, dome-shaped pustules or erythematous papules located in hair follicles, with superficial, limited inflammatory reaction in the surrounding tissue and is predominantly caused by *S. aureus.* **Furuncles (boils)** are deeper hair follicle infections that manifest as nodules with intense surrounding inflammatory reaction. These occur most frequently on the neck, trunk, axillae, and buttocks. A **carbuncle** represents the deepest of hair follicle infections and is characterized by multiseptate, loculated abscesses. Boils and carbuncles frequently require incisional drainage. Superficial folliculitis can be treated with topical therapy, such as an antibacterial chlorhexidine wash or an antibacterial lotion or solution such as clindamycin 1%, applied twice a day for 7–10 days, or mupirocin ointment applied three times daily for 5–7 days. Oral antibiotics *may* be necessary for unresponsive cases or for furuncles and carbuncles.

P. aeruginosa folliculitis **(hot tub folliculitis)** presents as pruritic papules, pustules, or deeper, purple-red nodules predominantly on skin areas covered by a swimsuit after bathing in hot tubs. Folliculitis develops 8–48 hours after exposure, usually without associated systemic symptoms, and resolves in 1–2 weeks without treatment.

Perianal Dermatitis

Perianal dermatitis (perianal streptococcal disease) is caused by group A streptococcus and is characterized by well-demarcated, very tender, marked perianal erythema extending 2 cm from the anus. Manifestations include anal pruritus and painful defecation, sometimes with blood-streaked stools. The differential diagnosis includes diaper dermatitis, candidiasis, pinworm infection, and anal fissures. Optimal treatment is oral penicillin or amoxicillin.

SUPERFICIAL FUNGAL INFECTIONS

Cutaneous fungal infections are common in children (Table 99.1). The estimated lifetime risk of developing **dermatophytosis** is 10–20%. Diagnosis is usually established by visual inspection and may be confirmed by potassium hydroxide (KOH) examination or fungal culture of skin scrapings from the margins of the lesion. Recommended tinea treatment is usually for 4–6 weeks duration and is continued for 2 weeks after resolution of symptoms; topical antifungal creams (e.g., miconazole, clotrimazole, ketoconazole, tolnaftate) are appropriate for tinea corporis, tinea pedis, and tinea cruris, whereas tinea capitis requires oral treatment. The diagnosis of **onychomycosis** should be confirmed by KOH examination and fungal culture. Recommended treatment is terbinafine or itraconazole for at least 12 weeks.

SUPERFICIAL VIRAL INFECTIONS

Herpes Simplex Virus

Primary herpetic infections can occur after inoculation of the virus at any mucocutaneous site. Herpes simplex virus type 1 (HSV-1) is common in children and classically causes gingivostomatitis, whereas HSV-2 classically infects the genitalia as a sexually transmitted infection (see Chapter 117), though HSV-1 may cause approximately 30% of genital herpes, and HSV-2 can cause gingivostomatitis. For the cutaneous manifestations of neonatal HSV infection, see Chapter 65.

Herpes gingivostomatitis involves the gingivae and may spread throughout the oropharynx. Herpes labialis **(cold sores or fever blisters)** is limited to the vermilion border involving skin and mucous membranes. Clinical manifestations of *primary* HSV gingivostomatitis include typical oropharyngeal vesicular lesions with high fever, malaise, stinging mouth pain, drooling, fetid breath, and cervical lymphadenopathy.

Herpetic skin lesions are quite painful and characteristically begin as erythematous papules that quickly progress to the characteristically grouped, 2- to 4-mm, fluid-filled vesicles on an erythematous base. Removal of the vesicle roof reveals a small, sharply demarcated ulcer with a punched-out appearance. The characteristic grouped vesicles distinguish HSV from chickenpox (see Chapter 98). Within several days, the vesicles become pustular, rupture, and encrust. Diagnosis is made clinically or with polymerase chain reaction (PCR). Scarring is uncommon, but there may be residual hyperpigmentation. After primary infection, the virus remains latent in nerve dorsal root ganglia. About 20–40% of adults experience *recurrent* oral episodes of HSV labialis throughout life. Recurrences occur in roughly the same location and may be preceded by prodromal symptoms of tingling or burning without fever or lymphadenopathy.

TABLE 99.1 Superficial Fungal Infections

NAME	ETIOLOGY	MANIFESTATIONS	DIAGNOSIS	THERAPY
DERMATOPHYTES				
Tinea capitis (ringworm)	*Microsporum audouinii, Trichophyton tonsurans, Microsporum canis*	Prepubertal infection of scalp, hair shafts; black dot alopecia	*M. audouinii* fluorescence: blue-green with Wood lamp*; +KOH, culture	Griseofulvin; terbinafine, itraconazole
Kerion	Inflammatory reaction to tinea capitis	Swollen, boggy, crusted, purulent, tender scalp mass with lymphadenopathy; secondary distal id reaction common	As above	As above, plus steroids for *id* reactions
Tinea corporis (ringworm)	*M. canis, Trichophyton rubrum,* others	Slightly pruritic ringlike, erythematous papules, plaques with scaling and slow outward expansion of the border; check cat or dog for *M. canis*	+KOH, culture; *M. canis* fluorescence: blue-green with Wood lamp; differential diagnosis: granuloma annulare, pityriasis rosea, nummular eczema, psoriasis	Topical miconazole, clotrimazole, terbinafine, tolnaftate, ciclopirox, oxiconazole, or butenafine
Tinea cruris (jock itch)	*Epidermophyton floccosum, Trichophyton mentagrophytes, T. rubrum*	Symmetric, pruritic, scrotal sparing, scaling plaques	+KOH, culture; differential diagnosis: erythrasma *(Corynebacterium minutissimum)*	See tinea corporis, therapy; wear loose cotton underwear
Tinea pedis (athlete's foot)	*T. rubrum, T. mentagrophytes*	Moccasin or interdigital distribution, dry scales, interdigital maceration with secondary bacterial infection	+KOH, culture; differential diagnosis: *C. minutissimum* erythrasma	Medications as above; wear cotton socks
Tinea unguium (onychomycosis)	*T. mentagrophytes, T. rubrum, Candida albicans*	Uncommon before puberty; peeling of distal nail plate; thickening, splitting of nails	+KOH, culture	Oral terbinafine or itraconazole
Tinea versicolor	*Malassezia furfur*	Tropical climates, steroids or immunosuppressive drugs; uncommon before puberty; chest, back, arms; oval hypopigmented or hyperpigmented in Black people, red-brown in white people; scaling patches	+KOH; orange-gold fluorescence with Wood lamp; differential diagnosis: pityriasis alba	Topical selenium sulfide, oral ketoconazole
YEAST				
Candidiasis	*C. albicans*	Diaper area, intense erythematous plaques or pustules, isolated or confluent	+KOH, culture	Topical nystatin; oral nystatin treats concomitant oral thrush

**Wood lamp examination uses an ultraviolet source in a completely darkened room. Trichophyton usually has no fluorescence.*
KOH, Potassium hydroxide.

Viral paronychia (**herpetic whitlow**) is a painful, localized infection of a digit, usually of the distal pulp space, with erythematous and occasionally vesiculopustular eruption. It occurs in children who suck their thumbs or bite their nails and those with herpetic gingivostomatitis. **Herpes gladiatorum** occurs in wrestlers and rugby players who acquire cutaneous herpes from close body contact with other players' cutaneous infections. Cutaneous HSV infection in persons with an underlying skin disorder (e.g., atopic dermatitis) can result in **eczema herpeticum (Kaposi varicelliform eruption)**, a disseminated cutaneous infection. There may be hundreds of herpetic vesicles over the body, usually concentrated in the areas of skin affected by the underlying disorder.

Treatment with oral valacyclovir or famciclovir may shorten duration of disease for primary and recurrent infection. Prophylactic antiviral therapy may be warranted in those with frequent recurrences. Neonates, persons with eczema, and persons with immunodeficiency are at increased risk for disseminated and severe HSV disease and should receive intravenous acyclovir therapy.

Human Papillomaviruses (Warts)

Warts are caused by the human papillomaviruses (HPVs), nonenveloped, double-stranded DNA viruses that infect skin and mucous membrane keratinocytes. More than 100

HPV serotypes have been identified, with different serotypes accounting for the variation in location and clinical presentations. There are 15–20 **oncogenic (high-risk)** types, of which HPV types 16 and 18 are associated with 70% of cases of cervical cancer as well as vulvar and vaginal cancers. Regardless of the infecting serotype, all warts are associated with hyperplasia of the epidermal cells.

Warts occur at all ages. **Common warts (verruca vulgaris)**, associated with HPV types 1 and 2, are the most frequent form (71%). They occur in school-age children, with a prevalence of 4–20%. They are transmitted by direct contact or by fomites and have an incubation period of approximately 1 month before clinical presentation. The common wart is a painless, well-circumscribed, small (2–5 mm) papule with a papillated or verrucous surface typically distributed on the fingers, toes, elbows, and knees. They also may be found on the nose, ears, and lips. **Filiform warts** are verrucous, exophytic, 2-mm papules that have a narrow or pedunculated base. **Flat warts (verruca plana)** are associated with HPV types 3 and 10 and are multiple, flat-topped, 2- to 4-mm papules clustered on the dorsal surface of the hands, on the soles of the feet **(plantar warts)**, or on the face. Plantar warts may be painful because of the effect of pressure and friction on the lesions. **Genital warts (condylomata acuminata)** are associated with the HPV types 6 and 11 (90%). They are flesh-colored, hyperpigmented, or erythematous lesions that are filiform, fungating, or plaque-like in appearance and involve multiple sites on the vulva, vagina, penis, or perineum. Genital warts are the most common sexually transmitted infection, with 1 million new cases annually.

Warts typically are self-limited and resolve spontaneously over years without specific treatment. Treatment options are available for common and flat warts as well as condylomata acuminata. Topical preparations for common and flat warts disrupt infected epithelium (using salicylic acid, liquid nitrogen, or laser therapy) and result in the cure of approximately 75% of patients. Treatment of anogenital warts requires assessment of size, number, patient preference, cost, convenience, and adverse effects (see Chapter 117). Medications may include topical podophyllotoxin or imiquimod. Additional treatment methods include laser ablation and immunotherapy with intralesional interferon; immunotherapy may result in significant toxicities.

The most serious consequence of HPV infection is **cervical cancer** (>12,000 new cases annually) as well as vulvar, vaginal, penile, anal, and head and neck cancers. Three HPV vaccines are licensed for use in the United States: a quadrivalent vaccine (which protects against serotypes 6, 11, 16, and 18), a bivalent vaccine (types 16 and 18), and a 9-valent vaccine (types 6, 11, 16, 18, 31, 33, 45, 52, and 58), though only the 9-valent vaccine is currently available in the United States. The two- to three-dose regimen of these vaccines (based on age) has more than a 98% efficacy in preventing the precancerous dysplasia that precedes cervical cancer.

Molluscum Contagiosum

Molluscum contagiosum virus, a poxvirus that replicates in host epithelial cells, produces discrete, small (2–4 mm), pearly flesh-colored or pink, nontender, dome-shaped papules with central umbilication. Papules occur most commonly in intertriginous regions, such as the axillae, groin, and neck. They rarely occur on the face or in the periocular region. The infection typically affects toddlers and young children and is acquired through direct contact with infected individuals. Spread occurs by autoinoculation. Infection with molluscum contagiosum may be complicated by a surrounding dermatitis. Severely immunocompromised persons or persons with extensive atopic dermatitis often have widespread lesions.

Diagnosis is clinical. Lesions are self-limited, resolving over months to years, and usually no specific treatment is recommended. Available treatment options are limited to destructive modalities, such as cryotherapy with topical liquid nitrogen, vesicant therapy with topical 0.9% cantharidin, or removal by curettage, and should be reserved for extensive disease.

PEARLS FOR PRACTITIONERS

See Infectious Diseases: Pearls for Practitioners at the end of this section.

REVIEW QUESTIONS

Available online.

CHAPTER 100

Lymphadenopathy

ETIOLOGY

Lymphoid tissue steadily enlarges until puberty and subsequently undergoes progressive atrophy. Lymph nodes are most prominent in children 4–8 years of age. Normal lymph node size is less than 10 mm in diameter, with the exceptions of 15 mm for inguinal nodes, 5 mm for epitrochlear nodes, and 2 mm for supraclavicular nodes, which are usually not palpable. **Lymphadenopathy** is enlargement of lymph nodes and occurs in response to a wide variety of infectious, inflammatory, and malignant processes. **Generalized lymphadenopathy** is enlargement of two or more noncontiguous lymph node groups, whereas **regional lymphadenopathy** involves one lymph node group only.

Lymphadenitis is acute or chronic inflammation of lymph nodes. Acute lymphadenitis usually results when bacteria and toxins from a site of acute inflammation are carried via lymph to regional nodes. Numerous infections cause lymphadenopathy and lymphadenitis (Tables 100.1 and 100.2). Causes of inguinal regional lymphadenopathy also include sexually transmitted infections (see Chapter 117). Regional lymphadenitis associated with a characteristic skin lesion at the site of inoculation defines various **lymphocutaneous syndromes**. **Lymphangitis** is an inflammation of subcutaneous lymphatic channels that presents as an acute bacterial infection, usually caused by *Staphylococcus aureus* and group A streptococci.

Cervical lymphadenitis is the most common regional lymphadenitis among children and is commonly associated with pharyngitis caused by group A streptococcus (see Chapter 104), respiratory viruses, and Epstein-Barr virus (EBV). Other common infectious causes of cervical

TABLE 100.1 Infectious Causes of Generalized Lymphadenopathy

VIRAL
Epstein-Barr virus (infectious mononucleosis)
Cytomegalovirus (infectious mononucleosis-like syndrome)
HIV (acute retroviral syndrome and chronic disease)
Hepatitis B virus
Hepatitis C virus
Varicella
Adenoviruses
Rubeola (measles)
Rubella
BACTERIAL
Endocarditis
Brucella (brucellosis)
Leptospira interrogans (leptospirosis)
Streptobacillus moniliformis (bacillary rat-bite fever)
Mycobacterium tuberculosis (tuberculosis)
Treponema pallidum (secondary syphilis)
FUNGAL
Coccidioides immitis (coccidioidomycosis)
Histoplasma capsulatum (histoplasmosis)
PROTOZOAL
Toxoplasma gondii (toxoplasmosis)
Trypanosoma cruzi (Chagas disease)

TABLE 100.2 Infectious Causes of Regional Lymphadenopathy

CERVICAL CHAIN
Staphylococcus aureus
Group A streptococcus
Group B streptococcus (in infants)
Bartonella henselae (cat-scratch disease)
Yersinia pestis (plague)
Francisella tularensis (glandular tularemia)
Mycobacterium tuberculosis
Nontuberculous mycobacteria
Sporothrix schenckii (sporotrichosis)
Fusobacterium necrophorum
Epstein-Barr virus
Toxoplasma gondii
SEXUALLY TRANSMITTED INFECTIONS (PRIMARILY INGUINAL LYMPHADENOPATHY)
Neisseria gonorrhoeae (gonorrhea)
Treponema pallidum (syphilis)
Herpes simplex virus
Haemophilus ducreyi (chancroid)
Chlamydia trachomatis serovars L_{1-3} (lymphogranuloma venereum)
LYMPHOCUTANEOUS SYNDROMES
Bacillus anthracis (anthrax)
F. tularensis (ulceroglandular tularemia)
B. henselae (cat-scratch disease)
Pasteurella multocida (dog or cat bite)
Rickettsialpox
Spirillum minus (spirillary rat-bite fever)
Y. pestis (plague)
Nocardia (nocardiosis)
Cutaneous diphtheria *(Corynebacterium diphtheriae)*
Cutaneous coccidioidomycosis *(Coccidioides immitis)*
Cutaneous histoplasmosis *(Histoplasma capsulatum)*
Cutaneous leishmaniasis
Cutaneous sporotrichosis *(S. schenckii)*
Tinea capitis

lymphadenitis include *Bartonella henselae* (cat-scratch disease) and nontuberculous mycobacteria; tularemia, endemic mycoses, tuberculosis, *Nocardia,* and *Actinomyces* are less common causes.

EPIDEMIOLOGY

Acute cervical lymphadenitis as a complication of group A streptococcal infection parallels the incidence of streptococcal pharyngitis (see Chapter 104). Many cases are caused by *S. aureus.* EBV and cytomegalovirus (CMV) are ubiquitous, with most infections occurring in young children, who may often be asymptomatic or only mildly symptomatic. Risk factors for other specific causes of lymphadenopathy may be indicated by past medical and surgical history; preceding trauma; exposure to animals; contact with persons infected with tuberculosis; sexual history; travel history; food and ingestion history, especially of undercooked meat or unpasteurized dairy products; and current medications.

CLINICAL MANIFESTATIONS

The exact location and detailed measurement of the size, shape, characteristics, and number of involved nodes should be noted, including their consistency, mobility, tenderness, warmth, fluctuance, firmness, and adherence to adjacent tissues. Important findings include presence or absence of dental disease, oropharyngeal or skin lesions, ocular disease, other nodal enlargement, and any other signs of systemic illness, including hepatosplenomegaly and skin lesions.

Acute cervical lymphadenopathy associated with pharyngitis is characterized by small and rubbery lymph nodes in the anterior cervical chain with minimal to moderate tenderness. **Suppurative cervical lymphadenitis**, frequently caused by *S. aureus* or group A streptococcus, shows erythema and warmth of the overlying skin with moderate to exquisite tenderness.

EBV is the primary cause of **infectious mononucleosis**, a clinical syndrome characterized by fever, fatigue and malaise, cervical or generalized lymphadenopathy, tonsillitis, and pharyngitis. The pharynx shows enlarged tonsils with exudate and, sometimes, an enanthem with pharyngeal petechiae. Lymphadenopathy is typically bilateral and is most prominent in the anterior and posterior cervical and submandibular lymph nodes and less commonly involves axillary and inguinal lymph nodes. Other findings include splenomegaly in 50% of cases, hepatomegaly in 10–20%, and maculopapular or urticarial rash in 5–15%. A diffuse, erythematous rash develops in approximately 80% of mononucleosis patients treated with amoxicillin. EBV, a member of the herpesvirus family, infects B lymphocytes and is spread by salivary secretions. After primary infection, EBV is maintained latently in multiple episomes in the cell nucleus of resting B lymphocytes and establishes a lifelong infection that remains clinically inapparent. Most people shed EBV intermittently, with approximately 20% of healthy individuals shedding EBV at any given time.

CMV, *Toxoplasma gondii,* adenoviruses, hepatitis B virus, hepatitis C virus, and acute HIV infection (also known as **acute**

retroviral syndrome) can cause an infectious mononucleosis-like syndrome with lymphadenopathy. Compared with EBV infection, infectious mononucleosis-like illness caused by CMV has minimal pharyngitis and often more prominent splenomegaly; it often presents with fever only. The most common manifestation of toxoplasmosis is asymptomatic cervical lymphadenopathy, but approximately 10% of cases of acquired toxoplasmosis develop chronic posterior cervical lymphadenopathy and fatigue, usually without significant fever.

The cause of **cat-scratch disease** is *Bartonella henselae,* a small, pleomorphic, gram-negative bacillus that stains with Warthin-Starry silver stain. *B. henselae* causes apparently asymptomatic bacteremia in cats; kittens under 1 year of age are more likely to harbor the organism. *B. henselae* is transmitted to humans by bites and scratches, which may be minor. *B. henselae* also causes bacillary angiomatosis and peliosis hepatis in people with HIV infection (see Chapter 126). Cat-scratch disease typically presents with a cutaneous papule or conjunctival granuloma at the site of bacterial inoculation, followed by lymphadenopathy of the draining regional nodes. The nodes are tender with suppuration in approximately 10% of cases. Lymphadenopathy may persist for 1–4 months. Less common features of cat-scratch disease include erythema nodosum, osteolytic lesions, encephalitis, oculoglandular (Parinaud) syndrome, hepatic or splenic granulomas, endocarditis, polyneuritis, and transverse myelitis.

Lymphadenitis caused by **nontuberculous mycobacteria** usually is unilateral in the cervical, submandibular, or preauricular nodes and is more common in toddlers. The nodes are relatively painless and firm initially but gradually soften, rupture, and may drain over time. The local reaction is circumscribed, and overlying skin may develop a violaceous discoloration without warmth. Fever and systemic symptoms are minimal or absent. Nontuberculous mycobacteria are ubiquitous in soil, vegetation, dust, and water. *Mycobacterium* species commonly causing lymphadenitis in children include *M. avium* complex, *M. scrofulaceum,* and *M. kansasii. M. tuberculosis* can also cause cervical lymphadenitis in children with appropriate epidemiologic exposures or risk factors.

LABORATORY AND IMAGING STUDIES

Initial laboratory tests of regional lymphadenopathy include a complete blood count and inflammatory markers. Infectious mononucleosis is characterized by lymphocytosis with **atypical lymphocytes**; thrombocytopenia and elevated hepatic enzymes are common.

Cultures of infected skin lesions and tonsillar exudates should be obtained. Isolation of group A streptococci from the oropharynx suggests, but does not confirm, streptococcal cervical lymphadenitis. A blood culture should be obtained from children with systemic signs and symptoms of bacteremia.

Serologic testing (or polymerase chain reaction) for EBV and for *Bartonella henselae* should be obtained if there are appropriate findings. The most reliable test for diagnosis of acute EBV infection is the immunoglobulin M (IgM) antiviral capsid antigen (Fig. 100.1). Heterophile antibody is also diagnostic but is not reliably positive in children younger than 4 years with infectious mononucleosis.

Extended diagnostic work-up for lymphadenopathy is guided by the specific risk factors in the history and physical

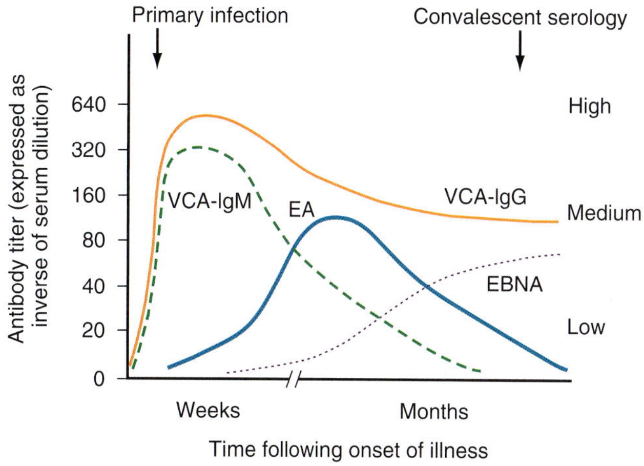

FIGURE 100.1 Idealized time course for the development of antibody to different Epstein-Barr virus antigens after primary infection with the virus. *IgM,* Immunoglobulin M; *VCA,* viral capsid antigen. (From Katz BZ, Muller WJ. Epstein-Barr virus [mononucleosis and lymphoproliferative disorders]. In: Long SS, Prober CG, Fischer M, eds. *Principles and Practice of Pediatric Infectious Diseases.* 6th ed. Philadelphia: Elsevier; 2023:fig. 208-3.)

examination findings. Chest radiograph, throat culture, antistreptolysin O titer, and serologic tests for CMV, HIV, toxoplasmosis, syphilis, tularemia, *Brucella,* histoplasmosis, and coccidioidomycosis may be indicated. Genital tract evaluation and specimens should be obtained with regional inguinal lymphadenopathy (see Chapter 117). Screening for tuberculosis can be performed using the standard tuberculin skin test (which may be positive with atypical mycobacterial infection) or an interferon-γ release assay (which is uncommonly positive with atypical mycobacterial infection, based on the infecting species).

Aspiration is indicated for acutely inflamed, fluctuant cervical lymph nodes, especially those larger than 3 cm in diameter or not responding to antibiotic treatment. Ultrasound or computed tomography may help in establishing the extent of lymphadenopathy and defining whether the mass is solid, cystic, or suppurative with abscess formation. Pus from fluctuant lesions should be examined by Gram and acid-fast stains and cultured for aerobic and anaerobic bacteria and mycobacteria. Biopsy should be performed if **lymphoma** is suspected because of firm, matted, nontender nodes and other systemic findings.

If the diagnosis remains uncertain and lymphadenopathy persists despite empirical antibiotic therapy for presumed *S. aureus* and group A streptococcus, excisional biopsy of the entire node should be performed, if possible. This is curative for nontuberculous mycobacterial lymphadenitis. Biopsy material should be submitted for histopathology as well as Gram, acid-fast, Giemsa, periodic acid-Schiff, Warthin-Starry silver *(B. henselae),* and methenamine silver stains. Cultures for aerobic and anaerobic bacteria, mycobacteria, and fungi should be performed.

DIFFERENTIAL DIAGNOSIS

Noninfectious causes of cervical swelling and/or lymphadenopathy include congenital (branchial cleft) and acquired cysts, Kawasaki disease, autoimmune diseases (e.g., sarcoidosis, autoimmune lymphoproliferative syndrome [ALPS], or

Kikuchi-Fujimoto disease), benign neoplasms, and malignancies. The differential diagnosis for generalized lymphadenopathy includes juvenile idiopathic arthritis, systemic lupus erythematosus, and serum sickness and other adverse drug reactions, especially with phenytoin and other antiepileptic medications, allopurinol, isoniazid, antithyroid medications, and pyrimethamine. Leukemia, lymphoma, and occasionally neuroblastoma may have lymph nodes that are usually painless, uninflamed, matted, and firm (see Chapters 156, 157, and 159). A syndrome of **periodic fever, aphthous stomatitis, pharyngitis, and adenitis (PFAPA)** is an occasional cause of recurrent fever and cervical lymphadenitis (see Chapter 104).

TREATMENT

Management of *lymphadenopathy* and *lymphadenitis* depends on patient age, associated findings, node size and location, and severity of the acute systemic symptoms. In children, most cases of cervical lymphadenopathy, without other signs of acute inflammation, require no specific therapy and usually regress within 2–3 weeks. Progression to lymphadenitis or development of generalized lymphadenopathy requires further evaluation.

The specific treatment of cervical lymphadenitis depends on the underlying etiology. Empirical treatment targeting *S. aureus* and group A streptococcus includes a penicillinase-resistant penicillin (e.g., oxacillin) or first-generation cephalosporin (e.g., cefazolin or cephalexin). For patients with hypersensitivity to β-lactam antibiotics, or if community-acquired methicillin-resistant *S. aureus* is suspected, clindamycin or trimethoprim-sulfamethoxazole is appropriate. Response to empirical antibiotic therapy for suppurative cervical lymphadenitis obviates the need for further evaluation. Absence of a clinical response within 48–72 hours is an indication for further laboratory evaluation, imaging, and possible aspiration or excisional biopsy and culture.

There is no specific treatment for infectious mononucleosis. Localized cat-scratch disease often may not require treatment because the lymphadenopathy typically resolves in 2–4 months without sequelae. Azithromycin may hasten resolution and reduces node size at 30 days, but no benefit is evident at 90 days. Aspiration and drainage are indicated for suppurative nodes. The recommended treatment of cervical lymphadenitis caused by nontuberculous mycobacteria is complete surgical excision. Antimycobacterial drugs are necessary only if there is recurrence or inability to excise infected nodes completely or if *M. tuberculosis* is identified, which requires 6 months of antituberculous chemotherapy (see Chapter 125).

COMPLICATIONS AND PROGNOSIS

Most acute infections caused by *S. aureus* and group A streptococcus respond to treatment and have an excellent prognosis. Complications such as abscess formation, cellulitis, and rarely bacteremia may occur. Abscess formation is treated with incision and drainage in conjunction with appropriate antibiotic therapy.

Infectious mononucleosis usually resolves in 2–4 weeks, but fatigue and malaise may wax and wane for several weeks to months. EBV also is associated with numerous complications during the acute illness. Neurologic complications include seizures, aseptic meningitis syndrome, Bell palsy, transverse myelitis, encephalitis, and Guillain-Barré syndrome. Hematologic complications include Coombs-positive hemolytic anemia, antibody-mediated thrombocytopenia, hemophagocytic lymphohistiocytosis, and, rarely, aplastic anemia. Corticosteroids have been used for respiratory compromise resulting from tonsillar hypertrophy, which responds rapidly, and for thrombocytopenia, hemolytic anemia, and neurologic complications. Splenic rupture is very rare. **X-linked lymphoproliferative disease**, which results from a pathologic gene variant, manifests as fulminant infectious mononucleosis with primary EBV infection and progresses to malignant lymphoproliferative disease or dysgammaglobulinemia.

EBV infection, as with other herpesviruses, persists for life, but no symptoms are attributed to intermittent reactivation in immunocompetent hosts. EBV is causally associated with nasopharyngeal carcinoma, Burkitt lymphoma, Hodgkin disease, leiomyosarcoma in immunocompromised persons, and EBV lymphoproliferative disease, especially in posttransplant patients and in those with advanced HIV infection.

Lymphadenitis caused by nontuberculous mycobacteria has an excellent prognosis. Surgical excision of cervical lymphadenitis caused by nontuberculous mycobacteria is curative in over 97% of cases, and even patients managed without surgery or antimicrobials are able to resolve the infection over time.

PREVENTION

The incidence of suppurative regional lymphadenitis reflects the incidence of predisposing conditions, such as dental disease, streptococcal pharyngitis, otitis media, impetigo, and other infections involving the face and scalp. There are no guidelines to prevent lymphadenitis caused by nontuberculous mycobacteria.

PEARLS FOR PRACTITIONERS

See Infectious Diseases: Pearls for Practitioners at the end of this section.

REVIEW QUESTIONS

Available online.

CHAPTER 101
Meningitis

ETIOLOGY

Meningitis, inflammation of the leptomeninges, can be caused by bacteria, viruses, or—rarely—fungi. The term **aseptic meningitis** principally refers to viral meningitis, but meningitis with negative cerebrospinal fluid (CSF) bacterial cultures may be seen with other infectious organisms (Lyme disease, syphilis, tuberculosis), parameningeal infections (brain abscess, epidural abscess, subdural empyema), chemical exposure (nonsteroidal antiinflammatory drugs, intravenous immunoglobulin), autoimmune disorders, and other diseases, including Kawasaki disease.

The organisms commonly causing bacterial meningitis (Table 101.1) before the availability of current conjugate vaccines were *Haemophilus influenzae* type b, *Streptococcus pneumoniae,* and *Neisseria meningitidis.* In the United States, the rates of *H. influenzae* type b and *Streptococcus pneumoniae* meningitis have declined substantially after the introduction of targeted vaccines. The bacteria causing neonatal meningitis are the same as those causing neonatal sepsis including *Streptococcus agalactiae* (Group B streptococcus, GBS), *Escherichia coli* and *Listeria monocytogenes* (see Chapter 64). In older children, *S. pneumoniae* and *N. meningitidis* remain the most common causes of bacterial meningitis. Staphylococcal meningitis primarily occurs after neurosurgery or penetrating head trauma.

Partially treated meningitis refers to bacterial meningitis complicated by antibiotic treatment before the lumbar puncture (LP), which may result in negative CSF cultures, although other CSF findings suggestive of bacterial infection persist. In this case, the etiology can sometimes be confirmed by polymerase chain reaction (PCR) of the CSF.

The most common viruses causing meningitis are enteroviruses and parechoviruses. In neonates, evaluation for herpes simplex virus (HSV) should be considered based on risk factors and presentation. Other viruses that less commonly cause meningitis include Epstein-Barr virus (EBV), cytomegalovirus (CMV), lymphocytic choriomeningitis virus (LCMV), many arboviruses (see Chapter 102), and HIV. The mumps virus can cause meningitis in unvaccinated children. Other infectious causes of meningitis or meningoencephalitis include *Borrelia burgdorferi* (Lyme disease), *Bartonella henselae* (cat-scratch disease), syphilis, *Mycobacterium tuberculosis, Mycoplasma pneumoniae, Toxoplasma*, fungi (*Cryptococcus, Histoplasma, Blastomycosis,* and *Coccidioides*), and parasites (*Angiostrongylus cantonensis, Naegleria fowleri, Baylisascaris,* and *Acanthamoeba*).

TABLE 101.1 Bacterial Causes of Meningitis

AGE	MOST COMMON	LESS COMMON
Neonatal	Group B streptococcus *Escherichia coli* Other enteric gram-negative bacilli	*Listeria monocytogenes* *Enterococcus faecalis* *Neisseria meningitidis* *Streptococcus pneumoniae* Other streptococci *Citrobacter* species *Salmonella* *Pseudomonas aeruginosa* *Haemophilus influenzae* *Staphylococcus aureus* (NICU only)
>1–3 months	*S. pneumoniae* Gram-negative bacilli Group B streptococcus	*N. meningitidis* *Salmonella*
>3 months	*S. pneumoniae* *Neisseria meningitidis*	Gram-negative bacilli Group B streptococcus *Haemophilus influenzae* type b (unimmunized), other serotypes

NICU, Neonatal intensive care unit.

EPIDEMIOLOGY

The incidence of bacterial meningitis is highest among children under 1 year of age, especially infants under 2 months of age. Extremely high rates are found in people identifying as Native American, Alaskan Native, and Australian aboriginal, suggesting that genetic factors more prevalent in these populations may play a role in susceptibility. Other risk factors include acquired or congenital immunodeficiencies, functional or anatomic asplenia, cochlear implantation, penetrating head trauma, recent neurosurgical procedure, and crowding, such as that which occurs in some daycare centers or college and military dormitories. A CSF leak (fistula), resulting from congenital anomaly or following a basilar skull fracture, increases the risk of meningitis, especially that caused by *S. pneumoniae.*

Enteroviruses and parechoviruses cause meningitis, with peaks during summer and fall in temperate climates. These infections are more prevalent among infants, school-age children, and immunocompromised persons. The prevalence of arboviral meningitis or encephalitis is determined by geographic distribution and seasonal activity of the arthropod (mosquito) vectors. In the United States, most arboviral infections occur during the summer and fall. Both the windows of timing and geography may be expanding with climate change and its impact on viral vectors.

CLINICAL MANIFESTATIONS

Preceding upper respiratory tract symptoms may occur; however, rapid onset is typical of infections with *S. pneumoniae* and *N. meningitidis.* Indications of meningeal inflammation include headache, irritability, nausea, nuchal rigidity, lethargy, photophobia, and vomiting. Fever is usually present. Kernig and Brudzinski signs of meningeal irritation are often positive in children older than 12 months. In young infants, signs of meningeal inflammation may be minimal, with only irritability, depressed mental status, temperature instability, and/or poor feeding present. Focal neurologic signs, seizures, arthralgia, myalgia, petechial or purpuric lesions, sepsis, shock, and coma may occur. Symptoms of increased intracranial pressure include headache, diplopia, ptosis, and vomiting; a bulging fontanelle may be present in infants. Papilledema is uncommon unless there is occlusion of the venous sinuses, subdural empyema, or brain abscess.

LABORATORY AND IMAGING STUDIES

If bacterial meningitis is suspected, an LP should be performed unless there is evidence of cardiovascular instability or of increased intracranial pressure (due to the risk of herniation). Routine CSF examination includes a white blood cell count with differential, protein and glucose levels, and Gram stain (Table 101.2). CSF should be cultured for bacteria and, when appropriate, fungi and/or mycobacteria. Multiplex PCR panels are often used to diagnose bacterial as well as viral meningitis, especially in the setting of prior antibiotic exposure. Peripheral leukocytosis is common, and blood cultures may be positive depending on the organism and whether there was antibiotic pretreatment. Ideally, CSF should be obtained prior to empirical therapy; however, antibiotics should not be delayed if there is an inability to perform an LP. If imaging is required prior to the LP, blood cultures should be sent and

TABLE 101.2 Cerebrospinal Fluid Findings in Various Central Nervous System Disorders

CONDITION	PRESSURE (CM H_2O)	LEUKOCYTES (CELLS/µL)	PROTEIN (mg/dL)/ GLUCOSE (mg/dL)	COMMENTS
Normal	10–20	<5; 60–70% lymphocytes, 30–40% monocytes, 1–3% neutrophils	20–45/>50% of serum glucose	WBC up to 10–20 cells/µL can be normal in neonates
Acute bacterial meningitis	Usually elevated (>25)	>100; usually thousands; PMNs predominate	100–500/usually <40 or <40% of serum glucose	Organisms may be seen on Gram stain and recovered by culture
Partially treated bacterial meningitis	Normal or elevated	1–10,000; PMNs usual but mononuclear cells may predominate if pretreated for extended period	>100/depressed or normal	Pretreatment may render CSF sterile, but bacteria may be detected by PCR
Tuberculous meningitis	Usually elevated; may be low because of CSF block in advanced stages	10–500; PMNs early but lymphocytes and monocytes predominate later	100–500; may be higher in presence of CSF block/usually <50	Acid-fast smear and culture or mycobacteria PCR may be positive. Adenine deaminase can be used to aid in the diagnosis
Fungal	Usually elevated	10–500; PMNs early; mononuclear cells predominate later	20–500/usually <50	Organisms may be seen on smear, in culture, or by India ink preparation, and antigen may be positive in cryptococcal disease
Viral meningitis or meningoencephalitis	Normal or slightly elevated	10–1,000; PMNs early; mononuclear cells predominate later	<50/normal or depressed	Viruses may be detected by PCR
Abscess (parameningeal infection)	Normal or elevated	0–100 PMNs unless rupture into CSF	20–200/normal	Profile may be completely normal

CSF, Cerebrospinal fluid; *PCR*, polymerase chain reaction; *PMN*, polymorphonuclear leukocyte; *WBC*, white blood cell.

antibiotics started prior to a CT scan or MRI. Interpretation of CSF in children who received prior antibiotics is complicated. In meningococcal meningitis, CSF can rapidly become sterile, often within 1–2 hours, and most commonly with a single dose of therapy. Sterilization of the CSF in *S. pneumoniae* meningitis may also occur within a few hours. In these cases, PCR is useful in identifying causative bacteria.

DIFFERENTIAL DIAGNOSIS

Many disorders other than meningitis and encephalitis may show signs of meningeal irritation and increased intracranial pressure, including trauma, intracranial hemorrhage, rheumatic diseases, and malignancies. Seizures can be associated with CNS infection or can be the sequelae of brain edema, cerebral infarction or hemorrhage, or vasculitis.

TREATMENT

Treatment of bacterial meningitis should be prompt and focus on sterilization of the CSF by antibiotics (Table 101.3) and maintenance of adequate cerebral and systemic perfusion. Due to increasing *S. pneumoniae* resistance, an empiric third-generation cephalosporin *plus* vancomycin or linezolid should be administered until culture results and antibiotic susceptibility testing are available. Ceftazidime, cefepime, or ceftriaxone are also adequate to treat *N. meningitidis, H. influenzae,* and most *E. coli.* For infants younger than 2 months, ampicillin is added to cover *L. monocytogenes.* Duration of treatment is 5–7 days for *N. meningitidis,* 7–10 days for *H. influenzae,* and 10–14 days for *S. pneumoniae.* Meningitis caused by gram-negative bacilli should generally be treated a minimum of 21 days or 14 days beyond the first negative CSF culture, whichever is longer.

Dexamethasone as **adjunctive therapy** initiated just before or concurrently with the first dose of antibiotics significantly diminishes the incidence of hearing loss resulting from *H. influenzae* meningitis. The role of adjuvant steroids for diminishing neurologic sequelae and mortality for pneumococcal and meningococcal meningitis in children is less clear.

Supportive therapy involves treatment of dehydration, shock, disseminated intravascular coagulation, syndrome of inappropriate antidiuretic hormone (SIADH), seizures, increased intracranial pressure, apnea, arrhythmias, and coma. Adequate cerebral perfusion must be maintained in the presence of cerebral edema.

COMPLICATIONS AND PROGNOSIS

SIADH may complicate meningitis and necessitates monitoring of serum sodium levels. Persistent fever is common during treatment but also may be related to ineffective treatment or immune complex–mediated pericardial or joint effusions, thrombophlebitis, drug fever, or nosocomial infection. A

TABLE 101.3 Initial Antimicrobial Therapy by Age for Presumed Bacterial Meningitis

AGE	RECOMMENDED TREATMENT	ALTERNATIVE TREATMENTS
Newborns (0–28 days)	Ceftazidime plus ampicillin with or without gentamicin	Ampicillin plus gentamicin
Infants and toddlers (1 mo–4 yr)	Ceftriaxone plus vancomycin or linezolid	Cefepime plus vancomycin or linezolid
Children and adolescents (5–13 yr) and adults	Ceftriaxone plus vancomycin or linezolid	Cefepime plus vancomycin or linezolid

repeat LP after 48 hours of therapy should be considered for those whose condition has not improved or has worsened, for gram-negative meningitis, and for those who received adjunct steroids, which can interfere with the ability to monitor clinical response. CNS imaging should be considered in children who demonstrate focal neurologic signs or symptoms, or persistently positive CSF cultures. CT with contrast or MRI is used to detect subdural effusions with *S. pneumoniae* and *H. influenzae* meningitis or brain abscess associated with gram-negative organisms. *Citrobacter* species are associated with a high incidence of brain abscess formation. Neurosurgery should be consulted to consider drainage if a brain abscess is present.

With current management, the mortality rate for bacterial meningitis in children remains significant, up to 15% depending on the organism. Of survivors, up to 30% have sequelae, including deafness, seizures, blindness, paresis, ataxia, or hydrocephalus. All children with meningitis should have a hearing evaluation before discharge and at follow-up. Learning disabilities and behavioral problems may be more subtle, long-term consequences of infection. Careful developmental follow-up is important. Poor prognosis is associated with young age, long duration of illness before effective antibiotic therapy, seizures, coma at presentation, shock, low or absent CSF white blood cell count in the presence of visible bacteria on CSF Gram stain, and immunocompromised status.

Rarely, relapse may occur 3–14 days after treatment, possibly from parameningeal foci or resistant organisms. Recurrence may indicate an underlying immunologic or anatomic defect that predisposes the patient to meningitis.

PREVENTION

Routine immunizations against *H. influenzae* type b and *S. pneumoniae* are recommended for all children beginning at 2 months of age. Quadrivalent vaccines against *N. meningitidis* (serotypes A, C, Y, and W-135) are recommended at age 11 or 12 years with a booster dose at 16 years and for children older than 2 months who are at high risk of infection, including functional asplenia, complement deficiencies, and travelers to or residents of hyperendemic areas (Figs. 95.1 and 95.2). A vaccine specifically targeting *N. meningitidis* serotype B is recommended for high-risk patients 10 years and older, including those with asplenia and complement deficiencies. **Chemoprophylaxis** with rifampin, ciprofloxacin, azithromycin, or ceftriaxone to eradicate the carrier state and decrease transmission is recommended both for index cases with *N. meningitidis* and for their close contacts. For invasive *H. influenzae* type B, prophylaxis consists of rifampin.

PEARLS FOR PRACTITIONERS

See Infectious Diseases: Pearls for Practitioners at the end of this section.

REVIEW QUESTIONS

Available online.

CHAPTER 102

Encephalitis

ETIOLOGY

Encephalitis is an inflammatory process of the brain parenchyma, which usually presents with fever, headache, and mental status changes. Encephalitis is a challenging diagnosis in many aspects, because determining its etiology is difficult and treatment options are quite limited. The term **meningoencephalitis** is used when meningeal inflammation is also present. Encephalitis may be diffuse or localized and is usually an acute infectious process, but it also may be postinfectious, autoimmune, part of a systemic disorder or the result of an indolent viral infection. Organisms cause encephalitis by one of two mechanisms: (1) direct infection of the brain parenchyma via an extension of meningitis, secondary to viremia, or retrograde spread via peripheral nerves or (2) a postinfectious, immune-mediated response in the central nervous system (CNS) that usually begins several days to weeks after clinical manifestations of the infection.

Viruses are the principal infectious causes of acute infectious encephalitis (Table 102.1). The most common viral causes of encephalitis in the United States are enteroviruses, arboviruses, and herpesviruses. HIV is also an important cause of subacute encephalitis in children and adolescents and may present as an acute febrile illness, but more commonly it is insidious in onset (see Chapter 126). Other less common viral causes of encephalitis include measles, JC virus, lymphocytic choriomeningitis virus (LCMV), rabies, influenza, and Japanese encephalitis. Numerous other infectious etiologies for encephalitis or meningoencephalitis are possible in the appropriate setting, including prion diseases (e.g., Creutzfeldt-Jakob disease) and parasites such as amoeba and *Baylisascaris,* as well as *Bartonella henselae, Mycobacterium tuberculosis, Plasmodium falciparum,* and *Mycoplasma pneumoniae.* Encephalitis also may result from metabolic,

TABLE 102.1 Causes of Acute Infectious Encephalitis

VIRUSES	BACTERIA
Enteroviruses	*Borrelia burgdorferi* (Lyme disease)
Parechoviruses	*Bartonella henselae* (cat-scratch disease)
Herpes simplex viruses (types 1 and 2)	*Mycoplasma pneumoniae*
EBV	*Rickettsia rickettsii* (Rocky Mountain spotted fever)
Arboviruses (West Nile virus, St. Louis, Japanese, La Crosse, Powassan, and equine encephalitis viruses)	**PARASITES**
Cytomegalovirus	*Plasmodium falciparum*
Human immunodeficiency virus	*Naegleria fowleri*
Rabies virus	*Acanthamoeba* spp.
LCMV	*Baylisascaris*
VZV	**FUNGI**
Influenza virus	*Cryptococcus neoformans*
Mumps virus	*Coccidioides* species
Measles virus	*Histoplasma capsulatum*

EBV, Epstein-Barr virus; *LCMV,* lymphocytic choriomeningitis virus; *VZV,* varicella-zoster virus.

toxic, and neoplastic disorders. In many cases, the cause remains unknown.

Acute disseminated encephalomyelitis (ADEM) is the abrupt development of multiple neurologic signs related to an inflammatory, demyelinating disorder of the brain and spinal cord. ADEM can follow childhood viral infections (such as an upper respiratory tract infection) or vaccinations and can clinically resemble multiple sclerosis. Symptoms most commonly begin within 2 weeks of the preceding infection and can last for several weeks.

Autoimmune encephalitis is a relatively common cause of encephalitis and is associated with specific autoantibodies directed to brain antigens, such as anti-*N*-methyl-D-aspartate receptor (NMDAR) and antimyelin oligodendrocyte glycoprotein (MOG) antibodies. The presentation is often subacute with psychiatric manifestations, cortical dysfunction, movement disorders, autonomic dysfunction, and seizures.

EPIDEMIOLOGY

Travel and other exposure history should be obtained for all patients with encephalitis. Arboviral and enteroviral encephalitides characteristically appear in clusters or epidemics that occur from midsummer to early fall, although sporadic cases of enteroviral encephalitis occur throughout the year. Herpesviruses and other infectious agents account for additional sporadic cases throughout the year.

Arboviruses tend to be limited to certain geographic areas, reflecting the reservoir and mosquito vector. In North America, West Nile virus and La Crosse encephalitis occur in the summertime, resulting in a range of manifestations from asymptomatic infection to severe neurologic involvement. La Crosse virus is found in the Midwest and Southeastern United States, whereas West Nile virus is more disseminated across the country. The principal vectors for West Nile virus are *Culex* mosquitoes, and a broad range of birds serves as its major reservoir.

Herpes simplex virus (HSV) encephalitis can occur in neonates with or without skin lesions via perinatal or postnatal transmission. Beyond the neonatal period, HSV encephalitis (without skin lesions) can result from primary or reactivated infection with HSV type 1. In the immunocompromised host, other herpes viruses, such as cytomegalovirus (CMV), Epstein-Barr virus (EBV), human herpesvirus 6 (HHV-6), and varicella-zoster virus (VZV), as well as *Toxoplasma gondii* and JC viruses, can reactivate and cause encephalitis. Fungal infections of the CNS are rare but can also cause disease in this patient population.

CLINICAL MANIFESTATIONS

Acute infectious encephalitis may be preceded by a prodrome of several days of nonspecific symptoms, such as sore throat, fever, headache, and abdominal complaints followed by the characteristic symptoms of progressive lethargy, behavioral changes, altered mental status, and neurologic deficits. Seizures are common at presentation. Children with encephalitis also may have a nonspecific maculopapular rash; severe complications include fulminant coma, transverse myelitis, anterior horn cell disease, or peripheral neuropathy.

Neonates with HSV encephalitis can present with fever, lethargy, and/or seizures. Vesicular skin lesions typical of cutaneous infection may or may not be present.

DIFFERENTIAL DIAGNOSIS

The diagnosis is established presumptively by the presence of characteristic neurologic signs, typical epidemiologic findings, and evidence of infection by cerebrospinal fluid (CSF) analysis, electroencephalogram (EEG), and brain imaging techniques. Encephalitis may result from infections with bacteria, *Mycoplasma, Rickettsia,* fungi, and parasites and from many noninfectious diseases, including autoimmune, inflammatory, metabolic diseases (encephalopathy) such as Reye syndrome, hypoglycemia, collagen vascular disorders, drugs, hypertension, and malignancies.

Elucidating a careful history, including immunization record, travel to endemic regions, animal exposures, and geographic and social risk factors, may help to establish the etiology of encephalitis in a patient. If the patient is known to be or found to be immunocompromised, the differential diagnosis must be broadened.

LABORATORY AND IMAGING STUDIES

The diagnosis of viral encephalitis is supported by examination of the CSF, which typically shows a lymphocytic pleocytosis, a slight elevation in protein content, and a normal glucose level. CSF occasionally may be normal. Extreme elevations of protein and reductions of glucose suggest tuberculosis, cryptococcal infection, or meningeal carcinomatosis. Blood can be sent for a complete blood count with differential and culture, as well as autoimmune encephalitis antibodies, liver function tests, and infectious serologies.

Neuroimaging studies are often required prior to a lumbar puncture (LP) in these children because they generally have altered mental status. MRI is generally the study of choice in the diagnosis of encephalitis; however, CT may be used to exclude contraindications to LP or if MRI is unavailable in a timely manner. Brain imaging may be normal or may show diffuse cerebral swelling of the parenchyma or focal abnormalities. EEG is often abnormal and can show diffuse, slow wave activity, although focal changes may be present. A temporal lobe focus on EEG or brain imaging is a characteristic feature of HSV infection.

Serum and CSF testing may help determine an infectious etiology for encephalitis. Depending on the risk factors, serologic studies should be obtained as indicated by time of year, geography as well as travel, social, and medical history for arboviruses, HIV, EBV, *M. pneumoniae, B. henselae,* and Lyme disease. In most cases of viral encephalitis, the virus is difficult to isolate from the CSF. A CSF multiplex PCR panel should be sent and will often include HSV, enteroviruses, West Nile virus, and other viruses. Viral cultures of stool or throat may also be obtained though they have less utility and are less likely to be available. Even with extensive testing and the use of PCR assays, the cause of encephalitis remains undetermined in one-third of cases. Next-generation sequencing tests from the CSF, when available, can sometimes add additional noninvasive diagnostic information. Both blood and CSF should be sent to detect brain-specific antibodies present in approximately 95% of patients with autoimmune encephalitis.

Brain biopsy is seldom performed and is generally recommended only if the etiology remains unknown, and a patient continues to deteriorate. Rabies encephalitis and prion-related diseases (Creutzfeldt-Jakob disease and kuru) may be routinely diagnosed by culture or pathologic examination of brain biopsy tissue. Brain tissue can be sent for pathology, culture, and PCR testing and may be helpful to identify arbovirus and enterovirus infections, tuberculosis, fungal infections, and noninfectious illnesses, particularly primary CNS vasculopathies and malignancies.

TREATMENT

With the exception of HSV, VZV, CMV, HHV-6, and HIV, there is no specific therapy for *viral* encephalitis. Management is supportive and frequently requires intensive care unit admission to facilitate aggressive therapy for seizures, timely detection of electrolyte abnormalities, and, when necessary, airway monitoring and protection or reduction of increased intracranial pressure and maintenance of adequate cerebral perfusion pressure.

Intravenous acyclovir is the treatment of choice for HSV and VZV infections. CMV is treated with ganciclovir in immunocompromised patients. HHV-6 encephalitis in patients who are post–bone marrow transplant can also be treated with ganciclovir or foscarnet. HIV infections may be treated with a combination of antiretroviral agents. *M. pneumoniae* infections may be treated with doxycycline, fluoroquinolones, or macrolides, although the clinical value of treating encephalitis associated with *Mycoplasma* disease is uncertain.

ADEM has been treated with high-dose intravenous corticosteroids, but it is unclear whether improved outcomes reflect milder cases recognized by MRI, fewer cases caused by measles (which can cause severe ADEM), or improved supportive care. Autoimmune encephalitis has been treated with steroids, intravenous immunoglobulin, and rituximab.

COMPLICATIONS AND PROGNOSIS

Prognosis of encephalitis depends on neurologic findings, pathogen, and age, among other factors. Among survivors, symptoms usually resolve over several days to 2–3 weeks. Although most patients with epidemic forms of infectious encephalitis (St. Louis, California, West Nile, and enterovirus infections) in the United States recover without sequelae, severe cases leading to death or substantial neurologic sequelae can occur with virtually any of these neurotropic viruses. Sequelae can include paresis or spasticity, cognitive impairment, weakness, ataxia, and recurrent seizures. Most patients gradually recover some or all their function. The overall mortality for infectious encephalitis is low but depends on the etiology.

Disease caused by HSV, need for ICU care, focal neurologic findings, seizures, or coma are associated with a worse prognosis, especially in children younger than 5 years of age. Rabies, with very rare exceptions, is fatal.

PREVENTION

The best prevention for arboviral encephalitis is to avoid mosquito-borne or tick-borne exposures and to remove ticks carefully (see Chapter 123). There are no vaccines in use in the United States for the prevention of arboviral infection or for enteroviruses except for poliomyelitis. There are no specific preventive measures for HSV encephalitis except for cesarean section for mothers with active genital lesions (see Chapter 65). Rabies can be prevented by pre-exposure or postexposure vaccination. Influenza encephalitis can be prevented by use of influenza vaccination.

PEARLS FOR PRACTITIONERS

See Infectious Diseases: Pearls for Practitioners at the end of this section.

REVIEW QUESTIONS

Available online.

CHAPTER 103

The Common Cold

ETIOLOGY

Upper respiratory tract infection (URI), also known as the common cold, is a self-limited viral process with prominent symptoms of rhinorrhea and nasal congestion, absent or mild fever, and few systemic manifestations. URIs are the most common cause of human disease and are often a cause of missed work or school, as well as visits to primary care pediatricians. Young children are at highest risk for frequent URI due to their lack of immunity from previous infection and close contact with others who frequently shed viruses.

The viruses most commonly associated with colds are rhinoviruses. Other viruses that cause URIs include respiratory syncytial virus (RSV), human metapneumovirus, coronaviruses (including the SARS-CoV-2 virus that causes COVID-19 and other human coronaviruses), coxsackieviruses, influenza, parainfluenza, and adenoviruses. Viral infection of nasal epithelium causes an acute inflammatory response with mucosal infiltration by inflammatory cells and release of cytokines. The host inflammatory response is partly responsible for many of the symptoms.

EPIDEMIOLOGY

URIs occur throughout the year, with peak incidence from fall through late spring, reflecting the seasonal prevalence of viral pathogens and confined habitation during colder months. Young children have an average of seven to eight viral infections each year. The number decreases with age, to two to three colds each year by adulthood. Children in out-of-home day care during the first year of life have 50% more URIs than children cared for at home only. With preschool attendance, it is not unusual for children to experience one infection per month of the respiratory virus season. This difference diminishes during subsequent years in day care.

CLINICAL MANIFESTATIONS

URI symptoms typically develop 1–3 days after viral infection and include nasal congestion, rhinorrhea, sore or scratchy throat, and occasional nonproductive cough. Fever, although uncommon in adults, may occur in infants and young children. Symptoms usually persist for approximately 5–7 days, although it can be longer in young children. Constitutional symptoms such as fever, myalgia, and headaches generally are present only early in the illness. Respiratory symptoms tend to persist for the duration of the illness. There is often a change in the color or consistency of nasal secretions, which is not necessarily indicative of sinusitis or bacterial superinfection. Examination of the nasal mucosa may reveal swollen, erythematous nasal turbinates.

LABORATORY AND IMAGING STUDIES

Laboratory studies often are not helpful. A nasopharyngeal swab for respiratory virus polymerase chain reaction (PCR) may be obtained in the inpatient setting in immunocompromised patients or for infection prevention reasons. Skin testing, specific immunoglobulin E (IgE) testing, or a nasal smear for eosinophils is not routinely performed but may be useful in the evaluation for allergic rhinitis (see Chapter 80).

DIFFERENTIAL DIAGNOSIS

The differential diagnosis of URI includes allergic rhinitis, foreign body (especially with unilateral nasal discharge), sinusitis, pertussis, and pharyngitis. Allergic rhinitis is characterized by absence of fever, eosinophils in the nasal discharge, and other manifestations, such as allergic shiners, nasal polyps, a transverse crease on the nasal bridge, and pale, edematous, nasal turbinate mucosa. Other rare causes of chronic rhinorrhea are choanal atresia or stenosis, cerebrospinal fluid fistula, diphtheria, tumor, congenital syphilis (with *snuffles*), nasopharyngeal malignancy, and granulomatosis with polyangiitis.

TREATMENT

There is no specific therapy for URIs. Antibacterial therapy is not beneficial and instead may cause harm. Management consists of symptomatic therapies. Antihistamines and decongestants are *not* recommended for the management of URIs in children younger than 6 years of age because of adverse effects and lack of benefits. Similarly, cough suppressants and expectorants have *not* been shown to be beneficial. Vitamin C and inhalation of warm, humidified air are no more effective than placebo. The benefit of zinc lozenges or sprays has been inconsistent in children.

COMPLICATIONS AND PROGNOSIS

Otitis media is the most common complication and occurs in about 5% of children with a URI (see Chapter 106). Other complications include bacterial sinusitis, which should be considered if rhinorrhea or daytime cough persists without improvement for at least 10–14 days or if severe signs of sinus involvement develop, such as high fever for more than 3 days, facial pain, or facial swelling (see Chapter 105). Viral infections may lead to exacerbation of asthma and may result in inappropriate antibiotic treatment. In immunocompromised patients viral URIs can progress to lower respiratory tract infections and cause more severe disease.

PREVENTION

There are no proven methods for prevention of colds other than good handwashing and avoiding contact with infected persons. No significant effect of vitamin C or echinacea for prevention of URIs has been confirmed.

PEARLS FOR PRACTITIONERS

See Infectious Diseases: Pearls for Practitioners at the end of this section.

REVIEW QUESTIONS

Available online.

CHAPTER 104

Pharyngitis

ETIOLOGY

Many infectious agents can cause pharyngitis (Table 104.1), with viruses being the most common. **Group A streptococcus** *(Streptococcus pyogenes)* is the most common important bacterial cause of pharyngitis. Other bacterial organisms less often associated with pharyngitis include groups C and G streptococci (also β-hemolytic) and rarely *Arcanobacterium haemolyticum* (β-hemolytic, gram-positive rod) and *Francisella tularensis* (gram-negative coccobacillus and cause of tularemia). *Chlamydophila pneumonia* is associated with lower respiratory disease but can also cause sore throat. *Mycoplasma pneumoniae* is associated with atypical pneumonia and may cause mild pharyngitis without distinguishing clinical manifestations. *Neisseria gonorrhoeae* should be considered in a sexually active adolescent or adult with pharyngitis. Other bacteria, including *Staphylococcus aureus, Haemophilus influenzae,* and *S. pneumoniae,* are cultured frequently from the throats of children, but their role in causing pharyngitis is unclear.

TABLE 104.1 Major Microbial Causes of Acute Pharyngitis

AGENT	SYNDROME OR DISEASE	ESTIMATED PROPORTION OF ALL PHARYNGITIS (%)
BACTERIAL		
Group A streptococcus (*Streptococcus pyogenes*)	Pharyngitis, tonsillitis, scarlet fever	15–30
Group C and G streptococcus	Pharyngitis, tonsillitis	1–5
Arcanobacterium haemolyticum	Pharyngitis (scarlet fever–like syndrome)	0.5–3
Fusobacterium necrophorum	Lemierre syndrome	Unknown
Mycoplasma pneumoniae	Pharyngitis, pneumonia	Unknown
Other (e.g., *Neisseria gonorrhoeae, Corynebacterium diphtheriae, Francisella tularensis*)	Pharyngitis, laryngitis, tularemia	<5
VIRAL		
Rhinoviruses (>100 types)	URI	20
Coronaviruses (>4 types, including COVID-19)	URI, acute respiratory distress	>5
Adenoviruses (types 3, 4, 7, 14, 21)	Pharyngoconjunctival fever, acute respiratory disease	5
Herpes simplex viruses (types 1 and 2)	Gingivitis, stomatitis, pharyngitis	4
Parainfluenza viruses (types 1–4)	URI, croup	2
Influenza viruses (types A and B)	Influenza	2
Epstein-Barr virus	Mononucleosis	Unknown
Cytomegalovirus	Mononucleosis	Unknown
Coxsackie virus	Herpangina, hand, foot and mouth disease	Unknown
Unknown		40

URI, Upper respiratory tract infection.
Modified from Hayden GF, Hendley JO, Gwaltney JM Jr. Management of the ambulatory patient with a sore throat. Curr Clin Top Infect Dis. *1988;9:62–75.*

Many viruses cause acute pharyngitis. Some viruses, such as adenoviruses, are more likely than others to cause pharyngitis as a prominent symptom, whereas other viruses, such as rhinoviruses, are more likely to cause pharyngitis as a minor part of an illness that primarily features other symptoms, such as rhinorrhea or cough. Epstein-Barr virus (EBV), enteroviruses (herpangina), herpes simplex virus (HSV), and primary HIV infection can also produce pharyngitis.

EPIDEMIOLOGY

Sore throat is the primary symptom in approximately one-third of upper respiratory tract illnesses. Streptococcal pharyngitis is relatively uncommon before 2–3 years of age, but the incidence increases in young school-age children and then declines in late adolescence and adulthood. Streptococcal pharyngitis occurs throughout the year in temperate climates. The illness often spreads to siblings and classmates. Viral infections generally spread via close contact with an infected person and peak during winter and spring. EBV or cytomegalovirus-related **mononucleosis** (see Chapter 100) can feature pharyngitis as a prominent symptom and is most common in adolescents and young adults.

CLINICAL MANIFESTATIONS

Pharyngeal inflammation causes cough, sore throat, dysphagia, and fever. If involvement of the tonsils is prominent, the term **tonsillitis** or **tonsillopharyngitis** is often used.

The onset of streptococcal pharyngitis is often rapid and associated with prominent sore throat and moderate to high fever. Headache, nausea, vomiting, and abdominal pain are frequent. In a typical case, the pharynx is distinctly red. The tonsils are enlarged and may be covered with a yellow, blood-tinged exudate. There may be petechiae on the soft palate and posterior pharynx, and the uvula may be red, stippled, and swollen. Anterior cervical lymph nodes are enlarged and tender to touch. However, some children present with only mild pharyngeal erythema without tonsillar exudate or cervical lymphadenitis. Compared with classic streptococcal pharyngitis, the onset of viral pharyngitis is typically more gradual, and symptoms more often include rhinorrhea, cough, and diarrhea. Conjunctivitis, coryza, or oral ulcerations also suggest a viral etiology. The diagnosis of streptococcal pharyngitis cannot be made on clinical features alone.

In addition to sore throat and fever, some patients with streptococcal pharyngitis exhibit the stigmata of **scarlet fever**: circumoral pallor, strawberry tongue, and a fine diffuse erythematous macular-papular rash. The tongue initially has a white coating, but red and edematous lingual papillae later project through this coating, producing a **white strawberry tongue**. When the white coating peels off, the resulting **red strawberry tongue** is beefy red with prominent papillae. Patients infected with *A. haemolyticum* may present with similar findings.

Gingivostomatitis is characteristic of HSV type 1 primary infection. **Herpangina** is an enteroviral infection with sudden onset of high fever, vomiting, headache, malaise, myalgia, poor intake, drooling, sore throat, and dysphagia. The oral lesions of herpangina may be nonspecific, but classically there are one or more small, tender, papular, or pinpoint vesicular lesions on an erythematous base scattered over the soft palate, uvula, and tongue. These vesicles enlarge from 1–4 mm over 3–4 days, rupture, and produce small, punched-out ulcers that persist for several days. Similar oral lesions may be seen in **hand-foot-and-mouth disease** caused by coxsackieviruses.

LABORATORY EVALUATION

The principal challenge is to distinguish pharyngitis caused by group A streptococcus from pharyngitis caused by viral organisms. A rapid streptococcal antigen test, a throat culture, or both should be performed to improve diagnostic precision and to identify children most likely to benefit from antibiotic therapy. Antigen-based rapid diagnostic tests for streptococcal pharyngitis have excellent specificity of 95–99%. However, the sensitivity of these rapid tests varies, and negative rapid tests should be confirmed by a throat culture or polymerase chain reaction (PCR) because these are the definitive diagnostic tests to establish the presence of streptococcal pharyngitis. However, as many as 20% of positive cultures in children represent chronic **streptococcal carriage** and not acute pharyngitis, and thus children with symptoms more consistent with viral pharyngitis such as rhinorrhea or cough should generally not have throat swabs obtained for streptococcus due to the increased likelihood of identifying the carrier state and providing unnecessary antibiotics in response.

The predictive values of white blood cell count, erythrocyte sedimentation rate, and C-reactive protein are not sufficient to distinguish streptococcal from nonstreptococcal pharyngitis, and these tests are not routinely recommended. The white blood cell count in patients with infectious mononucleosis usually shows a predominance of atypical lymphocytes.

DIFFERENTIAL DIAGNOSIS

The differential diagnosis of infectious pharyngitis includes other local infections of the oral cavity, retropharyngeal abscesses (*S. aureus,* streptococci, anaerobes), diphtheria (if unimmunized), peritonsillar abscesses (streptococci, anaerobes, or, rarely, *S. aureus*), and epiglottitis. In addition, neutropenic mucositis (leukemia, aplastic anemia), thrush (candidiasis secondary to T-cell immune deficiency), autoimmune ulceration (systemic lupus erythematosus, Behçet disease), and Kawasaki disease may cause pharyngitis. Pharyngitis can be a feature of the acute retrovirus syndrome associated with primary HIV infection (see Chapter 126).

Acute necrotizing ulcerative gingivitis (ANUG) and Vincent angina refer to virulent forms of anaerobic gingivitis and pharyngitis, respectively; gray pseudomembranes are found on the tonsils. **Lemierre syndrome** is acute pharyngitis complicated by suppurative thrombophlebitis of the internal jugular vein and septic pulmonary emboli. It primarily occurs in adolescents and is caused by *Fusobacterium necrophorum* (obligate anaerobic gram-negative bacilli). **Ludwig angina** is a mixed anaerobic bacterial cellulitis of the submandibular and sublingual regions. It is typically due to spreading from an abscess of the second or third mandibular molar. It also has been associated with tongue piercing. A propensity for rapid spread, glottic and lingual swelling, and consequent airway obstruction makes prompt intervention imperative.

A syndrome of **periodic fever, aphthous stomatitis, pharyngitis, and cervical adenitis (PFAPA)** is a rare cause of recurrent fever in children. The fevers begin at a young age (usually <5 years). Episodes last approximately 5 days, with a mean of 28 days between episodes. Episodes are shorter with oral prednisone and do not respond to nonsteroidal antiinflammatory medications or antibiotics. Long-term sequelae do not develop.

TREATMENT

Even if untreated, most episodes of streptococcal pharyngitis resolve uneventfully over a few days. Early antimicrobial therapy accelerates clinical recovery by 24–48 hours. The major benefit of antimicrobial therapy is the prevention of acute rheumatic fever (see Chapter 147) and prevention of spread to other sites. Because the latent (incubation) period of **acute rheumatic fever** is relatively long (1–3 weeks), treatment instituted within 9 days of illness onset is virtually 100% successful in preventing rheumatic fever. Treatment begun after this period, although less than 100% successful, has some preventive value. Therefore antibiotic therapy should be started promptly in children with a positive rapid antigen test, throat culture, or PCR for group A streptococcus or a diagnosis of scarlet fever. In addition, a child who has symptomatic pharyngitis and a history of rheumatic fever or a recent family history of rheumatic fever or whose sibling has documented streptococcal infection should be treated.

A variety of antimicrobial agents can be used to treat streptococcal pharyngitis (Table 104.2). Penicillin or amoxicillin remains first-line therapy. Ten days of treatment is recommended to prevent rheumatic fever. Intramuscular penicillin G can be used for children who cannot tolerate oral therapy. Cephalosporins have superior pharyngeal bacterial eradication rates compared to penicillin; however, they are only recommended as an alternative option. Five days of azithromycin is also an alternate treatment option for group A streptococcal pharyngitis, although rates of resistance to azithromycin are higher than those to penicillins. Test of cure for patients who respond clinically to treatment is not required. Children with

TABLE 104.2 Antimicrobial Treatment of Group A Streptococcal Pharyngitis

Oral penicillin V (2–3 times daily for 10 days) 250 mg/dose for children <27 kg, or 500 mg/dose for children ≥ 27 kg, × 10 days
Intramuscular benzathine penicillin G–for children ≤27 kg: 600,000 U; for larger children and adults: 1.2 million U, given as a single dose
Oral amoxicillin as a single daily dose (50 mg/kg; maximum, 1,000–1,200 mg) × 10 days
For persons allergic to penicillin:
Cephalexin 25 mg/kg/dose BID, maximum dose 500 mg/dose × 10 days
Clindamycin 6–7 mg/kg/dose TID, maximum dose 300 mg/dose × 10 days
For persons allergic to β-lactams:
Azithromycin, children: 12 mg/kg (maximum: 500 mg/dose) on day 1 followed by 6 mg/kg/dose (maximum: 250 mg/dose) OD on days 2–5

BID, Twice daily; *OD,* once daily; *TID,* three times daily.

recurrent episodes of group A streptococcal pharyngitis pose a problem, but true treatment failure is rare. Recurrent infection may represent nonadherence, chronic streptococcal carriage in the setting of a new viral pharyngitis, or reinfection. A second course of treatment can be administered. Clindamycin can be effective for eliminating streptococcal carriage.

Specific antiviral therapy is unavailable for most cases of viral pharyngitis. Patients with primary herpetic gingivostomatitis benefit from early treatment with oral acyclovir.

COMPLICATIONS AND PROGNOSIS

Pharyngitis caused by streptococci or respiratory viruses usually resolves completely. The complications of group A streptococcal pharyngitis include local suppurative complications, such as peritonsillar abscess, parapharyngeal abscess, and other infections of the deep fascial spaces of the neck, and nonsuppurative complications, such as acute rheumatic fever and acute postinfectious glomerulonephritis. Viral upper respiratory tract infections, including infections caused by influenza A, adenoviruses, parainfluenza type 3, and rhinoviruses, may predispose the patient to bacterial middle ear infections.

PREVENTION

Antimicrobial prophylaxis with daily oral penicillin V prevents recurrent streptococcal infections and is recommended following an episode of acute rheumatic fever to prevent recurrences.

PEARLS FOR PRACTITIONERS

See Infectious Diseases: Pearls for Practitioners at the end of this section.

REVIEW QUESTIONS

Available online.

CHAPTER 105

Sinusitis

ETIOLOGY

Sinusitis is a suppurative infection of the paranasal sinuses and most commonly occurs as a complication of an upper respiratory tract infection (URI). Only the maxillary and ethmoid sinuses are present at birth, whereas the sphenoid sinuses are present by 5 years of age. Frontal sinuses develop between 7 years of age and adolescence. The ostia draining the sinuses are narrow (1–3 mm) and drain into the middle meatus in the **ostiomeatal complex**. The mucociliary transport system maintains the sinuses as normally sterile. Indwelling nasogastric and nasotracheal tubes predispose to nosocomial sinusitis.

Obstruction to mucociliary flow, such as mucosal edema resulting from a URI, impedes sinus drainage and predisposes to bacterial proliferation. Most cases of pediatric sinusitis are caused by viral etiologies. **Acute bacterial rhinosinusitis (ABRS)** is typically caused by *Streptococcus pneumoniae,* nontypable *Haemophilus influenzae,* and *Moraxella catarrhalis. Staphylococcus aureus* and anaerobes emerge as important pathogens in subacute and chronic sinusitis. Fungal sinusitis can occur in immunocompromised patients, especially those with prolonged and/or profound neutropenia.

EPIDEMIOLOGY

The true incidence of sinusitis is unknown. In addition to predisposing URIs, other risk factors include allergic rhinitis, cystic fibrosis, immunodeficiency, HIV infection, nasogastric or nasotracheal intubation, primary ciliary dyskinesia, nasal polyps, and nasal foreign body.

CLINICAL MANIFESTATIONS

The most common presentation of ABRS is persistent rhinorrhea, nasal congestion, and cough, especially at night. Symptoms should be persistent and not improving for more than 10 days to distinguish ABRS from a URI. Less common symptoms include halitosis, headache, facial swelling, and tenderness. Alternate presentations of ABRS include high fever and purulent nasal discharge for at least 3 days or a biphasic illness where a patient has typical URI symptoms for up to a week but then worsens with increasing respiratory symptoms and new or recurrent fever.

Chronic sinusitis includes upper respiratory symptoms for more than 30 days, often accompanied by sore throat and/or headache. Fever is rare.

LABORATORY AND IMAGING STUDIES

Culture of the nasal mucosa is not useful. Sinus aspirate culture is the most accurate method of determining etiology but is not practical or necessary in immunocompetent patients.

Routine imaging is not recommended in uncomplicated infections. Plain x-ray, CT, and MRI may reveal sinus clouding, mucosal thickening, or air-fluid levels in the sinuses. However, abnormal radiographic findings do not differentiate infection from allergic disease and often show abnormalities in the sinuses of children with a simple viral URI. Conversely, normal imaging can have a high negative predictive value for bacterial sinusitis. Bony erosion may be seen on imaging studies in immunocompromised hosts, especially in the setting of fungal sinusitis.

TREATMENT

Amoxicillin for 5–7 days can be used as first-line therapy of uncomplicated ABRS in children. Broadening therapy to amoxicillin-clavulanate is appropriate if there is no clinical response to amoxicillin within 2–3 days, if risk factors for resistant organisms are present (antibiotic treatment in the preceding 1–3 months, daycare attendance), if there is chronic sinusitis, or if any amount of eye swelling is present.

COMPLICATIONS AND PROGNOSIS

Complications of bacterial sinusitis include orbital cellulitis, epidural or subdural empyema, brain abscess, dural sinus thrombosis, osteomyelitis of the frontal sinus (**Pott puffy tumor**), and meningitis. These all should be managed with sinus drainage and initial broad-spectrum parenteral antibiotics.

Orbital (postseptal) cellulitis is a serious complication of sinusitis that follows bacterial spread into the orbit through the wall of the infected sinus. It typically begins as ethmoid sinusitis and spreads through the **lamina papyracea**, a thin, bony plate that separates the medial orbit and the ethmoid sinus. Orbital involvement can lead to subperiosteal abscess, cavernous sinus thrombosis, and vision loss. Clinical manifestations of orbital cellulitis include a swollen edematous eye, eye pain, proptosis, chemosis, and limitations and pain with extraocular muscle motion, diplopia, and reduced visual acuity. Infection of the orbit must be differentiated from that of the preseptal (anterior to the palpebral fascia) or periorbital space. **Preseptal (periorbital) cellulitis** is common in young children; these patients do not have proptosis or ophthalmoplegia. Preseptal cellulitis may be associated with a skin lesion or trauma and usually is caused by *S. aureus* or group A streptococcus.

The diagnosis of orbital cellulitis is confirmed by a CT scan of the orbit, which helps determine the extent of orbital infection. Therapy for orbital cellulitis involves broad-spectrum parenteral antibiotics, such as vancomycin or clindamycin with ceftriaxone or amoxicillin-sulbactam. An orbital abscess may need surgical drainage. Preseptal cellulitis may be treated with oral antibiotics in children with mild disease.

PREVENTION

The best means of prevention is good handwashing to minimize acquisition of URIs and management of allergic rhinitis.

PEARLS FOR PRACTITIONERS

See Infectious Diseases: Pearls for Practitioners at the end of this section.

REVIEW QUESTIONS

Available online.

CHAPTER 106 Otitis Media

ETIOLOGY

Otitis media (OM) is a suppurative infection of the middle ear cavity. Bacteria gain access to the middle ear when the normal patency of the eustachian tube is blocked by upper airway infection or hypertrophied adenoids. Air trapped in the middle ear is resorbed, creating negative pressure in this cavity and facilitating reflux of nasopharyngeal bacteria.

Bacteria are the most common pathogens in OM, most frequently as a co-infection with viruses. Viruses can be the sole pathogen in OM, but this is less common (<20%). The common bacterial pathogens are nontypable *Haemophilus influenzae, Streptococcus pneumoniae, Moraxella catarrhalis,* and, less frequently, group A streptococcus. *S. pneumoniae* that is **intermediate or resistant** to penicillin is isolated with increasing frequency from young children, particularly those who attend daycare or have recently received antibiotics.

EPIDEMIOLOGY

Diseases of the middle ear account for approximately one third of office visits to pediatricians. The peak incidence of acute otitis media (AOM) is between 6 and 15 months of life. By the third birthday, 80% of children will have experienced at least one episode of symptomatic or asymptomatic OM. OM is more common in younger children, children exposed to other young children, and those with a positive family history. In most of the United States, OM is a seasonal disease with a distinct peak in late winter/early spring, which corresponds to the respiratory viral season.

Approximately 10% of children in the general population have **recurrent OM**, as defined by the presence of three or more AOM episodes in the preceding 6 months or four or more episodes in the preceding 12 months. Craniofacial anomalies (cleft palate) and immunodeficiencies often are associated with recurrent OM, although most children with recurrent AOM are otherwise healthy.

CLINICAL MANIFESTATIONS

In infants, the most frequent symptoms of AOM are nonspecific and include fever, irritability, and poor feeding. In older children and adolescents, AOM usually is associated with fever and **otalgia** (acute ear pain). AOM also may present with **otorrhea** (ear drainage) after spontaneous rupture of the tympanic membrane. Signs of a common cold, which predisposes to AOM, are often present (see Chapter 103). A bulging tympanic membrane, air fluid level, or visualization of purulent material by otoscopy are reliable signs of infection (Table 106.1).

Examination of the ears is essential for diagnosis and should be part of the physical examination of any child with fever. The hallmark of OM is the presence of effusion in the middle ear cavity (see Table 106.1). The presence of an effusion does not confirm the presence of a bacterial OM, but it does define the need for appropriate diagnosis and therapy.

Pneumatic otoscopy, using an attachment to an otoscope, allows evaluation of ventilation of the middle ear and is a standard for clinical diagnosis. The tympanic membrane of the normal, air-filled middle ear has much greater compliance than if the middle ear is fluid filled. With AOM, the tympanic membrane is often characterized by **hyperemia**, or red color rather than the normal pearly gray color, but may appear pink, white, or yellow depending on the degree of bulging (Fig. 106.1). The light reflex is lost, and the middle ear structures are obscured and difficult to distinguish. There should be poor or absent mobility to negative and positive pressure; this is a necessary finding for the diagnosis of OM. A hole in the tympanic membrane or purulent drainage confirms perforation. Occasionally, bullae are present on the lateral aspect of the tympanic membrane, which characteristically are associated with severe ear pain.

LABORATORY AND IMAGING STUDIES

Routine laboratory studies are not useful in the evaluation of OM. Bacteria recovered from the nasopharynx do not correlate with bacteria isolated by tympanocentesis. Tympanocentesis and middle ear exudate culture are not necessary, but they are required for accurate identification of bacterial pathogens and may be useful in neonates, immunocompromised patients, and patients not responding to therapy.

DIFFERENTIAL DIAGNOSIS

An important distinction is differentiation of AOM from **OM with effusion (OME)**. AOM is accompanied by signs of acute illness, such as fever, pain, and upper respiratory tract inflammation. OME is the presence of effusion without any of the other signs and symptoms. OME may occur either as the sequela of AOM or eustachian tube dysfunction secondary to an upper respiratory tract infection. It may also predispose to the development of AOM. Because OME is not an acute infectious process, it is important to be able to differentiate between OME and AOM accurately to prevent overprescribing of antibiotics.

TABLE 106.1 Definition of Acute Otitis Media

A diagnosis of AOM requires:
History of acute onset of signs and symptoms Presence of middle ear effusion Signs and symptoms of middle ear inflammation
The definition of AOM includes all of the following:
Recent, usually abrupt, onset of signs and symptoms of middle ear inflammation and middle ear effusion
The presence of middle ear effusion that is indicated by any of the following:
Bulging of the TM Limited or absent mobility of the TM Air-fluid level behind the TM Abnormal TM color (white, yellow, amber) Otorrhea
Signs or symptoms of middle ear inflammation as indicated by either:
Distinct erythema of the TM Distinct otalgia (discomfort clearly referable to the ear that results in interference with or precludes normal activity or sleep)

AOM, Acute otitis media; *TM*, tympanic membrane.

TREATMENT

Recommendations for treatment are based on age, certainty of diagnosis, and severity of illness (Table 106.2). The recommended first-line therapy for most children meeting criteria for antibiotic therapy is amoxicillin (80–90 mg/kg/day in two divided doses). Some children with mild illness or uncertain diagnosis may be observed initially with delayed initiation of antibiotic therapy if appropriate follow-up within 48–72 hours can be arranged. Antibiotics are initiated if symptoms do not self-resolve (see Table 106.2). The failure of initial therapy with amoxicillin at 3 days suggests infection with β-lactamase-producing *H. influenza, M. catarrhalis,* or resistant *S. pneumoniae.* Recommended next-step treatments include high-dose amoxicillin-clavulanate (amoxicillin 80–90 mg/kg/day), cefdinir, or ceftriaxone (50 mg/kg intramuscularly in daily doses for 3 days). Intramuscular ceftriaxone is especially appropriate for children with vomiting that precludes oral treatment. Tympanocentesis may be required for patients who are difficult to treat or who do not respond to therapy. Acetaminophen and ibuprofen are recommended for fever or pain. Decongestants or antihistamines are not effective.

COMPLICATIONS AND PROGNOSIS

The complications of OM are tympanic membrane perforation, chronic effusion, chronic otorrhea, hearing loss, **cholesteatoma** (mass-like keratinized epithelial growth), facial palsy, petrositis, intracranial extension (brain abscess, subdural empyema, or venous thrombosis), and mastoiditis. **Acute mastoiditis** is a suppurative complication of OM with inflammation and potential destruction of the mastoid air spaces.

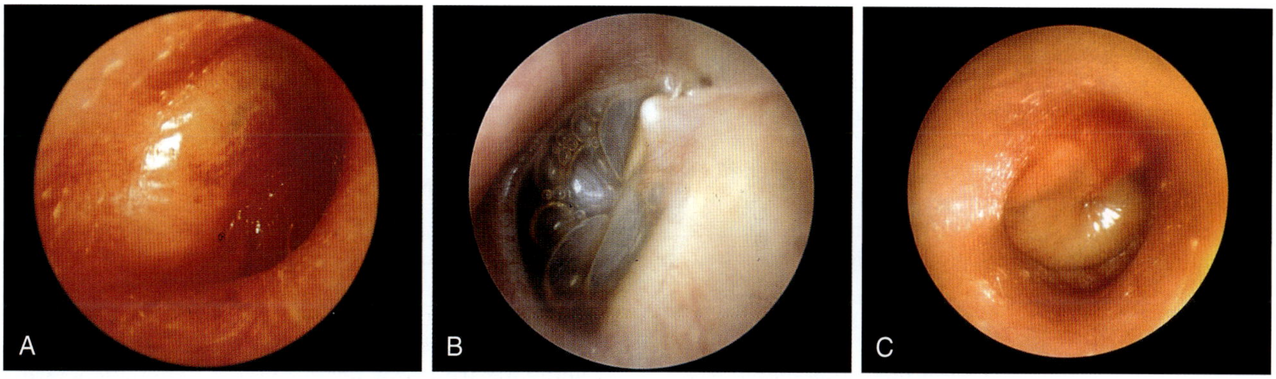

FIGURE 106.1 Acute otitis media. **(A)** This is the classic picture—an erythematous, opaque, bulging tympanic membrane. The light reflex is reduced, and the landmarks are partially obscured. Mobility is markedly reduced. **(B)** In this acutely febrile child who complained of otalgia, the presence of both air and fluid formed bubbles separated by grayish-yellow menisci. Even though the drum was not injected, this finding, combined with fever and otalgia, is consistent with acute infection. **(C)** In this child, the tympanic membrane was injected at the periphery, and a yellow purulent effusion caused the inferior portion to bulge outward. Mobility was markedly reduced. (From Chi DH, Tobey A. Otolaryngology. In: Zitelli BJ, McIntire SC, Nowalk AJ, Garrison J eds. *Zitelli and Davis' Atlas of Pediatric Physical Diagnosis.* 8th ed. Philadelphia: Saunders; 2023:873–922, fig. 24.24.)

TABLE 106.2 Recommendations for Initial Management of Confirmed Acute Otitis Media*

AGE	AOM WITH OTORRHEA	AOM WITH SEVERE SYMPTOMS†	BILATERAL AOM WITHOUT OTORRHEA	UNILATERAL AOM WITHOUT OTORRHEA
6 mo to 2 yr	Antibiotics	Antibiotics	Antibiotics	Antibiotics or additional observation‡
≥2 yr	Antibiotics	Antibiotics	Antibiotics or additional observation	Antibiotics or additional observation

*Applies only to children with well-documented AOM with high certainty of diagnosis.
†A toxic-appearing child, persistent otalgia for >48 hr, temperature ≥39°C (102.2°F) in the past 48 hr, or if there is uncertain follow-up.
‡Requires shared decision making with parents and close follow-up within 48–72 hr.
AOM, Acute otitis media.
Reproduced with permission from Lieberthal AS, Carroll AE, Chonmaitree T, et al. American Academy of Pediatrics clinical practice guideline: the diagnosis and management of acute otitis media. Pediatrics. *2013;131:e964–e999. Copyright 2013 by the AAP.*

The disease progresses from a periostitis to an osteitis with mastoid abscess formation. Posterior auricular tenderness, swelling, and erythema, in addition to the signs of OM, are present. The pinna is displaced downward and outward. Computed tomography scan of the mastoid reveals clouding of the air cells, demineralization, or bone destruction. Treatment includes systemic antibiotics and drainage if the disease has progressed to abscess formation.

OME is the most frequent sequela of AOM and occurs most frequently in the first 2 years of life (up to 30–50% of children with AOM). **Persistent middle ear effusion** may last for many weeks or months in some children but usually resolves by 3 months following infection. Evaluating young children for this condition is an important part of all well child examinations because, although not an infectious process, it is associated with hearing loss.

Conductive hearing loss should be assumed to be present with persistent middle ear effusion; the loss is mild to moderate and often is transient or fluctuating. In children at developmental risk or with frequent episodes of recurrent AOM, 3 months of persistent effusion with significant bilateral hearing loss is a reasonable indicator of need for intervention with insertion of pressure equalization tubes (tympanostomy tubes).

PREVENTION

Parents should be encouraged to continue exclusive breastfeeding as long as possible and should be cautioned about the risks of *bottle-propping* and of children taking a bottle to bed. The home should be a smoke-free environment, and pacifier use should be limited.

The conjugate *S. pneumoniae* vaccine reduces pneumococcal OM caused by vaccine serotypes by 50%, all pneumococcal OM by 33%, and all OM by 6–10%. Annual immunization against influenza virus may be helpful in high-risk children.

PEARLS FOR PRACTITIONERS

See Infectious Diseases: Pearls for Practitioners at the end of this section.

REVIEW QUESTIONS

Available online.

CHAPTER 107

Otitis Externa

ETIOLOGY

Otitis externa, also known as **swimmer's ear**, is defined by inflammation and exudate in the external auditory canal in the absence of other disorders, such as otitis media or mastoiditis. The most common bacterial pathogens are *Pseudomonas aeruginosa*, especially in association with swimming in pools or lakes, and *Staphylococcus aureus*. Otitis externa develops in approximately 20% of children with **tympanostomy tubes**, associated with *S. aureus, Streptococcus pneumoniae, Moraxella catarrhalis, Proteus, Klebsiella,* and, occasionally, anaerobes. Coagulase-negative staphylococci and *Corynebacterium* are isolated frequently from cultures of the external canal but represent normal flora. **Malignant otitis externa** is caused by *P. aeruginosa* in immunocompromised persons and adults with diabetes.

EPIDEMIOLOGY

Otitis externa cases peak in summer, in contrast to otitis media, which occurs primarily in colder seasons in association with viral upper respiratory tract infections. Cleaning of the auditory canal, swimming, and, in particular, diving disrupt the integrity of the cutaneous lining of the ear canal and local defenses, such as cerumen, predisposing to otitis externa.

CLINICAL MANIFESTATIONS

Pain, tenderness, and aural discharge are the characteristic clinical findings of otitis externa. Fever is notably absent. Hearing is typically normal, but conductive hearing loss may be present if edema of the canal is severe. Tenderness with movement of the pinna, especially the tragus, and with chewing is particularly characteristic; symptoms which are notably absent in otitis media. Inspection usually reveals that the lining of the auditory canal is inflamed with mild to severe erythema and edema. Scant to copious discharge from the auditory canal may obscure the tympanic membrane. The most common symptoms of **malignant otitis**

externa are similar, but facial nerve palsy, vertigo, and/or sensorineural hearing loss may also occur. The most common physical findings are swelling and granulation tissue in the canal, usually with a discharge from the external auditory canal.

LABORATORY AND IMAGING STUDIES

The diagnosis of uncomplicated otitis externa usually is established solely on the basis of the clinical symptoms and physical examination findings without the need for additional laboratory or microbiologic evaluation. Cultures are required to identify the etiologic agent and the antimicrobial susceptibility but typically are reserved for severe disease or recurrent cases.

DIFFERENTIAL DIAGNOSIS

Otitis media with tympanic perforation and discharge into the auditory canal may be confused with otitis externa; pain on movement of the pinnae or tragus, typical of otitis externa, is absent. Local and systemic signs of **mastoiditis** (Chapter 106) indicate a process more extensive than otitis externa. Malignancies or cholesteatoma presenting in the auditory canal are rare in children but may present with discharge, unusual pain, or hearing loss.

TREATMENT

Topical antimicrobial/corticosteroid otic preparations (such as ofloxacin, ciprofloxacin with hydrocortisone or dexamethasone, and polymyxin B-neosporin-hydrocortisone) are sufficient in most cases of otitis externa. These preparations are equally effective and are active against *S. aureus* and most gram-negative bacteria, including *P. aeruginosa*. Use of aminoglycosides such as neomycin should be avoided in cases of tympanic membrane rupture due to their ototoxicity. **Tympanostomy tube otorrhea** is best treated with topical quinolone otic drugs, which are considered less likely to be ototoxic.

Treatment with topical otic analgesics and cerumenolytics is usually unnecessary. It is important with any topical therapy to remove purulent discharge from the external auditory canal with a swab or with suction to permit instillation of the solution. Excess water should be removed after bathing and the ear canal dried using a hairdryer. The predisposing activity, such as swimming or diving, should be avoided until the inflammation has resolved.

Fungi such as *Aspergillus, Candida,* and dermatophytes are occasionally isolated from the external ear. It may be difficult to determine whether they represent normal flora or are the cause of inflammation. In most cases, local therapy and restoration of normal pH as recommended for bacterial otitis externa are sufficient.

Malignant otitis externa is treated by parenteral antimicrobials with activity against *P. aeruginosa,* such as an extended-spectrum penicillin (piperacillin-tazobactam), a cephalosporin with activity against *P. aeruginosa* (ceftazidime, cefepime), or a fluoroquinolone (ciprofloxacin).

COMPLICATIONS AND PROGNOSIS

Acute otitis externa usually resolves promptly without complications within 1–2 days of initiating treatment. Persistent pain, especially if severe or if accompanied by other symptoms (e.g., fever), should prompt re-evaluation for other conditions.

Complications of malignant otitis externa include invasion of the bones at the base of the skull, which may cause cranial nerve palsies. A mortality of 15–20% occurs in adults with malignant otitis externa. Relapses within the first year after treatment are common.

PREVENTION

Overly vigorous cleaning of an asymptomatic auditory canal should be avoided. Drying the auditory canals with acetic acid (2%) or diluted isopropyl alcohol (rubbing alcohol) after swimming may be used prophylactically to help prevent the maceration that facilitates bacterial invasion. There is no role for prophylactic otic antibiotics.

PEARLS FOR PRACTITIONERS

See Infectious Diseases: Pearls for Practitioners at the end of this section.

REVIEW QUESTIONS

Available online.

CHAPTER 108
Croup (Laryngotracheobronchitis)

ETIOLOGY AND EPIDEMIOLOGY

Croup, or laryngotracheobronchitis, is the most common infection of the middle respiratory tract. The most common causes of croup are parainfluenza viruses (types 1, 2, and 3), respiratory syncytial virus (RSV), influenza, adenovirus, and SARS-CoV-2. Laryngotracheal airway inflammation disproportionately affects children because a small decrease in diameter secondary to mucosal edema and inflammation exponentially increases airway resistance and work of breathing. During inspiration, the walls of the subglottic space are drawn together, aggravating the obstruction and producing the **stridor** characteristic of croup. Croup is most common in children 6 months to 3 years of age, with a peak in fall and early winter. It typically follows a common cold. Symptomatic reinfection is common and is usually mild. In adolescents, it manifests as laryngitis.

CLINICAL MANIFESTATIONS

The manifestations of croup are a harsh cough described as **barking** or **brassy**, hoarseness, inspiratory stridor, low-grade fever, and respiratory distress. **Stridor** is a harsh, high-pitched respiratory sound produced by turbulent airflow. It is usually inspiratory, but it may be biphasic and is a sign of upper airway obstruction. Signs of upper airway obstruction, such as labored breathing, cyanosis, and marked suprasternal, intercostal, and subcostal retractions, may be evident on examination (see Chapter 136). Wheezing may be present if there is lower airway involvement. Symptoms of croup are characteristically worse at night and are exacerbated with crying or agitation.

LABORATORY AND IMAGING STUDIES

Croup is a clinical diagnosis and does not require routine radiology or laboratory studies. If obtained, anteroposterior radiographs of the neck often show the diagnostic subglottic narrowing of croup known as the **steeple sign** (Fig. 108.1). Leukocytosis is uncommon and suggests epiglottitis or bacterial tracheitis. Many rapid tests (using polymerase chain reaction [PCR]) are available for viral causes of croup.

DIFFERENTIAL DIAGNOSIS

The infectious differential diagnosis includes epiglottitis, bacterial tracheitis, and parapharyngeal abscess. Noninfectious causes of stridor include mechanical and anatomic causes (foreign body aspiration, laryngomalacia, subglottic stenosis, hemangioma, vascular ring, vocal cord paralysis). Stridor in infants younger than 4 months of age, positional stridor, or persistence of symptoms for longer than 1 week indicates an increased probability of another lesion and the need for imaging and direct laryngoscopy (see Chapter 136).

Epiglottitis is a medical emergency because of the risk of sudden airway obstruction. Following the introduction of the *Haemophilus influenzae* type b vaccine, this illness is rare and usually caused by group A streptococcus, *Staphylococcus aureus,* or *H. influenzae* type b in unimmunized patients. Patients typically prefer sitting, often with the head held forward, the mouth open, and the jaw thrust forward **(sniffing position)**, and they may appear distressed and toxic. Lateral radiograph reveals thickened and bulging epiglottis **(thumb sign)** and swelling of the aryepiglottic folds. The diagnosis is confirmed by direct observation of the inflamed and swollen supraglottic structures and swollen, cherry red epiglottis. Direct observation of the larynx should only be performed in the operating room with an anesthesiologist and a surgeon prepared to place an endotracheal tube or perform a tracheostomy if needed. Epiglottitis requires antibiotic therapy and endotracheal intubation to maintain the airway. Both onset and clinical recovery are rapid, and most children can be extubated safely within 48–72 hours.

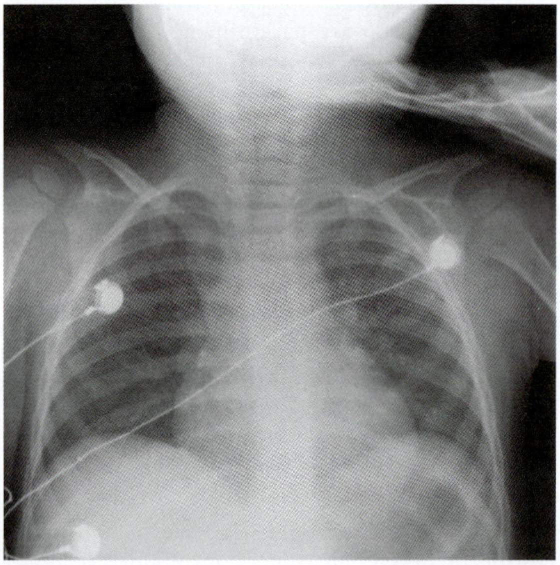

FIGURE 108.1 Croup (laryngotracheobronchitis). Radiograph of the airway and chest of a patient with croup, demonstrating the typical subglottic narrowing ("steeple sign"). (From Rodrigues KK, Roosevelt GE. Acute inflammatory upper airway obstruction [croup, epiglottitis, laryngitis, and bacterial tracheitis]. In: Kliegman RM, St. Geme III JW, eds. *Nelson Textbook of Pediatrics.* 22nd ed. Philadelphia: Elsevier; 2025: fig. 433-1.)

Bacterial tracheitis is a rare but serious superinfection of the trachea that may follow viral croup and is most commonly caused by *S. aureus.* Patients may appear toxic, and intubation may be required. **Spasmodic croup** describes sudden onset of croup symptoms, usually at night, but without a significant upper respiratory tract prodrome. These episodes may be recurrent and severe but usually are of short duration. Spasmodic croup has a milder course than viral croup and responds to relatively simple therapies, such as exposure to cool or humidified air. The etiology is not well understood and may be allergic.

TREATMENT

Oral or intramuscular dexamethasone for children with viral croup reduces symptoms and the need for hospitalization and shortens hospital stays. Dexamethasone (0.6 mg/kg) may be given once intramuscularly or orally. Alternatively, prednisolone (2 mg/kg/day) may be given orally for 3 days. For significant airway compromise, administration of aerosolized racemic (D- and L-) epinephrine reduces subglottic edema by adrenergic vasoconstriction, temporarily producing marked clinical improvement. The peak effect is within 10–30 minutes and fades within 60–90 minutes. A rebound effect may occur, with worsening of symptoms as the effect of the drug dissipates. Aerosol treatment may need to be repeated as needed in severe cases.

Children should be kept as calm as possible to minimize forceful inspiration. One useful calming method is for a child with croup to sit on the parent's lap. Heliox (a combination of helium and oxygen) may be considered in patients who have persistent respiratory distress despite racemic epinephrine but evidence to support its use is limited.

Hospitalization is often required for children with cyanosis or stridor at rest. Children receiving aerosol treatment should be hospitalized or observed for at least 2–3 hours because of the risk of rebound airway obstruction. Decreased symptoms may indicate improvement or fatigue and impending respiratory failure.

COMPLICATIONS AND PROGNOSIS

The most common complication of croup is viral pneumonia, which occurs in 1–2% of children. Parainfluenza virus pneumonia and secondary bacterial pneumonia are more common in immunocompromised patients. Bacterial tracheitis may also be a complication of croup.

The prognosis for croup is excellent. Illness usually lasts approximately 5 days. As children grow, they become less susceptible to the airway effects of viral infections of the middle respiratory tract.

PREVENTION

There are no licensed vaccines for parainfluenza or adenovirus. There is an RSV monoclonal antibody, nirsevimab, available for all infants under 8 months of age and licensed RSV vaccines for pregnant people and adults age 60 and older. Annual influenza vaccine and SARS-CoV-2 vaccination is recommended for all children 6 months of age and older.

PEARLS FOR PRACTITIONERS

See Infectious Diseases: Pearls for Practitioners at the end of this section.

REVIEW QUESTIONS

Available online.

CHAPTER 109

Pertussis

ETIOLOGY

Pertussis **(whooping cough)** is caused by *Bordetella pertussis,* a gram-negative pleomorphic bacillus with fastidious growth requirements. *B. pertussis* infects only humans and is transmitted from person to person by coughing.

EPIDEMIOLOGY

The typical incubation period is 7–10 days but can range between 5 and 21 days. Patients are most contagious during the first 2 weeks of cough. The annual rate of pertussis was approximately 100–200 cases per 100,000 population in the prevaccination era; worldwide, there continues to be an estimated 20 million cases of pertussis and 200,000 childhood deaths annually. In the United States, the incidence of pertussis decreased after the introduction of vaccine, but it has increased steadily since the 1980s, with more than 17,500 cases reported in 2024. Pertussis incidence peaks among those less than 6 months of age, ranging from 40 to 160 cases per 100,000 population in the United States. These infants are too young to be completely immunized and are most likely to have severe complications. Infection in late childhood and adolescence is likely due to a combination of waning immunity from previous vaccines, underimmunization, exposure to infected family members, and improved diagnostics. Epidemics can occur in fully immunized patients because vaccine-induced immunity wanes.

CLINICAL MANIFESTATIONS

Classic pertussis is seen in children between 1 and 10 years old. The progression of the disease is divided into catarrhal, paroxysmal, and convalescent stages. The **catarrhal stage** is marked by nonspecific signs (increased nasal secretions and low-grade fever) lasting 1–2 weeks. The **paroxysmal stage** is the most distinctive stage of pertussis and lasts 2–4 weeks. Coughing occurs in **paroxysms** during expiration, causing young children to lose their breath. This pattern of coughing is needed to dislodge plugs of necrotic bronchial epithelial tissues and thick mucus. The forceful inhalation against a narrowed glottis that follows this paroxysm of cough produces the characteristic **whoop**. Posttussive emesis is common. The **convalescent stage** is marked by gradual resolution of symptoms over 1–2 weeks. Coughing becomes less severe, and the paroxysms and whoops slowly disappear. Although the disease typically lasts 6–8 weeks, residual cough may persist for months, especially with physical stress or respiratory irritants.

Infants may not display the classic findings, and the first sign in the neonate may be apnea. Young infants are unlikely to have the classic whoop, more likely to have central nervous system damage due to hypoxia, and more likely to have secondary bacterial pneumonia. Adolescents and adults with pertussis usually present with persistent, nonproductive cough that often begins as a nonspecific upper respiratory tract infection. In general, adolescents and adults do not have a whoop with the cough, although they may have severe paroxysms.

LABORATORY AND IMAGING STUDIES

The diagnosis depends on isolation of *B. pertussis* or detection of its nucleic acids. Culture on specialized media can be performed during the early phases of illness on specimens from nasopharyngeal swabs or aspirates, but this can be difficult to accomplish given the organism's fastidious nature. Polymerase chain reaction is also available; false-positive results can occur. Serologic tests are not useful for diagnosing acute infection but can be confirmatory in the convalescent phase of illness, though there are no commercial kits approved by the U.S. Food and Drug Administration.

Lymphocytosis is present in 75–85% of infants and young children but is not diagnostic. The white blood cell count may increase from 20,000/mm^3 to more than 50,000/mm^3, consisting primarily of mature lymphocytes. Physical examination and radiographic signs of segmental lung atelectasis may develop during pertussis, especially during the paroxysmal stage. Perihilar infiltrates are common and are similar to those seen in viral pneumonia.

DIFFERENTIAL DIAGNOSIS

For a young child with classic pertussis, the diagnosis based on the pattern of illness is quite accurate. The paroxysmal stage is the most distinctive part of the syndrome. Other causes of pertussis-like prolonged cough illnesses include *Bordetella parapertussis* and *Bordetella holmesii,* which cause a similar but milder illness and are not prevented by *B. pertussis* vaccination, as well as *Mycoplasma pneumoniae, Chlamydophila pneumoniae,* adenoviruses, and respiratory syncytial virus.

TREATMENT

Macrolide antibiotics (azithromycin, clarithromycin, or erythromycin) are recommended for treatment. Azithromycin is preferred in neonates due to the association between erythromycin treatment and the development of pyloric stenosis. Treatment during the catarrhal phase eradicates nasopharyngeal carriage of organisms within 3–4 days and may lessen symptom severity. Treatment in the paroxysmal stage does not alter the course of illness but decreases the potential for spread to others. Trimethoprim-sulfamethoxazole is an alternative therapy among children older than 2 months.

COMPLICATIONS AND PROGNOSIS

Major complications are most common among infants and young children and include hypoxia, apnea, pneumonia, seizures, encephalopathy, dehydration, malnutrition, and death. The most frequent complication is pneumonia caused by *B. pertussis* itself or resulting from secondary bacterial infection with *Streptococcus pneumoniae, Haemophilus influenzae,* and *Staphylococcus aureus.* Atelectasis may develop secondary to mucus plugs. The force of the paroxysm may produce pneumomediastinum, pneumothorax, or interstitial or subcutaneous emphysema; epistaxis; hernias; and retinal and subconjunctival hemorrhages. Otitis media and sinusitis may occur.

Most children recover normal pulmonary function with complete healing of the respiratory epithelium. Most permanent disability is a result of encephalopathy.

PREVENTION

Active immunity is induced with acellular pertussis components given as a vaccine in combination with the tetanus and diphtheria toxoids (DTaP). DTaP vaccine is recommended at 2, 4, 6, and 15–18 months, with a booster at 4–6 years, and has an efficacy of 70–90%. A single booster dose of Tdap vaccine is recommended at 11–12 years or every 10 years (as Tdap or Td) for all adults. A booster dose of Tdap vaccine is recommended for pregnant women with each pregnancy, preferably in the third trimester, to provide higher levels of antibodies to the infant via transplacental transfer.

Macrolides are effective in preventing secondary cases in contacts exposed to pertussis. Underimmunized close contacts under 7 years of age should receive a booster dose of DTaP (unless a booster dose has been given within the preceding 3 years), whereas those 7–10 years of age should receive Tdap. All close contacts should receive prophylactic antibiotics for 5 days (azithromycin) or 7–14 days (clarithromycin or erythromycin, duration based on age).

PEARLS FOR PRACTITIONERS

See Infectious Diseases: Pearls for Practitioners at the end of this section.

REVIEW QUESTIONS

Available online.

CHAPTER 110

Bronchiolitis

ETIOLOGY

Bronchiolitis is a disease of small bronchioles with edema, increased mucus production, and occasional bronchospasm, sometimes leading to airway obstruction. It is commonly caused by a viral lower respiratory tract infection. Bronchiolitis is commonly seen in infants and young children, with most severe cases occurring among infants; it is potentially life-threatening.

Respiratory syncytial virus (RSV) is a primary cause of bronchiolitis, followed in frequency by human metapneumovirus, parainfluenza viruses, influenza viruses, adenoviruses, rhinoviruses, coronaviruses, and, infrequently, *Mycoplasma pneumoniae.* Viral bronchiolitis is extremely contagious and is spread by contact with infected respiratory secretions. Although coughing produces aerosols, hand carriage of contaminated secretions is the most frequent mode of transmission.

EPIDEMIOLOGY

Bronchiolitis is a leading cause of hospitalization of infants. Bronchiolitis occurs almost exclusively during the first 2 years of life, with a peak age at 2–6 months. Many healthy children with bronchiolitis can be managed as outpatients; however, premature infants and children with chronic lung disease of prematurity, hemodynamically significant congenital heart disease, neuromuscular weakness, or immunodeficiency are at increased risk of severe, potentially fatal disease. Children acquire infection after exposure to infected family members, who typically have symptoms of an upper respiratory tract infection, or from infected children in daycare. In most regions of the United States, annual peaks are usually in the late fall through winter months (from November through March).

CLINICAL MANIFESTATIONS

Bronchiolitis caused by RSV typically has an incubation period of 4–6 days and classically presents as a progressive respiratory illness similar to the common cold in its early phase, with cough and rhinorrhea. It progresses over 3–7 days to noisy, raspy breathing and audible wheezing. There is usually a low-grade fever accompanied by irritability, which may reflect the increased work of breathing. In contrast to the classic progression of disease, young infants infected with RSV may not have prodromal symptoms and may have apnea as the first or only sign of infection.

Physical signs of bronchiolar obstruction include prolongation of the expiratory phase of breathing, nasal flaring, intercostal retractions, suprasternal retractions, and air trapping with hyperexpansion of the lungs. During the wheezing phase, percussion of the chest usually reveals only hyperresonance, but auscultation usually reveals diffuse wheezes and crackles throughout the breathing cycle. With more severe disease, grunting and cyanosis may be present.

LABORATORY AND IMAGING STUDIES

Routine laboratory tests are not required to confirm the diagnosis. It is important to assess oxygenation in severe cases of bronchiolitis. **Pulse oximetry** is adequate for monitoring oxygen saturation. Frequent, regular assessments and cardiorespiratory monitoring of infants are necessary because respiratory failure may develop precipitously in very tired infants even though blood gas values taken before rapid decompensation are reassuring.

Rapid viral diagnosis of nasopharyngeal secretions performed by polymerase chain reactions for RSV, human metapneumovirus, parainfluenza viruses, influenza viruses, coronaviruses, and adenoviruses are sensitive tests to confirm the infection. Identifying the viral agent is helpful for cohorting children with the same infection but is not necessary to make the diagnosis of bronchiolitis.

Chest radiographs are not always necessary but frequently show signs of lung hyperinflation, including increased lung lucency and flattened or depressed diaphragms. Areas of increased density may represent either viral pneumonia or localized atelectasis.

DIFFERENTIAL DIAGNOSIS

The major difficulty in the diagnosis of bronchiolitis is differentiating other diseases associated with wheezing. It may be difficult to differentiate asthma from bronchiolitis by physical examination, but age of presentation, presence of fever, and absence of personal or family history of asthma are the major differential factors. Bronchiolitis occurs primarily in the first year of life and is accompanied by fever, whereas asthma usually presents in older children with previous wheezing episodes and is typically unaccompanied by fever unless a respiratory tract infection is the trigger for the asthma exacerbation.

Wheezing may also be due to an airway foreign body, congenital airway obstructive lesion, cystic fibrosis, exacerbation of chronic lung disease, viral or bacterial pneumonia, and other lower respiratory tract diseases (see Chapter 79). **Cardiogenic asthma**, which can be confused with bronchiolitis in infants, is wheezing associated with pulmonary congestion secondary to left-sided heart failure. Wheezing associated with gastroesophageal reflux is likely to be chronic or recurrent, and the patient may have a history of frequent emesis. Cystic fibrosis is associated with poor growth, chronic diarrhea, and a positive family history. A focal area on radiography that remains inflated despite changes in position suggests **foreign body aspiration**.

TREATMENT

Bronchiolitis treatment consists of supportive therapy, including respiratory monitoring, control of fever, hydration, upper airway suctioning, and, if needed, oxygen administration. Indications for hospitalization include moderate to marked respiratory distress, hypoxemia, apnea, inability to tolerate oral feeding, and lack of appropriate care available at home. Hospitalization of high-risk children with bronchiolitis should be considered. Among hospitalized infants, supplemental oxygen by nasal cannula is often necessary, but intubation and ventilatory assistance for respiratory failure or apnea are required in less than 10% of these infants. Bronchodilators, corticosteroids, chest physiotherapy, and hypertonic saline are seldom effective and are not generally recommended. Likewise, antibiotics should be avoided unless there is strong suspicion for concomitant bacterial infection.

COMPLICATIONS AND PROGNOSIS

Most hospitalized children show marked improvement in 2–5 days with supportive treatment alone. The course of the wheezing phase varies, however. Tachypnea and hypoxia may progress to respiratory failure requiring assisted ventilation. Apnea is a major concern for very young infants with bronchiolitis.

Most cases of bronchiolitis resolve completely, although minor abnormalities of pulmonary function and bronchial hyperreactivity may persist for several years. Recurrence is common but tends to be mild and should be assessed and treated similarly to the first episode. The incidence of asthma seems to be higher in children hospitalized for bronchiolitis as infants, but it is unclear whether this is causal or whether children prone to asthma are more likely to be hospitalized with bronchiolitis. There is a 1–2% mortality rate, highest among infants with preexisting cardiopulmonary or immunologic impairment.

PREVENTION

One-time injection of **nirsevimab**, an RSV-specific monoclonal antibody, is indicated for all infants under 8 months of age entering their first RSV season and is effective in reducing the risk of hospitalization for bronchiolitis. Previously, only certain infants were given monthly injections of **palivizumab**, an RSV-specific monoclonal antibody, just before the onset of the RSV season. Palivizumab was indicated for infants with prematurity (born before 29 weeks gestation), those with chronic lung disease of prematurity, and those with hemodynamically significant congenital heart disease in the first year of life, and, rarely, in the second year of life. Additionally, an RSV vaccine is approved for pregnant people during 32–36 weeks of gestation to prevent severe RSV disease in infants. Infants whose birthing parent has received an RSV vaccine in the recommended time frame prior to birth do not need additional RSV monoclonal antibody. Providers should consult CDC updates to RSV prevention for most current recommendations. Immunization with influenza vaccine is recommended for all children older than 6 months and may prevent influenza-associated disease.

PEARLS FOR PRACTITIONERS

See Infectious Diseases: Pearls for Practitioners at the end of this section.

REVIEW QUESTIONS

Available online.

CHAPTER 111

Pneumonia

ETIOLOGY

Pneumonia is an infection of the lower respiratory tract that involves the airways and parenchyma, with consolidation of the alveolar spaces. The term **lower respiratory tract infection** is often used to encompass bronchitis, bronchiolitis (see

Chapter 110), pneumonia, or any combination of the three. **Pneumonitis** is a general term for lung inflammation that may or may not be associated with consolidation. **Lobar pneumonia** describes pneumonia localized to one or more lobes of the lung. **Atypical pneumonia** describes patterns typically more diffuse or interstitial than lobar pneumonia. **Bronchopneumonia** refers to inflammation of the lung that is centered in the bronchioles and leads to the production of a mucopurulent exudate that obstructs some of these small airways and causes patchy consolidation of the adjacent lobules. **Interstitial pneumonitis** refers to inflammation of the interstitium, which is composed of the walls of the alveoli, the alveolar sacs and ducts, and the bronchioles. Interstitial pneumonitis is characteristic of acute viral infections but may also be a chronic inflammatory or fibrosing process (**childhood interstitial lung diseases**).

Defects in host defenses increase the risk of pneumonia. Airway contaminants are caught in the mucus secreted by the goblet cells. Cilia on epithelial surfaces, composing the ciliary elevator system, beat synchronously to move particles upward toward central airways and into the throat, where they are swallowed or expectorated. Polymorphonuclear neutrophils from the blood and tissue macrophages ingest and kill microorganisms. IgA secreted into the upper airway fluid protects against invasive infections and facilitates viral neutralization.

Infectious agents that commonly cause community-acquired pneumonia vary by age (Table 111.1). *Streptococcus pneumoniae* is the most common bacterial cause of pneumonia (particularly **lobar pneumonia**) and occurs in children of any age outside the neonatal period. Other common causes include respiratory syncytial virus (RSV) in infants (see Chapter 110), other respiratory viruses (parainfluenza viruses, influenza viruses, human metapneumovirus, adenoviruses, coronaviruses) in children younger than 5 years old, and *Mycoplasma pneumoniae* in children older than age 5 years. *M. pneumoniae* and *Chlamydophila pneumoniae* are principal causes of **atypical pneumonia**.

Chlamydia trachomatis and, less commonly, *Mycoplasma hominis, Ureaplasma urealyticum,* and cytomegalovirus (CMV) cause a respiratory syndrome in infants 2 weeks to 3 months of age, with subacute onset of an **afebrile pneumonia**; cough and hyperinflation are the predominant signs. These infections are difficult to diagnose and distinguish from each other. In adults these organisms are carried primarily as part of the genital mucosal flora. Women who harbor these agents may transmit them perinatally to newborns.

Additional agents occasionally cause pneumonia. **Severe acute respiratory syndrome (SARS)** is due to SARS-associated coronavirus (SARS-CoV) or SARS-CoV-2, the cause of the coronavirus infectious disease (COVID-19) pandemic. SARS-CoV-2 causes less mortality in children than in adults; in addition to respiratory disease, it is also associated with a postinfectious multisystem inflammatory syndrome (MIS) similar to, but distinct from, Kawasaki disease (Chapter 89). SARS-CoV-2 is a highly contagious, airborne (cough, sneeze, talking, breathing) virus that presents within a broad spectrum of symptoms. Many pediatric patients are asymptomatic (but contagious) or have mild to moderate symptoms that do not require hospitalization. A minority of patients develop a severe or critical illness.

Avian influenza (bird flu) is a highly contagious viral disease of poultry and other birds caused by **influenza A (H5N1)**. There were outbreaks among humans in Southeast Asia in 1997 and 2003–2004, with high mortality rates; outbreaks among poultry and dairy cows occurred in the United States in 2024. A novel influenza A (H1N1) of swine origin began circulating in 2009. Other etiologic agents to consider, based on specific exposure history, include *Staphylococcus aureus* and *Streptococcus pyogenes* (especially after influenza infection), *Mycobacterium tuberculosis, Francisella tularensis, Brucella* spp., *Coxiella burnetii, Chlamydophila psittaci, Legionella pneumophila,* hantavirus, *Histoplasma capsulatum, Coccidioides immitis, Blastomyces dermatitidis,* and oral flora or gram-negative bacilli (after aspiration).

Causes of pneumonia in immunocompromised persons include gram-negative enteric bacteria, mycobacteria (*M. avium* complex), fungi (aspergillosis), viruses (CMV), and *Pneumocystis jirovecii.* Pneumonia in patients with cystic fibrosis is usually caused by *S. aureus* in infancy and *Pseudomonas aeruginosa* or *Burkholderia cepacia* in older patients.

EPIDEMIOLOGY

Immunizations have markedly reduced the incidence of pneumonia caused by pertussis, diphtheria, measles, *Haemophilus influenzae* type b, and *S. pneumoniae.* Where used, bacille Calmette-Guérin (BCG) immunization for tuberculosis has also had some impact. Pneumonia is the single largest contributor of childhood mortality worldwide, with an estimated 1 million deaths in children under 5 years of age annually. Risk factors for lower respiratory tract infections include exposure to infected persons, gastroesophageal reflux, neurologic impairment (aspiration), immunocompromised states, anatomic abnormalities of the respiratory tract, residence in residential care facilities, and hospitalization, especially in an intensive care unit.

CLINICAL MANIFESTATIONS

Age is a determinant in the clinical manifestations of pneumonia. Neonates may have fever or hypoxia only, with subtle or absent physical examination findings (see Chapter 64). With a young infant, apnea may be the first sign of pneumonia. Fever, chills, tachypnea, cough, malaise, pleuritic chest pain, retractions, and apprehension—because of difficulty breathing or shortness of breath—are common in older infants and children.

Dominant features of the pulmonary symptoms of **COVID-19** include cough, fever, dyspnea, and myalgias; other common features include abdominal pain and diarrhea, headache, sore throat, as well as loss of taste or smell sensations. *Severe* involvement includes worsening dyspnea, hypoxia, and greater than 50% lung infiltrates on imaging. *Critical* illness includes respiratory failure requiring mechanical ventilation or extracorporeal membrane oxygenation (ECMO) and multiorgan system dysfunction (myocarditis, hypercoagulability, acute kidney injury).

Physical examination findings cannot reliably distinguish viral and bacterial pneumonias, but complete physical examination may help identify other foci of disease or associated findings to suggest an etiology.

Viral pneumonias are generally associated more often with cough, wheezing, or stridor; fever is less prominent than with bacterial pneumonia. Mucosal congestion and upper

TABLE 111.1 Etiologic Agents and Empirical Antimicrobial Therapy for Pneumonia in Patients Without History of Recent Antibiotic Therapy, Prior to Microbiologic Diagnostic Result Availability

AGE GROUP	COMMON PATHOGENS* (IN APPROXIMATE ORDER OF FREQUENCY)	LESS COMMON PATHOGENS	OUTPATIENTS (5 DAYS TOTAL DURATION OF TREATMENT)†	PATIENTS REQUIRING HOSPITALIZATION (5–7 DAYS TOTAL DURATION OF TREATMENT)‡	PATIENTS REQUIRING INTENSIVE CARE (10–14 DAYS TOTAL DURATION OF TREATMENT)*,‡
Neonates (up to 1 mo of age)	Group B streptococcus, *Escherichia coli*, other gram-negative bacilli, *Streptococcus pneumoniae*	Cytomegalovirus, herpes simplex virus, *Listeria monocytogenes*, *Treponema pallidum*, *Haemophilus influenzae* (type b,§ nontypable)	Outpatient management not recommended	Ampicillin *plus* ceftazidime or an aminoglycoside *plus* an antistaphylococcal agent if *Staphylococcus aureus* is suspected	Ampicillin *plus* ceftazidime or an aminoglycoside *plus* an antistaphylococcal agent if *S. aureus* is suspected
1–3 mo					
Febrile pneumonia	Respiratory syncytial virus, other respiratory viruses (parainfluenza viruses, influenza viruses, adenoviruses, coronaviruses), *S. pneumoniae*, *H. influenzae* (type b,§ nontypable)		Initial outpatient management not recommended	Amoxicillin or ampicillin if fully immunized for age for *S. pneumoniae* and *H. influenzae* type b. Alternatives: ceftriaxone if not fully immunized or local *S. pneumoniae* penicillin resistance is significant, with clindamycin if MRSA suspected	Ceftriaxone; consider adding nafcillin, oxacillin, clindamycin, vancomycin, or linezolid if necrotizing pneumonia or *S. aureus* is suspected
Afebrile pneumonia	*Chlamydia trachomatis*, *Mycoplasma hominis*, *Ureaplasma urealyticum*, cytomegalovirus *Bordetella pertussis*		Consider testing for atypical pathogens with close follow-up prior to prescribing macrolides, given their association with pyloric stenosis in this age group	As above; consider testing for atypical pathogens prior to prescribing macrolides, given their association with pyloric stenosis in this age group	As above; consider testing for atypical pathogens prior to prescribing macrolides, given their association with pyloric stenosis in this age group
3 mo–5 yr	Respiratory syncytial virus, other respiratory viruses (parainfluenza viruses, influenza viruses, human metapneumovirus, adenoviruses, coronaviruses), *S. pneumoniae*, *H. influenzae* (type b,§ nontypable)	*C. trachomatis*, *Mycoplasma pneumoniae*, *Chlamydophila pneumoniae*, group A streptococcus, *S. aureus*, *Mycobacterium tuberculosis*	Amoxicillin	Ampicillin or amoxicillin. Alternatives: ceftriaxone if not fully immunized or local *S. pneumoniae* penicillin resistance is significant, with clindamycin if MRSA suspected	Cefuroxime or ceftriaxone *with or without* clindamycin, vancomycin, or linezolid
5–21 yr	*M. pneumoniae*, *S. pneumoniae*, *C. pneumoniae*	*H. influenzae* (type b,§ nontypable), influenza viruses, adenoviruses, coronaviruses, other respiratory viruses	Amoxicillin**	Ampicillin or amoxicillin**	Cefuroxime or ceftriaxone *with or without* clindamycin, vancomycin, or linezolid**

Severe pneumonia, from Streptococcus pneumoniae, Staphylococcus aureus, *group A streptococcus,* Haemophilus influenzae, *or* Mycoplasma pneumoniae *requiring admission to an intensive care unit. Antipseudomonal agents should be added if* Pseudomonas *is suspected. **Depending on the local epidemiology and clinical suspicion for* M. pneumoniae *infection add azithromycin.*

†*Oral administration.*

‡*Intravenous administration for inpatients except for the macrolides (erythromycin, azithromycin, and clarithromycin), which are given orally.*

§Haemophilus influenzae *type b infection is uncommon with universal* H. influenzae *type b immunization. Pandemic viruses vary from influenza to coronaviruses (location and year dependent).*

MRSA, Methicillin-resistant *Staphylococcus aureus.*

airway inflammation suggest a viral infection. Bacterial pneumonias are typically associated with higher fever, chills, cough, dyspnea, and auscultatory findings of lung consolidation. Atypical pneumonia in young infants is characterized by tachypnea, cough, and crackles on auscultation. Concomitant conjunctivitis may be present in infants with chlamydial or adenoviral pneumonia. Other signs of respiratory distress include nasal flaring, intercostal and subcostal retractions, and grunting.

Asymmetry or shallow breathing may be due to splinting from pain. Hyperexpansion, common in asthma but also frequently accompanying viral lower respiratory infections, may cause a low diaphragm seen on a chest x-ray. Poor diaphragmatic excursion may indicate hyperexpanded lungs or an inability for expansion due to a large consolidation or effusion. Dullness to percussion may be due to lobar or segmental infiltrates or pleural fluid. Auscultation may be normal in early or very focal pneumonia, but the presence of localized crackles, rhonchi, and wheezes may help one detect and locate pneumonia. Distant breath sounds may indicate a large, poorly ventilated area of consolidation or pleural fluid.

LABORATORY AND IMAGING STUDIES

Bacterial flora of the upper respiratory tract does not accurately reflect flora present in lower respiratory tract infections, and high-quality sputum is rarely obtainable from children. In otherwise healthy children without life-threatening disease, invasive procedures to obtain lower respiratory tissue or secretions are seldom indicated. Serologic tests are not useful for the most common causes of bacterial pneumonia.

The white blood cell (WBC) count with viral pneumonias is often normal or mildly elevated, with a predominance of lymphocytes, whereas with bacterial pneumonias the WBC count can be elevated (>15,000–20,000/mm^3) and with a predominance of neutrophils. Mild eosinophilia is characteristic of infant *C. trachomatis* pneumonia. Blood cultures should be performed on moderately to severely ill hospitalized children to attempt to diagnose a bacterial cause of pneumonia. Blood cultures identify a bacterial respiratory pathogen in approximately 2–5% of children hospitalized for pneumonia (and up to 10–20% of those with pneumonia with empyema or large effusion). Urinary antigen tests are especially useful for *L. pneumophila* (Legionnaires disease).

Viral respiratory pathogens can be diagnosed using polymerase chain reaction (PCR) or rapid viral antigen detection. *M. pneumoniae* can be confirmed by *Mycoplasma* PCR. CMV pneumonitis can be diagnosed with PCR from bronchoalveolar lavage fluid. The diagnosis of *M. tuberculosis* is established by the tuberculin skin test or serum interferon-γ release assay, in conjunction with analysis of sputum or gastric aspirates by culture, antigen detection, or PCR.

The need to establish an etiologic diagnosis of pneumonia is greater in immunocompromised patients, patients with recurrent pneumonia, or those with pneumonia unresponsive to empirical therapy. For these patients, bronchoscopy with bronchoalveolar lavage and brush mucosal biopsy, needle aspiration of the lung, and open lung biopsy are methods of obtaining material for microbiologic diagnosis.

When there is a pleural **effusion or empyema**, a thoracentesis to obtain pleural fluid can be diagnostic and therapeutic. Evaluation differentiates between empyema and a sterile parapneumonic effusion caused by irritation of the pleura contiguous with the pneumonia. Gram stain, bacterial culture, or broad-range bacterial PCR may lead to microbiologic diagnosis. The pleural fluid can also be cultured for mycobacteria and fungi. Removal of grossly purulent pleural fluid reduces the patient's toxicity and associated discomfort and may facilitate more rapid recovery. Drainage of large pleural accumulations also improves pulmonary mechanics and gas exchange by increasing the ability of the lung to expand.

Frontal and lateral radiographs are required to localize disease and adequately visualize retrocardiac infiltrates; they are recommended for diagnosis among hospitalized children but are not necessary to confirm the diagnosis in well-appearing outpatients. Although there are characteristic radiographic findings of pneumonia, radiography alone cannot provide a definitive microbiologic diagnosis. Bacterial pneumonia characteristically shows lobar consolidation or a round pneumonia, with pleural effusion in 10–30% of cases (Fig. 111.1). Viral pneumonia characteristically shows diffuse, streaky infiltrates of bronchopneumonia (Fig. 111.2) and hyperinflation. Atypical pneumonia, as with *M. pneumoniae* and *C. pneumoniae,* shows increased interstitial markings or bronchopneumonia. Chest radiographs may be normal in early pneumonia, with infiltrates appearing during treatment as hydration is restored. Hilar lymphadenopathy is uncommon with bacterial pneumonia but may be a sign of tuberculosis, endemic mycoses, autoimmune conditions, or an underlying malignant neoplasm. Decubitus views or ultrasound should be used to assess the size of pleural effusions and whether they are freely mobile. CT is used to evaluate serious disease, lung abscesses, bronchiectasis, and effusion characteristics. Unusual etiologies or recurrent pneumonias require special considerations (Table 111.2). Lung abscesses and pneumatoceles usually do not require surgical management. Empyema requires chest tube drainage.

DIFFERENTIAL DIAGNOSIS

Pneumonia must be differentiated from other acute pulmonary diseases, including allergic hypersensitivity pneumonitis, e-cigarette, or vaping product use–associated lung injury (EVALI), asthma, and cystic fibrosis; cardiac diseases, such as pulmonary edema caused by heart failure; and autoimmune diseases, such as certain vasculitides and systemic lupus erythematosus. Radiographically, pneumonia must be differentiated from lung trauma and contusion, hemorrhage, foreign body aspiration, and sympathetic effusion due to subdiaphragmatic inflammation.

TREATMENT

Therapy for pneumonia includes supportive and specific treatment and depends on the degree of illness, complications, and knowledge of the infectious agent likely causing the pneumonia. Most cases of pneumonia in healthy children can be managed on an outpatient basis. However, children with hypoxemia, inability to maintain adequate hydration, or moderate to severe respiratory distress should be hospitalized.

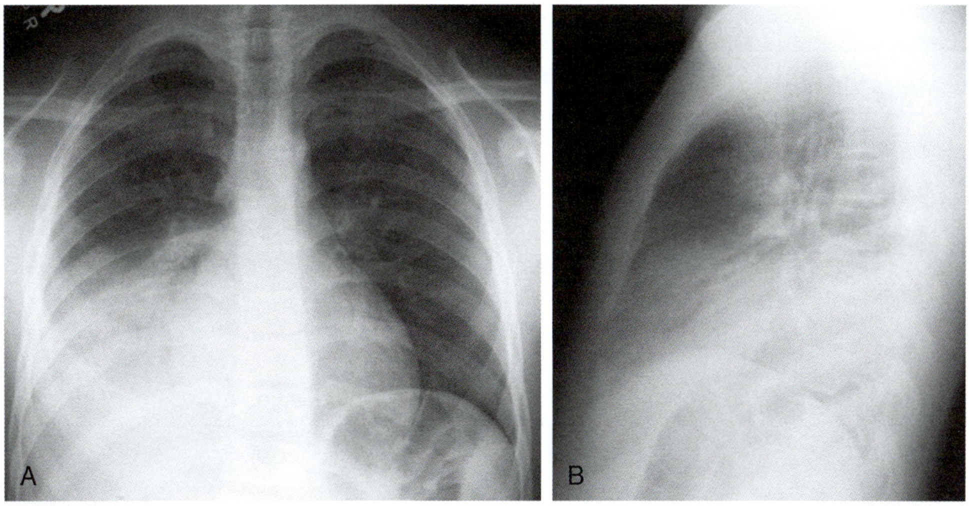

FIGURE 111.1 Acute lobar pneumonia of the right lower lobe in a 14-year-old child with fever and cough. **(A)** Posteroanterior and **(B)** lateral chest radiographs demonstrate right-lower-lobe airspace consolidation, which obliterates the silhouette of the right diaphragm. (From Kelly MS, Sandora TJ. Community-acquired pneumonia. In: Kliegman RM, St. Geme III JW, eds. *Nelson Textbook of Pediatrics*. 22nd ed. Philadelphia: Elsevier; 2025:fig. 449.3.)

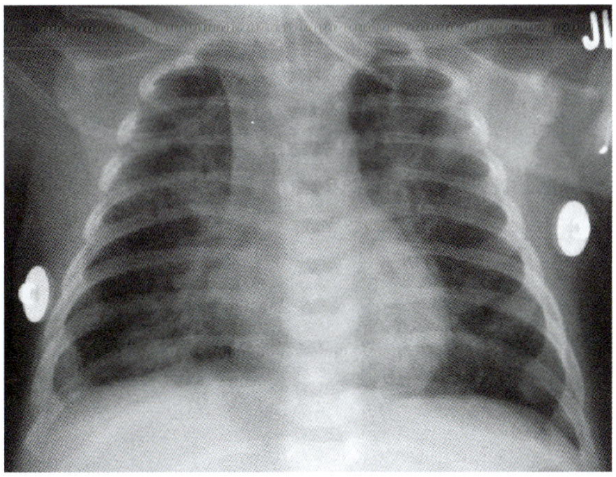

FIGURE 111.2 Diffuse respiratory syncytial virus pneumonia in a 6-month-old infant with tachypnea and fever. Anteroposterior chest radiograph shows bilateral, perihilar, peribronchial thickening and fine airspace disease with hyperinflation. (From Kelly MS, Sandora TJ. Community-acquired pneumonia. In: Kliegman RM, St. Geme III JW, eds. *Nelson Textbook of Pediatrics*. 22nd ed. Philadelphia: Elsevier; 2025:fig. 449.2A.)

Hospitalization should be considered in infants under 6 months with suspected bacterial pneumonia or those in whom there is a concern for substantial respiratory symptom progression.

Because viruses cause many community-acquired pneumonias in young children, not all children require empiric antibiotic treatment for pneumonia. Recommended empiric therapies in those without recent antibiotic exposure are listed in Table 111.1. A 5-day therapy course is appropriate in stable outpatients. Exceptional situations include lack of response to empirical therapy, unusually severe presentations, nosocomial pneumonia, and immunocompromised children susceptible to infections with opportunistic pathogens (Table 111.3). Presumed pneumococcal pneumonia can be treated with high-dose ampicillin or amoxicillin therapy. Ceftriaxone and/or vancomycin can be used if the isolate shows high-level resistance and/or the patient is severely ill. For infants 2–18 weeks old with afebrile pneumonia most likely caused by *C. trachomatis*, a macrolide is the recommended treatment. School-age and adolescent children with high suspicion for atypical pneumonia should be tested for *Mycoplasma* and *Chlamydophila*; macrolide therapy

TABLE 111.2 Differential Diagnosis of Recurrent Pneumonia

HEREDITARY DISORDERS
Cystic fibrosis Sickle cell disease
DISORDERS OF IMMUNITY
AIDS Bruton agammaglobulinemia Complement deficiency Selective IgG subclass deficiencies Common variable immunodeficiency syndrome Severe combined immunodeficiency syndrome
DISORDERS OF LEUKOCYTES
Chronic granulomatous disease Hyperimmunoglobulin E syndrome (Job syndrome) Leukocyte adhesion defect
DISORDERS OF CILIA
Primary ciliary dyskinesia Kartagener syndrome
ANATOMIC DISORDERS
Sequestration Lobar emphysema Foreign body Tracheoesophageal fistula (H type) Congenital pulmonary airway malformation (cystic adenomatoid malformation) Gastroesophageal reflux Bronchiectasis Aspiration (oropharyngeal incoordination)
NONINFECTIOUS MIMICS OF PNEUMONIA
Autoimmune diseases (e.g., granulomatosis with polyangiitis) Hypersensitivity pneumonitis Interstitial lung diseases

TABLE 111.3 Antimicrobial Therapy for Pneumonia Caused by Specific Pathogens*

PATHOGEN	RECOMMENDED TREATMENT	ALTERNATIVE TREATMENT
Streptococcus pneumoniae with MIC for penicillin ≤2.0 mcg/mL	Ampicillin or penicillin IV; amoxicillin PO	Ceftriaxone, clindamycin, or vancomycin IV; cefuroxime, cefprozil, cefpodoxime, levofloxacin,† or linezolid PO
S. pneumoniae with MIC for penicillin ≥4.0 mcg/mL	Ceftriaxone IV; levofloxacin† or linezolid PO	Ampicillin, levofloxacin,† linezolid, or vancomycin IV; clindamycin IV or PO
Group A streptococcus	Penicillin or ampicillin IV; amoxicillin or penicillin PO	Ceftriaxone IV, or clindamycin PO or IV
Group B streptococcus	Penicillin or ampicillin IV; amoxicillin or penicillin PO	Ceftriaxone IV, or clindamycin PO or IV
Haemophilus influenzae	Ampicillin IV or amoxicillin PO if β-lactamase negative; ceftriaxone IV or amoxicillin-clavulanate PO if β-lactamase positive	Ciprofloxacin† or levofloxacin† IV; cefixime or cefpodoxime PO
Mycoplasma pneumoniae, Chlamydophila pneumoniae, or *Chlamydia trachomatis*	Azithromycin PO	Clarithromycin, erythromycin, doxycycline,† or a fluoroquinolone† PO
MSSA	Cefazolin, oxacillin, or nafcillin IV; cephalexin PO	Clindamycin IV or PO, vancomycin IV, or linezolid IV or PO
MRSA	Clindamycin IV or PO; linezolid IV or PO; vancomycin IV	TMP-SMX IV or PO
Gram-negative aerobic bacilli (except *P. aeruginosa*)	Ceftriaxone with or without an aminoglycoside IV; amoxicillin-clavulanate or cefixime PO	Piperacillin-tazobactam plus an aminoglycoside‡; fluoroquinolone† PO
P. aeruginosa	Ceftazidime or cefepime IV with or without an aminoglycoside‡; ciprofloxacin† if susceptible PO	Piperacillin-tazobactam or a carbapenem IV
Herpes simplex virus	Acyclovir IV	

*Oral outpatient therapy may be used for mild illness or mild inpatient illness. Intravenous inpatient therapy should be used for moderate to severe illness.

†Appropriate respiratory fluoroquinolones include moxifloxacin, gatifloxacin, levofloxacin, and gemifloxacin. Fluoroquinolones are not recommended for pregnant or lactating women.

‡Aminoglycoside dosing should be guided by serum antibiotic concentrations after a steady state has been reached.

IV, Intravenous; *MIC*, minimum inhibitory concentration; *MRSA*, methicillin-resistant *Staphylococcus aureus*; *MSSA*, methicillin-susceptible *Staphylococcus aureus*; *PO*, per os (orally); *TMP-SMX*, trimethoprim-sulfamethoxazole.

can be offered if positive. Oseltamivir or zanamivir should be used if influenza is identified or suspected, ideally within 48 hours of symptom onset.

Severe or *critical* COVID-19 is typically treated with oxygen, dexamethasone, remdesivir, and respiratory support.

COMPLICATIONS AND PROGNOSIS

Bacterial pneumonias frequently cause inflammatory fluid to collect in the adjacent pleural space, causing a **parapneumonic effusion** or, if grossly purulent, an **empyema**. Small effusions typically do not require any targeted therapy. Large effusions may restrict breathing and require drainage. Air dissection within lung tissue results in a **pneumatocele**. Scarring of the airways and lung tissue may leave dilated bronchi, resulting in **bronchiectasis** and increased risk for recurrent infection.

Pneumonia that causes necrosis of lung tissue may evolve into a **lung abscess**. Lung abscess is an uncommon problem in children and is usually caused by aspiration, infection behind an obstructed bronchus, or certain virulent organisms. Anaerobic bacteria usually predominate, along with various streptococci, *Escherichia coli, Klebsiella pneumoniae, P. aeruginosa*, and *S. aureus*. Chest radiograph or CT scan reveals a cavitary lesion, often with an air-fluid level, surrounded by parenchymal inflammation. If the cavity communicates with the bronchi, organisms may be isolated from sputum. Diagnostic bronchoscopy may be indicated to exclude a foreign body and obtain microbiologic specimens. Lung abscesses usually respond to appropriate antimicrobial therapy with clindamycin or ampicillin-sulbactam.

Most children recover from pneumonia rapidly and completely, although radiographic abnormalities may persist for 6–8 weeks. In a few children, symptoms may last longer than 1 month or may be recurrent. In such cases, the possibility of underlying disease must be investigated further, such as with the tuberculin skin test, sweat chloride determination for cystic fibrosis, serum immunoglobulin (Ig) and IgG subclass determinations, CT or bronchoscopy to identify anatomic abnormalities or foreign body, and barium swallow for gastroesophageal reflux.

Severe adenovirus pneumonia may result in **bronchiolitis obliterans**, a subacute inflammatory process in which the small airways are replaced by scar tissue, resulting in a reduction in lung volume and lung compliance. **Unilateral hyperlucent lung**, or **Swyer-James syndrome**, is a focal sequela of severe necrotizing pneumonia in which all or part of a lung has increased translucency radiographically; it has been linked to adenovirus type 21.

PREVENTION

Annual influenza and SARS-CoV-2 **vaccines** are recommended for all children over 6 months of age (see Chapter 95).

Trivalent or quadrivalent, inactivated influenza vaccines are licensed for use beginning at 6 months of age; live-attenuated vaccine can be used for persons 2–49 years of age. Universal childhood vaccination with conjugate vaccines for *H. influenzae* type b and *S. pneumoniae* has greatly diminished the incidence of these pneumonias. RSV infections can be prevented by use of palivizumab or nirsevimab in some populations (see Chapter 110).

Reducing the duration of mechanical ventilation and administering antibiotics judiciously reduces the incidence of **ventilator-associated pneumonias**. The head of the bed should be raised to 30–45 degrees for intubated patients to minimize risk of aspiration, and all suctioning equipment and saline should be sterile. Handwashing before and after every patient contact and use of gloves for invasive procedures are important measures to prevent nosocomial transmission of infections. Hospital staff with respiratory illnesses or who are carriers of certain organisms, such as methicillin-resistant *S. aureus* (MRSA), should comply with infection control policies to prevent transfer of organisms to patients. Treating sources of aerosols, such as air coolers, can prevent *L. pneumonia*.

PEARLS FOR PRACTITIONERS

See Infectious Diseases: Pearls for Practitioners at the end of this section.

REVIEW QUESTIONS

Available online.

CHAPTER 112 Infective Endocarditis

ETIOLOGY

Infective endocarditis (IE) is an infection on the endothelial surface of the heart, including the heart valves. The management of infections on the endothelial surfaces of blood vessels **(endovascular infections)** is very similar. Turbulent flow from congenital heart disease or an indwelling central venous catheter can result in endothelial damage. Fibrin and platelets gather at the site, forming a thrombus. In the setting of transient bacteremia, this lesion can become infected and can result in a **vegetation**, which usually occurs on a valve leaflet and is composed of microorganisms trapped in a fibrin mesh that extends into the bloodstream.

Many microorganisms have been reported to cause endocarditis, although there are only a few common causes in children (Table 112.1). Viridans group streptococci (*S. mutans, S. sanguinis,* others) are the principal cause in children with congenital heart diseases without previous surgery. *Staphylococcus aureus* and coagulase-negative staphylococci (CONS) are important causes of endocarditis, especially following cardiac surgery and in the presence of prosthetic cardiac and endovascular materials. Less common causes of indolent or culture negative endocarditis include the HACEK organisms (*Haemophilus* spp., *Aggregatibacter* spp., *Cardiobacterium hominis, Eikenella corrodens,* and *Kingella kingae*), *Bartonella, Brucella, Coxiella,* and *Mycoplasma*. Gram-negative endocarditis is rare. *Candida* species can cause fungal endocarditis, especially in premature infants with central venous catheters and/or receiving parenteral nutrition.

EPIDEMIOLOGY

Rheumatic heart disease used to be a major risk factor for IE but has become much less common. Patients at highest risk for IE include those with prosthetic cardiac valves and children who have cyanotic congenital heart disease, either with or without repair. The risk in these patients is increased after dental and oral procedures or procedures of the respiratory, genitourinary, or gastrointestinal tracts. Use of central vascular catheters is a significant risk factor for native valve endocarditis. Approximately 10–15% of IE in children occurs without structural heart disease (normal native valve) or other obvious risk factors. *S. aureus* is the most likely infective organism in these cases.

CLINICAL MANIFESTATIONS

The most common early symptoms of IE are nonspecific and include fever, malaise, and weight loss. Tachycardia and a new or changed heart murmur are common findings. The subtle and nonspecific findings underscore the need to obtain blood cultures if endocarditis is suspected, especially for children with congenital heart disease and for unexplained illness after dental or surgical procedures. Endocarditis is often a subacute, slowly progressive process, but it can also present acutely with high fevers and a sepsis-like picture. Heart failure, splenomegaly, petechiae, glomerulonephritis, and embolic (Osler nodes, Janeway lesions, and splinter hemorrhages) or immunologic phenomena (Roth spots) may be present. In neonates, the signs and symptoms of IE may be especially subtle and variable, including feeding issues, respiratory distress, and hypotension, in addition to changes in the cardiac exam.

LABORATORY STUDIES AND IMAGING

The key to diagnosis is confirming continuous bacteremia or fungemia by culturing the blood. Multiple blood cultures should be obtained before initiating antibiotic therapy. For optimal sensitivity, adequate volumes of blood should be obtained: 1–3 mL for infants and young children and at least 5–7 mL for older children. If volumes are not adequate, emphasis should be placed on obtaining aerobic blood cultures, because anaerobic organisms rarely cause IE. If possible, in patients who are not critically ill, empirical antibiotic therapy should be held until at least three sets of blood cultures (from different venipuncture sites) are obtained. Patients who have recently been treated with antibiotics or who are currently receiving antibiotics should have additional serial cultures performed. Despite adequate blood culture techniques, the microbiologic diagnosis is not confirmed in 5–15% of cases; this is known as **culture-negative endocarditis**.

The agent in culture-negative endocarditis may be identified by antibody testing and examination of the valve tissue (following surgery) by polymerase chain reaction (PCR) for bacterial (16 S) or fungal (18 S) ribosomal RNA. Metagenomic next-generation sequencing of cell free bacterial DNA in blood samples may improve the diagnosis of culture-negative endocarditis.

Erythrocyte sedimentation rate and C-reactive protein are often elevated. Leukocytosis, anemia, and hematuria are common laboratory findings.

TABLE 112.1 Pathogens Causing Infective Endocarditis in Children

BACTERIA
Viridans Streptococcus groups: *S. sanguis, S. mitis, S. mutans, S. anginosus, S. salivarius, S. bovis* *Staphylococcus aureus* *Enterococcus* Coagulase-negative staphylococci Streptococci: groups A, B (in neonates and elderly), *Streptococcus pneumoniae* Gram-negative enteric bacilli HACEK organisms (i.e., *Haemophilus* spp., *Aggregatibacter* spp., *Cardiobacterium hominis, Eikenella corrodens*, and *Kingella kingae*) *Chlamydophila* *Coxiella burnetii* (Q fever)
FUNGI
Candida species
CULTURE NEGATIVE
Fastidious organisms (*Abiotrophia* or *Granulicatella* sp.) *Bartonella* sp. *Tropheryma whipplei* *Coxiella burnetii* (Q fever)

Echocardiography should be performed in all cases where IE is suspected. It can be used to visualize vegetations and assess valvular regurgitation and conduit flow. Transesophageal echocardiography (TEE) is more sensitive than transthoracic echocardiography (TTE) for adolescents and adults and for patients with prosthetic valves, but it is often unnecessary in children. Positron emission tomography (PET) with 18F-fluorodeoxyglucose combined with CT scanning has been used in adults to diagnose endocarditis; data for this approach in children are limited.

DIFFERENTIAL DIAGNOSIS

IE must be differentiated from other causes of bacteremia and other cardiac conditions. The **Duke criteria** (revised in 2023) can be used to assist in the diagnosis of IE (Table 112.2). Noninfectious causes of endocardial vegetations must be excluded, such as sterile clots or lupus. Prolonged bacteremia can be caused by infectious endothelial foci outside the heart, often associated with congenital vascular malformations, vascular trauma, an infected venous thrombosis, or previous vascular surgery.

TREATMENT

Severely ill patients must be stabilized with supportive therapies for cardiac failure, pulmonary edema, and low cardiac output (see Chapter 146). Empirical antibiotic therapy may be started for acutely ill patients after blood cultures are obtained. With subacute disease, awaiting results of blood cultures to confirm the diagnosis is recommended to direct therapy according to the susceptibility of the isolate. Because

TABLE 112.2 2023 Duke Criteria for Infective Endocarditis

DEFINITE ENDOCARDITIS	POSSIBLE ENDOCARDITIS	REJECTED ENDOCARDITIS
Pathologic criteria OR 2 major criteria, or 1 major and 3 minor criteria, or 5 minor criteria	1 major and 1 minor criterion, or 3 minor criteria	Firm alternate diagnosis, or Lack of recurrence despite antibiotics for <4 days, or No pathologic evidence of endocarditis with antibiotic therapy for <4 days, or Does not meet criteria for possible endocarditis
MAJOR CRITERIA		
A. Microbiologic criteria • Positive blood cultures (2 sets of typical microorganisms or 3 sets of atypical organisms), or • Certain positive laboratory tests by PCR or antibody testing for *Bartonella, Coxiella,* or *Tropheryma* B. Imaging major criteria • Echocardiogram or cardiac CT supportive of infective endocarditis, or • 18F PET/CT supportive of infective endocarditis C. Surgical major criteria • Evidence of endocarditis by direct inspection during surgery without meeting subsequent pathologic or microbiologic criteria		
MINOR CRITERIA		
A. Predisposing condition B. Fever ≥38.0°C (100.4°F) C. Vascular phenomena D. Immunologic phenomena E. Microbiologic evidence not meeting major criterion F. Imaging criteria G. Physical examination criteria		

From Fowler VG, Durack DT, Selton-Suty C, et al. The 2023 Duke-International Society for Cardiovascular Infectious Diseases Criteria for Infective Endocarditis: Updating the Modified Duke Criteria. Clin Infect Dis. *2023;77(4):518–526.*

antibiotics must reach the organisms by passive diffusion through the fibrin mesh, high doses of bactericidal antibiotics are required for an extended period of treatment (4–6 weeks). Exact duration of therapy varies depending on the presence of prosthetic material and the causative organism. Historically all antibiotic therapy was delivered intravenously, but randomized trials and observational studies in adults support the use of oral step-down therapy in certain cases. *Staphylococcus aureus* bacteremia can be persistent, and if associated with an indwelling catheter it requires line removal in most cases. Surgery is indicated if medical treatment is unsuccessful, if bacteremia is persistent, or if the pathogen is unusual or difficult to treat (e.g., fungal endocarditis). Surgical intervention may also be required with the presence of a valve annulus or myocardial abscess, rupture of a valve leaflet, valvular insufficiency with acute or refractory heart failure, recurrent serious embolic complications, or refractory prosthetic valve disease (Table 112.3).

COMPLICATIONS AND PROGNOSIS

The major complications of IE are direct damage to cardiac tissue and function, and distant complications secondary to **septic emboli** from vegetations. Damage to cardiac valves may cause regurgitation, defects in valve leaflets, abscess of the valve ring, or myocardial abscess. Cardiac function can decline, resulting in heart failure. These complications should be monitored by physical examination and echocardiography. Septic emboli can result in pneumonia, osteomyelitis, and abscesses in the brain, kidneys, and spleen.

The prognosis of IE varies depending on causative organism and underlying cardiac condition. Cardiovascular infections with gram-negative bacilli and fungi have the poorest prognosis.

TABLE 112.3 2015 American Heart Association Recommendation for Surgical Management of Left-Sided Native Valve Endocarditis

- Early surgery (during initial hospitalization and before completion of a full course of antibiotics) is indicated in patients with IE who present with valve dysfunction resulting in symptoms or signs of heart failure.
- Early surgery should be considered particularly in patients with IE caused by fungal or highly resistant organisms (e.g., vancomycin-resistant *Enterococcus*, multidrug-resistant gram-negative bacilli).
- Early surgery is indicated in patients with IE complicated by heart block, annular or aortic abscess, or destructive penetrating lesions.
- Early surgery is indicated for evidence of persistent infection (manifested by persistent bacteremia or fever lasting >5–7 days and provided that other sites of infection and fever have been excluded) after the start of appropriate antimicrobial therapy.
- Early surgery is reasonable in patients who present with recurrent emboli and persistent or enlarging vegetations despite appropriate antibiotic therapy.
- Early surgery is reasonable in patients with severe valve regurgitation and mobile vegetations >10 mm.
- Early surgery may be considered in patients with mobile vegetations >10 mm, particularly when involving the anterior leaflet of the mitral valve and associated with other relative indications for surgery.

IE, Infective endocarditis.
From El-Dalati S, Cronin D, Shea M, et al. Clinical practice update on infectious endocarditis. Am J Med. *2020;133:44–49, table 2.*

PREVENTION

Good oral hygiene should be emphasized in all patients at risk for IE. In certain high-risk patients (unrepaired cyanotic heart disease, previous IE, prosthetic cardiac valve, repaired congenital heart disease with residual defects, cardiac transplantation), prophylactic antibiotics may be considered before certain dental and other invasive procedures of the respiratory tract and/or infected skin or muscle.

PEARLS FOR PRACTITIONERS

See Infectious Diseases: Pearls for Practitioners at the end of this section.

REVIEW QUESTIONS

Available online.

CHAPTER 113 Acute Gastroenteritis

ETIOLOGY AND EPIDEMIOLOGY

Acute gastroenteritis refers to a clinical syndrome of diarrhea (defined as more than three loose or liquid stools in 24 hours) with or without vomiting that usually lasts for several days. In general, diarrhea is caused by a variety of infectious or inflammatory processes in the intestine that directly affect enterocyte secretory and absorptive functions. Gastroenteritis or enteritis has many infectious causes, including viruses, bacteria, and parasites (Table 113.1). Based on pathogenesis, diarrhea can be classified as invasive or inflammatory producing bloody stools with abdominal cramping and fever, or it can be classified as secretory manifesting with large quantities of watery stool without other significant symptoms (Table 113.2).

Infectious diarrhea is a leading cause of morbidity and mortality in children around the world. Rates of disease and death vary with age and access to health care, clean water, and sanitation. Gastrointestinal infections are generally acquired via fecal-oral transmission or through ingestion of contaminated food or water. The patient's immune status and environmental exposures (i.e., food, water, travel, antibiotics, childcare) help guide the differential diagnosis in the presence of acute gastrointestinal symptoms. The severity and duration of these symptoms can vary based on host risk factors including immune and nutritional status, pathogen inoculum, and presence of prior immunity to the specific infection.

Viral gastroenteritis is the most common cause of diarrhea in children. These illnesses may be associated with vomiting as well as diarrhea, have incubation periods of hours to days, and are usually self-limited illnesses lasting 3–7 days. **Rotavirus** has historically been the most frequent cause of diarrhea in young children. Primary infection with rotavirus may

TABLE 113.1 Common Pathogenic Organisms Causing Diarrhea and Their Virulence Mechanisms

ORGANISMS	PATHOGENIC MECHANISM(S)
VIRUSES	
Rotaviruses	Damage to microvilli
Caliciviruses (noroviruses)	Mucosal lesion
Astroviruses	Mucosal lesion
Enteric adenoviruses (serotypes 40 and 41)	Mucosal lesion
BACTERIA	
Campylobacter jejuni	Invasion, enterotoxin
Clostridioides difficile	Cytotoxin, enterotoxin
Escherichia coli	
Enteropathogenic (EPEC)	Adherence, effacement
Enterotoxigenic (ETEC) (traveler's diarrhea)	Enterotoxins (heat stable or heat labile)
Enteroinvasive (EIEC)	Invasion of mucosa
Enterohemorrhagic (EHEC) (includes O157:H7 causing HUS)	Adherence, effacement, cytotoxin
Enteroaggregative (EAEC)	Adherence, mucosal damage
Salmonella	Invasion, enterotoxin
Shigella	Invasion, enterotoxin, cytotoxin
Vibrio cholerae	Enterotoxin
Vibrio parahaemolyticus	Invasion, cytotoxin
Yersinia enterocolitica	Invasion, enterotoxin
PARASITES	
Entamoeba histolytica	Invasion, enzyme and cytotoxin production; cyst resistant to physical destruction
Giardia lamblia	Adheres to mucosa; cyst resistant to physical destruction
Spore-forming intestinal protozoa *Cryptosporidium parvum* *Isospora belli* *Cyclospora cayetanensis*	Adherence, inflammation
Microsporidia (*Enterocytozoon bieneusi, Encephalitozoon intestinalis*)	

HUS, Hemolytic uremic syndrome.

cause moderate to severe disease in infancy but is less severe later in life. The rotavirus vaccine has resulted in significant reductions in the incidence of acute gastroenteritis and hospitalizations due to rotavirus. **Norovirus** occurs in people of all ages, year-round, and is the most common cause of outbreaks of acute gastroenteritis because it is highly contagious. Other viral causes of acute gastroenteritis include astroviruses, sapovirus, and enteric adenoviruses (serotypes 40 and 41).

Food-borne and water-borne diseases are important causes of acute gastroenteritis both for individual and public health reasons. In the United States, common bacterial food-borne causes of gastroenteritis include nontyphoidal *Salmonella, Campylobacter, Shigella, Escherichia coli* O157:H7, *Yersinia,* and *Listeria monocytogenes.* Food-borne diarrhea can also result from ingestion of preformed enterotoxins produced by bacteria, such as *Staphylococcus aureus* and *Bacillus cereus,* which multiply in contaminated foods, and nonbacterial toxins such as from fish, shellfish, and mushrooms. After a short incubation period, vomiting and cramps are prominent symptoms, and diarrhea may or may not be present. Heavy metals that leach into canned food or drinks cause gastric irritation and emetic syndromes that may mimic symptoms of acute infectious enteritis. **Traveler's diarrhea** occurs frequently, especially within the first 1–2 weeks of arrival to endemic areas. Epidemiology varies with destination, but in general children are at risk for the same illnesses that affect adult travelers.

Nontyphoidal *Salmonella* produces diarrhea by invading the intestinal mucosa. The organisms are transmitted through contact with infected animals (chickens, iguanas, other reptiles, turtles) or from contaminated food products, such as dairy products, eggs, and poultry. A large inoculum of organisms is required for disease because *Salmonella* is killed by gastric acidity. The incubation period for *Salmonella* gastroenteritis ranges from 6 to 72 hours but is usually less than 24 hours. *Shigella dysenteriae* may cause disease by producing **Shiga toxin**. The incubation period is 1–7 days. Infected adults may shed organisms for up to 1 month. Infection is spread by person-to-person contact or by the ingestion of contaminated food with 10–100 organisms. The colon is selectively affected. High fever and febrile seizures may occur in addition to diarrhea.

Only certain strains of *E. coli* produce diarrhea. Strains associated with enteritis are classified by the mechanism of diarrhea. **Enterotoxigenic (ETEC)** strains produce heat-labile (cholera-like) and/or heat-stable enterotoxin that adhere to the epithelial cells in the small intestine and produce disease by liberating toxins that induce intestinal secretion and limit absorption. ETEC is a frequent cause of **traveler's diarrhea**. **Enterohemorrhagic (EHEC)** or **Shiga toxin–producing (STEC)** strains, especially the *E. coli* O157:H7 strain, produce a **Shiga-like toxin** that is responsible for a hemorrhagic colitis and most cases of **hemolytic uremic syndrome (HUS)**, which presents with microangiopathic hemolytic anemia, thrombocytopenia, and kidney failure (see Chapter 165). STEC is associated with contaminated food, including unpasteurized fruit juices and especially undercooked beef, and can present with nonbloody diarrhea that then becomes bloody. **Enteroinvasive *E. coli* (EIEC)** invades the colonic mucosa, producing widespread mucosal damage with acute inflammation similar to *Shigella.* EIEC diarrhea is usually watery and is often associated with fever. **Enteropathogenic (EPEC)** strains cause mild watery diarrhea but can cause severe dehydration in young children in resource-limited settings in sporadic or epidemic patterns.

Campylobacter jejuni is spread by person-to-person contact and by contaminated water and food, especially poultry, raw milk, and cheese. The organism invades the mucosa of the jejunum, ileum, and colon. ***Yersinia enterocolitica*** is transmitted by pets and contaminated food, classically chitterlings. Infants and young children characteristically have diarrheal disease, whereas older children usually have acute lesions of

TABLE 113.2 Mechanisms of Infectious Diarrhea

PRIMARY MECHANISM	DEFECT	STOOL EXAMINATION	EXAMPLES	COMMENTS
Secretory	Decreased absorption, increased secretion: electrolyte transport	Watery, normal osmolality	Cholera, toxigenic *Escherichia coli* (EPEC, ETEC); carcinoid, *Clostridioides difficile*, cryptosporidiosis (in AIDS)	Persists during fasting; bile salt malabsorption also may increase intestinal water secretion; no stool leukocytes
Mucosal invasion	Inflammation, decreased mucosal surface area and/or colonic reabsorption, increased motility	Blood and increased WBCs in stool	*Salmonella* infection, shigellosis, amebiasis, yersiniosis, *Campylobacter* infection	Dysentery (blood, mucus, and WBCs)

EPEC, Enteropathogenic; *ETEC*, enterotoxigenic; *WBC*, white blood cell; infection may also contribute to increased motility.
Adapted from Maqbool A, Liacouras CA. Major symptoms and signs of digestive tract disorders. In: Kliegman RM, St. Geme III JW, eds. Nelson Textbook of Pediatrics. *22nd ed. Philadelphia: Elsevier; 2025:table 332.10.*

the terminal ileum or acute mesenteric lymphadenitis mimicking appendicitis or Crohn disease. Postinfectious arthritis, rash, and spondylopathy may develop.

Clostridioides difficile causes diarrhea and/or colitis and is usually associated with prior antibiotic exposure. The organism produces spores that spread from person to person and as fomites on surfaces. Infection is generally health care acquired, but community acquisition of infection is increasingly reported. Diagnosis is made by detection of toxin in the stool. Infants younger than 12 months should not be tested for *C. difficile* because they are frequently asymptomatically colonized with the organism in their stool, possibly due to a lack of the receptor required for infection. Of note, patients on antibiotics often experience diarrhea related to alterations in their intestinal flora that are unrelated to *C. difficile* infection.

Important enteric parasites found in North America include *Giardia lamblia, Cryptosporidium parvum,* and *Entamoeba histolytica* (amebiasis). ***G. lamblia*** is transmitted through ingestion of cysts, either from contact with an infected individual or from food or water contaminated with infected feces. The organism adheres to the microvilli of the duodenal and jejunal epithelium. Insidious onset of progressive anorexia, nausea, gaseousness, abdominal distention, watery diarrhea, secondary lactose intolerance, and weight loss is characteristic of giardiasis. ***Cryptosporidium*** causes mild, watery diarrhea in immunocompetent persons that resolves without treatment. It can produce severe, prolonged diarrhea in persons with AIDS (see Chapter 126). ***E. histolytica*** infects the colon; amebae may pass through the bowel wall and invade the liver, lung, and brain. Diarrhea is of acute onset, is bloody, and contains leukocytes. Amebiasis occurs in warmer climates, whereas giardiasis is endemic throughout the United States and is common among young children in daycare centers.

CLINICAL MANIFESTATIONS

Gastroenteritis may be accompanied by systemic findings, such as fever, lethargy, myalgias, and abdominal pain. **Viral diarrhea** is characterized by watery stools with no blood or mucus. Vomiting may be present, and dehydration may be prominent, especially in infants and younger children. Fever, when present, is generally low grade.

Dysentery is enteritis involving the colon and rectum; it presents with stools that contain blood and/or mucus and is often associated with fever. *Shigella* is the prototypical cause of dysentery, which must be differentiated from infection with EIEC, EHEC, *E. histolytica* **(amebic dysentery)**, *C. jejuni, Y. enterocolitica,* and nontyphoidal *Salmonella.* Gastrointestinal bleeding and blood loss may be significant.

A chief consideration in the management of a child with diarrhea *is assessing the degree of dehydration* which will dictate the urgency of the situation, the volume of fluid needed for rehydration, and the potential need for hospitalization. Mild to moderate dehydration can usually be treated with oral rehydration; severe dehydration usually requires intravenous rehydration and may even require admission to an intensive care unit.

LABORATORY AND IMAGING STUDIES

Initial laboratory evaluation of moderate to severe diarrhea primarily focuses on the assessment of degree of dehydration and can include electrolytes, blood urea nitrogen, creatinine, and urinalysis for specific gravity. Stool specimens can be examined for mucus, blood, and leukocytes, which indicate colitis in response to bacteria that diffusely invade the colonic mucosa. Patients infected with Shiga toxin–producing *E. coli* and *E. histolytica* generally have minimal fecal leukocytes.

Polymerase chain reaction (PCR)—also called the nucleic acid amplification test (NAAT)—assays may be used if the diagnosis alters management. Multiplex PCR panels for gastroenteritis have replaced bacterial stool cultures. Stool evaluation for parasitic agents should be considered for acute dysenteric illness, especially in travelers returning from endemic areas, and in protracted cases of diarrhea in which no bacterial agent is identified. The diagnosis of *E. histolytica* is based on identification of the organism in the stool. Serologic tests are useful for diagnosis of extraintestinal amebiasis, including amebic hepatic abscess. Giardiasis can be diagnosed by identifying trophozoites or cysts in stool, but this may require three specimens. More specific and sensitive fecal immunoassays and NAATs are the diagnostic tests of choice.

Positive blood cultures are uncommon with bacterial enteritis except for *Salmonella* and *E. coli* enteritis in very young infants. In typhoid fever, blood cultures are more likely to be positive than stool cultures.

DIFFERENTIAL DIAGNOSIS

Diarrhea can be caused by infection, toxins, medications, gastrointestinal allergy (including allergy to milk or soy proteins), malabsorption defects, inflammatory bowel disease, celiac disease, or any injury to enterocytes. Acute enteritis may mimic other diseases, such as intussusception and acute appendicitis, which are best identified by diagnostic imaging. Many noninfectious causes of diarrhea produce chronic diarrhea, with persistence for more than 14 days. Persistent or chronic symptoms may require tests for malabsorption or invasive studies, including endoscopy and small bowel biopsy.

TREATMENT

Most infectious causes of diarrhea in children are self-limited. Antibiotics are not generally useful and may be a risk factor in the development of HUS when *E. coli* O157:H7 is present. Management of viral and most bacterial causes of diarrhea is primarily supportive and consists of preventing or correcting dehydration and ongoing fluid and electrolyte deficits. Therapy for severe fluid and electrolyte losses involves intravenous hydration. Less severe degrees of dehydration (<10%) in the absence of excessive vomiting or shock may be managed with oral rehydration solutions containing glucose and electrolytes. Ondansetron may be administered to reduce emesis when this is persistent.

Antibiotic therapy may be necessary for high-risk patients or those with severe disease or bacteremia. Antibiotic treatment of *Shigella* may reduce the duration of symptoms and decrease transmission of infection. Azithromycin is first-line oral therapy for children; ciprofloxacin and third generation cephalosporins may also be used. Many *Shigella sonnei* isolates, the predominant strain affecting children, are resistant to amoxicillin and trimethoprim-sulfamethoxazole. Fluoroquinolone resistance in *Salmonella* and many other gram-negative organisms is increasing in many parts of the world. *Salmonella* should be treated with antibiotics in children less than 3 months of age due to risk of bacteremia and extraintestinal infection.

Treatment of traveler's diarrhea is generally supportive, although antibiotics can be indicated in instances of bloody diarrhea or a febrile illness, in which case azithromycin is a recommended choice for children. Due to lack of consistent access to health care in many areas, providing a prescription to a family in advance of travel to a high-risk area such as in Asia, Africa, or South America may be considered.

Treatment of *C. difficile* (pseudomembranous colitis) depends on the severity but includes discontinuation of the inciting antibiotic and administration of oral metronidazole, fidaxomicin, or vancomycin. *E. histolytica* dysentery is treated with metronidazole followed by a luminal agent, such as iodoquinol. Options for the treatment of *G. lamblia* are metronidazole, tinidazole, or nitazoxanide.

COMPLICATIONS AND PROGNOSIS

The major complication of gastroenteritis is dehydration and hypovolemic shock. Seizures may occur with high fever, especially with *Shigella*. Intestinal abscesses can form with *Shigella, Yersinia,* and *Salmonella* infections, leading to intestinal perforation. Severe vomiting associated with gastroenteritis can cause esophageal tears or aspiration pneumonia. *Salmonella* can cause bacteremia, osteomyelitis, and CNS infection in young infants and some immunocompromised patients.

Deaths resulting from diarrhea reflect the principal problem of disruption of fluid and electrolyte homeostasis, which can lead to dehydration, electrolyte imbalance, hemodynamic instability, and shock. Although significant progress has been made, diarrheal diseases cause a huge number of deaths globally (approximately 1.2 million in 2021). Children under 5 years of age account for most of these deaths. Children who are malnourished and/or have impaired immunity, including those with HIV, are at highest risk for life-threatening diarrhea.

PREVENTION

The most important means of preventing childhood diarrhea is the provision of clean, uncontaminated water and proper hygiene in growing, collecting, and preparing foods. Good hygienic measures, especially appropriate handwashing with soap and water, are the best means of controlling person-to-person spread of most organisms causing gastroenteritis. Poultry products should be considered potentially contaminated with *Salmonella* and should be handled and cooked appropriately. Families should also be aware of the risk of acquiring salmonellosis from household reptile pets and should practice thorough handwashing after handling the animals or their cages. Children under 5 years of age and immunocompromised persons should avoid contact with reptiles.

Immunization against rotavirus infection is recommended for all children beginning at 6 weeks of age, with the first dose by 15 weeks and the last dose by 8 months of age (see Chapter 95). Two typhoid vaccines are licensed in the United States: an oral live-attenuated vaccine (Ty21a) for children 6 years of age and older and a capsular polysaccharide vaccine (ViCPS) for intramuscular administration for children 2 years of age and older. These are recommended for travelers to endemic areas of developing countries or for household contacts of *S. typhi* chronic carriers. Newer typhoid vaccines are now available in other parts of the world, especially South Asia.

The risk for traveler's diarrhea, caused primarily by ETEC, may be minimized by avoiding uncooked food and untreated drinking water. Symptomatic self-treatment for mild diarrhea with an **oral rehydration solution** is recommended, and self-treatment of moderate diarrhea and fever with azithromycin can be considered for children. Prompt medical evaluation is indicated for disease persisting more than 3 days, bloody stools, fever above 102°F (38.9°C) or chills, persistent vomiting, or moderate to severe dehydration.

PEARLS FOR PRACTITIONERS

See Infectious Diseases: Pearls for Practitioners at the end of this section.

REVIEW QUESTIONS

Available online.

CHAPTER 114
Viral Hepatitis

ETIOLOGY

Acute hepatitis can be the result of many infectious and noninfectious etiologies. Among infectious causes of hepatitis, viruses have an important role. The primary hepatotropic viruses, hepatitis A to G, differ in their virologic characteristics, transmission, severity, likelihood of persistence, and subsequent risk of causing hepatocellular carcinoma (Table 114.1). Several other viruses can also cause hepatitis in children including EBV, CMV, HSV, enteroviruses, and adenovirus. The cause of 10–15% of cases of acute hepatitis is unknown.

EPIDEMIOLOGY

Hepatitis A virus (HAV) is the most common cause of acute viral hepatitis and is spread by fecal-oral transmission. HAV is common in children globally, especially in areas of poor sanitation. Among U.S. children, infection due to HAV was often associated with childcare settings; rates have decreased since the introduction of routine vaccination. Hepatitis B virus (HBV), hepatitis C virus (HCV), and hepatitis D virus (HDV) infections can result in chronic hepatitis, or a chronic carrier state, which facilitates spread. HDV, also known as the **delta agent**, is a defective virus that requires HBV for spread and causes either co-infection with HBV or superinfection in chronic carriers of hepatitis B surface antigen (HBsAg). Routine vaccination has also been effective in reducing the rates of HBV infection, especially in children.

The major risk factors for HBV and HCV are injectable drug use, frequent exposure to blood products, unprotected sexual exposure, and perinatal transmission from maternal infection. Hepatitis E virus (HEV) infection occurs following travel to endemic areas (South Asia) outside of the United States. Hepatitis G virus (HGV) is prevalent in persons with HIV. HBV and HCV cause chronic infection, which may lead to cirrhosis and hepatocellular carcinoma and represents a persistent risk of transmission.

In 2021 and 2022, clusters of severe hepatitis of unknown etiology were reported in previously healthy pediatric patients from many countries including the United States. Studies have found that human adenoviruses were often found in the blood of these patients, sometimes associated with other viruses such as EBV or HHV-6. In several of these

TABLE 114.1 Characteristics of Hepatitis Viruses

FEATURE	HAV	HBV	HCV	HDV	HEV	HGV
Viral structure	27-nm ssRNA virus	42-nm dsDNA virus	30- to 60-nm ssRNA virus	36-nm circular ssRNA hybrid particle with HBsAg coat	27- to 34-nm ssRNA virus	50- to 100-nm ssRNA virus
Family	Picornavirus	Hepadnavirus	Flavivirus	Satellite	Flavivirus	Flavivirus
Transmission	Fecal-oral, rarely parenteral	Transfusion, sexual, inoculation, perinatal	Parenteral, transfusion, perinatal	Similar to HBV	Fecal-oral (endemic and epidemic)	Parenteral, transfusion
Incubation period	15–30 days	60–180 days	14–160 days	Co-infection with HBV	35–60 days	Unknown
Serum markers	Anti-HAV	HBsAg, HBeAg, anti-HBs, anti-HBc, anti-HBe	Anti-HCV (IgG, IgM), RIBA, PCR assay for HCV RNA	Anti-HDV, RNA	Anti-HEV	RNA by RT-PCR assay
Fulminant liver failure	Rare	<1% unless co-infection with HDV	Uncommon	2–20%	20%	Unlikely
Persistent infection	No	5–10% (90% with perinatal infection)	85%	2–70%	No	Persistent infection common; chronic disease rare
Increased risk of hepatocellular carcinoma	No	Yes	Yes	No	No	Unknown
Prophylaxis	Vaccine, immune serum globulin	Vaccine, hepatitis B immunoglobulin (HBIG)				

dsDNA, Double-stranded DNA; *HAV*, hepatitis A virus; *HBV*, hepatitis B virus; *HCV*, hepatitis C virus; *HDV*, hepatitis D virus; *HEV*, hepatitis E virus; *HGV*, hepatitis G virus; *Ig*, immunoglobulin; *PCR*, polymerase chain reaction; *RIBA*, recombinant immunoblot assay; *RT-PCR*, reverse transcriptase–polymerase chain reaction; *ssDNA/ssRNA*, single-stranded DNA/RNA.

patients, adeno-associated virus type 2 (AAV2) was detected by PCR testing.

CLINICAL MANIFESTATIONS

Asymptomatic or mild, nonspecific illness without icterus is common with HAV, HBV, and HCV, especially in young children. When present, symptoms of acute infection include malaise, nausea, vomiting, and diarrhea, followed by jaundice, and are difficult to distinguish between these viruses. Fulminant HAV infection is rare, and chronic infection does not occur. In acute HBV infection the likelihood of symptoms increases with age, ranging from 1% of infants younger than 12 months to 30–50% of people older than 5 years. In HBV infection, the **preicteric phase**, which lasts ~1 week, is characterized by headache, anorexia, malaise, abdominal discomfort, nausea, and vomiting; it usually precedes the onset of clinically detectable disease. Extrahepatic manifestations such as arthralgia, arthritis, rash, thrombocytopenia, glomerulonephritis, or papular acrodermatitis **(Gianotti-Crosti syndrome)** can occur early in the illness. Jaundice and tender hepatomegaly occur later and characterize the **icteric phase**. Prodromal symptoms, particularly in children, may abate during the icteric phase. Hepatic enzymes may increase 15- to 20-fold. Resolution of the hyperbilirubinemia and normalization of the transaminases may take 6–8 weeks.

LABORATORY AND IMAGING STUDIES

Alanine aminotransferase (ALT) and aspartate aminotransferase (AST) levels are elevated and generally reflect the degree of parenchymal inflammation. Alkaline phosphatase and total and direct (conjugated) bilirubin levels indicate the degree of cholestasis, which results from hepatocellular and bile duct damage. The prothrombin time (INR: international normalized ratio) is a good predictor of severe hepatocellular injury and progression to fulminant hepatic failure (see Chapter 131).

The diagnosis of viral hepatitis is confirmed by serologic testing (see Table 114.1; Fig. 114.1). The presence of immunoglobulin M (IgM)–specific antibody to HAV with low or absent IgG antibody is presumptive evidence of acute HAV infection.

The presence of HBsAg signifies acute or chronic infection with HBV. Antigenemia appears early in the illness and is usually transient but is characteristic of chronic infection. Maternal HBsAg status should always be determined when HBV infection is diagnosed in children younger than 1 year of age because of the likelihood of vertical transmission. Of note, transient HbsAg positivity can also occur following hepatitis B vaccination but should resolve over time. Hepatitis B early antigen (HBeAg) appears in the serum with acute HBV. The continued presence of HBsAg and HBeAg in the absence of antibody to e antigen (anti-HBe) indicates high risk of transmissibility that is associated with ongoing viral replication. Clearance of HBsAg from the serum precedes a variable **window period**, followed by the emergence of the antibody to surface antigen (anti-HBs), which indicates development of lifelong immunity and is also a marker of immunization. Antibody to core antigen (anti-HBc) is a useful marker for recognizing HBV infection during the window phase (when HBsAg has disappeared but before the appearance of anti-HBs). Anti-HBe is useful in predicting a low degree of infectivity during the carrier state.

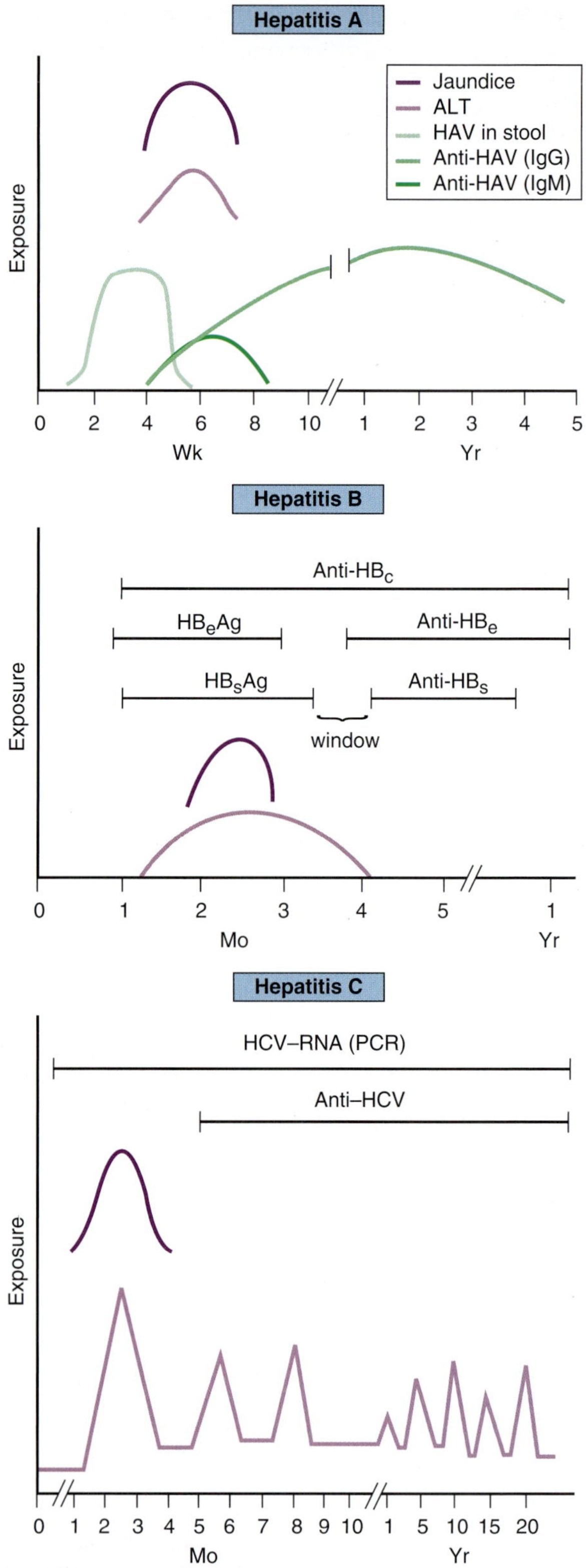

FIGURE 114.1 Clinical course and laboratory findings associated with hepatitis A, hepatitis B, and hepatitis C. *ALT,* Alanine aminotransferase; *HAV,* hepatitis A virus; *anti-HBc,* antibody to hepatitis B core antigen; *HBeAg,* hepatitis B early antigen; *anti-HBe,* antibody to hepatitis B early antigen; *HBsAg,* hepatitis B surface antigen; *anti-HBs,* antibody to hepatitis B surface antigen; *HCV,* hepatitis C virus; *PCR,* polymerase chain reaction.

Seroconversion after HCV infection may occur 6 months after infection. A positive result of HCV enzyme-linked immunosorbent assay (ELISA) should be confirmed with the more specific recombinant immunoblot assay, which detects antibodies to multiple HCV antigens. Detection of HCV RNA by polymerase chain reaction (PCR) is a sensitive marker for active infection, and results may be positive just 3 days after inoculation.

DIFFERENTIAL DIAGNOSIS

In addition to the many viruses that may cause hepatitis as a component of systemic infection, bacterial sepsis can also cause hepatic inflammation and dysfunction. Patients with cholecystitis, cholangitis, and choledocholithiasis may present with acute symptoms and jaundice. Other causes of acute liver disease in childhood include drugs (isoniazid, phenytoin, valproic acid, carbamazepine, oral contraceptives, acetaminophen), parenteral nutrition, toxins (ethanol, poisonous mushroom), Wilson disease, metabolic disease (galactosemia, tyrosinemia, mitochondrial disorders), α_1-antitrypsin deficiency, tumor, shock, anoxia, autoimmune hepatitis, hemophagocytic syndromes, and graft-versus-host disease (see Chapter 131).

TREATMENT

The treatment of acute hepatitis is largely supportive and involves rest, hydration, and adequate nutrition. Hospitalization is indicated for children with severe vomiting and dehydration, a prolonged prothrombin time, or signs of hepatic encephalopathy. When the diagnosis of viral hepatitis is established, attention should be directed toward preventing its spread to close contacts. For HAV, hygienic measures include handwashing and careful disposal of excreta, contaminated diapers or clothing, needles, and other blood-contaminated items.

The treatment of chronic HBV and HCV infections includes the use of direct-acting antivirals, nucleotide and nucleoside analogues (HBV), or protease and polymerase inhibitors (HCV). Pan-genotypic antivirals for HCV are available for children 3 years and older; most children in this age group are recommended to receive therapy.

COMPLICATIONS AND PROGNOSIS

Most cases of acute viral hepatitis resolve without specific therapy, with less than 0.1% of cases progressing to fulminant hepatic necrosis. HAV and HEV cause acute infection only. HBV, HCV, and HDV may persist as chronic infection, with chronic inflammation, fibrosis, and cirrhosis and the associated risk of hepatocellular carcinoma.

Perinatal transmission of HBV infection is marked by an initial phase of immune tolerance with high levels of viremia and HBeAg positivity, but no liver disease. This phase can last for many years to decades. Chronic HBsAg carriers are usually HBeAg negative and have no clinical, biochemical, or serologic evidence of active hepatitis unless there is superinfection with HDV. Approximately 10–15% of HBsAg carriers eventually clear HBsAg.

Approximately 85% of untreated persons infected with HCV remain chronically infected, which is characterized by fluctuating transaminase levels (see Fig. 114.1). There is poor correlation of symptoms with ongoing liver damage. Approximately 20% of persons with chronic infection develop cirrhosis, and approximately 25% of those develop hepatocellular carcinoma. HIV infection and ethanol use increase the risk of HCV progression.

PREVENTION

Good hygienic practices significantly reduce the risk of fecal-oral transmission of HAV. HAV vaccine is recommended for routine immunization of all children beginning at 12 months. Unvaccinated household and sexual contacts of persons with HAV should receive postexposure prophylaxis as soon as possible and within 2 weeks of the last exposure. HAV vaccine at the age-appropriate dose is preferred for persons 6 months to 40 years of age. Immunoglobulin (0.1 mL/kg for travel lasting up to 1 month, and 0.2 mL/kg for travel lasting up to 2 months, repeating 0.2 mL/kg doses every 2 months thereafter if risk continues) given intramuscularly (IGIM) is preferred for children under 6 months of age, persons over 40 years of age, and immunocompromised persons. For pre-exposure prophylaxis, unvaccinated travelers to endemic regions who are 12 months of age or older should receive a single dose of HAV vaccine administered at any time before departure. Older adults, immunocompromised people, or those with chronic liver disease or other chronic medical conditions who are traveling to an endemic area in less than 2 weeks' time should receive IGIM along with the HAV vaccine dose to optimize protection.

HBV vaccine is recommended for routine immunization of all infants beginning at birth and for all children and adolescents through 18 years of age who have not been immunized previously (see Fig. 95.1). It is also recommended as a pre-exposure vaccination for older children and adults at increased risk of sexual, percutaneous, or mucosal exposure to HBV as well as those with chronic liver disease or HIV and travelers to areas of endemic HBV infection. Routine prenatal screening for HBsAg is recommended for all pregnant women in the United States. Infants born to HBsAg-positive mothers should receive HBV vaccine and hepatitis B immunoglobulin (HBIG; 0.5 mL) within 12 hours of birth, with subsequent vaccine doses at 1 and 6 months of age followed by testing for HBsAg and anti-HBs at 9–15 months of age. Infants born to mothers whose HBsAg status is unknown should receive vaccine within 12 hours of birth. If maternal testing is positive for HBsAg, the infant should receive HBIG as soon as possible (no later than 1 week of age). The combination of HBIG and vaccination is 99% effective in preventing vertical transmission of HBV. Vaccination alone without HBIG may prevent 75% of cases of perinatal HBV transmission and approximately 95% of cases of symptomatic childhood HBV infection.

Postexposure prophylaxis of unvaccinated persons using HBIG and vaccine is recommended following needle-stick injuries with blood from an HBsAg-positive patient and for sexual or needle-sharing contacts or victims of sexual abuse by an HBsAg-positive person. The screening of blood donors significantly reduces the risk of blood-borne transmission.

PEARLS FOR PRACTITIONERS

See Infectious Diseases: Pearls for Practitioners at the end of this section.

REVIEW QUESTIONS

Available online.

CHAPTER 115

Urinary Tract Infection

ETIOLOGY

Urinary tract infections (UTIs) include **cystitis** (infection localized to the bladder), **pyelonephritis** (infection of the renal parenchyma, calyces, and renal pelvis), and **renal abscess**, which may be intrarenal or perinephric. *Escherichia coli*, ascending from bowel (perineum) flora, accounts for 85% of first infections. Other bacteria commonly causing infection include *Klebsiella, Proteus, Enterococcus, Pseudomonas,* and *Enterobacter. Staphylococcus saprophyticus* is associated with UTI in some children and accounts for 15% or more of UTIs in adolescent females. *Staphylococcus aureus* is an uncommon cause of UTI and usually represents hematogenous seeding of the urinary tract.

EPIDEMIOLOGY

Approximately 3% of females and 1% of males have a UTI during their prepubertal years, with the highest incidence in the first year of life. It is only during the first year of life that the incidence of UTIs in males exceeds that in females; during this period uncircumcised males are at 10-fold greater risk of developing a UTI compared to circumcised males. After 12 months of age, UTI in healthy children usually is seen predominantly in females.

A short urethra predisposes females to UTIs. Obstruction to urine flow and urinary stasis is the major risk factor and may result from anatomic abnormalities, nephrolithiasis, kidney tumor, indwelling urinary catheter, ureteropelvic junction obstruction, megaureter, extrinsic compression, and pregnancy. Severe vesicoureteral reflux, whether primary or secondary to urinary tract obstruction, predisposes to chronic infection and kidney scarring. Scarring may also develop in the absence of reflux. Constipation or withholding urine also increases the risk of UTI.

CLINICAL MANIFESTATIONS

The symptoms and signs of UTI vary markedly with age. Few have high positive predictive value in neonates, with fever, feeding problems, and growth faltering as suggestive symptoms. Infants 1 month to 2 years of age may present with fever, feeding problems, growth faltering, or diarrhea and vomiting. The symptoms may masquerade as gastrointestinal illness, with colic, irritability, and crying periods. At 2 years of age, children begin to show the classic signs of UTI, such as urgency, dysuria, frequency, and abdominal or back pain. *The presence of UTI should be suspected in all infants and young children with unexplained fever and in patients of all ages with fever and congenital anomalies of the urinary tract.*

LABORATORY AND IMAGING STUDIES

The diagnosis of UTI in infants and young children requires the presence of both pyuria (see below) and significant bacteriuria (bacteria in the urine) on urine culture. The threshold for significant bacteriuria varies based on urine collection method. It is appropriate to obtain urine cultures by midstream, clean-catch technique for older children and adolescents, whereas transurethral catheterization (and less commonly, suprapubic bladder aspiration) is the appropriate method for younger children and infants. Greater than 100,000 CFU/mL on a clean catch urine culture and greater than 50,000 CFU/mL of a single pathogenic organism indicates significant bacteriuria.

Perineal bags for urine collection are prone to contamination and are not recommended for urine collection for culture. If there is uncertainty about diagnosis of UTI in a younger child or infant, urine can be collected by the most convenient method for urinalysis, and if suggestive of infection, urine can then be collected by catheterization prior to starting antibiotics.

Urinalysis showing **pyuria** (leukocyturia of >10 white blood cells [WBCs]/mm^3) suggests infection but is also consistent with urethritis, vaginitis, nephrolithiasis, glomerulonephritis, and interstitial nephritis. Other urinalysis findings suggestive of infection include any bacteria per high-power field in the unstained uncentrifuged urinary sediment, positive urinary leukocyte esterase test, and positive urinary nitrite test. Combined testing for leukocyte esterase, nitrite, and microscopic bacteria has almost 100% sensitivity for detecting UTI by positivity of one or more of the three tests. The negative predictive value of a urinalysis is about 100% if all three tests are negative and may obviate the need for culture except in neonates, where urinalysis results are less reliable predictors of infection.

Ultrasonography of the bladder and kidneys is recommended for infants and non–toilet-trained children with first-time febrile UTIs to exclude structural abnormalities or detect hydronephrosis. Voiding cystourethrogram (VCUG) is indicated if the ultrasound is abnormal (hydronephrosis, scarring, or other findings suggesting obstruction or congenital abnormality). Vesicoureteral reflux is the most common abnormality found and is ranked from grade I (ureter only) to grade V (complete gross dilation of the ureter and obliteration of caliceal and pelvic anatomy) (see Chapter 168). A technetium-99m dimercaptosuccinic acid (DMSA) scan can identify acute pyelonephritis and is most useful to define kidney scarring as a late effect of UTI.

DIFFERENTIAL DIAGNOSIS

The diagnosis of a UTI is confirmed by a positive urine culture, but this does not distinguish between upper and lower tract infection. Localization of a UTI is important because pyelonephritis is associated more frequently with bacteremia and anatomic abnormalities than uncomplicated cystitis. The clinical manifestations of UTI do not reliably distinguish the site of infection in neonates, infants, and toddlers. Fever and abdominal pain may occur with either lower or upper UTI, although high fever, vomiting, costovertebral tenderness, leukocytosis on complete blood count (CBC), and bacteremia each suggest upper tract involvement.

The manifestations of UTI overlap with signs of sepsis seen in young children and with enteritis, appendicitis, mesenteric lymphadenitis, and pneumonia in older children. Dysuria may indicate pinworm infection, hypersensitivity to soaps or detergents, vaginitis, or sexual abuse and infection.

TREATMENT

Therapy should be initiated for symptomatic children and for all children with a urine culture and pyuria confirming UTI. For infants and children who do not appear ill but have a positive urine culture, oral antibiotic therapy should be initiated. For all young infants and any child with suspected UTI who appears toxic, appears dehydrated, or is unable to retain oral fluids, initial antibiotic therapy should be administered parenterally.

Neonates with UTI are treated initially with parenteral antibiotics. Often, if there is rapid clinical improvement and initial blood cultures are negative, newborn patients can eventually be transitioned to enteral antibiotics to complete a 10- to 14-day total course of therapy. Older children with febrile UTI are treated for 7–10 days of enteral antibiotics or a combination of parenteral followed by enteral antibiotic therapy. Initial treatment with parenteral antibiotics in this age group is determined by clinical status. Parenteral antibiotics should be continued until there is clinical improvement (typically 24–48 hours), defined as resolution of fever and improved oral intake. Isolated cystitis can be treated with shorter durations of antibiotics of 3–5 days. Empirical antibiotic therapy should be guided by the local antimicrobial susceptibility patterns and the results of the patient's prior urine cultures because of increasing problems related to antimicrobial resistance. Definitive antibiotic therapy should be guided by the patient's urine culture results. Commonly used empirical parenteral antibiotics include cefazolin, ceftriaxone, or ampicillin plus gentamicin. Oral regimens include cephalexin, amoxicillin plus clavulanic acid, trimethoprim-sulfamethoxazole, or fluoroquinolones (older children). Infants and children who do not show the expected clinical response within 2–3 days of starting antimicrobial therapy should be re-evaluated, have another urine specimen obtained for culture, and undergo prompt imaging to evaluate for kidney abscess.

The degree of toxicity, dehydration, and ability to retain oral intake of fluids should be assessed carefully. Restoring or maintaining adequate hydration, including correction of electrolyte abnormalities that are often associated with vomiting or poor oral intake, is important.

COMPLICATIONS AND PROGNOSIS

Bacteremia occurs in approximately 5% of patients with pyelonephritis and is more likely in infants than in older children. Focal renal abscesses are an uncommon complication. Parents should be counseled to follow up for evaluation for subsequent fevers to determine the possibility of a recurrence of UTI. If a recurrent UTI is diagnosed, further imaging studies (VCUG) are indicated, if not already performed, to evaluate the possibility of vesicoureteral reflux (see Chapter 168).

PREVENTION

Primary prevention is achieved by promoting good perineal hygiene and managing underlying risk factors for UTI, such as chronic constipation, encopresis, and daytime and nighttime urinary incontinence. There is evidence that antibiotic prophylaxis may prevent more severe symptomatic recurrent infections, although the effect is small and is associated with the development of resistant organisms. The impact of secondary prophylaxis to prevent renal scarring is unknown. Acidification of the urine with cranberry juice is not recommended as the sole means of preventing UTI in children at high risk.

PEARLS FOR PRACTITIONERS

See Infectious Diseases: Pearls for Practitioners at the end of this section.

REVIEW QUESTIONS

Available online.

CHAPTER 116

Vulvovaginitis

ETIOLOGY

Vulvovaginitis, inflammation of the vulva or vagina or both, is the *most common gynecologic problem in prepubertal females.* Suboptimal hygienic practices, proximity of the vagina to the rectum, and low levels of estrogen predispose prepubertal females to vulvovaginal irritation. Low levels of estrogen result in thin, atrophic vaginal epithelium that is susceptible to bacterial invasion. At puberty, estrogen increases, and the pH of the vagina becomes more acidic. Vulvovaginitis can be due to nonspecific and specific causes. **Nonspecific vaginitis** results from overgrowth of normal aerobic vaginal flora that is associated with **suboptimal** hygiene. There are several specific causes of vulvovaginitis (Table 116.1), including sexually transmitted infections such as *Trichomonas vaginalis* and herpes simplex virus (see Chapter 117). **Bacterial vaginosis** is the most common cause of vaginitis in postpubertal females and represents disruption of the normal vaginal flora with reduction in *Lactobacillus* and overgrowth of organisms including *Gardnerella vaginalis, Bacteroides, Mobiluncus,* and *Peptostreptococcus.*

EPIDEMIOLOGY

Nonspecific vaginitis is the most common cause of vulvovaginitis in prepubertal females. *G. vaginalis* is often present as part of the normal vaginal flora in prepubertal females, and its role as a cause of vaginitis in this age group is uncommon. *Candida* is much less common in prepubertal females than in postpubertal females.

CLINICAL MANIFESTATIONS

The primary symptoms of vulvovaginitis are vaginal discharge, erythema, foul smell, dysuria, and pruritus. Characteristics of specific etiologies are outlined in Table 116.1.

LABORATORY AND IMAGING STUDIES

Wet mount microscopic examination, prepared by mixing vaginal secretions with normal saline solution, and culture may be used to confirm a specific diagnosis (see Table 116.1). **Clue cells** are vaginal epithelial cells that are covered with *G.*

TABLE 116.1 Characteristics of Vulvovaginitis

ETIOLOGY CONDITION/ DISORDER	PRESENTATION	DIAGNOSIS	TREATMENT
Physiologic vaginal discharge (physiologic leukorrhea)	Minimal, clear, thin discharge without pruritus or inflammation; occurs soon after birth and again at 6–12 mo before menarche	No pathogenic organisms on culture	Reassurance
Nonspecific vulvovaginitis	Vaginal discharge, dysuria, pruritus; fecal soiling of underwear	Evidence of poor hygiene; no pathogenic organisms on culture	Improved hygiene, sitz baths 2–3 times/day
Bacterial vaginosis	Often asymptomatic; possible thin vaginal discharge with a "fishy" odor	≥3 of the following criteria: (1) thin, homogeneous vaginal discharge; (2) vaginal pH >4.5; (3) a fishy odor of volatile amines on the addition of a drop of 10% potassium hydroxide to a drop of vaginal discharge (the "whiff test"); and (4) the presence of clue cells on a saline wet mount of vaginal discharge	Metronidazole or clindamycin
Candidiasis	Pruritus, dysuria, white vaginal discharge that is usually not malodorous	*Candida* on KOH preparation of vaginal discharge	Topical antifungal (e.g., butoconazole, clotrimazole, miconazole, nystatin) Single oral dose fluconazole
Enterobiasis (pinworms)	Perineal pruritus (nocturnal); gastrointestinal symptoms; variable vulvovaginal contamination from feces; often recurrent symptoms	Adult worms in stool or eggs on perianal skin ("Scotch tape test")	Pyrantel pamoate, mebendazole, or albendazole
Molluscum contagiosum	Vulvar lesions, nodules with central umbilication; white core of curdlike material	Clinical appearance; isolation of poxvirus	Generally self-limited; dermal curettage of umbilicated area
Pthirus pubis infection (pediculosis pubis)	Pruritus, excoriation, sky-blue macules; inner thigh or lower abdomen	Nits on hair shafts, lice on skin or clothing	1% permethrin
Sarcoptes scabiei infection (scabies)	Nocturnal pruritus, pruritic vesicles, pustules in runs	Mites; ova, black dots of feces (microscopic)	5% permethrin
Shigella infection	Bloody vaginal discharge; fever, malaise, fecal contamination, diarrhea; blood and mucus in stool, abdominal cramps	Stools: white blood cells and red blood cells, NAAT positive for *Shigella*	TMP-SMX, azithromycin, or oral third-generation cephalosporin
Staphylococcus, Streptococcus infection	Vaginal discharge, possibly bloody; hyperemic vulvar mucosa; spread from primary lesion	Isolation of causative organism on bacterial culture	First-generation cephalosporin or dicloxacillin; penicillin or amoxicillin for group A streptococcus infection
Foreign body	Foul-smelling vaginal discharge, sometimes bloody	Foreign body on physical examination	Removal of foreign body

KOH, Potassium hydroxide; *NAAT*, nucleic acid amplification test; *TMP-SMX*, trimethoprim-sulfamethoxazole.

vaginalis and have a granular appearance (Fig. 116.1). Vaginal cultures for *G. vaginalis* are not useful. *Candida* may be identified by KOH stain or by culture.

DIFFERENTIAL DIAGNOSIS

Noninfectious causes of vulvovaginitis include physical agents (foreign body, sand), chemical agents (bubble bath, soap, detergent), and vulvar skin disease (atopic dermatitis, seborrhea, psoriasis). Physiologic vaginal discharge or **physiologic leukorrhea** of desquamated vaginal cells and mucus occurs normally in females soon after birth, with discharge lasting about 1 week, and appears again at 6–12 months before menarche. The discharge is minimal, clear, and thin without pruritus or inflammation. No treatment is necessary.

TREATMENT

The treatment of vulvovaginitis depends on the etiology (see Table 116.1). Treatment of nonspecific vaginitis focuses on improving perineal hygiene. Douching or vaginal irrigation is not beneficial and is not recommended.

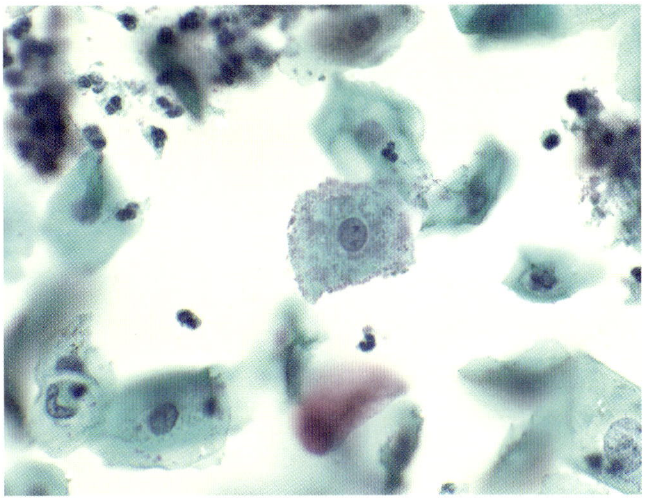

FIGURE 116.1 A film of coccobacilli covers squamous cells in a cervical cytology sample. This aspect is commonly referred to as "clue cells" and is associated with bacterial vaginosis (Papanicolaou stain, ×100). (From Tambouret R. Gynecologic infections. In: Kradin RL, ed. *Diagnostic Pathology of Infectious Diseases*. 2nd ed. Philadelphia: Elsevier; 2018:fig 17.9.)

COMPLICATIONS AND PROGNOSIS

Complications of nonspecific vulvovaginitis are rare, and prognosis is excellent. Bacterial vaginosis is associated with birth complications such as chorioamnionitis and preterm labor, but evidence regarding treatment of bacterial vaginosis to prevent these complications is conflicting.

PREVENTION

There are no recognized prophylactic measures for bacterial vaginosis or nonspecific vaginitis other than maintaining good perineal hygiene. Females should wear cotton underwear and limit time spent in tights, leggings, and wet swimsuits. Douching is not protective and reduces normal vaginal flora, which are protective against pathogenic organisms.

PEARLS FOR PRACTITIONERS

See Infectious Diseases: Pearls for Practitioners at the end of this section.

REVIEW QUESTIONS

Available online.

CHAPTER 117

Sexually Transmitted Infections

Adolescents and young adults have the highest rates of sexually transmitted infections (STIs). Compared with adults, sexually active adolescents are more likely to believe they will not contract an STI, more likely to come into contact with an infected sexual partner, less likely to receive health care when an STI develops, and less likely to complete treatment for an STI.

Although numerous organisms cause STIs, the diseases can be grouped by their characteristic clinical presentations. **Urethritis** and **endocervicitis** (Table 117.1) are characteristic of *Neisseria gonorrhoeae* and *Chlamydia trachomatis.* Seventy percent of new genital chlamydial infections occur in people aged 15–24 years, and most infections are asymptomatic. **Genital ulcers** (Table 117.2) are characteristic of syphilis *(Treponema pallidum),* genital herpes simplex virus (HSV) infections, chancroid *(Haemophilus ducreyi),* lymphogranuloma venereum (LGV; *C. trachomatis*), and granuloma inguinale, also known as *donovanosis (Klebsiella granulomatis).* **Vaginal discharge** (Table 117.3) is a symptom of trichomoniasis *(Trichomonas vaginalis)* and is part of the spectrum of vulvovaginitis (see Chapter 116), which is not always associated with sexual activity. Human papillomavirus (HPV) causes **condylomata acuminata**, or **genital warts** (Table 117.4), and is the major risk factor for cervical, vulvar, and vaginal cancers.

STIs are associated with significant physiologic and psychological morbidity. Early diagnosis and treatment are important for preventing medical complications and infertility. All STIs are preventable; primary prevention of STIs should be a goal of all health care providers for adolescents. Diagnosis of an STI necessitates evaluation or treatment for concomitant STIs and notification and treatment of sexual partners; some STIs are reportable to local and state health departments.

Many infections that are not traditionally considered STIs are sexually transmissible, including those caused by HIV, human T-cell leukemia viruses types I and II, cytomegalovirus, Epstein-Barr virus, human herpes virus (HHV-6, HHV-7), hepatitis B virus, molluscum contagiosum virus, Mpox, and *Sarcoptes scabiei.* The presence of any STI suggests behavior that increases risk for HIV (see Chapter 126), and HIV counseling and testing (and pre-exposure prophylaxis [PrEP] if indicated) should be provided to all adolescents with STIs. Acquisition of gonorrhea, chlamydia, syphilis, genital HSV, and trichomoniasis in prepubertal children beyond the neonatal period indicates sexual contact and signifies the need to investigate for possible sexual abuse (see Chapter 21); diagnosis of STIs in infants can represent abuse or perinatal acquisition. The association of sexual abuse with vulvovaginitis and genital HPV infection, which may result from skin or genital HPV types, is less certain.

PELVIC INFLAMMATORY DISEASE

Direct extension of *N. gonorrhoeae* and/or *C. trachomatis* to the endometrium, fallopian tubes, and peritoneum causes **pelvic inflammatory disease (PID)**. Complications of PID include tubo-ovarian abscess, perihepatitis (**Fitz-Hugh-Curtis syndrome**, an inflammation of the liver capsule), and infertility. The differential diagnosis of PID includes ectopic pregnancy, septic abortion, ovarian cyst torsion or rupture, urinary tract infection, appendicitis, mesenteric lymphadenitis, and inflammatory bowel disease. Pelvic ultrasound may detect thickened adnexal structures and is the imaging study of choice to exclude other possible diagnoses. Minimum clinical criteria for diagnosis of PID are pelvic or lower abdominal tenderness with uterine, adnexal, or cervical motion tenderness. Additional criteria that support the diagnosis are fever, mucopurulent cervical discharge or cervical friability,

TABLE 117.1 Features of Sexually Transmitted Infections Caused by *Chlamydia trachomatis* and *Neisseria gonorrhoeae**

FEATURE	*C. TRACHOMATIS*	*N. GONORRHOEAE*
Incubation period	7–21 days	2–7 days
Possible presentations	Conjunctivitis (including neonatal conjunctivitis), pneumonia, urethritis, cervicitis, proctitis, epididymitis, perihepatitis, lymphogranuloma venereum, reactive arthritis (arthritis, urethritis, and bilateral conjunctivitis)	Pharyngitis, conjunctivitis (including neonatal conjunctivitis), urethritis, cervicitis, proctitis, epididymitis, perihepatitis, disseminated disease (arthritis, dermatitis, endocarditis, meningitis)
SIGNS/SYMPTOMS OF COMMON SYNDROMES		
Urethritis	*Female* Dysuria, frequency >10 PMNs/hpf *Male* Penile discharge >10 PMNs/hpf *Both* Mucoid, watery discharge, negative Gram stain	*Female* Dysuria, frequency, painful, >10 PMNs/ hpf *Male* Mucopurulent discharge, dysuria, frequency, >10 PMNs/hpf *Both* Positive Gram stain
Mucopurulent cervicitis	Cervical erythema, friability, with thick creamy discharge	Cervical edema, erythema, or friability with purulent or mucopurulent discharge
	>10 PMNs/hpf	>10 PMNs/hpf
	Mild cervical tenderness	Mild cervical tenderness
	Gram-negative intracellular diplococci	Gram-negative diplococci
Pelvic inflammatory disease	Lower abdominal pain	
	Adnexal tenderness, mass (5–50%)	
	Pain on cervical motion (>95%)	
	Fever (35%)	
	Vaginal discharge (55%)	
	Mucopurulent cervical discharge (80%)	
	Menstrual irregularities (variable)	
	Nausea, vomiting (variable)	
	Weakness, syncope, dizziness (variable)	
	Perihepatitis (5%)	
DIAGNOSTIC TESTS	NAAT, culture	NAAT, culture
TREATMENT	Ceftriaxone *plus* doxycycline OR ceftriaxone *plus* doxycycline *plus* metronidazole If PID: cefotetan or cefoxitin *plus* doxycycline OR ceftriaxone *plus* doxycycline *plus* metronidazole	

**Co-infection is common, and clinical presentations have significant overlap.*
hpf, High power field; *NAAT,* nucleic acid amplification test; *PID,* pelvic inflammatory disease; *PMN,* polymorphonuclear cell.

presence of abundant numbers of white blood cells (WBCs) on saline microscopy of vaginal fluid, elevated inflammatory markers, and documented infection with *N. gonorrhoeae* or *C. trachomatis*. Adolescents should be hospitalized for treatment if there is uncertainty about the diagnosis, pregnancy, no clinical response to oral therapy within 72 hours, inability to adhere to or tolerate oral therapy, tubo-ovarian abscess, or severe illness with high fever, nausea, and vomiting. The recommended parenteral treatment for hospitalized patients is intravenous (IV) ceftriaxone plus doxycycline (oral [PO] or IV) plus metronidazole (PO or IV) or either cefotetan or cefoxitin IV plus doxycycline IV. The recommended ambulatory treatment of PID is ceftriaxone 500 mg in a single intramuscular (IM) dose (or cefoxitin 2 g IM plus probenecid 1 g PO), plus doxycycline (100 mg PO twice a day) for 14 days, with metronidazole (500 mg PO twice a day) for 14 days. Follow-up examination should be performed within 72 hours.

GONORRHEA *(NEISSERIA GONORRHOEAE)*

N. gonorrhoeae, a gram-negative coccus, is often seen microscopically as diplococci. Gonorrhea is a common STI among adolescents. The highest incidence in the United States is in 15- to 24-year-olds, and incidence rates differ by race and gender, with more cases in men than in women. The organism causes infection at the site of acquisition, which commonly results in mucopurulent cervicitis and urethritis (see Table 117.1), but infection of the rectum and pharynx can also

TABLE 117.2 Features of Sexually Transmitted Infections Characterized by Genital Ulcers

	SYPHILIS	GENITAL HERPES	CHANCROID	GRANULOMA INGUINALE (DONOVANOSIS)
Agent	*Treponema pallidum*	HSV-1, HSV-2	*Haemophilus ducreyi*	*Klebsiella granulomatis*
Incubation	10–90 days	2–14 days	1–10 days	8–80 days
Systemic findings	Primary syphilis: uncommon Secondary syphilis: fever, rash, malaise, anorexia, arthralgia, lymphadenopathy	Headache, fever, malaise, myalgia (40–70%)	None	Local spread only
Inguinal lymphadenopathy	Late, bilateral, nontender, no suppuration	Early, bilateral, tender, no suppuration	Early, rapid, tender, and unilateral; suppuration likely (bubo)	Lymphatic obstruction
Primary lesion	Papule	Vesicle	Papule to pustule	Subcutaneous nodule
ULCER CHARACTERISTICS				
Number	Usually 1	Multiple	<3	>1, may coalesce
Edges	Distinct	Reddened, ragged	Sharply demarcated, serpiginous borders	Rolled, distinct
Depth	Shallow	Shallow	Shallow	Raised
Base	Red, smooth	Red, smooth	Necrotic	Beefy red, clean
Secretion	Serous	Serous	Purulent	None
Induration	Firm	None	None	Firm
Pain	None	Usual	Often	None
EVALUATION AND MANAGEMENT				
Serology	MHA-TP or FTA-ABS; VDRL or RPR	Seroconversion (primary infection only)	None	None
Isolation	No in vitro test; rabbit testes inoculation	PCR, culture	Swab of ulcer on selective medium, node aspirates usually sterile	None
Microscopic	Dark-field examination	PCR or fluorescent antibody staining	Gram-negative coccobacilli	Staining of ulcer biopsy material for Donovan bodies
Treatment	*Early (primary, secondary and early latent):* benzathine penicillin G (50,000 U/kg, up to adult dose of 2.4 million U IM) once	Acyclovir *or* famciclovir *or* valacyclovir	Aspirate or excise fluctuant nodes	Recommended: Azithromycin Alternative: Doxycycline or erythromycin or trimethoprim-sulfamethoxazole
	Late latent (>1 yr duration): benzathine penicillin G (50,000 U/kg, up to adult dose of 2.4 million U IM) weekly × 3 doses		Incision and drainage of buboes >5 cm Azithromycin *or* ceftriaxone *or* ciprofloxacin *or* erythromycin	

FTA-ABS, Fluorescent treponemal antibody–absorption; *HSV,* herpes simplex virus; *IM,* intramuscular; *MHA-TP,* microhemagglutination assay–*Treponema pallidum*; *PCR,* polymerase chain reaction; *RPR,* rapid plasma reagin; *VDRL,* Venereal Disease Research Laboratory.

occur. **Disseminated gonococcal infections** can occur with hematogenous spread and results in petechial or pustular acral skin lesions, asymmetric polyarthralgia, tenosynovitis or oligoarticular septic arthritis, and, occasionally, endocarditis or meningitis. Perinatal transmission of maternal infection can lead to neonatal sepsis (see Chapter 64), meningitis (see Chapter 101), and ophthalmia neonatorum (see Chapter 120).

Gonococcal infection is diagnosed by either culture of endocervical or urethral swab specimens or nucleic acid amplification tests (NAATs) of endocervical swabs, vaginal swabs, urethral swabs, throat specimens, and urine. Culture should be performed in cases of possible treatment failure to allow for antimicrobial susceptibility testing. In cases of suspected sexual abuse, culture is the preferred diagnostic method due

TABLE 117.3 Features of Sexually Transmitted Infections Characterized by Vaginal Discharge

FEATURE	PHYSIOLOGIC LEUKORRHEA (NORMAL)	TRICHOMONIASIS	BACTERIAL VAGINOSIS
Agent	Normal flora	*Trichomonas vaginalis*	Reduction in *Lactobacillus* and overgrowth organisms including *Gardnerella vaginalis, Bacteroides, Mobiluncus*, and *Peptostreptococcus*
Incubation	—	5–28 days	Not necessarily sexually transmitted
Predominant Symptoms			
Pruritus	None	Mild to moderate	None to mild
Discharge	Minimal	Moderate to severe	Mild to moderate
Pain	None	Mild	Uncommon
Vulvar inflammation	None	Common	Uncommon
Characteristics of Discharge			
Amount	Small	Profuse	Moderate
Color	Clear, milky	Yellow-green or gray	Gray
Consistency	Flocculent	Frothy	Homogeneous
Viscosity	Thin	Thin	Thin
Foul odor	None	Possible	Yes
Odor with KOH	None	Possible	Characteristic fishy odor (amine)
pH	<4.5	>5.0	>4.5
Diagnosis			
Saline drop	Squamous and few WBCs	WBC; motile flagellates, slightly larger than WBCs	Squamous cells studded with bacteria ("clue cells") and WBCs
Gram stain	Gram-positive and gram-negative rods and cocci	*Trichomonas*	Predominance of gram-negative rods and cocci with paucity of gram-positive rods
Culture	Mixed flora with *Lactobacillus* predominant	Culture generally not indicated; antibody and nucleic acid tests available	Culture not useful
Treatment	Reassurance	Recommended: Metronidazole Alternative: tinidazole	Metronidazole or clindamycin

KOH, Potassium hydroxide; *WBC*, white blood cell.

to concerns regarding NAAT false-positive results from cross reaction with nongonococcal *Neisseria* species.

Increasing rates of resistance to fluoroquinolones limit treatment options. A single IM dose of ceftriaxone (500 mg for patients 45–150 kg and 1 g for patients >150 kg) is recommended for uncomplicated gonococcal infections of the cervix, urethra, and rectum. If chlamydial infection has not been ruled out, empirical treatment for *C. trachomatis* with doxycycline should also be given. For patients with disseminated gonococcal infections, hospitalization is warranted; gonorrhea culture and antimicrobial susceptibility testing should be performed to guide therapy in these cases.

CHLAMYDIA (*CHLAMYDIA TRACHOMATIS*)

Chlamydiae are obligate intracellular bacteria. Chlamydia infects nonciliated squamocolumnar cells and the transitional epithelial cells that line the mucosa of the urethra, cervix, rectum, and conjunctiva. The incidence of chlamydial infections is highest among people younger than 25 years, and annual screening is recommended for all sexually active women in this age group.

There are at least 18 *C. trachomatis* serovars. Serovars A through C cause trachoma, an ocular infection eventually leading to blindness from extensive local scarring; serovars B and D through K cause urethritis, cervicitis, PID, inclusion conjunctivitis in newborns, and infant pneumonia; serovars L1–3 cause LGV, a less frequent STI characterized by an ulcerative genital lesion followed by unilateral, painful inguinal lymphadenitis.

Chlamydia is the most frequently diagnosed bacterial STI in adolescents and accounts for most cases of **nongonococcal urethritis and cervicitis** (see Table 117.1). There is a 2.5:1 female:male ratio. Males often have dysuria and mucopurulent

TABLE 117.4 Features of Sexually Transmitted Infections Characterized by Nonulcerative External Genital Symptoms

FEATURE	GENITAL WARTS	VULVOVAGINAL CANDIDIASIS	PEDICULOSIS PUBIS (CRABS)
Agent	Human papillomavirus	*Candida albicans*	*Pthirus pubis*
Incubation/transmission	Variable	Uncommon sexual transmission	5–10 days for eggs to hatch
Presenting complaints	Genital warts are seen or felt	Vulvar itching or discharge	Pubic itching; live organisms may be seen; sexual partner has "crabs"
Signs	Firm, gray-to-pink, single or multiple, fimbriated, painless excrescences on vulva, introitus, vagina, cervix, penis, perineum, anus	Inflammation of vulva, with thick, white, "cottage cheese" discharge, pH <4.5; friable mucosa that easily bleeds	Eggs (nits) at base of pubic hairs, lice may be visible; excoriated, red skin secondary to infestation
Clinical associations	Cervical neoplasia, dysplasia	Oral contraceptives, diabetes, antibiotics	—
Diagnosis	Clinical appearance; most infections asymptomatic; acetowhite changes on colposcopy; enlarged cells with perinuclear halo and hyperchromatic nuclei	KOH (10%): pseudohyphae; Gram stain: gram-positive pseudohyphae; Nickerson or Sabouraud medium for culture	History and clinical appearance
Treatment	*Patient-applied therapies:* podofilox solution or gel *or* imiquimod cream *Provider-applied therapies:* cryotherapy with liquid nitrogen or cryoprobe *or* topical podophyllin resin *or* trichloroacetic acid or bichloracetic acid *or* surgical removal	*Intravaginal agents:* butoconazole *or* clotrimazole *or* miconazole *or* nystatin *Oral agent:* fluconazole	Permethrin 1% cream *or* pyrethrin with piperonyl butoxide

KOH, Potassium hydroxide.

discharge, although asymptomatic infection also occurs. Females are more often asymptomatic or may have minimal symptoms, including dysuria, mild abdominal pain, or vaginal discharge. Prepubertal females may have vaginitis. At least 30% of persons with gonococcal cervicitis, urethritis, proctitis, or epididymitis have *C. trachomatis* co-infection.

Chlamydia infection is usually diagnosed by NAAT detection of vaginal, cervical, urethral, and early-morning first-voided urine specimens. Amplification tests have supplanted less sensitive culture and enzyme-linked immunosorbent assay (ELISA) tests. NAAT can be used for vaginal and urine specimens from females in the evaluation of sexual abuse.

Recommended treatment for *C. trachomatis* infection is oral doxycycline 100 mg twice daily for 7 days; azithromycin and levofloxacin are alternatives. Individuals should be advised to avoid unprotected intercourse until all their sexual partners have been tested and treated. Tests of cure are not recommended unless therapeutic adherence is in question, symptoms persist, or reinfection is suspected.

SYPHILIS *(TREPONEMA PALLIDUM)*

Syphilis is caused by *T. pallidum*, a long, slender, coiled spirochete. It cannot be cultivated routinely in vitro but can be observed by dark-field microscopy. Untreated infection progresses through several clinical stages (see Table 117.2). **Primary syphilis** manifests as a single, *painless* genital ulcer, or **chancre**, usually on the genitalia, that appears approximately 3 weeks after inoculation and spontaneously heals in a few weeks. **Secondary syphilis** follows 4–8 weeks later and is manifested as fever, generalized lymphadenopathy, and a disseminated maculopapular rash that is also present on the palms and soles. Plaque-like skin lesions, **condylomata lata**, and mucous membrane lesions occur, particularly in moist areas around the vulva and anus, and are infectious. Secondary syphilis resolves spontaneously within 3–12 weeks. **Tertiary syphilis** is a slowly progressive disease involving the cardiovascular, neurologic, and musculoskeletal systems that manifests 15–30 years after initial infection. **Latent syphilis** is an asymptomatic infection detected by serologic testing. Early latent syphilis indicates acquisition within the preceding year; all other cases of latent syphilis are designated as either late latent syphilis or latent syphilis of unknown duration. Infection can be passed from pregnant people to infect their infants, resulting in **congenital syphilis** (see Chapter 65).

The diagnosis of syphilis is based on serologic testing. There are different types of serologic tests for syphilis, and both are required to make a diagnosis:

- **nontreponemal antibody tests:** the **Venereal Disease Research Laboratory (VDRL)** test, the **rapid plasma reagin (RPR)** test
- specific **treponemal antibody tests:** the **microhemagglutination assay–T. pallidum** (MHA-TP), the **fluorescent treponemal antibody-absorption** (FTA-ABS) test, various enzyme immunoassays (EIAs), and chemiluminescence immunoassays.

The syphilis traditional screening algorithm starts with a screening nontreponemal antibody test followed by a specific treponemal antibody test. Screening with nontreponemal antibody tests indicates a presumptive diagnosis but needs to be confirmed by one of the specific treponemal tests to exclude false-positive results. The nontreponemal antibody test titer can then help guide management because it increases with increasing duration of infection and decreases in response to therapy. A **reverse-sequence screening** approach to diagnose syphilis starts with a specific treponemal test followed by a confirmatory nontreponemal test if the specific treponemal test is positive. A nonquantitative VDRL test can be performed on cerebrospinal fluid but is insensitive. Rheumatic disease and other infectious diseases may cause false-positive VDRL results. Dark-field examination of chancres, mucous membranes, or cutaneous lesions may reveal motile organisms but is usually unnecessary.

The treatment of choice for all stages of syphilis is parenteral penicillin G. Primary syphilis, secondary syphilis, and early latent syphilis are treated with a single IM dose of benzathine penicillin G. Tertiary, late latent, and latent syphilis of unknown duration are treated with three doses at 1-week intervals. Neurosyphilis is treated with IV aqueous crystalline penicillin G for 10–14 days. A systemic, febrile **Jarisch-Herxheimer reaction** can occur within the first 24 hours of penicillin initiation in patients being treated for syphilis.

HERPES SIMPLEX VIRUS INFECTION

HSV-1 and HSV-2 are large, double-stranded DNA viruses of the herpesvirus family. The virus initially infects mucosal surfaces and enters cutaneous neurons, where it migrates along the axons to sensory ganglia. Because viral replication occurs in the ganglia, infectious virus moves along the axon to infect and destroy epithelial cells. Infection may disseminate to other organs in immunocompromised patients. Virus latency is maintained in the ganglia where it undergoes periodic reactivation and replication. Although either virus can be found in any site, HSV-1 more commonly occurs in the central nervous system, eyes, and mouth, whereas HSV-2 more commonly involves the genitalia. Reinfection can occur with exposure to the other type or even a second strain of the same type.

Primary genital herpes is characterized by multiple painful, grouped vesicles or ulcerative and crusted external genital lesions on an erythematous base (see Table 117.2). In females, the cervix may also be involved. Symptoms may include fever, regional lymphadenopathy, discharge, and dysuria. Primary illness lasts 10–20 days. Asymptomatic primary infection also occurs. **Secondary**, **recurrent**, or **reactivation eruptions** are not as dramatic and are not associated with systemic symptoms. In primary infection, viral shedding lasts an average of 11 days, and the entire course from vesicle and ulcer onset resolves over 20 days. In recurrent disease, virus shedding lasts for an average of 4 days, and the course resolves over 9–10 days. Many persons experience four to six recurrences per year. Some primary and many recurrent episodes are asymptomatic.

Viral cultures and polymerase chain reaction (PCR) are the preferred methods of diagnosis; culture typically shows cytopathic effect in 1–3 days and seldom takes longer than 5 days. PCR assays have increased sensitivity over culture. Viral shedding is intermittent after primary infection, so both culture and PCR can fail to detect latent infection. Serologic testing is useful for primary infection only (to show seroconversion between acute and convalescent sera), and positive serologies persist lifelong. Titers are not helpful in guiding management of recurrences.

Oral acyclovir, famciclovir, and valacyclovir are effective treatments in reducing the severity and duration of symptoms in primary cases and may reduce recurrences. Once-daily suppressive therapy reduces the frequency of genital herpes recurrences by more than 75%, and lesions tend to be mild when they do occur. Local hygiene and sitz baths may relieve discomfort. The use of condoms provides some protection against sexual transmission of HSV.

TRICHOMONIASIS *(TRICHOMONAS VAGINALIS)*

Trichomoniasis is caused by the protozoan *T. vaginalis* and often is associated with other STIs, such as gonorrhea and *Chlamydia*. Infection is asymptomatic in as many as 70–85% of infected persons. Symptomatic males can have urethritis. Symptomatic females have vaginitis, with thin, malodorous, frothy yellow-green discharge, vulvar irritation, and cervical "strawberry hemorrhages" (see Table 117.3). Diagnosis is based on visualization of motile, flagellated protozoans in the urine or in a saline wet mount, which has a sensitivity of only 60–70% among symptomatic women. *T. vaginalis*–specific NAAT is available for testing vaginal, endocervical, and urine samples and is highly sensitive (95–100%) and specific (95–100%). Rapid point-of-care testing has become available in recent years, with a turnaround time of approximately 10 minutes. Treatment with oral metronidazole or tinidazole in a single dose is recommended for adolescents and adults; sexual partners should also be treated to prevent reinfection.

GENITAL WARTS (HUMAN PAPILLOMAVIRUSES)

HPV, the cause of genital warts **(condylomata acuminata)**, is the most common STI in the United States, with the highest prevalence rates among 15- to 24-year-olds. Most HPV infections are asymptomatic or subclinical (90%) and self-resolve within 2 years. HPV types 6 and 11 cause 90% of genital warts and are nononcogenic. HPV types 16 and 18 are associated with 70% of cases of cervical cancer. HPV types 31, 33, 35, 39, 45, 51, 52, 56, 58, 59, 66, and 68 are also oncogenic. Three HPV vaccines are licensed for use in the United States: a quadrivalent vaccine (types 6, 11, 16, and 18), a bivalent vaccine (types 16 and 18), and a 9-valent vaccine (types 6, 11, 16, 18, 31, 33, 45, 52, and 58), though only the 9-valent vaccine is currently available in the United States. Vaccination is recommended for all adolescents at age 11–12 years (though can be started at age 9). It is important that children be vaccinated before becoming sexually active because the rate of HPV acquisition is high shortly after the onset of sexual activity.

Genital warts can occur on the squamous epithelium or mucous membranes of the genital and perineal structures of females and males (see Table 117.4). Genital warts are usually multiple, firm, gray-to-pink excrescences. Untreated genital warts may remain unchanged, increase in size or number, or resolve spontaneously. Warts can become tender if macerated or secondarily infected. The diagnosis is usually established by appearance without biopsy. The differential diagnosis includes condylomata lata (secondary syphilis) and tumors.

The goal of treatment is removal of symptomatic warts to induce wart-free periods. Treatment modalities involve destruction of infected epithelium; patient-applied therapies include podofilox, sinecatechins, or imiquimod, and provider-applied therapies include cryotherapy with liquid nitrogen or cryoprobe and trichloroacetic acid or bichloroacetic acid. An alternative is surgical removal. Intralesional interferon and laser surgery have also been effective. Factors that may influence selection of treatment include wart number, size, anatomic sites, wart morphology, patient preference, treatment cost, convenience, adverse effects, and provider experience. Recurrences after treatment are common and are frequently asymptomatic.

MPOX

Mpox (formerly monkeypox) virus is a *Poxviridae* family member of the genus *Orthopoxvirus* and has two clades (I, II). Mpox is spread by person-to-person direct contact and has been a cause of a global outbreak among men who have sex with men (clade II), but children younger than 15 (clade I) have also been infected perhaps from household contacts.

The **clinical presentation** may have few and mild prodromal symptoms (fever, malaise, lymphadenopathy) before the appearance of the rash, which progresses from macules to papules to vesicles to pustules, eventually forming scabs. The disease is usually self-limited and diagnosed by NAAT testing of the lesions. Most patients require only supportive care, but severe infection may be treated with tecovirimat. Vaccination is available for high-risk patients.

PUBIC LICE *(PTHIRUS PUBIS)*

Pubic lice, or pediculosis pubis, are caused by infestation with *Pthirus pubis,* the **pubic crab louse**. The louse is predominantly sexually transmitted and lives out its life cycle on pubic hair, where it causes characteristic, intense pruritus (see Table 117.4). Diagnosis can be made clinically; lice are visible to the naked eye. Erythematous papules and **egg cases (nits)** are not seen before puberty. Treatment consists of education regarding personal and environmental hygiene and the application of an appropriate pediculicide, such as permethrin 1% cream or pyrethrins with piperonyl butoxide. Bedding and clothing should be decontaminated (machine washed and machine dried using the heat cycle or dry cleaned) or removed from body contact for at least 72 hours. Fumigation of living areas is not necessary.

PEARLS FOR PRACTITIONERS

See Infectious Diseases: Pearls for Practitioners at the end of this section.

REVIEW QUESTIONS

Available online.

CHAPTER 118

Osteomyelitis

ETIOLOGY

Acute hematogenous osteomyelitis is the most common manifestation of osteomyelitis in children and evolves secondary to bacteremia. **Subacute osteomyelitis** may follow local inoculation by penetrating trauma and is not associated with systemic symptoms; **chronic osteomyelitis** results from an untreated or inadequately treated (usually subacute) osteomyelitis.

In children beyond the newborn period and without hemoglobinopathies, bone infections occur most commonly in the metaphyses of long bones due to sluggish blood flow through tortuous vascular loops unique to this site. Preceding nonpenetrating trauma is often reported and may lead to local bone injury that predisposes to infection. Bone infections in children with sickle cell disease typically occur in the diaphyseal portion of the long bones, probably as a consequence of antecedent focal infarction. In children younger than 12–18 months of age, capillaries perforate the epiphyseal growth plate, permitting spread of infection across the epiphysis and leading to suppurative arthritis, whereas in older children, infection is contained in the metaphysis because these vessels no longer cross the epiphyseal plate (Fig. 118.1).

Staphylococcus aureus is responsible for more than 80% of acute skeletal infections in which an organism can be identified. Group A streptococcus is another common cause, and *Streptococcus pneumoniae* is occasionally identified. Group B streptococcus and enteric gram-negatives are other major causes in neonates. Sickle cell disease and other hemoglobinopathies predispose to osteomyelitis caused by *Salmonella* and *S. aureus. Pasteurella multocida* osteomyelitis may follow cat or dog bites. The use of polymerase chain reaction (PCR) testing reveals that a significant proportion of **culture-negative osteomyelitis** is due to *Kingella kingae,* particularly in children under 5 years of age. Conjugate vaccine has greatly reduced the incidence of *Haemophilus influenzae* type b infections.

Subacute focal bone infections caused by *Pseudomonas aeruginosa* and *S. aureus* usually occur in ambulatory persons who sustain **puncture wounds** of the foot. *Pseudomonas* **chondritis** is strongly associated with puncture wounds through sneakers, which harbor *Pseudomonas* in the foam insole. *S. aureus* is the most common cause of chronic osteomyelitis. **Chronic recurrent multifocal osteomyelitis** (also known as **chronic nonbacterial osteomyelitis**) is an *autoinflammatory noninfectious* syndrome characterized by recurrent episodes of fever, bone pain, and radiographic findings of osteomyelitis. Bones uncommonly involved in acute hematogenous osteomyelitis—such as the clavicle, scapula, or small bones of the hands or feet—are often affected. Pathogens are not identified on culture, and histopathology demonstrates plasmacytic infiltrates.

EPIDEMIOLOGY

Osteomyelitis may occur at any age but is most common in children 3–12 years of age; it affects males twice as frequently as females. Osteomyelitis from penetrating trauma or peripheral vascular disease is more common in adults.

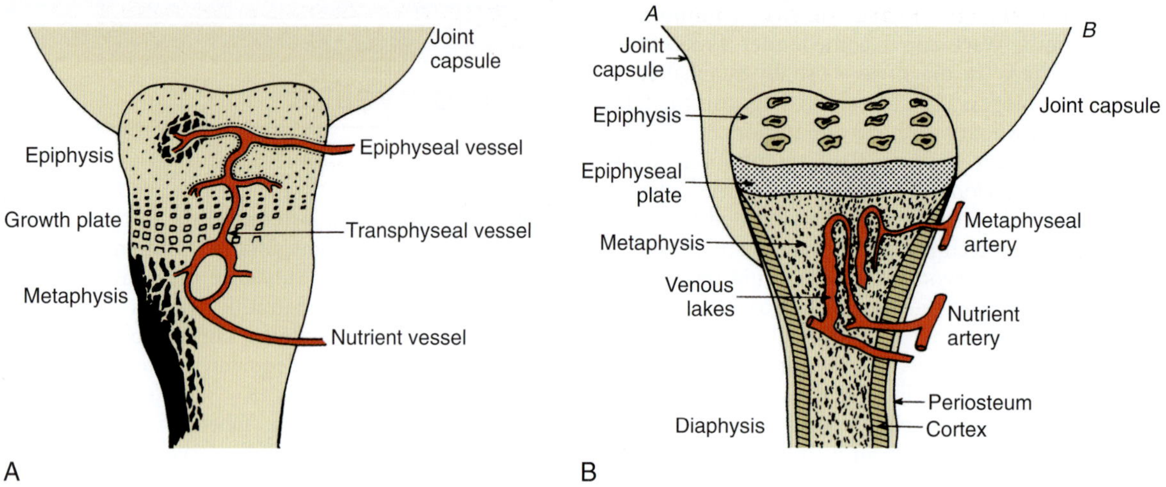

FIGURE 118.1 **(A)** Major structures of the bone of an infant before maturation of the epiphyseal growth plate. Note the transphyseal vessel, which connects the vascular supply of the epiphysis and metaphysis, facilitating spread of osteomyelitis between these two areas. **(B)** Major structures of the bone of a child. Joint capsule A inserts below the epiphyseal growth plate, as in the hip, elbow, ankle, and shoulder. Rupture of a metaphyseal osteomyelitis abscess in these bones is likely to produce the pyarthrosis of suppurative arthritis. Joint capsule B inserts at the epiphyseal growth plate, as in other tubular bones. Rupture of a metaphyseal abscess in these bones is likely to lead to a subperiosteal abscess but seldom to an associated pyarthrosis. (From Gutman LT. Acute, subacute, and chronic osteomyelitis and pyogenic arthritis in children. *Curr Probl Pediatr*. 1985;15:1–72.)

CLINICAL MANIFESTATIONS

The most common presenting complaints are focal pain, exquisite point tenderness over the bone, warmth, erythema, and swelling. Fever, anorexia, irritability, and lethargy may accompany the focal findings. Weight bearing and active and passive motion of the affected extremity are decreased, mimicking paralysis **(pseudoparalysis)**. Muscle spasm may make the extremity difficult to examine. The adjacent joint space may be involved in young children, suggested by pain with minimal joint range of motion (see Chapter 119).

Usually only one bone is involved. The femur, tibia, or humerus is affected in approximately 65% of patients. Approximately 15% of cases involve the bones of the hands or feet, and 10% involve the pelvis. Vertebral osteomyelitis is notable for an insidious onset, vague symptoms, backache, occasional spinal cord compression, and, usually, little associated fever or systemic toxicity. Patients with osteomyelitis of the pelvis may present with fever, limp, and vague abdominal, hip, groin, or thigh pain. **Pyomyositis** of pelvic muscles may mimic osteomyelitis.

LABORATORY AND IMAGING STUDIES

The presence of leukocytosis is inconsistent. Blood cultures are important but are negative in more than half of cases. Elevated acute phase reactants including erythrocyte sedimentation rate (ESR) and C-reactive protein (CRP) are sensitive but nonspecific findings. Serial determinations of inflammatory markers can be helpful in monitoring the course of the illness and response to treatment. Direct subperiosteal or metaphyseal needle aspiration can definitively establish the diagnosis. Identification of bacteria in aspirated material by Gram stain can establish the diagnosis within hours of clinical presentation.

Plain radiographs can demonstrate soft tissue swelling such as the **loss of the periosteal fat line** within the first 3 days of symptoms, but bony lesions such as **periosteal elevation** and **bone destruction** are absent until after 10–14 days of symptoms. **Brodie abscess** is a subacute intraosseous abscess that does not drain into the subperiosteal space and is classically located in the distal tibia. **Sequestra**, portions of avascular bone that have separated from adjacent bone, frequently are covered with a thickened sheath, or **involucrum**, both of which are hallmarks of chronic osteomyelitis.

MRI is sensitive to the inflammatory marrow changes even during the earliest stages of osteomyelitis and is the diagnostic study of choice (Fig. 118.2). Whole-body rapid short tau inversion recovery (STIR) MRI is useful for identifying multifocal disease.

DIFFERENTIAL DIAGNOSIS

Osteomyelitis must be differentiated from infectious arthritis (see Chapter 119), cellulitis, pyomyositis, fasciitis, bursitis, spondylodiscitis, trauma, juvenile idiopathic arthritis, bone cysts, Langerhan cell histiocytosis, and malignancy.

TREATMENT

Initial antibiotic therapy for osteomyelitis is based on the likely organism for the age of the child, Gram stain of bone aspirate, and associated diseases (Table 118.1). Initial therapy includes an antibiotic that targets *S. aureus* and *Kingella,* such as cefazolin. Clindamycin, vancomycin, or linezolid should be used if methicillin-resistant *S. aureus* is suspected based on patient factors or local *S. aureus* epidemiology. For patients with sickle cell disease, initial therapy should include an antibiotic with activity against *Salmonella* and *S. pneumoniae.*

Response to IV antibiotics usually occurs within 48 hours. Lack of improvement after 48 hours indicates that surgical drainage may be necessary or that an unusual pathogen may be present. Surgical drainage is indicated for presence of extensive, severe, chronic, or atypical disease; presence of abscess; hip joint involvement; or **sequestrum** or spinal cord compression. Antibiotics are typically administered for 3–4 weeks. After initial inpatient treatment and adequate clinical

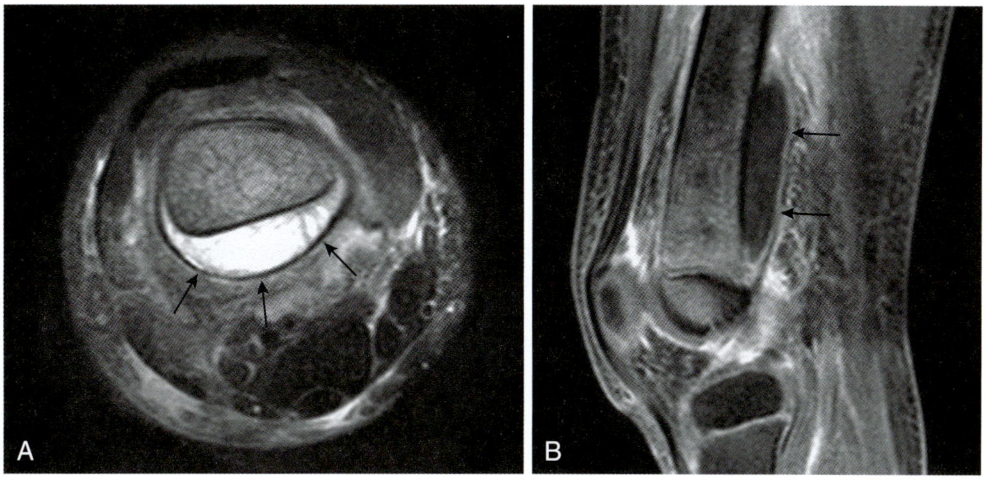

FIGURE 118.2 Acute osteomyelitis of the distal femur in a 5-year-old child. **(A)** T2 weighted fat-saturated axial magnetic resonance imaging (MRI) shows a large subperiosteal abscess *(arrows)* at the posterior femur. Increased signal is seen within the bone, along with adjacent soft tissue edema. **(B)** T1 weighted fat-saturated post-gadolinium sagittal MRI demonstrates the longitudinal extent of the same subperiosteal abscess and its enhancing wall *(arrows)*. (From Kan JH, Meyers AB, Azouz EM. Musculoskeletal infections. In: Coley BD, ed. *Caffey's Pediatric Diagnostic Imaging*. 13th ed. Philadelphia: Saunders; 2019:fig. 137.13.)

TABLE **118.1** Recommended Antibiotic Therapy for Osteomyelitis in Children

COMMON PATHOGEN	RECOMMENDED TREATMENT*
ACUTE HEMATOGENOUS OSTEOMYELITIS	
Staphylococcus aureus	
Methicillin-sensitive	Nafcillin (or oxacillin) or cefazolin
Methicillin-resistant	Clindamycin or trimethoprim-sulfamethoxazole or vancomycin or linezolid
Streptococcus pyogenes (group A streptococci)	Ampicillin/amoxicillin
Streptococcus pneumoniae	Ampicillin/amoxicillin or ceftriaxone or vancomycin
SUBACUTE FOCAL OSTEOMYELITIS	
Pseudomonas aeruginosa	Cefepime or piperacillin-tazobactam or ciprofloxacin
Kingella kingae	Cephalosporin (first or second generation) or ampicillin-sulbactam

Optimal specific therapy is based on susceptibilities of the organism that is isolated.

response, including decreases in inflammatory markers, transition to home therapy with oral antibiotic is standard for most patients. Home IV antibiotics are reserved for those with especially complicated disease and are associated with increased adverse event rates and need for unscheduled medical visits.

COMPLICATIONS AND PROGNOSIS

Complications of acute osteomyelitis are uncommon and usually arise because of inadequate or delayed medical or surgical therapy or concomitant bacteremia. Vascular insufficiency, which affects delivery of antibiotics, and trauma are associated with higher rates of complications.

Hematogenous osteomyelitis has an excellent prognosis if treated promptly and if surgical drainage is performed when appropriate. The poorest outcomes are in neonates and in infants with involvement of the hip or shoulder joints (see Chapter 119). Approximately 2–4% of acute infections recur despite adequate therapy, and ~25% of these fail to respond to extensive surgical debridement and prolonged antimicrobial therapy, ultimately resulting in bone loss, sinus tract formation, or amputation (although rare). Sequelae related to skeletal growth disturbance are most common with neonatal osteomyelitis or if the growth plate has been extensively disrupted.

PREVENTION

There are no effective means of preventing hematogenous *S. aureus* osteomyelitis. Universal immunization of infants with conjugate *H. influenzae* type b vaccine has practically eliminated serious bacterial infections from this organism, including bone and joint infections.

Children with puncture wounds to the foot should receive prompt irrigation, cleansing, debridement, removal of any visible foreign body or debris, and tetanus prophylaxis. The value of oral prophylactic antibiotics for preventing osteomyelitis after penetrating injury is uncertain.

PEARLS FOR PRACTITIONERS

See Infectious Diseases: Pearls for Practitioners at the end of this section.

REVIEW QUESTIONS

Available online.

CHAPTER 119

Infectious Arthritis

ETIOLOGY

Infectious arthritis (**suppurative** or **septic arthritis**) is a serious bacterial infection of the joint space resulting from hematogenous bacterial dissemination. Infectious arthritis less often results from contiguous spread of infection from surrounding soft tissues or direct inoculation into the joint (penetrating trauma). Spread of osteomyelitis into the joint space is more common in children under 18 months of age and occurs via organisms passing through transphyseal vessels to the epiphysis (see Fig. 118.1A). The bacteria causing infectious arthritis are similar to those causing osteomyelitis (Table 119.1). Lyme disease may also cause arthritis (see Chapter 123).

The arthritis of **disseminated gonococcal infections** includes both reactive and suppurative forms in early and late gonococcal disease, respectively. With untreated genital infection, gonococcemia may occur with fever and a polyarticular, symmetric arthritis and rash, known as the **arthritis-dermatitis syndrome**. Bacterial cultures of the synovium are sterile at this stage, despite a relatively high prevalence of bacteremia. Monoarticular arthritis of large, weight-bearing joints develops days to weeks later. Cultures of affected synovial fluid at this stage often yield the pathogen.

Reactive arthritis is immune-mediated synovial inflammation that follows a bacterial or viral infection, especially with *Chlamydia trachomatis, Yersinia,* and other enteric infections. Reactive arthritis of the hip joints in children 3–6 years of age is known as **toxic** or **transient synovitis** (see Chapter 201).

TABLE 119.1 Pathogenic Organisms Causing Arthritis in Children

COMMON	UNCOMMON
YOUNG INFANT (<2 MO)	
Group B streptococci	*Neisseria gonorrhoeae*
Staphylococcus aureus	*Candida*
Escherichia coli	
Klebsiella pneumonia	
OLDER INFANTS AND CHILDREN (2 MO TO MATURITY)	
S. aureus	Anaerobic bacteria
Streptococcus pneumoniae	*Pseudomonas aeruginosa*
Group A streptococci	*Enterobacteriaceae*
Kingella kingae	*Haemophilus influenzae* type b*
N. gonorrhoeae	*Mycobacterium tuberculosis*
Borrelia burgdorferi (Lyme disease)	
REACTIVE ARTHRITIS	
Yersinia enterocolitica	
Campylobacter jejuni	
Shigella flexneri	
Chlamydia trachomatis	
Salmonella	
Group A streptococci	
Neisseria meningitidis	
Coccidioides immitis	
Rubella virus	

The incidence of invasive infections caused by Haemophilus influenzae *type b has diminished greatly with universal childhood Hib vaccination.*

EPIDEMIOLOGY

Infectious arthritis occurs most commonly in children younger than 5 years of age and adolescents.

CLINICAL MANIFESTATIONS

The typical features of suppurative arthritis include monoarticular involvement with erythema, warmth, swelling, and tenderness over the affected joint with a palpable effusion and markedly decreased range of movement secondary to pain. The onset may be sudden or insidious with symptoms noted only when the joint is moved, such as during a diaper change, or if parents become aware of decreased voluntary movement of a joint or limb. Toddlers may exhibit a limp or refuse to walk. In septic arthritis of the hip, the lower limb may be preferentially held in external rotation and flexion to minimize pain from pressure on the joint capsule. Similarly, the knee and elbow joints are usually held in flexion. The joints of the lower extremity are most often involved: knees (40%), hips (20%), and ankles (14%). Small joints, such as those of the hand, are usually involved after penetrating trauma or closed fist injuries.

Minor genital tract symptoms that have been ignored may precede development of the early arthritis-dermatitis syndrome associated with disseminated gonococcal infection. A history of febrile illness preceding the development of monoarticular arthritis characterizes late gonococcal arthritis.

Reactive arthritis is typically symmetric and polyarticular, and it usually involves the large joints, especially the hips. Patients may have had a preceding episode of gastroenteritis or urethritis. Urethritis may appear with the arthritis.

LABORATORY AND IMAGING STUDIES

Leukocytosis and elevated inflammatory markers such as C-reactive protein (CRP) or erythrocyte sedimentation rate (ESR) are common. Arthrocentesis is important to distinguish among the causes of arthritis (Table 119.2). Adolescents with acute infectious arthritis should have urethral, cervical, rectal, and pharyngeal examinations and cultures or nucleic acid amplification tests performed for *Neisseria gonorrhoeae.*

Either blood or joint cultures are positive in approximately 50% of cases. Joint fluid that exhibits the characteristics of pyogenic infection may not reveal bacterial pathogens, even in the absence of preceding antibiotic therapy because of the bacteriostatic effects of synovial fluid. Gram stain should be performed and is often informative even if the cultures are negative. PCR testing for *Kingella* is useful in culture-negative samples.

TABLE 119.2 Synovial Fluid Findings in Various Joint Diseases

CONDITION	APPEARANCE	WBC COUNT MM³/L (MEAN)	PMNS (%)	MUCIN CLOT	SYNOVIAL FLUID–BLOOD GLUCOSE DIFFERENCE (MG/DL)	COMMENTS
Normal	Clear, yellow	0–200 (200)*	<10	Good	No difference	—
Trauma	Clear, turbid, or hemorrhagic	50–4,000 (600)	<30	Good	No difference	Common in hemophilia
Systemic lupus erythematosus	Clear or slightly turbid	0–9,000 (3,000)	<20	Good to fair	No difference	LE cell positive, complement decreased
Juvenile idiopathic arthritis, reactive arthritis, inflammatory bowel disease	Turbid	250–80,000 (19,000)	>70	Poor	30	Decreased complement
Infectious pyogenic infection	Turbid	10,000–250,000 (80,000)	>90	Poor	50–90	Positive culture result, positive Gram stain
Tuberculosis	Turbid	2,500–100,000 (20,000)	>60	Poor	40–70	Positive results on culture, PPD or interferon-γ release assay testing, and acid-fast stain
Lyme arthritis	Turbid	500–100,000 (20,000)	>60	Poor	70	History of tick bite or erythema migrans and appropriate travel risk factors

*Average in parentheses.
LE, Lupus erythematosus; *PMN*, polymorphonuclear cell; *PPD*, purified protein derivative; *WBC*, white blood cell.

Ultrasound is especially helpful for identifying joint effusions and is the initial diagnostic procedure of choice for evaluating suppurative infections of the hip. Plain radiographs typically add little information to the physical findings. Radiographs may show joint capsule swelling, a widened joint space, and displacement of adjacent normal fat lines. Magnetic resonance imaging is helpful to confirm the diagnosis and exclude concurrent bone infection or deep abscesses.

DIFFERENTIAL DIAGNOSIS

The differential diagnosis of infectious arthritis in infants, children, and adolescents includes other infectious diseases, autoimmune disorders, rheumatic fever, malignancy, and trauma.

Suppurative arthritis must be distinguished from Lyme disease (Chapter 123), osteomyelitis, suppurative bursitis, fasciitis, myositis, cellulitis, and soft tissue abscesses. Psoas muscle abscess often presents with fever and pain on hip flexion and rotation. Juvenile idiopathic arthritis, Kawasaki syndrome, IgA vasculitis, other rheumatic disorders, and Crohn disease must be differentiated from infectious arthritis. In most of these diseases, the presence of symmetric or multiple joint involvement often excludes infectious arthritis. **Suppurative bursitis** with *Staphylococcus aureus* occurs most often in older males and is usually a consequence of trauma or, less commonly, a complication of bacteremia.

TREATMENT

Initial antibiotic therapy for infectious arthritis is based on the likely organism for the age of the child and the Gram stain of joint fluid. Suppurative arthritis of the hip joint or shoulder joint necessitates prompt surgical drainage. With insertion of the joint capsule below the epiphysis in these ball-and-socket joints, increased pressure in the joint space can adversely affect the vascular supply to the head of the femur or humerus, leading to avascular necrosis. Infections of the other joints may be treated with repeated arthrocenteses in addition to appropriate parenteral antibiotics.

Several antimicrobial agents provide adequate antibiotic levels in joint spaces (Table 119.3). Initial therapy for neonates should include antibiotics with activity against *S. aureus*, group B streptococcus, and aerobic gram-negative rods such as *E. coli*, based on local susceptibility patterns. Initial therapy for children 3 months to 5 years old should include antibiotics with

TABLE 119.3 Recommended Antibiotic Therapy for Infectious Arthritis in Children

AGE GROUP	COMMON PATHOGENS	RECOMMENDED TREATMENT*
Infants (<2 mo of age)	Group B streptococci	Ampicillin *plus* aminoglycoside
	Escherichia coli	Ceftazidime or ceftriaxone *with or without* aminoglycoside
	Klebsiella pneumoniae	Ceftazidime or ceftriaxone *with or without* aminoglycoside
	Staphylococcus aureus	Nafcillin (*or* oxacillin *or* cefazolin), *or* clindamycin *or* vancomycin
Older infants and children	*S. aureus*	Nafcillin (*or* oxacillin *or* cefazolin), *or* clindamycin *or* vancomycin *or* linezolid
	Streptococcus pneumoniae	Ampicillin *or* ceftriaxone *or* vancomycin *or* linezolid
	Group A streptococci	Penicillin G or ampicillin
	Kingella kingae	First or second generation cephalosporin or ampicillin-sulbactam
	Haemophilus influenzae type b†	Ampicillin *or* ceftriaxone
	Neisseria gonorrhoeae: disseminated gonococcal infection	Ceftriaxone

**Use the narrowest-spectrum agent available based on organism's susceptibilities.*
†The incidence of invasive infections caused by Haemophilus influenzae *type b has diminished greatly with universal childhood* Haemophilus influenzae *type b vaccination.*

activity against *S. aureus*. Confirmed methicillin-susceptible *S. aureus* infections are best treated with cefazolin, nafcillin, or oxacillin initially; methicillin-resistant *S. aureus* infections are best treated with clindamycin if susceptible, or vancomycin or linezolid otherwise.

The duration of therapy depends on clinical resolution of fever and pain and decline of the CRP. Duration of therapy can be as short as 10–14 days for patients with quick improvement on therapy; courses may need to be extended to 21 days or longer for those with slow symptom resolution or complicated disease. Treatment may be transitioned to oral antibiotics after initial improvement on IV therapy; first-line oral agents with excellent, narrow-spectrum activity against *S. aureus* include cephalexin and clindamycin. Amoxicillin-clavulanate and trimethoprim-sulfamethoxazole can also be used but may have spectra of activity broader than is required for this infection.

COMPLICATIONS AND PROGNOSIS

The prognosis for the common forms of infectious arthritis encountered in infants and children is excellent. The major complications of neonatal, childhood, and gonococcal arthritis are loss of joint function resulting from damage to the articular surface. The highest incidence of these complications occurs with hip and shoulder infections, presumably resulting from avascular necrosis, and in those with delay in therapy of 4 or more days from symptom onset. The high incidence of concurrent suppurative arthritis with adjacent osteomyelitis in neonates places the epiphyseal growth plate at high risk for growth abnormalities. Neonates with osteomyelitis have an approximately 40–50% likelihood of growth disturbances with loss of longitudinal bone growth and ultimate limb shortening.

PREVENTION

There are no effective means of preventing hematogenous *S. aureus* arthritis. Universal immunization of infants with conjugate Hib vaccine has practically eliminated serious bacterial infections from this organism, including bone and joint infections.

PEARLS FOR PRACTITIONERS

See Infectious Diseases: Pearls for Practitioners at the end of this section.

REVIEW QUESTIONS

Available online.

CHAPTER 120

Ocular Infections

ETIOLOGY

Acute conjunctivitis is usually a viral or bacterial infection of the eye characterized by a rapid onset of symptoms that persist for a few days. Nontypable *Haemophilus influenzae, Streptococcus pneumoniae, Staphylococcus aureus,* and *Moraxella catarrhalis* account for approximately two thirds of bacterial causes (Table 120.1). Other causes include *Neisseria gonorrhoeae* and *Pseudomonas aeruginosa*; the latter is associated with extended-wear soft contact lenses. *Bartonella henselae* can cause granulomatous conjunctivitis associated with preauricular lymphadenopathy or **Parinaud oculoglandular syndrome.** Viral conjunctivitis most commonly is caused by adenoviruses, which cause **epidemic keratoconjunctivitis**, and less frequently by coxsackieviruses and other enteroviruses. **Keratitis**, or inflammation of the cornea, is not commonly associated with conjunctivitis but occurs with *N. gonorrhoeae,* herpes simplex virus (HSV), and adenovirus infections.

Neonatal conjunctivitis, or **ophthalmia neonatorum**, is purulent conjunctivitis during the first month of life, usually acquired during birth. The common causes of neonatal conjunctivitis, in order of decreasing prevalence, are chemical conjunctivitis secondary to antibiotic gonococcal prophylaxis, *Chlamydia trachomatis, Staphylococcus aureus, Escherichia coli,* other gram-negative enteric bacilli, HSV, and *N. gonorrhoeae.*

EPIDEMIOLOGY

Conjunctivitis is common in young children, especially if they come in contact with other children with conjunctivitis. Predisposing factors for bacterial infection include nasolacrimal duct obstruction, sinus disease, ear infection, and allergic disease when children rub their eyes frequently. Conjunctivitis occurs in 1–12% of neonates. Approximately 50% of infants born vaginally to infected mothers have neonatal acquisition of *C. trachomatis,* with which the risk of chlamydial conjunctivitis **(inclusion conjunctivitis)** is 25–50%.

CLINICAL MANIFESTATIONS

Symptoms of ocular infection include redness, discharge, matted eyelids, and mild photophobia. Physical examination findings include chemosis, injection of the conjunctiva, and edema of the eyelids. Corneal involvement suggests gonococcal or herpetic infection. Herpetic corneal lesions appear as dendritic or ameboid ulcers or, more commonly in recurrent infection, as a deep keratitis. Unilateral conjunctivitis with ipsilateral otitis media is often caused by nontypable *H. influenzae.*

The timing and manifestations of neonatal conjunctivitis are helpful in identifying the cause (Table 120.2). *N. gonorrhoeae* causes severe conjunctivitis with profuse purulent discharge. Chlamydial conjunctivitis usually occurs in the second week of life but may appear 3 days to 6 weeks after delivery. There is mild to moderate inflammation with purulent discharge issuing from one or both eyes.

LABORATORY AND IMAGING STUDIES

Cultures are not routinely obtained because bacterial conjunctivitis is usually self-limited or responds quickly to topical antibiotic treatment. If gonococcal conjunctivitis is suspected, especially in neonates, Gram stain and culture must be obtained. In these infants, blood and other sites of infection (such as cerebrospinal fluid) should also be cultured. Additional testing for *Chlamydia,* HIV, and syphilis should be performed on the mother and infant as necessary.

DIFFERENTIAL DIAGNOSIS

Distinguishing bacterial from viral conjunctivitis by presentation and appearance is difficult (see Table 120.1). Vesicular lid lesions, if present, suggest HSV. **Hyperpurulent conjunctivitis** characterized by reaccumulation of purulent discharge within minutes is characteristic of *N. gonorrhoeae* infection. The differential diagnosis is delineated in Table 120.3.

Blepharitis is associated with staphylococcal infections, seborrhea, and meibomian gland dysfunction. The child complains

TABLE 120.1 Manifestations of Acute Conjunctivitis in Children

	CLINICAL CHARACTERISTICS	
FEATURE	**BACTERIAL**	**VIRAL**
Common pathogens	*Haemophilus influenzae* (usually nontypable)	Adenoviruses types 8, 19
	Streptococcus pneumoniae	Enteroviruses
	Moraxella catarrhalis	Herpes simplex virus
Incubation	24–72 hr	1–14 days
SYMPTOMS		
Photophobia	Mild	Moderate to severe
Blurred vision	Common with discharge	If keratitis is present
Foreign body sensation	Unusual	Yes
SIGNS		
Discharge	Purulent discharge	Mucoid/serous discharge
Palpebral reaction	Papillary response	Follicular response
Preauricular lymph node	Unusual for acute (<10%)	More common (20%)
Chemosis	Moderate	Mild
Hemorrhagic conjunctivae	Occasionally with pneumococcus or *Haemophilus* sp.	Frequent with enteroviruses
Treatment (topical)	Polymyxin B–trimethoprim *or* erythromycin or ofloxacin or ciprofloxacin	Adenovirus: self-limited Herpes simplex virus: trifluridine 1% solution *or* ganciclovir 0.15% gel *or* acyclovir; ophthalmologic consultation
End of contagious period	24 hr after start of effective treatment	Varies by pathogen

TABLE 120.2 Clinical Manifestations and Treatment of Neonatal Conjunctivitis

ETIOLOGIC AGENT	CASES (%)	DISCHARGE AND EXTERNAL EXAMINATION	TYPICAL AGE AT ONSET	DIAGNOSIS	ASSOCIATED MANIFESTATIONS	TREATMENT
Chemical: silver nitrate	Variable (1%), depending on use of silver nitrate	Watery discharge	1–3 days	No organisms on smear or culture	None	None
Chlamydia trachomatis (inclusion conjunctivitis)	2–40	Scant discharge; mild swelling; hyperemia; follicular response; late corneal staining	4–19 days	Test of discharge with a DFA or PCR assay	May precede *C. trachomatis* pneumonia (at 3 wk to 3 mo of age)	Recommended: Erythromycin (oral) Alternate: azithromycin
Bacterial: *Staphylococcus, Streptococcus, Pseudomonas, E. coli*	30–50	Purulent moderate discharge; mild lid and conjunctival swelling; corneal involvement with risk for perforation	2–7 days	Gram stain; culture on blood agar		Topical therapy
Neisseria gonorrhoeae	<1	Copious, purulent discharge; swelling of lids and conjunctivae; corneal involvement common; risk for perforation and corneal scar	1–7 days	Gram stain (gram-negative intracellular diplococci); culture on chocolate agar. Culture other sites including blood and CSF	May be associated with severe disseminated gonococcal infection	Ceftriaxone Hospitalize patient
HSV	<1	Clear or serosanguineous discharge; lid swelling; keratitis with cloudy cornea; dendrite formation	3 days to 3 wk	Viral culture; DFA test, PCR assay	May be associated with disseminated perinatal HSV infection	Acyclovir (intravenous) and topical trifluridine or ganciclovir

CSF, Cerebrospinal fluid; *DFA*, direct fluorescent antibody; *HSV*, herpes simplex virus; *PCR*, polymerase chain reaction.

of photophobia, burning, irritation, and a foreign body sensation that causes the child to rub the eyes. Eyelid hygiene with an **eyelid scrub** routine is the initial step in treatment.

Hordeola are acute suppurative nodular inflammatory lesions of the eyelids associated with pain and redness. **External hordeola** or **styes** occur on the anterior eyelid, in the Zeis glands, or in the lash follicles and usually are caused by staphylococci. **Internal hordeola** occur in the meibomian glands and may be infected with staphylococci or may be sterile. If the meibomian gland becomes obstructed, the gland secretions accumulate, and a **chalazion** develops. Hordeola usually respond spontaneously to local treatment measures but may recur.

Dacryocystitis is an infection or inflammation of the lacrimal sac, which is usually obstructed, and is commonly caused by *Staphylococcus aureus* or coagulase-negative staphylococci. A mucopurulent discharge can be expressed with gentle pressure on the nasolacrimal sac. Treatment usually requires probing of the nasolacrimal system to establish communication.

Endophthalmitis is an emergent, sight-threatening infection that usually follows trauma, surgery, or hematogenous spread from a distant focus. Causative organisms include coagulase-negative staphylococci, *S. aureus, S. pneumoniae, Bacillus cereus,* and *Candida albicans.* Examination is difficult because of severe blepharospasm and extreme photophobia. A **hypopyon** and haze in the anterior chamber may be visible on examination.

TREATMENT

The lids should be treated as needed with warm compresses to remove accumulated discharge. Acute bacterial conjunctivitis is frequently self-limited. Topical antibiotics may modestly hasten resolution but are generally not recommended in otherwise healthy patients that do not wear contact lenses. Antibiotics are instilled between the eyelids four times a day until the discharge and chemosis subside. Recommended treatment includes topical trimethoprim-polymyxin B solution or erythromycin ointment (see Table 120.1). Ciprofloxacin solution should be restricted to corneal infections and resistant gram-negative infections in hospitalized patients. Gonococcal conjunctivitis in adolescents and adults is treated with a single IM dose of ceftriaxone (1 g).

The treatment of **ophthalmia neonatorum** depends on the cause (see Table 120.2). Gonococcal ophthalmia neonatorum is treated with a single dose of ceftriaxone (25–50 mg/kg IV or IM; maximum dose 250 mg). These infants should be hospitalized. Antibiotic treatment also is recommended for infants born to mothers with untreated gonorrhea. Chlamydial

TABLE 120.3 Differential Diagnosis of Ocular Infections

CONDITION	ETIOLOGIC AGENTS	SIGNS AND SYMPTOMS	TREATMENT
Bacterial conjunctivitis	*Haemophilus influenzae, Haemophilus aegyptius, Streptococcus pneumoniae, Neisseria gonorrhoeae*	Mucopurulent unilateral or bilateral discharge, normal vision, photophobia, conjunctival injection and edema (chemosis); gritty sensation	Topical antibiotics, parenteral ceftriaxone for gonococcus
Viral conjunctivitis	Adenovirus, echovirus, coxsackievirus	Same as for bacterial infection; may be hemorrhagic, unilateral	Self-limited
Neonatal conjunctivitis	*Chlamydia trachomatis,* gonococcus, chemical (silver nitrate), *Staphylococcus aureus,* HSV	Palpebral conjunctival follicle or papillae; same as for bacterial infection	Ceftriaxone for gonococcus and oral erythromycin for *C. trachomatis* (HSV; see Table 120.2)
Allergic conjunctivitis	Seasonal pollens or allergen exposure	Itching, incidence of bilateral chemosis (edema) greater than that of erythema, tarsal papillae	Antihistamines, steroids, cromolyn
Keratitis	Herpes simplex, adenovirus, *S. pneumoniae, S. aureus, Pseudomonas, Acanthamoeba,* chemicals	Severe pain, corneal swelling, clouding, limbus erythema, hypopyon, cataracts; contact lens history with amebic infection	Specific antibiotics for bacterial/fungal infections; keratoplasty, acyclovir for herpes
Endophthalmitis	*S. aureus, S. pneumoniae, Candida albicans,* associated surgery or trauma	Acute onset, pain, loss of vision, swelling, chemosis, redness; hypopyon and vitreous haze	Specific antibiotics for bacterial/fungal infections
Anterior uveitis (iridocyclitis)	JIA, reactive arthritis, sarcoidosis, Behçet disease, inflammatory bowel disease	Unilateral/bilateral; erythema, ciliary flush, irregular pupil, iris adhesions; pain, photophobia, small pupil, poor vision	Topical steroids, plus therapy for primary disease
Posterior uveitis (choroiditis)	Toxoplasmosis, histoplasmosis, *Toxocara canis*	No signs of erythema, decreased vision	Specific therapy for pathogen
Episcleritis/scleritis	Idiopathic autoimmune disease (e.g., SLE, IgA vasculitis)	Localized pain, intense erythema, unilateral; blood vessels bigger than in conjunctivitis; scleritis may cause globe perforation	Episcleritis is self-limiting; topical steroids for fast relief
Foreign body	Occupational or other exposure	Unilateral, red, gritty feeling; visible or microscopic size	Irrigation, removal; check for ulceration
Blepharitis	*S. aureus, Staphylococcus epidermidis,* seborrheic, blocked lacrimal duct; rarely molluscum contagiosum, *Pthirus pubis, Pediculus capitis*	Bilateral, irritation, itching, hyperemia, crusting, affecting lid margins	Topical antibiotics, warm compresses
Dacryocystitis	Obstructed lacrimal sac: *S. aureus, H. influenzae, S. pneumoniae*	Pain, tenderness, erythema, and exudate in areas of lacrimal sac (inferomedial to inner canthus); tearing (epiphora); possible orbital cellulitis	Systemic, topical antibiotics; surgical drainage
Dacryoadenitis	*S. aureus, S. pneumoniae,* CMV, measles, EBV, enteroviruses; trauma, sarcoidosis, leukemia	Pain, tenderness, edema, erythema over gland area (upper temporal lid); fever, leukocytosis	Systemic antibiotics; drainage of orbital abscesses
Orbital cellulitis (postseptal cellulitis)	Paranasal sinusitis: *S. anginosus, S. aureus, S. pneumoniae, H. influenzae,* other streptococci Trauma: *S. aureus* Fungi: *Aspergillus, Mucor* if immunodeficient	Rhinorrhea, chemosis, vision loss, painful extraocular motion, proptosis, ophthalmoplegia, fever, lid edema, leukocytosis	Systemic antibiotics; drainage of orbital abscesses

(Continued)

TABLE 120.3 Differential Diagnosis of Ocular Infections—cont'd

CONDITION	ETIOLOGIC AGENTS	SIGNS AND SYMPTOMS	TREATMENT
Periorbital cellulitis (preseptal cellulitis)	Direct skin inoculation or trauma: *S. aureus, S. pyogenes* Adjacent sinusitis: *S. pneumoniae, H. influenzae, M. catarrhalis* Bacteremia (rare): *S. pyogenes*	Cutaneous erythema, warmth, normal vision, minimal involvement of orbit; fever, leukocytosis, toxic appearance	Systemic antibiotics

CMV, Cytomegalovirus; *EBV*, Epstein-Barr virus; *HSV*, herpes simplex virus; *Ig*, immunoglobulin; *JIA*, juvenile idiopathic arthritis; *SLE*, systemic lupus erythematosus.

conjunctivitis is treated with oral erythromycin for 14 days, partly to reduce the risk of subsequent chlamydial pneumonia.

COMPLICATIONS AND PROGNOSIS

The prognosis for bacterial and viral conjunctivitis is excellent. The major complication is keratitis, which can lead to ulcerations and perforation, and is uncommon except with *N. gonorrhoeae* and HSV infections. Chlamydial conjunctivitis may progress in infants to chlamydial pneumonia, which typically develops from 2–18 weeks of age (see Chapter 111).

PREVENTION

Careful handwashing is important to prevent the spread of conjunctivitis. Decreased transmission of bacterial conjunctivitis has not been demonstrated with the use of antibiotics. Further, the American Academy of Pediatrics advises against requiring antibiotics prior to returning to school or child care.

All newborns, whether delivered vaginally or by cesarean section, should receive prophylaxis for gonococcal ophthalmia neonatorum as soon as possible after delivery. A single application of erythromycin 0.5% ointment is used most often; an alternative method is tetracycline 1% ointment, which is equally effective. Erythromycin ointment does not prevent chlamydial ophthalmia.

PEARLS FOR PRACTITIONERS

See Infectious Diseases: Pearls for Practitioners at the end of this section.

REVIEW QUESTIONS

Available online.

CHAPTER 121

Infection in the Immunocompromised Person

See also Section 13 (Immunology).

ETIOLOGY

Many diseases or their treatments adversely affect the immune system, including primary immunodeficiencies, HIV infection and AIDS, cancer, stem cell and organ transplantation, and immunosuppressive drugs used to treat cancer and autoimmune diseases. These patients are at significant risk of life-threatening infections from invasive bacterial or fungal flora of the oropharynx, skin, and gastrointestinal tract; acquisition of exogenous infection from infected persons or the environment; and reactivation of latent infections until their immune function recovers (Table 121.1).

The infections seen in immunocompromised persons can often be predicted by which component of the immune system is abnormal. Episodes of fever and **neutropenia**, commonly defined as an **absolute neutrophil count (ANC)** of less than 500/mm^3, are especially common in patients with cancer and transplant recipients and increase the risk for bacterial and fungal infections. The use of **corticosteroids** and potent immunosuppressive drugs that impair the activation of T lymphocytes increases the risk for pathogens normally controlled by T-cell–mediated responses, such as *Pneumocystis jirovecii* and *Toxoplasma gondii,* as well as intracellular pathogens, such as *Salmonella, Listeria,* and *Mycobacterium.* Lymphopenia also increases the risk of viral infections, due to either primary acquisition or reactivation of latent infection.

Immunocompromised patients may also have increased risk for bacterial infection due to the presence of central indwelling catheters. Organisms most isolated in this case include coagulase-negative staphylococci, *S. aureus,* gram-negative bacteria, *Enterococcus,* and *Candida* (see Chapter 122).

Fungal pathogens account for approximately 10% of all infections associated with childhood cancer. *Candida* species are the most common cause of all fungal infections, with *Aspergillus* species being the second most common pathogen. Risk factors for fungal infections include oropharyngeal and gastrointestinal mucositis facilitating systemic fungal invasion, presence of long-term indwelling intravascular catheters, parenteral nutrition, hyperglycemia, extreme prematurity, and broad-spectrum antibacterial therapy that promotes fungal colonization as a precursor to infection.

Infection with *T. gondii* represents reactivation of quiescent infection facilitated by cancer-associated or therapy-associated cellular immunodeficiency. *P. jirovecii* primarily causes pneumonitis in patients with cancer or HIV or those who are posttransplantation or on long-term corticosteroids.

Viral opportunistic infections in patients with cancer usually represent symptomatic reactivation from latency facilitated by cancer or therapy-associated cellular immunodeficiency. Herpes simplex virus (HSV) can cause severe and prolonged mucocutaneous infection or disseminated disease. Cytomegalovirus (CMV) can also cause focal or systemic disease in immunocompromised persons, especially in

TABLE 121.1 Immunodeficiencies and Associated Prevalent Pathogens

DEFECT	PATHOGEN
Neutropenia	**GRAM-POSITIVE COCCI**
	Staphylococcus aureus Coagulase-negative staphylococci (*S. epidermidis, S. haemolyticus, S. hominis*) Viridans group streptococci (*S. mitis, S. oralis*) *Granulicatella* and *Abiotrophia* spp. (formerly nutritionally variant streptococci) Enterococci (*E. faecalis, E. faecium*)
	GRAM-NEGATIVE BACILLI
	Escherichia coli *Pseudomonas aeruginosa* *Klebsiella pneumoniae* *Enterobacter* and *Citrobacter* spp.
	FUNGI
	Candida sp. *Aspergillus* sp. *Zygomycetes*
Damaged integument	
Skin and central venous catheter related	Coagulase-negative staphylococci (*S. epidermidis, S. haemolyticus, S. hominis*) *Staphylococcus aureus* *Stenotrophomonas maltophilia* *Pseudomonas aeruginosa* *Acinetobacter* spp. Corynebacteria *Candida* spp. (*C. albicans, C. parapsilosis*)
Oral mucositis	Viridans group streptococci (*S. mitis, S. oralis*) *Abiotrophia* and *Granulicatella* spp. (nutritionally variant streptococci) *Capnocytophaga* spp. *Fusobacterium* spp. *Rothia mucilaginosa* *Candida* spp. (*C. albicans, C. tropicalis, C. glabrata*) Herpes simplex virus
Gut mucosal barrier injury	*Escherichia coli* *Pseudomonas aeruginosa* Coagulase-negative staphylococci Enterococci (*E. faecalis, E. faecium*) *Candida* spp. Viridans-group streptococci (*S. oralis, mitis*)
Neutropenic enterocolitis	*Clostridium* spp. (*C. septicum, C. tertium*) *Staphylococcus aureus* *Pseudomonas aeruginosa*
Impaired cellular immunity	Herpesviruses (HSV, VZV, EBV, CMV) Adenovirus *Listeria monocytogenes* *Nocardia* spp. *Salmonella* sp. *Mycobacterium tuberculosis* Nontuberculous mycobacteria *Pneumocystis jirovecii* *Aspergillus* spp. *Candida* sp. *Cryptococcus* spp. *Histoplasma capsulatum* *Coccidioides* spp. *Toxoplasma gondii*
Impaired humoral immunity	*Streptococcus pneumoniae* *Haemophilus influenzae* Norovirus Hepatitis B virus Polyoma virus (JC) *Campylobacter/Helicobacter*
COMPROMISED ORGAN FUNCTION	
Splenectomy	*Streptococcus pneumoniae* *Haemophilus influenzae* *Neisseria meningitidis* *Capnocytophaga canamorsus* Babesiosis

From Blijlevens NMA, van der Velden WJFM. Infections in the immunocompromised host: general principles. In: Mandell GL, Bennett JE, Dolin R, eds. Mandell, Douglas, and Bennett's Principles and Practice of Infectious Diseases. *9th ed. Philadelphia: Elsevier; 2020:3617, table 305.1.*

transplant recipients. Manifestations of CMV disease include retinitis, hepatitis, pneumonitis, esophagitis, encephalitis, and colitis. Reactivation of Epstein-Barr virus (EBV) is associated with **posttransplant lymphoproliferative disorder (PTLD)**. Varicella-zoster virus (VZV) can cause serious primary infection in susceptible persons, sometimes with accompanying encephalitis, hepatitis, or pneumonitis. VZV can also reactivate as shingles during chemotherapy and may cause disseminated infection.

EPIDEMIOLOGY

Chemotherapeutic agents target rapidly dividing cells, especially myeloproliferative cells, which causes myelosuppression. Children receiving allogeneic stem cell (bone marrow) transplants are at greater risk for infection than children receiving autologous transplants. Prolonged time to hematologic engraftment is a significant risk factor for infection in these patients (Fig. 121.1). Foreign bodies (shunts, central venous catheters) and mucositis interfere with cutaneous barriers against infection and, together with neutropenia and/or lymphopenia, increase the risk of bacterial or fungal infections. Multiple antimicrobial exposures put these patients at risk for resistant bacterial, fungal, and viral infections.

Infections are both more frequent and more severe in immunocompromised patients and are a significant contributor to cancer-related deaths. The most frequently infected sites are the respiratory tract (lung, sinuses), the bloodstream, surgical wounds, and the urinary tract.

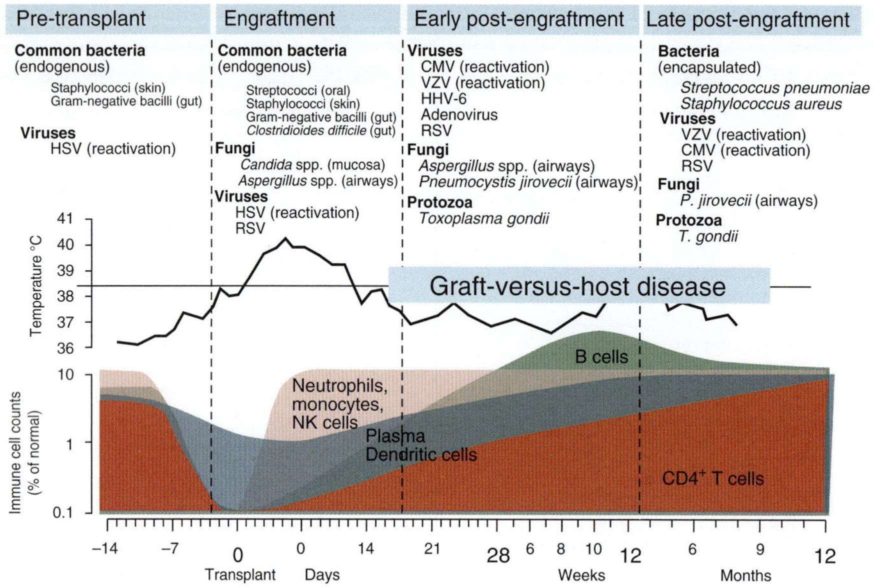

FIGURE 121.1 Infectious phases after transplant. The infectious complications that occur most commonly are set against the phases before and after an allogeneic hematopoietic stem cell transplant. Note the timescale progresses from days to weeks and then to months. The fluctuations in the different components of the immune system are represented at the bottom of the figure and show when severe deficiency coincides with the time of engraftment and begins to recover thereafter. The various classes of microorganism change during the different phases, but note that viruses and fungi can cause infections throughout the entire period. *CMV,* Cytomegalovirus; *HHV-6,* human herpesvirus 6; *HSV,* herpes simplex virus; *NK,* natural killer; *RSV,* respiratory syncytial virus; *VZV,* varicella-zoster virus. (From Blijlevens NMA, van der Velden WJFM. Infections in the immunocompromised host: general principles. In: Bennett JE, Dolin R, Blaser MJ, eds. *Mandell, Douglas, and Bennett's Principles and Practice of Infectious Diseases.* 9th ed. Philadelphia: Elsevier; 2020:fig. 305.5.)

CLINICAL MANIFESTATIONS

Fever is the most common, and sometimes the only, presenting symptom of serious infection in cancer and transplant patients. The presence of *fever with neutropenia,* even in the absence of other signs or symptoms, demands prompt evaluation and empiric antimicrobial therapy because of the potential for life-threatening infection. All symptoms and signs should be evaluated thoroughly. However, some symptoms may be absent based on the underlying immunodeficiency and in the absence of neutrophils to induce localized signs of inflammation; determination of the source of infection by physical examination is often difficult. For instance, chest findings may be absent, despite pneumonia, and revealed only by chest radiograph at presentation or when the neutrophil count recovers.

LABORATORY TESTS AND IMAGING

Evaluation of fever and neutropenia in immunocompromised persons requires comprehensive evaluation including detailed physical examination and screening for symptoms. Blood cultures for bacterial and fungal pathogens should be obtained by peripheral venipuncture and from all lumens of any indwelling vascular catheters (Table 121.2). A complete blood count with manual differential, C-reactive protein, culture of urine, and Gram staining/culture of potential sites of specific infection should be performed. Chest radiographs are important to assess for the presence of pulmonary infiltrates. Specialized imaging studies, such as CT or MRI, can be useful in selected cases, such as with suspected sinusitis or intraabdominal infection, or to further delineate the location and extent of abnormalities seen on plain radiographs. Sinus infection with bacteria, *Aspergillus,* or Zygomycetes is common in neutropenic hosts and may be detected only on the CT scan. Further investigation with bronchoscopy or sinus scope may be required if imaging is suspicious for infection. Viruses can be detected in blood, respiratory samples, urine, stool, cerebrospinal fluid, and skin lesions by polymerase chain reaction.

TABLE 121.2 Initial Diagnostic Evaluation of Children With Fever and Neutropenia

- Careful medical history
- Physical examination with attention to the skin, perirectal area, and other mucosal sites (which should be repeated at least daily in febrile neutropenic patients)
- Specimens for culture
  - Blood: peripheral venipuncture and specimens from every lumen or access port of intravascular catheters
  - Urine
  - Respiratory secretions: for bacteria and viruses if symptoms are present
  - Any site with clinical signs of infection, including *C. difficile* toxin assay if diarrhea present and cerebral spinal fluid if headache, meningismus, or mental status change
- Chest imaging
- Other imaging studies or diagnostic procedures as clinically indicated
  - Sinus radiograph or CT
  - Abdominal ultrasonography or CT
  - Head CT or magnetic resonance imaging with contrast

Modified from Ardura MI, Koh AY. Risk factors and infectious agents in children with cancer: Fever and granulocytopenia. In: Long SS, Prober CG, Fischer M, eds. Principles and Practice of Pediatric Infectious Diseases. *6th ed. Philadelphia: Elsevier; 2023:97, box 97.1.*

DIFFERENTIAL DIAGNOSIS

Initially, the patient should have a complete physical examination, including careful scrutiny of the oropharynx, nares, external auditory canals, skin and axilla, groin, perineum, and rectal area. The exit site and subcutaneous tunnel of any indwelling vascular catheter should be examined closely for erythema and palpated for tenderness and expression of purulent material. Perirectal abscess is a potentially serious infection in neutropenic hosts, with tenderness being the only clue on examination. Any presumptive infection identified during the evaluation should direct appropriate cultures and tailor antiinfective therapy.

TREATMENT

Treatment should be provided as appropriate for focal infections identified by physical examination or diagnostic imaging. Select *low-risk* patients may be managed as outpatients and/or with enteral antibiotics. Empirical treatment of fever and neutropenia without an identified source should include an extended-spectrum penicillin or cephalosporin with activity against gram-negative bacilli, including *P. aeruginosa.* If the patient has an indwelling vascular catheter and is ill-appearing, vancomycin or linezolid may be added because of the risk of methicillin-resistant *S. aureus* (MRSA) but can be discontinued if *S. aureus* is not cultured after 48 hours. Specific antibiotic regimens should be guided by local antibiotic resistance patterns at each institution.

If no microbiologic cause is isolated, empirical broad-spectrum antibiotics are generally continued as long as the patient remains neutropenic, regardless of whether the fever resolves. Studies are ongoing to understand the safety of potentially stopping therapy prior to resolution of neutropenia if no infection is identified and the patient remains clinically well. Antimicrobial and diagnostic stewardship strategies are important to balance against the risk of severe infection in these patients. Antimicrobial therapy should be modified as indicated by new findings or if the patient's clinical status deteriorates. Further investigation for fungal infection and empirical treatment with antifungal agents is instituted in patients who have neutropenia and persistent fever without a focus, despite broad-spectrum antibacterial therapy after approximately 5 days.

PREVENTION

Current guidelines discourage the use of broad-spectrum *prophylactic* antibiotics to prevent fever and neutropenia because of lack of efficacy and concerns about development of antibiotic resistance, although in some specific high-risk populations, prophylaxis may be utilized in the setting of prolonged neutropenia. Administration of trimethoprim-sulfamethoxazole or an alternate agent to prevent *P. jirovecii* infection is routine for patients undergoing intensive chemotherapy or immunosuppression for transplantation. Prophylaxis against *P. jirovecii* generally starts with initiation of chemotherapy and continues until 6 months after it has been completed. In select populations, such as patients undergoing hematopoietic stem cell transplantation, prophylactic antifungals such as fluconazole or mold-acting agents, such as voriconazole or posaconazole, are beneficial. Patients at risk for viral reactivation with HSV, VZV, and/or CMV may be placed on antiviral prophylaxis with acyclovir or ganciclovir. Immunocompromised susceptible persons exposed to chickenpox within 2 days before the onset of rash until 5 days after the onset of rash in the index case should receive varicella-zoster immune globulin (VZIG). Infection after VZIG may not result in protective immunity, and persons who receive VZIG prophylaxis should be considered still at risk with any subsequent exposures.

An evaluation for infectious risks specific to an individual patient can be very useful prior to performing hematopoietic cell transplantation, solid organ transplantation, and cellular immunotherapy. This allows for tailored prophylactic strategies, vaccination planning, and infection prevention guidance for both the patient and their family.

PEARLS FOR PRACTITIONERS

See Infectious Diseases: Pearls for Practitioners at the end of this section.

REVIEW QUESTIONS

Available online.

CHAPTER 122

Health Care–Associated Infections

Infections are a common and important complication of indwelling medical devices and are a major part of health care–associated infections.

VASCULAR DEVICE INFECTIONS

Vascular catheters are inserted in many inpatients and are sometimes used for outpatients. The use of catheters for long-term access to the bloodstream has been an important advance for the care of people who require parenteral nutrition, chemotherapy, or extended parenteral antibiotic therapy. The major complication of such catheters is infection. Short, peripheral IV catheters used for short-term access in stable patients are associated with a low rate of infection, especially in children. **Peripherally inserted central catheters (PICC)** are commonly used for medium-term venous access. **Central venous catheters** are commonly placed for extended vascular access, such as for chemotherapy, using tunneled silicone elastomer catheters (**Broviac** or **Hickman catheters**) that are surgically inserted into a central vein, passed through a subcutaneous tunnel before exiting the skin, and anchored by a subcutaneous cuff. Contamination of the catheter hub or any connection of the IV tubing is common and is a major predisposition to catheter-associated infection. Totally implanted venous access systems **(Port-a-Cath, Infuse-a-Port)** have a silicone elastomer catheter tunneled beneath the skin to a reservoir implanted in a subcutaneous pocket. Implanted catheters or ports decrease, but do not eliminate, the opportunity for microbial entry at the skin site.

Catheter-related thrombosis and catheter-related infection can develop separately or together. Ultrasound can identify thrombi, but infection can only be identified by culture. **Thrombophlebitis** is inflammation with thrombosis in a blood vessel. **Septic thrombophlebitis** is thrombosis with organisms embedded in the clot. **Central line–associated bloodstream infection (CLABSI)** implies isolation of the same organism from a catheter and from peripheral blood of a patient with clinical symptoms of bacteremia and no other apparent source of infection. Confirmation requires quantitative colony counts of both samples, which is not routinely performed. Possible sources of the bacteremia include the infusate, contamination via tubing and catheter connections, or transient bacteremia seeding the catheter, which may or may not be clinically apparent. Infection may be associated with an **exit site infection** limited to the insertion site or may extend along the catheter tunnel of buried catheters to cause a **tunnel infection**. Given the proximity of central venous catheters to cardiac valves, persistent central infections can also be complicated by endocarditis. An echocardiogram should be considered in patients with persistent bacteremia related to a central line (see Chapter 112).

Many microorganisms cause catheter-related infections (Table 122.1). Gram-positive cocci, primarily staphylococci, cause more than 50% of CLABSIs and exit site infections. Other skin flora, such as coagulase-negative staphylococci, diphtheroids, and *Bacillus,* are often involved. Gram-negative organisms also commonly cause infection. Polymicrobial infections of central venous catheters are common. Fungal catheter infections, usually *Candida* species, are most common among persons receiving broad-spectrum antibiotics or parenteral nutrition.

Risk factors for CLABSI include prematurity, burns, and skin disorders that adversely affect the skin integrity, neutropenia, and other immunodeficiencies (see Chapter 121). Infection rates are lower for tunneled and implanted catheters. Catheters inserted in emergency settings are more likely to be infected than catheters placed electively.

Clinical signs of catheter-associated bacteremia or fungemia range from mild fever to overwhelming sepsis. Infection at the site of the central catheter entrance is manifested as a localized cellulitis with warmth, tenderness, swelling, erythema, and discharge. Tunnel infection is manifested by similar findings along the tunnel route. Thrombophlebitis is classically manifested as a warm, erythematous, tender palpable cord originating at the IV catheter site but may be subclinical or manifested only by persistent fever without signs of local inflammation.

TABLE **122.1** Organisms Causing Catheter-Related Infections

CLASSIFICATION OF PATHOGEN	COMMON	UNCOMMON
Gram-positive organisms	Coagulase-negative staphylococci, *Staphylococcus aureus, Enterococcus*	Diphtheroids, *Bacillus, Lactobacillus, Micrococcus*
Gram-negative organisms	*Escherichia coli, Klebsiella, Pseudomonas aeruginosa*	*Acinetobacter, Enterobacter, Neisseria*
Fungi	*Candida* sp.	*Malassezia furfur*
Miscellaneous		Nontuberculous mycobacteria

The treatment of catheter-related infection depends on the site of the infection and the pathogen involved. CLABSI is optimally treated with catheter removal; however, in a stable patient or with certain organisms, antibiotic therapy alone may suffice. Infection with organisms of low virulence may be manifested by fever alone, and removal of the catheter frequently is followed by prompt defervescence and complete resolution of infection. Empirical initial therapy for suspected infection should generally include antibiotics active against gram-negative organisms and against *S. aureus* and coagulase-negative staphylococci, such as a broad-spectrum cephalosporin in combination with vancomycin or linezolid. Subsequently, antibiotic regimens should be tailored to the specific organism identified. If the patient is not critically ill and the pathogen is a lower virulence organism, a trial of antibiotics given through the infected catheter can be considered. Catheter removal is indicated with sepsis, septic thrombophlebitis, clinical deterioration (despite appropriate therapy), persistently positive blood culture results after 48–72 hours of appropriate antimicrobial therapy, embolic lesions, or fungal infection because of poor response to antifungal therapy alone. Catheter removal is also recommended for infection with *Staphylococcus aureus* and *Pseudomonas aeruginosa.* Infection of the pocket around an implanted port is unlikely to respond to antibiotics alone, and removal of the foreign body is usually necessary.

The total duration of therapy is variable depending on the pathogen, line retainment or removal, and the duration of positive cultures. For example, coagulase negative staphylococci can be treated for ranges of 3–7 days, depending on line removal. Other pathogens may require longer durations of up to 10–14 days after sterilization of the bloodstream (or longer for cases of complicated or disseminated infection).

Antibiotic-lock therapy is a method of sterilizing intravascular catheters by using high concentrations of antibiotics or ethanol infused into the portion of the catheter between the hub and the vessel entry. The solution is allowed to dwell within the catheter segment for several hours. It may be useful for treatment of catheter-associated infections in which line salvage is desired and/or for prevention of infection in patients at high risk.

Aseptic technique is essential during catheter insertion. Catheters that are placed during emergency situations should be replaced as soon as medically feasible. Care of indwelling catheters involves meticulous attention to sterile technique whenever the system is entered. Care of the catheter entry site commonly involves a topical antibiotic or disinfectant. Catheters that are no longer necessary should be removed.

VENTILATOR-ASSOCIATED PNEUMONIA

Intubation of the airway provides direct access to the lungs and bypasses normal host defenses. Organisms enter the lungs directly through the lumen of the tube or by descending around the tube, which may result in **ventilator-associated pneumonia**. Contaminated respiratory equipment, humidification systems, or condensate introduces bacteria directly into lower airways. The continuously open upper airway increases the risk of aspiration of oropharyngeal flora and reflux of gastric contents and interferes with clearance of the airway because an effective cough requires a closed glottis.

URINARY CATHETERS

The most important risk factors for urinary tract infections (UTIs) are the presence of catheters, instrumentation, and anatomic abnormalities (see Chapter 115). Organisms enter the bladder through the catheter by instillation of contaminated irrigation fluids, backflow of contaminated urine from the drainage bag, or ascent of bacteria around the meatus along the outside of the catheter. Indwelling catheters facilitate direct access to the bladder and should have a closed drainage system. After simple, straight catheterization, the incidence of UTI is 1–2%. Organisms that cause catheter associated UTIs include fecal flora, such as gram-negative enteric bacilli, most commonly *Escherichia coli* and *Klebsiella* species. With concomitant antibiotic treatment, resistant organisms can predominate, and fungi may emerge as pathogens.

The most important aspect of prevention is to minimize the duration and use of catheterization. Intermittent catheterization is preferred over indwelling catheter drainage whenever feasible. Insertion of catheters must be performed with aseptic technique, and the drainage system must remain closed at all times, with sterile technique used whenever the system is entered. Drainage bags always should be dependent to avoid backflow of urine into the bladder.

PERITONEAL DIALYSIS–ASSOCIATED INFECTIONS

Indwelling catheters used for peritoneal dialysis may develop exit site infections or tunnel infections or lead to peritonitis. The usual route of infection is from the skin surface along the tunnel and into the peritoneum. The most common pathogens are skin flora, including *Staphylococcus* species; organisms that contaminate water, such as *Pseudomonas* and *Acinetobacter*; enteric flora, such as *E. coli* and *Klebsiella*; and fungi, such as *C. albicans*. Peritonitis may present with fever, vague abdominal pain, and cloudy dialysate. The diagnosis is established on clinical manifestations and confirmed by culture of the dialysate. Prevention of infection requires careful planning of the location of the exit site to minimize contamination, aseptic insertion of the catheter, meticulous care of the catheter site, securing of the catheter to avoid tension and motion, and aseptic technique during dialysis.

CENTRAL NERVOUS SYSTEM SHUNTS

Important risk factors of health care–associated CNS infections are surgery, presence of a ventriculoperitoneal shunt (VPS), and cerebrospinal fluid (CSF) leaks. Infection of a VPS results from contamination of the system at the time of placement, breakdown of overlying skin, or from hematogenous seeding. Externalized ventricular drains and subdural bolts allow direct access of skin flora to the CSF. For these devices, the rates of infection increase with the duration of catheterization, especially beyond 5 days. Device-related CNS infections can be diagnosed in the same way as other types of meningitis or ventriculitis with assessment of the CSF for pleocytosis, protein, glucose, and Gram stain and culture.

The most common pathogens causing shunt infections are coagulase-negative staphylococci and *S. aureus*. After skull fracture or cranial surgery, a CSF leak may facilitate ascending infection from the nasopharynx, especially with *Streptococcus pneumoniae*, which frequently colonizes the nasopharynx. Patients with shunt infections may present with only fever and headache or may present with typical signs and symptoms of meningitis (see Chapter 101). Infections caused by coagulase-negative staphylococci or *Cutibacterium acnes* typically present with insidious onset of fever, malaise, headache, and vomiting. Empirical therapy is often with vancomycin and a third-generation cephalosporin.

Antibiotics frequently are used perioperatively during placement of shunts and other neurosurgical procedures. It is not clear that antibiotics decrease infection rates in these clean procedures, especially beyond one dose. External ventricular drains should be maintained as closed systems with aseptic technique and removed as soon as possible. Drainage bags always should be dependent to avoid backflow.

PEARLS FOR PRACTITIONERS

See Infectious Diseases: Pearls for Practitioners at the end of this section.

REVIEW QUESTIONS

Available online.

CHAPTER 123

Zoonoses and Vector-Borne Infections

Zoonoses are classically defined as infections that are transmitted in nature between vertebrate animals and humans. Many zoonotic pathogens are maintained in nature by means of an **enzootic cycle**, in which mammalian hosts and arthropod vectors reinfect each other. Humans frequently are only incidentally infected. Many zoonoses are spread by ticks, including Lyme disease, Rocky Mountain spotted fever (RMSF), ehrlichiosis, tularemia, tick typhus, and babesiosis. Of the more than 150 different human zoonotic and vector-borne diseases that have been described (Table 123.1; Fig. 123.1), Lyme disease *(Borrelia burgdorferi)* is the most common tick-borne infection in the United States. Other common zoonotic pathogens include *Rickettsia rickettsii* (RMSF), *Ehrlichia* spp. (ehrlichiosis), West Nile virus, and *Anaplasma* spp. (anaplasmosis). Transmission of infection seems to be most efficient after 24–48 hours of nymphal tick attachment for human granulocytic ehrlichiosis, after 36 hours for *B. burgdorferi,* and after 36–48 hours for *Babesia*. The epidemiology of zoonoses is related to the geographic distribution of the hosts and, if vector-borne, the distribution and seasonal life cycle of the vector. Climate change has shifted and expanded the distribution of vector-borne illnesses.

LYME DISEASE *(Borrelia Burgdorferi)*

Etiology

Lyme disease is a tick-borne infection caused by the spirochete *B. burgdorferi.* The vector in the Eastern and Midwestern United States is *Ixodes scapularis,* the **black-legged tick** that is

TABLE 123.1 Diseases Transmitted by Animals (Zoonoses)

DISEASE AND/OR ORGANISM	ANIMAL SOURCES/RESERVOIRS	VECTOR OR MODES OF TRANSMISSION
BACTERIAL DISEASES		
Aeromonas species	Aquatic animals, especially shellfish, medical leeches; has also been isolated from feces of horses, pigs, sheep, and cows	Wound infection, ingestion of contaminated food or water, direct contact with infected animal or their environment
Anthrax *(Bacillus anthracis)*	Herbivores (cattle, goats, horses, sheep) Outbreaks associated with heavy rainfall, flooding, or drought; spores remain viable in soil or animal products, such as wool or hides, for decades	Direct contact with infected animals or their carcasses, or contact with products from infected animals (e.g., meat, hides, hair, or wool) contaminated with *B. anthracis* spores; ingestion of contaminated meat; inhalation of contaminated dust
Bartonellosis *(Bartonella quintana, Bartonella bacilliformis)*	Cats, dogs, ruminants, rodents, human body louse	Bites from human body louse, sand flies
Brucellosis (*Brucella* species)	Cattle, coyotes, hares, chickens, goats, sheep, pigs, dogs, elk, bison, deer, camels, desert rats and other rodents, marine mammals	Direct or indirect contact with aborted fetuses, tissues, or fluids of infected animals; inoculation through mucous membranes or cuts or abrasions of the skin; inhalation of contaminated aerosols; ingestion of unpasteurized dairy products
Campylobacteriosis *(Campylobacter jejuni)*	Poultry, dogs (especially puppies), kittens, ferrets, pigs, nonhuman primates, pet rodents, cattle, sheep, birds	Ingestion of contaminated food or water, direct contact (particularly with animals with diarrhea), person-to-person (fecal-oral), fomites
Capnocytophaga canimorsus	Dogs, rarely cats	Bites, scratches, and prolonged contact with dogs
Cat-scratch disease *(Bartonella henselae)*	Cats and other felids, infrequently other animals (<10%)	Scratches, bites; fleas play a role in cat-to-cat transmission (evidence for transmission from cat fleas to humans is lacking)
Erysipeloid *(Erysipelothrix rhusiopathiae)*	Pigs, horses, dogs, cats, rats, sheep, cattle, wild and domestic birds (including poultry), fresh and saltwater fish, shellfish	Direct contact with animal or contaminated animal product, or water
Hemolytic-uremic syndrome (e.g., Shiga toxin–producing *Escherichia coli* [STEC])	Cattle, sheep, goats, deer, dogs, pigs, poultry	Ingestion of undercooked contaminated ground beef, unpasteurized milk, or other contaminated foods (e.g., alfalfa sprouts and other vegetable products, mayonnaise, apple cider, and cheddar) or water; contact with infected animals or their environments (e.g., farms and ranches); contact with animals in public settings including petting zoos and agricultural fairs (fecal-oral)
Leptospirosis (*Leptospira* species)	Cattle, sheep, goats, pigs, horses, dogs, rodents, and all other mammals, but rare in cats	Contact with or ingestion of water, food, or soil contaminated with urine or fluids from rodents or other infected animals, or direct contact with infected animals or their organs
Lyme disease *(Borrelia burgdorferi, Borrelia mayonii)*	White-footed mice, squirrels, shrews, and other small rodents; opossums, raccoons, birds; white-tailed deer	Tick bite (blacklegged/deer tick [*Ixodes scapularis* or *Ixodes pacificus*] in the United States, castor bean tick *[Ixodes ricinus]* in Europe)
Mycobacterium marinum	Found in brackish water, fresh water, and saltwater; fish (and cleaning aquaria)	Contaminated water sources; skin injury or contamination of existing wound
Mycobacterium bovis and *Mycobacterium tuberculosis*	Cattle, elephants, giraffes, rhinoceroses, bison, deer, elk, feral pigs, badgers, possums, nonhuman primates	*M. tuberculosis* is uncommon in nonhuman species, although when it is identified it is typically found in nonhuman primates and elephants Sporadic cases of *M. tuberculosis* have been reported in other species including cattle Transmission is by the airborne route
Pasteurellosis *(Pasteurella multocida)*	Cats, dogs, rabbits, pigs, other animals, birds	Bites, scratches, licks, saliva, respiratory droplets from animals (primarily cats and dogs), and contaminated meat

(Continued)

TABLE 123.1 Diseases Transmitted by Animals (Zoonoses)—cont'd

DISEASE AND/OR ORGANISM	ANIMAL SOURCES/RESERVOIRS	VECTOR OR MODES OF TRANSMISSION
Plague *(Yersinia pestis)*	Rodents (e.g., prairie dogs, chipmunks, squirrels, mice, voles, rats), cats, dogs, rabbits, wild carnivores (e.g., bobcats, coyotes)	Bite of infected rodent fleas (especially Oriental rat fleas—*Xenopsylla cheopis*); in the United States, the most common vector is *Oropsylla montana*, a flea found on rodents including prairie dogs and squirrels; direct contact with infected animal tissues, airborne from other human or animal (e.g., cat) with pneumonic plague
Q fever *(Coxiella burnetii)*	Sheep, goats, cows, cats, dogs, rabbits, rodents, horses, pigs, buffalo, camels, pigeons, geese, other wild fowl, ticks	Contact with excreta (birth products, urine, feces, milk) of infected animals, inhalation of pathogen-contaminated dust, ingestion of unpasteurized milk, and fomite transmission (possible role of ticks not well defined); rarely by blood transfusions, sexual contact in humans, or from a pregnant woman to her fetus
Rat-bite fever *(Streptobacillus moniliformis, Spirillum minus)*	Rodents (especially rats, occasionally squirrels), gerbils	Bites, scratches, contact with secretions, aerosol spread, direct contact with rodent; contaminated food or water; unpasteurized, contaminated milk
Relapsing fever (tick-borne) (*Borrelia* species)	Wild rodents	Soft tick bites (*Ornithodoros* species); bites from blacklegged ticks (*I. scapularis* and *I. pacificus*) transmit *B. miyamotoi*
Salmonellosis (*Salmonella* species)	Cattle, poultry, turtles, frogs, lizards, snakes, salamanders, geckos, iguanas, fish, invertebrates, dogs, cats, pigs, sheep, horses, hedgehogs, hamsters, guinea pigs, mice, rats and other rodents, ferrets, other wild and domestic animals	Fecal-oral transmission most common; ingestion of contaminated food (e.g., meat, poultry, dairy, eggs, produce, processed foods), unpasteurized milk and other raw dairy products, or contaminated water; contact with infected animals or their environments (including healthy reptiles); contaminated animal products including dry dog and cat food and pet treats
Streptococcus iniae	Fish from many regions of the world	Skin wound during handling and preparation of infected fish
Tetanus *(Clostridium tetani)*	Any animal indirectly via soil containing animal feces	Wound infection, skin injury or soft tissue injury with inoculation of bacteria (as from soil or a contaminated object)
Tularemia *(Francisella tularensis)*	Sheep, dogs, cats, pigs, horses, wild rabbits, hares, voles, squirrels, beaver, lemmings, muskrats, moles, hamsters, birds, reptiles, fish	Tick bites (wood tick *[Dermacentor andersoni]*, dog tick *[D. variabilis]*, lone star tick *[Amblyomma americanum]*), deerfly bites; direct contact with infected animal, ingestion of contaminated water or meat, mechanical transmission from claws or teeth (cats/dogs), aerosolization of tissues or excreta
Vibrio species	Shellfish	Ingestion of contaminated food or water; skin injury or contamination of existing wound
Yersiniosis *(Yersinia enterocolitica, Yersinia pseudotuberculosis)*	Pigs, deer, elk, horses, goats, sheep, cattle, rodents, birds, rabbits	Ingestion of contaminated food (particularly raw or undercooked pork products), raw or unpasteurized milk or other dairy products, contaminated water; rarely direct contact
FUNGAL DISEASES		
Cryptococcosis *(Cryptococcus neoformans)*	Excreta of birds including pigeons, canaries, parakeets, and chickens	Inhalation of aerosols from accumulations of bird feces; can also be isolated from fruit and vegetables, house dust, air conditioners, air, and sawdust; can enter body through skin as well as inhalation
Histoplasmosis *(Histoplasma capsulatum)*	Excreta of bats, birds such as pigeons and starlings	Inhalation of aerosolized spores from accumulations of bat or bird feces; spores can also be ingested
Ringworm/tinea corporis (*Microsporum* and *Trichophyton* species)	Cats, dogs, chickens, pigs, mice, moles, horses, rodents, cattle, monkeys, goats	Direct contact; pathogenic fungi found worldwide; hot and humid climates generally increase incidence

(Continued)

TABLE 123.1 Diseases Transmitted by Animals (Zoonoses)—cont'd

DISEASE AND/OR ORGANISM	ANIMAL SOURCES/RESERVOIRS	VECTOR OR MODES OF TRANSMISSION
PARASITIC DISEASES		
Angiostrongylus cantonensis (rat lungworm)	Rodents and mollusks (e.g., slugs and snails)	Ingestion of larvae in raw or undercooked snails or slugs, freshwater shrimp, land crabs, frogs or on contaminated raw produce
Anisakiasis (*Anisakis* species) (herring worm disease)	Crustaceans eat infective larvae from marine mammal feces; fish or squid eat the infected crustaceans	Ingestion of larvae in raw or undercooked fish or squid (e.g., sushi)
Babesiosis (several *Babesia* species)	Mice and various other rodents and small mammals; wildlife	Tick bite (in the United States, *Babesia microti* is transmitted mainly by *I. scapularis*; in Europe, *Babesia divergens* is transmitted mainly by *Ixodes* tick bites)
Balantidiasis *(Balantidium coli)*	Pigs	Ingestion of contaminated food or water
Baylisascariasis *(Baylisascaris procyonis)*	Raccoons	Ingestion of eggs shed in raccoon feces found in dirt or animal waste
Clonorchiasis/opisthorchiasis (*Clonorchis/Opisthorchis* species)	Fish, crabs, crayfish, snails, cats, dogs	Ingestion of metacercariae in raw or undercooked fish, crabs, or crayfish
Cryptosporidiosis (*Cryptosporidium* species)	*Cryptosporidium parvum* can infect all mammals; common in calves and other young ruminants; seen in pigs, rarely occurs in cats, dogs, and horses; other *Cryptosporidium* species can infect birds and reptiles	Fecal-oral route; ingestion of contaminated water (especially groundwater) or foods; infection by inhaling aerosols can also occur
Cutaneous larva migrans (primarily *Ancylostoma* species hookworms)	Dogs, cats	Penetration of skin by larvae, which develop in soil contaminated with animal feces
Dog tapeworm *(Dipylidium caninum)*	Dogs are definitive hosts; cats and other animals (e.g., foxes) can also be hosts	Ingestion of fleas infected with cysticercoid stage
Dwarf tapeworm *(Hymenolepis nana)* and rat tapeworm *(Hymenolepis diminuta)*	Rodents (humans are more important reservoirs than rodents for *H. nana*; for *H. diminuta*, rodents are primary and human infection is infrequent); arthropods including beetles and fleas can serve as intermediate hosts	Ingestion of eggs in contaminated food or water; animal-to-person (fecal-oral); person-to-person (fecal-oral); infection can occur after ingestion of cysticercoid-infected arthropods Autoinfection may also occur in humans if eggs remain in intestine *(H. nana)*
Echinococcosis, hydatid disease (*Echinococcus* species)	Definitive hosts are canids including dogs, coyotes, foxes, dingoes, jackals, hyenas, and wolves; intermediate hosts encompass many domestic and wild animals including herbivores such as sheep, goats, cattle, and deer	Ingestion of eggs shed in animal feces
Fascioliasis (*Fasciola* species)	Sheep, cattle	Ingestion of larvae in contaminated water, in raw watercress and other contaminated water plants, or eating raw or undercooked sheep or goat liver
Fish tapeworm *(Diphyllobothrium latum)*	Saltwater and freshwater fish	Ingestion of larvae in raw or undercooked fish (e.g., sushi)
Giardiasis *(Giardia duodenalis)*	Wild and domestic animals including dogs, cats, cattle, pigs, beavers, muskrats, rats, pet rodents, rabbits, nonhuman primates	Ingestion of contaminated water or foods, and animal-to-person (fecal-oral)
Myiasis (*Dermatobia, Cochliomyia, Chrysomya, Cuterebra,* and *Wohlfahrtia* species)	Flies	Exposure of flies to broken or wounded skin; with *Chrysomya* screwworm flies, exposure of flies to unbroken soft skin
Taeniasis/beef tapeworm *(Taenia saginata)*	Cattle (intermediate host)	Ingestion of larvae in raw or undercooked beef; cysticercosis in cattle is caused by ingestion of embryonated eggs excreted by humans with *Taenia* infection

(Continued)

TABLE 123.1 Diseases Transmitted by Animals (Zoonoses)—cont'd

DISEASE AND/OR ORGANISM	ANIMAL SOURCES/RESERVOIRS	VECTOR OR MODES OF TRANSMISSION
Taeniasis and cysticercosis/pork tapeworm (*Taenia solium; Taenia asiatica* less common)	Pigs (intermediate host)	Ingestion of larvae in raw or undercooked pork resulting in intestinal infection in humans with adult tapeworms (taeniasis); porcine cysticercosis (infection in pigs) is caused by ingestion of embryonated eggs excreted by humans with *Taenia* infection; human cysticercosis is caused by ingestion of eggs through fecal contamination of food or water, or by autoinfection
Toxoplasmosis *(Toxoplasma gondii)*	Members of the Felidae family (including domestic cats) are definitive hosts; many mammals (e.g., sheep, goats, and swine) and birds can serve as intermediate hosts	Transmission can be food-borne, zoonotic, congenital, or in rare instances through organ transplantation; zoonotic transmission can occur through ingestion of infective oocysts from hands after cleaning litter boxes or gardening (soil), or ingestion of vegetables/low growing fruits, or ingestion of anything that has become contaminated with cat feces; consumption of cysts in raw or undercooked meat (such as lamb, pork, venison) or shellfish (clams, mussels, oysters); drinking unpasteurized goat milk; drinking contaminated water
Trichinellosis (*Trichinella spiralis* and other *Trichinella* species)	Pigs, bears, seals, walruses, rodents, horses, foxes, wolves	Ingestion of larvae in raw or undercooked meat, particularly pork or wild game meat
Ocular or visceral toxocariasis/ larva migrans (*Toxocara canis* and *Toxocara cati*)	Dogs, cats; puppies are a major source of environmental contamination	Ingestion of infected, larvated eggs, usually from soil, dirty hands, or food contaminated by animal feces
CHLAMYDIAL AND RICKETTSIAL DISEASES		
Human ehrlichiosis (*Ehrlichia chaffeensis, Ehrlichia ewingii,* and *Ehrlichia muris eauclairensis*)	Dogs, red foxes, deer, coyotes, goats, lemurs *(E. chaffeensis)*; dogs may be reservoir hosts along with wolves and jackals (*Ehrlichia canis* and *E. ewingii*)	Tick bites (Lone star tick *[Amblyomma americanum]* for *E. chaffeensis, E. ewingii;* blacklegged tick *[I. scapularis]* for *E. muris eauclairensis*); in rare cases, *Ehrlichia* species have been spread through blood transfusion and organ transplantation
Human anaplasmosis *(Anaplasma phagocytophilum)*	Small mammals including wood rats and deer mice; deer may also be involved	Tick bites (*I. scapularis* and *I. pacificus*)
Psittacosis *(Chlamydia psittaci)*	Most birds (especially psittacine birds such as parakeets, parrots, macaws, and cockatoos) and poultry	Inhalation of aerosols from feces of infected birds as well as fecal-oral transmission
Rickettsialpox *(Rickettsia akari)*	House mice	Mite bites (house mouse mite, *Liponyssoides sanguineus*)
Rocky Mountain spotted fever *(Rickettsia rickettsii)*	Dogs, wild rodents, rabbits	Tick bites (American dog tick, *Dermacentor variabilis;* Rocky Mountain wood tick, *D. andersoni;* and brown dog tick, *Rhipicephalus sanguineus*)
Rickettsia parkeri infection (maculatum disease, American boutonneuse fever)	Unknown; perhaps cattle, dogs, small wild rodents	Tick bites (Gulf coast tick *[Amblyomma maculatum]*)
Typhus, flea-borne endemic typhus, Murine typhus *(Rickettsia typhi)*	Rats, opossums, cats, dogs	Infected flea feces scratched into abrasions; oriental rat fleas *(Xenopsylla cheopis)* and cat fleas *(Ctenocephalides felis)* are vectors
Typhus, louse-borne epidemic typhus *(Rickettsia prowazekii)*	Flying squirrels (sylvatic typhus)	Person-to-person via infected body louse, contact with flying squirrels, their nests, or ectoparasites (role and species of ectoparasites undefined)
VIRAL DISEASES		
B virus (formerly herpes B, monkey B virus, herpesvirus simiae, or herpesvirus B)	Macaque monkeys	Bite or exposure to secretions or tissues
Colorado tick fever virus	Rodents (e.g., squirrels, chipmunks)	Tick bites (Rocky Mountain wood tick *[Dermacentor andersoni]*)

(Continued)

TABLE 123.1 Diseases Transmitted by Animals (Zoonoses)—cont'd

DISEASE AND/OR ORGANISM	ANIMAL SOURCES/RESERVOIRS	VECTOR OR MODES OF TRANSMISSION
Crimean Congo hemorrhagic fever *(Nairovirus)*	Many wild and domestic animals including cattle, hares, goats, sheep	Infectious blood and body fluids from animal slaughter; ixodid (hard) ticks, genus *Hyalomma,* are reservoir and vector; person-to-person via contact (droplet, contact) with infectious blood or body fluids; improperly sterilized medical equipment
Eastern equine encephalitis virus	Birds	Mosquito bites (*Coquillettidia* species, *Aedes* species, *Culex* species, *Ochlerotatus* species); rarely through organ transplantation
Ebola virus	Fruit bats; nonhuman primates may become infected	Direct contact through broken skin or mucous membranes (eyes, nose, mouth) with blood or body fluids, contaminated needles, prolonged presence in semen of infected individuals (possible sexual transmission), infected fruit bats or nonhuman primates
Hantaviruses	Wild and peridomestic rodents	Inhalation of aerosols of infected secreta and excreta; contact with infected rodents or infected droppings and urine
Hendra virus	Flying foxes (*Pteropus* genus) are the natural reservoir; horses can become infected	Contact with body fluids of infected horses; close contact with fruit bats
Novel influenza (e.g., H5N1, H7N9, H9N2, H3N2 variant)	Chickens, birds, pigs	Contact with infected animals or aerosols (markets, slaughterhouse)
Jamestown Canyon virus	Deer	Mosquito bites (*Aedes* species, *Anopheles* species, and *Culiseta* species)
Japanese encephalitis virus	Pigs, birds	Mosquito bites *(Culex tritaeniorhynchus)*
Kyasanur forest disease/Alkhurma hemorrhagic fever	Monkeys, rodents, and shrews are common hosts after being bitten by infected ticks	Primarily tick bites *(Haemaphysalis spinigera),* contact with infected animal
La Crosse virus	Rodents (e.g., chipmunks and squirrels)	Mosquito bites *(Aedes triseriatus)*
Lassa fever	Multimammate rat *(Mastomys natalensis)*	Inhalation of aerosols or direct contact with infected secreta or excreta; consumption of food contaminated by rodents
Lymphocytic choriomeningitis virus	Rodents, particularly house mice and pet hamsters (includes feeder rodents used as reptile food), guinea pigs	Direct contact, inhalation of aerosols, ingestion of food contaminated with rodent excreta
Marburg hemorrhagic fever	African fruit bat *(Rousettus aegyptiacus),* infected nonhuman primates	Contact with fruit bats or their excreta (e.g., entering caves or mines inhabited by bats); contact with infectious blood or tissue of infected monkeys
Middle East respiratory syndrome (MERS coronavirus)	Uncertain; virus found in camels in several countries	Respiratory droplets from infected individuals (possible airborne transmission in some cases), direct contact
Monkeypox (Mpox)	Natural reservoir unknown; African rodent species play a role in transmission	Animal-to-human direct contact, bite, or scratch; contact with infected body fluids or contaminated bedding
Nipah virus	Fruit bats; pigs can become infected	Close contact with bats; consumption of bat-contaminated fruit/sap; direct contact with infected pigs
Omsk hemorrhagic fever	Infected rodents including muskrats and voles	Handling infected muskrats (e.g., hunting, trapping, skinning), and bites from infected ticks *(Dermacentor reticulatus, Ixodes persulcatus, Dermacentor marginatus)*
Orf (pox virus of sheep)	Sheep, goats, and occasionally other ruminants	Contact with infected saliva, infected fomites
Powassan virus	Small to medium-sized rodents (e.g., groundhogs, squirrels, mice)	Tick bites *(Ixodes cookei, Ixodes marxi, I. scapularis)* and rarely blood transfusion

(Continued)

TABLE 123.1 Diseases Transmitted by Animals (Zoonoses)—cont'd

DISEASE AND/OR ORGANISM	ANIMAL SOURCES/RESERVOIRS	VECTOR OR MODES OF TRANSMISSION
Rabies *(Lyssavirus)*	In the United States, primarily mammalian wildlife (bats, raccoons, skunks, foxes, coyotes, mongooses) or, less frequently, domestic animals (dogs, cats, cattle, horses, sheep, goats, ferrets)	Bites; rarely contact of open wounds, abrasions (including scratches), or mucous membranes with saliva or other infectious materials (e.g., neural tissue), corneal and organ transplantation
Rift Valley fever	Domesticated livestock (e.g., cattle, sheep, goats, buffalo, and camels)	Contact with blood, body fluids, or tissues of infected animals; bites from infected mosquitoes; rarely bites from other insects with virus on their mouthparts
Severe acute respiratory virus-1 (SARS-CoV-1)	Bats, civet cats, potentially other animal species	Respiratory droplets (airborne transmission believed to occur in some cases), direct contact
Severe acute respiratory virus-2 (SARS-CoV-2)	Unknown	Respiratory droplets and aerosols
South American arenaviruses (Junin, Machupo, Guanarito, Sabia, Chapare, Lujo)	Rodents	Inhalation of aerosols of infected secretions or excreta, consumption of food or water contaminated with infected secretions or excreta, direct contact of abraded or broken skin with rodent excrement
St. Louis encephalitis virus	Birds	Mosquito bites (*Culex* species) and rarely blood transfusion
Tick-borne encephalitis virus	Small rodents are primary reservoirs; large animals such as cows, goats and sheep become infected but do not play a role in virus maintenance	Tick bites (*Ixodes* species), consumption of infected raw milk products, and rarely blood transfusion or organ transplantation
Venezuelan equine encephalitis virus	Sylvatic rodents, possibly birds; horses are dead-end hosts	Mosquito bites (*Aedes* species, *Anopheles* species, *Culex* species, *Deinocerites* species, *Mansonia* species, and *Psorophora* species)
West Nile virus	Birds	Mosquito bites (*Culex* species) and rarely blood transfusion, organ transplantation
Western equine encephalitis virus	Birds	Mosquito bites *(Culex tarsalis)*
Yellow fever virus	Nonhuman primates	Mosquito bites (*Haemagogus* species, *Sabethes* species, *Aedes [Stegomyia]* species)

From Kimberlin DW, Banerjee R, Barnett ED, et al., eds. Appendix VII: Diseases transmitted by animals (zoonoses). In: Red Book: 2024–2027 Report of the Committee on Infectious Diseases. *Itasca, IL: American Academy of Pediatrics; 2024:1157.*

commonly known as the **deer tick**. The vector on the Pacific Coast is *Ixodes pacificus,* the **western black-legged tick**. Ticks usually become infected by feeding on the white-footed mouse *(Peromyscus leucopus),* which is a natural reservoir for *B. burgdorferi.* The larvae are dormant over winter and emerge the following spring in the nymphal stage, the stage of the tick that is most likely to transmit the infection to humans.

Epidemiology

In 2023 over 89,000 cases of Lyme disease were reported by state health departments, with more than 90% of cases reported from New England and the eastern parts of the Middle Atlantic states (Fig. 123.2). In Europe most cases occur in Scandinavian countries and Central Europe. Because exposure to ticks is more common in warm months, Lyme disease is noted predominantly in spring and summer. The incidence is highest among children 5–9 years old and adults aged 65–79.

Clinical Manifestations

The clinical manifestations are divided into early and late stages. Early infection may be localized or disseminated. **Early localized disease** develops 7–14 days after a tick bite as the site forms an erythematous papule that expands to form a red, raised border, often with central clearing (Fig. 123.3). The lesion, **erythema migrans**, is occasionally pruritic or painful, harbors *B. burgdorferi,* and, without treatment, may expand to as much as 15 cm in diameter. Systemic manifestations may include malaise, lethargy, fever, headache, arthralgias, stiff neck, myalgias, and lymphadenopathy. The skin lesions and early manifestations resolve without treatment over 2–4 weeks. Not all patients with Lyme disease recall a tick bite or develop erythema migrans.

Approximately 25% of children with Lyme disease are initially diagnosed with **early disseminated disease**, which is a consequence of bacteremic dissemination of *B. burgdorferi* to multiple sites. Early disseminated disease is characterized by multiple secondary skin lesions, aseptic meningitis, increased

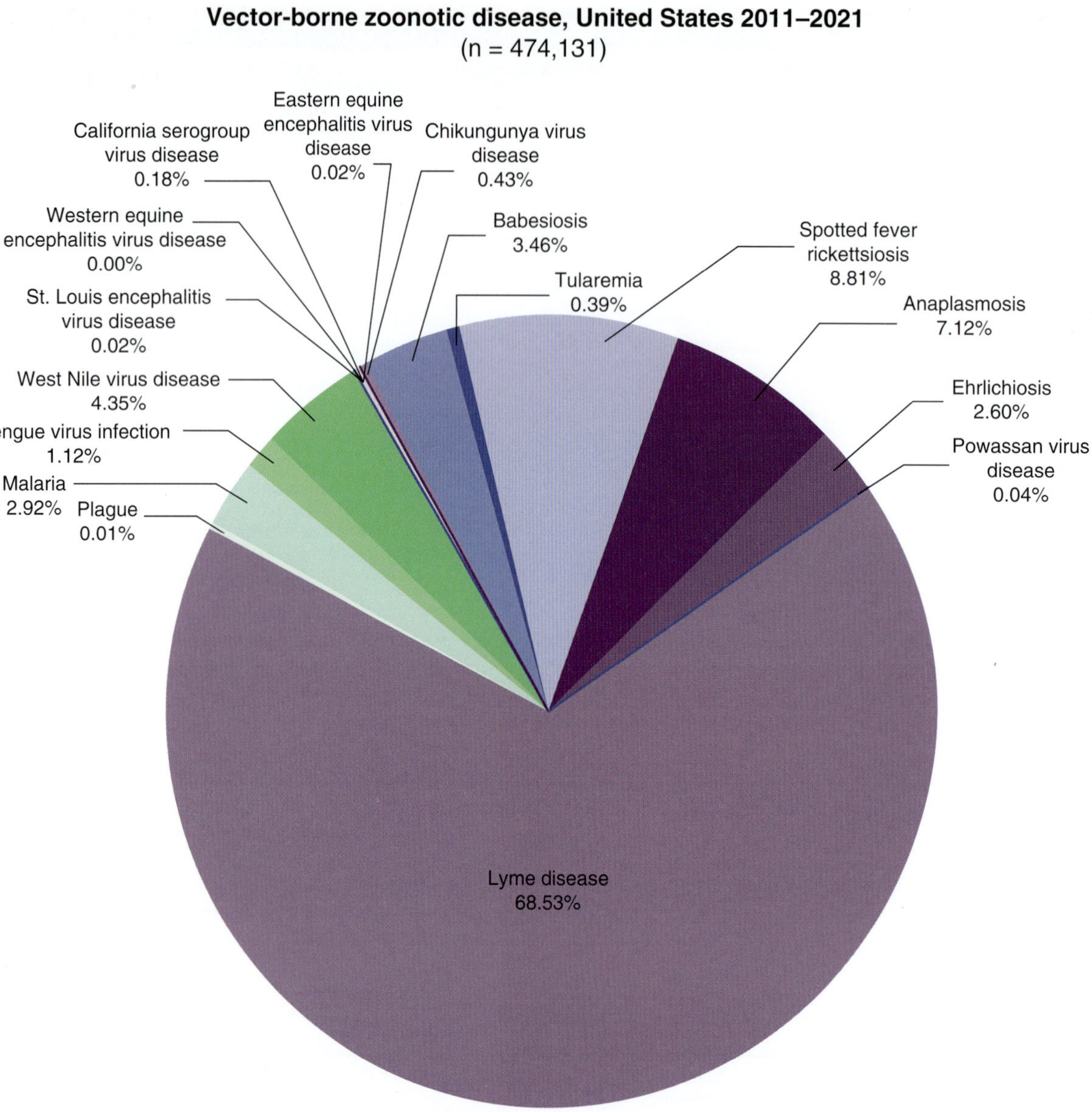

FIGURE 123.1 Proportion of vector-borne zoonoses by pathogenic agent as reported to the U.S. Centers for Disease Control and Prevention in the United States between 2011 and 2021; *N* = 474,131 cases. (From Reller ME, Dumler JS. Zoonoses. In: Goldman L, Cooney KA, eds. *Goldman-Cecil Medicine*. 27th ed. Philadelphia: Elsevier; 2024:2063, fig. 303-2.)

intracranial pressure, papilledema, neuropathies including Bell palsy, polyradiculitis, peripheral neuropathy, mononeuritis multiplex, or transverse myelitis. Carditis with various degrees of heart block may develop during this stage.

Late disease begins weeks to months after infection and is diagnosed in approximately 7% of children at initial presentation. Arthritis is the usual manifestation and may develop in 50–60% of untreated patients. The knee is involved in greater than 90% of cases, but any or more than one joint may be affected. Symptoms may resolve over 1–2 weeks.

LABORATORY AND IMAGING STUDIES

Antibody tests during early, localized Lyme disease may be negative and are not useful. Additionally, patients appropriately treated for their early, localized Lyme disease may not develop a positive antibody test. The diagnosis of late disease is confirmed by serologic tests specific for *B. burgdorferi.* The sensitivity and specificity of serologic tests for Lyme disease vary by type of assay and stage of disease. A positive enzyme-linked immunosorbent assay (ELISA) or immunofluorescence assay result must be confirmed by immunoblot showing antibodies against at least either two to three (for immunoglobulin M [IgM]) or five (for IgG) proteins of *B. burgdorferi.* The sensitivity of this 2-tiered testing approaches 100% for late stage disease.

In Lyme arthritis, joint fluid shows an inflammatory response with total white blood cell count of 25,000–125,000 cells/mm^3, often with a polymorphonuclear predominance (see Table 119.2). With CNS involvement, the cerebrospinal fluid analysis shows lymphocytic pleocytosis with normal glucose and slightly elevated protein.

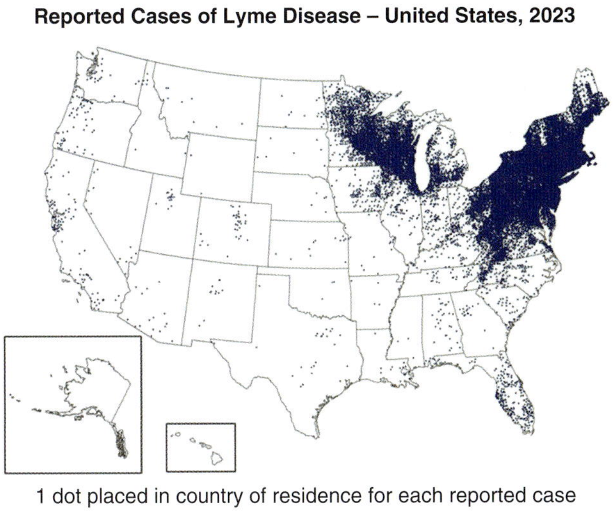

FIGURE 123.2 Reported cases of Lyme disease—United States, 2023. Each dot represents one case of Lyme disease and is placed randomly in the patient's county of residence. The presence of a dot in a state does not necessarily mean that Lyme disease was acquired in that state. People travel between states, and the place of residence is sometimes different from the place where the patient became infected. Many high-incidence states have modified surveillance practices. Contact your state health department for more information. (From Centers for Disease Control and Prevention. https://www.cdc.gov/lyme/media/images/2025/02/2023-Lyme-map-for-website-annotated.jpg.)

Differential Diagnosis

A history of a tick bite and the classic rash is helpful but is not always present. Erythema migrans of early, localized disease may be confused with nummular eczema, tinea corporis, granuloma annulare, an insect bite, or cellulitis. **Southern tick-associated rash illness (STARI)**, which is similar to erythema migrans but not associated with any of the disseminated complications of Lyme disease, occurs in southeastern and south-central states and is associated with the bite of *Amblyomma americanum,* the **lone star tick**, which is abundant in the southern states and incapable of transmitting *B. burgdorferi.*

During early, disseminated Lyme disease, multiple lesions may appear as erythema multiforme or urticaria. The aseptic meningitis is similar to viral meningitis, and the seventh nerve palsy is indistinguishable from idiopathic Bell palsy. Lyme carditis is similar to viral myocarditis. Monoarticular or pauciarticular arthritis of late Lyme disease may mimic suppurative arthritis, juvenile idiopathic arthritis, or rheumatic fever (see Chapter 90). The differential diagnosis of neuroborreliosis includes degenerative neurologic illness, encephalitis, and depression.

Treatment

Erythema migrans (early localized disease) and carditis with first-degree or second-degree heart block (early disseminated disease) are treated with doxycycline for 10 days or amoxicillin for 14 days. Doxycycline for 14 days is the preferred regimen for children of any age with facial nerve palsy. Early disseminated disease with severe carditis with third-degree heart block is treated with IV or IM ceftriaxone for 14–21 days. Lyme meningitis or radiculoneuritis is treated with doxycycline (PO) or ceftriaxone (IV) for 14–21 days. Arthritis is treated with doxycycline (for children ≥8 years of age)

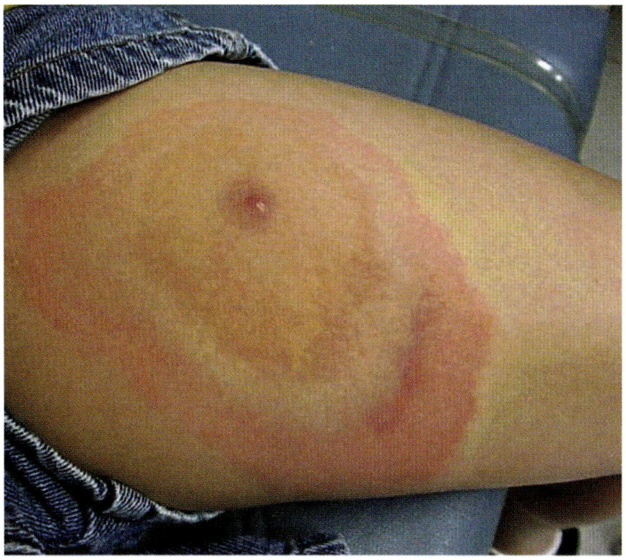

FIGURE 123.3 Expanding annular lesion of erythema migrans at the site of a tick bite. (Courtesy Dr. Jay Capra, Abilene, TX.)

or amoxicillin for 28 days. If there is recurrence, treatment should be with a repeated oral regimen or with the regimen for late neurologic disease. Patients with persistent synovitis may require treatment with nonsteroidal antiinflammatory agents or intraarticular steroids (in consultation with a rheumatologist).

Complications and Prognosis

Carditis, especially conduction disturbances, and arthritis are the major complications of Lyme disease. Lyme disease is readily treatable and curable. The long-term prognosis is excellent when early and late disease are treated. Early treatment of erythema migrans almost always prevents progression to later stages. Recurrences of arthritis after treatment occur in 5–10% of patients. The most common reason patients "recur" or do not respond to treatment is that the initial diagnosis was incorrect.

Prevention

Measures to minimize exposure to tick-borne diseases are the most reasonable means of preventing Lyme disease. Preventive measures to avoid tick-borne diseases include using insect repellents that contain **DEET** (*N,N*-diethyl-*m*-toluamide) on skin and insect repellents that contain **permethrin** on clothing, avoiding tick-infested habitats (thick scrub oak, briar, poison ivy sites), avoiding excretory products of wild animals, wearing appropriate protective clothing (closed-toe shoes, long pants), and promptly removing ticks.

Ticks are best removed using blunt forceps or tweezers to grasp the tick as close to the skin as possible to pull the tick steadily outward. Squeezing, twisting, or crushing the tick should be avoided because the tick's bloated abdomen can act like a syringe if squeezed.

Postexposure prophylaxis is not routinely recommended because the overall risk of acquiring Lyme disease after a tick bite is only 1–3% even in endemic areas, and treatment of the infection, if it develops, is highly effective. Nymphal stage ticks must feed for more than 36 hours before the risk of transmission of *B. burgdorferi* from infected ticks becomes substantial. In hyperendemic regions, prophylaxis of adults and children with doxycycline, single dose (or 4.4 mg/kg for children weighing less than 45 kg), within 72 hours of a nymphal tick that was attached for over 36 hours is effective in preventing Lyme disease.

ROCKY MOUNTAIN SPOTTED FEVER *(Rickettsia Rickettsii)*

Etiology

The cause of RMSF is *R. rickettsii,* a gram-negative, intracellular, coccobacillary bacterium. *R. rickettsii* invades and proliferates within the endothelial cells of blood vessels of all major organs and tissues, causing vasculitis and resulting in increased vascular permeability, edema, and, eventually, decreased vascular volume, altered tissue perfusion, and widespread organ failure. Many tick species are capable of transmitting *R. rickettsii.* The principal ticks are the **American dog tick** *(Dermacentor variabilis)* in the Eastern United States and Canada, the **wood tick** *(Dermacentor andersoni)* in the Western United States and Canada, the **brown dog tick** *(Rhipicephalus sanguineus)* in Mexico and Southwestern United States, and *Amblyomma cajennense* in Central and South America.

Epidemiology

RMSF is the most common rickettsial illness in the United States, occurring primarily in the eastern coastal, southeastern, and south-central states. Most cases occur from April to September after outdoor activity in wooded areas. RMSF occurs more commonly in adults, but the case fatality rate is highest in children under 10 years of age. In approximately 50% of pediatric cases of RMSF there is no recall of a tick bite.

Clinical Manifestations

The incubation period of RMSF is 2–14 days, with an average of 7 days. The onset is nonspecific with headache, malaise, and fever. An initial pale, rose red macular or maculopapular rash appears in 90% of cases usually 2–5 days after fever onset. The *early* rash blanches on pressure and is accentuated by warmth. It progresses over hours or days to a petechial and purpuric eruption that appears first on the feet and ankles, then the wrists and hands, and progresses centripetally to the trunk and head. A hallmark feature is the involvement of the palms and soles (Fig. 123.4). Myalgias, especially of the lower extremities, and intractable headaches are common. Severe cases progress with splenomegaly, myocarditis, acute kidney injury, pneumonitis, and shock.

Laboratory and Imaging Studies

Thrombocytopenia, anemia, hyponatremia, hypoalbuminemia, and elevated hepatic transaminase levels are common laboratory findings. Organisms can be detected in skin biopsy specimens by fluorescent antibodies or polymerase chain reaction (PCR), although this test is not widely available. Serologic testing is used to confirm the diagnosis. Approximately 50% of patients will not have detectable antibody until the second week of illness, but treatment should not be withheld pending confirmation.

Differential Diagnosis

The differential diagnosis includes meningococcemia, bacterial sepsis, toxic shock syndrome, leptospirosis, ehrlichiosis, measles, enteroviruses, infectious mononucleosis, collagen vascular diseases, IgA vasculitis, COVID-19–associated multisystem inflammatory syndrome in children (MIS-C), and idiopathic thrombocytopenic purpura. The diagnosis of RMSF should be suspected with fever and petechial rash, especially with a history of a tick bite or outdoor activities during spring and summer in endemic regions. Delayed diagnosis and late treatment usually result from atypical initial symptoms and late appearance of the rash.

Treatment

Therapy for suspected RMSF should not be postponed pending results of diagnostic tests. Doxycycline is the drug of choice. Short courses of doxycycline are not associated with dental staining.

Complications and Prognosis

In severe infections, capillary leakage results in noncardiogenic pulmonary edema (acute respiratory distress syndrome), hypotension, disseminated intravascular coagulation, circulatory collapse, and multiple organ failure, including encephalitis, myocarditis, hepatitis, and kidney failure.

Untreated illness may persist for 3 weeks and progress to multisystem involvement. The mortality rate is as high as 40% without treatment, which is reduced to 1–3% with treatment. Permanent sequelae are common after severe disease.

Prevention

Preventive measures to avoid tick-borne infections and careful removal of ticks are recommended. There are no data to support antibiotic prophylaxis for RMSF after a tick bite.

EHRLICHIOSIS *(Ehrlichia Chaffeensis)* AND ANAPLASMOSIS *(Anaplasma Phagocytophilum)*

Etiology

The term **ehrlichiosis** often is used to refer to all forms of infection with *Ehrlichia.* **Human monocytic ehrlichiosis** is caused by *E. chaffeensis,* which infects predominantly monocytic cells and is transmitted by the tick *A. americanum* (lone star tick). Disease may also be caused by *Ehrlichia ewingii* (granulocytes) and *Ehrlichia muris*–like agent (unknown, suspected monocytes). **Human anaplasmosis** is caused by *A. phagocytophilum* and is transmitted by the tick *I. scapularis* (black-legged tick) or *I. pacificus* (western black-legged tick).

Epidemiology

Human monocytic ehrlichiosis occurs in broad areas across the Southeastern, South-Central, and Mid-Atlantic United

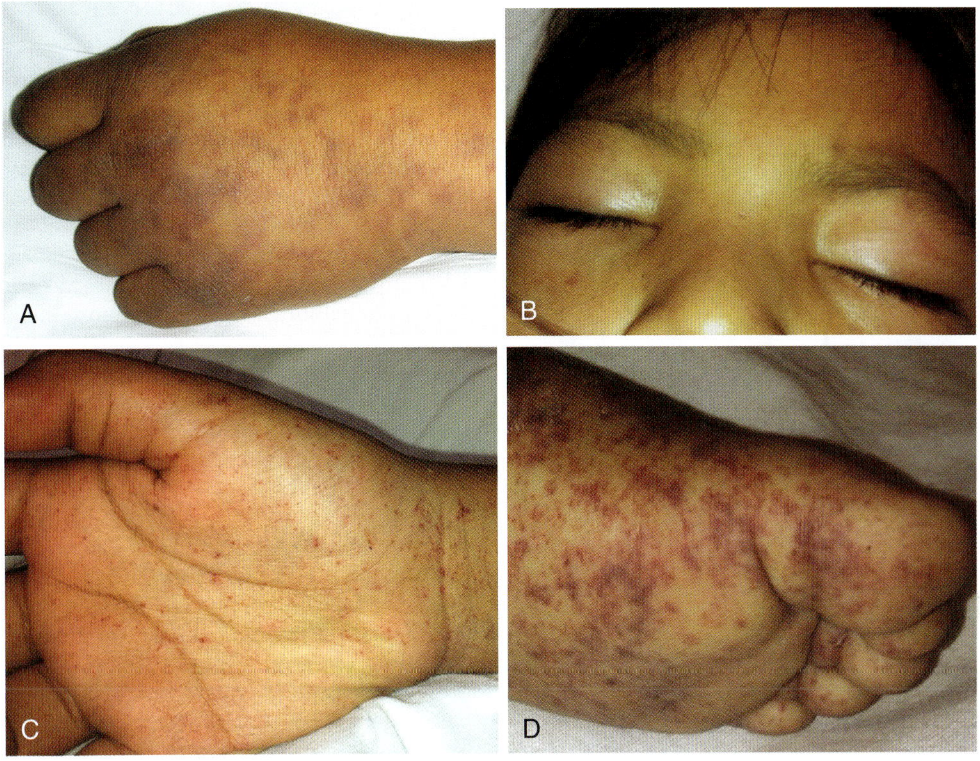

FIGURE 123.4 Clinical signs identified in children with Rocky Mountain spotted fever. **(A)** Edema of the dorsum of the hand. **(B)** Periorbital edema. (**C** and **D**) Petechial rashes involving the palm and sole. (From Paddock CD, Alvarez-Hernández G. *Rickettsia rickettsii* [Rocky Mountain spotted fever]. In: Long SS, Prober CG, Fischer M, eds. *Principles and Practice of Pediatric Infectious Diseases.* 6th ed. Philadelphia: Churchill Livingstone; 2023:fig. 178.3.)

States in a distribution that parallels that of RMSF. Anaplasmosis is found mostly in the Northeastern and Upper Midwestern United States, but infections have been identified in Northern California, the Mid-Atlantic states, and broadly across Europe. Ehrlichiosis due to *E. muris*–like agents has been reported only from Wisconsin and Minnesota.

Clinical Manifestations

Human monocytic ehrlichiosis, anaplasmosis, and *Ehrlichiosis ewingii* cause similar acute febrile illnesses characterized by fever, malaise, headache, myalgias, anorexia, and nausea. Rash occurs more commonly in ehrlichiosis than anaplasmosis; rash is uncommon in adults. In contrast to adult patients, ~65% of children with human monocytic ehrlichiosis present with a macular or maculopapular rash, although petechial lesions may occur. Symptoms usually last for 1–2 weeks.

Laboratory and Imaging Studies

Characteristic laboratory findings include leukopenia, lymphocytopenia, thrombocytopenia, anemia, and elevated hepatic transaminases. Hyponatremia is common. Morulae are found infrequently in circulating monocytes of persons with human monocytic ehrlichiosis but are found in 20–60% of persons with anaplasmosis (Fig. 123.5). Seroconversion or fourfold rise in antibody titer confirms the diagnosis; this requires acute and convalescent samples and is not helpful during the acute illness. PCR tests for both ehrlichiosis and anaplasmosis are available and can confirm diagnosis during the acute illness.

Differential Diagnosis

Ehrlichiosis is clinically similar to other arthropod-borne infections, including RMSF, tularemia, babesiosis, early Lyme disease, murine typhus, relapsing fever, and Colorado tick fever. The differential diagnosis also includes infectious mononucleosis, Kawasaki disease, COVID-19–associated MIS-C, endocarditis, viral infections, hepatitis, leptospirosis, Q fever, collagen vascular diseases, and leukemia.

Treatment

Therapy for suspected ehrlichiosis should not be postponed pending results of diagnostic tests. Ehrlichiosis and anaplasmosis are treated with doxycycline.

Complications and Prognosis

Severe pulmonary involvement with acute respiratory distress syndrome has been reported in several cases. Other reported severe complications include meningoencephalitis and myocarditis. Most patients improve within 48 hours of initiating antibiotics. Failure to respond to doxycycline within 3 days suggests either misdiagnosis or co-infection with another organism.

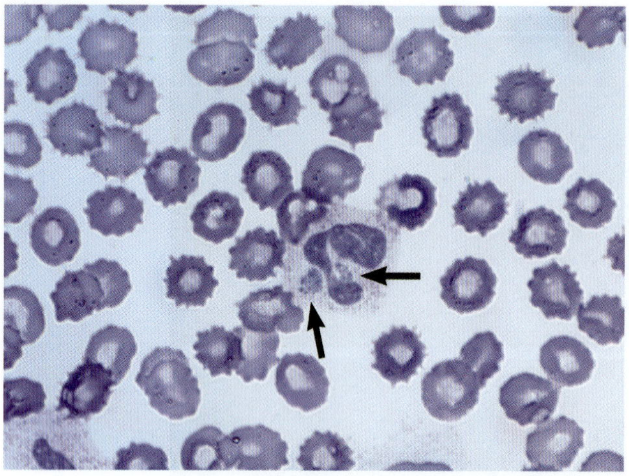

FIGURE 123.5 Human monocytotropic ehrlichiosis. Peripheral blood smear (buffy coat preparation) showing intracellular inclusions *(arrows)* in mononuclear cells of a patient with human monocytotropic ehrlichiosis (Wright stain, ×400). (From Dumler JS, Walker DH. *Ehrlichia chaffeensis* [human monocytotropic ehrlichiosis], *Anaplasma phagocytophilum* [human granulocytotropic anaplasmosis], and other Anaplasmataceae. In: Bennett JE, Dolin R, Blaser MJ, eds. *Mandell, Douglas, and Bennett's Principles and Practice of Infectious Diseases.* 9th ed. Philadelphia: Elsevier; 2020:fig. 192.1.)

Prevention

Preventive measures to avoid tick-borne infections and careful removal of ticks are recommended. There are no data to support antibiotic prophylaxis for ehrlichiosis or anaplasmosis after a tick bite.

WEST NILE VIRUS (SEE CHAPTER 102)

Dengue Fever

There are four dengue fever virus types (flaviviruses) transmitted to humans predominantly by the *A. aegypti* mosquito vector. Enzootic transmission via monkeys may occur, but person (viremic) to mosquito to person is the most frequent mechanism of viral infection. Dengue virus is most prevalent in tropical climates, and endogenous infections have been reported in Florida, Texas, and Puerto Rico.

Infected patients may have subclinical disease or a self-limited febrile illness. Dengue hemorrhagic fever, the most severe manifestation of the illness, occurs in patients who have had a previous dengue virus infection (different serotype) and who manifest an exaggerated immunologic response to the new dengue virus serotype.

Dengue viremia usually precedes the influenza-like illness characterized by fever, myalgias, musculoskeletal pain **(break-bone fever)**, headaches, macular rash, elevated liver enzymes, acute respiratory distress syndrome, and peripheral cytopenias. Shock may occur with third space fluid losses, which may be associated with an increasing hematocrit. Epistaxis, hemoptysis, gastrointestinal, and uterine bleeding may occur.

Diagnosis is based on geographic epidemiology, clinical presentation, and detection of dengue virus by PCR. Therapy requires good supportive care with fluid and blood replacement as needed. Vaccination is recommended in endemic areas.

Ebola Virus

Ebola virus is a filovirus producing a severe and often lethal hemorrhagic fever syndrome. It is transmitted by direct person-to-person contact, particularly body fluids; the fruit bat may be the animal reservoir for Ebola and the related Marburg virus. Ebola is most often seen in central Africa, although imported cases have been reported in persons traveling from endemic or epidemic regions.

Clinical manifestations may begin with a sudden onset of fever, myalgias, diarrhea, and malaise but are then followed by significant hemorrhagic manifestations. Leukopenia, lymphopenia, thrombocytopenia, elevated liver enzymes, and prolonged clotting times are common. The diagnosis is confirmed by the presence of IgM and IgG antibodies to the virus. Treatment is supportive, including replacement of blood and fluid losses. The fatality rate is approximately 50%.

Chikungunya Virus

Chikungunya virus is an alphavirus in the togavirus family and is transmitted by most *Aedes* species of mosquitos in Africa, Latin America, and Asia. Nonhuman primates may be the animal reservoir.

Chikungunya fever is characterized by a sudden illness with high fever, rash, and severe arthralgias. Fever may abate but return for 1–2 days after an extended afebrile period of 4–10 days (termed the "saddleback" pattern). Polyarthralgias involve the small joints, which are exquisitely tender, and may persist for several weeks. The rash appears as facial flushing but evolves to a maculopapular occasionally pruritic eruption on the trunk, extremities, soles, and palms. Children may have CNS symptoms (irritability, seizures). Leukopenia, lymphocytosis, and elevated laboratory markers of inflammation are common.

The diagnosis is confirmed by PCR or antibody responses. Treatment is supportive, particularly for the incapacitating joint manifestations. Tumor necrosis factor (TNF)–blocking agents may be beneficial for severe and persistent arthritis.

Zika Virus

Zika virus, a member of the flavivirus group, is transmitted by many *Aedes* mosquito species and is prevalent in equatorial regions of South America and Asia. Humans are the reservoir. Zika virus infection manifests with fever, rash, arthralgia, nonpurulent conjunctivitis, and headache. Infection in children and adults is usually self-limited; the greatest concern is infection during pregnancy resulting in transplacental transmission to the fetus with subsequent severe microcephaly and other congenital malformations. Diagnosis is confirmed by Zika virus antibody titers or PCR.

PEARLS FOR PRACTITIONERS

See Infectious Diseases: Pearls for Practitioners at the end of this section.

REVIEW QUESTIONS

Available online.

CHAPTER 124 Parasitic Diseases

PROTOZOAL DISEASES

Protozoa are the simplest organisms of the animal kingdom. They are unicellular. Most are free-living, but some have a commensal or parasitic existence. Protozoal diseases include malaria, toxoplasmosis, babesiosis, and the intestinal protozoal diseases amebiasis, cryptosporidiosis, and giardiasis.

Malaria

Etiology

Malaria is caused by obligate intracellular protozoa of the genus *Plasmodium,* including *P. falciparum, P. malariae, P. ovale, P. vivax,* and *P. knowlesi. Plasmodium* has a complex life cycle that enables survival in different cellular environments in the human host and in the mosquito vector. There are two major phases in the life cycle, an **asexual phase (schizogony)** in humans and a **sexual phase (sporogony)** in mosquitoes. The **erythrocytic phase** of *Plasmodium* asexual development begins when the merozoites released from exoerythrocytic schizonts in the liver penetrate erythrocytes. When inside the erythrocyte, the parasite transforms into the **ring form**, which enlarges to become a **trophozoite**. These latter two forms can be identified with Giemsa stain on blood smear, which is the primary means of confirming the diagnosis of malaria.

The parasites usually are transmitted to humans by female *Anopheles* mosquitoes. Malaria also can be transmitted through blood transfusion, via contaminated needles, and transplacentally to a fetus.

Epidemiology

Malaria is an important cause of fever, morbidity, and mortality globally, with transmission in more than 100 countries with a combined population of over 3.2 billion people. Endemic areas include sub-Saharan Africa, southern Asia, Southeast Asia, and Central and South America. Approximately 1,500–2,000 imported cases are recognized annually in the United States, with most cases occurring among infected people traveling or returning to the United States from endemic areas.

Clinical Manifestations

The clinical manifestations of malaria range from asymptomatic infection to fulminant illness and death, depending on the virulence of the infecting species and the host immune response. The typical incubation period ranges from 7 to 30 days, depending on the *Plasmodium* species (Table 124.1). The most characteristic clinical feature of malaria, which is seldom noted with other infectious diseases, is **febrile paroxysms** alternating with periods of fatigue but otherwise relative wellness. The classic symptoms of the febrile paroxysms of malaria include high fever, rigors, sweats, and headache. Paroxysms coincide with the ruptures of schizonts that occur every 48 hours with *P. vivax* and *P. ovale* **(tertian periodicity)**, every 72 hours with *P. malariae* **(quartan periodicity)**, and every 24 hours with *P. knowlesi.* Periodicity can be tertian with *P. falciparum* infections but is often irregular.

Short-term relapse describes the recurrence of symptoms after a primary attack that is due to the survival of erythrocyte forms in the bloodstream. **Long-term relapse** describes the renewal of symptoms long after the primary attack, usually due to the release of merozoites from an exoerythrocytic source in the liver. Long-term relapse occurs with *P. vivax* and *P. ovale* because of persistence in the liver (Fig. 124.1).

Laboratory and Imaging Studies

The diagnosis of malaria is established by the identification of organisms on stained smears of peripheral blood. In nonimmune persons, symptoms typically occur 1–2 days before parasites are detectable on blood smear. Although *P. falciparum* is most likely to be identified from blood during a febrile paroxysm, the timing of the smears is less important than obtaining three sets of smears every 12–24 hours. Both thick and thin blood smears should be examined. The concentration of erythrocytes on a **thick smear** is approximately 20–40 times greater than that on a **thin smear**. Thick smears are used to scan large numbers of erythrocytes quickly. Thin smears allow for positive identification of the malaria species and determination of the percentage of infected erythrocytes, called parasitemia, which also is useful in following the response to therapy. **Rapid diagnostic tests** are available as point-of-care tests. Such tests provide results in 15–20 minutes and are particularly useful in areas where reliable microscopic diagnosis is not available. The rapid tests are able to detect *P. falciparum* but are unable to differentiate between *P. vivax, P. ovale,* and *P. malariae.* Sensitivity is lower for non-*falciparum* species and in patients with low-level parasitemia. For these reasons, as well as to guide management decisions, all rapid tests should be followed by microscopic examination regardless of the results.

Differential Diagnosis

The most important aspect of diagnosing malaria in children is to consider the possibility of malaria in any child who has fever, chills, splenomegaly, anemia, or decreased level of consciousness with a history of recent travel or residence in an endemic area, regardless of the use of chemoprophylaxis. The differential diagnosis is broad and includes many infectious diseases, such as typhoid fever, dengue, tuberculosis, brucellosis, relapsing fever, infective endocarditis, influenza, yellow fever, trypanosomiasis, kala-azar, and amebic liver abscess.

Treatment

Specific treatment should be guided by where the patient acquired the infection, chemoprophylactic regimen, and the local resistance patterns. Patients with malaria often require hospitalization and may require intensive care unit admission. Artemisinin combination therapy (ACT) is the recommended first-line treatment (if accessible) for uncomplicated malaria, even for chloroquine-susceptible *P. falciparum.* ACTs include artemether-lumefantrine (preferred because of its fast onset of action), artesunate-amodiaquine, and artesunate-mefloquine. Artesunate is the first-line treatment for severe malaria and is available as a commercial product, but it is not consistently stocked in all hospitals. Patients presenting with severe malaria to a hospital where artesunate is not in stock should be treated with an effective oral antimalarial until intravenous artesunate is obtained. Atovaquone-proguanil, quinine sulfate plus doxycycline or tetracycline or clindamycin, and mefloquine

TABLE 124.1 Characteristics of *Plasmodium* Species Causing Malaria

CHARACTERISTIC	*P. FALCIPARUM*	*P. VIVAX*	*P. OVALE*	*P. MALARIAE*	*P. KNOWLESI*
Exoerythrocytic cycle	5.5–7 days	6–8 days	12 days	9 days	16 days
Erythrocytic cycle	43–52 hr	48 hr	48 hr	72 hr	24 hr
Usual incubation period (range)	13–14 days	13–14 days	13–14 days	35 days	12–16 days
Erythrocyte preference	Can infect all	Reticulocytes	Reticulocytes	Older red cells	Can infect all
Usual parasite load (% erythrocytes infected)	High	Low	Low	Low	May be high
Secondary exoerythrocytic cycle (hypnozoites) and relapses	Absent	Present	Present	Absent	Absent
Severity of primary attack	Can be severe	Mild to severe	Mild	Mild—severe disease in a patient suspected of having *P. malariae* should raise the suspicion of *P. knowlesi*	Mild to severe
Usual periodicity of febrile attacks	43–52 hr	48 hr	48 hr	72 hr	24 hr

Modified from Ansong D, Seydel KB, Taylor TE. Malaria. In: Ryan ET, Hill DR, Solomon T, et al., eds. Hunter's Tropical Medicine and Emerging Infectious Disease. *10th ed. Philadelphia: Saunders; 2020.*

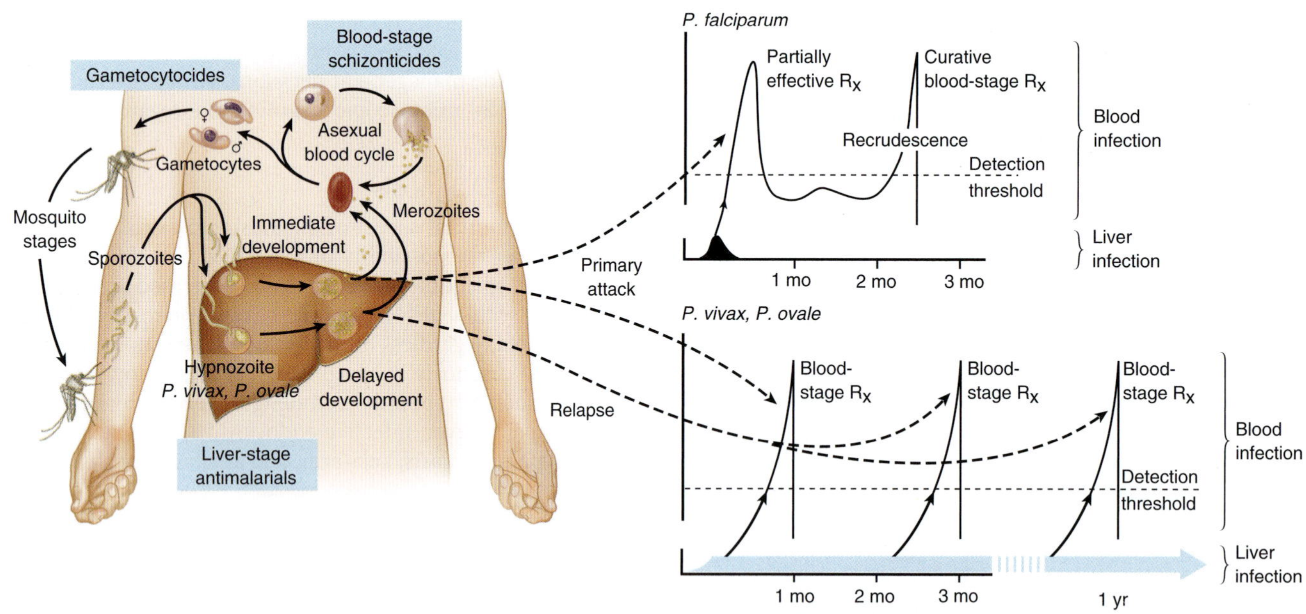

FIGURE 124.1 The *Plasmodium* life cycle and disease patterns of recrudescence and relapse. Anopheline mosquitoes transmit malaria by injecting sporozoites into the human host. The sporozoites then invade hepatocytes, in which they develop into schizonts. Each infected hepatocyte ruptures to liberate 10,000–30,000 merozoites that invade circulating erythrocytes. Growth and development of the parasites in red cells result in subsequent waves of merozoite invasion. This asexual blood cycle repeats every 24 *(Plasmodium knowlesi)*, 48 *(Plasmodium falciparum, Plasmodium vivax, Plasmodium ovale)*, or 72 *(Plasmodium malariae)* hours, leading to amplification of parasite density; paroxysms of chills, fevers, and sweats; and other manifestations of disease. Malaria symptoms are typically experienced 2–4 weeks after the mosquito bite. If the parasites are not cleared (e.g., patient receives partially effective therapy), recrudescence of parasitemia and malaria symptoms can occur. Eradicating parasites with an effective drug regimen cures malaria. Some *P. vivax* and *P. ovale* parasites can postpone their development in the liver, persisting as latent forms called hypnozoites. Hypnozoites are not eradicated by standard therapy (e.g., chloroquine) directed against blood stages. Resumption of hypnozoite development months to years after initial infection can lead to malaria relapse that requires an additional round of drug therapy to treat recurrent symptoms and eradicate blood-stage parasites. A course of primaquine can prevent relapses of malaria, but this treatment may not always be successful because of inadequate patient compliance, interindividual variations of drug metabolism, or variable parasite responses to low or high drug doses. (From Fairhurst RM, Wellems TE. Malaria [*Plasmodium* species]. In: Bennett JE, Dolin R, Blaser MJ, eds. *Mandell, Douglas, and Bennett's Principles and Practice of Infectious Diseases.* 9th ed. Philadelphia: Elsevier; 2020:fig. 274.2.)

are appropriate second-line therapies for malaria acquired in areas of chloroquine resistance.

Complications and Prognosis

Cerebral malaria is a complication of *P. falciparum* infection and a frequent cause of death (10–40% of cases), especially among children and nonimmune adults. Similar to other complications, cerebral malaria is more likely to occur among patients with intense parasitemia (>5% of erythrocytes on a blood smear). Other complications include splenic rupture, kidney failure, severe hemolysis **(blackwater fever)**, pulmonary edema, hypoglycemia, thrombocytopenia, and **algid malaria** (sepsis syndrome with vascular collapse).

Death may occur with any of the malarial species but is most frequent with complicated *P. falciparum* malaria. The likelihood of death is increased in children with preexisting health problems, such as measles, intestinal parasites, schistosomiasis, anemia, and malnutrition. Death is much more common in developing countries.

Prevention

There are two components of malaria prevention: reduction of exposure to infected mosquitoes and chemoprophylaxis. Mosquito protection is necessary because no prophylactic regimen can guarantee protection in every instance due to the widespread development of resistant organisms.

Chemoprophylaxis is necessary for all visitors to, and residents of, the tropics who have not lived there since infancy. Children of women from endemic areas have passive immunity until 3–6 months of age, after which they are increasingly likely to acquire malaria. Specific chemoprophylaxis should be guided by the distribution of resistance pattern and determined before making specific recommendations (http://www.cdc.gov/malaria/travelers/country_table/a.html). Mefloquine, doxycycline, chloroquine, and atovaquone-proguanil are commonly prescribed medications. Two vaccines, RTS,S/AS01 and R21/Matrix-M, were recommended by the World Health Organization in 2021 and 2023 respectively for children living in malaria endemic areas. Roll-out of these vaccines has been ongoing while multiple other vaccine candidates are also in development or trial phase.

Toxoplasmosis

Toxoplasmosis is a zoonosis caused by *Toxoplasma gondii,* an intracellular protozoan parasite. Infection is acquired by oocysts, such as those excreted by newly infected cats, which play an important role in amplifying the organism in nature, or from ingesting cysts in contaminated, undercooked meat. Less commonly, transmission occurs transplacentally during acute infection of pregnant women. In the United States, the incidence of congenital infection is 1–10 per 10,000 live births.

Acquired toxoplasmosis is usually asymptomatic. Symptomatic infection is typically a febrile syndrome that presents similar to mononucleosis with lymphadenopathy, fever, and hepatosplenomegaly. Disseminated infection, including myocarditis, pneumonia, and CNS toxoplasmosis, is more common among immunocompromised persons, especially persons with AIDS. Among women infected during pregnancy, 50–60% give birth to an infected infant. The later in pregnancy infection occurs, the more likely it is that the fetus will be infected but the less severe the illness (see Chapter 65). Serologic diagnosis can be established by a fourfold increase in antibody titer or seroconversion, a positive immunoglobulin M (IgM) antibody titer, or positive polymerase chain reaction for *T. gondii* in peripheral white blood cells, cerebrospinal fluid (CSF), serum, or amniotic fluid.

Treatment includes pyrimethamine and sulfadiazine, which act synergistically against *Toxoplasma.* Because these compounds are folic acid inhibitors, they are used in conjunction with folinic acid. Spiramycin, which can be obtained from the U.S. Food and Drug Administration, is also used in therapy of pregnant women with toxoplasmosis. Corticosteroids are reserved for patients with acute CNS or ocular infection.

Ingesting only well-cooked meat and avoiding cats or soil in areas where cats defecate are prudent measures for pregnant or immunocompromised persons. Administration of spiramycin to infected pregnant women has been associated with lower risks of congenital infection in their offspring.

HELMINTHIASES

Helminths are divided into three groups: roundworms, or nematodes, and two groups of flatworms, the trematodes (flukes) and the cestodes (tapeworms).

Hookworm Infections

Hookworms are nematodes, with infection caused by several species of hookworms, with *Ancylostoma duodenale* and *Necator americanus* being the most important (Table 124.2). There are more than 600 million humans worldwide infected with hookworms. *A. duodenale* is the predominant species in the Mediterranean region, northern Asia, and certain areas of South America. *N. americanus* predominates in the Western Hemisphere, sub-Saharan Africa, and Southeast Asia. Optimal soil conditions and fecal contamination are found in many agrarian tropical countries and in the southeastern United States. Infection typically occurs in young children, especially during the first decade of life. The larvae are found in warm, damp soil and infect humans by penetrating the skin. They migrate to the lungs, ascend the trachea, are swallowed, and reside in the intestine. The worms mature and attach to the intestinal wall, where they suck blood and shed eggs.

Infections are usually asymptomatic. Intense pruritus *(ground itch)* occurs at the site of larval penetration, usually the soles of the feet or between the toes, and physical examination may show papules and vesicles. Migration of larvae through the lungs usually is asymptomatic. Symptoms of abdominal pain, anorexia, indigestion, fullness, and diarrhea occur with hookworm infestation. The major finding of infection is anemia and eosinophilia. Examination of fresh stool for hookworm eggs is diagnostic. Therapy includes anthelmintic treatment with albendazole, mebendazole, or pyrantel pamoate and treatment for anemia. Eradication depends on sanitation of the patient's environment and treatment with antiparasitics.

Ascariasis

Ascariasis is caused by *Ascaris lumbricoides,* a large nematode. It is the most prevalent helminthiasis, affecting more than 800 million people (see Table 124.2). After humans ingest the eggs, larvae are released and penetrate the intestine, migrate to the lungs, ascend the trachea, and are swallowed. On entering the intestines again, they mature and produce eggs that are

TABLE 124.2 Major Pediatric Syndromes Caused by Parasitic Nematodes

SYNDROME	ETIOLOGIC AGENT	TRANSMISSION	TREATMENT
Hookworm iron deficiency	*Ancylostoma duodenale*	Larval ingestion and penetration	Albendazole *or* mebendazole *or* pyrantel pamoate
	Necator americanus	Larval penetration	
Cutaneous larva migrans	*Ancylostoma braziliense* (a zoonotic hookworm)	Larval penetration (and failure to migrate)	Generally self-limited; albendazole *or* ivermectin
Trichuris dysentery or colitis	*Trichuris trichiura*	Egg ingestion	Mebendazole *or* albendazole *or* ivermectin
Intestinal ascariasis	*Ascaris lumbricoides*	Ingestion of *Ascaris* eggs	Albendazole *or* mebendazole *or* ivermectin
Visceral larva migrans	*Toxocara canis* *T. cati* *Baylisascaris procyonis*	Egg ingestion	Albendazole *or* mebendazole *or* ivermectin
Ocular larva migrans	*Toxocara canis* *T. cati* *Baylisascaris procyonis*	Egg ingestion	Albendazole *or* mebendazole *or* ivermectin
Diarrhea, malabsorption (celiac-like)	*Strongyloides stercoralis*	Larval penetration	Ivermectin
Pinworm	*Enterobius vermicularis*	Egg ingestion	Albendazole *or* mebendazole *or* pyrantel pamoate
Trichinellosis	*Trichinella spiralis*	Ingestion of infected undercooked meat	Albendazole *or* mebendazole *plus* corticosteroids for severe symptoms
Abdominal angiostrongyliasis	*Angiostrongylus costaricensis*	Ingestion of contaminated food	Albendazole *or* mebendazole
Eosinophilic meningitis	*Angiostrongylus cantonensis* (rat lungworm)	Ingestion of undercooked snails or slugs; contaminated produce	Albendazole

excreted in the stool and are deposited in the soil, where they survive for prolonged periods.

Manifestations may be the result of migration of the larvae to other sites of the body or the presence of adult worms in the intestine. **Pulmonary ascariasis** occurs as the larvae migrate through the lung, producing cough, blood-stained sputum, eosinophilia, and transient infiltrates on chest x-ray films. Adult larvae in the small intestine may cause abdominal pain and distention. Intestinal obstruction from adult worms can occur, particularly in children due to the small diameter of their intestinal lumens and their propensity to acquire large worm burdens. Migration of worms into the bile duct may rarely cause acute biliary obstruction. Examination of fresh stool for characteristic eggs is diagnostic. Effective control depends on adequate sanitary treatment and disposal of infected human feces.

Visceral Larva Migrans

Visceral larva migrans is a systemic nematodiasis caused by ingestion of the eggs of the dog tapeworm, *Toxocara canis,* or, less commonly, the cat tapeworm, *Toxocara cati,* or the raccoon tapeworm, *Baylisascaris procyonis* (see Table 124.2). These organisms also cause **ocular larva migrans**.

Visceral larva migrans is most common in young children with pica who have dogs or cats as pets. Ocular toxocariasis occurs in older children. The eggs of these roundworms are produced by adult worms residing in the dog and cat intestine. Ingested eggs hatch into larvae that penetrate the gastrointestinal tract and migrate to the liver, lung, eye, CNS, and heart, where they die and calcify.

Symptoms of visceral larva migrans are the result of the number of migrating larvae and the associated immune response. Light infections are often asymptomatic. Symptoms include fever, cough, wheezing, and seizures. Physical findings may include hepatomegaly, lung crackles, rash, and lymphadenopathy. Visual symptoms may include decreased acuity, strabismus, periorbital edema, or blindness. Eye examination may reveal granulomatous lesions near the macula or disc. Ocular larva migrans is generally characterized by isolated, unilateral ocular disease and no systemic findings.

Eosinophilia and hypergammaglobulinemia associated with elevated isohemagglutinin levels suggest the diagnosis, which is confirmed by serology (enzyme-linked immunosorbent assay) or, less commonly, by biopsy. This is usually a self-limited illness. In severe disease, albendazole or mebendazole is used, often with adjunctive corticosteroids to limit the inflammatory response of *Toxocara* antigens by dying parasites. Deworming puppies and kittens, major excreters of eggs, decreases the risk of infection.

Enterobiasis (Pinworm)

Pinworm is caused by *Enterobius vermicularis,* a nematode that is distributed worldwide. Enterobiasis affects individuals at all socioeconomic levels, especially children. Crowded living conditions predispose to infection. Humans ingest the eggs carried on hands, which are present in house dust or on bedclothes. The eggs hatch in the stomach, and the larvae migrate to the cecum and mature. At night, the females migrate to the perianal area to lay their eggs (up to 10,000 eggs), which remain infective in the indoor environment for 2–3 weeks.

The most common symptoms are nocturnal anal pruritus **(pruritus ani)** and sleeplessness, presumably resulting from the migratory female worms. Vaginitis and salpingitis may develop secondary to aberrant worm migration. The eggs are detected by microscopically examining adhesive cellophane tape pressed against the anus in the morning to collect eggs. Less commonly, a worm may be seen in the perianal region. Treatment is with albendazole, mebendazole, or pyrantel pamoate each given as a single oral dose and repeated in 2–3 weeks.

Schistosomiasis

Schistosomiasis (bilharziasis) is caused by flukes that parasitize the bloodstream, including *Schistosoma haematobium, S. mansoni, S. japonicum,* and, rarely, *S. intercalatum* and *S. mekongi* (Table 124.3). Schistosomiasis affects more than 200 million people worldwide. Humans are infected by cercariae in contaminated water that emerge in an infectious form from snails and penetrate intact skin. Each adult worm migrates to specific sites: *S. haematobium* to the **bladder plexus** and *S. mansoni* and *S. japonicum* to the **mesenteric vessels**. The eggs are deposited by the adult flukes in urine *(S. haematobium)* or stool (*S. mansoni* and *S. japonicum*). *S. haematobium* is prevalent in Africa and the Middle East; *S. mansoni* in Africa, the Middle East, the Caribbean, and South America; *S. japonicum* in China, the Philippines, and Indonesia; *S. mekongi* in Cambodia and Laos; and *S. intercalatum* in West and Central Africa.

The manifestations of schistosomiasis result from eggs that are trapped at the site of deposition or at metastatic locations. Within 4–8 weeks of infection, while the worms are maturing, a syndrome of fever, malaise, cough, abdominal pain, hepatosplenomegaly, eosinophilia, and rash can occur **(Katayama fever)**. This syndrome is followed by a resultant inflammatory response that leads to further symptoms. Eggs may be found in the urine *(S. haematobium)* or stool (*S. mansoni* and *S. japonicum*) of infected individuals. Sanitary measures, molluscacides, and therapy (praziquantel) for infected individuals may help control the illness.

Echinococcosis

Echinococcosis includes **hydatid or unilocular cyst disease**, caused by *Echinococcus granulosus* (the **minute dog tapeworm**); polycystic disease, caused by *Echinococcus vogeli*; and **alveolar cyst disease**, caused by *Echinococcus multilocularis* (Table 124.4). Dogs become infected with tapeworms by eating infected sheep or cattle viscera and excrete eggs in their stools. Humans acquire echinococcosis by ingesting eggs and become an intermediate host. The eggs hatch in the intestinal tract, and the larva **(oncospheres)** penetrate the mucosa

TABLE 124.3 Major Pediatric Syndromes Caused by Parasitic Trematodes

SYNDROME	ETIOLOGIC AGENT	TRANSMISSION	TREATMENT
Schistosomiases		Freshwater contact with penetration through the skin	
Intestinal or hepatic schistosomiasis	*Schistosoma mansoni* *Schistosoma japonicum* *Schistosoma mekongi*		Praziquantel *or* oxamniquine
Urinary schistosomiasis	*Schistosoma haematobium*		
Parasitoses due to Other Trematodes		Ingestion of raw or inadequately cooked foods	
Clonorchiasis	*Clonorchis sinensis* (Chinese liver fluke)		Praziquantel *or* albendazole
Fascioliasis	*Fasciola hepatica* (sheep liver fluke)		Triclabendazole
Fasciolopsiasis	*Fasciolopsis buski*		Praziquantel
Heterophyiasis	*Heterophyes heterophyes*		Praziquantel
Metagonimiasis	*Metagonimus yokogawai*		Praziquantel
Metorchiasis	*Metorchis conjunctus* (North American liver fluke)		Praziquantel
Nanophyetiasis	*Nanophyetus salmincola* (salmon fluke)		Praziquantel
Opisthorchiasis	*Opisthorchis viverrini* (Southeast Asian liver fluke)		Praziquantel *or* albendazole
Paragonimiasis	*Paragonimus westermani, P. kellicotti, P. uterobilateralis, P. skrjabini, P. heterotremus, P. africanus* (lung flukes)		Praziquantel *or* triclabendazole

TABLE 124.4 Major Pediatric Syndromes Caused by Parasitic Cestodes

SYNDROME	ETIOLOGIC AGENT	TRANSMISSION	TREATMENT
Echinococcosis		Ingestion of *Echinococcus* eggs	
Unilocular	*E. granulosus*		Surgical resection *plus* albendazole
Alveolar echinococcosis	*E. multilocularis*		Surgical resection is only reliable means of treatment; some reports suggest adjunct use of albendazole or mebendazole
Neurocysticercosis	Larval stage of *Taenia solium* (cysticerci)	Ingestion of eggs through direct fecal-oral contact or ingestion of fecally contaminated foods	Albendazole *or* praziquantel
Adult tapeworm infections	*T. solium* (pork tapeworm)	Ingestion of contaminated raw/undercooked pork	Praziquantel
	Hymenolepis diminuta	Ingestion of infected insect	Praziquantel
	Hymenolepis nana	Fecal-oral	Praziquantel

and enter the circulation to pass to the liver and other visceral organs, forming cysts.

E. granulosus has a worldwide distribution and is endemic in sheep-raising and cattle-raising areas of Australia, South America, South Africa, the former Soviet Union, and the Mediterranean region. The prevalence is highest in children. Symptoms caused by *E. granulosus* result from space-occupying cysts. Pulmonary cysts may cause hemoptysis, cough, dyspnea, and respiratory distress. Brain cysts appear as tumors; liver cysts cause problems as they compress and obstruct blood flow. Ultrasonography identifies cystic lesions, and the diagnosis is confirmed by serologic testing. Large or asymptomatic granulosa cysts are removed surgically. Treatment with albendazole has shown benefit.

Neurocysticercosis

Neurocysticercosis is caused by infection with the embryonated eggs of the **pork tapeworm**, *Taenia solium,* and is the most frequent helminthic infection of the CNS (see Table 124.4). Humans are infected after consuming cysticerci in raw or undercooked larva-containing pork. Infected humans then pass *T. solium* eggs in their feces. Fecal-oral transmission of eggs, to either the originally infected host or other individuals, then results in cysticerci development in organs; in particular, in subcutaneous tissues, brain, and eyes. *T. solium* is endemic in Asia, Africa, and Central and South America.

Cysts typically enlarge slowly, causing no or minimal symptoms for years or decades until the organism begins to die. The cyst then begins to swell, and leakage of antigen incites an inflammatory response, resulting in the presenting signs of focal or generalized seizures and calcified cerebral cysts identified by computed tomography or magnetic resonance imaging. The CSF shows lymphocytic or eosinophilic pleocytosis. The diagnosis is confirmed by serologic testing. Neurocysticercosis is treated with albendazole or praziquantel, along with corticosteroids for concomitant cerebral inflammation from cyst death, and anticonvulsant drugs.

PEARLS FOR PRACTITIONERS

See Infectious Diseases: Pearls for Practitioners at the end of this section.

REVIEW QUESTIONS

Available online.

CHAPTER 125
Tuberculosis

ETIOLOGY

Mycobacterium tuberculosis bacilli are pleomorphic, weakly gram-positive curved rods that are **acid fast**, which is the capacity to form stable mycolate complexes with arylmethane dyes. *M. tuberculosis* grows slowly; culture from clinical specimens on solid synthetic media usually takes 3–6 weeks. Drug susceptibility testing can require an additional 4 weeks. Growth can be detected in 1–3 weeks in selective liquid media using radiolabeled nutrients. Polymerase chain reaction (PCR) of clinical specimens may allow rapid diagnosis and some limited susceptibility testing in many laboratories.

EPIDEMIOLOGY

It is estimated that one-third of the world's population is infected with tuberculosis (TB). Most of these are latent infections. Without treatment, tuberculosis *disease* develops in 5–10% of immunologically normal adults with tuberculosis *infection* at some time during their lives; the risk is higher in infants and those who are immunocompromised, especially HIV-positive individuals. According to the World Health Organization (WHO), an estimated 10 million new cases of TB occur each year worldwide, including 11% of cases in children. One to 2 million deaths are attributed to the disease annually. Greater than 10,000 TB cases were reported in the United States in 2024.

Transmission of *M. tuberculosis* is from person to person, usually by respiratory droplets that become airborne when a symptomatic individual coughs, sneezes, laughs, or even breathes. Infected droplets dry and become droplet nuclei, which may remain suspended in the air for hours, long after the infectious person has left the environment.

Several patient-related factors are associated with an increased chance of transmission. Of these, a positive acid-fast smear of the sputum most closely correlates with infectivity. Children with primary pulmonary tuberculosis disease rarely, if ever, infect others because tubercle bacilli are relatively sparse in the endobronchial secretions of young children with pulmonary tuberculosis. In addition, when young children cough, they rarely produce sputum, lacking the tussive force necessary to project and suspend infectious particles of the requisite size. Hospitalized patients with suspected pulmonary tuberculosis should be initially placed in airborne isolation. Most infectious patients become noninfectious within 2 weeks of starting effective treatment. *Cavitary disease, nonadherence to treatment, and resistant infection increase the risk of transmission.*

In North America, TB rates are highest in foreign-born persons from high-prevalence countries, residents of prisons or nursing homes, unhoused persons, users of illegal drugs, people with limited health care access, health care workers, and children exposed to adults in high-risk groups. Most children are infected with *M. tuberculosis* from household contacts, but outbreaks of childhood tuberculosis centered in schools, daycares, churches, school buses, and stores still occur. A high-risk adult working in the area has been the source of the outbreak in most cases. Certain biologic response modifiers (anti–tumor necrosis factor [TNF] antibodies), often used for treatment of inflammatory conditions, can increase risk of development of tuberculosis disease. Genes involved in **Mendelian susceptibility to mycobacterial diseases (MSMD)** increase the risk of infection for environmental *(atypical)* mycobacterium and dissemination of **bacille Calmette-Guérin (BCG)** vaccine and possibly *M. tuberculosis*. These pathogenic gene variants affect the interleukin 12 (IL-12)/interferon-γ (IFN-γ)–mediated immunity pathway.

CLINICAL MANIFESTATIONS

TB infection (latent TB) describes the asymptomatic stage of infection with *M. tuberculosis*. The **tuberculin skin test (TST)** or **interferon**-γ release assay (IGRA) is positive, but the chest radiograph is normal or shows healed infection (calcification). **TB disease** occurs when there are clinical signs and symptoms and/or an abnormal chest radiograph or extrapulmonary manifestation. The interval between TB infection and the onset of disease may be several weeks in children or many decades in adults. In young children, TB usually develops as an immediate complication of the primary infection, and the distinction between infection and disease may be less obvious.

Primary TB (initial infection) in children is often an asymptomatic infection. Often it is manifested by a positive TST or IGRA with mild abnormalities on the chest radiograph, such as atelectasis or a nonspecific infiltrate accompanied by hilar or other adenopathy **(Ghon complex)**. Malaise, low-grade fever, erythema nodosum, or symptoms resulting from lymph node enlargement may occur after the development of delayed hypersensitivity. **Progressive primary disease** is characterized by a primary pneumonia that develops shortly after initial infection. Progression to disseminated **miliary disease** or CNS infection occurs most commonly in the first year of life. Cavitation is rare in children but more typical with reactivation pulmonary TB in adolescents and adults.

Tuberculous pleural effusion, which may accompany primary infection, generally represents the immune response to the organisms and most commonly occurs in older children or adolescents. Pleurocentesis reveals lymphocytes and an increased protein level, but the pleural fluid usually does not contain bacilli.

Reactivation pulmonary tuberculosis, common in adolescents and typical in adults, usually is confined to apical segments of upper lobes or superior segments of lower lobes. There is usually little lymphadenopathy and no extrathoracic infection. This is a manifestation of a secondary expansion of infection at a site seeded years previously during primary infection. Advanced disease is associated with cavitation and endobronchial spread of bacilli. Symptoms include fever, night sweats, malaise, and weight loss. A productive cough and hemoptysis often herald cavitation and bronchial erosion.

Miliary tuberculosis refers to widespread hematogenous dissemination to multiple organs. The lesions are of roughly the same size as a millet seed, from which the name *miliary* is derived. Miliary TB is characterized by fever, general malaise, weight loss, lymphadenopathy, night sweats, and hepatosplenomegaly. Diffuse bilateral pneumonitis is common, and meningitis is often present. The chest radiograph reveals bilateral miliary infiltrates, showing overwhelming infection. The TST may be nonreactive as a result of **anergy**.

Tuberculous meningitis most commonly occurs in children younger than 5 years or immunocompromised patients, often within 6 months of primary infection or during miliary TB. Tubercle bacilli that seed the meninges during the primary infection replicate, triggering an inflammatory response. This condition may have an insidious onset, initially characterized by low-grade fever, headache, and subtle personality change. Progression of the infection results in basilar meningitis with impingement of the cranial nerves and is manifested by meningeal irritation and, eventually, increased intracranial pressure, deterioration of mental status, and coma. CT scans show hydrocephalus, edema, periventricular lucencies, and infarctions. Cerebrospinal fluid (CSF) analysis reveals pleocytosis (50–500 leukocytes/mm^3), which early in the course of disease may be either lymphocytes or polymorphonuclear leukocytes. Glucose is low, and protein is significantly elevated. Acid-fast bacilli are not detected frequently in the CSF by either routine or fluorescent staining procedures. Although culture is the standard for diagnosis, PCR for *M. tuberculosis* may be useful to confirm meningitis but lacks sensitivity.

Skeletal tuberculosis results from either hematogenous seeding or direct extension from a caseous lymph node. This is usually a chronic disease with an insidious onset that may be mistaken for chronic osteomyelitis. Radiographs reveal cortical destruction. Biopsy and culture are essential for proper diagnosis. Tuberculosis of the spine, **Pott disease**, is the most common skeletal site.

Other forms of TB include **abdominal tuberculosis** that occurs from swallowing infected material. This is a relatively uncommon complication in developed nations where dairy herds are inspected for bovine tuberculosis. Gastrointestinal TB can present with signs and symptoms similar to inflammatory bowel disease. **Tuberculous peritonitis** is associated with abdominal TB and presents as fever, anorexia, ascites, and abdominal pain. **Urogenital tuberculosis** is a late reactivation complication and is rare in children. Symptomatic illness presents as dysuria, frequency, urgency, hematuria, and *sterile* pyuria or infertility. TB may also result in extrathoracic lymphadenitis in the cervical, supraclavicular, and submandibular areas **(scrofula)**.

Congenital tuberculosis can mimic neonatal sepsis or more commonly present at weeks to months of age with hepatosplenomegaly and respiratory disease.

LABORATORY AND IMAGING STUDIES

Two types of tests are used to detect the immune response to *M. tuberculosis* and are used to screen patients for TB infection and investigation of active TB. The TST response to tuberculin antigen is a manifestation of a T-cell–mediated delayed hypersensitivity. The **Mantoux test**, an intradermal injection of **purified protein derivative standard (PPD-S)**, usually on the volar surface of the forearm, is the standard TST. It is usually positive 2–6 weeks after onset of infection (up to 3 months) and at the time of symptomatic illness. False-negative responses may occur early in the illness, with overwhelming TB infection, with concomitant viral infection, or as a result of immunosuppression (secondary to underlying illness, HIV, or malnutrition). Tests with questionable results should be repeated after several weeks. All internationally adopted children from TB endemic regions with an initially negative TST should have a repeat TST after 3 months in the United States. The TST is interpreted based on the host status and size of induration (Tables 125.1 and 125.2). In general, interpretation of TST in people who have had previous BCG vaccine can be difficult, given the cross-reaction of TST with antigens present in the vaccine. However, in situations when a TB exposure has occurred, the TST should be read and interpreted as if no BCG vaccine had been given.

An interferon gamma release assay (IGRA) is a whole-blood test that measures INF-γ production by T lymphocytes in response to antigens from the *M. tuberculosis* complex, which includes *M. bovis* but not antigens found in the BCG vaccine. An IGRA is the recommended diagnostic test for persons older than 2 years of age in the United States. It has similar sensitivity to the TST but improved specificity because it is unaffected by prior BCG vaccination. It is also practically easier to obtain, because it requires only one visit to complete. As with the TST, in immunocompromised persons and in active tuberculosis, IGRA findings may be indeterminate. Though the PPD has traditionally been preferred for young children, currently either TST or IGRA testing is acceptable for children of any age.

The ultimate diagnostic confirmation relies on culture of the organism. Sputum is an excellent source for diagnosis in pulmonary disease in adults but is difficult to obtain in young children. Induced sputum or gastric fluid obtained via an indwelling nasogastric tube with samples taken before or immediately on waking contains swallowed sputum and provides alternate samples in young children. Large volumes of fluid (CSF, pericardial fluid) yield a higher rate of recovery of organisms, but slow growth of the mycobacteria makes culture less helpful in acute illness. Even with optimal collection, cultures are positive in less than half of children with TB. When the organism is grown, drug susceptibilities should be determined because of the increasing incidence of resistant organisms. Utilization of culture and susceptibility results from the source case is often necessary given the difficulty of obtaining timely results.

PCR testing for mycobacteria has expedited diagnosis, especially with CNS disease. However, these assays have limited sensitivity and provide no susceptibility data. Most experts would recommend that infants younger than 12 months with suspected TB undergo lumbar puncture for evaluation of CNS involvement regardless of the presence of neurological symptoms.

TABLE 125.1 TST and IGRA Recommendations for Infants, Children, and Adolescents*

Children for Whom Immediate TST or IGRA Is Indicated†: • Contacts of people with confirmed or suspected contagious tuberculosis (contact investigation) • Children with radiographic or clinical findings suggesting tuberculosis disease • Children immigrating from countries with endemic infection (e.g., Asia, Middle East, Africa, Latin America, countries of the former Soviet Union), including international adoptees • Children with history of significant‡ travel to countries with endemic infection who have substantial contact with the resident population§
Children Who Should Have Annual TST or IGRA: • Children living with HIV infection
Children at increased risk of progression of TBI to TB disease: Infants <1 year of age and children with other medical conditions, including diabetes mellitus, chronic renal failure, malnutrition, or congenital or acquired immunodeficiencies, and children receiving TNF antagonists, deserve special consideration. Underlying immune deficiencies associated with these conditions theoretically would enhance the possibility for rapid progression to severe disease. Initial histories of potential exposure to tuberculosis should be included for all these patients. If these histories or local epidemiologic factors suggest a possibility of exposure, immediate and periodic TST or IGRA should be considered.
A TST or IGRA should be performed before initiation of immunosuppressive therapy, including prolonged systemic corticosteroid administration, organ transplantation, use of TNF-α antagonists or blockers, or other immunosuppressive therapy in any child requiring these treatments.

**Bacille Calmette-Guérin (BCG) immunization is not a contraindication to a TST; IGRA is generally preferred for BCG-vaccinated children.*
†Beginning as early as 3 months of age for TST; IGRA may be used at any age.
‡Some experts define significant travel as birth, travel, or residence in a country with an elevated tuberculosis rate for at least 1 month.
§If the child is well and has no history of exposure, the TST or IGRA should be delayed for 8 to 10 weeks after return.
HIV, Human immunodeficiency virus; *IGRA,* interferon-gamma release assay; *TB,* tuberculosis; *TBI, Mycobacterium tuberculosis* infection; *TNF,* tumor necrosis factor; *TST,* tuberculin skin test;
From American Academy of Pediatrics. Tuberculosis. In: Kimberlin DW, Banerjee R, Barnett ED, et al., eds. Red Book: 2024–2027 Report of the Committee on Infectious Diseases. *Itasca, IL: American Academy of Pediatrics; 2024;894.*

Diagnostic Imaging

Because many cases of pulmonary tuberculosis in children may be clinically silent, radiography is a cornerstone for the diagnosis of disease (Figs. 125.1 and 125.2). All lobar segments of the lung are at equal risk of being the focus of the

TABLE 125.2 Definitions of Positive TST Results in Infants, Children, and Adolescents*,†

INDURATION ≥5 MM
Children in close contact with known or suspected contagious people with TB disease
Children suspected to have TB disease: • Findings on chest radiograph consistent with active or previous TB disease • Clinical evidence of TB disease‡
Children receiving immunosuppressive therapy§ or with immunosuppressive conditions, including HIV infection
INDURATION ≥10 MM
Children at increased risk of disseminated TB disease: • Children <4 yr • Children with other medical conditions, including Hodgkin disease, lymphoma, diabetes mellitus, chronic renal failure, or malnutrition (see Table 125.1) • Children born in high-prevalence regions of the world • Children with significant travel to high-prevalence regions of the world¶ • Children frequently exposed to adults who are living with HIV, lacking housing, or incarcerated, or to people who inject or use drugs
INDURATION ≥15 MM
Children without any risk factors

*See www.cdc.gov/tb/publications/guidelines/pdf/ciw778.pdf.
†These definitions apply regardless of previous bacille Calmette-Guérin immunization; erythema alone at TST site does not indicate a positive test result. Tests should be read at 48–72 hours after placement.
‡Evidence by physical examination or laboratory assessment that would include TB in the working differential diagnosis (e.g., meningitis).
§Including immunosuppressive doses of corticosteroids or tumor necrosis factor-α antagonists or blockers or immunosuppressive drugs used in transplant recipients.
¶Some experts define significant travel as travel or residence in a country with an elevated TB rate for at least 1 month.
HIV, Human immunodeficiency virus; *TB,* tuberculosis; *TST,* tuberculin skin test.
From American Academy of Pediatrics. Tuberculosis. In: Kimberlin DW, Banerjee R, Barnett ED, et al., eds. Red Book: 2024–2027 Report of the Committee on Infectious Diseases. Itasca, IL: American Academy of Pediatrics; 2024;890.

initial infection. In 25% of cases, two or more lobes of the lungs are involved, although disease usually occurs at one site only. Spread of infection to regional lymph nodes occurs early. Hilar lymphadenopathy is inevitably present with childhood TB. Partial bronchial obstruction caused by external compression from the enlarging nodes can cause air trapping, hyperinflation, and lobar emphysema. Occasionally, children have a picture of lobar pneumonia without impressive hilar lymphadenopathy. If the infection is progressively destructive, liquefaction of the lung parenchyma leads to formation of a thin-walled primary tuberculous cavity. Adolescents with pulmonary tuberculosis may develop segmental lesions with hilar lymphadenopathy or the apical infiltrates, with or without cavitation, that are typical of adult reactivation tuberculosis.

Radiographic studies aid greatly in the diagnosis of **extrapulmonary tuberculosis** in children. Plain radiographs, CT, and MRI of the tuberculous spine usually show collapse and destruction of the vertebral body with narrowing of the involved disk spaces. Radiographic findings in bone and joint TB range from mild joint effusions and small lytic lesions to massive destruction of the bone. CT or MRI of the brains of patients with CNS involvement may be normal during early stages of the infection. As disease progresses, basilar enhancement and communicating hydrocephalus with signs of cerebral edema or early focal ischemia are the most common findings.

Caseating granulomas on tissue pathology can also help to establish the diagnosis of TB on samples from lymph nodes and other biopsies.

DIFFERENTIAL DIAGNOSIS

The differential diagnosis of TB includes a multitude of diagnoses because TB may affect any organ, and in early disease the symptoms and signs may be nonspecific. In pulmonary disease, TB may appear similar to bacterial or fungal pneumonia, malignancy, and any systemic disease in which generalized lymphadenopathy occurs. The diagnosis of TB should be suspected if the TST or IGRA is positive and/or if there is history of TB exposure.

The differential diagnosis of tuberculous lymphadenopathy includes infections caused by atypical mycobacteria, *Bartonella,* fungi, viruses, and bacteria, as well as toxoplasmosis, sarcoidosis, drug reactions, and malignancy.

TREATMENT

Combination therapy is the backbone of therapy for tuberculosis disease to prevent the emergence of resistance. The treatment of TB is affected by the presence of naturally occurring drug-resistant organisms in large bacterial populations, even before therapy is initiated, and the fact that mycobacteria replicate slowly and can remain dormant in the body for prolonged periods. Several regimens are available for treatment of TB infection in children and in recent years have been shortened and simplified. One recommended option is **rifampin (RIF)** for 4 months. For children over age 2 years, combination therapy with once-weekly **isoniazid (INH)** and **rifapentine (RPT)** for 3 months is another option. Alternate options include INH and RIF daily for 3 months or INH alone for 9 months. Therapy for TB infection is aimed at eradicating organisms sequestered within macrophages and suppressed by normal T-cell activity.

Children with both pulmonary and extrapulmonary tuberculosis are treated with combination therapy (Table 125.3) for a prolonged course, traditionally 6–9 months, depending on the type of disease. INH and RIF are bactericidal for *M. tuberculosis.* Along with pyrazinamide ± ethambutol, they form the backbone of the antimicrobial treatment of tuberculosis. Other drugs and prolonged regimens are used in special circumstances, such as CNS infection and multidrug-resistant **(MDR)** or extensively drug-resistant **(XDR)** tuberculosis, which are unfortunately increasing in prevalence in some parts of the world and are associated with increased treatment failure and mortality.

In the United States, drug-susceptible pulmonary tuberculosis is traditionally treated with 2 months of four drugs and then completed with INH and RIF for an additional 4 months. In some circumstances this regimen can be shortened to a total 4-month course. Longer courses are used for extrapulmonary disease. Steroids are often used in conjunction with antiinfective therapy for CNS TB. Noncompliance or nonadherence is a major problem in TB control because of the long-term nature of treatment and the sometimes difficult social circumstances

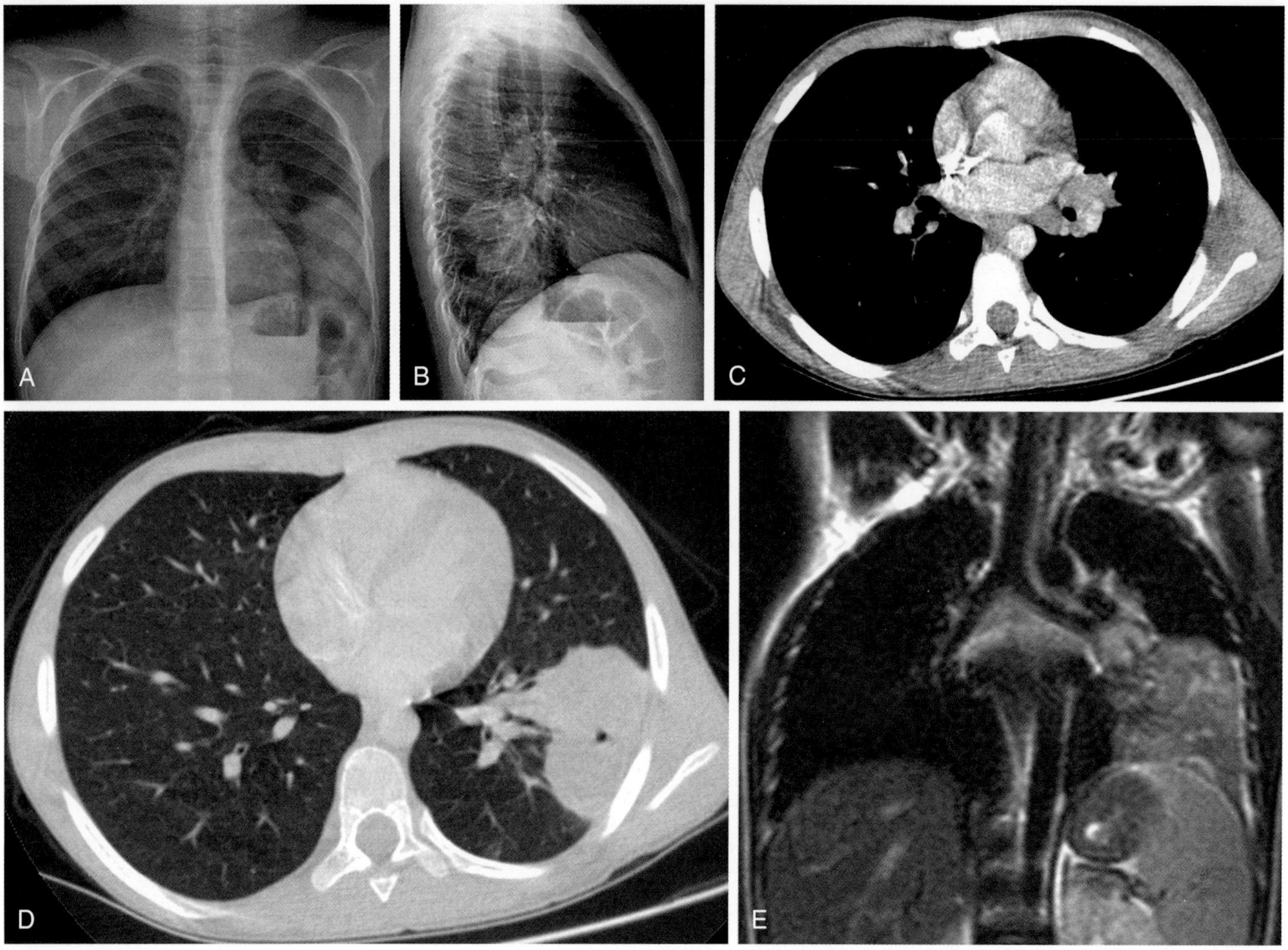

FIGURE 125.1 Primary tuberculosis (TB) in an 8-year-old child who presented with cough, abdominal pain, and fatigue. (**A** and **B**) Radiographs show nodular consolidation in the left lower lung zone and an enlarged left hilum. (**C** and **D**) Contrast-enhanced computed tomography demonstrates a peripheral consolidation in the left lower lobe, associated with enlarged left hilar lymph nodes. **(E)** On coronal T2 weighted magnetic resonance imaging, the consolidation and lymph nodes exhibit high signal intensity. The parenchymal consolidation and associated ipsilateral lymph nodes constitute the primary Ghon complex in TB. Culture of bronchial lavage fluid confirmed the diagnosis. (From Westra SJ, Yikilmaz A, Lee EY. Pulmonary Infection. In: Coley BD, ed. *Caffey's Pediatric Diagnostic Imaging*. 13th ed. Philadelphia: Elsevier; 2019:e-fig. 54.18.)

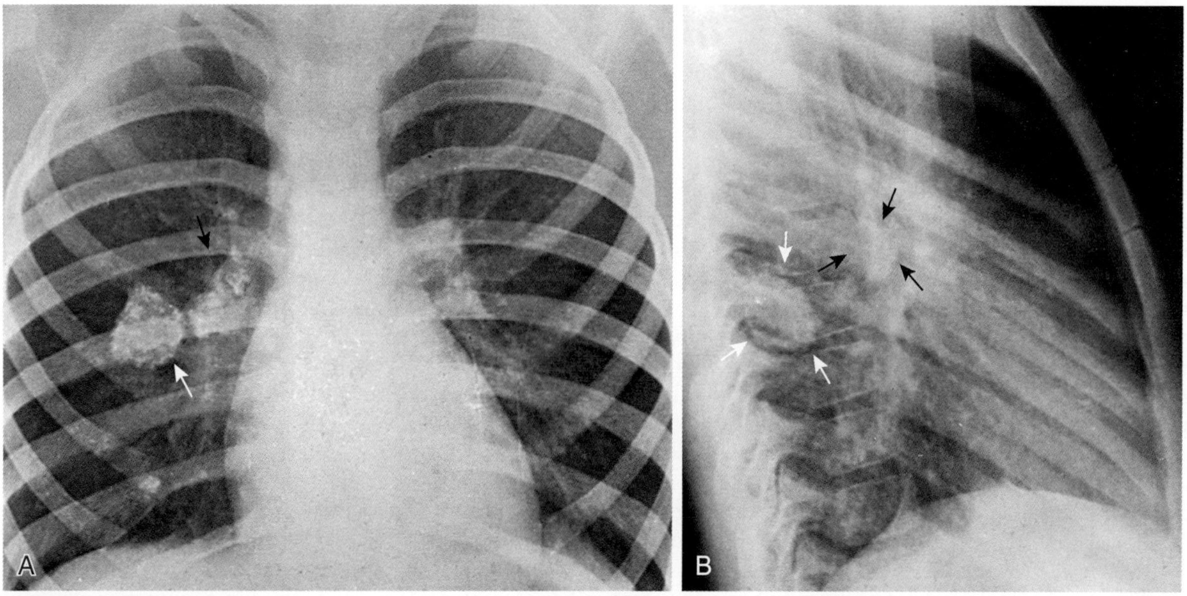

FIGURE 125.2 A large calcified primary tuberculous focus in the right lower lobe That Dwarfs the Rest of the Complex in an Asymptomatic 6-Year-Old Child. The healing and calcification of this huge necrotic focus *(white arrow)* without manifest clinical disease at any time shows the often benign clinical aspects of severe structural tuberculous disease. The *black arrow* shows calcified hilar adenopathy. In the frontal projection **(A)**, the large calcifying focus appears to be perihilar. **(B)** In the lateral projection, this focus lies posterior to right hilar nodes *(black arrows)* in the apical segment of the right lower lobe *(white arrows)* near the dorsal pleura. (From Westra SJ, Yikilmaz A, Lee EY. Pulmonary Infection. In: Coley BD, ed. *Caffey's Pediatric Diagnostic Imaging*. 13th ed. Philadelphia: Elsevier; 2019:e-fig. 54.21.)

TABLE 125.3 Recommended Usual Treatment Regimens for Drug-Susceptible TB Infection and TB Disease in Infants, Children, and Adolescents

INFECTION OR DISEASE CATEGORY	REGIMEN	REMARKS
Mycobacterium tuberculosis infection		Evidenced by positive TST or IGRA result, without disease*
Isoniazid susceptible	3 months of isoniazid plus rifapentine (3HP), once a week	Not for children <2 years
	or	
	4 mo of rifampin (4R), once a day	Continuous daily therapy is required. Check for drug interactions
	or	
	3 mo of isoniazid plus rifampin, once a day	To be considered if above 2 regimens are not feasible.
	or	
	6 or 9 mo of isoniazid, once a day	If daily therapy is not possible, DOT twice a week can be used; medication doses differ with daily and twice-weekly regimens.
Isoniazid resistant	4 mo of rifampin, once a day	Continuous daily therapy is required.
Isoniazid-rifampin resistant	Consult a TB specialist	Moxifloxacin or levofloxacin with or without ethambutol or pyrazinamide are most commonly given.
Pulmonary disease†	2 mo of rifampin, isoniazid, pyrazinamide, and ethambutol (RIPE) daily, followed by 2–4 mo of isoniazid and rifampin by DOT‡ for drug-susceptible *M. tuberculosis*	Some experts recommend a 3-drug initial regimen (isoniazid, rifampin, and pyrazinamide) if the risk of drug resistance is low. DOT is highly desirable.
Extrapulmonary disease or meningitis	2 mo of isoniazid, rifampin, pyrazinamide, and ethionamide or a fluoroquinolone, once a day,§ followed by 4–10 mo of isoniazid and rifampin once daily or 3 times a week (6–12 mo total) for drug-susceptible *M. tuberculosis*	See text for information on corticosteroids for CNS disease.

**See text for comments and additional acceptable/alternative regimens.*
†Duration of therapy may be longer for people living with HIV infection, and additional drugs and dosing intervals may be indicated.
‡If initial chest radiograph shows pulmonary cavities and/or sputum culture after 2 months of therapy remains positive, the continuation phase is extended to 7 months, for a total treatment duration of 9 months.
§When susceptibility to first-line drugs is established, the ethionamide or fluoroquinolone can be discontinued.
DOT, Directly observed therapy; *IGRA,* interferon-gamma release assay; *TB,* tuberculosis; *TST,* tuberculin skin test.
From American Academy of Pediatrics. Tuberculosis. In: Kimberlin DW, Banerjee R, Barnett ED, et al., eds. Red Book: 2024–2027 Report of the Committee on Infectious Diseases. *Itasca, IL: American Academy of Pediatrics; 2024;899–901.*

of the patients. As treatment regimens become shorter, adherence assumes an even greater importance. Improvement in compliance occurs with **directly observed therapy (DOT)**, which requires a health care worker to witness the administration of medications and is the standard of care in most settings.

COMPLICATIONS AND PROGNOSIS

The prognosis of TB in infants, children, and adolescents is excellent with early recognition and effective chemotherapy. In most children with pulmonary tuberculosis, the disease completely resolves, and ultimately radiographic findings are normal. The prognosis for children with bone and joint tuberculosis and tuberculous meningitis depends directly on the stage of disease at the time antituberculosis medications are started. Tuberculosis of the spine may result in angulation or **gibbus** formation that requires surgical correction after the infection is cured. Most childhood tuberculous meningitis occurs in developing countries, where the prognosis is poor. Resistant organisms are more difficult to treat and worsen prognosis.

PREVENTION

TB control programs work on case finding and treatment, which interrupts secondary transmission of infection from close contacts. Infected close contacts are identified by positive TST or IGRA testing and can be started on appropriate treatment to prevent transmission.

Prevention of transmission in health care settings involves appropriate physical ventilation of the air around the source case. Offices, clinics, and hospital rooms used by adults with possible TB should have adequate ventilation, with air exhausted to the outside **(negative-pressure ventilation)**. The only currently available vaccine against TB is the **BCG vaccine**. The original vaccine organism was a strain of attenuated *Mycobacterium bovis.* The preferred route of administration is intradermal injection with a syringe and needle because this is the only method that permits accurate measurement of an individual dose. The official recommendation of the WHO is a single dose administered during infancy. This vaccine is not routinely used in the United States. Studies show BCG provides up to 80–90% protection from miliary disease and TB meningitis in infants. Many who receive BCG vaccine never have a positive TST reaction. When a reaction does occur, the induration size is usually less than 10 mm, and it variably wanes after several years. BCG vaccination does not affect results of an IGRA.

PEARLS FOR PRACTITIONERS

See Infectious Diseases: Pearls for Practitioners at the end of this section.

REVIEW QUESTIONS

Available online.

CHAPTER 126

Human Immunodeficiency Virus and Acquired Immunodeficiency Syndrome

ETIOLOGY

The cause of acquired immunodeficiency syndrome (AIDS) is the human immunodeficiency virus (HIV), a single-stranded RNA virus of the retrovirus family. HIV-1 causes 99% of all human cases. HIV-2, which is less virulent, causes 1–9% of cases in parts of Africa and is very rare in the United States.

HIV infects **helper T cells (CD4 cells)** and cells of monocyte-macrophage lineage via interaction of viral protein gp120 with the CD4 molecule and chemokines (CXCR4 and CCR5) that serve as co-receptors. Interaction with these molecules facilitates membrane fusion and cell entry by the virus. HIV infection directly and indirectly depletes CD4 T cells. Helper T cells are important for delayed hypersensitivity, T-cell–dependent B-cell antibody production, and T-cell–mediated lymphokine activation of macrophages; their destruction produces a profound combined (B- and T-cell) immunodeficiency. A lack of T-cell regulation and unrestrained antigenic stimulation result in polyclonal hypergammaglobulinemia with nonspecific and ineffective globulins. Other cells bearing CD4, such as microglia, astrocytes, oligodendroglia, and placental tissues, also may be infected with HIV.

HIV infection is a continuously progressive process with a variable period of clinical latency before development of **AIDS-defining conditions**. All untreated patients have evidence of ongoing viral replication and progressive CD4 lymphocyte depletion. There are no overt manifestations of immunodeficiency until CD4 cell numbers decline to critical threshold levels. Quantitation of the viral load (HIV-1 RNA level) is an important parameter in management.

Horizontal transmission of HIV is by sexual contact (vaginal, anal, or orogenital), percutaneous contact (from contaminated needles or other sharp objects), or mucous membrane exposure to contaminated blood or body fluid. Transmission by contaminated blood and blood products has been nearly eliminated in developed countries by screening donated blood products but still occurs in developing countries. **Vertical transmission** of HIV from mother to infant may occur transplacentally in utero, during birth, or via breast-feeding. Risk factors for perinatal transmission include prematurity, prolonged rupture of membranes, and high maternal HIV viral load at delivery. In non–breast-feeding infants, perinatal transmission can be decreased from approximately 25% to less than 8% with administration of IV zidovudine during labor and postnatal treatment of the infant with PO zidovudine. Maternal treatment during pregnancy with combination antiretroviral therapy (cART) can reduce the risk of transmission to less than 1%. Breast-feeding by mothers with HIV increases the risk of vertical transmission. Breast-feeding may be considered with continued administration of cART for the mother and postnatal prophylactic ART for the infant if viral suppression (<200 copies/mL blood) in the mother is achieved. In developing countries, breast-feeding by an HIV-positive mother may outweigh the endemic risks of infant diarrhea, other infections, and malnutrition. In untreated infants, the mean incubation interval for development of an AIDS-defining condition after vertical transmission is 5 months (range of 1–24 months) compared with a longer incubation period after horizontal transmission of 7–10 years.

EPIDEMIOLOGY

The WHO states that worldwide as of 2024, approximately 40.8 million persons are living with HIV, and 1.4 million of them are children. There were 1.3 million new infections in 2024 with approximately 120,000 new infections in children. Approximately 65% of all people living with HIV reside in sub-Saharan Africa. Worldwide, 630,000 people died from HIV-related illnesses in 2024. Per HIV.gov, in 2022 the estimated number of people over the age of 13 years and living with HIV in the United States was 1.2 million. Vertical transmission is decreasing, with less than 100 infants each year in the United States acquiring HIV perinatally. Most pediatric cases in the United States occur in adolescents who engage in unprotected sexual activities. Worldwide the number of deaths related to HIV and the numbers of children infected with HIV have steadily decreased in large part due to treatment with ART.

CLINICAL MANIFESTATIONS

In adolescents and adults, primary infection results in the **acute retroviral syndrome** (resembling mononucleosis) that develops after an incubation period of 2–6 weeks and consists of fever, malaise, weight loss, pharyngitis, lymphadenopathy, and often a maculopapular rash. The risk of opportunistic infections and other AIDS-defining conditions is related to the depletion of CD4 T cells. A combination of CD4 cell count and percentage and clinical manifestations is used to classify HIV infection in children (Tables 126.1 and 126.2).

Initial symptoms with vertical transmission vary and may include growth faltering, neurodevelopmental delay, lymphadenopathy, hepatosplenomegaly, chronic or recurrent diarrhea, interstitial pneumonitis, or oral thrush. These findings may be subtle and remarkable only by their persistence. Manifestations that are more common in children than adults with HIV infection include recurrent bacterial infections, lymphoid hyperplasia, chronic parotid swelling, lymphocytic interstitial pneumonitis, and earlier onset of progressive neurologic

TABLE 126.1 HIV Infection Stage Based on Age-Specific CD4 Count or Percentage

	AGED <1 YR		AGED 1–<6 YR		AGED ≥6 YR	
STAGE	CELLS/MM³	%	CELLS/MM³	%	CELLS/MM³	%
1	≥1,500	≥34	≥1,000	≥30	≥500	≥26
2	750–1,499	26–33	500–999	22–29	200–499	14–25
3	<750	<26	<500	<22	<200	<14

From the Panel on Antiretroviral Therapy and Medical Management of HIV-Infected Children. Guidelines for the use of antiretroviral agents in pediatric HIV infection [table 5]. https://clinicalinfo.hiv.gov/en/guidelines/pediatric-arv/appendix-c-cdc-pediatric-hiv-cd4-cell?guideline%5B0%5D=title_bookpart%3AHIV+Clinical+Guidelines%3A+Pediatric+ARV&redirected=1.

TABLE 126.2 HIV–Related Symptoms and Conditions

MILDLY SYMPTOMATIC

Children with two or more of the conditions listed but none of the conditions listed in Moderate Symptoms category are considered mildly symptomatic:

- Lymphadenopathy (≥0.5 cm at more than two sites; bilateral at one site)
- Hepatomegaly
- Splenomegaly
- Dermatitis
- Parotitis
- Recurrent or persistent upper respiratory tract infection, sinusitis, or otitis media

MODERATELY SYMPTOMATIC

- Anemia (hemoglobin <8 g/dL), neutropenia (white blood cell count <1,000/µL), and/or thrombocytopenia (platelet count <100 × 10³/µL) persisting for ≥30 days
- Bacterial meningitis, pneumonia, or sepsis (single episode)
- Candidiasis, oropharyngeal (thrush), persisting (>2 mo) in children >6 mo of age
- Cardiomyopathy
- Cytomegalovirus infection, with onset before 1 mo
- Diarrhea, recurrent or chronic
- Hepatitis
- HSV stomatitis, recurrent (>2 episodes within 1 yr)
- HSV bronchitis, pneumonitis, or esophagitis with onset before 1 mo
- Herpes zoster (shingles) involving at least 2 distinct episodes or more than 1 dermatome
- Leiomyosarcoma
- Lymphoid interstitial pneumonia or pulmonary lymphoid hyperplasia complex
- Nephropathy
- Nocardiosis
- Persistent fever (lasting >1 mo)
- Toxoplasmosis, onset before 1 mo
- Varicella, disseminated (complicated chickenpox)

AIDS-DEFINING CONDITIONS

- Bacterial infections, multiple or recurrent*
- Candidiasis of bronchi, trachea, or lungs
- Candidiasis of esophagus
- Cervical cancer, invasive†
- Coccidioidomycosis, disseminated or extrapulmonary
- Cryptococcosis, extrapulmonary
- Cryptosporidiosis, chronic intestinal (>1 mo duration)
- Cytomegalovirus disease (other than liver, spleen, or nodes), onset at age >1 mo
- Cytomegalovirus retinitis (with loss of vision)
- Encephalopathy attributed to HIV
- HSV: chronic ulcers (>1 mo duration) or bronchitis, pneumonitis, or esophagitis (onset at age >1 mo)
- Histoplasmosis, disseminated or extrapulmonary
- Isosporiasis, chronic intestinal (>1 mo duration)
- Kaposi sarcoma
- Lymphoma, Burkitt (or equivalent term)
- Lymphoma, immunoblastic (or equivalent term)
- Lymphoma, primary, of brain
- *Mycobacterium avium* complex or *Mycobacterium kansasii*, disseminated or extrapulmonary
- *Mycobacterium tuberculosis* of any site, pulmonary, disseminated, or extrapulmonary
- *Mycobacterium*, other species or unidentified species, disseminated or extrapulmonary
- *Pneumocystis jirovecii* (previously known as *Pneumocystis carinii*) pneumonia
- Pneumonia, recurrent†
- Progressive multifocal leukoencephalopathy
- *Salmonella* septicemia, recurrent
- Toxoplasmosis of brain, onset at age >1 mo
- Wasting syndrome attributed to HIV

*Only among children aged <6 years.
†Only among adults, adolescents, and children aged ≥6 years.
HIV, Human immunodeficiency virus; *HSV*, herpes simplex virus.
What's New: Pediatric OIs HIV Clinical Guidelines NIH: https://clinicalinfo.hiv.gov/en/guidelines/hiv-clinical-guidelines-pediatric-opportunistic-infections/whats-new.
HIV Clinical Guidelines: Pediatric ARV—What's New in the Guidelines Clinicalinfo.HIV.gov: https://clinicalinfo.hiv.gov/en/guidelines/pediatric-arv/whats-new.
From the Panel on Antiretroviral Therapy and Medical Management of HIV-Infected Children. Guidelines for the use of antiretroviral agents in pediatric HIV infection [table 6].

deterioration. Pulmonary manifestations of HIV infection are common and include *Pneumocystis jirovecii* pneumonia, which can present early in infancy as a primary pneumonia characterized by hypoxia, tachypnea, retractions, elevated serum lactate dehydrogenase, and fever.

In the United States, most pregnant people are screened and, if positive, treated for HIV infection. Pregnant people with high HIV viral loads at delivery will be offered a cesarean section. All infants born to HIV-positive mothers are bathed prior to receiving their newborn hepatitis B vaccine and vitamin K injection, receive antiretroviral prophylaxis, are recommended to be exclusively formula fed (unless maternal viral suppression has been achieved), and are prospectively tested for infection. The diagnosis of HIV infection in most infants born in the United States is confirmed before development of clinical signs of infection.

LABORATORY AND IMAGING STUDIES

HIV infection can be diagnosed definitively in non–breast-fed infants by 1 month of age and in virtually all infected infants by 6 months of age using viral diagnostic assays (RNA polymerase chain reaction [PCR] or DNA PCR). Maternal antibodies may be detectable until 12–15 months of age, and a positive serologic test in the infant is not considered diagnostic until 18 months of age. HIV PCR (RNA or DNA) is the preferred method for diagnosing HIV infection during infancy and identifies ~50% of infected newborns at 48 hours and ~90% at 28 days. The timing of diagnostic viral testing varies depending on specific risk factors but typically involves testing at 2–3 weeks of age, at 1–2 months of age, and at 4–6 months of age. Testing at birth and 2–6 weeks after cessation of antiretroviral prophylaxis should be considered for infants at high risk for in utero infection (high maternal HIV viral load at delivery). HIV infection of an exposed infant is confirmed if virologic tests are positive on two separate occasions. HIV infection can be reasonably excluded in non–breast-fed infants with at least two virologic tests performed at older than 1 month of age, with one test being performed after 4 months of age. Loss of HIV antibody combined with negative HIV DNA PCR confirms absence of HIV infection. Persistence of a positive HIV antibody test after 18 months of age indicates HIV infection.

DIFFERENTIAL DIAGNOSIS

The differential diagnosis of AIDS in infants includes primary immunodeficiency syndromes and intrauterine infections such as cytomegalovirus (CMV) and syphilis. Prominence of individual symptoms, such as diarrhea, may suggest other etiologies.

TREATMENT

Management of HIV infection in children and adolescents is evolving and complex. It should be directed by a specialist in the treatment of HIV infection. Rapid initiation of cART is recommended for all HIV-positive children, irrespective of age or immune status.

Effective cART significantly reduces viral loads and leads to the amelioration of clinical symptoms and opportunistic infections. Combination therapy that includes either a nonnucleoside reverse transcriptase inhibitor (NNRTI), a protease inhibitor (PI), or an integrase inhibitor depending on the child's age plus a dual-nucleoside/nucleotide reverse transcriptase inhibitor (NRTI) backbone is recommended for initial treatment of all HIV-positive children. The goal of therapy is to reduce the HIV viral load to below the level of detection and normalize or preserve the patient's immune status. The most recent specific recommendations for treatment regimens (https://clinicalinfo.hiv.gov/en/guidelines) should be consulted before initiating therapy for any patient.

The ability of HIV to develop resistance to antiretroviral agents rapidly and the development of cross-resistance to several classes of agents simultaneously are major problems. Determination of HIV viral load, CD4 cell count, and HIV resistance genotype is essential for initiating, monitoring, and modifying antiretroviral treatment.

Routine immunizations are recommended but may result in suboptimal immune responses. Additional vaccines are also recommended, such as the 23-valent pneumococcal polysaccharide vaccine for children aged 2 years and older who have not received a 20-valent pneumococcal conjugate vaccine and the MenACWY vaccine beginning at age 2 months. Because of the risk of fatal measles in children with AIDS, children without severe immunosuppression should receive their first dose of measles, mumps, rubella (MMR) at 12 months of age and the second dose at 4–6 years of age. Varicella-zoster virus (VZV) vaccine should be given only to asymptomatic, nonimmunosuppressed children beginning at 12 months of age as two doses of vaccine at least 3 months apart. Inactivated influenza virus vaccine should be administered annually to all HIV-infected children at or after 6 months of age.

COMPLICATIONS

The approach to the numerous opportunistic infections in HIV-positive patients involves treatment and prophylaxis for infections likely to occur as CD4 cells are depleted. With potent ART and immune reconstitution, routine prophylaxis for common opportunistic infections depends on the child's age and CD4 count. Infants born to HIV-positive mothers should receive prophylaxis for *P. jirovecii* pneumonia with trimethoprim-sulfamethoxazole (TMP-SMX) until HIV infection has been excluded; if they are found to be HIV positive, TMP-SMX is continued until 1 year of age regardless of CD4 cell counts. TMP-SMX prophylaxis for *P. jirovecii* pneumonia for children aged >6 years is provided if CD4 cell counts are less than 200 cells/mm^3 or CD4 percentage is less than 15% and for children 1 to less than 6 years of age, if CD4 cell counts are less than 500 cells/mm^3 or CD4 percentage is less than 15%. Clarithromycin or azithromycin prophylaxis for *Mycobacterium avium* complex infection is provided if CD4 cell counts are below certain thresholds dependent on age.

PROGNOSIS

The availability of cART has improved the prognosis for HIV and AIDS dramatically. Risk of death is directly related to the degree of immunosuppression, viral load, and young age. Children less than 1 year of age with very low CD4 percentiles and high viral loads have the poorest prognosis.

PREVENTION

Identification of HIV-positive women before or during pregnancy is crucial to providing optimal therapy for infected women and their infants and to prevent perinatal transmission. Prenatal HIV counseling and testing with consent should be provided for all pregnant women in the United States.

Administration of maternal cART throughout pregnancy to achieve viral suppression (viral load <200 copies/mL) with postnatal antiretroviral prophylaxis to the infant reduces the risk of transmission even further to less than 1% in non–breastfeeding infants. The current recommendations for the United States include a 4- to 6-week prophylactic regimen with zidovudine for the infant in combination with maternal intrapartum therapy. The maternal regimen includes continuation or initiation of ART. In high-risk situations (e.g., mother's viral load is >1,000 copies/mL or is unknown, mother did not receive cART during pregnancy), IV zidovudine during delivery is administered and additional antiretrovirals may be given to the infant postnatally (https://clinicalinfo.hiv.gov/en/guidelines/perinatal/intrapartum-antiretroviral-therapyprophylaxis?view=full).

Scheduled cesarean section at 38 weeks to prevent vertical transmission is recommended for women with HIV RNA levels greater than 1,000 copies/mL but is not routinely recommended in pregnant people receiving cART with viral load less than 1,000 copies/mL or when membranes have already ruptured unless other obstetric indications for cesarean delivery or induction of labor are present.

Preventing HIV infection in adults decreases the incidence of infection in children. Adolescent and adult prevention results from behavior changes such as safe-sex practices, decrease in IV drug use, **pre-exposure prophylaxis (PREP)**, and needle exchange programs. Screening of blood donors has almost eliminated the risk of HIV transmission from blood products. HIV infection is almost never transmitted in a casual or nonsexual household setting.

PEARLS FOR PRACTITIONERS

See Infectious Diseases: Pearls for Practitioners at the end of this section.

REVIEW QUESTIONS

Available online.

Suggested Readings

Bennett JE, Dolin V, Blaser MJ, eds. *Mandell, Douglas, and Bennett's Principles and Practice of Infectious Diseases.* 9th ed. Philadelphia: Elsevier; 2020.

Cherry JD, Kaplan SL, Harrison GJ, et al., eds. *Textbook of Pediatric Infectious Diseases.* 9th ed. Philadelphia: Elsevier; 2024.

Isaacs D. *Evidence-Based Pediatric Infectious Disease.* Malden, MA: Blackwell Publishing; 2007.

Kimberlin DW, Banerjee R, Barnett ED, et al., eds. *Red Book: 2024-2027 Report of the Committee on Infectious Diseases.* Itasca, IL: American Academy of Pediatrics; 2024.

Kliegman RM, St. Geme J, eds. *Nelson Textbook of Pediatrics.* 22nd ed. Philadelphia: Elsevier; 2025.

Long SS, Prober CG, Fischer M, Kimberlin DW. *Principles and Practice of Pediatric Infectious Diseases.* 6th ed. Philadelphia: Elsevier; 2023.

PEARLS FOR PRACTITIONERS

CHAPTER 94

Infectious Disease Assessment

- A complete infectious diseases history should include environmental exposures, sick contacts, travel to endemic areas, immune status, and immunization history.
- Depending on the situation, standard tests may include complete blood count with differential, inflammatory markers, transaminases, urinalysis and culture, lumbar puncture, or blood culture.
- A microbiologic diagnosis of infection may be confirmed or suggested by rapid antigen tests, cultures, serologic tests, or molecular tests (e.g., polymerase chain reaction).

CHAPTER 95

Immunization and Prophylaxis

- Purified polysaccharide vaccines are poor immunogens for children younger than 2 years. Conjugation of a polysaccharide to a protein carrier creates immunogenic vaccines for *Haemophilus influenzae* type b, *Streptococcus pneumoniae,* and *Neisseria meningitidis* for this age group.
- Contraindications to vaccination include anaphylaxis to prior immunization and immunocompromised patients (live-virus vaccines).
- Administration of blood products and immunoglobulin can diminish response to live-virus vaccines if administered before the recommended interval.

CHAPTER 96

Antimicrobial Therapy

- Obtain relevant cultures and diagnostic samples prior to initiating empiric antibiotics.
- Use of broad-spectrum empiric therapy is recommended for critically ill or immunocompromised patients.
- Sites with poor antimicrobial drug penetration may need drainage (abscess, osteomyelitis).
- Use targeted antimicrobial therapy to employ the least toxic, most narrow-spectrum agent effective against the causative pathogen.

CHAPTER 97

Fever Without a Focus

- Children younger than 21 days with fever should have a complete evaluation of blood, urine, and cerebrospinal fluid and should receive empirical antibiotics.
- Urinary tract infection is the most common serious bacterial infection in children younger than 6 months.
- Children 2–36 months with fever should have a careful history and physical exam. Those without localizing signs or symptoms may need urine and blood cultures.
- Children with sickle cell anemia are at increased risk of bacteremia with encapsulated organisms.
- Children with unexplained fevers lasting more than 14 days have fever of unknown origin (FUO). Among these

episodes of FUO, infections cause ~40–50%, inflammatory diseases ~20%, and malignancy ~10%.

CHAPTER 98
Infections Characterized by Fever and Rash

- Common childhood infectious causes of febrile illnesses with rash include measles, rubella, human herpesvirus type 6 (HHV-6), parvovirus B19, and varicella.
- Chickenpox is characterized by fever and a pruritic vesicular rash that comes in crops; secondary staphylococcal or streptococcal skin infection is a common complication.
- Measles is characterized by cough, coryza, conjunctivitis, fever, rash, and Koplik spots on the buccal mucosa and is extremely contagious.
- Congenital rubella syndrome is characterized by intrauterine growth restriction, retinitis, blueberry muffin rash, and patent ductus arteriosus.
- Roseola (due to HHV-6 and HHV-7) is characterized by an abrupt onset of a rash that appears after defervescence of 4–5 days of fever.
- Erythema infectiosum (due to parvovirus B19) is characterized by fever, malaise, a slapped-cheek rash, and transient aplastic crisis in children with sickle cell anemia.

CHAPTER 99
Cutaneous Infections

- Many childhood cutaneous infections are caused by *Staphylococcus aureus* or group A streptococci.
- Local epidemiology of methicillin-resistant *S. aureus* infections often guides treatment.
- Crusted impetigo is often caused by *S. aureus.*
- Necrotizing fasciitis is a surgical emergency and is suggested by rapid extension of lesions, pain out of proportion to lesions, toxic appearance, or crepitus.
- Common viral causes of superficial skin infections include herpes simplex virus (HSV), human papillomavirus (HPV), and molluscum contagiosum virus.

CHAPTER 100
Lymphadenopathy

- Cervical lymphadenitis is the most common childhood regional lymphadenitis; common causes include streptococcal pharyngitis, respiratory viruses, Epstein-Barr virus (EBV), and cytomegalovirus (CMV).
- The differential diagnosis of cervical adenitis should include Kawasaki disease, cat-scratch disease, atypical tuberculosis, mononucleosis, HIV, and lymphoma.
- Hilar or mediastinal lymphadenopathy can suggest tuberculosis, endemic mycoses, lymphoma, or autoimmune diseases.

CHAPTER 101
Meningitis

- The organisms that most commonly cause neonatal meningitis are group B streptococcus, *Escherichia coli,* and *Listeria monocytogenes.* Older children are more likely to have *Streptococcus pneumoniae* and *Neisseria meningitidis* as a cause of meningitis.
- Partially treated bacterial meningitis may decrease the ability to grow the organism; polymerase chain reaction (PCR) is useful to detect the pathogen but does not provide antimicrobial pathogen sensitivities.
- Enteroviruses and parechovirus are common causes of viral meningitis.
- Herpes simplex may produce meningoencephalitis and requires treatment with intravenous acyclovir.
- Presumptive therapy for neonatal meningitis includes ampicillin and ceftazidime; for older children (non-neonates), ceftriaxone and vancomycin or linezolid should be used.

CHAPTER 102
Encephalitis

- Viruses are the most common infectious cause of aseptic meningitis and encephalitis. Intravenous acyclovir should be used empirically if HSV or varicella-zoster virus is suspected.
- Acute flaccid myelitis appears to be seasonal, presents with acute weakness in the affected limb, and is associated with multiple viral infections including enteroviruses.

CHAPTER 103
The Common Cold

- Young children typically have multiple upper respiratory tract infections (URIs) each year, up to 8–12. Antibiotics are not beneficial in treating these episodes and may instead cause harm.
- Complications of URIs include otitis media, sinusitis, and exacerbation of asthma.

CHAPTER 104
Pharyngitis

- Viruses are the most common cause of pharyngitis. However, if group A streptococcus is isolated by rapid antigen test, PCR, or culture, it should be treated to prevent acute

rheumatic fever. Penicillin or amoxicillin is the choice of first-line therapy.
- Approximately 20% of school-age children are colonized with group A streptococcus without symptoms.
- A major reason to treat streptococcal pharyngitis is to prevent rheumatic fever.
- Streptococcal pharyngitis is relatively uncommon in young children under 3 years of age.

CHAPTER 105
Sinusitis

- The bacterial causes of acute sinusitis mirror those of otitis media and are *Streptococcus pneumoniae,* nontypable *Haemophilus influenzae,* and *Moraxella catarrhalis.*
- Complications of sinusitis include orbital cellulitis, Potts puffy tumor, and brain abscess.

CHAPTER 106
Otitis Media

- Poor or absent tympanic membrane mobility to negative and positive pressure using pneumatic otoscopy is a finding consistent with the diagnosis of acute otitis media (AOM).
- Complications of AOM include persistent middle ear effusion, hearing loss, mastoiditis, brain abscess, perforated tympanic membrane, and cholesteatoma.
- OM with effusion is the most frequent sequela of AOM and may result in persistent middle ear effusion, which may be associated with hearing loss.
- Not all episodes of AOM require antibiotic treatment.

CHAPTER 107
Otitis Externa

- Otitis externa is most frequently caused by *Pseudomonas aeruginosa.*
- Topical antibiotic/corticosteroid preparations are effective treatments.

CHAPTER 108
Croup (Laryngotracheobronchitis)

- Croup (laryngotracheobronchitis) is the most common infection of the middle respiratory tract; it is typically caused by parainfluenza virus and presents with stridor.
- The differential diagnosis of croup includes a foreign body, tracheitis, epiglottitis, tracheomalacia, and a vascular ring.
- Treatment includes use of cool mist, oral steroids, and nebulized racemic epinephrine.

CHAPTER 109
Pertussis

- Pertussis typically lasts 6–8 weeks; it is marked by catarrhal, paroxysmal, and convalescent stages and can lead to apnea and severe respiratory distress in infants.
- Vaccination with DTaP and Tdap have reduced the incidence of pertussis, but pertussis remains a common infection among infants younger than 6 months.
- Pertussis is associated with lymphocytosis and posttussive emesis.

CHAPTER 110
Bronchiolitis

- Bronchiolitis is a common lower respiratory infection in children younger than 2 years, is most commonly caused by respiratory syncytial virus (RSV), and requires only supportive treatment.
- The differential diagnosis of bronchiolitis includes asthma, heart failure, pneumonia, foreign body, and congenital airway or lung anomalies.
- The RSV monoclonal antibody nirsevimab is recommended for all infants to prevent bronchiolitis.

CHAPTER 111
Pneumonia

- *Streptococcus pneumoniae* is the most common bacterial cause of pneumonia outside the neonatal period and is the target of antibiotic selection for community-acquired pneumonia.
- Diagnostic evaluation for children hospitalized for pneumonia often includes complete blood count, blood culture, chest radiography, and occasionally rapid viral diagnostic testing.
- Amoxicillin and ampicillin are first-line antibiotic selections for community-acquired pneumonia in children.
- Short duration therapies (e.g., 5 days) have been shown in randomized trials to be effective for stable outpatients.

CHAPTER 112
Infective Endocarditis

- Streptococci are the most common cause of native valve endocarditis in children, whereas staphylococci are more common in those with prosthetic material.
- If infectious endocarditis is suspected, multiple optimal-volume blood cultures should be obtained prior to starting antimicrobial therapy.
- The 2023 modified Duke Criteria are used to make the diagnosis.

- Treatment is typically begun parenterally and is guided by the pathogen identified.

CHAPTER 113
Acute Gastroenteritis

- Management of acute gastroenteritis should include supportive care (correcting dehydration and electrolyte abnormalities) and not antibiotics in most circumstances.
- Enterohemorrhagic *Escherichia coli*–producing Shiga toxin is associated with hemolytic uremic syndrome (HUS), characterized by microangiopathic hemolytic anemia, thrombocytopenia, and acute kidney injury.
- Nucleic acid amplification tests (NAAT) are the tests of choice for the most common causes of viral and bacterial gastroenteritis.
- When antibiotics are indicated, first-line therapy for traveler's diarrhea in children is azithromycin.

CHAPTER 114
Viral Hepatitis

- Various types of viral hepatitis are difficult to distinguish during acute infection; most have a nonspecific prodromal phase followed by an icteric phase. Often acute illness with hepatitis A virus (HAV), HBV, and HCV is mild or even asymptomatic in children.
- Vaccines are recommended for all infants to prevent HAV and HBV infections.
- HBV and HCV infection may become chronic with a later risk for cirrhosis or hepatic cancer.
- Treatment of HBV or HCV infection is treated with direct-acting antiviral medications.

CHAPTER 115
Urinary Tract Infection

- *Escherichia coli* accounts for most pediatric urinary tract infections (UTIs).
- A renal ultrasound should be performed in young children to detect scarring, reflux, and congenital renal anomalies.
- UTI diagnosis requires a positive urine culture.
- Urine leukocyte esterase and nitrite testing aids in the diagnosis of a UTI.

CHAPTER 116
Vulvovaginitis

- Bacterial vaginosis represents disruption of the normal vaginal flora with reduction in lactobacillus and overgrowth of other organisms.
- Nonspecific vaginitis is the most common cause of vulvovaginitis in prepubertal females.

CHAPTER 117
Sexually Transmitted Infections

- There is increasing antibiotic resistance in *Neisseria gonorrhoeae.* Outpatient treatment of gonococcal urethritis or endocervicitis should include a single intramuscular dose of ceftriaxone. If concurrent *Chlamydia trachomatis* infection has not been ruled out, the patient should also be treated with doxycycline.
- Chlamydia is the most frequently diagnosed bacterial sexually transmitted infection in adolescents and accounts for most cases of nongonococcal urethritis and cervicitis.
- Chlamydial cervicitis is often asymptomatic.

CHAPTER 118
Osteomyelitis

- *Staphylococcus aureus* is the most common bacterial cause of osteomyelitis and is the target of antibiotic selection for this condition.
- Magnetic resonance imaging is the most sensitive diagnostic imaging test for osteomyelitis and will identify lesions early in the course of disease.
- An antistaphylococcal agent (nafcillin, oxacillin, or cefazolin) is the preferred initial empirical therapy for osteomyelitis in areas where methicillin-resistant *S. aureus* rates are low.
- Most patients are transitioned to oral therapy at hospital discharge to complete 3–4 total weeks of therapy.

CHAPTER 119
Infectious Arthritis

- *Staphylococcus aureus* is the most common bacterial cause of septic arthritis and is the target of antibiotic selection for this condition.
- Diagnostic evaluation for septic arthritis should include joint aspirate for cell count, Gram stain, and culture.
- Polymerase chain reaction evaluation for *Kingella kingae* is sometimes useful.
- An antistaphylococcal agent (nafcillin, oxacillin, or cefazolin) is the preferred empirical therapy for septic arthritis in areas where methicillin-resistant *S. aureus* rates are low.

CHAPTER 120
Ocular Infections

- All newborns should receive prophylaxis for ophthalmia neonatorum, typically with erythromycin 0.5% ointment, which will prevent gonococcal but not chlamydial ophthalmia.

- *Chlamydia* conjunctivitis in the newborn is treated with oral antibiotics to prevent chlamydial pneumonia.
- Neonatal conjunctivitis due to gonococcus is treated with intramuscular or intravenous ceftriaxone.
- Conjunctivitis and/or keratitis in patients who use contact lenses may be due to *Pseudomonas.*

CHAPTER 121
Infection in the Immunocompromised Person

- The presence of fever with neutropenia, even in the absence of other symptoms, demands prompt and thorough evaluation and empirical antimicrobial therapy.
- Fever is often the only sign of serious infection in immunocompromised patients.
- Rectal tenderness or pain on defecation may suggest a perianal abscess.
- The central line exit site and subcutaneous track should be inspected and blood drawn for culture from each lumen to detect line infections.
- Fungal infection should be considered and empirically treated in patients with persistent fever and neutropenia.

CHAPTER 122
Health Care–Associated Infections

- A major complication of indwelling medical devices such as central lines, ventriculoperitoneal shunts, and urinary catheters is infection (health care–associated infections).
- Antibiotic lock therapy may be used to aid in treatment or prevention of catheter line infections.

CHAPTER 123
Zoonoses and Vector-Borne Infections

- Lyme disease *(Borrelia burgdorferi)* is the most common tick-borne infection in the United States.
- Early treatment of erythema migrans almost always prevents progression to later stages of Lyme disease.
- Ehrlichiosis and anaplasmosis present like Rocky Mountain spotted fever (RMSF).
- RMSF is a severe life-threatening illness that has a high case fatality rate if untreated.
- Dengue hemorrhagic fever is seen in patients with a previous infection with dengue virus.

CHAPTER 124
Parasitic Diseases

- Chemoprophylaxis for malaria is necessary for all visitors to and residents of the tropics who have not lived there since infancy.
- Malaria is characterized by febrile paroxysms.
- Long-term relapse with malaria occurs because of persistent hepatic infection with either *Plasmodium vivax* or *P. ovale.*

CHAPTER 125
Tuberculosis

- The diagnosis of *Mycobacterium tuberculosis* infection can be difficult. Children of any age should have a purified protein derivative (PPD) test or interferon-γ release assay. A negative or indeterminate result does not exclude active infection.
- Pulmonary tuberculosis (TB) initially presents as a pulmonary infiltrate with hilar adenopathy.
- Bone or brain involvement with TB occurs due to hematogenous spread following primary pulmonary TB.
- Reactivation of TB occurs most often in adolescents and patients exposed to corticosteroids or anti–tumor necrosis factor antibodies.

CHAPTER 126
Human Immunodeficiency Virus and Acquired Immunodeficiency Syndrome

- Vertical transmission of HIV from mother to child is an uncommon occurrence in the United States due to the effectiveness of preventative measures including early maternal diagnosis, maternal treatment during pregnancy and delivery, postnatal prophylactic treatment of the infant, and avoidance of breast-feeding for people with HIV who are not on cART and/or do not have a suppressed viral load.
- Perinatally acquired HIV presents with growth faltering, lymphadenopathy, hepatosplenomegaly, parotitis, diarrhea, and opportunistic infections.

SECTION 17

THE DIGESTIVE SYSTEM

Dawn R. Ebach | Sussette Szachowicz

CHAPTER 127

Digestive System Assessment

HISTORY

After identifying the major gastrointestinal (GI) symptoms, the onset and progression should be determined (improved, unchanged, worsening, involvement of other organ systems). Characterization of signs and symptoms should identify factors that trigger, aggravate, or alleviate the symptoms; the timing, frequency, and duration of symptoms; relationship to meals and defecation; and associated symptoms (e.g., fever or weight loss). Other key history includes exposure to others (family, school contacts, pets), travel, environmental exposure, and impact of illness on the child (school absences, weight loss).

PHYSICAL EXAMINATION

The history may suggest a diagnosis and direct the evaluation, which should include a full examination as well as a thorough abdominal examination. Extraintestinal disorders may produce GI manifestations (e.g., emesis with group A streptococcal pharyngitis, abdominal pain with lower lobe pneumonia, respiratory distress with COVID-19). The examination should begin with a careful external visual inspection for abdominal distention, bruising or discoloration, abnormal abdominal veins, jaundice, surgical scars, and ostomies. Abnormalities of intensity and pitch of bowel sounds can occur with bowel obstruction. When palpating for tenderness, the examiner should note location, facial expression, guarding, and rebound tenderness. Palpation can also detect enlargement of the liver or spleen as well as feces and masses. If detected, organomegaly should be measured (with a tape measure), noting tenderness, abnormal firmness, or contour. A rectal examination, including inspection for fissures, skin tags, abscesses, and fistulous openings, may be performed for children with history suggesting constipation, GI bleeding, abdominal pain, chronic diarrhea, and suspicion of inflammatory bowel disease (IBD). Digital rectal examination should include assessment of anal sphincter tone, anal canal size and elasticity, tenderness, extrinsic masses, presence of fecal impaction, and caliber of the rectum. Stool should be tested for occult blood.

SCREENING TESTS

A **complete blood count** may provide evidence for inflammation (white blood cell [WBC] and platelet count), poor nutrition or bleeding (hemoglobin, red blood cell [RBC] volume, reticulocyte count), and infection (WBC number and differential, presence of toxic granulation). Serum electrolytes, blood urea nitrogen, and creatinine help define hydration status. Tests of liver dysfunction include total and direct bilirubin, alanine aminotransferase, aspartate aminotransferase for evidence of hepatocellular injury, and γ-glutamyltransferase or alkaline phosphatase for evidence of bile duct injury. **Hepatic synthetic function** can be assessed by coagulation factor levels, prothrombin time, and albumin level. Pancreatic enzyme tests (amylase, lipase) provide evidence of pancreatic injury or inflammation. Urinalysis can gage dehydration and identify a possible source of protein loss. Stool may be examined for blood or calprotectin (inflammation).

DIAGNOSTIC IMAGING

Radiology

A plain abdominal x-ray to document excessive retained stool when history is consistent with constipation and encopresis is not necessary, as physical examination alone can confirm the diagnosis. An abdominal x-ray (both anteroposterior and decubitus) should be completed if there is concern for bowel obstruction or perforation. A kidney-ureter-bladder x-ray may demonstrate lower lobe pneumonia.

Endoscopy

Endoscopy permits the direct visualization of the interior of the gut. **Video endoscopes** may be used even in very small infants by pediatric gastroenterologists. **Wireless capsule endoscopy** (Fig. 127.1) enables visualization of lesions beyond the reach of conventional endoscopes.

Consultation with a pediatric gastroenterologist for endoscopy is recommended for further evaluation of suspected esophageal or gastric inflammation unresponsive to medications, to confirm the diagnosis of eosinophilic esophagitis or celiac disease, to evaluate GI bleeding, to investigate suspected IBD, or to screen for polyp disorders. In addition, a trained endoscopist can remove esophageal and gastric foreign bodies, place feeding tubes, obtain biopsies, and treat bleeding ulcers or varices.

COMMON MANIFESTATIONS OF GASTROINTESTINAL DISORDERS

Abdominal Pain

General Considerations

Abdominal pain can result from injury to or inflammation of the intraabdominal organs or overlying somatic structures

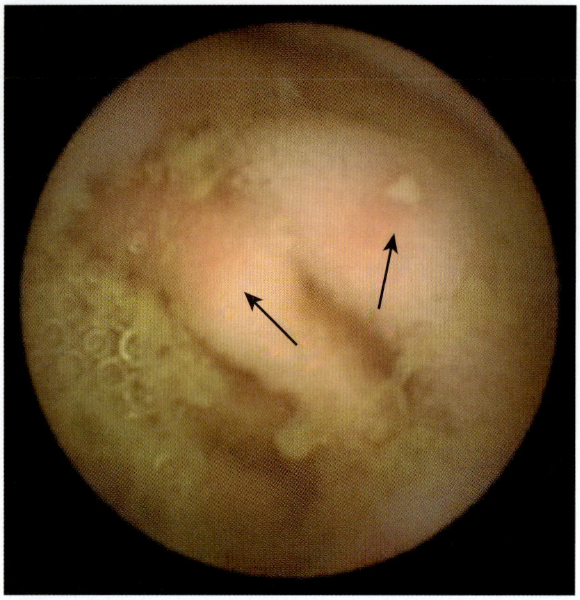

FIGURE 127.1 Wireless capsule endoscopy. Aphthous ulcers *(arrows)* in jejunum diagnostic of Crohn disease in patient with negative findings on upper endoscopy and colonoscopy.

in the abdominal wall or from extraabdominal diseases. **Visceral pain** results when autonomic nerves within the gut detect injury, transmitting sensation by nonmyelinated fibers. The pain is vague, dull, slow in onset, and poorly localized. A variety of stimuli, including normal peristalsis and various intraluminal chemical and osmotic states, activate these fibers to some degree. Regardless of the stimulus, visceral pain is perceived when a threshold of intensity or duration is crossed. Lower degrees of activation may result in perception of nonpainful or perhaps vaguely uncomfortable sensations, whereas more intensive stimulation of these fibers results in pain. Overactive sensation may be the basis of some kinds of abdominal pain, the disorders of brain-gut interaction, such as **functional abdominal pain, disorders of gut-brain interaction**, and **irritable bowel syndrome (IBS)**.

In contrast to visceral pain, **somatic pain** results when overlying body structures are injured. Somatic structures include the parietal peritoneum, fascia, muscles, and skin of the abdominal wall. In contrast to pain emanating from visceral injury, somatic nociceptive fibers are myelinated and are capable of rapid transmission of well-localized painful stimuli. When intraabdominal processes cause inflammation or injury to the parietal peritoneum or abdominal wall structures, poorly localized visceral pain becomes well-localized somatic pain. In acute appendicitis, the initial activation of visceral nociceptive fibers yields poorly localized discomfort in the mid-abdomen. When the inflammatory process extends to the overlying parietal peritoneum, the pain becomes severe and localizes to the right lower quadrant. This is called ***somatoparietal pain***.

Referred pain is a painful sensation in a body region distant from the true source of pain. The location of referred pain is predictable based on the locus of visceral injury. Stomach pain is referred to the epigastric and retrosternal regions, and liver and pancreas pain is referred to the epigastric region. Gallbladder pain often is referred to the region below the right scapula. Somatic pathways stimulated by small bowel visceral afferents affect the periumbilical area, and colonic injury results in infraumbilical referred pain.

Acute Abdominal Pain

Distinguishing Features

Acute abdominal pain can signal the presence of a dangerous intraabdominal process (e.g., appendicitis or bowel obstruction) or may originate from extraintestinal sources (e.g., lower lobe pneumonia or urinary tract stone). Not all episodes of acute abdominal pain require emergency intervention. Appendicitis and volvulus, however, must be ruled out expeditiously. Few patients presenting with acute abdominal pain have a surgical emergency, but they must be separated from cases that can be managed conservatively.

Initial Diagnostic Evaluation

Table 127.1 lists a diagnostic approach to acute abdominal pain in children. Events that occur with a discrete, abrupt onset, such as passage of a stone, perforation of a viscus, or vascular infarction, result in a sudden onset of pain. Gradual onset of pain is common with infectious or inflammatory causes, such as appendicitis and IBD.

A standard group of laboratory tests usually is performed for acute abdominal pain (see Table 127.1). An abdominal x-ray series evaluates for bowel obstruction, fecalith, or nephrolithiasis. Ultrasound, computed tomography (CT), or magnetic resonance imaging can visualize the appendix if appendicitis is suspected but the diagnosis remains in doubt. If the initial evaluation suggests intussusception, ultrasound, followed by a barium or pneumatic (air) enema, may be used to initially diagnose and then treat this condition (see Chapter 130).

Differential Diagnosis

Table 127.2 lists the differential diagnoses of acute abdominal pain in children. The urgent task of the clinician is to rule out surgical emergencies. In infants, malrotation with volvulus, incarcerated hernia, congenital anomalies, and intussusception are concerns. In older children and teenagers, appendicitis is more common. An acute surgical abdomen is characterized by signs of peritonitis, including tenderness, abdominal wall rigidity, guarding, and absent or diminished bowel sounds. Helpful characteristics of onset, location, referral, and quality of pain are noted in Table 127.3.

Recurrent Abdominal Pain

Recurrent abdominal pain is a common problem, affecting more than 10% of all children. The peak incidence occurs between ages 7–12 years. Although the differential diagnoses of recurrent abdominal pain are fairly extensive (Table 127.4), most children do not have a serious underlying illness causing the pain.

Differential Diagnosis

Children with **functional abdominal pain (disorders of gut-brain interaction [DGBI])** characteristically have pain almost daily. The pain is not associated with meals or relieved by defecation and may be associated with a tendency toward anxiety and perfectionism. Symptoms are often exacerbated by stress at school or novel social situations. The pain often is worst in the morning and often prevents or delays children from attending school. **IBS** is a subset of DGBI,

TABLE 127.1 Diagnostic Approach to Acute Abdominal Pain

HISTORY	
Onset	Sudden or gradual, prior episodes, association with meals, history of injury
Nature	Sharp vs. dull, colicky or constant, burning
Location	Epigastric, periumbilical, generalized, right or left lower quadrant, change in location over time
Associated symptoms	Fever, vomiting (bilious?), diarrhea (bloody?), abdominal distention
Extraintestinal symptoms	Cough, dyspnea, dysuria, urinary frequency, flank pain, hematuria
Course of symptoms	Worsening or improving, change in nature or location of pain, aggravating and alleviating factors, last menstrual period
PHYSICAL EXAMINATION	
General position	Growth and nutrition, general appearance, hydration, degree of discomfort, body position
Abdominal	Tenderness, distention, bowel sounds, rigidity, guarding, mass
Genitalia	Testicular torsion, hernia, pelvic inflammatory disease, ectopic pregnancy
Surrounding structures	Breath sounds, rales, rhonchi, wheezing, flank tenderness, tenderness of abdominal wall structures, ribs, costochondral joints
Rectal examination	Perianal lesions, stricture, tenderness, fecal impaction, blood
LABORATORY	
CBC, C-reactive protein, ESR	Evidence of infection or inflammation
AST, ALT, GGT, bilirubin	Biliary or liver disease
Amylase, lipase	Pancreatitis
Urinalysis	Urinary tract infection; bleeding due to stone, trauma, or obstruction
Pregnancy test	Ectopic pregnancy
RADIOLOGY	
Plain flat and upright abdominal films	Bowel obstruction, appendiceal fecalith, free intraperitoneal air, kidney stones, constipation, mass, lower lobe pneumonia
CT or MRI scan ± PET scan	Intraabdominal or pelvic abscess, appendicitis, Crohn disease, pancreatitis, gallstones, kidney stones
Barium enema	Intussusception, malrotation
Ultrasound	Gallstones, appendicitis, intussusception, pancreatitis, kidney stones
Colonoscopy	Colitis
Upper endoscopy	Suspected peptic ulcer or esophagitis

ALT, Alanine aminotransferase; *AST,* aspartate aminotransferase; *CBC,* complete blood count; *CT,* computed tomography; *ESR,* erythrocyte sedimentation rate; *GGT,* γ-glutamyltransferase; *MRI,* magnetic resonance imaging; *PET,* positron emission tomography.

TABLE 127.2 Differential Diagnoses of Acute Abdominal Pain

TRAUMATIC
Duodenal hematoma Ruptured spleen Perforated viscus Traumatic pancreatitis
FUNCTIONAL
Constipation* Irritable bowel syndrome* Dysmenorrhea* Mittelschmerz (ovulation)* Infantile colic* Abdominal migraine
INFECTIOUS
Appendicitis* Viral or bacterial gastroenteritis/mesenteric adenitis* Abscess Spontaneous bacterial peritonitis Pelvic inflammatory disease Cholecystitis Urinary tract infection* Pneumonia Bacterial typhlitis Hepatitis/perihepatitis
GENITAL
Testicular torsion/epididymitis Ovarian torsion Ruptured ovarian cyst Ectopic pregnancy
GENETIC
Sickle cell crisis* Familial Mediterranean fever Porphyria Hereditary angioedema
METABOLIC
Diabetic ketoacidosis Fabry disease
INFLAMMATORY
Inflammatory bowel disease* Vasculitis IgA vasculitis* Pancreatitis
OBSTRUCTIVE
Intussusception* Malrotation with volvulus Ileus* Incarcerated hernia Postoperative adhesion Distal intestinal obstruction syndrome (cystic fibrosis) Duplication cyst Congenital stricture
BILIARY
Gallstone Gallbladder hydrops Biliary dyskinesia
PEPTIC
Gastric or duodenal ulcer Gastritis* Esophagitis

Continued

TABLE 127.2 Differential Diagnoses of Acute Abdominal Pain—cont'd

KIDNEY
Kidney stone Hydronephrosis/ureteropelvic junction obstruction

**Common.*
Ig, Immunoglobulin.

characterized by an association of abdominal discomfort with a change in stool frequency or consistency and relief of pain with defecation. Symptoms in IBS are linked to gut motility. Pain is commonly accompanied in both groups of children by school avoidance, secondary gains, anxiety about imagined causes, lack of coping skills, and disordered peer relationships (Table 127.5).

TABLE 127.3 Distinguishing Features of Abdominal Pain in Children

DISEASE	ONSET	LOCATION	REFERRAL	QUALITY	COMMENTS
DGBI/irritable bowel syndrome	Recurrent	Periumbilical, splenic, and hepatic flexures	None	Dull, crampy, intermittent; duration 2 hr	Family stress, school phobia, diarrhea and constipation; hypersensitive to pain from distention
Gastroesophageal reflux	Recurrent, after meals, at bedtime	Substernal	Chest	Burning	Sour taste in mouth; Sandifer syndrome
Duodenal ulcer	Recurrent, before meals, at night	Epigastric	Back	Severe burning, gnawing	Relieved by food, milk, antacids; family history important; gastrointestinal bleeding
Pancreatitis	Acute	Epigastric-hypogastric	Back	Constant, sharp, boring	Nausea, emesis, marked tenderness
Intestinal obstruction	Acute or gradual	Periumbilical–lower abdomen	Back	Alternating cramping (colic) and painless periods	Distention, obstipation, bilious emesis, increased bowel sounds
Appendicitis	Acute	Periumbilical or epigastric; localizes to right lower quadrant	Back or pelvis if retrocecal	Sharp, steady	Nausea, emesis, local tenderness, ± fever, avoids motion
Meckel diverticulum	Recurrent	Periumbilical–lower abdomen	None	Sharp	Hematochezia; painless unless intussusception, diverticulitis, or perforation
Inflammatory bowel disease	Recurrent	Depends on site of involvement		Dull cramping, tenesmus	Fever, weight loss, ± hematochezia
Intussusception	Acute	Periumbilical–lower abdomen	None	Cramping, with painless periods	Guarded position with knees pulled up, currant jelly stools, lethargy
Lactose intolerance	Recurrent with milk products	Lower abdomen	None	Cramping	Distention, gaseousness, diarrhea
Urolithiasis	Acute, sudden	Back	Groin	Severe, colicky pain	Hematuria
Pyelonephritis	Acute, sudden	Back	None	Dull to sharp	Fever, costochondral tenderness, dysuria, urinary frequency, emesis
Cholecystitis and cholelithiasis	Acute	Right upper quadrant	Right shoulder	Severe, colicky pain	Hemolysis ± jaundice, nausea, emesis

DGBI, Disorders of gut-brain interaction.
Modified from Andreoli TE, Carpenter CJ, Plum F, et al. Cecil Essentials of Medicine. *Philadelphia: WB Saunders; 1986.*

TABLE 127.4 Differential Diagnoses of Recurrent Abdominal Pain

Functional abdominal pain/DGBI*
Irritable bowel syndrome*
Chronic pancreatitis
Gallstones
Peptic disease
Duodenal ulcer
Gastric ulcer
Esophagitis
Lactose intolerance*
Fructose malabsorption
Inflammatory bowel disease*
Crohn disease
Ulcerative colitis
Constipation*
Obstructive uropathy
Congenital intestinal malformation
Malrotation
Duplication cyst
Stricture or web
Celiac disease*
Abdominal migraine
Eosinophilic esophagitis*

**Common.*
DGBI, Disorders of gut-brain interaction.

Distinguishing Features

One needs to distinguish between DGBI and more serious underlying disorders. **Warning signs** for underlying illness are listed in Table 127.6. If present, further investigation is necessary. Some laboratory evaluation is warranted even in the absence of warning signs. The initial evaluation recommended in Table 127.7 is a sensible approach, avoiding unnecessary testing and providing ample sensitivity for most serious underlying disorders. While waiting for laboratory and ultrasound results, a 3-day trial of a lactose-free diet can evaluate for lactose intolerance. If tests are normal and no warning signs are present, testing should be stopped. If there are warning signs, progression of symptoms, or laboratory abnormalities that suggest a specific diagnosis, additional investigation may be warranted.

Treatment of Disorders of Gut-Brain Interaction

A child who is repeatedly kept home from school because of pain receives reinforcement in the form of being excused from responsibilities and withdraws from full social functioning. This tends to both increase anxiety and prolong the course. To break the cycle of pain and disability, the child with functional pain must be assisted in **returning to normal activities** immediately. Instead of being sent home from school with stomachaches, a child may be allowed to take a short break from class until symptoms abate. The child and parents should be informed that pain is likely to be worse on the day the child returns to school as anxiety worsens dysmotility and enhances pain perception. Medications may be helpful. Probiotics and peppermint oil can be beneficial in treating IBS. Dietary changes such as the low FODMAP (fermentable olio-di-monosaccharides and polyols) diet (reducing highly fermentable sugars in the diet) can be beneficial in a subset of patients. In difficult and persistent cases, cognitive behavioral therapy, amitriptyline, or a selective serotonin reuptake inhibitor may be helpful. Auriculotherapy (acupuncture) is being used in some centers to treat abdominal pain associated with

TABLE 127.5 Rome IV Criteria for Pediatric Functional Gastrointestinal Syndromes/Disorders of Brain-Gut Interaction

A. DIAGNOSTIC CRITERIA FOR CHILDHOOD FUNCTIONAL ABDOMINAL PAIN
Must be fulfilled for at least 2 months before diagnosis; must be met at least 4 times per month and include all of the following: 1. Episodic or continuous abdominal pain that does not occur solely during physiological events such as eating and menses 2. Insufficient criteria for other functional gastrointestinal diseases including irritable bowel syndrome, functional dyspepsia, or abdominal migraine 3. After appropriate evaluation, the abdominal pain cannot be fully explained by another medical condition
B. DIAGNOSTIC CRITERIA FOR IRRITABLE BOWEL SYNDROME
Must include all of the following:* 1. Abdominal pain at least 4 days per month associated with one or more of the following: a. Related to defecation b. A change in the frequency of stool c. A change in the form (appearance of stool) 2. In children with constipation, the pain does not resolve with resolution of the constipation 3. After appropriate evaluation, the symptoms cannot be fully explained by another medical condition
*Criteria fulfilled at least 2 months before diagnosis
C. DIAGNOSTIC CRITERIA FOR ABDOMINAL MIGRAINE
Must include all of the following occurring at least twice:* 1. Paroxysmal episodes of intense, acute periumbilical midline or diffuse abdominal pain lasting 1 hour or more (should be the most severe and distressing symptom) 2. Episodes are separated by weeks to months 3. The pain is incapacitating and interferes with normal activities 4. Stereotypical pattern and symptoms in the individual patient 5. The pain is associated with 2 or more of the following: a. anorexia b. nausea c. vomiting d. headache e. photophobia f. pallor 6. After appropriate evaluation, the symptoms cannot be fully explained by another medical condition
*Criteria fulfilled for at least 6 months before diagnosis
D. DIAGNOSTIC CRITERIA FOR CYCLIC VOMITING SYNDROME
Must include all of the following: 1. The occurrence of 2 or more periods of intense, unremitting nausea and paroxysmal vomiting, lasting hours to days within a 6-month period 2. Episodes are stereotypical in each patient 3. Episodes are separated by weeks to months with return to baseline health between episodes 4. After appropriate medical evaluation, the symptoms cannot be attributed to another condition
E. FUNCTIONAL CONSTIPATION
Must include 2 or more of the following occurring at least once per week for a minimum of 1 month with insufficient criteria for the diagnosis of irritable bowel syndrome: 1. 2 or fewer defecations in the toilet per week in a child of developmental age of at least 4 years 2. At least 1 episode of fecal incontinence per week 3. History of retentive posturing or excessive volitional stool retention 4. History of painful or hard bowel movements 5. Presence of a large fecal mass in the rectum 6. History of large diameter stools that can obstruct the toilet After appropriate evaluation, the symptoms cannot be fully explained by another medical condition

Courtesy of the Rome Foundation.

TABLE 127.6 Warning Signs of Underlying Illness in Recurrent Abdominal Pain

Vomiting
Abnormal screening laboratory study (anemia, hypoalbuminemia, inflammatory markers)
Fever
Bilious emesis
Growth failure
Pain awakening child from sleep
Weight loss
Location away from periumbilical region
Blood in stools or emesis
Delayed puberty
Nocturnal diarrhea
Dysphagia
Arthritis
Perianal disease
Family history of inflammatory bowel disease, celiac disease, or peptic ulcer disease

TABLE 127.7 Suggested Evaluation of Recurrent Abdominal Pain

INITIAL EVALUATION	FOLLOW-UP EVALUATION*
Complete history and physical examination Ask about "warning signs" (see Table 127.6) Determine degree of functional impairment (e.g., missing school) CBC ESR Amylase, lipase Urinalysis Abdominal ultrasound—examine liver, bile ducts, gallbladder, pancreas, kidneys, ureters Trial of 3-day lactose-free diet	CT or MRI scan of the abdomen and pelvis with oral and/or intravenous contrast Celiac disease serology—tissue transglutaminase IgA antibody Fecal calprotectin or lactoferrin Endoscopy of the esophagus, stomach, and duodenum Colonoscopy

**Consider using one or more of these to investigate warning signs, abnormal laboratory tests, or specific or persistent symptoms.*

CBC, Complete blood count; *CT*, computed tomography; *ESR*, erythrocyte sedimentation rate; *IgA*, immunoglobulin A; *MRI*, magnetic resonance imaging.

IBS. When significant anxiety or social dysfunction persists, a mental health professional should be consulted.

Vomiting

Vomiting is a coordinated, sequential series of events that leads to forceful oral emptying of gastric contents. It is a common problem in children and has many causes. Vomiting should be distinguished from **regurgitation** of stomach contents, also known as gastroesophageal reflux (GER). Although the results of vomiting and regurgitation are similar, they have completely different characteristics. Vomiting is usually preceded by nausea and is accompanied by forceful gagging and retching. Regurgitation, on the other hand, is effortless and not preceded by nausea.

Differential Diagnosis

In neonates with true vomiting, congenital obstructive lesions must be considered. Allergic reactions to formula in the first 2 months of life may present with vomiting. **Infantile GER** ("spitting up") occurs in up to half of infants and can be large in volume, but is effortless, and these infants do not appear ill. **Pyloric stenosis** occurs in the first 1–2 months of life and is characterized by steadily worsening, forceful vomiting that occurs immediately after feedings. A visibly distended stomach, often with visible peristaltic waves, is often seen before vomiting. Pyloric stenosis is more common in male infants; the family history may be positive. Other congenital obstructive lesions, such as intestinal duplication cysts, atresias, webs, and midgut volvulus with malrotation, should be considered. Metabolic disorders (e.g., organic acidemias, galactosemia, urea cycle defects, adrenogenital syndromes) may present with vomiting in infants. In older children with acute vomiting, viruses and food poisoning are common. Other infections, especially streptococcal pharyngitis, urinary tract infections, and otitis media, commonly result in vomiting. When vomiting is chronic, central nervous system causes (increased intracranial pressure, migraine) must be considered. **Cyclic vomiting syndrome** or abdominal migraine may be the etiology of recurrent vomiting. When abdominal pain or bilious emesis accompanies vomiting, evaluation for intestinal obstruction, peptic disorders, and appendicitis must be immediately initiated.

Distinguishing Features

Table 127.8 lists common diagnoses that must be considered and their important historical features. Given the frequency of viral gastroenteritis as the etiology, it is important to be alert for unusual features that suggest another diagnosis. Viral gastroenteritis usually is not associated with severe abdominal pain or headache and does not recur at frequent intervals.

Physical examination should include assessment of the child's hydration status, including examination of vital signs as well as capillary refill, moistness of mucous membranes, and skin turgor (see Chapter 39). The chest should be auscultated for evidence of rales or other signs of pulmonary involvement. The abdomen must be examined carefully for distention, organomegaly, bowel sounds, tenderness, and guarding. Testing stool for occult blood should be considered if ulcer disease or severe esophagitis is suspected.

Laboratory evaluation of vomiting should include serum electrolytes, tests of kidney function, complete blood count, amylase, lipase, and liver function tests. Additional testing may be required immediately when history and examination suggest a specific etiology. Urinalysis should be done if there is a history of dysuria. Urine pregnancy testing needs to be considered in adolescent females. Ultrasound is useful to look for pyloric stenosis, gallstones, kidney stones, hydronephrosis, biliary obstruction, pancreatitis, malrotation, intussusception, and other anatomic abnormalities. CT may be indicated to rule out appendicitis or to observe structures that cannot be visualized well by ultrasound. Barium studies can show obstructive or inflammatory lesions of the gut and can be therapeutic, as in the use of contrast enemas for intussusception (see Chapter 130).

Treatment

Treatment needs to address the consequences and the causes of the vomiting. Dehydration must be treated with fluid resuscitation. This can be accomplished in most cases with oral fluid-electrolyte solutions, but intravenous (IV) fluids may be required. Electrolyte imbalances should be corrected by appropriate choice of fluids. Underlying causes should be treated when possible.

TABLE 127.8 Differential Diagnoses and Historical Features of Vomiting

DIFFERENTIAL DIAGNOSES	HISTORICAL CLUES
Viral gastroenteritis	Fever, diarrhea, sudden onset, absence of pain
Gastroesophageal reflux	Effortless, not preceded by nausea, chronic
Hepatitis	Jaundice, history of exposure
Extra-GI infections	
Otitis media	Fever, ear pain
Urinary tract infection	Dysuria, unusual urine odor, frequency, incontinence
Pneumonia	Cough, fever, chest discomfort
Allergic	
Milk or soy protein intolerance (infants)	Associated with particular formula or food, blood in stools
Other food allergy (older children)	
FPIES	Acute onset vomiting, diarrhea, dehydration, shock
Peptic ulcer or gastritis	Epigastric pain, blood or coffee-ground material in emesis, pain relieved by acid blockade
Appendicitis	Fever, abdominal pain migrating to the right lower quadrant, tenderness
Pancreatitis	Severe epigastric abdominal pain
Anatomic obstruction	
Intestinal atresia	Neonate, usually bilious, polyhydramnios
Midgut malrotation	Pain, bilious vomiting, GI bleeding, shock
Intussusception	Colicky pain, lethargy, vomiting, currant jelly stools, mass occasionally
Duplication cysts	Colic, mass
Pyloric stenosis	Nonbilious vomiting, postprandial, <4 mo old, hunger, progressive weight loss
Hirschsprung disease	Abdominal distention, lack of stools
Bacterial gastroenteritis	Fever, often with bloody diarrhea
CNS	
Increased intracranial pressure	Headaches, neurologic changes
Hydrocephalus	Large head, altered mental status, bulging fontanelle
Meningitis	Fever, stiff neck
Migraine syndrome	Attacks scattered in time, relieved by sleep; headache
Cyclic vomiting syndrome	Similar to migraine, usually no headache
Brain tumor	Morning vomiting, accelerating over time, headache, diplopia
Motion sickness	Associated with travel in vehicle
Labyrinthitis	Vertigo
Metabolic disease	Presentation early in life, worsens when catabolic or when exposed to substrate
Pregnancy	Morning, sexually active, cessation of menses
Drug reaction or side effect	Associated with increased dose or new medication
Cancer chemotherapy	Temporarily related to administration of chemotherapeutic drugs
Eosinophilic esophagitis	May have dysphagia or abdominal pain

CNS, Central nervous system; *FPIES,* food protein–induced enterocolitis syndrome; *GI,* gastrointestinal.

Antiemetic medications should not be prescribed until the etiology of the vomiting is known, and then only for severe symptoms. Drugs that block serotonin 5-HT_3 receptors, such as ondansetron, are frequently used for viral gastroenteritis and can improve tolerance of oral rehydration therapy. They are helpful for chemotherapy-induced vomiting, often combined with dexamethasone. No antiemetic should be used in patients with surgical emergencies or when a specific treatment of the underlying condition is possible. Correction of dehydration, ketosis, and acidosis is helpful to reduce vomiting in most patients with viral gastroenteritis.

Acute and Chronic Diarrhea

Diarrhea is a major cause of childhood morbidity and mortality worldwide. Deaths from diarrhea are rare in industrialized countries but are common elsewhere. **Acute diarrhea** is a major problem when it occurs in children with malnutrition or in the absence of basic medical care (see Chapter 28). In North America, most acute diarrhea is viral and is self-limited, requiring no diagnostic testing or specific intervention. Bacterial agents tend to cause much more severe illness and typically are seen in food-associated outbreaks or in regions with poor public sanitation. Bacterial enteritis should be suspected when there is **dysentery** (bloody diarrhea with fever) and whenever severe symptoms are present. These infections can be diagnosed by stool culture or nucleic acid assays for specific pathogens. **Chronic diarrhea** lasts more than 2 weeks and has a wide range of possible causes, including serious and benign conditions that are more difficult to diagnose.

Parents use the word *diarrhea* to describe loose or watery stools, excessively frequent stools, or stools that are large in volume. Constipation with overflow incontinence can be mislabeled as diarrhea. A more exact definition of diarrhea is excessive daily stool liquid volume (>10 mL stool/kg body weight/day or >200 mL/day for adults). Stool texture, volume, and frequency help to characterize the episode of diarrhea.

Differential Diagnosis

Diarrhea may be classified by etiology or by physiologic mechanisms (secretory or osmotic) and chronicity (acute vs. chronic). Etiologic agents include viruses, bacteria or their toxins, chemicals, parasites, malabsorbed substances, and inflammation. Table 127.9 lists common causes of diarrhea in childhood. **Secretory diarrhea** occurs when the intestinal mucosa directly secretes fluid and electrolytes into the stool. Secretion is stimulated by mediators of inflammation and by various hormones, such as vasoactive intestinal peptide secreted by a neuroendocrine tumor. Cholera is a secretory diarrhea stimulated by the enterotoxin of *Vibrio cholerae*, which causes increased levels of cyclic adenosine monophosphate within enterocytes and leads to secretion into the small-bowel lumen.

Osmotic diarrhea occurs after malabsorption of an ingested substance, which "pulls" water into the bowel lumen. A classic example is the diarrhea of lactose intolerance. Osmotic diarrhea also can result from generalized maldigestion, such as that seen with pancreatic insufficiency or with intestinal injury. Certain nonabsorbable laxatives, such as polyethylene glycol and milk of magnesia, also cause osmotic diarrhea. Fermentation of malabsorbed substances (e.g., lactose) often occurs, resulting in gas, cramps, and acidic stools. A common cause of chronic loose stools in early childhood is

TABLE 127.9 Differential Diagnoses of Diarrhea

	INFANT	CHILD	ADOLESCENT
ACUTE			
Common	Gastroenteritis* Systemic infection Antibiotic associated	Gastroenteritis* Food poisoning Systemic infection Antibiotic associated	Gastroenteritis* Food poisoning Antibiotic associated
Rare	Primary disaccharidase deficiency Food protein–induced enterocolitis syndrome Hirschsprung toxic colitis Adrenogenital syndrome Opiate withdrawal (neonate)		Hyperthyroidism Appendicitis
CHRONIC			
Common	Postinfectious secondary lactase deficiency Cow's milk/soy protein intolerance Chronic nonspecific diarrhea of infancy (toddler's diarrhea) Celiac disease Cystic fibrosis	Postinfectious secondary lactase deficiency Irritable bowel syndrome Celiac disease Lactose intolerance Giardiasis Inflammatory bowel disease	Irritable bowel syndrome Inflammatory bowel disease Lactose intolerance Giardiasis Laxative abuse (anorexia nervosa) Celiac disease
Rare	Primary immune defects Familial villous atrophy Secretory tumors Congenital chloride diarrhea Acrodermatitis enteropathica Lymphangiectasia Abetalipoproteinemia Eosinophilic gastroenteritis Short-bowel syndrome Autoimmune enteropathy/IPEX-like disorders Malabsorption syndromes Factitious	Acquired immune defects Secretory tumor Pseudoobstruction Factitious AIDS enteropathy Eosinophilic gastroenteritis	Secretory tumors Primary bowel tumor AIDS enteropathy Addison disease Parasitic infections

*Gastroenteritis includes viral (rotavirus, norovirus, astrovirus) and bacterial (*Salmonella, Shigella, Escherichia coli, Clostridium difficile, Yersinia, Campylobacter*, other) agents.
IPEX, Immune dysregulation, polyendocrinopathy, enteropathy, X-linked.

functional diarrhea, commonly known as ***toddler's diarrhea***. This condition is defined by frequent watery stools in the setting of normal growth and weight gain. The cause is likely a combination of excessive intake of fluids (especially of sweetened liquids) or high osmolar foods (fruit drinks, popsicles), increased gastrointestinal motility, and low-fat diet. Diarrhea may improve with decreased fluid and simple carbohydrate intake as well as increasing fat intake. Reassurance should be provided that the diarrhea will improve with time.

Distinguishing Features

Stools are isosmotic, even in osmotic diarrhea, because of the relatively free exchange of water across the intestinal mucosa. Osmoles present in the stool are a mixture of electrolytes and other osmotically active solutes. To determine whether the diarrhea is osmotic or secretory, the **osmotic gap** is calculated:

$$\text{Osmotic gap} = 290 - 2\left(\left[\text{Na}^+\right] + \left[\text{K}^+\right]\right)$$

Assuming the stool is isosmotic (an osmolarity of 290 mOsm/L), the measured stool sodium and potassium (and their associated anions, accounting for an equal amount) account for much of the osmolality. Secretory diarrhea is characterized by an osmotic gap of less than 50. A number significantly higher than 50 defines osmotic diarrhea and indicates that malabsorbed substances other than electrolytes account for fecal osmolarity.

Another way to differentiate between osmotic and secretory diarrhea is to stop all feedings (in hospitalized patients receiving IV fluids). If the diarrhea stops completely while the child is NPO (nothing by mouth), the patient has osmotic diarrhea. A child with a pure secretory diarrhea would continue to have massive stool output. Neither method for classifying diarrhea works perfectly because most diarrheal illnesses are a mixture of secretory and osmotic components. Viral enteritis damages the intestinal lining, causing malabsorption and osmotic diarrhea. The associated inflammation results in release of mediators that cause excessive secretion. A child with viral enteritis may have decreased stool volume while NPO, but the secretory component of the diarrhea persists until the inflammation resolves.

The **history** should include the onset of diarrhea, number and character of stools, estimates of stool volume, and presence of other symptoms, such as blood in the stool, fever, and weight loss. Recent travel and exposures should be documented, dietary factors should be investigated, and a list of medications recently used should be obtained. Factors that seem to worsen or improve the diarrhea should be determined. **Physical examination** should be thorough, evaluating for abdominal distention, tenderness, quality of bowel sounds, presence of blood in the stool or a large fecal mass on rectal examination, and anal sphincter tone.

Laboratory testing should include stool culture and/or stool enteric pathogen polymerase chain reaction panel and complete blood count if bacterial enteritis is suspected. If diarrhea occurs after a course of antibiotics, a *Clostridium difficile* toxin assay should be ordered. If stools are reported to be oily or fatty, fecal fat content or fecal elastase to test for pancreatic insufficiency should be measured. Tests for specific diagnoses should be sent when appropriate (e.g., serum antibody tests for celiac disease; fecal calprotectin and/or colonoscopy for suspected IBD). A trial of lactose restriction for several days or lactose breath hydrogen testing is helpful in the evaluation of lactose intolerance.

Constipation and Encopresis

Constipation is a common problem in childhood. When a child is thought to be constipated, the parents may be concerned about straining or pain with defecation, hard stool consistency, large stool size, decreased stool frequency, fear of passing stools, or any combination of these. Constipation is defined as *fewer than three bowel movements per week, stools that are hard, dry, or lumpy or are difficult to pass, or a feeling that not all stool has passed.* A common pattern of constipation is **functional constipation**, which is characterized by two or fewer stools per week, voluntary withholding of stool, and infrequent passage of large-diameter, often painful stools. Children with functional fecal retention often exhibit "retentive posturing" (standing or sitting with legs extended and stiff or crossed legs) and have associated fecal incontinence caused by leakage of retained stool (**encopresis**).

Differential Diagnosis

The differential diagnoses are listed in Table 127.10. **Functional constipation** commonly occurs during toilet training, when the child is unwilling to defecate on the toilet. Retained stool becomes harder and larger over time, leading to painful defecation. This aggravates voluntary withholding of stool, with perpetuation of the constipation.

Hirschsprung disease is characterized by delayed meconium passage in newborns, abdominal distention, vomiting, occasional fever, and foul-smelling stools. This condition is caused by failure of ganglion cells to migrate into the distal bowel, resulting in spasm and functional obstruction of the aganglionic segment. Only about 6% of infants with Hirschsprung disease pass meconium in the first 24 hours of life, compared with 95% of normal infants. Most affected babies rapidly become ill with symptoms of enterocolitis or obstruction. Affected older children do not pass large-caliber stools because of inability of the anal sphincter to relax, and they do not have encopresis. Other causes of constipation include spinal cord abnormalities, hypothyroidism, medications, cystic fibrosis, intestinal pseudoobstruction syndromes, and anorectal malformations (see Table 127.10). A variety of systemic disorders affecting metabolism or muscle function can result in constipation. Children with **developmental disabilities** have a great propensity for constipation because of diminished capacity to cooperate with toileting, reduced effort or control of pelvic floor muscles during defecation, and diminished perception of the need to pass stool.

Distinguishing Features

Table 127.10 includes typical characteristics of the common causes of constipation. Congenital malformations usually cause symptoms from birth. Functional constipation is overwhelmingly the most common diagnosis in older patients. Constipation in older children often begins after starting school, when free and private access to toilets may be restricted. Use of some drugs, especially opiates and some psychotropic medications, also is associated with constipation.

For a few specific causes of constipation, directed diagnostic testing can make the diagnosis. A narrowed, aganglionic distal bowel and dilated proximal bowel on barium enema

TABLE 127.10 Common Causes of Constipation and Characteristic Features

CAUSES OF CONSTIPATION	CLINICAL FEATURES
Hirschsprung disease	*History:* Failure to pass stool in first 24 hr, abdominal distention, vomiting, symptoms of enterocolitis (fever, foul-smelling diarrhea, megacolon). Not associated with large-caliber stools or encopresis *Examination:* Snug anal sphincter; empty, contracted rectum. May have explosive release of stool as examiner's finger is withdrawn *Laboratory:* Absence of ganglion cells on rectal suction biopsy specimen, absent relaxation of the internal sphincter, "transition zone" from narrow distal bowel to dilated proximal bowel on barium enema
Functional constipation	*History:* No history of significant neonatal constipation, onset at potty training, large-caliber stools, retentive posturing, may have encopresis *Examination:* Normal or reduced sphincter tone, dilated rectal vault, fecal impaction, soiled underwear, palpable fecal mass in left lower quadrant *Laboratory:* No abnormalities, barium enema would show dilated distal bowel
Anorectal, intestinal, and colonic malformations/syndromes Anal stenosis Anteriorly displaced anus Imperforate anus Colonic stricture Intestinal pseudoobstruction	*History:* Constipation from birth due to abnormal anatomy *Examination:* Anorectal abnormalities are shown easily on physical examination Anteriorly displaced anus is found chiefly in females, with a normal-appearing anus located close to the posterior fourchette of the vagina *Laboratory:* Barium enema shows the anomaly Genetic or idiopathic decreased or absent peristalsis
Multisystem disease Muscular dystrophy Cystic fibrosis Diabetes mellitus Developmental delay Celiac disease	*History:* Presence of other symptoms or prior diagnosis *Examination:* Specific abnormalities may be present that directly relate to the underlying diagnosis *Laboratory:* Tests directed at suspected disorder confirm the diagnosis
Spinal cord abnormalities Meningomyelocele Tethered cord Sacral teratoma or lipoma	*History:* History of swelling or exposed neural tissue in the lower back, history of urinary incontinence *Examination:* Lax sphincter tone due to impaired innervation, visible or palpable abnormality of lower back usually (but not always) present *Laboratory:* Bony abnormalities often present on plain x-ray. Magnetic resonance imaging of spinal cord reveals characteristic abnormalities
Drugs Narcotics Psychotropics	*History:* Recent use of drugs known to cause constipation (lead poisoning, opiates) *Examination:* Features suggest functional constipation *Laboratory:* No specific tests available

suggests Hirschsprung disease. Rectal suction biopsy confirms the absence of ganglion cells in the rectal submucosal plexus, with hypertrophy of nerve fibers. Lack of internal anal sphincter relaxation can be shown by anorectal manometry in Hirschsprung disease. Hypothyroidism is diagnosed by examination and by thyroid function testing. Anorectal malformations are easily detected by rectal examination. Cystic fibrosis (meconium ileus) is diagnosed by sweat chloride determination or *CFTR* gene analysis (see Chapter 138). Most children with constipation have functional constipation and do not have any laboratory abnormality. Examination reveals normal or reduced anal sphincter tone (owing to stretching by passage of large stools). Fecal impaction is usually present, but a large-caliber, empty rectum may be found if a stool has just been passed.

Evaluation and Treatment of Functional Constipation

In most cases of constipation, the history is consistent with functional constipation—absence of neonatal constipation, active fecal retention, and infrequent, large stools with soiling. In these patients, no testing other than a good physical examination is necessary. Young children with painful defecation must have a prolonged course of stool softener therapy to alleviate fear of defecation. The child should be asked to sit on the toilet for a few minutes on awakening in the morning and immediately after meals, when the colon is most active and it is easiest to pass a stool. Use of a stepstool under the feet improves the passage of stool through the rectum by mimicking the natural squatting position. Use of a positive reinforcement system for taking medication and sitting on the toilet is helpful for younger children. The stool softener chosen should be non–habit forming, safe, and palatable. Polyethylene glycol and milk of magnesia are the most commonly used osmotic agents.

Gastrointestinal Bleeding

GI tract bleeding can be an emergency when large-volume bleeding is present, but even the presence of small amounts of blood in stool or emesis is sufficient to cause concern. Evaluation of bleeding should include confirmation that blood truly is present, estimation of the amount of bleeding, checking for anemia, stabilization of the patient's intravascular blood volume, localization of the source of bleeding, and appropriate treatment of the underlying cause. When bleeding is massive, it is crucial that the patient receive adequate resuscitation with fluid and blood products before proceeding with diagnostic testing.

Differential Diagnosis

GI bleeding has different causes at different ages (Table 127.11).

Distinguishing Features

Red substances in foods, beverages, or medications (such as cefdinir) occasionally can be mistaken for blood. A test for occult blood is worth performing whenever the diagnosis is in doubt.

The GI tract may not be the source of the observed fecal blood. A history of cough and examination of the mouth, nostrils, and lungs is needed to exclude these as a source of swallowed blood and hematemesis. Blood in the toilet or diaper may be coming from the urinary tract, vagina, or a severe diaper rash. If the bleeding is GI, it is important to determine the source as the upper GI tract or distal to the ligament of Treitz. Vomited blood is always proximal. Rectal bleeding may be coming from anywhere in the gut. When dark clots or melena are seen mixed with stool, a higher location is suspected,

TABLE 127.11 Causes and Distinguishing Characteristics of Gastrointestinal Bleeding

AGE	TYPE OF BLEEDING	CHARACTERISTICS
NEWBORN		
Ingested maternal blood*	Hematemesis or rectal, large	Apt test indicates adult hemoglobin is present, cracked maternal nipples
Peptic disease	Hematemesis, amount varies	Blood found in stomach on lavage
Coagulopathy	Hematemesis or rectal, bruising, other sites	History of home birth (no vitamin K)
Allergic colitis*	Streaks of bloody mucus in stool	Eosinophils in feces and in rectal mucosa
Necrotizing enterocolitis	Rectal	Sick infant with tender and distended abdomen
Duplication cyst	Hematemesis	Cystic mass in abdomen on imaging study
Volvulus	Hematemesis, hematochezia	Acute tender, distended abdomen
INFANCY TO 2 YEARS OLD		
Peptic disease	Usually hematemesis, rectal possible	Epigastric pain, coffee-ground emesis
Esophageal varices	Hematemesis	History or evidence of liver disease
Intussusception*	Rectal bleeding	Crampy pain, distention, mass
Meckel diverticulum*	Rectal	Massive, bright red or maroon blood; no pain
Bacterial enteritis*	Rectal	Bloody diarrhea, fever
NSAID injury	Usually hematemesis, rectal possible	Epigastric pain, coffee-ground emesis
>2 YEARS OLD		
Peptic disease	See above	See above
Esophageal varices	See above	See above
NSAID injury*	See above	See above
Inflammatory bowel disease	Usually rectal	Crampy pain, poor weight gain, diarrhea
Bacterial enteritis*	See above	See above
Pseudomembranous colitis	Rectal	History of antibiotic use, bloody diarrhea
Juvenile polyp	Rectal	Painless, bright red blood in stool; not massive
Meckel diverticulum*	See above	See above
Nodular lymphoid hyperplasia	Rectal	Streaks of blood in stool, no other symptoms
Angiodysplasia	Rectal	Difficult to diagnosis, often requires capsule endoscopy
Mallory-Weiss syndrome*	Hematemesis	Bright red or coffee-ground, follows retching
Hemolytic uremic syndrome	Rectal	Thrombocytopenia, anemia, uremia
IgA vasculitis	Rectal	Purpuric rash, nephritis, arthritis, colitis
Hemorrhoids	Rectal	Dilated external veins, blood with wiping

*Common.
IgA, Immunoglobulin A; *NSAID*, nonsteroidal antiinflammatory drug.

TABLE 127.12 Evaluation of GI Bleeding

LABORATORY INVESTIGATION	INITIAL RADIOLOGIC EVALUATION
All Patients	**All Patients**
CBC and platelet count Coagulation tests: prothrombin time, partial thromboplastin time Tests of liver dysfunction: AST, ALT, GGT, bilirubin Occult blood test of stool or vomitus Blood type and crossmatch	Abdominal x-ray series
Evaluation of Bloody Diarrhea	**Evaluation of Hematemesis**
Stool culture or PCR, *Clostridium difficile* toxin Sigmoidoscopy or colonoscopy CT or MRI enterography	Barium upper GI series if endoscopy not available
Evaluation of Rectal Bleeding With Formed Stools	**Evaluation of Bleeding With Pain and Vomiting (Bowel Obstruction)**
External and digital rectal examination Sigmoidoscopy or colonoscopy Meckel scan Mesenteric arteriogram Video capsule endoscopy	Abdominal x-ray series Pneumatic or contrast enema Upper GI series Abdominal CT

ALT, Alanine aminotransferase; *AST,* aspartate aminotransferase; *CBC,* complete blood count; *CT,* computed tomography; *GGT,* γ-glutamyltransferase; *GI,* gastrointestinal; *MRI,* magnetic resonance imaging; *PCR,* polymerase chain reaction.

whereas bright red blood on the surface of stool probably is coming from lower in the colon. When upper GI tract bleeding is suspected, a nasogastric tube may be placed and gastric contents aspirated for evidence of recent bleeding.

The location and hemodynamic significance of the bleeding can also be assessed by history and examination. The parents should be asked to quantify the bleeding. Details of associated symptoms should be sought, as well as any pertinent medical history (e.g., liver disease). Assessment of the vital signs, including orthostatic changes when bleeding volume is large, pulses, capillary refill, and assessment of pallor of the mucous membranes, provides valuable information. Laboratory assessment and imaging studies should be ordered as indicated (Table 127.12).

Treatment

Treatment of GI bleeding should begin with an initial assessment, rapid stabilization, and a logical sequence of diagnostic tests. When a treatable cause is identified, specific therapy should be started. In many cases, the amount of blood is small, and no resuscitation is required. For children with large-volume bleeds, the **ABCs** of resuscitation (**A**irway, **B**reathing, **C**irculation) should be addressed first (see Chapter 39). Oxygen should be administered, and the airway should be protected with an endotracheal tube if massive hematemesis is present. Fluid boluses and transfusion with packed RBCs as required should be administered through two large-bore IVs. Frequent reassessment should continue to ensure maintenance of physiologic stability.

PEARLS FOR PRACTITIONERS

See The Digestive System: Pearls for Practitioners at the end of this section.

REVIEW QUESTIONS

Available online.

CHAPTER 128
Oral Cavity

EFFECTS OF SYSTEMIC DISEASE ON THE ORAL CAVITY

Medications taken for a variety of conditions may cause oral abnormalities. Drugs with anticholinergic properties diminish saliva production and increase the risk of dental caries and parotitis. Tetracyclines taken before the eruption of the permanent teeth stain the enamel. Excessive fluoride in vitamin preparations or in drinking water can result in mottled teeth. Gingival hypertrophy may be caused by cyclosporine, phenytoin, and calcium channel blockers.

Gastroesophageal reflux disease (GERD) can lead to substantial enamel erosion and caries. Neonatal hyperbilirubinemia can result in discoloration of the deciduous teeth. Kidney failure is associated with mottled enamel of the permanent teeth. Congenital syphilis causes marked abnormalities in the shape of teeth, especially incisors and molars. Celiac disease can result in enamel defects. Crohn disease is associated with oral aphthous ulcers. Abnormal pigmentation of the lips and buccal mucosa is seen with Peutz-Jeghers syndrome (freckling) and Addison disease (hyperpigmented macules). Candidiasis is seen commonly with immunodeficiency disorders and diabetes. Leukemic infiltrates result in gum hyperplasia and bleeding; treatment of neoplastic conditions can cause severe mucositis. Some tumors, including lymphoma, may present as mass lesions of the buccal cavity.

Osteogenesis imperfecta is associated with abnormal dentin and risk of caries. Children with *ectodermal dysplasias* commonly have malformed or missing teeth. Pierre Robin and Stickler syndromes are associated with micrognathia and cleft palate. Disorders resulting in facial dysmorphism can have a profound effect on dental occlusion and mandibular function. Examples include mandibulofacial dysostosis, Crouzon syndrome, conditions associated with skeletal dysplasias, and others.

DECIDUOUS AND PRIMARY TEETH

Most infants are born without teeth. *Natal teeth*, present at birth, are usually supernumerary, and may be poorly attached. Usually, no treatment is necessary, but removal by a dentist may be needed if they are causing difficulties with feeding or injuries to the tongue. Table 128.1 presents the ages when normal **deciduous teeth** are acquired. The lower central incisors are typically the first to erupt, followed by the upper central incisors, lateral incisors, first molars, and bicuspids. **Delayed eruption** may occur in association with hypopituitarism, hypothyroidism, osteopetrosis, Gaucher disease, Down syndrome, cleidocranial dysplasia, and rickets. Deciduous teeth begin to be replaced by the permanent teeth at around age 6 years. The sequence of replacement is similar to that of the appearance of deciduous teeth.

DENTAL CARIES

Etiology

Dental caries, commonly referred to as *cavities,* occur as a result of interactions between the tooth enamel, dietary carbohydrates, and oral flora. There is increased susceptibility if the enamel is abnormal or hypoplastic. Bacteria *(Streptococcus mutans)* can adhere to and colonize the teeth, survive at low pH, and produce acids during fermentation of carbohydrates that cause dental caries. The diet has a significant role. A classic example is "bottle mouth," or **baby bottle caries**. This condition results when infants are allowed to have a bottle in the mouth for prolonged periods, especially during sleep, and with sweet beverages or milk in the bottle. Bacteria then have continuous substrate for acid production and can destroy multiple teeth, especially the upper incisors. Sticky sweet foods, such as candy, have the same effect.

Epidemiology and Treatment

Risk of caries is associated with lack of dental care and poor socioeconomic status and is greatest in developing countries. Treatment of caries is with dental restorative surgery. The carious portion of the tooth is removed and filled with silver amalgam or plastic. If the damage is severe, a protective crown may be required; extraction of the tooth may be necessary when not salvageable. If not properly treated, dental decay results in inflammation and infection of the dental pulp and surrounding alveolar bone, which can lead to abscess and facial space infections.

TABLE 128.1 Time of Eruption of the Primary and Permanent Teeth

	PRIMARY, AGE (MO)		PERMANENT, AGE (YR)	
TOOTH TYPE	UPPER	LOWER	UPPER	LOWER
Central incisor	6 ± 2	7 ± 2	7–8	6–7
Lateral incisor	9 ± 2	7 ± 2	8–9	7–8
Cuspids	18 ± 2	16 ± 2	11–12	9–10
First bicuspids	—	—	10–11	10–12
Second bicuspids	—	—	10–12	11–12
First molars	14 ± 2	12 ± 2	6–7	6–7
Second molars	24 ± 2	20 ± 2	12–13	11–13
Third molars	—	—	17–21	17–21

Prevention

Avoiding inappropriate use of bottles and excessive sweets is a commonsense remedy for baby bottle caries. Oral hygiene offers some protection, but young children (<8 years old) do not have the ability to brush their own teeth adequately; brushing should be done by the parents. Fluoride supplementation of community water supplies to a concentration of 1 ppm is highly effective in reducing dental caries. Home water supplies, such as from a well, should have the fluoride content tested before supplements are prescribed. If the child spends part of the day at another location, the total fluoride concentration from all sources must be considered before prescribing any oral supplements. Excessive fluoride supplementation causes fluorosis, a largely cosmetic defect of chalky white marks and brown staining of the teeth.

The American Academy of Pediatrics recommends that primary care physicians apply fluoride varnish to the teeth of all children every 3–6 months, starting at the emergence of the first tooth. Fluoride varnish is a concentrated fluoride preparation that adheres to the teeth on contact with saliva. It is painted onto the teeth with a small brush, after first drying the tooth with a gauze pad, and has a prolonged cavity-prevention effect.

CLEFT LIP AND PALATE

Epidemiology

Cleft lip and palate occur separately or together and affect approximately 1 in 700 infants. Clefting occurs with two possible patterns: isolated soft tissue cleft palate or cleft lip with or without associated clefts of the hard palate. Isolated cleft palate is associated with a higher risk of other congenital malformations. The combined cleft lip/palate type has a male predominance.

Etiology

Cleft lip is due to hypoplasia of the mesenchymal tissues with subsequent failure of fusion. There is a strong genetic component; the risk is highest in children with affected first-degree relatives. Monozygotic twins are affected with only 60% concordance, suggesting other nongenomic factors. Environmental factors during gestation also increase risk, including medications (phenytoin, valproic acid, thalidomide), maternal alcohol and tobacco use, dioxins and other herbicides, and possibly high altitude. Chromosomal and nonchromosomal syndromes are associated with clefting, as are specific genes in some families.

Clinical Manifestations and Treatment

Cleft lip can be unilateral or bilateral and associated with cleft palate and defects of the alveolar ridge and dentition. When present, palatal defects allow direct communication between the nasal and oral cavities, creating problems with speech and feeding. Management includes squeeze-bottle feedings, special nipples, nipples with attached shields to seal the palate, and gastrostomy in severe cases. Surgical closure of the cleft lip is usually done by 3 months of age. Closure of the palate follows, usually before 1 year of age. Missing teeth are replaced by prostheses. Cosmetic results are often good, but they depend on the severity of the defect.

Complications

Speech is nasal as a result of the cleft palate. Surgical treatment is effective, but it sometimes does not restore palatal function completely. Speech therapy or, occasionally, the use of a speech-assisting appliance may help. Frequent episodes of otitis media are common, as are defects of teeth and the alveolar ridge.

THRUSH

Epidemiology

Oropharyngeal *Candida albicans* infection, or thrush, is common in healthy neonates. The organism may be acquired in the birth canal or from the environment. Persistent infection is common in breast-fed infants as a result of colonization or infection of the mother's nipples. Thrush in older patients can occur but should suggest the possibility of an immunodeficiency, broad-spectrum antibiotic or inhaled steroid use, or diabetes.

Clinical Manifestations

Thrush is easily visible as white plaques, often with a "fuzzy" appearance, on oral mucous membranes. When scraped with a tongue depressor, the plaques are difficult to remove, and the underlying mucosa is inflamed and friable. Clinical diagnosis is usually adequate but may be confirmed by fungal culture or potassium hydroxide smear. Oropharyngeal candidiasis is sometimes painful (especially if associated with esophagitis) and can interfere with feeding.

Treatment

Thrush is treated with topical nystatin or an azole antifungal agent such as fluconazole. When the mother's breasts are infected and painful, consideration should be given to treating the mother at the same time. Because thrush is commonly self-limited in newborns, withholding therapy in asymptomatic infants and treating only persistent or severe cases is a reasonable approach.

PEARLS FOR PRACTITIONERS

See The Digestive System: Pearls for Practitioners at the end of this section.

REVIEW QUESTIONS

Available online.

CHAPTER 129

Esophagus and Stomach

GASTROESOPHAGEAL REFLUX

Etiology and Epidemiology

Gastroesophageal reflux (GER) is defined as the effortless retrograde movement of gastric contents upward into the esophagus or oropharynx. **Physiologic GER** ("spitting up") is normal in infants. Nearly half of all infants are reported to spit up between 2–4 months of age. Infants who regurgitate meet the criteria for physiologic GER so long as they maintain adequate nutrition and have no signs of respiratory complications or esophagitis. Contributing factors of infantile GER include liquid diet; horizontal body position; short, narrow esophagus; small, noncompliant stomach; frequent, relatively large-volume feedings; and an immature lower esophageal sphincter (LES). As infants grow, they spend more time upright, eat more solid foods, develop a longer and larger diameter esophagus, have a larger and more compliant stomach, and experience lower caloric needs per unit of body weight. As a result, most infants stop spitting up by 9–12 months of age; however, physiologic GER may persist until 14 months of age.

Gastroesophageal reflux disease (GERD) occurs when GER leads to troublesome symptoms or complications such as poor growth, pain, or breathing difficulties. GERD occurs in a minority of infants but is often implicated as the cause of fussiness. GERD is seen in fewer than 5% of older children. In older children, normal protective mechanisms against GER include antegrade esophageal motility, tonic contraction of the LES, and the geometry of the gastroesophageal junction. Abnormalities that cause GER in older children and adults include reduced tone of the LES, transient relaxations of the LES, esophagitis (which impairs esophageal motility), increased intraabdominal pressure, cough, respiratory difficulty (asthma or cystic fibrosis), and hiatal hernia.

Clinical Manifestations

The presence of GER is easy to observe in an infant who spits up. In older children, the refluxate is usually kept down by reswallowing, but GERD may be suspected by associated symptoms, such as heartburn, cough, epigastric abdominal pain, dysphagia, wheezing, aspiration pneumonia, hoarse voice, growth faltering, and recurrent hiccoughs or belching. In severe cases of esophagitis, there may be laboratory evidence of anemia and hypoalbuminemia secondary to esophageal bleeding and inflammation.

When esophagitis develops as a result of acid reflux, esophageal motility and LES function are impaired further, creating a cycle of reflux and esophageal injury.

Laboratory and Imaging Studies

A clinical diagnosis is often sufficient in children with classic effortless regurgitation and no complications. Diagnostic studies are indicated if there are persistent symptoms or complications or if other symptoms suggest the possibility of GERD in the absence of regurgitation. A child with recurrent pneumonia, chronic cough, or apneic spells without overt emesis may have occult GERD. A **barium upper gastrointestinal (GI) series** helps to rule out gastric outlet obstruction, malrotation, or other anatomic contributors to GERD. Because of the brief nature of the examination, a negative barium study does *not* rule out GERD, nor does it rule it in as it is normal to have some reflux into the esophagus many times per day. A **24-hour esophageal pH probe monitoring** uses a pH electrode placed transnasally into the distal esophagus, with continuous recording of esophageal pH. Data typically are gathered for 24 hours and analyzed for the number and temporal pattern of acid reflux events. **Esophageal impedance monitoring** records the migration of electrolyte-rich gastric fluid in the esophagus. **Endoscopy** is useful to evaluate for esophagitis, esophageal stricture, and anatomic abnormalities.

Treatment

In otherwise healthy young infants, no treatment is necessary. For infants with complications of GER, an H_2 blocker or proton pump inhibitor may be offered (Table 129.1), but these have shown little benefit in infants with uncomplicated GER and/or fussiness. Prokinetic medications, such as metoclopramide, occasionally are helpful by enhancing gastric emptying and increasing LES tone, but they have limited efficacy and may lead to complications. When severe symptoms persist despite medication, or if life-threatening aspiration is present, surgical intervention may be required. Fundoplication procedures, such as the Nissen operation, are designed to enhance the antireflux anatomy of the LES. In children with a severe neurologic defect who cannot tolerate oral or gastric tube feedings, placement of a feeding jejunostomy may be considered as an alternative to fundoplication. In older children, lifestyle changes should be discussed, including cessation of smoking, weight loss, not eating or exercising before bed, and limiting intake of caffeine, carbonation, and high-fat foods. If lifestyle changes are ineffective in reducing symptoms, proton pump inhibitor therapy is effective in reducing symptoms and supports healing.

TABLE 129.1 Treatment of Gastroesophageal Reflux

THERAPIES	COMMENTS
CONSERVATIVE THERAPIES	
Towel on caregiver's shoulder	Cheap, effective; useful only for physiologic reflux
Thickened feedings	Reduces number of episodes, enhances nutrition
Smaller, more frequent feedings	Can help some; be careful not to *underfeed* child
Avoidance of tobacco smoke and alcohol	Always a good idea; may help reflux symptoms
Abstaining from caffeine	Inexpensive, offers some benefit
Positional therapy—upright in seat, elevate	Prone positioning with head of crib or bed up is helpful, but *not* for young infants because of risk of SIDS
Weight loss when indicated	Increased weight (especially abdominal) increases intraabdominal pressure, leading to reflux
MEDICAL THERAPY	
Proton pump inhibitor	Effective medical therapy for heartburn and esophagitis
H_2-receptor antagonist	Reduces heartburn, less effective for healing esophagitis
Metoclopramide	Enhances stomach emptying and LES tone; real benefit is often minimal
SURGICAL THERAPY	
Nissen endoscopic laparoscopic fundoplication procedure	For life-threatening or medically unresponsive cases
Feeding jejunostomy	Useful in child requiring tube feeds; delivering feeds downstream eliminates GERD

GERD, Gastroesophageal reflux disease; *LES*, lower esophageal sphincter; *SIDS*, sudden infant death syndrome.

EOSINOPHILIC ESOPHAGITIS

Etiology and Epidemiology

This chronic immune-mediated disorder is characterized by infiltration of eosinophils into the mucosa of the esophagus. It is thought to be triggered by non–immunoglobulin E (IgE)–mediated allergic reactions to ingested foods or aeroallergens. Eosinophilic esophagitis (EoE) may have a familial component. Incidence appears to be increasing with estimated prevalence of more than 50 per 100,000 children. It is more common in males than females and in patients with history of atopy.

Clinical Manifestations

The presentation of EoE often varies with age. In young children, it may present with oral aversion, vomiting, and growth faltering. In school-age children, it may present with vague abdominal pain or vomiting. In adolescents and adults, it presents with dysphagia and food impactions. These symptoms are attributed to the inflammatory response in the esophagus leading to edema, poor esophageal motility, or obstruction.

Laboratory and Imaging Studies

Diagnosis requires multilevel esophageal biopsies via flexible endoscopy with the finding of more than 15 eosinophils per high-power field (Fig. 129.1). Gross findings at endoscopy may include normal appearance, esophageal linear furrowing, trachealization, and eosinophilic abscesses (Fig. 129.2). A barium study may reveal a food impaction in an acutely symptomatic patient or esophageal stricture in someone with chronic disease.

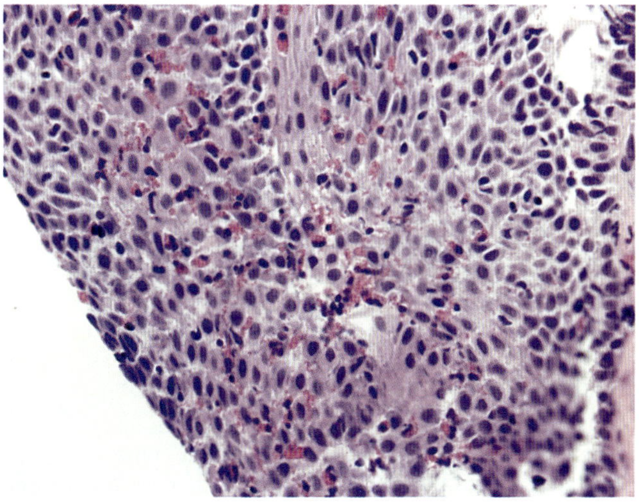

FIGURE 129.1 Histologic image of eosinophilic esophagitis. Note the large number of eosinophils within the lamina propria.

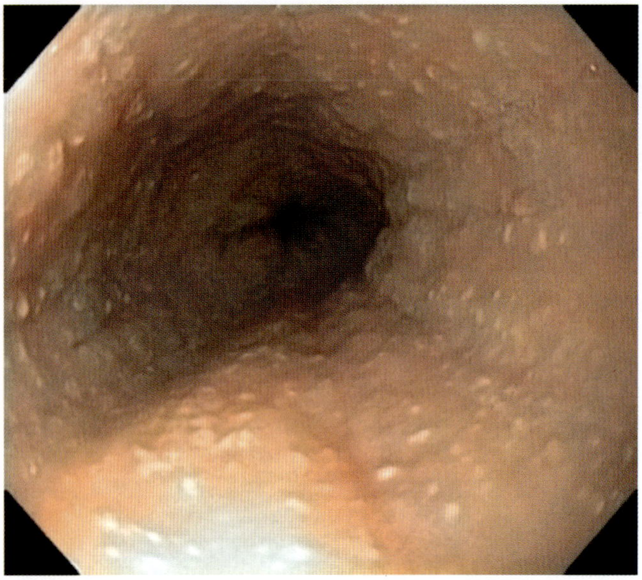

FIGURE 129.2 Endoscopic picture of eosinophilic esophagitis. White plaques on the surface are collections of eosinophils (eosinophilic abscesses). Linear furrowing is also seen.

Treatment and Prognosis

Treatment with high-dose proton pump inhibitor therapy can lead to resolution of esophageal eosinophilia in a subset of patients. Identification of causative antigens can be difficult, as typical allergy testing (skin prick, radioallergosorbent test, and immunocap assays) only identifies IgE-mediated antigens. One approach is to eliminate from the diet cow's milk, soy, wheat, eggs *(four-food elimination diet)* or additionally peanuts and fish/shellfish *(six-food elimination diet)*, as these are the most common causative dietary antigens. Alternatively, eliminating the most common allergen first (cow's milk) can be effective for a number of patients. Repeat endoscopies are often necessary to document efficacy of these eliminations. An elemental diet can also be used and is very effective, but it often requires either nasogastric or gastrostomy administration because of its poor palatability.

Systemic glucocorticoids can decrease symptoms, but long-term use is discouraged due to concerns for potential complications. Swallowed "topical" glucocorticoids administered via a metered-dose inhaler (fluticasone) or mixed as a slurry (budesonide) have shown benefit. *Candida* esophagitis or oral thrush are the most common side effects. Dupilumab is an injectable antibody to interleukin (IL)-4 and IL-13 signaling that is effective for EoE as well as other allergic disorders.

Endoscopy can be used to relieve food impactions and to dilate esophageal strictures secondary to EoE. The prognosis for EoE is largely unknown. Symptoms tend to wax and wane over time.

Complications

Growth faltering or weight loss may be seen due to difficulty in eating. Food impactions are a common complication in the older child and may require endoscopic removal. Chronic inflammation of the esophagus can predispose to esophageal strictures.

ESOPHAGEAL ATRESIA AND TRACHEOESOPHAGEAL FISTULA

Etiology and Epidemiology

The esophagus and trachea develop in proximity to each other during weeks 4–6 of fetal life. Defects in the mesenchyme separating these two structures result in a tracheoesophageal fistula (TEF), often in association with other anomalies (kidney, heart, spine, limbs). This defect occurs in about 1 in 3,000 live births. TEF is not thought to be a genetic defect.

Clinical Manifestations

The most common forms of TEF occur with esophageal atresia; the "H-type" TEF without atresia is uncommon, as is esophageal atresia without TEF (Fig. 129.3). Associated defects include the **VACTERL** association—**V**ertebral anomalies (70%), **A**nal atresia (imperforate anus) (50%), **C**ardiac anomalies (30%), **TE**F (70%), **R**enal anomalies (50%), and **L**imb anomalies (polydactyly, forearm defects, absent thumbs, syndactyly) (70%). A single umbilical artery is often present. Infants with esophageal atresia have a history of polyhydramnios, exhibit drooling, and have mucus and saliva bubbling from the nose and mouth. Patients with a TEF are vulnerable to aspiration pneumonia. When TEF is suspected, the first feeding should be delayed until a diagnostic study is performed.

Laboratory and Imaging Studies

The simplest test for TEF is to gently attempt to place a 10 F or larger tube via the mouth into the stomach. The passage of the tube is blocked at the level of the atresia. A chest x-ray reveals the tube coiled in the esophageal pouch. Air can be injected through the tube to outline the atretic pouch. Barium should not be used because of extreme risk of aspiration, but a tiny amount of dilute water-soluble contrast agent can be given carefully, then suctioned when the defect is clearly shown.

Treatment and Prognosis

The treatment of TEF is surgical. The fistula is divided and ligated. The esophageal ends are approximated and anastomosed. In some cases, primary anastomosis cannot be performed because of a long gap between the proximal and distal esophagus. Various techniques have been described to treat this problem, including pulling up the stomach, elongating the esophagus by myotomy, and simply delaying esophageal anastomosis and providing continuous suction to the upper pouch while allowing for growth.

Complications

The surgically reconstructed esophagus is not normal and is prone to poor motility, GER, anastomotic stricture, recurrent fistula, and leakage. The trachea also is malformed; tracheomalacia and wheezing are common.

ESOPHAGEAL FOREIGN BODIES

Etiology and Epidemiology

Young children often place nonfood items in the mouth. When these items are swallowed, they may become lodged in

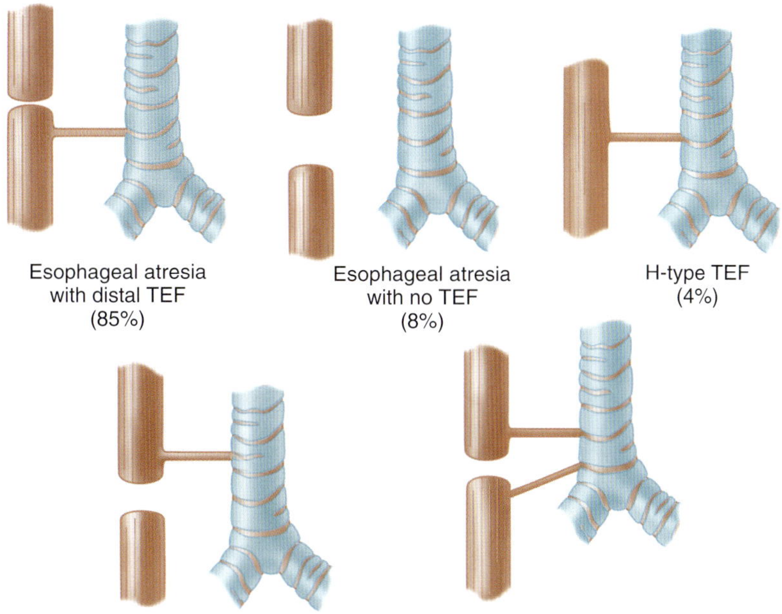

FIGURE 129.3 Various types of TEF with relative frequency (%). *TEF*, Tracheoesophageal fistula.

the esophagus at the thoracic inlet or at the LES. The most common objects are coins. Smaller coins may pass harmlessly into the stomach, where they rarely cause symptoms. Other common esophageal foreign bodies include food items, small toys or toy parts, button batteries, and other small household items. Children with a prior history of esophageal atresia or with poor motility secondary to GER or EoE are more prone to food impactions, which seldom occur in the normal esophagus.

Clinical Manifestations

Some children are asymptomatic, but most exhibit some degree of drooling, food refusal, or chest discomfort. Older children usually can point to the region of the chest where they feel the object to be lodged. Respiratory symptoms tend to be minimal, but cough or wheezing may be present, especially when the esophagus is completely blocked by a large object, such as a piece of meat, which presses on the trachea.

Diagnosis

Plain chest and abdominal radiographs should be taken when foreign body ingestion is suspected. Metallic objects are easily visualized. A plastic object often can be seen if the child is given a small amount of dilute x-ray contrast material to drink, although endoscopy is probably safer and more definitive.

Treatment

Endoscopy is ultimately necessary in most cases to remove a retained esophageal foreign body. Various devices can be used to remove the object, depending on its size, shape, and location. Coins usually are grasped with special-purpose forceps and removed. Nets, baskets, and snares also are available. Whenever objects that may threaten the airway are being recovered, endoscopy should be performed with endotracheal intubation and under general anesthesia. Removal is usually not necessary if the object is small and located in the stomach, as it will most likely pass without complication. Endoscopy is emergent for removal of any esophageal foreign body if the patient has airway compromise. Due to high risk of complications, emergent removal is required for esophageal button batteries (within 2 hours if possible) or multiple magnets. If a button battery ingestion is suspected (a double rim or halo is seen on x-ray) it is recommended to give 10 mL of honey every 10 minutes if child is >12 months and ingestion was within the last 12 hours.

Complications

Sharp objects may lacerate or perforate the esophagus; smooth objects present for a long time also may result in perforation due to ulceration. Corrosive objects, such as zinc-containing pennies and button batteries, can cause considerable local tissue injury and esophageal perforation. Magnets can lead to perforation and fistula formation when they connect between adjacent loops of bowel.

CAUSTIC INJURIES AND PILL ULCERS

Etiology and Epidemiology

In adolescents, caustic ingestion injuries are usually the result of suicide attempts. In toddlers, ingestion of household cleaning products typically is accidental. Injurious agents include drain cleaners, toilet bowl cleaners, dishwasher and laundry detergents, and powerful bleaching agents. Childproof lids for commercial products offer some protection but have not eliminated the problem. Lye-based drain cleaners, especially liquid products, cause the worst injuries because they are swallowed easily and liquefy tissue rapidly. Full-thickness burns can occur in seconds. Granular products are less likely to cause esophageal injury during accidental exposures because they burn the tongue and lips and often are expelled before swallowing. Less caustic agents, such as bleach and detergents, cause less serious injury. **Pill ulcers** occur when certain medications (tetracyclines and nonsteroidal antiinflammatory drugs) are swallowed without sufficient liquids, allowing prolonged direct contact of the pill with the esophageal mucosa.

Clinical Manifestations

Caustic burns cause immediate and severe mouth pain. The child cries out, drools, spits, and usually drops the container immediately. Burns of the lips and tongue are visible almost immediately. These burns clearly indicate the possibility of esophageal involvement, although esophageal injury can occur in the absence of oral burns. Symptoms may not be present; further evaluation by endoscopy usually is indicated with any significant history of caustic ingestion. Pill injury causes severe chest pain and often prominent odynophagia and dysphagia.

Laboratory and Imaging Studies

A chest x-ray should be obtained to rule out aspiration and to inspect for mediastinal air. The child should be admitted to the hospital and given intravenous (IV) fluids until endoscopy. The true extent of burns may not be endoscopically apparent immediately, but delayed endoscopy can increase the risk of perforation. Most endoscopists perform the initial endoscopy 12–24 hours after injury, when the patient has been stabilized. The extent of injury and severity of the burn should be carefully determined. Risk of subsequent esophageal strictures is related to the degree of burn and whether the injury is circumferential.

Treatment

A nasogastric tube can be placed over a guide wire at the time of the initial endoscopy to provide a route for feeding and to stent the esophagus. Systemic steroid use has not been found to be beneficial in reducing stricture formation. Broad-spectrum antibiotics should be prescribed if infection is suspected.

Complications

Esophageal strictures, if they occur, usually develop within 1–2 months and can be treated with endoscopic dilation. There is a risk of perforation during dilation. When esophageal injury is severe, surgical reconstruction of the esophagus using stomach or intestine may be necessary.

PYLORIC STENOSIS

Etiology and Epidemiology

Pyloric stenosis is an acquired condition caused by hypertrophy and spasm of the pyloric muscle, resulting in gastric outlet obstruction. It occurs in 6–8 per 1,000 live births, has a 5:1 male predominance, and is more common in first-born children. Its cause is unknown.

Clinical Manifestations

Infants with pyloric stenosis typically begin vomiting during the first weeks of life, but onset may be delayed. The emesis becomes increasingly frequent and forceful as time passes. Vomiting differs from spitting up because of its extremely forceful and often projectile nature. The vomited material never contains bile because the gastric outlet obstruction is proximal to the duodenum. This feature differentiates pyloric stenosis from most other obstructive lesions of early childhood. Affected infants are ravenously hungry early in the course of the illness but become more lethargic with increasing malnutrition and dehydration. The stomach becomes massively enlarged with retained food and secretions, and gastric **peristaltic waves** are often visible in the left upper quadrant. A hypertrophied pylorus (the "olive") may be palpated. As the illness progresses, very little of each feeding is able to pass through the pylorus, and the child becomes progressively thinner and more dehydrated.

Laboratory and Imaging Studies

Repetitive vomiting of purely gastric contents results in loss of hydrochloric acid; the classic laboratory finding is a **hypochloremic, hypokalemic metabolic alkalosis** with elevated blood urea nitrogen secondary to dehydration. Jaundice with unconjugated hyperbilirubinemia may also occur. Plain abdominal x-rays typically show an enlarged stomach and diminished or absent gas in the intestine (Fig. 129.4). Ultrasound examination shows marked elongation and thickening of the pylorus (Fig. 129.5). A barium upper GI series also may be obtained whenever doubt about the diagnosis exists; this shows a "string sign" caused by barium moving through an elongated, constricted pyloric channel.

Treatment

Treatment of pyloric stenosis includes IV fluid and electrolyte resuscitation followed by surgical pyloromyotomy. Before surgery, dehydration and hypochloremic alkalosis must be corrected, generally with an initial normal saline fluid bolus followed by infusions of half-normal saline containing 5% dextrose and potassium chloride when urine output is observed. In pyloromyotomy (often by laparoscope), the pyloric muscle is incised longitudinally to release the constriction.

PEPTIC DISEASE

Etiology and Epidemiology

Acid-related injury can occur in the esophagus, stomach, or duodenum. Table 129.2 lists risk factors for **peptic ulcer disease** in children. ***Helicobacter pylori*** is responsible for more than half of ulcers in the stomach and duodenum in adults. *H. pylori* plays a significant but lesser role in childhood ulcer disease. Risk factors for acquisition of *H. pylori* are low socioeconomic status and poor sanitation, with the highest incidence

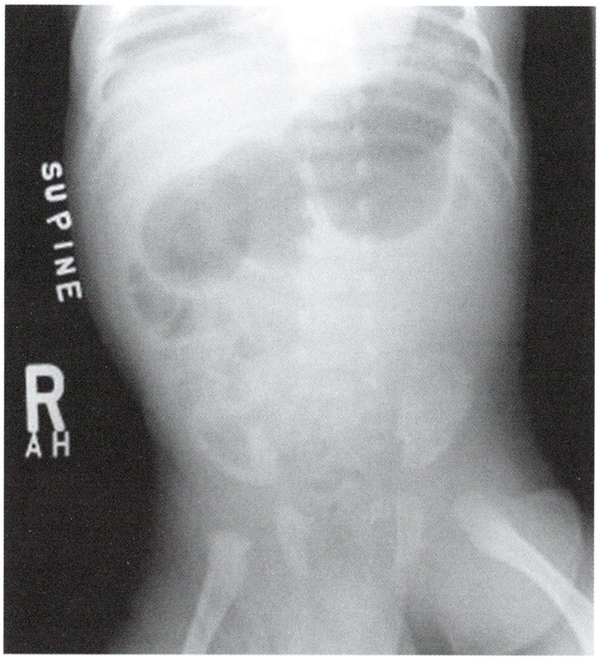

FIGURE 129.4 Pyloric stenosis. Note the huge, gas-filled stomach extending across the midline, with minimal air in the intestine downstream. (Courtesy Warren Bishop, MD.)

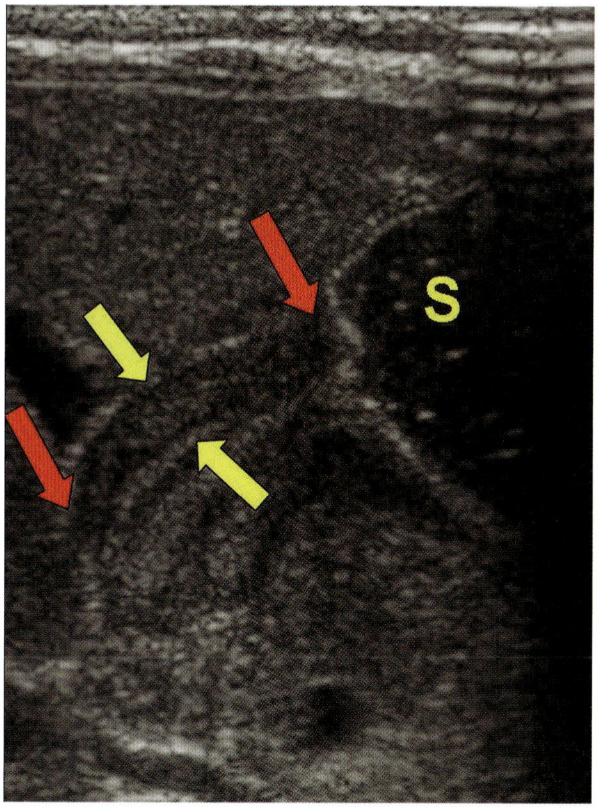

FIGURE 129.5 Ultrasound image of infant with pyloric stenosis. Large, fluid-filled stomach *(S)* is seen at right, with an elongated, thickened pylorus. The length of the pylorus is marked by the *red arrows*; the wall thickness is marked by the *yellow arrows*.

in developing countries. **Nonulcer dyspepsia** includes upper abdominal symptoms (pain, bloating, nausea, early satiety) in the absence of gastric or duodenal ulceration. Nonulcer dyspepsia is *not* associated with *H. pylori* infection. GER

TABLE 129.2 Risk Factors for Peptic Ulcer Disease

Helicobacter pylori infection
Drugs
NSAIDs, including aspirin
Tobacco use
Bisphosphonates
Potassium supplements
Family history
Sepsis
Head trauma
Burn injury
Hypotension

NSAIDs, Nonsteroidal antiinflammatory drugs.

(see Chapter 129) allows acidic gastric contents to injure the esophagus, resulting in **esophagitis**. Esophagitis is characterized by retrosternal and epigastric burning pain and is best diagnosed by endoscopy. It can range from minimal, with only erythema and microscopic inflammation on biopsy, to superficial erosions and, finally, to frank ulceration.

Clinical Manifestations

Typical symptoms are listed in Table 129.3. The presence of recurrent burning epigastric and retrosternal pain is a risk factor for esophagitis. With duodenal ulcers, pain typically occurs several hours after meals and often awakens patients at night. Eating tends to relieve the pain. Gastric ulcers differ in that pain is commonly aggravated by eating, resulting in weight loss. GI bleeding from either can occur. Many patients report symptom relief with antacids or proton inhibitors (reduces gastric acid secretion).

Laboratory and Imaging Studies

Endoscopy can be used to diagnose the underlying condition. Empiric therapy with H_2 blockers or proton pump inhibitors can be used but may delay diagnosis of conditions such as *H. pylori*. For patients with chronic epigastric pain, the possibilities of inflammatory bowel disease, anatomic abnormality such as malrotation, pancreatitis, and biliary disease should be ruled out by appropriate testing when suspected (see Chapter 127 and Table 129.3 for recommended studies). Testing for *H. pylori* can be performed by biopsy during endoscopy with use of a urease test or presence histologically on tissue. If endoscopy is not done, noninvasive tests for infection can be done with reasonable accuracy with *H. pylori* fecal antigen and ^{13}C urea breath tests.

Treatment

If *H. pylori* is present in association with ulcers, it should be treated with a multidrug regimen, such as omeprazole-clarithromycin-metronidazole (or amoxicillin). Other proton pump inhibitors may be substituted when necessary. Bismuth compounds are effective against *H. pylori* and can be considered in addition to the above-mentioned therapies. In North America, only the subsalicylate salt is available, the use of which raises some concerns about Reye syndrome and potential salicylate toxicity. Tetracycline is useful in adults but should be avoided in children less than 8 years of age. In the absence of *H. pylori*, esophagitis and

TABLE 129.3 Peptic Disorders, Symptoms, and Clinical Investigation

SYNDROME AND ASSOCIATED SYMPTOMS	CLINICAL INVESTIGATIONS
ESOPHAGITIS	
Retrosternal and epigastric location Burning pain Sensation of regurgitation Dysphagia, odynophagia	Endoscopy Therapeutic trial of acid-blocker therapy pH and/or impedance probe study
NONULCER DYSPEPSIA	
Upper abdominal location Fullness Bloating Nausea	Endoscopy Therapeutic trial of acid-blocker therapy Upper GI series to ligament of Treitz—rule out malrotation CBC, ESR, amylase, lipase, abdominal ultrasound
PEPTIC ULCER DISEASE	
"Alarm" symptoms: Weight loss Hematemesis Melena, heme-positive stools Chronic vomiting Microcytic anemia Nocturnal pain Other symptoms—same as for esophagitis and nonulcer dyspepsia	Endoscopy—mandatory with alarm symptoms Test for *Helicobacter pylori* CBC, ESR, amylase, lipase, abdominal ultrasound

CBC, Complete blood count; *ESR,* erythrocyte sedimentation rate; *GI,* gastrointestinal.

peptic ulcer disease are treated with a proton pump inhibitor, which yields higher rates of healing than H_2-receptor antagonists. Gastric and duodenal ulcers heal in 4–8 weeks in at least 80% of patients. Esophagitis requires several months of proton pump inhibitor treatment for optimal healing.

CYCLIC VOMITING SYNDROME

Etiology and Epidemiology

Cyclic vomiting syndrome (CVS) presents with intermittent episodes of prolonged nausea and vomiting with periods of health in between. It can occur at any age but is diagnosed most frequently in preschool to school-age children. It is thought to be a migraine variant; many patients have a positive family history of migraines, and some with CVS will eventually develop migraine headaches. Triggers for an episode often include viral illnesses, lack of sleep, stressful or exciting events (holidays, birthdays, vacations), physical exhaustion, and menses. Chronic cannabis use can also trigger CVS.

Clinical Manifestations

Episodes can start at any time but will often start in the early morning hours. Episodes are similar to each other in timing and duration. Repetitive vomiting can last hours to days. Patients may also have abdominal pain, diarrhea, and headaches. Those affected are typically pale, listless, and prefer to be left alone. They may have photo- or phonophobia. Use of frequent hot showers or baths may help relieve symptoms, particularly in those who use cannabis.

Laboratory and Imaging Studies

There are no specific tests for CVS, which is diagnosed based on the history and the exclusion of other disorders. Diagnoses that should be considered include malrotation with intermittent volvulus, uteropelvic junction obstruction, EoE, intracranial mass lesions, and metabolic disorders. Rome IV criteria for diagnosis are outlined in Table 127.5.

Treatment

For the acute episode, supportive treatment includes hydration; dark, quiet environment; and antiemetics such as ondansetron. In addition, abortive therapy using antimigraine medications such as triptans or antiemetics such as ondansetron can be used. For those with frequent or prolonged episodes, prophylactic therapy should be considered, such as cyproheptadine, tricyclic antidepressants, β blockers, or topiramate. For those triggered by cannabis use, haloperidol, lorazepam, and topical capsaicin can be effective for abortive therapy.

PEARLS FOR PRACTITIONERS

See The Digestive System: Pearls for Practitioners at the end of this section.

REVIEW QUESTIONS

Available online.

CHAPTER 130

Intestinal Tract

MALROTATION

Etiology and Epidemiology

During early fetal life, the midgut is attached to the yolk sac and loops outward into the umbilical cord. Beginning at around 10 weeks of gestation, the bowel re-enters the abdomen and rotates counterclockwise around the superior mesenteric artery until the cecum arrives in the right lower quadrant. The duodenum rotates behind the artery and terminates at the **ligament of Treitz** in the left upper quadrant. The base of the mesentery becomes fixed along a broad attachment posteriorly, running from the cecum to the ligament of Treitz (Fig. 130.1A). When rotation is incomplete or otherwise abnormal, "malrotation" is present. Incomplete rotation occurs when the cecum stops near the right upper quadrant and the duodenum fails to move behind the mesenteric artery; this results in an extremely narrow mesenteric root (see Fig. 130.1B) that makes the child susceptible to midgut **volvulus**, causing intestinal obstruction or mesenteric artery occlusion and intestinal infarction (Fig. 130.2). Abnormal mesenteric attachments **(Ladd bands)** can also cause partial obstruction by extending from the cecum across the duodenum.

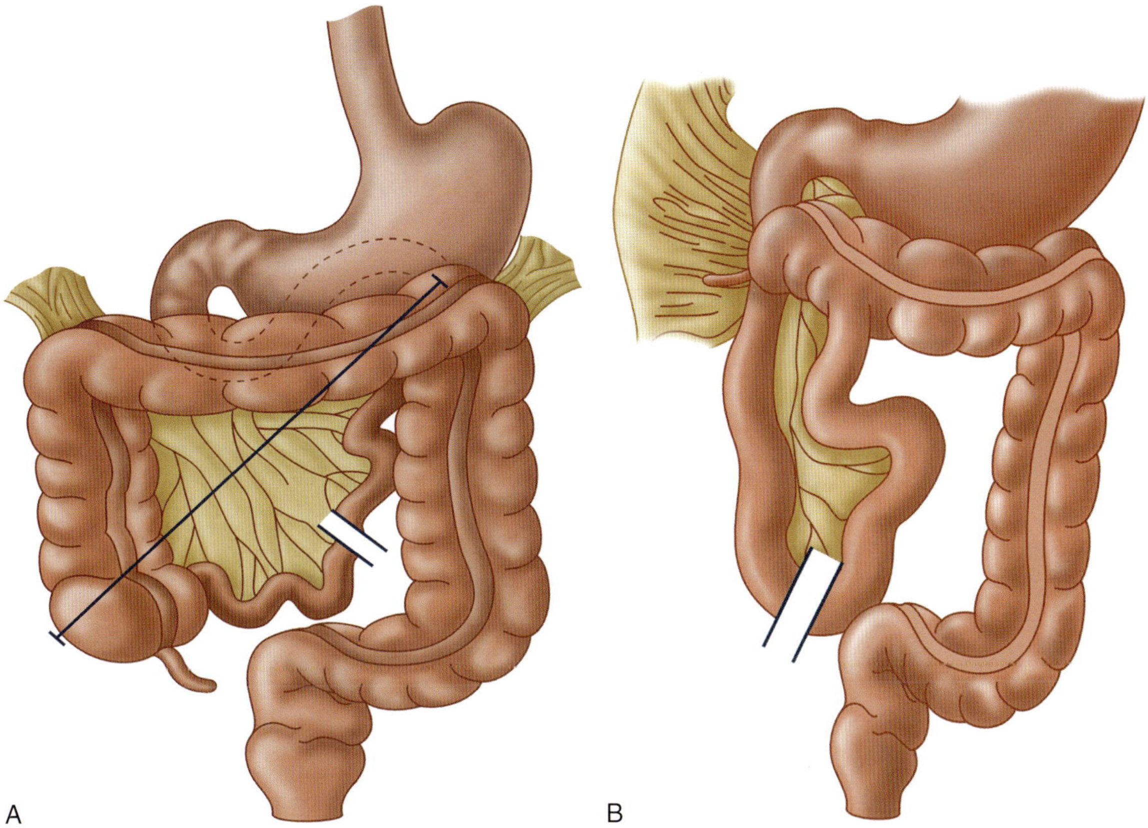

FIGURE 130.1 (A) Normal rotation of the midgut. Note the long axis of mesenteric attachment *(line)*. (B) Midgut malrotation. Note the narrow mesentery, which predisposes to volvulus, and the presence of Ladd bands extending across the duodenum from the abnormally elevated cecum. (From Donellan WJ, ed. *Abdominal Surgery of Infancy and Childhood*. Luxembourg: Harwood Academic; 1996:43/6, 43/8.)

Clinical Manifestations

About 60% of children with malrotation present with symptoms of bilious vomiting during the first month of life. The remaining 40% present later in infancy or childhood. The emesis initially may be due to obstruction by Ladd bands without volvulus. When midgut volvulus occurs, the venous drainage of the gut is impaired; congestion results in ischemia, pain, tenderness, and often bilious emesis and bloody stools. The bowel undergoes ischemic necrosis, and the child may appear septic. Physicians must be alert to the possibility of volvulus in patients with vomiting, fussiness, abdominal pain, or shock.

Laboratory and Imaging Studies

Plain abdominal x-rays generally show evidence of obstruction. Abdominal ultrasound may show evidence of malrotation. An upper gastrointestinal (GI) series shows the absence of a typical duodenal "C-loop," with the duodenum instead remaining on the right side of the abdomen. Abnormal placement of the cecum on follow-through (or by contrast enema) confirms the diagnosis. Laboratory studies are nonspecific, showing evidence of dehydration, electrolyte loss, or evidence of sepsis. A decreasing platelet count is a common indicator of bowel ischemia.

Treatment

Treatment is surgical. The bowel is untwisted, and Ladd bands and other abnormal membranous attachments are divided. The mesentery is spread out and flattened against the posterior wall of the abdomen by moving the cecum to the left side of the abdomen. Sutures may be used to hold the bowel in position, but postoperative adhesions tend to hold the mesentery in place, resulting in a broad attachment and eliminating the risk of recurrent volvulus. Necrotic bowel is resected and, at times, results in short gut syndrome.

INTESTINAL ATRESIA

Etiology and Epidemiology

Congenital partial or complete blockage of the intestine is a developmental defect that occurs in about 1 in 1,500 live births. Atresia occurs in several forms (Fig. 130.3). One or more segments of bowel may be missing completely, there may be varying degrees of obstruction caused by webs or stenosis, or there may be complete atresia of the lumen in cordlike bowel remnants. The result is obstruction with upstream dilation of the bowel and small, disused intestine distally. When obstruction is complete or high grade, bilious vomiting and abdominal distention are present in the newborn period. In lesser cases, as in "windsock" types of intestinal membranes or webs, the obstruction is partial, and symptoms are more subtle. Duodenal atresia is associated with other anomalies in more than half of infants. Down syndrome is the most common associated disorder, but it can also be associated with biliary, cardiac, kidney, or vertebral anomalies. Jejunal and ileal atresia can be seen in meconium ileus secondary to cystic fibrosis.

Clinical Manifestations

Intestinal atresia presents with a history of polyhydramnios, abdominal distention, and bilious vomiting in the neonatal period. If intestinal perforation is present, peritonitis and sepsis may develop.

Laboratory and Imaging Studies

Plain abdominal x-rays may localize the area of atresia and identify evidence of perforation, such as free air or calcifications typical of meconium peritonitis. **Duodenal atresia** appears as a double-bubble sign (gas in the stomach and enlarged proximal duodenum), with no gas distally. Atresias of the distal intestine are characterized by longer segments of dilated, air-filled bowel. Contrast studies are helpful if plain films are not sufficient. Atresia may be a complication of **meconium ileus** associated with cystic fibrosis. Laboratory evaluation for **cystic fibrosis** (see Chapter 138) should be considered in cases of small bowel atresia. A complete blood count, serum electrolytes, liver function tests, and lipase should be measured to identify dehydration, pancreatitis, and other complications.

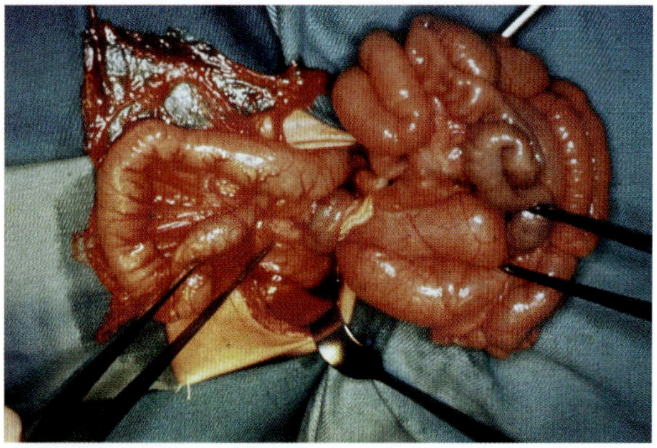

FIGURE 130.2 Malrotation with volvulus. Midgut is twisted around the mesentery, with an area of darker, ischemic intestine visible. (Courtesy Robert Soper, MD.)

Treatment

The treatment of intestinal atresia is surgical; surgery must be preceded by adequate hemodynamic stabilization of the patient. Intravenous (IV) fluids, nasogastric suction, and broad-spectrum antibiotics should be given.

OTHER CONGENITAL DISORDERS

Gastroschisis is an abdominal wall defect, not involving the umbilicus, through which intestinal contents have herniated. In contrast to omphalocele, the bowel is not covered by peritoneum or amniotic membrane. As a result, prolonged contact with the amniotic fluid typically causes a thick, exudative covering (a "peel") on the exposed bowel. Gastroschisis is not associated with extraintestinal anomalies, but segments of intestinal atresia are common. After surgical reduction of the defect, return of normal bowel function may be slow and require prolonged parenteral nutrition for infants with long atretic segments (short-bowel syndrome) and infants with a thick peel.

Omphalocele is an abdominal wall defect through the umbilicus caused by failure of the intestine to return to the

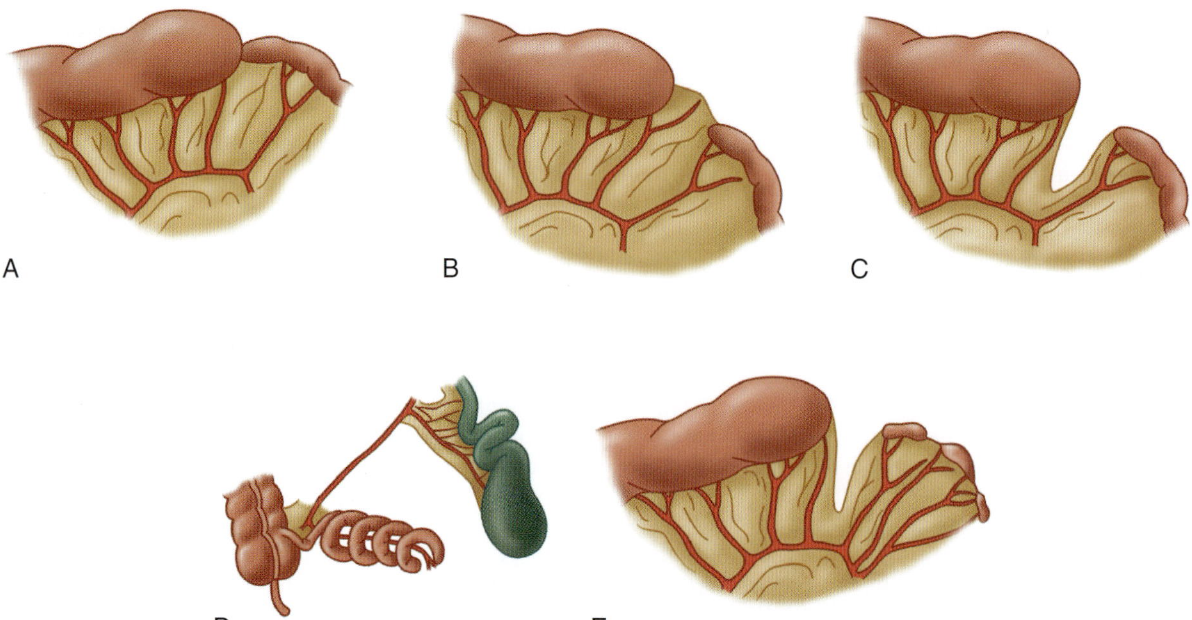

FIGURE 130.3 Types of intestinal atresia. **(A)** Internal web; **(B)** cordlike remnant connecting proximal and distal bowel; **(C)** interrupted bowel with V-shaped mesenteric defect; **(D)** "apple peel" atresia with surviving bowel spiraling around a marginal artery; **(E)** multiple atresias. (From Grosfeld JL, Ballantine TVN, Shoemaker R. Operative management of intestinal atresia based on pathologic findings. *J Pediatr Surg*. 1979;14:368–375.)

abdomen during fetal life. The bowel remains within the umbilical cord and is covered by peritoneum and amniotic membranes. This defect is associated with other congenital anomalies, especially cardiac defects, **Beckwith-Wiedemann syndrome**, and intestinal complications. Treatment is surgical closure, which sometimes must be performed in stages to fit the bowel into a congenitally small abdominal cavity.

Anorectal malformations, including imperforate anus and its variants, are embryologic defects recognized at birth by the absence of a normal anal opening. Evaluation of these infants should include observation for emergence of meconium from the vagina, urethra, or fistulas on the perineum. A urinary catheter should be placed if urinary distention is present. In low lesions, a fistulous opening that drains meconium is present on the perineum. Low lesions commonly are associated with fistulization between the bowel and bladder, vagina, or urethra. Lateral plain x-rays may show the level of the defect and show gas in the bladder caused by a fistula. Initial treatment is a colostomy to divert the fecal flow, with subsequent reconstruction. The internal sphincter muscle is functionally absent in high lesions, and continence after repair is difficult to achieve. All children with imperforate anus require magnetic resonance imaging (MRI) of the lumbosacral spinal cord because of high incidence of tethered spinal cord. Urologic dysfunction is common and should be evaluated.

Hirschsprung disease is a motility defect caused by failure of ganglion cell precursors to migrate into the distal bowel during fetal life. The aganglionic distal segment does not exhibit normal motility and is functionally obstructed secondary to spasm. In 75% of cases, the involved segment is limited to the rectosigmoid; total colonic involvement is seen in 8%. Rarely, long segments of small bowel also are aganglionic. An "ultrashort" segment involves only a few centimeters of distal rectum. About 95% of normal infants pass stool spontaneously by 24 hours of age; 95% of infants with Hirschsprung disease do not. Symptoms of distal bowel obstruction occur with distention and bilious vomiting. If the diagnosis is not made quickly, **enterocolitis** can result, associated with a high mortality rate. Diagnosis is based on examination and one or more diagnostic studies. Abdominal distention is present in most cases. Digital rectal examination reveals an empty rectum that clenches around the examiner's finger, giving the impression of an elongated sphincter. When the finger is withdrawn, a powerful gush of retained stool is often expelled. A deep **rectal biopsy** specimen obtained surgically or by using a suction biopsy instrument is required for diagnosis. When no ganglion cells are shown in the submucosal plexus, accompanied by nerve trunk hyperplasia, the diagnosis is certain. **Barium enema** and **anorectal manometry** may be used before biopsy, but false-negative and false-positive results can occur. Therapy is surgical. When the bowel is markedly distended or inflamed, an initial colostomy usually is performed above the aganglionic segment, followed weeks later by one of several definitive repair procedures. The transanal pull-through excises the aganglionic bowel and creates a primary colorectal anastomosis without laparotomy. This procedure can be considered in patients with uncomplicated involvement limited to the rectosigmoid region.

Meckel diverticulum is a remnant of the fetal omphalomesenteric duct and is an outpouching of the distal ileum present in 1–2% of the population. Although most diverticula are asymptomatic throughout life, some cause significant, painless GI bleeding. Ectopic gastric tissue within the diverticulum causes ulceration of mucosa in the adjacent ileum. Meckel diverticulum may be a lead point for intussusception or may enable twisting (volvulus) of neighboring bowel around its vascular supply. Diverticulitis mimics appendicitis. Diagnosis may be made in most cases by technetium scan (Meckel scan), which labels the acid-producing mucosa. Because not all diverticula are seen, ultrasound or video capsule endoscopy may be useful. When the level of suspicion is high, surgical or laparoscopic investigation is warranted. The treatment is surgical excision.

INFLAMMATORY BOWEL DISEASE

Epidemiology and Etiology

The peak incidence of inflammatory bowel disease (IBD) in children is in the second decade of life, but it may occur at any age. IBD includes Crohn disease (CD), which can involve any part of the gut, and ulcerative colitis (UC), which affects only the colon. The incidence of IBD is increasing, especially in industrialized countries, for reasons that are unclear. It is more common in northern latitudes. IBD is uncommon in tropical and Third World countries but is becoming more prevalent. It is more common in Jewish than in other ethnic populations. Genetic factors play a role in susceptibility, with significantly higher risk if there is a family history of IBD. Having a first-degree relative with IBD increases the risk about 30-fold. Susceptibility has been linked to some human leukocyte antigen subtypes, and linkage analysis has identified multiple other susceptibility loci on several chromosomes. Environmental factors also seem to play a role because there is often nonconcordance among monozygotic twins. Dietary and infectious triggers have been proposed but not yet proven. Smoking increases the risk as well as the severity of CD and decreases the risk for UC.

Very early-onset IBD occurring under the age of 6 years is rare and represents a wide genetic etiologic spectrum including congenital immune defects and other inflammatory disorders. IPEX (immune dysregulation, polyendocrinopathy, enteropathy, X-linked) and IPEX-like syndromes are the prototype disorders often associated with extraintestinal manifestations such as cytopenias, eczema, and eosinophilia.

Clinical manifestations depend on the region of involvement. UC involves only the colon, whereas CD can include the entire gut from mouth to anus. **Colitis** from either condition results in diarrhea; blood and mucus in the stool; urgency; and *tenesmus*, a sensation of incomplete emptying after defecation. When colitis is severe, the child often awakens from sleep to pass stool. **Toxic megacolon** is a life-threatening complication characterized by fever, abdominal distention and pain, massively dilated colon, anemia, and low serum albumin owing to intestinal protein losses. Symptoms of colitis always are present in UC and usually suggest the diagnosis early in its course. Extraintestinal manifestations of UC occur in a few patients and may include primary sclerosing cholangitis, arthritis, uveitis, and pyoderma gangrenosum (Table 130.1).

Symptoms can be subtle in CD. **Small bowel involvement** in CD is associated with loss of appetite, crampy postprandial pain, poor growth, delayed puberty, fever, anemia, and lethargy. Symptoms may be present for some time before the diagnosis is made. Severe CD with fibrosis may cause partial or complete small bowel obstruction. Perineal abnormalities,

TABLE 130.1 Comparison of Crohn Disease and Ulcerative Colitis

FEATURE	CROHN DISEASE	ULCERATIVE COLITIS
Malaise, fever, weight loss	Common	Sometimes
Rectal bleeding	Sometimes	Usual
Abdominal mass	Common	Rare
Abdominal pain	Common	Common
Perianal disease	Common	Rare
Ileal involvement	Common	None (except for backwash ileitis)
Strictures	Common	Unusual
Fistula	Common	Very rare
Skip lesions	Common	Not present
Transmural involvement	Usual	Not present
Crypt abscesses	Variable	Usual
Intestinal granulomas	Common	Rarely present
Risk of cancer*	Increased	Greatly increased
Erythema nodosum	Common	Less common
Mouth ulceration	Common	Rare
Osteopenia at onset	Yes	No
Autoimmune hepatitis	Rare	Yes
Sclerosing cholangitis	Rare	Yes

**Colonic cancer, cholangiocarcinoma, lymphoma in Crohn disease.*

including skin tags and fistulas, are another feature distinguishing CD from UC. Other extraintestinal manifestations of CD include arthritis, erythema nodosum, and uveitis.

Laboratory and Imaging Studies

Blood tests should include complete blood count, albumin, erythrocyte sedimentation rate, and C-reactive protein (Table 130.2). Anemia and elevated platelet counts are typical. Serologic testing for IBD may be considered but is not recommended for screening due to poor sensitivity. Elevated fecal calprotectin or positive lactoferrin testing indicates intestinal inflammation. These tests have a high negative predictive value but are not specific to IBD. Genetic testing is available for many causes of very early-onset IBD (e.g., *FOXP3* for IPEX).

In patients with suspected IBD, upper endoscopy and colonoscopy are used to determine location and severity of disease. Colonoscopic findings in UC include diffuse carpeting of the distal or entire colon with tiny ulcers and loss of haustral folds. Within the involved segment, no skip areas are present. In CD, ulcerations tend to be much larger and deeper with a linear, branching, or aphthous appearance; skip areas are usually present. **Upper endoscopy** cannot evaluate the jejunum and ileum but is more sensitive than contrast studies in identifying proximal CD involvement. Other methods to detect small bowel involvement include wireless **video capsule endoscopy**; computed tomography (CT) scanning, which can detect small bowel disease as well as abscesses; and **MR enterography**, which has the advantage of no radiation and good sensitivity for finding active bowel disease.

TABLE 130.2 Diagnostic Studies for Inflammatory Bowel Disease

STUDIES	INTERPRETATION
BLOOD TESTS	
CBC with WBC differential	Anemia, elevated platelets suggest IBD
ESR	Elevated in many but not all IBD patients
C-reactive protein	Elevated in many but not all IBD patients
Albumin	May be low in IBD due to fecal loss
ASCA	Found in about 50% of CD patients and few UC patients
Atypical p-ANCA	Found in most UC patients and few CD patients
Anti-OmpC	Found in some UC and CD patients, rare in non-IBD
Anti-C Bir1	Found in about 50% of CD patients
STOOL STUDIES	
Fecal calprotectin and lactoferrin	Elevated in IBD and can differentiate from functional disorders
IMAGING STUDIES	
Upper GI series with SBFT	Evaluate for ileal and jejunal CD
CT scan	Used to detect abscess, small bowel involvement
Magnetic resonance enterography	Used to detect bowel thickening, inflammation, and strictures as well as abscesses and fistulas
ENDOSCOPY	
Upper endoscopy	Evaluate for CD of esophagus, stomach, and duodenum; obtain tissue for histologic diagnosis
Colonoscopy	Show presence or absence of colitis and terminal ileal CD; obtain tissue for histology
Wireless video capsule endoscopy	Diagnosis of small bowel CD

anti-OmpC, Antibody to outer membrane protein C; *ASCA*, anti–saccharomyces cerevisiae antibody; *atypical p-ANCA*, atypical perinuclear staining by antineutrophil cytoplasmic antibody; *CBC*, complete blood count; *CD*, Crohn disease; *CT*, computed tomography; *ESR*, erythrocyte sedimentation rate; *GI*, gastrointestinal; *IBD*, inflammatory bowel disease; *SBFT*, small bowel follow-through; *UC*, ulcerative colitis; *WBC*, white blood cell.

Treatment

Ulcerative Colitis

UC is treated with aminosalicylate drugs, which deliver **5-aminosalicylic acid** (5-ASA) to the distal gut. Because it is rapidly absorbed, pure 5-ASA (mesalamine) must be specially packaged in coated capsules or pills or taken as a suppository to be effective in the colon. Other aminosalicylates (sulfasalazine, olsalazine, and balsalazide) use 5-ASA covalently linked to a carrier molecule. Sulfasalazine is the least expensive, but side effects resulting from its sulfapyridine component are common. When aminosalicylates alone cannot control the disease, steroid therapy may be required to induce remission. Whenever possible, steroids should not be used for long-term therapy. An immunosuppressive drug, such as **6-mercaptopurine** or **azathioprine**, is useful to spare excessive steroid use in difficult cases. Biological therapies, including anti–tumor necrosis factor (TNF) agents such as infliximab or adalimumab, may be used in moderate-to-severe UC. Other biologic therapies are being used (such as the antiintegrin vedolizumab or Janus kinase inhibitor tofacitinib) but are not yet Food and Drug Administration–approved in the pediatric patient who has failed anti-TNF therapy. Surgical colectomy with ileoanal anastomosis is an option for unresponsive severe disease or electively to end chronic symptoms and to reduce the risk of colon cancer, which is increased in patients with UC.

Crohn Disease

Systemic steroids or exclusive formula-based enteral nutrition is used to induce remission in CD. To avoid the need for repetitive steroid therapy, immunomodulator drugs such as azathioprine, 6-mercaptopurine, or methotrexate are often started soon after diagnosis; however, anti-TNF therapies are being used more frequently due to their efficacy and safety profile. Other biologic agents (such as vedolizumab and the anti-interleukin 12/23 drug ustekinumab) are being used but are not yet approved in the pediatric patient. Exclusive enteral nutrition is also an effective therapy for CD. Patients take formula as their sole source of nutrition for months as a steroid-sparing therapy. Surgery is sometimes necessary because of obstructive symptoms due to strictures, abscess, fistulas, or severe, unremitting symptoms. Because surgery is not curative in CD, its use must be limited, and the length of bowel resection must be minimized.

CELIAC DISEASE

Etiology and Epidemiology

Celiac disease is an injury to the mucosa of the small intestine caused by the ingestion of **gluten** (a protein component) from wheat, rye, barley, and related grains. In its severe form, celiac disease causes malabsorption and malnutrition. The availability of more sensitive and specific serologic testing has revealed many patients with few or no GI symptoms, but they may have extraintestinal manifestations and early, attenuated, or latent disease. Incidence of celiac disease is estimated at 1%. The disease is also seen in association with type 1 diabetes, autoimmune thyroiditis, Addison disease, Turner syndrome, and trisomy 21.

Clinical Manifestations

Symptoms can begin at any age when gluten-containing foods are given. Diarrhea, abdominal bloating, growth faltering, irritability, decreased appetite, and ascites caused by hypoproteinemia are classic findings. Children may be minimally symptomatic or may be severely malnourished. Constipation is found as a presenting finding in some patients. A careful inspection of the child's growth curve and evaluation for reduced subcutaneous fat and abdominal distention are crucial. Celiac disease should be considered in any child with chronic abdominal complaints, short stature, poor weight gain, or delayed puberty. Extraintestinal manifestations include osteopenia, arthritis or arthralgias, ataxia, dental enamel defects, elevated liver enzymes, nutritional anemias, dermatitis herpetiformis, and erythema nodosum.

Laboratory and Imaging Studies

Serologic markers include antiendomysial, deamidated antigliadin, and tissue transglutaminase immunoglobulin (Ig)A antibodies. Because IgA deficiency may be associated with celiac disease, total serum IgA also must be measured to document the accuracy of these tests. In the absence of IgA deficiency, any of these antibody tests yields a sensitivity and specificity of 95%. An endoscopic **small bowel biopsy** is essential to confirm the diagnosis and should be performed while the patient is still ingesting gluten. The biopsy specimen shows various degrees of villous atrophy (short or absent villi), mucosal inflammation, crypt hyperplasia, and increased numbers of intraepithelial lymphocytes. When there is any question about response to treatment, a repeat biopsy specimen may be obtained several months later; however, the antibodies should decrease with exclusion of gluten in the diet over time. Other laboratory studies should be performed to rule out complications, including complete blood count, calcium, phosphate, vitamin D, iron, total protein and albumin, and liver function tests. Mild elevations of the transaminases are common and should normalize with dietary therapy.

Treatment

Treatment consists of complete elimination of gluten from the diet. Consultation with a dietitian experienced in celiac disease is helpful, as is membership in a celiac disease support group. Lists of prepared foods that contain hidden gluten are particularly important for patients to use. Starchy foods that are safe include rice, soy, tapioca, buckwheat, potatoes, corn, and (pure) oats. Many resources also are available via the Internet to help families cope with the large changes in diet that are required. Most patients respond clinically within a few weeks with weight gain, improved appetite, and improved sense of well-being. Histologic improvement lags behind clinical response, requiring several months to normalize.

MILK AND SOY PROTEIN INTOLERANCE (ALLERGIC COLITIS)

See Chapter 85.

INTUSSUSCEPTION

Etiology and Epidemiology

Intussusception is the "telescoping" of a segment of proximal bowel (the intussusceptum) into downstream bowel (the intussuscipiens). Most cases occur in infants 1–2 years old; in this age group, nearly all cases are idiopathic. Viral-induced lymphoid hyperplasia may produce a lead point in these children. In older children, the proportion of cases caused by a pathologic lead point increases. In young children, symptomatic **ileocolonic** intussusception is common; the ileum invaginates into the colon, beginning at or near the ileocecal valve. When pathologic lead points are present, the intussusception may be ileoileal, jejunoileal, or jejunojejunal.

Clinical Manifestations

An infant with intussusception has sudden onset of crampy abdominal pain; the infant's knees draw up, and the infant cries out and exhibits pallor with a colicky pattern occurring every 15–20 minutes. Feedings are refused. As the intussusception progresses and obstruction becomes prolonged, bilious vomiting becomes prominent, and the dilated, fatigued intestine generates less pressure and less pain. As the intussuscepted bowel is pulled further and further into the downstream intestine by motility, the mesentery is pulled with it and becomes compressed. The venous outflow from the intussusceptum is obstructed, leading to edema, weeping of fluid, and congestion with bleeding. Third space fluid losses and "currant jelly" stools result. Another unexpected feature of intussusception is **lethargy**. Between episodes of pain, the infant is glassy-eyed and groggy and appears to have been sedated. A sausage-shaped mass caused by the swollen, intussuscepted bowel may be palpable in the right upper quadrant or epigastrium.

Laboratory and Imaging Studies

The diagnosis depends on the direct demonstration of bowel-within-bowel. A simple way of showing this is by abdominal ultrasound. If the ultrasound is positive, or if good visualization has not been achieved, a pneumatic or contrast enema under fluoroscopy is indicated. This is a potentially useful way to both identify and treat intussusception. Air and barium can show the intussusception quickly and, when administered with controlled pressure, usually can reduce it completely. The success rate for pneumatic reduction is higher than for hydrostatic reduction with barium and approaches 90% if done when symptoms have been present for less than 24 hours. The pneumatic enema has the additional advantages over barium of not preventing subsequent radiologic studies and having no risk of causing barium peritonitis if perforation occurs. Nonoperative reduction should not be attempted if the patient is unstable or has evidence of preexisting perforation or peritonitis.

Treatment

Therapy should begin with placement of an IV catheter and a nasogastric tube. Before radiologic intervention is attempted, the child must have adequate **fluid resuscitation** to correct dehydration caused by vomiting and third space losses. Ultrasound may be performed before the fluid resuscitation is complete. Surgical consultation should be obtained early as the surgeon may prefer to be present during nonoperative reduction. If pneumatic or hydrostatic reduction is successful, the child may be admitted to the hospital for overnight observation of possible recurrence (risk is 5–10%). If reduction is not complete, emergency surgery is often required. The surgeon attempts gentle manual reduction but may need to resect the involved bowel after failed radiologic reduction because of severe edema, perforation, a pathologic lead point (polyp, Meckel diverticulum), or necrosis.

APPENDICITIS

Etiology and Epidemiology

Appendicitis is the most common surgical emergency in childhood. The prevalence of appendicitis varies by age, with the peak in the second decade, but it may occur at any age. Appendicitis begins with obstruction of the lumen, most commonly by fecal matter (fecalith), but appendiceal obstruction also can occur secondary to hyperplasia of lymphoid tissue associated with viral infections or, rarely, the presence of neoplastic tissue, such as an appendiceal carcinoid tumor. Trapped bacteria proliferate and begin to invade the appendiceal wall, inducing inflammation and secretion. The obstructed appendix becomes engorged, its blood supply is compromised, and it may then rupture. The entire process is rapid, with appendiceal rupture usually occurring within 48 hours of the onset of symptoms.

Clinical Manifestations

Classic appendicitis begins with **visceral pain**, localized to the periumbilical region. Nausea and vomiting occur soon after, triggered by the appendiceal distention. As the inflammation begins to irritate the parietal peritoneum adjacent to the appendix, **somatic pain** fibers are activated, and the pain localizes to the right lower quadrant. Examination of the patient reveals a tender right lower quadrant. Voluntary guarding is present initially, progressing to rigidity, then to rebound tenderness with rupture and peritonitis. These classic findings may not be present, especially in young children or if the appendix is retrocecal, covered by omentum, or in another unusual location. Clinical prediction rules including the Alvarado (also known as *MANTRELS*) score and the Pediatric Appendicitis Score have been developed for the diagnosis of appendicitis (Table 130.3). When classic history and physical examination findings are present, the patient may be taken directly to the operating room. When doubt exists, imaging is helpful to confirm the diagnosis and to rule out complications (right lower quadrant abscess, liver disease) and other disorders (e.g., mesenteric adenitis and ovarian or fallopian tube disorders). If the evaluation is negative and some doubt remains, the child should be admitted to the hospital for close observation and serial examinations.

Laboratory and Imaging Studies

The history and examination are often enough to make the diagnosis, but laboratory and imaging studies are helpful when the diagnosis is uncertain. A white blood cell count greater than 10,000/mm^3 is found in 89% of patients with appendicitis and 93% with perforated appendicitis. This criterion is met by 62% of abdominal pain patients without appendicitis. Urinalysis is done to rule out urinary tract infection, and x-rays of the chest or the kidney-ureter-bladder rule out lower lobe pneumonia masquerading as abdominal pain. Amylase, lipase, and liver enzymes may be done to look for pancreatic or liver and gallbladder disease. The plain abdominal x-ray may reveal a calcified fecalith, which strongly suggests the diagnosis. Ultrasound is often the preferred imaging method in children due to its lack of ionizing radiation, but CT or MRI may also be used. Imaging may reveal the presence of an enlarged, thick-walled appendix with surrounding fluid; a diameter of more than 6 mm is considered diagnostic.

TABLE 130.3 Common Pediatric Appendicitis Clinical Decision Tools

PEDIATRIC APPENDICITIS SCORE		ALVARADO SCORE	
SIGNS/SYMPTOMS	POINTS	SIGNS/SYMPTOMS	POINTS
Fever >38°C (100.4°F)	1	Temperature ≥37.7°C (99.1°F)	1
Anorexia	1	Anorexia	1
Nausea/vomiting	1	Nausea/vomiting	1
Migration of pain	1	Migration of pain	1
Right lower quadrant tenderness	2	Right lower quadrant tenderness	2
Right lower quadrant pain with coughing/hopping/ percussion	2	Rebound pain	1
Leukocytosis >10,000 per μL	1	Leukocytosis >10,000 per μL	2
PMN ≥ 75%	1	PMN ≥ 75%	1
Total possible score*	10	Total possible score**	10
*Scores ≤ 3 have low likelihood of appendicitis, scores 4–6 indicate possible appendicitis, and scores ≥ 7 indicate probable appendicitis		**Scores ≤ 3 have low likelihood of appendicitis, scores 4–6 indicate possible appendicitis, and scores ≥ 7 indicate probable appendicitis	

PMN, Polymorphonuclear leukocyte.

Treatment

Treatment of appendicitis is usually surgical; however, non-operative treatment with antibiotics is also increasingly being done in low-risk patients. Laparoscopic appendectomy is curative if performed before perforation. With perforation, drainage of fluid is often done by interventional radiology along with a course of IV antibiotics followed by appendectomy weeks later. Broad-spectrum coverage is necessary to cover the mixed bowel flora.

PEARLS FOR PRACTITIONERS

See The Digestive System: Pearls for Practitioners at the end of this section.

REVIEW QUESTIONS

Available online.

CHAPTER 131

Liver Disease

CHOLESTASIS

Etiology and Epidemiology

Cholestasis is defined as reduced bile flow and is characterized by elevation of the conjugated, or direct, bilirubin fraction. This condition must be distinguished from physiologic neonatal jaundice, in which the direct bilirubin is not elevated (see Chapter 61). Neonatal jaundice that is secondary to unconjugated hyperbilirubinemia is the result of immature hepatocellular excretory function or hemolysis, which increases the production of bilirubin. When direct bilirubin is elevated, many potentially serious disorders must be considered (Fig. 131.1, Table 131.1). Emphasis must be placed on the rapid diagnosis of treatable and potentially lethal disorders, especially biliary atresia, sepsis, urinary tract infection, hemophagocytic or histiocytic syndromes, and treatable metabolic disorders, such as galactosemia or tyrosinemia.

Clinical Manifestations

The jaundice of **extrahepatic biliary atresia** (biliary atresia) usually is not evident immediately at birth but develops in the first week or two of life. The reason is that extrahepatic bile ducts are usually present at birth but are then destroyed by an idiopathic inflammatory process. Aside from jaundice, these infants do not initially appear ill. The liver injury progresses rapidly to cirrhosis; symptoms of portal hypertension with splenomegaly, ascites, muscle wasting, and poor weight gain are evident by a few months of age. If surgical drainage is not performed successfully early in the course (ideally by 2 months), progression to liver failure is inevitable.

Idiopathic neonatal hepatitis is defined as inflammation of the liver, occurring in infancy, without an identifiable cause. It is characterized clinically by an ill-appearing infant with an enlarged liver and jaundice. This diagnosis can only be made after thorough testing for identifiable infectious, anatomic, and metabolic/genetic causes of neonatal cholestasis have been performed and are negative (see later). If liver biopsy is performed, the presence of giant cells is characteristic. Hepatobiliary scintigraphy typically shows slow hepatic uptake with eventual excretion of isotope into the intestine. These infants have a good prognosis overall, with spontaneous resolution occurring in most.

α1-Antitrypsin deficiency presents with clinical findings indistinguishable from neonatal hepatitis. Only about 10–20% of all infants with the genetic pathogenic variant exhibit neonatal cholestasis. Of these affected infants, about 20–30% develop chronic liver disease, which may result in cirrhosis and liver failure. Life-threatening α_1-antitrypsin deficiency occurs in only 3–5% of affected pediatric patients.

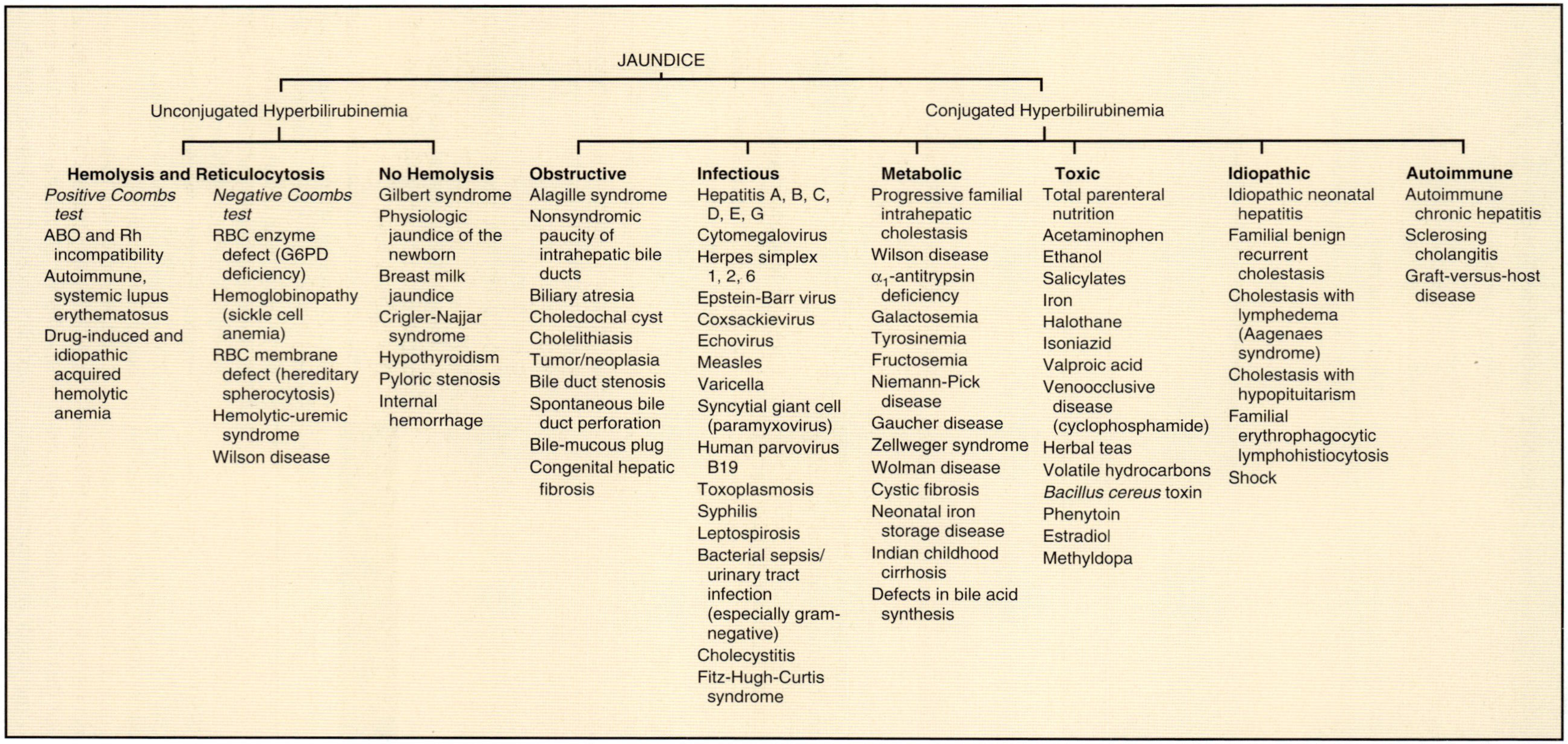

FIGURE 131.1 Differential diagnoses of jaundice in childhood. *G6PD*, Glucose-6-phosphate dehydrogenase; *GALD*, gestational alloimmune liver disease (neonatal hemochromatosis); *RBC*, red blood cell.

TABLE 131.1 Differential Diagnoses of Conjugated Hyperbilirubinemia in Infants

OBSTRUCTIVE/ANATOMIC DISORDERS	**DISORDERS OF BILE ACID SYNTHESIS AND METABOLISM**
Biliary atresia Choledochal cyst Caroli disease (cystic dilatation of intrahepatic ducts) Congenital hepatic fibrosis Neonatal sclerosing cholangitis Bile duct stenosis Spontaneous bile duct perforation Anomalous choledocho-pancreatico-ductal junction Cholelithiasis Inspissated bile or mucus Mass or neoplasia	**Primary Enzyme Deficiencies** 3β-hydroxy-Δ5-C27-steroid dehydrogenase/isomerase Δ4-3-oxosteroid 5β-reductase Oxysterol 7α-hydroxylase **Secondary** Zellweger syndrome (cerebrohepatorenal syndrome) Infantile Refsum disease Smith-Lemli-Opitz syndrome Other enzymopathies Mitochondrial disorders (respiratory chain)
INFECTIONS	**Intrahepatic Cholestasis**
Bacterial (gram negative) sepsis Urinary tract infection Listeriosis Syphilis Toxoplasmosis Tuberculosis Cytomegalovirus Herpesvirus (herpes simplex, herpes zoster, human herpesvirus 6) Rubella virus Hepatitis B virus HIV Coxsackievirus Echovirus Parvovirus B19 Adenovirus Measles	Alagille syndrome (arteriohepatic dysplasia) Nonsyndromic paucity of intrahepatic bile ducts PFIC Type 1: Byler disease Type 2: Defect in the bile salt export pump Type 3: Defect in canalicular phospholipid transporter Benign recurrent intrahepatic cholestasis North American Indian cirrhosis Hereditary cholestasis with lymphedema (Aagenaes syndrome) **Toxin or Drug-Related** Cholestasis associated with total parenteral nutrition Chloral hydrate Home remedies/herbal medicines Sinusoidal obstruction syndrome (venoocclusive disease)
METABOLIC DISORDERS	**Miscellaneous**
α_1-Antitrypsin deficiency Cystic fibrosis Citrin deficiency	Idiopathic neonatal hepatitis GALD Autoimmune hemolytic anemia with giant cell hepatitis Shock or hypoperfusion (including cardiac disease) Intestinal obstruction Langerhans cell histiocytosis Neonatal lupus erythematosus Dubin-Johnson syndrome Trisomies (18,21) Congenital disorders of glycosylation Kabuki syndrome Donahue syndrome (leprechaunism) Arthrogryposis, cholestatic pigmentary disease, kidney dysfunction syndrome Familial hemophagocytic lymphohistiocytosis
ENDOCRINE DISORDERS	
Panhypopituitarism Hypothyroidism	
DISORDERS OF CARBOHYDRATE METABOLISM	
Galactosemia Hereditary fructose intolerance (fructosemia) Glycogen storage disease type IV	
DISORDERS OF AMINO ACID METABOLISM	
Tyrosinemia Hypermethioninemia	
DISORDERS OF LIPID METABOLISM	
Wolman disease Cholesterol ester storage disease Farber disease Niemann-Pick disease Beta-oxidation defects Gaucher disease	

GALD, Gestational alloimmune liver disease; *PFIC*, progressive familial intrahepatic cholestasis.
Modified from Balistreri WF. Liver disease in infancy and childhood. In: Schiff ER, Sorrell MF, Maddrey WC, eds. Schiff's Diseases of the Liver. *8th ed. Philadelphia: Lippincott-Raven; 1999:1370; Suchy FJ. Approach to the infant with cholestasis. In: Suchy FJ, Sokol RJ, Balistreri WF, eds.* Liver Disease in Children. *2nd ed. Philadelphia: Lippincott Williams & Wilkins; 2001:188.*

α_1-Antitrypsin deficiency is the leading metabolic disorder requiring liver transplantation.

Alagille syndrome (ALGS) is characterized by chronic cholestasis with the unique liver biopsy finding of *paucity of bile ducts* in the portal triads. Associated abnormalities in some (syndromic) types include peripheral pulmonic stenosis or other cardiac anomalies; hypertelorism; unusual facies with deep-set eyes, prominent forehead, and a pointed chin; butterfly vertebrae; and a defect of the ocular limbus *(posterior embryotoxon)*. ALGS is due to pathogenic variants in either *JAG1* or *NOTCH2* and is autosomal dominant. Cholestasis is variable but is usually lifelong and associated with hypercholesterolemia and severe pruritus. Progression to end-stage liver disease is uncommon early in life. Liver transplantation sometimes is performed electively to relieve severe and uncontrollable pruritus; however, medications (maralixibat and odevixibat) that inhibit ileal bile acid transport can effectively improve pruritus. Alternative surgical treatments to prevent intestinal reabsorption of pruritus-inducing bile acids can also be effective. These include partial or complete drainage to an ostomy and bypass of the terminal ileum, the location of most bile acid reabsorption.

Laboratory and Imaging Studies

The laboratory approach to diagnosis of a neonate with cholestatic jaundice is presented in Table 131.2. Noninvasive studies may aid a rapid diagnosis. Early imaging studies are performed to evaluate for biliary obstruction and other anatomic lesions that may be surgically treatable. When necessary to rule out biliary atresia or to obtain prognostic information, liver biopsy can be very helpful; surgical exploration is a final option (Fig. 131.2). When cholestasis persists, biliary atresia has been ruled out, and routine testing fails to yield a diagnosis, genetic testing for rare etiologies should be considered.

Treatment

Treatment of extrahepatic biliary atresia is the surgical **Kasai hepatoportoenterostomy procedure**, in which the fibrotic extrahepatic bile duct remnant is removed and replaced with a Roux-en-Y loop of jejunum. This operation must be performed before 2 months of age to have the best chance of success. Even so, the success rate is not ideal, and many children require liver transplantation. Some metabolic causes of neonatal cholestasis are treatable by dietary manipulation (galactosemia) or medication (tyrosinemia); all affected patients require supportive care. This includes fat-soluble vitamin supplements (vitamins A, D, E, and K) and formula containing medium-chain triglycerides, which can be absorbed without bile salt–induced micelles. Choleretic agents, such as ursodeoxycholic acid, may improve bile flow in some conditions.

TABLE 131.2 Laboratory and Imaging Evaluation of Neonatal Cholestasis

EVALUATION	RATIONALE
INITIAL TESTS	
Total and direct bilirubin	Elevated direct fraction confirms cholestasis
AST, ALT	Hepatocellular injury
GGT	Biliary obstruction/injury
RBC galactose-1-phosphate uridyltransferase	Galactosemia
α_1-antitrypsin level and phenotype	α_1-antitrypsin deficiency
Urinalysis and urine culture	Urinary tract infection can cause cholestasis in neonates
Blood culture	Sepsis can cause cholestasis
Serum amino acids	Aminoacidopathies
Urine organic acids	Organic acidurias
Very-long-chain fatty acids	Zellweger syndrome, peroxisomal disorders
Carnitine profile	Mitochondrial and fatty acid oxidation disorders
Sweat chloride or CF gene pathogenic variant analysis	CF
VDRL or RPR	Congenital syphilis
Urine culture for cytomegalovirus	Congenital cytomegalovirus infection
GENETIC TESTING	
Rapidly advancing genetic diagnosis capabilities can identify Alagille syndrome, progressive familial cholestasis syndromes, α-1-AT deficiency, familial HLH, and bile acid synthesis disorders. Some laboratories offer PCR-based testing for most or all of these in a single panel.	
INITIAL IMAGING STUDY	
Abdominal ultrasound	Choledochal cyst, gallstones, mass lesion, Caroli disease
SECONDARY IMAGING STUDY	
Hepatobiliary scintigraphy	Evaluate for biliary atresia
Pathology	Liver; salivary gland (GALD)
Percutaneous liver biopsy	Biliary atresia, idiopathic giant cell hepatitis, α_1-antitrypsin deficiency

ALT, Alanine aminotransferase; *AST,* aspartate aminotransferase; *CF,* cystic fibrosis; *GALD,* gestational alloimmune liver disease; *GGT,* γ-glutamyltransferase; *HLH,* hemophagocytic lymphohistiocytosis; *PCR,* polymerase chain reaction; *RBC,* red blood cell; *RPR,* rapid plasma reagin; *VDRL,* Venereal Disease Research Laboratory.

VIRAL HEPATITIS

See Chapter 114.

FULMINANT LIVER FAILURE

Etiology and Epidemiology

Fulminant liver failure is defined as severe liver disease with onset of hepatic encephalopathy within 8 weeks after initial symptoms, in the absence of chronic liver disease. Etiology includes viral hepatitis, metabolic disorders, autoimmune hepatitis, ischemia, neoplastic disease, and toxins, but in ~50% no etiology is identified (Table 131.3).

Clinical Manifestations

Liver failure is a multisystem disorder with complex interactions among the liver, kidneys, vascular structures, gut, central nervous system (CNS), and immune function. Hepatic encephalopathy is characterized by varying degrees of impairment (Table 131.4). Respiratory compromise occurs as severity of the failure increases and requires early institution of ventilatory support. Hypoglycemia resulting from impaired glycogenolysis and gluconeogenesis must be prevented. Kidney function is impaired, and frank kidney failure, or **hepatorenal syndrome**, may occur. This syndrome is characterized by low urine output, azotemia, and low urine sodium content. Ascites develops secondary to hypoalbuminemia and disordered

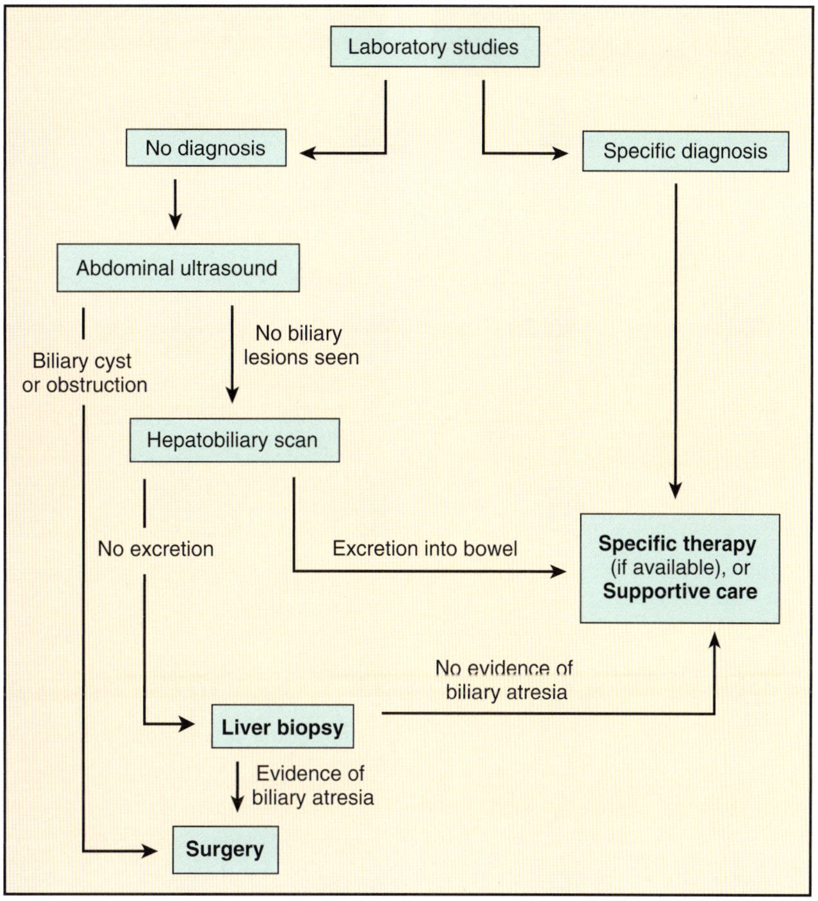

FIGURE 131.2 Algorithm for evaluation of neonatal cholestasis.

regulation of fluid and electrolyte homeostasis. Increased risk of infection occurs and may cause death. If portal hypertension is present, esophageal varices may cause significant hemorrhage, whereas hypersplenism may produce thrombocytopenia and other cytopenias.

Laboratory and Imaging Studies

Coagulation tests and serum albumin are used to follow hepatic synthetic function. These tests are confounded by administration of blood products and clotting factors. Vitamin K should be administered to maximize the liver's ability to synthesize factors II, VII, IX, and X. In addition to monitoring prothrombin time and partial thromboplastin time, many centers measure factor V serially as a sensitive index of hepatic synthetic function. The international normalized ratio reflects liver synthetic function and predicts the severity of hepatic failure. Kidney function tests, electrolytes, serum ammonia, blood counts, and urinalysis also should be followed. In the setting of acute liver failure, liver biopsy may be indicated to ascertain the nature and degree of injury and estimate the likelihood of recovery. In the presence of coagulopathy, biopsy must be done using a transjugular or surgical approach.

Treatment

Because of the life-threatening and complex nature of this condition, management must be carried out in an intensive care unit at a liver transplant center. Treatment of acute liver failure is supportive; the definitive lifesaving therapy is liver transplantation. Supportive measures are listed in Table 131.5. Efforts are made to treat metabolic derangements, avoid hypoglycemia, support respiration, minimize hepatic encephalopathy, and support kidney function.

CHRONIC LIVER DISEASE

Etiology and Epidemiology

Chronic liver disease in childhood is characterized by the development of cirrhosis and its complications and by progressive hepatic failure. Causative conditions may be congenital or acquired. Major congenital disorders leading to chronic disease include biliary atresia, tyrosinemia, untreated galactosemia, and α_1-antitrypsin deficiency. In older children, hepatitis B or C virus, autoimmune hepatitis, Wilson disease, primary sclerosing cholangitis, cystic fibrosis, and biliary obstruction secondary to choledochal cyst are leading causes.

Clinical Manifestations

Chronic liver disease is characterized by the consequences of portal hypertension, impaired hepatocellular function, and cholestasis. **Portal hypertension** caused by cirrhosis results in risk of gastrointestinal bleeding, ascites, and reduced hepatic blood flow. Blood entering the portal vein from the splenic and mesenteric veins is diverted to collateral circulation that

TABLE 131.3 Causes of Fulminant Liver Failure in Childhood

METABOLIC
Electron chain transport and other mitochondrial defects Disorders of fatty acid oxidation Galactosemia Tyrosinemia Hereditary fructose intolerance Bile acid synthesis disorders Wilson disease
CARDIOVASCULAR
Shock, hypotension Congestive heart failure Budd-Chiari syndrome
INFECTIOUS
Hepatitis virus A, B Echovirus Coxsackievirus Adenovirus Parvovirus Cytomegalovirus Sepsis Herpes simplex
NEOPLASTIC
Acute leukemia Lymphoproliferative disease
TOXIC
Acetaminophen Valproic acid Phenytoin Isoniazid Halothane *Amanita* mushrooms
IMMUNOLOGIC
Gestational alloimmune liver disease Autoimmune hepatitis Familial hemophagocytic lymphohistiocytosis Unknown

bypasses the liver, enlarging these previously tiny vessels in the esophagus, stomach, and abdomen. **Esophageal varices** are particularly prone to bleed, but bleeding also can occur from hemorrhoidal veins, engorged gastric mucosa, and gastric varices. **Ascites** develops as a result of transduction of a high-pressure ultrafiltrate from the surfaces of the viscera and is at risk of becoming infected **(spontaneous bacterial peritonitis)**; ascites can often be massive and interfere with patient comfort and respiration. The spleen enlarges secondary to impaired splenic vein outflow, causing excessive splenic entrapment of platelets and white blood cells; this increases the patient's susceptibility to bleeding and infection.

Impaired hepatocellular function is associated with coagulopathy unresponsive to vitamin K, low serum albumin, elevated ammonia, and **hepatic encephalopathy**. The diversion of portal blood away from the liver via collateral circulation worsens this process. Malaise develops and contributes to poor nutrition, leading to muscle wasting and other consequences.

Chronic cholestasis causes debilitating pruritus and deepening jaundice. The reduced excretion of bile acids impairs absorption of fat calories and fat-soluble vitamins, which

TABLE 131.4 Stages of Hepatic Encephalopathy

STAGE I
Alert and awake Agitated and distractible Infants and young children—irritable and fussy Normal reflexes Tremor, poor handwriting Obeys age-appropriate commands
STAGE II
Confused and lethargic Combative or inappropriate euphoria Hyperactive reflexes Asterixis present Purposeful movements, but may not obey commands
STAGE III
Stuporous but arousable Sleepy Incoherent speech Motor response to pain Hyperreflexic Hyperventilation Asterixis present
STAGE IV
Unconscious, not arousable Unresponsive or responds nonpurposefully to pain Reflexes hyperactive Irregular respirations Pupil response sluggish
STAGE V
Unconscious Hypoactive reflexes Flaccid muscle tone Apneic Pupils fixed

TABLE 131.5 Treatment of Fulminant Liver Failure

Hepatic encephalopathy	Avoid sedatives Lactulose via nasogastric tube—start with 1–2 mL/kg/day, adjust dose to yield several loose stools per day Rifaximin or neomycin Enemas if constipated Mechanical ventilation if stage III or IV
Coagulopathy	Administer intravenous vitamin K Fresh frozen plasma only if active bleeding, monitor coagulation studies frequently Platelet transfusions as required
Hypoglycemia	Intravenous glucose supplied with ≥10% dextrose solution, electrolytes as appropriate
Ascites	Restrict fluid intake to 50–60% maintenance Restrict sodium intake to 0.5–1 mEq/kg/day Monitor central venous pressure to maintain adequate intravascular volume (avoid kidney failure)
Kidney failure	Maintain adequate intravascular volume, give albumin only if low Diuretics Vasoconstrictors Dialysis or hemofiltration Exchange transfusion Liver transplantation

contributes to the poor nutritional state. Deficiency of vitamin K impairs production of clotting factors II, VII, IX, and X and increases the risk of bleeding. Vitamin E deficiency leads to hematologic and neurologic consequences unless corrected.

Laboratory and Imaging Studies

Laboratory studies include specific tests for diagnosis of the underlying illness and testing to monitor the status of the patient. Children presenting for the first time with evidence of chronic liver disease should have a standard investigation (Table 131.6). Monitoring should include coagulation tests, electrolytes and kidney function testing, complete blood count with platelet count, transaminases, alkaline phosphatase, and γ-glutamyltransferase at appropriate intervals. Frequency of testing should be tailored to the pace of the patient's illness. Ascites fluid can be tested for infection if suspected by culture and cell count and is generally found to have an albumin concentration lower than that of serum.

Treatment

Treatment of chronic liver disease is complex. Supportive care for each of the many problems encountered in these patients is outlined in Table 131.7. Ultimately, survival depends on the availability of a donor liver and the patient's candidacy for transplantation. When transplantation is not possible or is delayed, palliative procedures, such as portosystemic shunts to treat portal hypertension, can be considered. The transjugular intrahepatic portosystemic shunt is an expandable stent placed between the hepatic vein and a branch of the portal vein within the hepatic parenchyma. This procedure is performed using catheters inserted via the jugular vein and is entirely nonsurgical. All portosystemic shunts carry increased risk of hepatic encephalopathy.

SELECTED CHRONIC HEPATIC DISORDERS

Wilson Disease

Wilson disease is characterized by abnormal storage of copper in the liver, brain, and eyes, leading to hepatocellular injury and CNS dysfunction. It is an autosomal recessive trait caused by abnormalities in the *ATP7B* gene. The encoded protein of this gene functions as an adenosine triphosphate–driven copper pump. The **diagnosis** is made by identifying low serum levels of ceruloplasmin, elevated 24-hour urine copper excretion, the presence of Kayser-Fleischer rings in the iris, and elevated hepatic copper content. In any single patient, one or

TABLE 131.6 Laboratory and Imaging Investigation of Chronic Liver Disease

METABOLIC TESTING	ANATOMIC EVALUATION
Serum α_1-antitrypsin level and phenotype Serum ceruloplasmin and 24-hour urine copper if low ceruloplasmin Sweat chloride, CF gene tests if CF suspected Testing for other specific conditions as indicated by clinical/laboratory findings	Ultrasound of liver, pancreas, and biliary tree Consider magnetic resonance cholangiography or ERCP if evidence of biliary process Liver biopsy—as required for diagnosis or prognosis
VIRAL HEPATITIS	**TESTS TO EVALUATE NUTRITIONAL STATUS**
HBsAg Hepatitis B viral DNA, HBeAg if HBsAg positive Hepatitis C antibody Hepatitis C antibody confirmatory test if positive Hepatitis C viral RNA, genotype if antibody confirmed	Height, weight, skinfold thickness 25-hydroxyvitamin D level Vitamin A level Vitamin E level Prothrombin time and partial thromboplastin time before and after vitamin K administration Serum albumin and prealbumin
AUTOIMMUNE HEPATITIS	
Antinuclear antibody Liver-kidney microsomal antibody Anti–smooth muscle antibody Antineutrophil cytoplasmic antibody Total serum IgG (usually elevated)	
TESTS TO EVALUATE LIVER FUNCTION AND INJURY	
Prothrombin time and partial thromboplastin time Serum ammonia CBC with platelet count Serum albumin AST, ALT, GGT, alkaline phosphatase Total and direct bilirubin Serum cholylglycine or bile acids Serum cholesterol Ultrasound examination of liver and bile ducts Doppler ultrasound of hepatic vessels* Magnetic resonance cholangiography* Magnetic resonance angiography of hepatic vessels* Percutaneous or endoscopic cholangiography* Liver biopsy*	

Perform when indicated to obtain specific anatomical information.

ALT, Alanine aminotransferase; *AST*, aspartate aminotransferase; *CBC*, complete blood count; *CF*, cystic fibrosis; *ERCP*, endoscopic retrograde cholangiopancreatography; *GGT*, γ-glutamyltransferase; *HBeAg*, hepatitis B early antigen; *HBsAg*, hepatitis B surface antigen; *Ig*, immunoglobulin.

TABLE 131.7 Management of Chronic Liver Disease

PROBLEM	CLINICAL MANIFESTATIONS	DIAGNOSTIC TESTING	TREATMENT
Gastrointestinal variceal bleeding*	Hematemesis, rectal bleeding, melena, anemia	CBC, coagulation tests, Doppler ultrasound, magnetic resonance angiography, endoscopy	Somatostatin (octreotide) infusion, variceal band ligation or sclerotherapy, propranolol to reduce portal pressure, acid-blocker therapy, TIPSS or surgical portosystemic shunt if transplant not possible
Ascites	Abdominal distention, shifting dullness and fluid wave, respiratory compromise, spontaneous bacterial peritonitis	Abdominal ultrasound, diagnostic paracentesis; measure ascites fluid albumin (and serum albumin), cell count, WBC differential, culture fluid in blood culture bottles	Restrict sodium intake to 0.5–1 mEq/kg/day, restrict fluids, monitor kidney function, treat peritonitis and portal hypertension Central portosystemic shunt may be required
Nutritional compromise	Muscle wasting, fat-soluble vitamin deficiencies, poor or absent weight gain, fatigue	Coagulation studies, serum albumin, 25-hydroxyvitamin D level, vitamin E level, vitamin A level	Fat-soluble vitamin supplements: vitamins A, D, E, and K; use water-soluble form of vitamins Supplemental feedings—nasogastric or parenteral if necessary
Hepatic encephalopathy	Irritability, confusion, lethargy, somnolence, coma	Serum ammonia	Lactulose orally or via nasogastric tube, avoid narcotics and sedatives, liver transplantation

May also have peptic ulcerations.
CBC, Complete blood count; *TIPSS*, transjugular intrahepatic portosystemic shunt; *WBC*, white blood cell.

more of these measures may be normal. **Clinical presentation** varies but seldom occurs before age 3 years. Neurologic abnormalities may predominate, including tremor, decline in school performance, worsening handwriting, and psychiatric disturbances. Hepatic presentations include appearance of jaundice, spider hemangiomas, portal hypertension and its consequences, and fulminant hepatic failure, which may be characterized by the presence of acute hemolytic anemia and low alkaline phosphatase. **Treatment** consists of administration of copper-chelating drugs (penicillamine or trientine), with monitoring of urine copper excretion at intervals. Zinc salts often replace chelating agents after chelation therapy has successfully reduced excessive body copper stores. Adequate therapy must be continued for life to prevent liver and CNS deterioration. Patients whose initial presentation is with severe liver disease may require immediate transplantation.

Autoimmune Hepatitis

Immune-mediated liver injury may be primary or occur in association with other autoimmune disorders, such as inflammatory bowel disease or systemic lupus erythematosus. **Diagnosis** is made on the basis of elevated serum total immunoglobulin G and the presence of an autoantibody, most commonly antinuclear, anti–smooth muscle, or anti–liver-kidney microsomal antibody (see Table 131.6). Liver biopsy specimens show the presence of a plasma cell–rich portal infiltrate with piecemeal necrosis. **Treatment** consists of corticosteroids initially, usually with the addition of an immunosuppressive drug after remission is achieved. Steroids are tapered gradually as tolerated to minimize glucocorticoid side effects. Many patients require lifelong immunosuppressive therapy, but some may be able to stop medications after several years under careful monitoring for recurrence.

Metabolic-associated steatotic liver disease is characterized by the presence of macrovesicular fatty change in hepatocytes on biopsy. When accompanied by evidence of hepatic inflammation, the diagnosis is termed *MASH* (metabolic associated steatohepatitis). Varying degrees of inflammation and portal fibrosis may be present. This disorder chiefly occurs in obese children, sometimes in association with insulin-resistant (type 2) diabetes and hyperlipidemia. Children with marked obesity, with or without type 2 diabetes, who have elevated liver enzymes and no other identifiable liver disease are likely to have this condition. MASH can progress to cirrhosis. Treatment is weight loss and exercise. Efforts should be made to control blood glucose and hyperlipidemia and promote weight loss. The rate of progression to end-stage liver disease is slow.

PEARLS FOR PRACTITIONERS

See The Digestive System: Pearls for Practitioners at the end of this section.

REVIEW QUESTIONS

Available online.

CHAPTER 132
Pancreatic Disease

PANCREATIC INSUFFICIENCY

Etiology and Epidemiology

The cause of inadequate pancreatic digestive function in 95% of cases is **cystic fibrosis** (see Chapter 138). The defect in *CFTR* chloride channel function results in thick secretions in the lungs, intestines, pancreas, and bile ducts. In the pancreas, there is destruction of pancreatic function, often before birth. Some pathogenic variants result in less severe defects in *CFTR* function and later onset of lung disease and pancreatic insufficiency. Less common causes of pancreatic insufficiency are *Shwachman-Diamond syndrome* and *Pearson syndrome* in developed countries and severe malnutrition in developing countries.

Clinical Manifestations

Children with pancreatic exocrine insufficiency have multiple bulky, foul-smelling stools each day, usually with visible oil or fat. They typically have voracious appetites because of massive malabsorption of calories from fat, complex carbohydrates, and proteins. Protein-calorie malnutrition is uniformly present if diagnosis and treatment are not accomplished rapidly. It is important to distinguish children with malabsorption due to pancreatic disease from children with intestinal disorders that interfere with digestion or absorption. Appropriate testing should be performed to rule out conditions such as celiac disease and inflammatory bowel disease if any doubt about the state of pancreatic sufficiency exists.

Laboratory and Imaging Studies

Stools can be tested for the presence of maldigested fat, which usually indicates poor fat digestion. Measuring fecal fat can give either a qualitative assessment of fat absorption (fecal Sudan stain) or a semiquantitative measurement (72-hour fecal fat determination) of fat maldigestion. Another way to assess pancreatic function is to test for the presence of pancreatic enzymes in the stool. Of these, measuring **fecal elastase-1** by immunoassay seems to be the most accurate method of assessment. Depressed fecal elastase-1 concentration correlates well with the presence of pancreatic insufficiency. Imaging studies, such as ultrasound and computed tomography (CT), cannot accurately assess pancreatic function, but they may reveal evidence of injury or other alterations of the pancreas (such as fatty change) suggesting functional impairment.

Treatment

Replacement of missing pancreatic enzymes is the best available therapy. Pancreatic enzymes are available as capsules containing enteric-coated microspheres. The coating on these spheres is designed to protect the enzymes from gastric acid degradation. For children unable to swallow capsules, the contents may be sprinkled on a spoonful of soft food, such as applesauce. Excessive use of enzymes must be avoided because high doses (>6,000 U/kg/meal) can cause colonic fibrosis. In infants, typical dosing is 2,000–4,000 U of lipase/120 mL of formula. In children younger than 4 years old, 1,000 U/kg/meal is given. For older children, 500 U/kg/meal is usual. This dose may be adjusted upward as required to control steatorrhea, but a dose of 2,500 U/kg/meal should not be exceeded. Use of H_2-receptor antagonists or proton pump inhibitors can increase the efficacy of pancreatic enzymes by enhancing their release from the microspheres and reducing inactivation by acid.

ACUTE PANCREATITIS

Etiology and Epidemiology

The exocrine pancreas produces numerous proteolytic enzymes, including trypsin, chymotrypsin, and carboxypeptidase. These are produced as inactive proenzymes to protect the pancreas from autodigestion. Trypsin is activated after leaving the pancreas by enterokinase, an intestinal brush border enzyme. After activation, trypsin cleaves other proteolytic proenzymes into their active states. Protease inhibitors found in pancreatic juice inhibit early activation of trypsin, and the presence of self-digestion sites on the trypsin molecule allows for feedback by self-inactivation. Pancreatitis occurs when digestive enzymes are activated inside the pancreas, causing injury. Triggers for acute pancreatitis differ between adults and children. In the adult patient, most episodes are related to alcohol or gallstones. In children, most cases are idiopathic, with some due to physical injury, medications, hereditary pancreatitis, gallstones, or viral infection. There are other rare causes listed in Table 132.1.

TABLE 132.1 Causes of Acute Pancreatitis in Children

OBSTRUCTIVE
Cholelithiasis and biliary sludge
Choledochal cyst
Pancreas divisum
Anomalous junction of biliary and pancreatic ducts
Annular pancreas
Ampullary obstruction (mass, inflammation from Crohn disease)
Ascaris infection
MEDICATIONS AND TOXINS
L-asparaginase
Valproic acid
Azathioprine and 6-mercaptopurine
Didanosine
Pentamidine
Tetracycline
Opiates
Mesalamine
Sulfasalazine
Alcohol
Cannabis
SYSTEMIC DISEASES
Inflammatory bowel disease
Hemolytic uremic syndrome
Diabetic ketoacidosis
Collagen vascular disease
Kawasaki disease
Shock
Sickle cell disease
INFECTIOUS
Sepsis
Mumps
Coxsackievirus
Cytomegalovirus
Varicella-zoster
Herpes simplex
Mycoplasma
Ascaris
GENETIC
Cystic fibrosis—*CFTR* pathogenic variants
Hereditary pancreatitis—*SPINK*, *PRSS1*, and *CTRC* pathogenic variants
OTHER
Trauma
Hyperlipidemia
Hypercalcemia
Autoimmune

Clinical Manifestations

Acute pancreatitis presents with relatively rapid onset of pain, usually in the epigastric region. The pain may radiate to the back and is nearly always aggravated by eating. The patient moves frequently to find a position of comfort. Nausea and vomiting occur in most cases. Pain is typically continuous and quite severe, usually requiring narcotics. Severe pancreatitis can lead to hemorrhage, visible as ecchymoses in the flanks (Grey Turner sign) or periumbilical region (Cullen sign). Rupture of pancreatic ducts can lead to development of a pancreatic pseudocyst, characterized by persistent severe pain, tenderness, and a palpable mass. With necrosis and fluid collections, patients experiencing severe pancreatitis are prone to infectious complications (abscess), and the clinician must be alert for fever and signs of sepsis.

Laboratory and Imaging Studies

The diagnosis of acute pancreatitis is based on two of the following three criteria: abdominal pain consistent with the disease (severe epigastric pain typically), serum amylase and/or lipase greater than three times the upper limit of normal, and/or characteristic findings on imaging. Acute pancreatitis can be difficult to diagnose. Pancreatic enzymes are released into the blood during pancreatic injury. Nonspecific elevations of the enzymes are common. As acute pancreatitis progresses, the amylase level tends to decline faster than lipase, making the latter a good choice for diagnostic testing late in the course of the disease.

Because enzyme levels are not 100% sensitive or specific, imaging studies are important for the diagnosis of pancreatitis. In acute pancreatitis, edema is present in all but the mildest cases. Ultrasound can detect this edema and should be performed early as part of the overall diagnostic approach. If overlying bowel gas obscures the pancreas, a CT scan allows complete visualization of the gland. CT scans should be done with oral and intravenous contrast agents to facilitate interpretation. Ultrasound and CT also can be used to monitor for the development, progression, and resolution of **pseudocysts** and for evidence of ductal dilation secondary to obstruction. The other important reason to perform imaging studies early in the course of pancreatitis is to rule out gallstones; the liver, gallbladder, and common bile duct all should be visualized. **Magnetic resonance cholangiopancreatography (MRCP)** is superior to CT to detect anatomic variants causing pancreatitis, as it allows the best visualization of pancreatic and biliary ducts.

Treatment

There are no proven specific therapies for acute pancreatitis. If a predisposing etiology is found, such as a drug reaction or a gallstone obstructing the sphincter of Oddi, this should be specifically treated. Fluid resuscitation is necessary because of vomiting and third space losses. Pain relief should be provided as required. Oral, nasogastric, or nasojejunal feedings can begin early if tolerated, and these both shorten hospital course and improve outcome. If early enteral feeding is not possible, parenteral nutrition should be considered. Antibiotics should be considered if the patient is febrile, has extensive pancreatic necrosis, or has laboratory evidence of infection. A broad-spectrum antibiotic, such as carbapenem or quinolone, is considered the best choice. Percutaneous catheter drainage may be needed for severe necrosis.

CHRONIC PANCREATITIS

Etiology and Epidemiology

Chronic pancreatitis is defined as recurrent or persistent attacks of pancreatitis, which have resulted in irreversible morphologic changes in pancreatic structure. These include scarring of the ducts with irregular areas of narrowing and dilation (beading), fibrosis of parenchyma, and loss of acinar and islet tissue. Pancreatic exocrine insufficiency and diabetes mellitus may result from unremitting chronic pancreatitis. Most patients have discrete attacks of acute symptoms occurring repeatedly, but chronic pain may be present. The causes of chronic pancreatitis include hereditary pancreatitis and milder phenotypes of cystic fibrosis associated with pancreatic sufficiency. Familial disease is often caused by one of several known pathogenic variants in the trypsinogen gene, including pathogenic variants in the *SPINK1* gene, which codes for pancreatic trypsin inhibitor; *PRSS1*, a pathogenic variant of cationic trypsinogen; or *CTRC*, a pathogenic variant in chymotrypsin C. These variants favor intraglandular activation or loss of feedback inhibition of trypsinogen. Genetic testing is readily available for these variants. Genetic testing for cystic fibrosis must include screening for the less common variants associated with pancreatic sufficiency.

Clinical Manifestations

Children with chronic pancreatitis initially present with recurring attacks of acute pancreatitis. Injury to the pancreatic ducts predisposes these children to continued attacks owing to scarring of small and large pancreatic ducts, stasis of pancreatic secretions, stone formation, and inflammation. Loss of pancreatic exocrine and endocrine tissue over time can lead to exocrine and endocrine deficiency. More than 90% of the pancreatic mass must be destroyed before exocrine deficiency becomes clinically apparent; this is a late complication that does not occur in all cases. Chronic pain is a serious problem in most affected individuals.

Laboratory and Imaging Studies

Laboratory diagnosis of chronic pancreatitis is similar to acute pancreatitis, but with more severe loss of pancreatic tissue it becomes less likely that the patient presents with elevation of amylase or lipase. The diagnosis of chronic pancreatitis requires demonstration of chronic injury on imaging studies. Plain abdominal x-rays may show pancreatic calcifications. CT scan or magnetic resonance imaging may show fibrosis, glandular atrophy, and ductal strictures. MRCP can demonstrate details of ductular structure and is commonly performed before considering direct ductal imaging via endoscopic retrograde cholangiopancreatography (ERCP), in which dye is injected directly into the pancreatic and common bile ducts. When an accessible dominant ductal stricture or other obstruction of pancreatic discharge is found, ERCP does offer the possibility of therapeutic intervention. Diagnostic testing for the etiology of chronic pancreatitis should include genetic testing for hereditary pancreatitis and cystic fibrosis.

Treatment

Treatment is largely supportive. Interventional ERCP to dilate large strictures and remove stones and surgical pancreatic drainage procedures to decompress dilated pancreatic ducts by creating a side-to-side pancreaticojejunostomy may have some value.

PEARLS FOR PRACTITIONERS

See The Digestive System: Pearls for Practitioners at the end of this section.

REVIEW QUESTIONS

Available online.

CHAPTER 133
Peritonitis

ETIOLOGY AND EPIDEMIOLOGY

The peritoneum consists of a single layer of mesothelial cells that covers all intraabdominal organs. The portion that covers the abdominal wall is derived from the underlying somatic structures and is innervated by somatic nerves. The portion covering the viscera is derived from visceral mesoderm and is innervated by nonmyelinated visceral afferents. Inflammation of the peritoneum, or peritonitis, usually is caused by infection but may result from exogenous irritants introduced by penetrating injuries or surgical procedures, radiation, or endogenous irritants such as meconium or bile. Infectious peritonitis can be an acute complication of intestinal inflammation and perforation, as in appendicitis, or it can occur secondary to contamination of preexisting ascites associated with kidney, cardiac, or hepatic disease. In this setting, when there is no other intraabdominal source, it is referred to as ***spontaneous bacterial peritonitis***. Spontaneous bacterial peritonitis is usually due to pneumococcus and less often to *Escherichia coli*.

CLINICAL MANIFESTATIONS

Peritonitis is characterized on examination by marked abdominal tenderness. Rebound tenderness is generally quite pronounced. The patient tends to move very little owing to intense peritoneal irritation and pain. Fever is not always present; absence of fever should not be regarded as contradictory to the diagnosis. Patients who are taking corticosteroids for an underlying condition, such as nephrotic syndrome, are likely to have little fever and reduced tenderness.

LABORATORY AND IMAGING STUDIES

Blood tests should focus on identifying the nature of the inflammation and its underlying cause. An elevated white blood cell count, erythrocyte sedimentation rate, and C-reactive protein suggest infection. In children older than 5 years, appendicitis is the leading cause. Total serum protein, albumin, and urinalysis should be ordered to rule out nephrotic syndrome. Liver function tests should be performed to evaluate for chronic liver disease causing ascites. The best way to diagnose suspected peritonitis is to sample the peritoneal fluid with a needle or catheter (paracentesis). Peritoneal fluid in spontaneous bacterial peritonitis has a high neutrophil count of greater than 250 cells/mm^3. Other tests that should be completed on the peritoneal fluid include amylase (to rule out pancreatic ascites), culture, albumin, and lactate dehydrogenase concentration. For culture, a large sample of fluid should be placed into aerobic and anaerobic blood culture bottles immediately on obtaining the sample.

Appendicitis may be identified by ultrasound, magnetic resonance imaging, or computed tomography scan (Chapter 130). When other intraabdominal emergencies are suspected, such as midgut volvulus, meconium ileus, peptic disease, or any other condition predisposing to intestinal perforation, specific testing should be performed.

TREATMENT

Peritonitis caused by an intraabdominal surgical process, such as appendicitis or a penetrating wound, must be managed surgically. Spontaneous bacterial peritonitis should be treated with a broad-spectrum antibiotic with good coverage of resistant pneumococcus and enteric bacteria. Third-generation cephalosporins are generally effective as initial therapy while awaiting culture and sensitivity results. Anaerobic coverage with metronidazole should be added whenever a perforated viscus is suspected.

PEARLS FOR PRACTITIONERS

See The Digestive System: Pearls for Practitioners at the end of this section.

REVIEW QUESTIONS

Available online.

Suggested Readings

Brusaferro A, Farinelli E, Zenzeri L, Cozzali R, Esposito S. The management of paediatric functional abdominal pain disorders: latest evidence. *Paediatr Drugs*. 2018;20(3):235–247.

Chapin LM, Bass CA. Cirrhosis and portal hypertension in the pediatric population. *Clin Liver Dis*. 2018;22(4):735–752.

Clark MB, Slayton RL, Segura A, et al. Fluoride use in caries prevention in the primary care setting. *Pediatrics*. 2014;134(3):626–633.

Conrad MA, Rosh JR. Pediatric inflammatory bowel disease. *Pediatr Clin N Am*. 2017;65:577–591.

Fachler T, Shteyer E, Orlanski EM, et al. Pediatric gastrointestinal endoscopy: diagnostic yield and appropriateness of referral based on clinical presentation: a pilot study. *Front Pediatr*. 2021;9:607418.

Fawaz R, Baumann U, Ekong U, et al. Guideline for the evaluation of cholestatic jaundice in infants: joint recommendations of the North American Society for Pediatric Gastroenterology, Hepatology, and Nutrition and the European Society for Pediatric Gastroenterology, Hepatology, and Nutrition. *J Pediatr Gastroenterol Nutr*. 2017;64:154–168.

Gailey DG. Feeding infants with cleft and the postoperative cleft management. *Oral Maxillofac Surg Clin North Am*. 2016;28(2):153–159.

Hyams JS, Di Lorenzo C, Saps M, et al. Childhood functional gastrointestinal disorders: child/adolescent. *Gastroenterology*. 2016;150:1456–1468.

Jimenez J, Loveridge-Lenza B, Horvath K. Celiac disease in children. *Pediatr Clin North Am*. 2021;68(6):1205–1219.

Jones NL, Koletzko S, Goodman K, et al. Joint ESPGHAN/NASPGHAN guidelines for the management of Helicobacter pylori in children and adolescents (Update 2016). *J Pediatr Gastroenterol Nutr*. 2017;64:991–1003.

Khalaf R, Phen C, Karjoo S, et al. Cholestasis beyond the neonatal and infancy periods. *Pediatr Gastroenterol Hepatol Nutr*. 2016;19(1):1–11.
Kim JS. Acute abdominal pain in children. *Pediatr Gastroenterol Hepatol Nutr*. 2013;16(4):219–224.
Kocic M, Rasic P, Marusic V, et al. Age-specific causes of upper gastrointestinal bleeding in children. *World J Gastroenterol*. 2023;29(47):6095–6110.
Kulik DM, Uleryk EM, Maguire JL. Does this child have appendicitis? A systematic review of clinical prediction rules for children with acute abdominal pain. *J Emerg Med*. 2013;66(1):95–104.
Larson-Nath C, Vitola B. Pediatric acute liver failure. *Crit Care Clin*. 2022;38:301–315.
Li BU. Managing cyclic vomiting syndrome in children: beyond the guidelines. *Eur J Pediatr*. 2018;177(10):1435–1442.
Moyer VA. Prevention of dental caries in children from birth through age 5 years: U.S. Preventive Services Task Force recommendation statement. *Pediatrics*. 2014;133(6):1102–1111.
Papadopoulou A, Amil-Dias J, Karl-Heinz M, et al. Joint ESPGHAN/NASPGHAN guidelines on childhood eosinophilic gastrointestinal disorders beyond eosinophilic esophagitis. *J Pediatr Gastroenterol Nutr*. 2024;78(1).
Pham YH, Miloh T. Liver transplantation in children. *Clin Liver Dis*. 2018;22(4):807–821.
Rajindrajith S, Hathagoda W, Devanarayana NM. Functional diarrhea in children. *Indian J Pediatr*. 2024;91(6):584–589.
Rexwinkel R, Vlieger AM, Saps M, et al. A therapeutic guide on pediatric irritable bowel syndrome and functional abdominal pain-not otherwise specified. *Eur J Pediatr*. 2022;181(7):2603–2617.
Rosen R, Vandenplas Y, Singendonk M, et al. Pediatric gastroesophageal reflux clinical practice guidelines: joint recommendations of the North American Society for Pediatric Gastroenterology, Hepatology, and Nutrition and the European Society for Pediatric Gastroenterology, Hepatology, and Nutrition. *J Pediatr Gastroenterol Nutr*. 2018;66:516–554.
Sabri M, Saps M, Peters JM. Pathophysiology and management of pediatric ascites. *Curr Gastroenterol Rep*. 2003;5(3):240–246.
Sahn B, Bitton S. Lower gastrointestinal bleeding in children. *Gastrointest Endosc Clin N Am*. 2016;26(1):75–98.
Shaunak M, Byrne CD, Davis N, et al. Non-alcoholic fatty liver disease and childhood obesity. *Arch Dis Child*. 2021;106:3–8.
Somaraju UR, Solis-Moya A. Pancreatic enzyme replacement for people with cystic fibrosis. *Cochrane Database Syst Rev*. 2014;(10):CD008227.
Tabbers MM, DiLorenzo C, Berger MY, et al. Evaluation and treatment of functional constipation in infants and children: evidence-based recommendations from ESPGHAN and NASPGHAN. *J Pediatr Gastroenterol Nutr*. 2014;58(2):258–274.
Tukan A, Biank VF. Eosinophilic esophagitis for the general pediatrician. *Pediatr Ann*. 2021;50(8):e325–e329.
Uc A, Husain SZ. Pancreatitis in children. *Gastroenterology*. 2019;156(7):1969–1978.
van Heurn LW, Pakarinen MP, Wester T. Contemporary management of abdominal surgical emergencies in infants and children. *Br J Surg*. 2014;101(1):e24–e33.
Verkade HJ, Bezerra JA, Davenport M, et al. Biliary atresia and other cholestatic childhood diseases: advances and future challenges. *J Hepatol*. 2016;65(3):631–642.

PEARLS FOR PRACTITIONERS

CHAPTER 127

Digestive System Assessment

- Take a careful history and perform a thorough but focused physical examination, using your findings to form a diagnostic hypothesis and plan.
- Surgical emergencies, such as bowel obstruction or appendicitis, must be identified rapidly in children with acute abdominal pain. Common distinguishing characteristics include pain that is accompanied by vomiting, tenderness, abdominal wall rigidity, or guarding.
- Extraintestinal disorders (lower lobe pneumonia, pyelonephritis, streptococcal pharyngitis) may produce abdominal pain.
- When evaluating recurrent abdominal pain, a complete work-up must include not only a medical evaluation, but also assessment of functional impairment, such as missing school, and consideration of psychosocial factors influencing the pain.
- Recurrent abdominal pain is seen in 10% of school-age children and is often functional.
- For patients with emesis, remember to distinguish between true vomiting (forceful retching, usually preceded by nausea) from regurgitation (effortless, usually no nausea) when considering the differential diagnosis.
- Emesis in a neonate suggests a gastrointestinal (GI) obstruction such as pyloric stenosis or volvulus; an inborn error of metabolism should be considered in the presence of acidosis, hypoglycemia, or hyperammonemia.
- When treating a patient with significant GI bleeding, focus on fluid resuscitation and tissue oxygenation/perfusion as the first priority.
- Acute diarrhea is often due to viral gastroenteritis (rotavirus, norovirus). Dysentery often presents with fever, pain, and diarrhea with blood and mucus.
- Painless large volume rectal bleeding in a 2-year-old would suggest a Meckel diverticulum; older patients may also have a polyp.

CHAPTER 128

Oral Cavity

- Many systemic disorders affect the oral cavity, which careful examination can demonstrate. Examples include Peutz-Jeghers syndrome, Crohn disease, gastroesophageal reflux disease (GERD), Addison disease, and leukemia.
- Deciduous teeth erupt in a predictable sequence and at predictable ages. Significant delayed eruption may be associated with hypothyroidism, Down syndrome, and other disorders.
- Cleft lip and palate are common birth defects; combined cleft lip and palate is more common in males and isolated cleft palate is more likely to be associated with other congenital malformations.

CHAPTER 129

Esophagus and Stomach

- As many as half of infants will have physiologic reflux. The majority of these infants do not benefit from acid reduction therapy.

- Gastroesophageal reflux disease occurs when there are complications of reflux such as poor growth, esophagitis, abdominal or chest pain, or respiratory problems.
- Reflux cannot be diagnosed based on imaging as this is only a snapshot in time. Upper GI series evaluates for anatomic abnormalities.
- In an older child who has not improved with lifestyle changes, a trial with a proton pump inhibitor is recommended.
- Eosinophilic esophagitis should be considered in children with poor feeding or growth, chronic abdominal pain or vomiting, and in children with dysphagia or recurrent food impactions as well as atopy. Treatment includes dietary changes or topical (swallowed) glucocorticoid therapy.
- A neonate with poor feeding and drooling with a nasogastric tube on x-ray coiled in the neck most likely has a tracheoesophageal fistula.
- Button batteries in the esophagus must be removed emergently. Two or more ingested magnets should be removed as soon as possible due to risk of perforation.
- Infants with pyloric stenosis develop hypochloremic, hypokalemic metabolic alkalosis.
- The diagnosis of pyloric stenosis may be made with abdominal ultrasonography.
- *Helicobacter pylori* cannot be diagnosed by blood tests. Urea breath hydrogen testing, endoscopy with biopsies, and fecal antigen testing can be considered.
- Cyclic vomiting syndrome is a migraine variant that leads to repeated bouts of repetitive vomiting over hours to days.

CHAPTER 130
Intestinal Tract

- Bile-stained emesis in an infant may suggest a volvulus.
- Intestinal malrotation may lead to a volvulus with subsequent intestinal infarction.
- Delayed passage of first meconium after 24 hours of life should raise suspicion for Hirschsprung disease.
- Hirschsprung disease is diagnosed by suction or full thickness rectal biopsy.
- Duodenal atresia is associated with trisomy 21 and prematurity. There may also be polyhydramnios.
- Suspect Crohn disease in a child with poor growth, delayed puberty, fatigue, and abdominal pain. Initial testing may show anemia, thrombocytosis, elevated sedimentation rate and C-reactive protein, and hypoalbuminemia, but these can be normal.
- Fecal calprotectin is a marker of intestinal inflammation. Normal fecal calprotectin makes inflammatory bowel disease diagnosis unlikely.
- Recommended serologic testing for celiac disease is the tissue transglutaminase antibody immunoglobulin A (IgA). Confirmation by duodenal biopsy is recommended prior to initiating a gluten-free diet.
- Celiac disease is associated with type 1 diabetes, autoimmune thyroiditis, Turner syndrome, and trisomy 21.
- Intussusception is a cause of acute colicky abdominal pain in toddlers; there may also be rectal bleeding and intestinal obstruction.
- The diagnosis of intussusception is suggested by abdominal ultrasonography but confirmed and treated by barium or air enema.
- Appendicitis can occur at any age but is most common in adolescents and young adults.
- Periumbilical pain followed by nausea followed by right lower quadrant pain is suggestive of appendicitis.

CHAPTER 131
Liver Disease

- Infants with jaundice that persists beyond a few weeks of life should have both total and direct (conjugated) bilirubin measured to ensure that cholestasis is not missed.
- Cholestasis in infants requires prompt investigation to identify treatable causes such as biliary atresia, choledochal cyst, and certain disorders of metabolism.
- Neonatal giant cell hepatitis may be idiopathic or due to cytomegalovirus (CMV), herpes simplex, or syphilis.
- α_1-Antitrypsin deficiency may present as neonatal hepatitis.
- Alagille syndrome presents with chronic cholestasis due to paucity of bile ducts and is associated with pruritus, butterfly vertebra, triangular facies, congenital heart disease, and ocular posterior embryotoxon.
- Work-up of hepatitis in children requires consideration of more than just the classic hepatitis viruses and should include evaluation for autoimmune hepatitis, Wilson disease, and biliary obstruction, as well as measures of liver function.
- Wilson disease is associated with low serum ceruloplasmin and elevated 24-hour urine copper.
- Consultation with a major referral center with hepatology expertise should be sought for any child with acute severe hepatitis or chronic hepatitis.

CHAPTER 132
Pancreatic Disease

- Fecal elastase is the preferred test for pancreatic insufficiency.
- Cystic fibrosis is the most common cause of pancreatic insufficiency.
- The diagnosis of acute pancreatitis is based on symptoms of severe epigastric abdominal pain and tenderness, increase of amylase and/or lipase more than three times the upper limit of normal, and/or imaging findings of pancreatic inflammation.
- Complications of pancreatitis include shock, pancreatic pseudocyst formation, and pancreatic abscess.
- Patients with pancreatitis may feed enterally if tolerated.
- In patients with recurrent pancreatitis, consider hereditary disorders such as cystic fibrosis or familial pancreatitis involving pathogenic variants in *CFTR*, *PRSS1*, *SPINK1*, or *CTRC*.

CHAPTER 133

Peritonitis

- When peritonitis is suspected, appropriate laboratory and imaging studies should be ordered to reveal underlying conditions, such as appendicitis.
- Nephrotic syndrome, heart failure, and chronic liver disease are associated with an increased risk of spontaneous bacterial peritonitis due to chronic presence of ascites.
- Spontaneous bacterial peritonitis is most commonly caused by *Streptococcus pneumoniae* or *Escherichia coli.*
- Paracentesis is required to accurately diagnose spontaneous bacterial peritonitis.
- Analysis of ascites fluid should include culture, cell count with differential, amylase, albumin, and lactate dehydrogenase.

SECTION 18

THE RESPIRATORY SYSTEM

Erin W. MacKintosh | Sarah C. Hofman DeYoung | Susan G. Marshall

CHAPTER 134

Respiratory System Assessment

ANATOMY OF THE RESPIRATORY SYSTEM

Air enters the **nose** and passes over the large surface area of the **nasal turbinates**, which warm, humidify, and filter the inspired air. Secretions draining from the paranasal sinuses are carried to the **pharynx** by the mucociliary action of the ciliated respiratory epithelium. Enlarged lymphoid tissue can obstruct airflow through the nasopharynx (adenoids) or the posterior pharynx (palatine tonsils).

The **epiglottis** protects the larynx during swallowing by deflecting material toward the esophagus (Fig. 134.1). The **arytenoid cartilages**, which assist in opening and closing the vocal folds, are less prominent in children than in adults. The opening formed by the vocal folds (the **glottis**) is V shaped, with the apex of the V oriented anterior. Below the vocal folds, the walls of the **subglottic space** converge toward the cricoid portion of the trachea. The cricoid ring is the narrowest portion of the airway in children under 3 years of age; in older children and adults it is the glottis. The space from the nose through the thoracic inlet, where the neck meets the top of the thorax, is called the extrathoracic airway; all airways below the thoracic inlet are considered intrathoracic. C-shaped cartilage supports the **trachea** and **mainstem bronchi**, extending approximately 320 degrees around the airway circumference. The posterior wall of the trachea is membranous and bridged by the trachealis muscle, allowing airway caliber to change during inspiration and expiration. Beyond the lobar bronchi, cartilaginous support of the airways becomes discontinuous but persists until the terminal **bronchioles**. Airway formation and branching is complete at birth, although length and caliber continue to increase until final adult height is achieved.

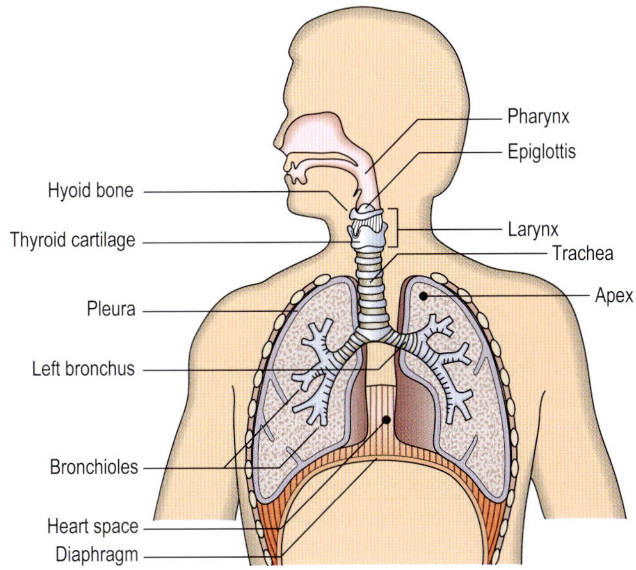

FIGURE 134.1 Anatomy of the respiratory tract. (From Rice A. Respiratory system. In Cross SS, ed. *Underwood's Pathology: A Clinical Approach*. 8th ed. Philadelphia: Elsevier; 2025. Fig. 14.1.)

The right lung has three lobes (upper, middle, lower) and comprises approximately 55% of the total lung volume. The left lung has two lobes (upper, lower); the inferior division of the left upper lobe (the lingula) is analogous to the right middle lobe. The **lung parenchyma**, where gas exchange occurs, is composed of the respiratory bronchioles, alveolar ducts, and alveoli. **Oxygen** (O_2) and **carbon dioxide** (CO_2) must traverse alveolar and capillary membranes and the **interstitium** to maintain adequate oxygenation and ventilation to meet metabolic demands.

The pediatric lung has tremendous capacity for growth. A full-term infant has approximately 25 million alveoli; an adult has nearly 300 million alveoli. The rapid growth of new alveoli occurs during the first 2 years of life and continues through adolescence. After this time, lung volume increases primarily by increases in alveolar dimensions, with new alveoli rarely formed.

PULMONARY PHYSIOLOGY

Pulmonary Mechanics

The major function of the lungs is to exchange O_2 and CO_2 between the atmosphere and the blood. The airways, alveolar-capillary interface, pulmonary circulation, tissue metabolism, respiratory mechanics, and neural control of breathing all impact gas exchange.

Air enters the lungs when intrathoracic pressure is less than atmospheric pressure. Negative intrathoracic pressure is generated by contraction and lowering of the **diaphragm** during normal inspiration. The accessory muscles of inspiration (**external intercostal**, **scalene**, and **sternocleidomastoid muscles**) are not used during quiet breathing but are recruited during exercise or in disease states to raise and enlarge the rib cage. Exhalation is normally passive, but with active exhalation the **abdominal** and **internal intercostal muscles** are recruited.

During normal breathing at rest, lung volumes are usually in the midrange of inflation (Fig. 134.2). **Tidal volume (V_T)** is

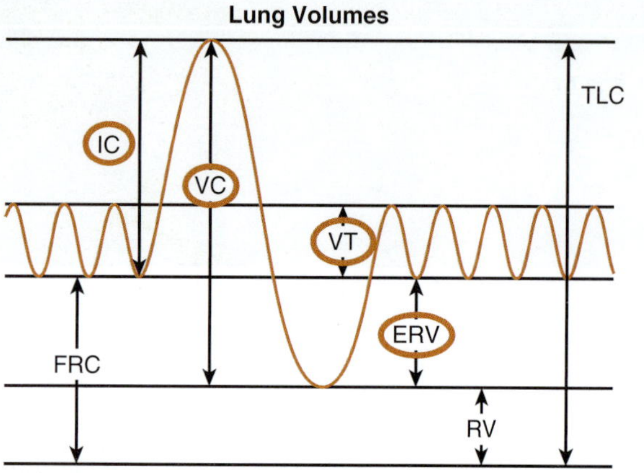

FIGURE 134.2 Lung volumes and capacities. Although spirometry can measure vital capacity and its subdivisions *(orange circles)*, calculation of residual volume (RV) requires measurement of functional residual capacity (FRC) by one of the following techniques: body plethysmography, helium dilution, or nitrogen washout. *ERV*, Expiratory reserve volume; *IC*, inspiratory capacity; *TLC*, total lung capacity; *VC*, vital capacity; *VT*, tidal volume. (From Koo P, McCool FD, Sethi JM. Evaluating lung structure and function. In Wing EJ, Schiffman FJ, eds. *Cecil Essentials of Medicine*. 10th ed. Philadelphia: WB Saunders; 2022:Fig. 15.19.)

the amount of air inspired with each *relaxed* breath. The volume of gas retained in the lung at the end of a *relaxed* exhalation is the **functional residual capacity (FRC)**. This retained gas volume maintains exchange of O_2 between breaths. **Total lung capacity (TLC)** is the volume of gas in the lungs at the end of *maximal* inhalation, and **residual volume (RV)** is the volume of gas left in the lungs at the end of a *maximal* exhalation. **Vital capacity (VC)** is the maximal amount of air that can be forcibly expelled from the lungs and is the difference between TLC and RV. **Inspiratory capacity (IC)** is the maximum volume of air that can be inspired after reaching the end of a normal expiration and **expiratory reserve volume (ERV)** is the extra volume of air that can be expired with maximum effort beyond the end of a normal, resting respiration.

Airway resistance is influenced by the diameter and length of the conducting airways, the viscosity of gas, and the nature of the airflow. During quiet breathing, airflow in the smaller airways is laminar (streamlined). At higher flow rates, turbulent flow increases resistance. Resistance is inversely proportional to the fourth power of the radius of the airway, so relatively small changes in airway diameter can result in large changes in airway resistance. Excessive airway secretions, bronchospasm, mucosal edema, stenosis, foreign bodies, loss of airway wall integrity (e.g. bronchiectasis), and airway compression may all produce symptomatic increases in airway resistance. Diseases that impact airway resistance, particularly lower airway resistance, fall into the category of **obstructive airway disease.**

Lung compliance (change in volume for a given change in pressure) is a measure of the ease with which the lung can be inflated. Processes that decrease lung compliance (e.g., surfactant deficiency, pulmonary fibrosis, pulmonary edema) may lead to **restrictive lung disease**. Restrictive physiology can also result from respiratory muscle weakness, pleural disease (e.g., effusion, inflammation, mass), thoracic stiffness (e.g., scoliosis), and abdominal distention.

Respiratory Gas Exchange

Alveolar ventilation is defined as the exchange of CO_2 between the alveoli and ambient air. Normally about 30% of each tidal breath fills the conducting airways, which do not participate in gas exchange **(anatomic dead space)**. Because this anatomic dead space is relatively constant, increasing the tidal volume generally increases the efficacy of ventilation. Conversely, if tidal volume decreases, then the *dead space:tidal volume ratio* (V_D/V_T) increases and alveolar ventilation decreases.

Gas exchange depends on **alveolar ventilation, pulmonary capillary blood flow**, and the **diffusion** of gases across the alveolar-capillary membrane. Exchange of CO_2 is determined primarily by alveolar ventilation, and the exchange of O_2 is influenced primarily by the regional matching of ventilation (V) with pulmonary blood flow (Q) (V/Q matching). V/Q matching is maintained, in part, by **hypoxic pulmonary vasoconstriction** (local constriction of the pulmonary vessels in areas that are underventilated). There are five causes of **hypoxemia** (Table 134.1). Disorders resulting in **V/Q mismatching** (such as pneumonia and atelectasis) are the most common causes of hypoxemia in children.

Lung Defense Mechanisms

The lungs are constantly exposed to particles and infectious agents. The **nose** is the primary filter for large particles. Particles less than 10 μm in diameter may reach the trachea and bronchi and deposit on the mucosa. Particles less than 1 μm may reach the alveoli. **Ciliated epithelium** lining the airways from the larynx to the bronchioles continuously propels a thin layer of mucus toward the pharynx to be expectorated or swallowed. **Alveolar macrophages** and **polymorphonuclear cells** engulf particles and pathogens that have been opsonized by locally secreted immunoglobulin A (IgA) antibodies or transudated serum antibodies.

Cough is a critically important mechanism for protecting the lungs from infectious processes. It may be voluntary or generated by reflex irritation of the nose, sinuses, pharynx, larynx, trachea, bronchi, or bronchioles. Cough is a rapid, forceful expiration intended to clear the airways of debris and secretions. Effective cough requires the ability to (1) inhale to near TLC, (2) close and open the glottis, and (3) contract abdominal muscles to forcibly exhale. Loss of the ability to cough (e.g., neuromuscular weakness) results in poor secretion clearance and predisposes to atelectasis and pneumonia. Persistent cough suggests chronic irritation at any of these sites, commonly due to infectious (e.g., chronic bronchitis), allergic (e.g., postnasal drip, asthma), or chemical (e.g., inhalation or aspiration) triggers.

HISTORY

Common respiratory complaints in children include cough, labored or noisy breathing, chest pain, and exercise intolerance. The complete respiratory history includes **onset, duration**, and **frequency** of symptoms. It is important to obtain information concerning severity (hospitalizations, missed school days, activity limitation) and pattern (acute, chronic, or intermittent), including factors leading to worsening or improvement. Exposure history is essential, including respiratory illness and **environmental factors** such as pet dander, smoking and vaping exposure (primary or secondhand), wildfire smoke, mold, or chemical fumes including secondhand occupational exposures. Key review of systems including growth history and nutritional status during infancy and

TABLE 134.1 Causes of Hypoxemia

CAUSE	EXAMPLE(S)	Pa_{O_2}	Pa_{CO_2}	Pa_{O_2} SIGNIFICANTLY IMPROVES WITH SUPPLEMENTAL OXYGEN
Ventilation-perfusion mismatch	Asthma Bronchopulmonary dysplasia Pneumonia Atelectasis	↓	Normal, ↓, or ↑	Yes
Hypoventilation	Apnea Drug overdose Neuromuscular disease	↓	↑	Yes
Extrapulmonary shunt	Cyanotic heart disease	↓	Normal or ↑	No
Intrapulmonary shunt	Pulmonary arteriovenous malformation Atelectasis	↓	Normal or ↑	No
Low FiO_2	High altitude	↓	↓	Yes
Diffusion defect	Scleroderma Hepatopulmonary syndrome Pulmonary fibrosis	↓	Normal	Yes

FiO_2, Fraction of inspired oxygen; *Pa_{CO_2}*, arterial partial pressure of carbon dioxide; *Pa_{O_2}*, arterial partial pressure of oxygen.

childhood may also contribute to diagnosis. For infants, a **feeding history** should be obtained, including questions of coughing or choking with eating or drinking. Family history should include questions about asthma and other atopy, immune deficiencies, cystic fibrosis (CF), or other chronic respiratory diseases.

A thorough history is essential in determining the etiology of cough. Morning cough may be due to the accumulation of excessive secretions during the night from sinusitis, allergic rhinitis, or bronchitis. Nighttime cough is a hallmark of asthma and can also be caused by gastroesophageal reflux disease or postnasal drip. Cough with wheeze is suggestive of asthma or bronchiolitis. Coughing with exercise is highly suggestive of exercise-induced asthma/bronchospasm. Habit cough can masquerade as organic disease but should disappear when children are distracted or during sleep. Acute paroxysmal cough (especially associated with cyanosis) suggests pertussis; a repetitive, staccato cough occurs in chlamydial pneumonia in infants. A harsh, brassy, seal-like cough suggests croup, tracheomalacia, or psychogenic (habit) cough. Sudden onset of cough after a choking episode suggests foreign body aspiration.

PHYSICAL EXAMINATION

Clothing should be removed from the upper half of the child's body as able so the thorax may be inspected while maintaining modesty for adolescents. It is optimal to observe the respiratory rate, pattern, and work of breathing while the child is quiet, noting the shape and symmetry of the chest wall including spine and the anteroposterior (AP) diameter.

Any factor that impairs respiratory mechanics is likely to increase the **respiratory rate**. Nonrespiratory causes of tachypnea include fever, pain, and stress/anxiety. Respiratory rates vary with age (Table 134.2).

TABLE 134.2 Normal Respiratory Rates by Age

AGE	RESPIRATORY RATE (BREATHS PER MINUTE)
Birth–9 mo	30–60
9 mo–2 yr	24–40
2–5 yr	20–36
5–12 yr	14–26
12 yr–adult	12–20

It is important to observe the respiratory **pattern** and **degree of effort** (work of breathing). Abnormal breathing patterns are detailed in Table 134.3. Increased work of breathing can be described as inspiratory (**nasal flaring**; supraclavicular, intercostal, or subcostal **retractions**) or expiratory (visible as active use of **abdominal muscles to exhale**). Causes of increased work of breathing during inspiration include extrathoracic airway obstruction (e.g., laryngomalacia, croup, subglottic stenosis) and/or decreased pulmonary compliance (e.g., pneumonia, pulmonary edema). Increased expiratory work of breathing usually indicates intrathoracic airway narrowing (e.g., asthma, tracheomalacia). **Grunting** (forced expiration against a partially closed glottis) is often seen in small children with respiratory distress but may also be a manifestation of pain.

When attempting to determine the cause of a respiratory complaint, it is useful to auscultate over all potential sites of pathology, including the nose and mouth, neck, large airways (central chest and back), and all lobes of both lungs (anterior and posterior, upper and lower, as well as lateral chest wall).

Stridor is a harsh, monophonic, often higher-pitched sound caused by a partially obstructed large airway, more commonly heard on inspiration and localized to the neck (extrathoracic) or upper central chest (intrathoracic). **Wheezing** is produced by partial obstruction of the smaller lower airways, more commonly heard during exhalation and localized to the chest. Wheezes can be monophonic and low-pitched (usually from large, central airways) or high-pitched and musical (from small peripheral airways). Secretions in the intrathoracic airways result in irregular sounds called **rhonchi**. Fluid or secretions in small airways may produce sounds characteristic of "ripping velcro" or "crackling tissue paper" (**crackles** or **rales**).

TABLE 134.3 Abnormal Breathing Patterns

PATTERN	FEATURES	CAUSES
Tachypnea	Respiratory rate > normal for age	Restrictive physiology, fever, increased metabolic demands, stress/anxiety
Bradypnea	Respiratory rate < normal for age	Sleep, sedating medications, CNS injury, metabolic alkalosis
Hyperpnea	Increased depth of breathing, normal rate	Stress/anxiety, exercise, metabolic acidosis
Periodic breathing	Brief pauses (<10 sec) followed by rapid, shallow breaths	Normal variant for preterm and term infants, prominent in sleep
Kussmaul respiration	Increased rate, increased tidal volume, regular deep respiration	Metabolic acidosis, especially diabetic ketoacidosis, uremia
Cheyne-Stokes respiration	Cyclic pattern of waxing and waning depth of breathing interposed with apnea	CNS injury (brainstem), elevated intracranial pressure, heart failure, uremia
Biot respiration	Rapid, deep respiration followed by apnea	CNS injury or infection
Apneustic respiration	Long inspiration with short or staccato expiration	Brainstem lesion
Agonal respiration	Slow rate, variable tidal volume	Shock, sepsis, or asphyxia

CNS, Central nervous system.

Having the child take a deep breath and exhale forcefully will accentuate abnormal lung sounds. **Decreased**, **absent**, or **asymmetric breath sounds** may be due to atelectasis, lobar consolidation (e.g., pneumonia), thoracic mass, or a pleural effusion. Observation of respiratory rate, work of breathing, and chest wall motion, combined with percussion and auscultation, help to identify intrathoracic disease (Table 134.4).

Digital clubbing (Fig. 134.3) can be seen in advanced CF as well as less common chronic pulmonary diseases such as interstitial lung disease. Clubbing is not associated with asthma; its presence should heighten concern for other diagnoses. Clubbing may also be present in nonpulmonary chronic diseases (cardiac, gastrointestinal, or hematologic) or, rarely, as a familial trait.

DIAGNOSTIC MEASURES

Imaging Techniques

Chest radiographs are useful in assessing respiratory disease in children. In addition to determining lung abnormalities, they provide information about the bony thorax (e.g., rib or vertebral abnormalities), the heart (e.g., cardiomegaly, pericardial effusion), the pleural space, and the great vessels (e.g., right aortic arch/vascular rings, rib notching). Chest radiographs should be obtained in both the posteroanterior (PA) and lateral projections and, if possible, following a full inspiration. Estimation of lung hyperinflation based on a single PA view is unreliable; flattened diaphragms and an increased AP diameter on lateral projection are better indicators of hyperinflation. Increased density on chest radiograph may represent *blood, water, mucus,* or *tissue.* **Expiratory** and **decubitus views** may be useful to detect partial bronchial obstruction due to an aspirated foreign body because the affected lung or lobe does not deflate on exhalation. Decubitus films can also help to differentiate pleural effusion from alveolar infiltrate.

TABLE 134.4 Physical Signs of Pulmonary Disease

DISEASE PROCESS	MEDIASTINAL DEVIATION	CHEST MOTION	VOCAL FREMITUS	PERCUSSION	BREATH SOUNDS	ADVENTITIOUS SOUNDS	VOICE SIGNS
Consolidation	No	Reduced over area	Increased	Dull	Bronchial or reduced	None or crackles	Egophony* Pectoriloquy†
Bronchospasm	No	Hyperexpansion with limited motion	Normal or decreased	Hyperresonant	Normal to decreased	Wheezes, crackles	Normal to decreased
Atelectasis	Shift toward affected side	Reduced over area	Decreased	Dull	Reduced	None or crackles	None
Pneumothorax	With tension: shift to the opposite side	Reduced over PMI	None	Resonant	None	None	None
Pleural effusion	If large: shift to opposite side	Reduced over area	None or reduced	Dull	None	Egophony Friction rub	Muffled
Interstitial process	No	Reduced	Normal to increased	Normal	Normal	Inspiratory crackles	None

*In egophony, e sounds like a (may be a sign of consolidation but also is associated with moderate-sized pleural effusions).
†In pectoriloquy, words/voice sounds clearer over the affected site (associated with consolidation and cavitary lesions).
PMI, Point of maximum impulse.
Modified from Andreoli TE, Bennett JC, Carpenter CJ, et al., eds. Cecil Essentials of Medicine. *4th ed. Philadelphia: WB Saunders; 1997:115.*

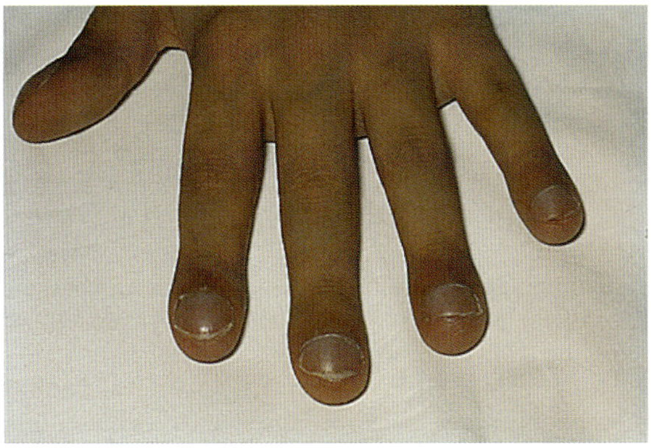

FIGURE 134.3 Clubbing of the fingers. There is increased curvature and loss of nail angle. This child has cystic fibrosis. (From Lissauer T, Clayden G, eds. *Illustrated Textbook of Pediatrics*. 4th ed. London: Mosby; 2012. Fig. 2.6a.)

A **barium esophagram** has value in diagnosing disorders of esophageal motility, vascular rings (esophageal compression), tracheoesophageal fistulas, and, to a lesser extent, gastroesophageal reflux. When evaluating for a tracheoesophageal fistula, contrast material must be instilled under pressure via a catheter with the distal tip situated in the esophagus (see Chapter 129). A **video fluoroscopic swallow study (VFSS)** can be used to diagnose swallowing disorders (dysphagia) or, alternatively, fiberoptic endoscopic evaluation of swallowing (FEES) can be used as a nonradiologic study particularly in infants.

Computed tomography (CT) of the chest is the imaging tool of choice for evaluating masses, interstitial lung disease, and bronchiectasis, as well as delineating pleural from parenchymal lesions. CT scans with intravenous contrast provide excellent information about the pulmonary vasculature and great vessels, allow distinction between adjacent radiodense structures within the mediastinum, characterize congenital pulmonary malformations, and can detect pulmonary embolism. The speed of current CT scanners makes it possible to scan most children without sedating them; sedation may be required in infants and toddlers to decrease motion artifact. **Magnetic resonance imaging (MRI)**, useful in visualizing cardiac and great vessel anatomy and mediastinal lesions, is less useful for evaluation of pulmonary parenchymal lesions. **Ultrasonography** can be used to delineate some intrathoracic masses and identify pneumothoraces and is the imaging procedure of choice for assessing size and character of parapneumonic effusion/empyema. It is also useful for assessing diaphragmatic motion in small children.

Measures of Respiratory Gas Exchange

A properly performed **arterial blood gas** analysis provides information about the effectiveness of both oxygenation and ventilation. Because arterial samples are difficult to obtain, capillary and venous blood samples are more commonly used, although they should not be used to assess oxygenation. The partial pressure of carbon dioxide (PCO_2) from a capillary sample is similar to that from arterial blood. The PCO_2 in venous samples is approximately 6 mm Hg higher than arterial PCO_2.

There are both respiratory and metabolic causes of acidosis (see Chapter 36). In the presence of an alkalosis or acidosis, respiratory compensation (altering PCO_2 to maintain a normal pH) can occur within minutes, but renal compensation (altering the serum bicarbonate level) may not be complete for several days. Because both the respiratory and metabolic compensation are incomplete, pH will remain on the side of the primary insult (whether acidosis or alkalosis).

Pulse oximetry measures the O_2 saturation of hemoglobin by measuring the blood absorption of two or more wavelengths of light. It is noninvasive and easy to use and generally reliable outside of several key limitations. Pulse oximetry may not accurately reflect true oxygen saturation in individuals with darker skin pigmentation, when abnormal hemoglobin is present (carboxyhemoglobin, methemoglobin), when perfusion is poor, or if no light passes through to the photodetector (e.g., nail polish). Given the sigmoidal shape of the oxyhemoglobin dissociation curve, O_2 saturation does not change significantly until the partial pressure of oxygen (PO_2) drops below approximately 60 mm Hg.

The measurement of PCO_2 is accomplished most reliably by blood gas analysis. There are noninvasive monitors that record exhaled PCO_2 **(end-tidal CO_2)**, which is representative of alveolar PCO_2. End-tidal PCO_2 measurements are most commonly used in intubated and mechanically ventilated patients, but some devices can measure PCO_2 at the nares. **Transcutaneous electrodes** can be used to monitor PCO_2 at the skin surface but are less reliable. Noninvasive techniques of CO_2 measurement are best suited for detecting trends rather than for providing absolute values.

Pulmonary Function Testing

Measurement of lung volumes and airflow rates is important in assessing pulmonary disease. Most children older than 6 years of age can perform **spirometry**. The patient inhales to TLC and then forcibly exhales until no more air can be expelled. During the forced expiratory maneuver, **forced vital capacity (FVC)**, **forced expired volume in the first second (FEV1)**, and **forced expiratory flow (FEF)** rates are measured. These values are compared to predicted values based primarily on patient height but also integrate age and gender. Severity of disease is quantified by *z*-scores as standard deviations from predicted values. The **peak expiratory flow rate (PEFR)** can be obtained with a simple hand-held device and may be useful for home monitoring of older children with asthma; it is *highly dependent on patient effort,* and values must be interpreted with caution. Measurement of **TLC**, **FRC**, and **RV** require **body plethysmography**. Helium dilution can also measure TLC and RV by determining the magnitude of dilution of inhaled helium in the air within the lung but may underestimate air trapping.

Abnormal results on pulmonary function testing can be used to categorize **obstructive** (low flow rates and/or increased RV) or **restrictive lung disease** (low FVC and TLC, with relative preservation of flow rates). When the FEV_1 is decreased to a greater extent than the FVC (**FEV1:FVC ratio** <80%), obstructive lung disease is diagnosed. The mean midexpiratory flow rate **($FEF_{25-75\%}$)** is a more sensitive measure of small airway disease than the FEV_1 but is also more variable. Spirometry can detect reversible airway obstruction characteristic of asthma when a significant improvement in FEV_1 (>12%) or in $FEF_{25-75\%}$ (>25%) following inhalation of a bronchodilator is measured. **Inhalation challenge tests** using methacholine, histamine, or cold, dry air are used to assess airway hyperreactivity; these require sophisticated equipment and special expertise and should only be performed in a pulmonary function laboratory with experienced technicians.

Endoscopic Evaluation of the Airways

Endoscopic evaluation of the upper airways **(nasopharyngoscopy)** is performed with a flexible fiberoptic nasopharyngoscope to assess airway patency, obstruction, and anatomic abnormalities of the nose, pharynx, and supraglottis. It is especially useful in evaluating stridor and is the diagnostic test of choice for assessing vocal cord motion/function as it does not require sedation. Drug-induced sleep endoscopy (DISE) of the upper airway instead occurs with a flexible scope under light anesthesia to guide options for sleep apnea surgical management. Endoscopic evaluation of the subglottic space and intrathoracic airways can be done with either a flexible or rigid bronchoscope under anesthesia. **Flexible bronchoscopy** is useful in identifying dynamic or static airway abnormalities (stenosis, malacia, endobronchial lesions, or excessive secretions) and to obtain airway samples for culture **(bronchoalveolar lavage)**. **Rigid bronchoscopy** is the method of choice for airway instrumentation, such as removing foreign bodies from the lower airways and airway dilation. Transbronchial biopsies are rarely performed in children; this can be pursued through advanced interventional flexible bronchoscopic techniques such as cryotherapy.

Examination of Sputum

Sputum specimens may be useful in evaluating lower respiratory tract infections but are difficult to obtain in children. Specimens containing large numbers of squamous epithelial cells or heavily contaminated with upper airway secretions may yield misleading results. Sputum in patients with lower respiratory tract bacterial infections often contains polymorphonuclear leukocytes and one predominant organism on culture. If sputum cannot be obtained, then bronchoalveolar lavage may be necessary for microbiologic diagnosis in selected situations. In patients with CF who are unable to expectorate sputum, specially processed throat cultures are used as surrogates for lower airway cultures.

Lung Biopsy

When less invasive methods fail to provide diagnoses in patients with pulmonary disease, a lung biopsy may be required. Concern for childhood interstitial lung disease (chILD), atypical infectious diseases (especially in an immunocompromised host), and evaluation of a mass/malformation are the most common indications for biopsy. CT-guided **needle biopsy** performed by an interventional radiologist is an option if limited histology is needed and the lesion is amenable to percutaneous approach (e.g., fungal nodules). Either a **thoracoscopic procedure** or a **thoracotomy** is preferred if thorough histologic evaluation is desired. The need for biopsy to diagnose chILD has decreased with genetic screening *(SFTPB, SFTPC, ABCA3, TTF1, COPA).*

THERAPEUTIC MEASURES

Oxygen Administration

The first treatment for children with hypoxemia is **supplemental oxygen** at a concentration sufficient to maintain *acceptable* O_2 saturation levels. Normal O_2 saturation is greater than 95%; lower saturations may be appropriate in certain clinical scenarios such as preterm birth or congenital heart disease. It is not necessary to achieve 100% saturation and supplementation in excess risks oxidative stress/damage, particularly in susceptible hosts. Patients requiring supplemental O_2 should be monitored with pulse oximetry, intermittently or continuously, or with arterial blood gas measurements of Po_2 to allow titration to the lowest required O_2 concentration. The actual fraction of inspired oxygen **(FiO_2)** delivered to the patient can be quite variable, affected by the delivery device used, device position, the child's size, and respiratory pattern.

For long-term administration of O_2, a **nasal cannula** is the most widely used device, because it enables patients to eat and speak unhindered by the O_2 delivery system. **Humidified high-flow nasal cannula** (HFNC) allows the provider to deliver greater flow rates of blended gas at a specific FiO_2. Depending on the size of the patient, the type of cannula, and device used, HFNC can deliver modest positive pressure, relieve dyspnea, and purge CO_2 from anatomic dead space to improve alveolar ventilation in addition to providing oxygenation. There are limited options for provision of HFNC outside the hospital. Supplemental O_2 may also be delivered by a variety of mask systems including a **simple mask** (delivers O_2 in L/min), a **Venturi mask** (blends to a specific Fio_2), and a **non-rebreather mask** (reservoir provides nearly 100% O_2).

Aerosol Therapy

Therapeutic agents such as bronchodilators, corticosteroids, and antibiotics can be delivered to the lower respiratory tract by **dry powder inhaler** (DPI), **metered-dose inhaler** (MDI), or **nebulizer**. These devices are designed to generate small particles that can bypass upper airway filtration and deposit in the lower airways. Factors influence drug deposition including patient technique, device used, age of the child, and breathing pattern. Nebulizers should be used with a face mask (infants) or mouthpiece (children and teens) to minimize loss of drug to ambient air. Plastic holding chambers **(spacers)** are available for all ages and should always be used with MDIs. DPIs require a single rapid, deep inhalation for optimal drug delivery, which is difficult for children under 6 years of age and those with developmental challenges or neuromuscular disorders. MDIs and nebulizers are equally effective in delivering medications only if the technique is correct; it is crucial to review this frequently and carefully with families (Fig. 134.4).

Chest Physiotherapy and Airway Clearance Techniques

When disease processes impair normal ciliary and cough function, **airway clearance therapy** may help maintain airway patency by mobilizing secretions toward the central airways, from which they can be expectorated. **Chest percussion** or **pneumatic vests** are often used in young or neurologically impaired children, and older children/adolescents with CF often use vests as part of their daily therapy. Older children can operate hand-held devices that generate expiratory back-pressure and vibration (e.g., TheraPEP, Flutter, Acapella, and Aerobika). Children who are too weak to generate an effective cough benefit from the use of a mechanical insufflation-exsufflation device (CoughAssist) in conjunction with chest physiotherapy. Chest physiotherapy may help

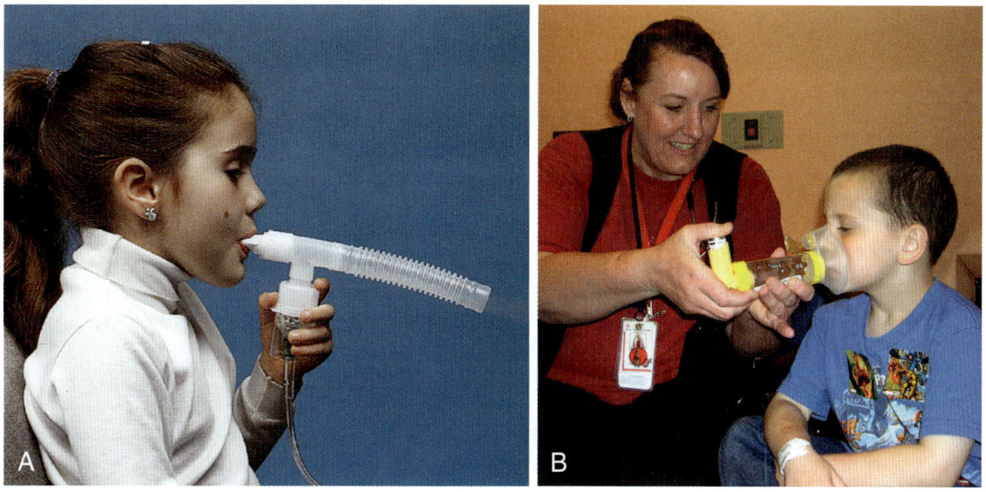

FIGURE 134.4 Inhaled drug delivery in children. **(A)** Proper use of a nebulizer with mouthpiece and **(B)** metered-dose inhaler with spacer and face mask. (A, From Hopper T. *Mosby's Pharmacy Technician*. 2nd ed. St. Louis: Mosby; 2007. Fig. 25.7; B, From Hockenberry MJ, Wilson D, eds. *Wong's Essentials of Pediatric Nursing*. 8th ed. St. Louis: Mosby; 2009. Fig. 23.5.)

with atelectasis; it is generally less beneficial for patients with asthma or pneumonia.

Intubation

If the upper airway is obstructed or mechanical ventilation is needed, it may be necessary to provide the patient with an **artificial airway**. This is best done by placing an endotracheal tube via the mouth or nose into the trachea **(intubation)**. **Endotracheal tubes** can damage the larynx and the airways if the tubes are of improper size and not carefully maintained. Because the cricoid ring is the narrowest segment of a child's airway and surrounded by cartilage, it is vulnerable to damage. Pressure created by the tube against the airway mucosa risks reactive subglottic stenosis and even mucosal ischemia/necrosis when the pressure exceeds capillary filling pressure. Therefore a small air leak should always be maintained around the endotracheal tube to minimize this risk. No clear, universally accepted guidelines are available regarding how long pediatric patients can be intubated without sustaining airway damage or when conversion to tracheostomy is indicated.

Intubation can negatively impact the physiology of the respiratory tract. It interferes with the humidification, warming, and filtration of inspired air and stimulates secretion production. Providing adequate humidification of inspired air and appropriate suctioning of the tube reduces the probability of occlusion by secretions. Alternatively, **laryngeal mask airway (LMA)** can be used to provide mechanical ventilation. This device consists of a tube with a soft mask at the distal end that is placed over the larynx, creating a seal without the trachea being instrumented. Although less invasive, the LMA is less secure, so its use is generally limited to procedural anesthesia.

Tracheostomy

Tracheostomy is the surgical placement of an artificial airway into the trachea below the larynx. The most common indication for tracheostomy in children is the ability to deliver mechanical ventilation for children with cardiopulmonary and neurologic indications; congenital or acquired upper airway obstruction may also be indications (see Chapter 136). If prolonged invasive mechanical ventilation is required or patients are reliant on near-continuous noninvasive positive pressure ventilation, elective tracheostomy can be performed to increase patient comfort, provide stable pressure delivery, and facilitate nursing care. Children with tracheostomy tubes can be cared for at home, provided the caregivers are well trained and adequately equipped. The tracheostomy tube can hamper the ability to phonate. More importantly, it can become accidentally dislodged or occluded with secretions, leading to life threatening airway obstruction, prompting recommendation for close monitoring by a trained caregiver.

Mechanical Ventilation

Patients who are unable to maintain adequate gas exchange may require **mechanical ventilation**. Most modes of mechanical ventilation involve inflation of the lungs with gas using positive pressure. The inspiratory phase is active (air is pushed in), and exhalation is passive.

Mechanical ventilation often requires an artificial airway, although it can be provided *noninvasively* via nasal or oronasal masks. **Noninvasive ventilation** is particularly useful in patients with obstructive sleep apnea and neuromuscular disease who require support only part of the day or night, but it can also be used to assist ventilation continuously for patients in acute respiratory failure from a variety of causes.

No method of mechanical ventilation perfectly simulates natural breathing. All methods have drawbacks and potential complications. Positive pressure is transmitted to the entire thorax and may impede venous return to the heart. The airways and lung parenchyma may be damaged by inflation pressures and high concentrations of inspired O_2. In general, inflation pressures should be limited to those necessary to provide sufficient lung expansion for adequate ventilation and the prevention of atelectasis. Pressure-cycled and volume-cycled ventilators (conventional ventilation) are the most widely used modalities in pediatrics. High-frequency jet ventilation and high-frequency oscillatory ventilation are used often in neonatology and may be used in patients with severe lung disease who are failing conventional mechanical ventilation.

PEARLS FOR PRACTITIONERS

See The Respiratory System: Pearls for Practitioners at the end of this section.

REVIEW QUESTIONS

Available online.

CHAPTER 135

Control of Breathing

Intrinsic respiratory drive is controlled by three distinct neuronal groups in the medulla and pons that coordinate to form the "pacemaker" of respiration. This rhythm is modulated by input from central and peripheral signals. **Central chemoreceptors** located throughout the brain respond to intracellular pH and Pco_2 levels (Fig. 135.1). **Peripheral receptors** located in the carotid and aortic bodies respond predominantly to changes in Po_2. Small acute changes in $Paco_2$ can result in significant changes in **minute ventilation**. The ventilatory drive response is blunted when the Pco_2 is chronically elevated, because the intracellular pH returns to normal levels following compensatory increases in the serum bicarbonate level. The peripheral receptors do not stimulate ventilation until the Pao_2 decreases to approximately 70 mm Hg (compared to normal Pao_2 of 100 mm Hg at sea level). These receptors become important in patients with chronic $Paco_2$ elevation who may have a blunted ventilatory response to CO_2. Mechanoreceptors in the thorax provide additional input to respiratory control.

The output of the central respiratory center can be modulated by reflex mechanisms. Full lung inflation temporarily inhibits inspiratory effort in infants **(Hering-Breuer reflex)** through vagal afferent fibers. Other reflexes from the airways and intercostal muscles may influence the depth and frequency of respiratory efforts (see Fig. 135.1).

APNEA

Etiology

Apnea is defined as the cessation of airflow due to either lack of respiratory effort **(central apnea)** or upper airway obstruction **(obstructive apnea)** (Table 135.1). Central apnea is more common in infants, whereas obstructive apnea, especially during sleep, is more common in older children.

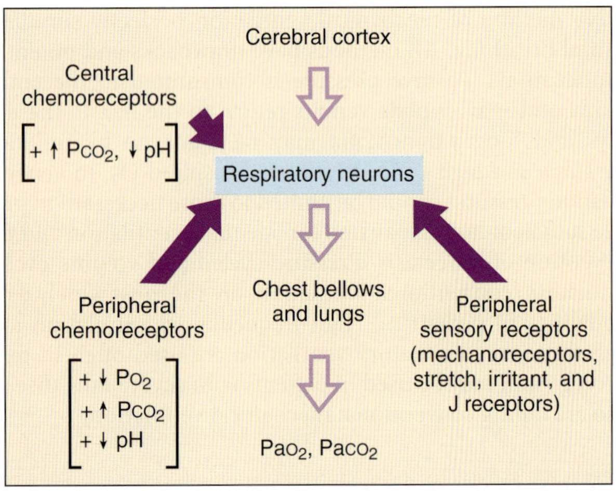

FIGURE 135.1 Schematic representation of the respiratory control system. The respiratory neurons in the brainstem receive information from the chemoreceptors, peripheral sensory receptors, and cerebral cortex. This information is integrated, and the resulting neural output is transmitted to the diaphragms and lungs. The sign denotes stimulation of the receptor. *J receptors*, Juxtacapillary receptors. (From Andreoli TE, Bennett JC, Carpenter CJ, et al., eds. *Cecil Essentials of Medicine*. 4th ed. Philadelphia: WB Saunders; 1997:171.)

Occasional central apnea lasting less than 10 seconds is common in healthy infants and can be present in normal children during sleep, especially after a sigh breath. Central pauses lasting longer than 15–20 seconds are considered abnormal. Premature infants can have **apnea of prematurity**, which consists of recurrent apneic episodes that are often of central origin, although they can be mixed central/obstructive. Apnea of prematurity should resolve by 44 weeks postconceptional age. Frequent central apnea outside of infancy is a rare occurrence and warrants evaluation.

Congenital central hypoventilation syndrome (CCHS) is a rare genetic disorder in which there is profound loss of respiratory control during sleep leading to primary central apnea, hypercarbia, and hypoxemia. Individuals with CCHS have a defect in the *PHOX2B* gene, which is necessary for autonomic nervous system development. Infants with CCHS most often have respiratory difficulties within the first several weeks of life, although it can also present later in childhood. Some *PHOX2B* pathologic variant types are associated with an increased risk of Hirschsprung disease and neural crest tumors (neuroblastoma). Other syndromes associated with abnormal central respiratory control include Rett, Joubert, and Prader-Willi syndromes and tuberous sclerosis complex. Secondary causes of central apnea and hypoventilation are more common and include medications impairing central respiratory drive (e.g., narcotics), increased intracranial pressure, central nervous system (CNS) tumors, myelomeningocele and/or Chiari malformation, and mitochondrial/metabolic disorders.

Breath-holding spells are a reflexive form of apnea occurring when a young child is awake, usually triggered by emotional stress or pain, and may be related to underlying autonomic dysfunction. Breath-holding spells usually occur in children under 3 years of age during periods of agitation or crying and can be associated with cyanosis and loss of consciousness. The return of spontaneous breathing usually occurs quickly. Most breath-holding spells are benign and lessen over time, but differential diagnoses of seizures and disorders of central respiratory control should be considered. Treatment of iron deficiency, when present, may partially or completely resolve frequency of spells.

Obstructive sleep apnea syndrome (OSA) affects 2–5% of young children, with peak prevalence at 2–8 years of age. It is caused by complete or partial upper airway obstruction during sleep. Respiratory drive is usually preserved, although infants and others with immature respiratory control may have obstructive and central apnea together. Restless sleep, behavioral problems, and inattention/hyperactivity are more common in young children than the classic adult findings of daytime hypersomnolence and loud snoring. Some children experience poor somatic growth due to interruption of normal growth hormone production during deep sleep. A small subset can have significant hypoxemia and hypercarbia leading to morning headaches and, if untreated, pulmonary hypertension and *cor pulmonale*. Not all children who snore have OSA, and not all children who have OSA snore. Thus, when the diagnosis is in question, it should be confirmed with a **polysomnogram** (PSG).

PSG is the definitive test for evaluation of obstructive and central sleep apnea. PSG involves continuous recording of electroencephalogram (EEG) and electrooculogram for sleep staging, oronasal airflow and pressure, audible snore, chest and abdominal wall excursion, leg and chin electromyogram,

TABLE 135.1 Categories of Apnea

DISEASE	RISK FACTORS	MECHANISM	SIGNS	TREATMENT
Apnea of prematurity	Prematurity (<36 wk corrected gestational age)	Immature central control, upper airway obstruction	Apnea, bradycardia	Caffeine, HFNC, CPAP, intubation
Central apnea/ hypoventilation	CCHS, Chiari malformation	Abnormal central control	Apnea	Mechanical ventilation or BiPAP
Obstructive sleep apnea	Adenotonsillar hypertrophy, obesity, Pierre Robin sequence, trisomy 21, cerebral palsy	Upper airway obstruction due to excess tissue, loss of pharyngeal tone, or crowded anatomy	Snoring, restless sleep, poor school performance, behavior problems, open-mouth breathing	Adenotonsillectomy, CPAP or BiPAP, sleep endoscopy–directed surgery, tracheostomy
Breath-holding spells	Iron deficiency, age <5 years, family history	Prolonged expiratory apnea; may involve dysfunction of the autonomic nervous system	Cyanosis, syncope, less commonly can see posturing or seizure activity after prolonged spells	Reassurance; condition is self-limiting. Must exclude seizure disorder

BiPAP, Bilevel positive airway pressure; *CCHS,* congenital central hypoventilation syndrome; *CPAP,* continuous positive airway pressure; *HFNC,* high flow nasal cannula.

electrocardiogram, pulse oximetry, and capnography. The most reported metric from a PSG is the **apnea-hypopnea index** (AHI) or number of times in an hour of sleep that the child has cessation or reduction of airflow of a significant magnitude to negatively affect oxygenation or sleep continuity. An obstructive AHI less than 1–2 is the generally accepted norm for pediatric patients, although the decision to treat often hinges on the severity of daytime impairment. Measured AHI is worse in rapid eye movement (REM) sleep and when the child is supine, so an ideal study captures all sleep stages and positions.

Adenotonsillar hypertrophy is the most common cause of OSA in otherwise healthy young children, with peak age 2–5 years. Other risk factors for OSA include obesity/increased body mass index, premature birth, craniofacial differences, trisomy 21, and neuromuscular diseases. The decision to treat is dependent on severity of daytime and nighttime symptoms as well as likelihood of spontaneous resolution with time, which is affected by obesity/increased body mass index and age at time of diagnosis. OSA may improve with the treatment of underlying respiratory conditions such as allergic rhinitis or asthma. Targeted treatment of OSA starts with determining whether the child will benefit from adenotonsillectomy. If surgical intervention is not indicated or fails to alleviate the problem, then the use of continuous positive airway pressure **(CPAP)** or bilevel positive airway pressure **(BiPAP)** via mask interfaces can be used to distend the upper airway during sleep. This requires a well-fitting mask, which may not be well tolerated in young children. Supplemental oxygen can blunt hypoxemia in milder cases of OSA but does not alter obstruction and sleep fragmentation. In extreme cases, especially those associated with craniofacial abnormalities or hypotonia, tracheostomy may be indicated.

BRIEF RESOLVED UNEXPLAINED EVENTS

A **brief resolved unexplained event (BRUE)** is defined as a short (usually <1 minute), self-limited episode with one or more of the following features: (1) cyanosis or pallor, (2) absent or irregular breathing, (3) change in tone, or (4) altered level of responsiveness in an infant under 1 year of age. The label BRUE should be used only when no other explanation for the event is identified with detailed history and physical examination. History and exam should focus on the most common identifiable causes of abnormal breathing episodes in infancy including gastroesophageal reflux, CNS pathology (seizures, intracranial bleeding from accidental or nonaccidental trauma), and respiratory disease (respiratory syncytial virus [RSV], pertussis, and pneumonia). Cardiovascular events (arrhythmia) and metabolic abnormalities are among diagnoses that may not be recognized on initial history and examination; these are uncommon.

Infants over 2 months of age and born at term or born at more than 32 weeks' gestation and currently 45 weeks gestational age who experience a single, brief (<1 minute), self-limited (no cardiopulmonary resuscitation [CPR] required) BRUE, with no concerning findings on exam or history, are considered at *low risk* for undiagnosed serious condition or repeat event. An electrocardiogram and pertussis screening may be considered in this low-risk group. Additional diagnostic tests (e.g., metabolic panel, complete blood count, imaging, PSG, and EEG) and hospital admission for cardiorespiratory monitoring are not recommended. Offering parents infant CPR instruction and attempting to alleviate anxiety surrounding the event are recommended. There is no consensus on evaluation and management of infants with BRUE who do not meet the *low-risk* criteria listed above, though there are unvalidated published frameworks for evaluation of these higher risk infants. Careful history and physical examination should be used to guide differential diagnosis and assessment. Cardiorespiratory monitoring for 12–24 hours in the hospital can provide more detailed information on respiratory and cardiac patterns while allowing time to gather additional history and perform repeat examinations. The evaluation can also occur in a coordinated manner in the outpatient setting, with a focus of the initial evaluation prioritizing time-sensitive conditions (i.e., nonaccidental trauma, cardiac arrhythmias, serious bacterial infections). Unless the clinical suspicion of OSA is high, PSG is not considered a useful tool for infants presenting with BRUE.

SUDDEN INFANT DEATH SYNDROME

Etiology and Epidemiology

Sudden infant death syndrome (SIDS) is defined as the *unexpected* death of an infant younger than 1 year of age in which

TABLE 135.2 Differential Diagnosis of Sudden Unexpected Infant Death

INFECTIOUS DISEASE
Fulminant infection*,† Infant botulism*
NEUROLOGIC
Seizure disorder† Brain tumor* Intracranial hemorrhage due to accidental or nonaccidental trauma*,† Drug intoxication‡
METABOLIC
Hypoglycemia† Medium-chain acyl-coenzyme A dehydrogenase deficiency† Carnitine deficiency*,† Urea cycle defect‡
RESPIRATORY
Laryngospasm Accidental suffocation† Hemosiderosis/pulmonary hemorrhage syndrome
CARDIOVASCULAR
Cardiac arrhythmia Congenital heart disease*
GASTROINTESTINAL
Gastroesophageal reflux*,† Midgut volvulus/shock*
OTHER
Sudden infant death syndrome

**Obvious or suspected at autopsy.*
†Relatively common.
‡Diagnostic test required.

the cause remains *unexplained* after autopsy, death scene investigation, and review of clinical history. The risk of SIDS is higher in male, premature, and low birthweight infants. Risk factors also include sleeping position, low socioeconomic status, and exposure to tobacco/alcohol/illicit drugs. The risk of SIDS is increased three- to fivefold in siblings of infants who have died of SIDS and is highest during the winter. SIDS is rare before 4 weeks or after 6 months of age and is most common between 2 and 4 months. The incidence of SIDS has decreased dramatically since the 1980s, largely due to the **back-to-sleep** campaign and modifications to infant sleep environments.

Proposed mechanisms for SIDS include cellular brainstem abnormalities and maturational delay related to neural or cardiorespiratory control; the exact mechanism of SIDS is unknown. Prone (chest down) position during sleep and exposure to maternal smoking both alter heart rate variability and arousal response, which may contribute to the risk of SIDS. A portion of SIDS deaths may be due to prolongation of the Q-T interval, abnormal CNS control of respiration, and CO_2 rebreathing from sleeping face down (especially in soft bedding). Importantly, there is no association between BRUE and SIDS.

Differential Diagnosis

Sudden unexpected infant death (SUID) is a term to describe any sudden and unexpected death occurring in the first year of life without an obvious cause before further investigation; this term includes those deaths caused by SIDS as well as those with subsequently identified explanation. See Table 135.2 for the differential diagnosis of SUIDs, including SIDS.

Prevention

SIDS is associated with prone position during sleep, especially with soft bedding, excessive bundling, and bed sharing. There has been a significant decline in SIDS with the back-to-sleep program and avoiding soft bedding. Thus all caregivers should be instructed to place their infants in the supine position (on their backs/chest up) unless there are medical contraindications. All loose, soft bedding should be excluded from the sleep space, and parents who share beds with their infants should be counseled on the risks, especially if consuming alcohol or sedating medications. Counseling for cessation of maternal cigarette smoking, both during and after pregnancy, is recommended. Breast-feeding, pacifier use, and sharing a room (in separate beds) have been identified as protective. There can be cultural and intergenerational factors that shape families' sleeping arrangements; understanding this context can help to provide appropriate and supportive guidance.

There are commercial devices marketed for SIDS prevention, such as sleep positioners and home oximeters, though none have been proven to reduce SIDS risk. PSG, home oximetry, and home cardiorespiratory monitoring are not helpful in predicting risk or preventing SIDS and should not be recommended for this purpose.

PEARLS FOR PRACTITIONERS

See The Respiratory System: Pearls for Practitioners at the end of this section.

REVIEW QUESTIONS

Available online.

CHAPTER 136
Upper Airway Obstruction

ETIOLOGY

Upper airway obstruction (UAO), which is defined as blockage of any part of the airway located above the thoracic inlet, ranges from nasal obstruction due to the common cold to life-threatening obstruction of the larynx or upper trachea. In children, nasal obstruction is usually more of a nuisance than a danger because the mouth can serve as an airway, but it may be a serious problem for neonates, who breathe predominantly through the nose. The differential diagnosis of airway obstruction varies with patient age and can be subdivided into **supraglottic**, **glottic**, and **subglottic** causes, with acute and subacute presentations (Tables 136.1, 136.2, and 136.3).

CLINICAL MANIFESTATIONS

UAO is more pronounced during inspiration because the negative pressure generated collapses the upper airway, increasing

TABLE 136.1 Age-Related Differential Diagnosis of Subacute Upper Airway Obstruction
NEWBORN
Choanal atresia Rhinitis neonatorum Micrognathia (Pierre Robin syndrome, Treacher Collins syndrome, DiGeorge syndrome) Macroglossia (Beckwith-Wiedemann syndrome, hypothyroidism, glycogen storage disease type II [GSD-II or Pompe disease], trisomy 21) Pharyngeal collapse Laryngeal web Vocal cord paralysis/paresis (idiopathic, birth trauma, or central nervous system pathology) Congenital subglottic stenosis Nasal encephalocele
INFANT
Chronic or recurrent rhinitis (infection, acid reflux, irritant) Laryngomalacia Subglottic stenosis (congenital or acquired; e.g., after intubation) Laryngeal web or cyst Laryngeal papillomatosis Airway hemangioma Vascular rings/slings
TODDLER
Chronic or recurrent rhinitis (infection, allergy, irritant) Hypertrophied tonsils and adenoids Croup (laryngotracheobronchitis) Laryngeal papillomatosis Vascular rings/slings
OLDER CHILDREN
Chronic or recurrent rhinitis (infection, allergic, irritants) Hypertrophied tonsils and adenoids (most common) Paradoxical vocal fold movement Infectious mononucleosis

resistance and turbulence of airflow that creates an inspiratory noise. Children with UAO may have increased inspiratory work of breathing manifested by **suprasternal retractions**. The respiratory noise most commonly associated with UAO is **stridor**, a harsh sound caused by the vibration of the airway structures. Stridor often decreases during sleep because of lower inspiratory flow rates and increases during feeding, excitement, and agitation because of higher flow rates. Occasionally stridor may also be present on exhalation. Hoarseness or aphonia with stridor suggests **vocal cord** involvement. **Stertor** is a low-pitched sound like a snore and suggests dynamic collapse of pharyngeal soft tissue structures.

DIAGNOSTIC STUDIES

Radiographic evaluation of a child with stridor is rarely helpful. On anteroposterior (AP) views of the neck taken with the head in extension, the subglottic space should be symmetrical with diameter continuing to increase down to the mid-trachea. Asymmetry suggests subglottic stenosis or a mass lesion, tapering suggests subglottic edema; these findings may be subtle. In a child with stertor or snoring, lateral views of the neck and nasopharynx may provide information about tonsil or adenoid hypertrophy. Computed tomography (CT) scans of the upper airway can help delineate the site of the obstruction when a soft tissue mass (e.g., tonsillar abscess) is suspected but may require sedation in younger children. Flexible nasopharyngoscopy/laryngoscopy, which can be done without sedation, is useful in assessing airway patency, the presence of adenoid tissue or vocal cord and other airway lesions, and laryngomalacia.

DIFFERENTIAL DIAGNOSIS

Choanal Stenosis (Atresia)

Choanal stenosis/atresia is a rare congenital problem presenting in the neonatal period; it may be bilateral or unilateral. Neonates are obligate nose breathers, so obstruction of nasal passages can cause significant respiratory distress, especially when feeding. Crying bypasses the obstruction as crying infants breathe through the mouth. Inability to easily pass a small catheter through the nostrils should raise the suspicion of choanal atresia. The diagnosis is confirmed by CT scan or by inspecting the area directly with a flexible nasopharyngoscope. An oral airway may be useful in the short term, but the definitive treatment is surgery.

Croup (Laryngotracheobronchitis)

See Chapter 108.

Epiglottitis

See Chapter 108.

Bacterial Tracheitis

See Chapter 108.

Laryngomalacia

Etiology

Laryngomalacia is due to exaggerated collapse of the supraglottic structures, especially the epiglottis and arytenoid cartilages, during inspiration. Laryngomalacia is the most common cause of stridor in infants. It may be due to decreased muscular tone of the larynx and surrounding structures or immature cartilaginous structures. It usually does not result in significant respiratory distress, but occasionally it is severe enough to cause apnea, hypoventilation, hypoxemia, and difficulty feeding.

Clinical Manifestations

The primary sign of laryngomalacia is **inspiratory stridor** with little or no expiratory component. The stridor is loudest when the infant is feeding or active and decreases when the infant is relaxed, placed prone, or when the neck is flexed. Any condition that increases upper airway inflammation will exacerbate laryngomalacia, including viral respiratory infections, dysphagia (swallowing dysfunction), and gastroesophageal reflux. Laryngomalacia peaks by 3–5 months of age and usually resolves between 6 and 12 months of age. Occasionally it can persist in otherwise healthy children up until 24 months of age and even longer in children with underlying conditions, especially those with neurologic diseases affecting control of upper airway muscles.

Diagnostic Studies

For infants with presumed laryngomalacia, the diagnosis can be tentatively established with history and physical

TABLE 136.2 Common Causes of Acute Upper Airway Obstruction

DIAGNOSIS	AGE	HISTORY	EXAM	RADIOGRAPH FINDINGS AND LABS	TREATMENT
INFECTIOUS					
Croup (parainfluenza and other viruses)	6 mo–3 yr	Fever, URI	Nontoxic, stridor, barky cough, hoarse	Steeple sign	Aerosolized epinephrine, systemic steroids, cool mist
Epiglottitis (*Streptococcus pneumoniae, Haemophilus influenzae*; respiratory viruses)	2–6 yr	High fever, rapid onset, no cough, unable to swallow	Toxic, agitated, tripod sitting, drooling, stridor	Thumb sign Leukocytosis	Intubation, antibiotics
Bacterial tracheitis (*Staphylococcus aureus, Moraxella catarrhalis)*	Any age	High fever, rapid onset, no URI symptoms	Toxic, anxious, ±stridor, ±cough	Ragged tracheal border Leukocytosis	Intubation, antibiotics
Retropharyngeal abscess (*S. aureus*, group A strep, oral anaerobes)	<6 yr	Fever, insidious onset, sore throat, no URI/cough	Ill-appearing, drooling, arched neck, inflamed pharynx	Thickened retropharyngeal space; better visualized on CT Leukocytosis	Antibiotics, surgical drainage
Peritonsillar abscess (group A strep, oral anaerobes)	>8 yr	Fever, sudden worsening, sore throat, trismus	Ill-appearing, "hot potato" voice, drooling, asymmetric tonsil swelling	Imaging not required Leukocytosis	Antibiotics, surgical drainage
NONINFECTIOUS					
Angioedema	Any age	No fever, sudden onset, urticarial, facial swelling, ±allergen exposure	Nontoxic (unless anaphylaxis), ±stridor, hoarse, facial edema	Steeple sign	Aerosolized or intramuscular epinephrine, systemic steroids, antihistamines
Spasmodic croup	6 mo–6 yr	Sudden onset, no fever/URI, recurrent, often nocturnal	Nontoxic, ±stridor, hoarse, barky cough	Often normal	Aerosolized epinephrine, antihistamines, antacids, systemic steroids
Foreign body	6 mo–5 yr	Sudden onset, cough, and choke	Nontoxic, anxious, stridor, aphonic, brassy cough	Radiopaque object may be seen	Rigid bronchoscopy

CT, Computed tomography; *URI*, upper respiratory tract infection (with coryza, sneezing).

TABLE 136.3 Differentiating Supraglottic From Subglottic Causes of Acute Airway Obstruction

FEATURE	SUPRAGLOTTIC OBSTRUCTION	SUBGLOTTIC OBSTRUCTION
Common clinical syndromes	Epiglottitis, peritonsillar and retropharyngeal abscess	Croup, angioedema, foreign body, bacterial tracheitis
Stridor	Quiet	Loud
Voice	Muffled	Hoarse
Dysphagia	Yes	No
Tripod or arching posture	Yes	No
Barking cough	No	Yes
Toxic	Yes	No, unless tracheitis
Trismus	Some	No
Drooling	Yes	No

Modified from Davis H, Gartner JC, Galvis AG, et al. Acute upper airway obstruction: croup and epiglottitis. Pediatr Clin North Am. *1981;28:859–880.*

examination. If the patient follows the typical course for laryngomalacia, no further work-up is necessary. To confirm the diagnosis, which is important in more severe or atypical cases, the patient should undergo flexible nasopharyngoscopy to assess the patency and dynamic movement (collapse) of the larynx and surrounding structures. This procedure can also identify vocal cord abnormalities and airway lesions above the vocal cords.

Treatment

In most cases, no therapy is required for laryngomalacia. The infant should be observed closely during times of respiratory viral infections for evidence of respiratory compromise. Medical management for moderate to severe laryngomalacia may include acid suppression for those infants with suspected gastroesophageal reflux, feeding therapy, and optimization of nutritional status. Infants with severe laryngomalacia resulting in hypoventilation, hypoxia, or growth failure may benefit from a surgical procedure (e.g., supraglottoplasty) or, in extreme cases, a tracheostomy to bypass the upper airway.

Subglottic Stenosis

Etiology

Subglottic stenosis is the narrowing of the portion of the trachea immediately below the vocal cords. It may be congenital but more often is acquired. Endotracheal intubation, especially prolonged or repeated intubation in premature infants, can lead to inflammation and scarring of the subglottic space.

Clinical Manifestations

Subglottic stenosis may present as stridor that is **biphasic** (on both inspiration and expiration) but usually is more prominent on inspiration. With increasing respiratory effort, the stridor becomes louder. Very small infants may not be able to breathe with enough force to generate a sound. Subglottic stenosis may also be associated with a barky cough similar to that noted with croup. Respiratory infections can cause subglottic edema, exacerbating the clinical manifestations of subglottic stenosis.

Diagnostic Studies

Definitive diagnosis requires endoscopic evaluation, by either flexible or rigid bronchoscopy.

Treatment

Mild subglottic stenosis can be managed conservatively and may improve sufficiently with airway growth alone. More severe cases require surgical intervention. A tracheostomy tube may be required to bypass the subglottic space until the airway is patent enough to allow adequate airflow.

Mass Lesions

Upper airway mass lesions are relatively uncommon in pediatrics. The most common laryngeal tumor in childhood is the **hemangioma**, which usually presents before 6 months of age, is benign, and is often able to be treated medically (see Chapter 195). Definitive diagnosis requires endoscopy, though imaging (CT angiography, MRI) can also be helpful to better describe extensive lesions. If the obstruction is severe, a tracheostomy tube may be needed until the lesion spontaneously involutes or improves with therapy.

Laryngeal webs are either the result of failed recanalization of the glottic airway in utero or secondary to airway trauma (intubation, traumatic injury, prior surgical manipulation). **Laryngeal cysts** most often occur due to airway trauma but can also be congenital. Laryngeal webs can present during infancy with a weak or high-pitched cry with respiratory distress. Both laryngeal webs and laryngeal cysts can produce biphasic stridor and are best identified by bronchoscopy.

Recurrent respiratory papillomatosis (also called **juvenile laryngeal papillomatosis**) is a rare condition of benign tumors caused by human papillomavirus (HPV, most commonly HPV-6 or HPV-11) acquired at birth via vertical transmission from maternal genital warts. Clinical manifestations can start in infancy and include biphasic stridor and hoarse voice/cry. The lesions are most commonly located in the larynx, but they can spread distally into the trachea, large bronchi, and even the lung parenchyma. Treatment options, which are rarely curative, include laser therapy, surgery, and interferon. Tracheostomy may be required to ensure an adequate airway but should be avoided if possible as there is risk of seeding of the distal airways with tumor.

Foreign Body

Foreign body should be considered in any infant or child capable of ingesting small objects who develops acute onset of stridor. Foreign bodies can lodge in the upper airway or in the lower airways (see Chapter 137).

Vocal Cord Paralysis

Etiology

Vocal cord paralysis is an important cause of laryngeal dysfunction. Paralysis may be unilateral or bilateral and is more often caused by damage to the recurrent laryngeal nerve than by a central lesion. The left recurrent laryngeal nerve passes around the aortic arch and is more susceptible to damage than the right laryngeal nerve. Peripheral nerve injury may be caused by trauma (neck traction during delivery of infants or thoracic surgical procedures) and mediastinal lesions. Central causes include Arnold-Chiari malformation, meningomyelocele, hydrocephalus, and intracranial hemorrhage. There are also congenital and idiopathic cases.

Clinical Manifestations

Vocal cord paralysis often presents as biphasic stridor and alterations in voice and cry, including a weak cry (in infants), hoarseness, and aphonia. Children with vocal cord paralysis are at risk for aspiration, often manifested as coughing/choking with drinking and coarse airway sounds audibly and by auscultation.

Diagnostic Studies

Diagnosis can be confirmed via nasopharyngoscopy in a spontaneously breathing, ideally awake, patient.

Treatment

Patients with traumatic injury to the recurrent laryngeal nerve often have spontaneous improvement over time, usually within

3–6 months. If the paralyzed vocal cord has not recovered within 1 year of the injury, it is likely to be permanently damaged. In some cases, injection of biocompatible material into a paralyzed vocal cord can reposition the cord to improve phonation and airway protection. In cases of bilateral vocal cord paralysis, surgical lateralization of one or both cords may be necessary for breathing, though this increases the risk of aspiration. Patients with vocal cord paralysis resulting in severe airway obstruction and aspiration may require tracheostomy tube placement. Patients with vocal cord paralysis are at higher risk for descending aspiration and should be evaluated by a video fluoroscopic swallow study (VFSS) to assess safety for oral feeding.

Adenoidal and Tonsillar Hypertrophy

Etiology

One of the most common causes of chronic UAO in normal children is hypertrophy of the adenoids and tonsils. Adenoidal and tonsillar hyperplasia may be aggravated by recurrent viral or bacterial infections, allergy, and inhaled irritants.

Clinical Manifestations

The signs of adenoidal and tonsillar hypertrophy are open-mouth breathing, snoring, and, in some patients, obstructive sleep apnea (see Chapter 135). The eustachian tubes enter the nasopharynx at the choanae and can be obstructed by enlarged adenoids, predisposing to recurrent or persistent otitis media.

Diagnostic Studies

Adenoidal hypertrophy is assessed by a lateral radiograph of the nasopharynx or by flexible nasopharyngoscopy.

Treatment

If the adenoids or tonsils are large and thought to be significantly contributing to UAO, the most effective treatment is removal. Because the adenoids are not a discrete organ but rather consist of lymphoid tissue, regrowth is possible, especially in preschool-age children. Refractory OSA is less common after adenotonsillectomy than adenoidectomy or tonsillectomy alone.

PEARLS FOR PRACTITIONERS

See The Respiratory System: Pearls for Practitioners at the end of this section.

REVIEW QUESTIONS

Available online.

CHAPTER 137

Lower Airway, Parenchymal, and Pulmonary Vascular Diseases

ETIOLOGY

There are several causes of lower airway diseases (Table 137.1). Lower airway diseases often result in airway obstruction. The most common chronic lower airway disease in children is **asthma**, which results in variable and recurring symptoms, diffuse bronchial obstruction from airway inflammation, and hyperresponsiveness of bronchial smooth muscle leading to airway constriction. Viral-induced wheezing episodes are common, especially in children under 3 years of age. Wheezing that is localized to one area of the chest suggests focal airway obstruction (e.g., foreign body aspiration or extrinsic compression).

TABLE 137.1 Causes of Wheezing in Childhood

ACUTE
Asthma
Exercise-induced asthma
Hypersensitivity reactions
Infection (e.g., acute bronchospasm with viral illness, bronchiolitis)
Inhalation of irritant gases or particulates
Descending aspiration
Foreign body (airway or esophageal)
Aspiration of gastric contents (ascending aspiration)
CHRONIC OR RECURRENT
Asthma
Hypersensitivity reactions, allergic bronchopulmonary aspergillosis (seen in children with either asthma or cystic fibrosis)
Vocal cord dysfunction
Recurrent aspiration/swallowing dysfunction (dysphagia)
Retained foreign body
Gastroesophageal reflux
Bronchopulmonary dysplasia
Bronchitis, bronchiectasis
Cystic fibrosis
Primary ciliary dyskinesia
Bronchiolitis obliterans
Pulmonary edema (congestive heart failure)
Bronchomalacia/tracheomalacia
Vascular ring
Pulmonary artery dilatation (absent pulmonary valve)
Bronchial or pulmonary cysts/masses
Enlarged lymph nodes (tuberculosis, lymphoma)
Endobronchial masses/tumors (carcinoid)
Bronchial or tracheal stenosis
Cardiomegaly

CLINICAL MANIFESTATIONS

A **wheeze** is a continuous sound that is produced by vibration of airway walls and generally has a more musical quality than stridor. In contrast to upper airway obstruction, obstruction below the thoracic inlet causes more wheezing on expiration than on inspiration. Intrathoracic pressure is increased relative to atmospheric pressure during exhalation, which results in collapse of the intrathoracic airways and accentuates airway narrowing on expiration. Expiratory airflow through these obstructed intrathoracic airways leads to wheeze, prolonged expiratory phase, and increased abdominal work of breathing. In patients with chronic airway infection (e.g., cystic fibrosis), the bronchi become permanently damaged and dilated (bronchiectasis). Patients with bronchiectasis have episodes of cough, often productive of purulent sputum, and may have inspiratory crackles.

DIAGNOSTIC STUDIES

When asthma is suspected, empiric trials of therapy are useful in arriving at a diagnosis; most commonly these include bronchodilators, short courses of oral corticosteroids, and use of inhaled corticosteroids. In children older than 6 years, **pulmonary function tests (spirometry)** can assess airflow obstruction and response to bronchodilators. **Radiographic evaluation** is not needed with each episode of wheezing, but those with significant respiratory distress, fever, history consistent with foreign body aspiration, or focal auscultatory findings should have posteroanterior (PA) and lateral chest radiographs obtained. Generalized *hyperinflation,* indicated by flattening of the diaphragms and an increased anteroposterior (AP) chest diameter, suggests diffuse obstruction of the small airways. Localized hyperinflation, especially on expiratory views, suggests localized bronchial obstruction (e.g., foreign body or an anatomic anomaly). Dysphagia leading to aspiration and airway inflammation can present with persistent wheezing. This is best assessed with a **video fluoroscopic swallowing study** or fiberoptic endoscopic evaluation of swallowing. Airway exposure to gastrointestinal contents (e.g., gastroesophageal reflux, tracheoesophageal fistula) may aggravate asthma and lead to wheezing in very young children, especially if it is associated with aspiration. Diagnostic pullback esophagram may be considered to evaluate for tracheoesophageal fistula. Infants with persistent wheezing despite empiric treatment with asthma therapy may benefit from an airway evaluation with **flexible bronchoscopy**.

DIFFERENTIAL DIAGNOSIS

Asthma

See Chapter 79.

Tracheomalacia

Etiology

Tracheomalacia is excessive collapsibility of the trachea due to lack of structural integrity of the tracheal wall (Fig. 137.1). The tracheal cartilaginous rings normally extend through a C-shaped arc of approximately 320 degrees, maintaining the rigidity of the trachea during changes in intrathoracic pressure. Structural cartilaginous changes predisposing to tracheomalacia include malformation, absence, damage, or incomplete extension around the airway circumference, with a resultant widened/broad-based membranous posterior trachea. These abnormalities can result in excessive compliance/collapsibility of the trachea, most pronounced during expiration. Tracheomalacia is the most common tracheal abnormality in infancy and may be congenital (e.g., tracheoesophageal fistula or bony dysplasia syndromes) or acquired (e.g., long-term mechanical ventilation). Tracheomalacia must be differentiated from extrinsic tracheal compression by masses or vascular structures. Localized tracheomalacia may persist after the trachea has been relieved of long-standing extrinsic compression (e.g., after vascular ring repair).

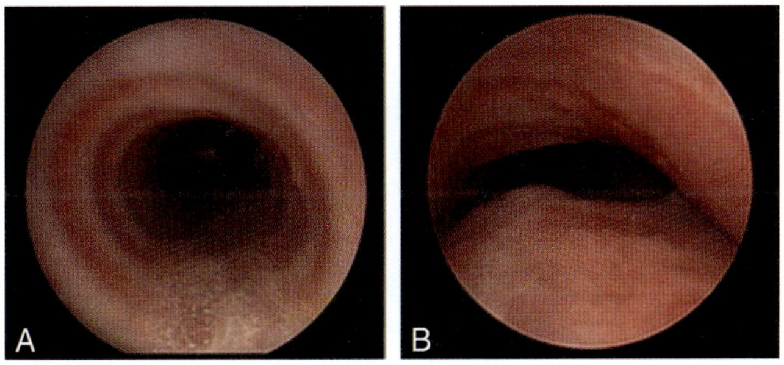

FIGURE 137.1 Normal tracheal anatomy **(A)** and tracheomalacia **(B)** showing loss of anterior tracheal ring integrity and collapse of the tracheal posterior wall membrane. (Courtesy Anne & Robert H. Lurie Children's Hospital of Chicago.)

Clinical Manifestations

With tracheomalacia, tracheal collapse may only be apparent during forced exhalation or with cough. It is commonly aggravated by respiratory infections. This collapse causes a harsh, monophonic wheeze compared to the polyphonic wheeze more often seen in small airway disease (e.g., asthma). Secretions may be retained behind the collapsible segment, predisposing to infection. Infants with severe tracheomalacia may completely collapse the trachea during agitation, resulting in cyanotic episodes that resemble breath-holding spells. The voice is normal, as is inspiratory effort. In older children, the hallmark sign is a brassy, barky cough due to the vibration of the tracheal walls. The expiratory noises of tracheomalacia are often mistakenly ascribed to asthma or bronchiolitis, and the barky cough is often misdiagnosed as croup.

Diagnostic Studies

The diagnosis of tracheomalacia lacks standardized diagnostic criteria, with conflicting universal definitions of severity. Diagnosis is established through a combination of clinical history, physical exam, pulmonary function testing, radiography, and airway endoscopy. Gold standard diagnosis is described as >50% tracheal caliber collapse under direct visualization with dynamic assessment.

Treatment

Infants with mild to moderate tracheomalacia usually require no intervention. Tracheomalacia improves with airway growth as the lumen increases in diameter and the tracheal wall strengthens. The treatment of older symptomatic children is geared toward treating the precipitating cause for cough and providing supportive care. Chest physiotherapy is essential to improve mucociliary clearance, and antibiotics are often necessary to treat concurrent infection. Pharmacotherapy such as muscarinic agonists (e.g., bethanechol) or low-dose ipratropium may be trialed to increase trachealis tone. Bronchodilators such as β-agonists can exacerbate collapsibility by decreasing central smooth airway tone.

Children, especially infants, with severe tracheomalacia may require tracheostomy tubes to administer continuous positive airway pressure (CPAP), which serves to stent open the airway. Custom-length tracheostomy tubes can be used to bypass the site of collapse if sufficiently proximal to the carina. Surgical techniques such as slide tracheoplasty may benefit short segments of severe malacia. Aortopexy has been used to limit the role of anterior collapse. Surgically placed airway stents can be problematic in children because airway stents may erode and migrate, do not grow with children, and serve as a source of fixed stenosis and obstruction. Three-dimensional printed absorbable airway external splints and internal stents can be used for severe pediatric tracheomalacia.

Tracheoesophageal Fistula

See Chapter 129.

Extrinsic Tracheal Compression

Compression of the trachea by vascular structures or masses can cause significant respiratory compromise. Tracheal compression by aberrant great vessels (e.g., aorta, innominate artery) may cause wheezing, stridor, cough, and dyspnea. Incomplete vascular rings are often asymptomatic and incidentally found, although an atypical distal origin of an **anomalous innominate artery** off the aortic arch can cause anterior tracheal compression. This usually results in mild respiratory symptoms. Surgical correction is rarely necessary. Complete vascular rings, which compress the esophagus posteriorly and the trachea anteriorly, include the double aortic arch and a right aortic arch with a persistent ligamentum arteriosum. Both lesions have right-sided aortic arches, which may be visible on chest radiograph. In addition to respiratory symptoms, complete vascular rings may cause *dysphagia lusoria* due to esophageal compression by an aberrant right subclavian artery. The diagnosis of vascular anomalies can often be made by a barium esophagram, which identifies the esophageal compression (Fig. 137.2). Bronchoscopy will identify a pulsatile compression of the airway, but the diagnostic procedures of choice are a computed tomography (CT) angiogram of the chest and great vessels or magnetic resonance angiogram (MRA). Definitive treatment of vascular rings requires surgical repair. Other causes of extrinsic tracheal compression include enlarged mediastinal lymph nodes (e.g., tuberculosis), mediastinal masses (e.g., teratoma, lymphoma, thymoma, germ cell tumors), and, rarely, cystic hygromas.

Foreign Body Aspiration

Epidemiology

Aspiration of foreign bodies into the trachea and bronchi is relatively common. Most children who aspirate foreign bodies are under 3 years of age. Patients with developmental delay and young children with older siblings are at increased risk. Given the less acute angle of the right mainstem bronchus takeoff compared to left, foreign bodies are more likely to lodge in right-sided airways. Some foreign bodies, especially nuts, can also lodge more proximally in the larynx or subglottic space, totally occluding the airway. Numerous foreign bodies are not radiopaque, which makes them difficult to detect radiographically. The most common foreign bodies aspirated by young children are food (especially nuts) and small toys. In younger children, coins and button batteries more often lodge in the esophagus than in the airways. Button batteries can cause airway, esophageal, and even surrounding vascular erosion and be life-threatening. Older children have been known to aspirate rubber balloons while attempting to inflate them, which also can be life-threatening.

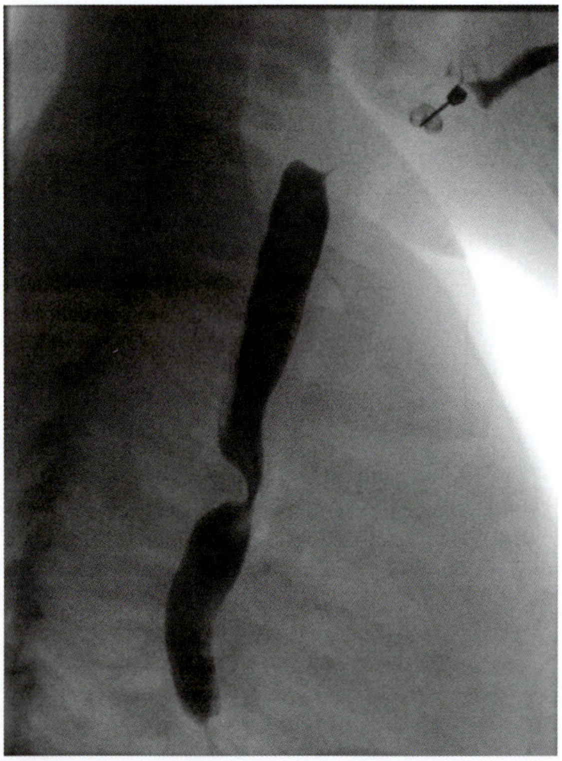

FIGURE 137.2 Vascular ring. Indentation of the posterior esophagus seen on barium swallow, lateral view. This child had a double aortic arch.

Clinical Manifestations

Some children who aspirate foreign bodies have clear histories of choking, witnessed aspiration, or physical or radiographic evidence of foreign body aspiration. A proportion of patients have a negative history because the aspiration went unrecognized. Physical findings observed with acute foreign body aspiration may include cough, localized wheezing, unilateral absence of breath sounds, stridor, and, rarely, bloody sputum.

Most foreign bodies are small and quickly expelled, but some may remain in the lung for long periods of time and may come to medical attention because of persistent cough, sputum production, or recurrent unilateral pneumonia. Foreign body aspiration should be in the differential diagnosis of patients with persistent wheezing unresponsive to bronchodilator therapy, persistent atelectasis, recurrent or persistent pneumonia, or chronic cough without another explanation. Foreign bodies may also lodge in the esophagus and compress the trachea, thus producing respiratory symptoms. Esophageal foreign bodies should be included in the differential diagnosis of infants or young children with persistent cough, stridor, or wheezing, particularly if dysphagia is present.

Diagnostic Studies

Radiographic studies will reveal the presence of radiopaque objects and can also identify focal air trapping, especially on expiratory views or decubitus films. Some foreign bodies are not radiopaque. Thus when foreign body aspiration is suspected, expiratory or lateral decubitus chest radiographs may help to identify air trapping on the affected, dependent side. If history or exam is suggestive of foreign body aspiration, the patient should undergo bronchoscopy. Flexible bronchoscopy can be used to locate an aspirated foreign body and may be useful when the presentation is not straightforward. Flexible bronchoscopic techniques such as cryoextraction may be trialed, but the gold standard for foreign body removal remains rigid bronchoscopy.

Prevention

Common foods, including peanuts or other nuts, popcorn, uncooked carrots, or any foods difficult to break into small pieces, have the potential to be aspirated by infants and children, particularly before molar teeth have erupted. Older siblings should be counseled to keep small toys separate and not present younger children with small parts.

Bronchiolitis

See Chapter 110.

Bronchopulmonary Dysplasia

See Chapter 60.

Congenital Lung Anomalies

Congenital lobar emphysema (congenital lobar overinflation) consists of hyperinflation of one or more lobes of the lung. This overdistention may cause severe respiratory distress in the neonatal period due to compression of surrounding normal lung tissue, but it can also be asymptomatic and remain undiagnosed for years. Radiographically, it may be mistaken for a pneumothorax. Lobectomy may be required if respiratory distress is severe or progressive, but surgical resection may not be indicated in asymptomatic patients.

Congenital pulmonary airway malformations (CPAMs) are a spectrum of lesions arising during early lung development with histologic appearance ranging from simplified bronchial to complex cystic alveolar tissue, connected to the tracheobronchial tree. They are often first identified on antenatal ultrasound and after birth can be inconspicuous on chest radiograph. CPAMs are nonfunctioning lung tissue and can have hybrid features of **pulmonary sequestration** (presence of systemic circulation connections). Although CPAMs can be stand-alone lesions, a substantial proportion of pulmonary sequestrations are hybrid CPAM lesions. Sequestrations without hybrid features are separate from the tracheobronchial tree and are classified as intrapulmonary (located in a normal lobe without its own pleura) and extrapulmonary (outside normal lung). CPAMs and sequestrations can coexist with other chest lesions including **congenital diaphragmatic hernia**. Sequestration is also associated with **Scimitar syndrome** (partial anomalous pulmonary venous return). Symptomatic neonates with respiratory distress, large lesions, sizeable cystic components, or family history of certain malignancies require further imaging. Although large malformations can cause neonatal respiratory distress, some are asymptomatic. Chest CT with contrast is the diagnostic test of choice (Fig. 137.3) but may be delayed if the child is asymptomatic with close clinical follow-up for symptom development. Surgical resection is curative, with greater compensatory alveolar growth of remaining healthy lobes achieved if performed within the first year of life; risk of infection or malignancy is not completely understood in these children to guide surgical intervention. With subspecialty consultation and follow-up, conservative management with observation may be a reasonable option for some patients.

Pulmonary hypoplasia, or a relative decrease in number and size of alveoli, may be the result of bronchopulmonary dysplasia or due to congenital differences such as congenital heart disease, trisomy 21, **congenital diaphragmatic hernia**, or unilateral congenital absence of a pulmonary artery. Alveolar growth after birth occurs rapidly within the first 3 years and is largely complete by 8 years of age though is believed to continue at a slow rate through adolescence.

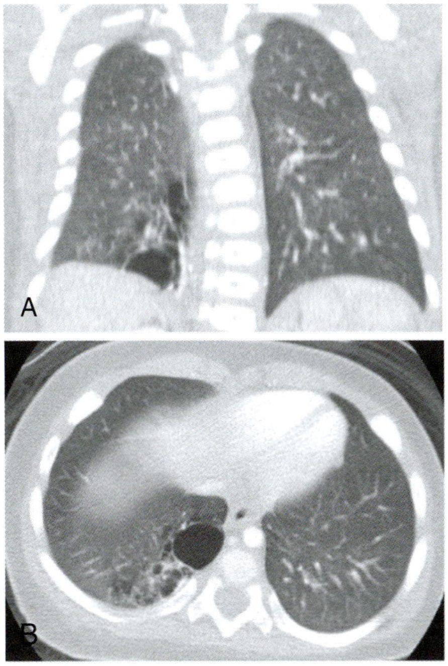

FIGURE 137.3 Congenital pulmonary airway malformation. Coronal **(A)** and axial **(B)** computed tomography images of a right lower lobe congenital pulmonary airway malformation in a child who presented with recurrent pneumonias. The entire left lung and upper and middle lobes of the right lung are normal.

Primary Ciliary Dyskinesia

Etiology

Primary ciliary dyskinesia (PCD) is a disorder of motile cilia and is characterized by a diverse array of clinical features, including chronic/recurrent upper and lower respiratory tract infections, risk for laterality defects (including *situs inversus totalis [SIT]* and heterotaxy), and male infertility. This disorder affects approximately 1 in 15,000–20,000 live births.

Clinical Manifestations

The clinical features of PCD reflect defective motile cilia function in the respiratory tract, sinuses, middle ear, and reproductive tract, as well as laterality defects. Early pediatric PCD clinical features include (1) history of unexplained neonatal respiratory distress, with supplemental oxygen requirement for more than 24 hours in term infants; (2) early-onset, year-round wet cough; (3) early onset, year-round nasal congestion; and (4) laterality defects. Patients develop progressive bronchiectasis that is universal by adulthood and can lead to end-stage lung disease. Cilia dysfunction in embryonic nodal cells can result in laterality defects and congenital heart disease. Other clinical manifestations include impaired growth, recurrent middle ear effusions with associated hearing loss, chronic sinusitis, nasal polyps, male infertility, and decreased female fertility. Genotype-phenotype relationships are emerging in PCD, particularly regarding variability in severity and progression of lung disease.

Diagnostic Studies

PCD diagnosis is a combination of clinical features and ultrastructural analysis of respiratory cilia by electron microscopy, obtained from scrapings/biopsy of nasal or airway epithelium. Results may be difficult to interpret because chronic infection and inflammation may also lead to ultrastructural abnormalities in nasal cilia. The most common ciliary ultrastructural defect is the absence of outer dynein arms (ODAs). A third of affected individuals have normal ciliary ultrastructure. The measurement of nasal nitric oxide is the most sensitive and specific diagnostic test for PCD, and a low nasal nitric oxide level (<77 nL/min) is consistent with PCD. PCD is usually autosomal recessive; it has been associated with X-linked cri du chat syndrome and other overlapping ciliopathies. Currently >50 distinct genes have been identified, where high-throughput genetic testing (e.g., genomic sequencing) can identify 70–80% of cases. High-speed video microscopy assesses ciliary beat frequency and pattern but requires specialized equipment, and there is currently an absence of standardized reporting methods.

Treatment

Treatment of PCD is geared toward treating infections and improving clearance of respiratory secretions. High-resolution chest CT scans are useful to confirm and monitor bronchiectasis. Surveillance cultures help identify organisms involved and guide antibiotic therapy. Chest physiotherapy and prompt treatment of bacterial infections are helpful, but the course of the lower airway disease tends to be slowly progressive. Inhaled hypertonic saline improves cough clearance and has been shown to improve lung function. Antiinflammatory antibiotics, such as low-dose macrolides, may reduce the number of exacerbations per year. Sinus surgical procedures are often done to manage chronic sinusitis, but their benefit is questionable. Most children require placement of pressure equalization (PE) tubes for management of recurrent otitis media. Multidisciplinary care with pulmonology, otolaryngology, audiology, respiratory therapy, and nutrition is recommended.

Pneumonia

See Chapter 111.

Pulmonary Edema

Etiology

Pulmonary edema is the seepage of fluid into the alveolar and interstitial spaces. Capillary hydrostatic forces and interstitial osmotic pressures contribute to fluid movement toward the air spaces; plasma osmotic pressures and tissue mechanical forces move fluid back toward the vasculature. Under normal circumstances, the sum of these forces favors absorption, so the alveolar and interstitial spaces remain dry. Fluid entering the alveoli is normally removed by pulmonary lymphatics. Pulmonary edema forms when transcapillary fluid flux exceeds lymphatic drainage. For example, reduced left ventricular function leads to pulmonary venous hypertension and increased capillary hydrostatic pressure, moving fluid into the interstitial space and alveoli. Fluid initially enters the interstitial space around the terminal bronchioles, alveoli, and arterioles **(interstitial edema)**, causing increased lung stiffness and premature closure of bronchioles on expiration. If the process continues, fluid then enters the alveoli, further reducing compliance and resulting in **intrapulmonary shunting** (alveolar units that are perfused but not ventilated). Decreased ventilation (hypercarbia) is a late finding.

Pulmonary edema is most commonly due to heart failure from left ventricular or biventricular dysfunction. **Pulmonary hypertension** (PH) and associated **cor pulmonale** (right ventricular dysfunction) do not usually cause pulmonary edema, because the increased vascular resistance is most often proximal to the capillary bed. Increased capillary permeability, seen in disease states such as sepsis and acute respiratory distress syndrome, can lead to pulmonary edema. Pulmonary edema may also occur with excessive swings in intrathoracic pressure, as seen after tracheal foreign body aspiration or severe obstruction from hypertrophied tonsils and adenoids **(postobstructive pulmonary edema)**. Pulmonary edema may also be present in conditions with decreased serum oncotic pressure (hypoalbuminemia); after administration of large volumes of intravenous (IV) fluids, especially if there is capillary injury; with ascent to high altitude **(high-altitude pulmonary edema)**; and after central nervous system injury **(neurogenic pulmonary edema)**.

Clinical Manifestations

The clinical manifestations of pulmonary edema are **dyspnea**, tachypnea, and cough (can occur with frothy, pink-tinged sputum). As the edema worsens, there is increased work of breathing and hypoxemia; diffuse inspiratory crackles can be heard on auscultation.

Diagnostic Studies

Chest radiographs may reveal diffuse hazy infiltrates, classically in a perihilar pattern, but these findings may be obscured by underlying lung disease. Interstitial edema *(Kerley B lines)* may be seen, especially at the lung bases.

Treatment

Treatment depends on the cause of the pulmonary edema and response to therapy. Patients should be positioned in an upright posture and given supplemental O_2. Diuretic therapy and rapidly acting IV inotropic agents may be helpful in cardiogenic pulmonary edema. CPAP or intubation with positive pressure ventilation using high positive end-expiratory pressures (PEEP) may be required.

Acute Respiratory Distress Syndrome

See Chapter 38.

Acute COVID

See Chapter 111.

E-cigarette or Vaping Product Use–Associated Lung Injury

Etiology

Use of electronic cigarettes (also known as vaping) has resulted in numerous associated medical complications. The most common consequence in pediatrics is second-hand and third-hand exposure to particulate matter from caregivers. Due to multiple reasons (perception of being less addictive and less harmful than traditional tobacco products, ease of accessibility, attractive flavors), e-cigarettes/vaping has rapidly risen to the most common form of tobacco used among adolescents and young adults. Although the long-term respiratory sequelae are incompletely understood, a distinct entity associated with acute lung injury within 90 days of e-cigarette use is e-cigarette or vaping product use–associated lung injury (EVALI). Injury to the distal airway and alveoli occurs with aerosolized oil deposition (most commonly vitamin E acetate), prompting an inflammatory cascade, pulmonary infiltration, and impaired gas exchange in the absence of alternative etiology (e.g., infection).

Clinical Manifestations and Diagnostic Studies

Symptoms of EVALI are widely variable, ranging from asymptomatic incidental discovery to acute hospitalization for cough, fever, dyspnea, chest pain, hypoxemia, and respiratory distress or failure. Diagnosis is one of exclusion, often through significant testing including labs, bronchoscopy with bronchoalveolar lavage, and radiography including chest CT. Chest x-ray most commonly shows bilateral infiltrates and ground-glass opacities that are more prominent at the lung bases; chest CT may also show subpleural sparing followed by small pleural effusions and centrilobular nodularity.

Treatment

Treatment includes respiratory support (ranging from supplemental oxygen to intubation), trials of IV systemic steroids, and e-cigarette/vaping cessation.

Pulmonary Hypertension and Cor Pulmonale

Etiology

Pulmonary hypertension (PH) is defined as a mean pulmonary artery pressure of 20 mm Hg or higher in children over 3 months of age at sea level. Pediatric PH is categorized into five groups based on the World Health Organization classification. Group 1 is pulmonary arterial hypertension (PAH) due to diseases within veins and small pulmonary muscular arteries such as persistent PH of the newborn, congenital heart disease (including those with excessive pulmonary blood flow due to left-to-right cardiac shunting), exposure to various drugs (e.g., cocaine, amphetamines), and **idiopathic pulmonary arterial hypertension (IPAH)**. Hereditary IPAH, also in this group, has been linked with the bone morphogenetic receptor-2 *(BMPR2)* gene. Group 2 is caused by dysfunction of the left heart such as valvular disease. Group 3 is secondary to lung disease or chronic hypoxia, including upper airway obstruction resulting in obstructive sleep apnea and hypoxemia. In group 4, PH is secondary to chronic pulmonary thromboembolism. Group 5 includes PH of unclear but multifactorial diseases, including some autoimmune diseases and metabolic diseases. The Panama classification is a pediatric-specific system that includes 10 categories to capture the heterogeneity of pulmonary hypertensive vascular disease.

Prolonged PH may lead to irreversible changes in the intima and media of the pulmonary arterioles. PH strains the right side of the heart, which leads to hypertrophy and dilation of the right ventricle. Altered structure and/or function of the right heart from PH is known as **cor pulmonale**. The most common causes of cor pulmonale in children are chronic lung diseases, especially severe bronchopulmonary dysplasia, and severe untreated obstructive sleep apnea (with chronic hypoxia).

Clinical Manifestations and Diagnostic Studies

PAH should be suspected with certain developmental anatomic abnormalities or historical exposures (e.g., congenital heart disease, bronchopulmonary dysplasia, congenital diaphragmatic hernia, prolonged hypoxemia). Exertional dyspnea and unexplained syncope are presenting symptoms. In addition to the other physical findings associated with pulmonary and cardiac diseases, an accentuated pulmonary component of the second heart sound may be heard. Definitive diagnosis is made by cardiac catheterization, but echocardiography may confirm the presence of right ventricular hypertrophy, ventricular dysfunction, interventricular septal flattening, and tricuspid insufficiency, which can be used to estimate the pulmonary artery pressures. Cardiac magnetic resonance imaging can be useful in diagnosis and to assess changes in ventricular function and size. Lung biopsy may be considered for children with PAH suspected to have diffuse lung disease, pulmonary veno-occlusive disease, or vasculitis.

Treatment

Treatment should focus on the underlying condition of known causes of PH, such as lung volume optimization in persistent PH of the newborn or therapy with diuretics and salt/fluid restriction in heart failure. In all conditions of PH and PAH (except when secondary to pulmonary venous obstruction), the relief of hypoxemia with supplemental O_2 therapy can be therapeutic as a pulmonary vasodilator. Medications for pulmonary vasodilation such as short-term inhaled nitric oxide may be helpful in some patients. Continuous infusions of prostacyclin may be utilized both acutely and chronically and is available in inhaled, subcutaneous, and IV forms. Endothelium antagonists may be beneficial. Unfortunately, some patients with the idiopathic form of PAH have progressive courses, and lung or heart-lung transplantation may be the only treatment option.

Pulmonary Hemorrhage

Etiology

Pulmonary hemorrhage is a rare but potentially life-threatening condition in children. It can be due to bleeding from the airways (hemangiomas, bronchial vessel bleeds) or from diffuse capillary bleeding (alveolar hemorrhage). Alveolar hemorrhage is usually due to diffuse capillary disruption/inflammation.

Clinical Manifestations

The presentation of pulmonary hemorrhage is variable with a spectrum of asymptomatic radiographic abnormalities to life-threatening respiratory failure. **Hemoptysis**, although experienced by most children with pulmonary hemorrhage, can be absent in a third of individuals. In addition to hemoptysis, presenting signs and symptoms include cough, wheeze, shortness of breath, pallor, fatigue, cyanosis, and fever. It is important to evaluate for extrapulmonary sources of bleeding, including hematemesis and bleeding from the nasopharynx or mouth, because these are more common than true pulmonary hemorrhage. Episodic pulmonary hemorrhage frequently manifests as recurrent respiratory symptoms associated with pulmonary infiltrates on chest radiographs. Symptomatic **airway hemorrhage** may result in significant hemoptysis with few radiographic changes; **alveolar bleeding** often causes profound respiratory symptoms, hypoxemia, diffuse infiltrates on radiographs, and minimal hemoptysis. Some patients experience a localized bubbling sensation in the chest, which may be helpful in differentiating local from diffuse sources of pulmonary bleeding. Physical examination findings may include locally or diffusely decreased breath sounds, cyanosis, and crackles on auscultation.

The differential diagnosis of pulmonary hemorrhage includes alveolar and airway bleeding. Airway bleeding can be due to airway hemangiomas, pulmonary arteriovenous malformations (e.g., hereditary hemorrhagic telangiectasia), and bronchial artery collaterals, which develop in some patients with chronic lung infections (e.g., cystic fibrosis). The causes of alveolar (capillary) bleeding can be divided into immune-mediated and non–immune-mediated categories. Immune-mediated causes include antineutrophil cytoplasmic autoantibodies (ANCA)–associated vasculitides, isolated pulmonary capillaritis, antiglomerular basement membrane disease, drug-induced vasculitis, and other connective tissue diseases. Non–immune-mediated causes include idiopathic pulmonary hemosiderosis, clotting disorders, infection, inhalation injury, and cardiac conditions associated with elevated pulmonary venous and capillary pressures (Table 137.2). Alveolar hemorrhage following bone marrow transplant can occur from immune-mediated causes and complications of diffuse alveolar damage. Rarely, a previously well infant will present with life-threatening acute alveolar hemorrhage. Often no cause is found, and, once the acute episode resolves, the infant returns to normal. Most of these infants never have a second bleeding episode. **Idiopathic pulmonary hemosiderosis** is a rare disorder characterized by recurrent alveolar bleeding, iron-deficiency anemia, and hemosiderin-laden macrophages in the lung, which can be identified microscopically with the use of special iron-staining techniques in bronchoalveolar lavage or lung biopsy specimens. Although the term *hemosiderosis* is sometimes used interchangeably with pulmonary hemorrhage, it is a pathologic finding that results from bleeding anywhere in the lung, airway, pharynx, nasopharynx, or mouth leading to hemosiderin accumulation in the lung.

TABLE 137.2 Differential Diagnosis of Hemoptysis-Pulmonary Hemorrhage

CARDIOVASCULAR DISORDERS
Heart failure with pulmonary edema Pulmonary hypertension with Eisenmenger syndrome (pulmonary vascular obstructive disease) Mitral stenosis Veno-occlusive disease Arteriovenous malformation (Osler-Weber-Rendu syndrome) Pulmonary embolism Portal vein obstruction
PULMONARY DISORDERS
Bronchogenic cyst Bronchopulmonary sequestration Pneumonia (bacterial, mycobacterial, fungal, parasitic, or viral) Bronchiectasis (cystic fibrosis, primary ciliary dyskinesia, immunodeficiency, retained foreign body) Tracheobronchitis Lung abscess Tumor (adenoma, carcinoid, hemangioma, metastasis) Trauma (contusion, laceration)
IMMUNE DISORDERS
IgA vasculitis Pulmonary capillaritis Idiopathic pulmonary hemosiderosis Antiglomerular basement membrane disease Granulomatosis with polyangiitis Systemic lupus erythematosus Polyarteritis nodosa
OTHER CONDITIONS/FACTORS
Coagulopathy (Von Willebrand factor) Toxic inhalation (nitrogen dioxide, pesticides, crack cocaine) Post–bone marrow transplantation Catamenial hemoptysis (females)

Diagnostic Studies

It is important to perform a thorough upper airway examination to evaluate for epistaxis. Sometimes this requires nasopharyngoscopy. If extrapulmonary sources of bleeding have been excluded, then a chest radiograph, CT angiogram of the chest, bronchoscopy, echocardiogram, and evaluation for rheumatologic/autoimmune diseases follow, especially to consider antiglomerular basement membrane disease, granulomatosis with polyangiitis, IgA vasculitis, and systemic lupus erythematosus. Approximately one-third of children with hemoptysis will have a normal chest radiograph, and additional diagnostic evaluation is warranted.

Treatment

The management of acute episodes of pulmonary bleeding includes the administration of supplemental O_2, blood transfusions, and, often with acute alveolar hemorrhages, mechanical ventilation with PEEP to tamponade the bleeding. Treatment is directed toward the underlying disorders and providing supportive care. In bronchial arterial bleeding, arteriography with vessel embolization has been shown to be successful.

Pulmonary Embolism

Etiology

Pulmonary embolism (PE) is rare in children. When it occurs, it is often associated with indwelling central venous catheters, oral contraceptives, or hypercoagulable states. Other risk factors, such as trauma, surgery, immobilization, systemic lupus erythematosus, systemic infection, and cancer, may lead to deep vein thromboses (DVTs) and pulmonary embolism.

Clinical Manifestations

In the distensible pulmonary vascular bed, small emboli may be asymptomatic unless they are infected (septic emboli). Large emboli may cause acute dyspnea, pleuritic chest pain, cough, and hemoptysis. Tachypnea, tachycardia, and hypoxia are common, as are nonspecific ST-segment and T-wave changes on the electrocardiogram (ECG). The P_2 heart sound may be increased. Unilateral calf swelling may be present in the setting of DVT.

Diagnostic Studies

Imaging plays an important role in the evaluation and management of acute PE. D-dimer testing and clinical prediction tools lack utility in the diagnosis of PE in children. CT pulmonary angiography (CTPA) is the standard of care and provides accurate diagnosis with rapid turnaround time. Although a chest CT or chest radiograph can provide information on other potential causes of acute chest pain, a chest radiograph has limited utility specific to PE, only occasionally showing findings of PE or infarction. Ventilation-perfusion scans may reveal defects in perfusion without matching ventilation defects, but they are difficult to perform in young children. Catheter pulmonary angiography is only for interventional management. Doppler or compression ultrasonography can be useful in assessing patients for lower extremity DVTs. Children with pulmonary embolism without an obvious cause should be evaluated for hypercoagulable states, the most common of which is factor V Leiden, an autosomal dominant blood clotting disorder caused by a pathogenic variant in the clotting factor V protein (see Chapter 152).

Treatment

Treatment includes anticoagulation, usually with low-molecular-weight heparin or unfractionated heparin. Although rare, if pulmonary embolism is extensive and hemodynamically compromising, catheter-directed thrombolytic agents such as tissue plasminogen activator (TPA) should be considered. All patients should receive supplemental oxygen, and it is important to treat the predisposing factors.

PEARLS FOR PRACTITIONERS

See The Respiratory System: Pearls for Practitioners at the end of this section.

REVIEW QUESTIONS

Available online.

CHAPTER 138

Cystic Fibrosis

ETIOLOGY AND EPIDEMIOLOGY

Cystic fibrosis (CF) is a life-shortening autosomal recessive disorder diagnosed in over 100,000 individuals worldwide. Although found predominantly in people of Northern European descent, CF is reported among all racial and ethnic groups. The gene for CF, on the long arm of chromosome 7, encodes for the **cystic fibrosis transmembrane conductance regulator (CFTR)**, a chloride channel located on the apical surface of epithelial cells. CFTR is important for the proper movement of salt and water across cell membranes and maintaining the appropriate composition of various secretions, especially in the airways, liver, and pancreas. The most common pathogenic variant is a deletion of three base pairs resulting in the absence of phenylalanine at the 508 position (Phe508del, F508del). Over 2,000 pathogenic variants of the *CFTR* gene have been identified, with 700 of those confirmed to be disease-causing variants.

The secretory and absorptive characteristics of epithelial cells are affected by abnormal CFTR, resulting in the clinical manifestations of CF. The altered chloride ion conductance in the sweat gland results in excessively high sweat sodium and chloride levels. This is the basis for the **sweat chloride test**, which is the diagnostic test of choice for this disorder. The sweat chloride test is positive (elevated sweat chloride ≥60 mEq/L) in 98% of patients with CF.

CLINICAL MANIFESTATIONS

CF is a chronic progressive disease that can present with protein and fat malabsorption (growth faltering, hypoalbuminemia, steatorrhea), liver disease (cholestatic jaundice), or chronic respiratory infection (Table 138.1). Most infants in the United States are diagnosed through newborn screening. Older children may present with pulmonary manifestations such as chronic cough, poorly controlled asthma, and chronic respiratory infections, but recurrent pancreatitis, **nasal polyps**, and chronic sinusitis can also be presenting manifestations. **Digital clubbing** is common in patients with CF, even in those without significant lung disease.

TABLE 138.1 Complications of Cystic Fibrosis

RESPIRATORY COMPLICATIONS
Bronchiectasis, bronchitis, bronchiolitis, pneumonia
Hemoptysis
Pneumothorax
Nasal polyps
Sinusitis
Cor pulmonale (associated with chronic hypoxemia)
Respiratory failure
Atypical mycobacterial infection
Allergic bronchopulmonary aspergillosis
GASTROINTESTINAL COMPLICATIONS
Pancreatic insufficiency
Meconium ileus/peritonitis (infants)
Intestinal atresia (infants)
Distal intestinal obstruction syndrome (non-neonatal obstruction)
Rectal prolapse
Fibrosing colonopathy (strictures)
Recurrent pancreatitis
Hepatic cirrhosis (portal hypertension, esophageal varices, hypersplenism)
Neonatal obstructive jaundice
Hepatic steatosis
Gastroesophageal reflux
Cholelithiasis
Growth failure (malabsorption)
Fat-soluble vitamin deficiency states (vitamins A, D, E, K)
Cystic fibrosis–related diabetes
Malignancy (rare)
OTHER COMPLICATIONS
Diabetes
Infertility
Delayed puberty
Dehydration–heat exhaustion
Electrolyte disturbances (hyponatremic hypochloremic metabolic alkalosis)
Hypertrophic osteoarthropathy–arthritis
Intracranial idiopathic hypertension
Digital clubbing

The respiratory epithelium of patients with CF exhibits marked impermeability to chloride and an excessive reabsorption of sodium. This leads to thicker airway secretions, resulting in airway obstruction and impaired mucociliary transport, leading to endobronchial colonization with bacteria, especially *Staphylococcus aureus* and *Pseudomonas aeruginosa*. Chronic bronchial infection results in **persistent or recurrent cough** that is often productive of sputum, especially in older children. Pulmonary infections with *P. aeruginosa, Burkholderia cepacia,* and other organisms are difficult to treat and may be associated with accelerated clinical deterioration. Chronic airway infection leads to airway obstruction and bronchiectasis and, eventually, to pulmonary insufficiency and premature death. Before the advent of diagnosis and prompt treatment with supportive therapies, individuals with CF did not survive beyond early childhood. The median age of survival is currently over 45 years, but expected survival continues to evolve with advances in care. Individuals born between 2019 and 2023 are predicted to live to a median age of 61 years.

Other possible respiratory complications of CF include increased risk of **allergic bronchopulmonary aspergillosis (ABPA)**, a hypersensitivity reaction to *Aspergillus* in the airways that causes airway inflammation/obstruction and aggravates CF lung disease. The treatment for ABPA is systemic corticosteroids and antifungal agents. Minor hemoptysis is usually due to airway infection, but major hemoptysis can be caused by bleeding from bronchial artery collateral vessels in damaged/chronically infected portions of the lung. Pneumothoraces can occur in patients with advanced lung disease.

In patients with CF, 85% are born with **exocrine pancreatic insufficiency**. The inspissation of mucus and subsequent destruction of the pancreatic ducts result in the inability to excrete pancreatic enzymes into the intestine. This leads to malabsorption of proteins, sugars (to a lesser extent), and especially fat. Fat malabsorption manifests clinically as **steatorrhea** (large, foul-smelling stools), deficiencies of fat-soluble vitamins (A, D, E, and K), and growth faltering. Protein malabsorption can present early in infancy as hypoproteinemia and peripheral edema. Approximately 10–20% of patients with CF are born with intestinal obstruction caused by inspissated meconium **(meconium ileus)**. In older patients, intestinal obstruction may result from thick inspissated mucus in the intestinal lumen **(distal intestinal obstruction syndrome [DIOS])**.

In adolescent patients, progressive pancreatic damage can lead to enough islet cell destruction to cause insulin deficiency. This initially presents as glucose intolerance, but true diabetes that requires insulin therapy **(CF-related diabetes)** may develop. The failure of the sweat ducts to conserve sodium and chloride may lead to hyponatremia and hypochloremic metabolic alkalosis, especially in infants.

Inspissation of mucus in the reproductive tract leads to reproductive dysfunction in both males and females. Though sperm is produced normally, **congenital bilateral absence of the vas deferens (CBAVD)** occurs in 95–98% of males with CF; advances in assisted reproductive technology (ART) have enabled males with CBAVD to have biological children. In females, secondary amenorrhea can be present due to chronic illness and reduced body weight. Fertility can be diminished by malnutrition and abnormal cervical mucus, but most women with CF can conceive and carry healthy pregnancies. Sexual health, fertility, and genetic counseling are important facets of CF care.

DIAGNOSTIC STUDIES

All infants with a positive newborn screen and/or with meconium ileus should be evaluated for CF. The diagnosis of CF should be seriously considered in any infant presenting with growth faltering, cholestatic jaundice, chronic respiratory symptoms, or electrolyte abnormalities (hyponatremia, hypochloremia, metabolic alkalosis). CF should be in the differential diagnosis of children with chronic respiratory or gastrointestinal symptoms, especially if there is digital clubbing. Any child with nasal polyps, especially those younger than 12 years, should be evaluated for CF. All siblings of patients with CF should also be evaluated.

Readily available commercial DNA tests detect numerous CF pathogenic variants, but DNA analysis will not detect all cases of CF. All states in the United States have newborn screening for CF based either on elevated immunoreactive trypsinogen (IRT) levels or DNA tests, identifying the majority of infants with CF, but there are both false-positive and false-negative results. The diagnostic test of choice is still the sweat test, with genetic testing and pathogenic variant analysis playing an increasing role. Indications for performing a **sweat test** are listed in Table 138.2. The following criteria should be met to establish the diagnosis of CF:

- The presence of one or more typical clinical features of CF (chronic pulmonary disease, characteristic gastrointestinal and nutritional abnormalities, salt loss syndromes, or obstructive azoospermia) AND one of the following:
- Two elevated sweat chloride tests performed at an accredited CF Foundation–certified laboratory (positive if the value is ≥60 mEq/L, borderline if 30–59 mEq/L, and negative if <30 mEq/L, with adequate sweat collection) OR
- Two pathogenic variants known to cause CF identified by DNA analysis OR
- A characteristic abnormality in ion transport across nasal epithelium demonstrated in vivo (nasal potential difference testing)

For those identified early by positive newborn screening or because a sibling has CF, positive sweat chloride testing or the presence of known disease-causing DNA pathogenic variants are the only criteria required for diagnosis, because clinical symptoms may not be manifested early in life.

Although the sweat test is both specific and sensitive for CF, it is subject to technical problems with both false-positive and false-negative results (Table 138.3). Cutoff diagnostic

TABLE 138.2 Indications for Sweat Testing
RESPIRATORY
Chronic or recurrent cough
Chronic or recurrent pneumonia
Recurrent bronchiolitis or bronchitis
Recurrent wheezing/difficult to control asthma
Recurrent or persistent atelectasis
Bronchiectasis
Hemoptysis
Pseudomonas aeruginosa in the respiratory tract (if not explained by other factors; e.g., tracheostomy or prolonged intubation)
GASTROINTESTINAL
Meconium ileus
Neonatal intestinal obstruction (meconium plug, atresia)
Steatorrhea, malabsorption
Hepatic cirrhosis in childhood (including any manifestations such as esophageal varices or portal hypertension)
Cholestatic jaundice in infancy
Pancreatitis
Rectal prolapse
Fat-soluble vitamin deficiency states (A, D, E, K)
Hypoproteinemia, hypoalbuminemia, peripheral edema unexplained by other causes
Prolonged, direct-reacting neonatal jaundice
MISCELLANEOUS
Positive newborn screen (sweat testing performed after 2 wk of age and >2 kg if asymptomatic)
Digital clubbing
Growth faltering
Family history of cystic fibrosis (e.g., in sibling or cousin)
Salty taste of skin (noted by parent on kissing affected child—from salt crystals formed after evaporation of sweat)
Hyponatremic hypochloremic alkalosis in infants
Nasal polyps
Recurrent sinusitis
Aspermia
Absent vas deferens

TABLE 138.3 Causes of False-Positive and False-Negative Results on Sweat Testing

FALSE POSITIVE
Adrenal insufficiency
Eczema
Ectodermal dysplasia
Nephrogenic diabetes insipidus
Hypothyroidism
Fucosidosis
Mucopolysaccharidosis
Dehydration
Malnutrition
Poor technique/inadequate sweat collection
Type I glycogen storage disease
Panhypopituitarism
Pseudohypoaldosteronism
Hypoparathyroidism
Prostaglandin E_1 administration
FALSE NEGATIVE
Edema
Poor technique/inadequate sweat collection

measurements evolve as more disease-causing DNA pathogenic variants are identified. Other supportive tests include the measurement of bioelectrical potential differences across nasal epithelium (not widely available) and measurement of fecal elastase levels. Low fecal elastase levels indicate exocrine pancreatic insufficiency. CF genotyping done by commercial laboratories identifies approximately 95% of patients with CF, but there are pathogenic variants that are not identified by standard testing. Not all pathogenic variants in CFTR are considered disease causing, and some have uncertain prognostic consequences. Some infants identified by newborn screening with borderline sweat tests and variants of uncertain consequence are considered to have CFTR-related metabolic syndrome (CRMS) or CF screen positive, inconclusive diagnosis (CFSPID). Older children that present with atypical clinical features and borderline sweat tests may be considered nonclassic CF or mild variant CF.

Identification of carriers (heterozygotes) and prenatal genetic screening for the most common pathogenic variants is offered at most medical centers. Prenatal testing techniques can identify more than 90% of carriers. Prenatal detection of a known CF genotype may be accomplished by amniocentesis or chorionic villus sampling.

TREATMENT

The treatment of CF is multifactorial. Most maintenance therapies are directed toward gastrointestinal and pulmonary complications. There is no single effective cure for CF, but advances in precision therapies have resulted in significant improvements for eligible patients. CFTR modulators target genotype-specific functional defects of the CFTR protein. As of late 2024 there are four U.S. Food and Drug Administration (FDA)-approved CFTR modulators, with additional therapies under investigation.

Modulators

Ivacaftor, the first CFTR modulator approved by the FDA, is a small molecule that potentiates CFTR function, holding the channel at the cell surface and holding the gate open. For the small group of individuals with specific CFTR pathogenic variants responsive to this, ivacaftor contributes to sustained health improvements including lung function. The second FDA-approved medication is a combination of ivacaftor and lumacaftor, which both potentiates and corrects protein folding. Approved for individuals with two copies of the most common CFTR pathogenic variant, F508del, it has been associated with a modest but significant improvement in lung function, improved body mass index, and a decrease in hospitalizations for pulmonary exacerbations. The third FDA-approved medication, a combination of ivacaftor and tezacaftor, also has both potentiating and correcting effects, with fewer drug interactions compared to lumacaftor-ivacaftor and available for a slightly larger number of individuals. The triple-drug combination elexacaftor-tezacaftor-ivacaftor is an important therapy that has demonstrated improvement in lung function and symptom-related quality of life and decreased sweat chloride compared to dual-therapy tezacaftor-ivacaftor. As of late 2024, it is approved for people with CF ages 2 and older with at least one of 178 specified pathogenic variants, including F508del, making approximately 90% of individuals with CF eligible. Clinical trials are ongoing for both triple-drug therapy in younger children and next-generation CFTR modulators.

Airway Clearance Therapies and Antibiotics

Treatment with CFTR modulator therapy does not preclude management of pulmonary complications. Management of pulmonary exacerbations is directed toward facilitating clearance of secretions from the airways and minimizing the effects of chronic bronchial infection. Airway secretion clearance techniques help remove mucus from the airways. Aerosolized DNAse and 7% hypertonic saline, both delivered by nebulizer, decrease the viscosity of mucus. **Chest physiotherapy** (therapy vest, oscillating therapies, postural drainage) mechanically promotes secretion clearance. **Antibiotic therapy** is important in controlling chronic infection and treating acute exacerbations. Patients may require 2- to 3-week courses of high-dose IV antibiotics and aggressive chest physiotherapy to treat pulmonary exacerbations. Antibiotics are selected based on organisms identified by sputum or throat culture. Common pathologic organisms include *P. aeruginosa* and *S. aureus*. Patients with symptomatic sinus disease and nasal polyps not responding to medical management may require surgical intervention.

Management of Gastrointestinal Manifestations

Exocrine pancreatic insufficiency is treated with enteric-coated pancreatic enzyme capsules, which contain lipase and proteases. Patients with CF are encouraged to follow high-calorie diets, often with the addition of nutritional supplements, as needed, to achieve normal weight trajectory. Even with optimal pancreatic enzyme replacement, stool losses of fat and protein may be high. Fat should not be withheld from the diet, even when significant steatorrhea exists. Rather, pancreatic enzyme doses should be titrated to optimize fat absorption, although there is a limit to the doses that should be used as excessive doses have been associated with **fibrosing colonopathy**. Fat-soluble vitamins (A, D, E, and K) are recommended, preferably in a water-miscible form.

Newborns with **meconium ileus** may require surgical intervention, but some can be managed with contrast (Gastrografin) enemas. Intestinal obstruction in patients with CF beyond the neonatal period is often due to DIOS, which may need to be treated with courses of oral laxatives (polyethylene glycol) or, in more refractory cases, with Gastrografin enemas. Pancreatic enzyme dosage adjustment, adequate hydration, and dietary fiber may help prevent recurrent episodes. Patients with CF-related diabetes are treated with insulin primarily to improve nutrition and prevent dehydration, because ketoacidosis is rare. Intermittent transaminase elevation is common in patients with CF. Although a minority (10–15%) will develop clinically significant CF-associated liver disease (CFLD), liver disease is the third leading specified cause of death in CF in the United States (2–3%, after lung disease and complications of lung transplantation). Portal hypertension and esophageal varices due to cirrhosis of the liver are managed, when necessary, with portal vein shunting procedures or liver transplantation.

The management of CF is complex and is best coordinated by medical teams at accredited CF centers. More than 50% of the CF population are now adults, highlighting the importance of a successful transition of pediatric patients to adult centers. As with other severe chronic diseases, management of patients with CF requires a multidisciplinary team working with patients and their families to maintain an optimistic, comprehensive, and aggressive approach to treatment.

PEARLS FOR PRACTITIONERS

See The Respiratory System: Pearls for Practitioners at the end of this section.

REVIEW QUESTIONS

Available online.

CHAPTER 139 Chest Wall and Pleura

Thoracic scoliosis, when severe (curve >50–60 degrees), can be associated with chest wall deformity and limitation of chest wall movement (see Chapter 203), resulting in decreased lung volumes (restrictive lung disease), ventilation-perfusion mismatching, hypoventilation, and even respiratory failure (see Chapter 38). Surgical correction of scoliosis may prevent further loss of lung function but rarely improves pulmonary function beyond presurgical levels. Neuromuscular weakness and hypotonia of the chest wall are also common causes of respiratory failure (see Chapter 38) and are classically associated with restrictive lung disease and hypoventilation. The differential diagnoses for weakness and hypotonia are extensive (see Chapter 183).

PECTUS EXCAVATUM AND CARINATUM

Pectus Excavatum

Sternal concavity **(pectus excavatum)**, a common chest wall deformity in children, is usually not associated with significant pulmonary compromise. Patients with pectus excavatum generally come to medical attention due to concerns over the appearance of the chest. Only in severe cases does it result in significant restrictive lung disease, obstructive defects, and/or decreased cardiac function. Adolescents with pectus excavatum may report exercise intolerance. Routine spirometry is often normal but can show decreased vital capacity consistent with restrictive lung disease. The most common reason for surgical correction is to improve appearance (cosmetic reasons), although in some cases surgical repair is used to improve cardiac function and exercise tolerance (diagnosed through a combination of chest CT, echocardiography, and cardiopulmonary exercise testing [CPET]).

Pectus Carinatum

Pectus carinatum is an abnormality of chest wall shape in which the sternum bows out. Though pectus carinatum does not cause abnormal pulmonary function, underlying pulmonary disease may contribute to the deformity. It can be observed after cardiac surgery performed via midsternal approach. Surgical correction of this condition is rarely indicated but occasionally is done for cosmetic purposes.

PNEUMOTHORAX

Etiology

Pneumothorax, which is the accumulation of air in the pleural space, may result from external trauma or through leakage of air from the lungs or airways. **Spontaneous primary pneumothorax** (no underlying cause) occurs in teenagers and young adults, more commonly in tall, thin males and smokers. Factors predisposing to **secondary pneumothorax** (underlying cause identified) include barotrauma from mechanical ventilation, asthma, cystic fibrosis, trauma to the chest, and severe necrotizing pneumonia.

Clinical Manifestations

The most common signs and symptoms of pneumothorax are chest and/or shoulder pain and dyspnea. If the pneumothorax is caused by air that enters the pleural space during inspiration and cannot escape, mediastinal shift and functional lung compression may occur, resulting in **tension pneumothorax** associated with severe respiratory distress and hemodynamic changes (reduced venous return to the heart). Subcutaneous emphysema may result when the air leak communicates with the mediastinum. Physical findings associated with pneumothorax include decreased breath sounds on the affected side, a tympanitic percussion note, and evidence of mediastinal shift (deviation of the *point of maximal impact* [PMI] and trachea away from the side of the pneumothorax). If the pneumothorax is small, there may be few or no clinical findings. The patient's clinical condition can deteriorate rapidly if the pneumothorax expands, especially if the air in the pleural space is under pressure (tension pneumothorax). This is a life-threatening condition that can result in death if the pleural space is not decompressed by evacuation of the pleural air.

Diagnostic Studies

The presence of a pneumothorax is confirmed by upright chest radiographs. Ultrasound imaging can augment sensitivity of diagnosis in supine subjects and is often used in trauma evaluations. CT scans are generally not necessary unless chest x-rays suggest the need for further evaluation. When indicated, CT scans of the chest can be useful in quantifying the size of pneumothoraces, for differentiating air within the lung parenchyma (cystic lung disease) from air in the pleural space, and for identifying subpleural blebs that may be present in spontaneous recurrent pneumothoraces. In infants, transillumination of the chest wall may be of some use in making a rapid diagnosis of pneumothorax.

Treatment

Treatment for pneumothorax depends on the size as well as the nature of the underlying disease. Small pneumothoraces (<20% of thorax occupied with pleural air) may not require intervention as they often resolve spontaneously. Inhaling high concentrations of supplemental O_2 may enhance reabsorption of pleural air by washing out nitrogen from the blood, although neonatal data recommends against this practice given lack of efficacy in enhancing absorption rate while inducing risk from hyperoxia. Larger pneumothoraces and any tension pneumothorax require immediate drainage of the air, preferably via chest tube. In an emergency, a simple needle aspiration may suffice, although placement of a chest tube is often required for resolution. In patients with recurrent or persistent pneumothoraces, sclerosing the pleural surfaces to obliterate the pleural space *(pleurodesis)* may be necessary. This can be done either chemically, by instilling talc or sclerosis agents (doxycycline) through the chest tube, or mechanically, by surgical abradement. Surgical approaches, such as open thoracotomy and **video-assisted thoracoscopic surgery (VATS)**, enable visualization of the pleural space and resection of pleural blebs, when indicated. Airline travel and spirometry may be restricted for a period of time (≥2 weeks) following radiographic resolution of the pneumothorax to minimize risk of recurrence. Scuba diving should be discouraged for patients who have had a pneumothorax.

PNEUMOMEDIASTINUM

Pneumomediastinum commonly results from the dissection of air from the pulmonary parenchyma into the mediastinum and less frequently from central airway or gastrointestinal sources. Pneumomediastinum is most often a mild, self-limited process that does not require aggressive intervention. The most common causes in children are abrupt Valsalva maneuvers (e.g., severe forceful coughing) and acute asthma exacerbations. Symptoms can include chest pain and dyspnea. There are often no physical findings, although a crunching noise over the sternum can sometimes be appreciated on auscultation, and subcutaneous emphysema may be detected in the neck. The diagnosis is confirmed by chest radiograph, and treatment is directed toward the underlying lung disease.

PLEURAL EFFUSION

Etiology

Fluid accumulates in the pleural space when the local hydrostatic forces pushing fluid out of the vascular space exceed the oncotic forces that are drawing fluid back. Pleural effusions can be transudates (intact membrane but abnormal hydrostatic or oncotic forces) or exudates (decreased integrity of the membrane due to inflammatory processes or impaired lymphatic drainage). There are relatively few causes of transudates, the most common being congestive heart failure and hypoproteinemia states; the causes of exudates are numerous. Almost any pulmonary inflammatory process can result in pleural fluid accumulation. Among the most common causes of exudates are infection (e.g., tuberculosis, bacterial pneumonia), collagen vascular diseases (e.g., systemic lupus erythematosus), and malignancy. Chylous pleural effusions (pleural fluid with elevated triglyceride levels) are seen with thoracic duct injury and abnormalities of lymphatic drainage (e.g., lymphangiomyomatosis, lymphangiectasia). Bacterial pneumonia can lead to an accumulation of pleural fluid **(parapneumonic effusion)**. When this fluid is purulent or infected, then it is called an **empyema**, although often the terms *parapneumonic effusion* and *empyema* are used interchangeably. Parapneumonic effusion/empyema is the most common reason for effusion in children. Most parapneumonic effusions are due to pneumonia caused by *Streptococcus pneumoniae,* group A streptococci, or *Staphylococcus aureus*

Clinical Manifestations

Pleural effusions may be asymptomatic when small but can cause dyspnea and tachypnea as they increase in size and compress lung tissue. Effusions due to infection are usually associated with fever, malaise, poor appetite, pleuritic chest pain, and splinting. Physical findings include tachypnea, decreased breath sounds, dullness to percussion, decreased tactile fremitus, and hypoxemia. Large effusions may occupy more than half the hemithorax and cause a mediastinal shift away from the affected side, compromising respiratory status, particularly in young children.

Diagnostic Studies

The presence of pleural fluid can often be confirmed by chest radiograph. Upright and decubitus chest radiograph (Fig. 139.1) can be useful to assess for layering of fluid; chest ultrasound or CT is necessary for accurate estimates of fluid volume and *loculations* (fibrous strands that compartmentalize the effusion). CT scans of the chest can help differentiate pleural fluid from parenchymal lesions and pleural masses.

The analysis of pleural fluid is useful in differentiating a transudate from an exudate. Thoracentesis for diagnostic purposes only is less commonly performed in pediatric patients; more often, these tests are obtained only if pursuing therapeutic surgical drainage. Routine tests on pleural fluid such as cell count, pH, protein, lactate dehydrogenase, and glucose characterize the effusions. Triglyceride levels, cytology, hematocrit, gram and acid-fast bacilli stain, culture, and adenosine deaminase levels can be useful in diagnosing chylous, malignant, and tuberculous effusions (Table 139.1). Nucleic acid amplification testing of pleural fluid can be used to detect the presence of a specific pathogen; the yield of pleural fluid cultures is low. Transudative pleural effusions have a low specific gravity (<1.015) and protein content, low lactate dehydrogenase activity, and a low white blood cell (WBC) count with few polymorphonuclear cells. In contrast, exudates are characterized by high specific gravity and high protein (>3 g/dL) and lactate dehydrogenase levels. They may also have a low pH

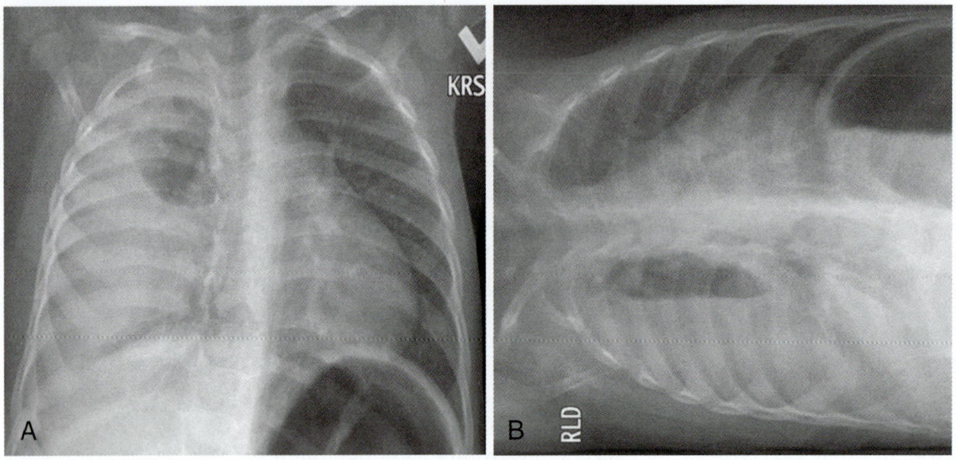

FIGURE 139.1 Parapneumonic effusion. **(A)** Posterior-anterior chest radiograph showing dense opacification of the right hemithorax. **(B)** On decubitus view, some of the density forms a horizontal layer indicating that there is pleural fluid in addition to pneumonia.

TABLE **139.1** Pleural Fluid Analysis

EXUDATIVE EFFUSION BY LIGHT TRADITIONAL CRITERIA
Pleural fluid protein/serum protein ratio >0.5 **OR** Pleural fluid LDH/serum LDH ratio >0.6 **OR** Pleural fluid LDH >two-thirds the upper limits of laboratory's normal serum LDH
CHYLOTHORAX
Triglycerides >110 mg/dL
TUBERCULOUS
Positive acid-fast bacilli stain, culture Pleural fluid protein >4 g/dL Pleural fluid adenosine deaminase level >35–50 U/L Pleural fluid glucose 30–50 mg/dL
HEMOTHORAX
Pleural fluid hematocrit/serum hematocrit >0.5

LDH, Lactate dehydrogenase.

(<7.2), low glucose level (<40 mg/dL), and a high WBC count with lymphocytes or polymorphonuclear leukocytes.

Treatment

Therapy is directed at the underlying condition causing the effusion and at relief of the mechanical consequences of the fluid collection. For small effusions, especially if they are transudates, no pleural drainage is required. Large effusions that are causing respiratory compromise should be drained with a **chest tube**. Approaches to parapneumonic effusions vary based on size. Small effusions can be managed conservatively with intravenous antibiotics alone. For medium-sized effusion without respiratory compromise management may include a trial empiric antibiotic therapy alone versus pursuing immediate drainage of fluid. With parapneumonic effusions/empyema, in addition to IV antibiotics, simple drainage with a chest tube is often not sufficient because the fluid may be thick and loculated. In such cases, pleural drainage is best achieved with either the administration of fibrinolytic agents via chest tubes or VATS. Both fibrinolytic therapy via chest tubes and VATS can reduce morbidity and length of hospital stay for complicated effusions.

PEARLS FOR PRACTITIONERS

See The Respiratory System: Pearls for Practitioners at the end of this section.

REVIEW QUESTIONS

Available online.

Suggested Readings

Levitzky MG. *Pulmonary Physiology*. 8th ed. New York: McGraw-Hill Education; 2018.

Merritt 2nd JL, Quinonez RA, Bonkowsky JL, et al. A Framework for Evaluation of the Higher-Risk Infant After a Brief Resolved Unexplained Event. *Pediatrics*. 2019;144(2):e20184101.

Sarniak AP, Clark JA, Heidemann SM. Respiratory system. In: RM, Kliegman RM, St, Geme J, eds. *Nelson Textbook of Pediatrics*. 22nd ed. Philadelphia: Elsevier; 2020.

Taussig LN, Landau LI. *Pediatric Respiratory Medicine*. 2nd ed. Philadelphia: Mosby; 2008.

Wilmott RW, Boat TF, Bush A, eds. *Kendig and Chernick's Disorders of the Respiratory Tract in Children*. 9th ed. Philadelphia: Elsevier; 2018.

PEARLS FOR PRACTITIONERS

CHAPTER 134

Respiratory System Assessment

- Airway branching is complete at birth; alveolar number increases through childhood.
- Resistance increases with reduction of airway diameter, leading to obstructive lung disease.
- Pulmonary compliance is reduced when lungs, pleura, or chest wall become stiff, causing restrictive lung disease.
- Ventilation-perfusion (V/Q) mismatch is the most common cause of hypoxemia in children.
- A chest radiograph can provide valuable information about parenchymal, pleural, and airway disease and is recommended as first-line imaging for most patients with respiratory complaints.
- Spirometry is the pulmonary function test of choice for diagnosing asthma and other obstructive lung diseases; body plethysmography is needed to confirm restrictive lung disease.
- Flexible bronchoscopy is useful for evaluation of airway anatomy and obtaining lower respiratory samples; rigid bronchoscopy is required for foreign body removal.

CHAPTER 135

Control of Breathing

- Ventilation and oxygenation are regulated by central and peripheral chemoreceptors, with signal origin in the deep brainstem.
- Central apnea is more often secondary (drugs, central nervous system tumor, trauma) than primary (genetic syndrome).
- Apnea of prematurity should resolve by 44 weeks postconceptual age.
- A brief resolved unexplained event (BRUE) is a short (generally <1 minute), self-limited episode with cyanosis or pallor, irregular breathing, change in tone, or altered level of responsiveness occurring in an infant younger than 1 year.
- The risk of sudden infant death syndrome (SIDS) is associated with preterm birth, maternal smoking, and prone sleep position.
- Obstructive sleep apnea is most commonly caused by adenotonsillar hypertrophy in children.
- Polysomnogram is the diagnostic test of choice for obstructive and central apnea.

CHAPTER 136

Upper Airway Obstruction

- Upper airway obstruction at the level of the glottis or subglottis produces stridor, worse when the child is awake and active.
- The most common cause of *noninfectious* stridor in infants is laryngomalacia.
- The most common cause of *infectious* stridor in infants and young children is croup (laryngotracheobronchitis).
- Upper airway obstruction at the level of the pharynx is usually due to soft tissue collapse or enlargement, leading to mouth breathing and snoring that is worse during sleep.
- The most common cause of *noninfectious* soft tissue upper airway obstruction in young children is adenotonsillar hypertrophy.
- The most common causes of *infectious* soft tissue upper airway obstruction include retropharyngeal abscess and peritonsillar abscess.

CHAPTER 137

Lower Airway, Parenchymal, and Pulmonary Vascular Diseases

- The most common cause of lower airway disease in children is asthma, a clinical disease of variable and recurring symptoms with airway inflammation and bronchial hyperresponsiveness.
- A wheeze is a continuous sound produced by small airway narrowing and is most pronounced on exhalation.
- Tracheomalacia is the most common tracheal abnormality, can be congenital or acquired, and often improves with growth.
- Vascular rings can be complete or incomplete, causing extrinsic tracheal compression, leading to wheezing, stridor, cough, or dyspnea.
- Foreign body aspiration most often occurs in children 1–4 years of age, often with nonradiopaque material such as food (e.g., nuts).
- Primary ciliary dyskinesia (PCD) is a heterogenous disorder of motile cilia with clinical features of neonatal respiratory distress, year-round productive cough, year-round nasal congestion, chronic sinusitis, chronic otitis media, and laterality defects. Late clinical manifestations include bronchiectasis and end-stage lung disease.
    - PCD diagnosis is multifactorial and involves compatible clinical phenotype, evaluation for cilia defects on electron microscopy, nasal nitric oxide testing, and genetic analysis.

- Pulmonary hypertension may lead to irreversible pulmonary vascular changes that strain the right heart and lead to cor pulmonale.
  - Cor pulmonale can be caused by chronic lung disease, particularly severe bronchopulmonary dysplasia, and untreated severe obstructive sleep apnea.
- Hemoptysis from pulmonary sources can occur from airway hemorrhage or alveolar bleeding.

CHAPTER 138

Cystic Fibrosis

- Cystic fibrosis (CF) is an autosomal recessive genetic disorder.
- The gene for CF encodes a polypeptide, the cystic fibrosis transmembrane conductance regulator (CFTR), a chloride channel located on the apical surface of epithelial cells.
  - Defects in the *CFTR* gene result in abnormal movement of salt and water across cell membranes leading to thick secretions impacting multiple organ systems.
- Clinical manifestations of CF in children include chronic cough, recurrent pulmonary infections, growth faltering, poor growth and weight gain, recurrent sinusitis, nasal polyposis, steatorrhea, recurrent pancreatitis, and rectal prolapse.
- Common pathogens in CF sputum are *Staphylococcus aureus* and *Pseudomonas aeruginosa.*
- Sweat chloride testing is the diagnostic test of choice and confirms diagnosis with newborn screening, genetic testing, and clinical symptoms.
- Management of CF includes enhancing airway clearance, medications to decrease mucus viscosity, treating airway infections, and improving nutritional status with pancreatic enzyme replacement therapy and nutritional supplements.
- Other therapies are genotype specific and improve the function of CFTR protein for individuals with CF.

CHAPTER 139

Chest Wall and Pleura

- Severe thoracic scoliosis can lead to chest wall deformity that limits lung volumes and causes restrictive lung disease.
- Pectus excavatum (sternal concavity) and pectus carinatum (sternal extrusion) are common chest wall deformities that are usually not associated with significant pulmonary compromise.
- Pneumothorax is an accumulation of air in the pleural space that can occur spontaneously from leakage of air from the lung or airways.
- Pleural effusions can be transudative (e.g., heart failure) or exudative (e.g., infection/empyema).
- Parapneumonic effusion/empyema in children is commonly associated with infection from *Streptococcus pneumoniae,* group A streptococci, or *Staphylococcus aureus.*

SECTION 19

THE CARDIOVASCULAR SYSTEM

Christopher Sumski

CHAPTER 140

Cardiovascular System Assessment

Assessment of the cardiovascular system in pediatric patients can be a daunting exercise, particularly in a busy exam room and with variable cooperation. Given the potential seriousness of cardiovascular disease, accurate and systematic assessment is crucial to facilitate timely diagnosis and treatment.

HISTORY

A **maternal history** of medication, substance or alcohol use, or tobacco/nicotine use may contribute to cardiac and other systemic findings. The **prenatal history** may reveal a maternal infection early in pregnancy (possibly teratogenic) or later in pregnancy (causing myocarditis or myocardial dysfunction in infants). Infants with heart failure exhibit **poor growth**, with weight being more significantly affected than height and head circumference.

Heart failure may present with fussiness, **fatigue**, or **diaphoresis** with feeds. **Tachypnea** without significant dyspnea may be present. Older children with heart failure may have easy fatigability, **shortness of breath** on exertion, and, sometimes, orthopnea. Not keeping up with other children during play or exercise is a sign of **exercise intolerance**. Heart failure may be misdiagnosed as recurrent pneumonia, bronchitis, wheezing, or asthma.

A history of a **heart murmur** is important, but many well children have a normal or innocent murmur at some time in their lives. Other cardiac symptoms include cyanosis, palpitations, chest pain, syncope, and near-syncope. A review of systems assesses for possible systemic diseases or congenital malformation syndromes that may cause cardiac abnormalities (Tables 140.1 and 140.2). Current and past medication use as well as history of drug use is important. **Family history** should be reviewed for hereditary diseases, early atherosclerotic heart disease, congenital heart disease, sudden unexplained deaths, thrombophilia, rheumatic fever, hypertension, and hypercholesterolemia.

PHYSICAL EXAMINATION

A complete cardiovascular examination starts in the supine position and includes evaluation in sitting and standing positions, when possible. **Inspection** is supplemented by **palpation** and **auscultation** to provide a complete examination.

The examination starts with vital signs. The normal **heart rate** varies with age and activity. Newborn resting heart rates are approximately 120 beats per minute, slightly higher in infants 3–6 months of age, and then gradually declining through adolescence to near 80 beats per minute. The range of normal for any given age is approximately 30 beats per minute above or below the average. Tachycardia may be a manifestation of anxiety, agitation, anemia, dehydration, shock, heart failure, or dysrhythmia. Bradycardia can be a normal finding in patients with high vagal tone (e.g., athletes) but may be a manifestation of atrioventricular block. The **respiratory rate** of infants is best assessed while the infant is quiet. Respiratory rate may be increased when there is a left-to-right shunt or pulmonary venous congestion.

Normal **blood pressure** also varies with age. A properly sized cuff should have a bladder width that is at least 40% and a length that is 80–100% of the arm circumference. Initially, blood pressure in the right arm is measured. If elevated, measurements in all four extremities are indicated to evaluate for coarctation of the aorta. The **pulse pressure** is determined by subtracting the diastolic pressure from the systolic pressure. It is normally below 50 mm Hg or half the systolic pressure, whichever is less. A wide pulse pressure may be seen with aortopulmonary connections (patent ductus arteriosus [PDA], truncus arteriosus, arteriovenous malformations), aortic insufficiency, or relative intravascular volume depletion (anemia, vasodilation with fever or sepsis). A narrow pulse pressure is seen with pericardial tamponade, aortic stenosis, and heart failure.

Inspection includes general appearance, nutritional status, circulation, and respiratory effort. Many chromosomal abnormalities and syndromes associated with cardiac defects have dysmorphic features or growth faltering (see Table 140.2). Skin color must be assessed for **cyanosis** and pallor. Central cyanosis (tongue, lips) is associated with arterial desaturation; isolated peripheral cyanosis (extremities, perioral) is associated with normal arterial saturation and increased peripheral extraction of oxygen. Perioral cyanosis is a common finding, especially in pale infants or when infants and toddlers become cold. Chronic arterial desaturation results in **clubbing** of the fingernails and toenails. Inspection of the chest may reveal asymmetry or a prominent left precordium, suggesting chronic cardiac enlargement.

After inspection, **palpation** of pulses in all four extremities, the precordial activity, and the abdomen is performed. Pulses are assessed for rate, regularity, intensity, symmetry, and timing between upper and lower extremities. A good pedal pulse with normal right arm blood pressure effectively rules out

TABLE 140.1 Cardiac Manifestations of Systemic Diseases

SYSTEMIC DISEASE	CARDIAC COMPLICATIONS
Hunter-Hurler syndrome	Valvular insufficiency, heart failure, hypertension
Duchenne muscular dystrophy	Cardiomyopathy, heart failure
Pompe disease	Short PR interval, cardiomegaly, heart failure, arrhythmias
Kawasaki disease	Coronary artery aneurysm, thrombosis, myocardial infarction, myocarditis
Marfan syndrome	Aortic and mitral insufficiency, dilated aortic root and/or ascending aorta, dissecting aortic aneurysm
Juvenile idiopathic arthritis	Pericarditis
Systemic lupus erythematosus	Pericarditis, Libman-Sacks endocarditis, congenital AV block
Lyme disease	Arrhythmias, myocarditis, heart failure
Graves disease (hyperthyroidism)	Tachycardia, arrhythmias, heart failure
Tuberous sclerosis	Cardiac rhabdomyoma
Neurofibromatosis	Pulmonic stenosis, coarctation of aorta
Rheumatic fever	Carditis (inflammation of the pericardium, myocardium, or heart valves), heart failure. If untreated, may progress to rheumatic heart disease with permanent valvular damage.

AV, Atrioventricular.

TABLE 140.2 Congenital Malformation Syndromes Associated With Congenital Heart Disease

SYNDROME	CARDIAC FEATURES
Trisomy 21 (Down syndrome)	Endocardial cushion defect, VSD, ASD, PDA
Trisomy 18	VSD, ASD, PDA, PS
Trisomy 13	VSD, ASD, PDA, dextrocardia
XO (Turner syndrome)	Coarctation of aorta, aortic stenosis
CHARGE syndrome (coloboma, heart, atresia choanae, retardation, genital and ear anomalies)	TOF, aortic arch and conotruncal anomalies*
22q11 deletion (DiGeorge) syndrome	Aortic arch anomalies, conotruncal anomalies*
VACTERL association† (vertebral, anal, cardiac, tracheoesophageal, radial, renal, limb anomalies)	VSD
Marfan syndrome	Dilated and dissecting aorta, aortic valve regurgitation, mitral valve prolapse
Williams syndrome	Supravalvular aortic stenosis, peripheral pulmonary stenosis
Infant of diabetic mother	Hypertrophic cardiomyopathy, VSD, conotruncal anomalies
Asplenia syndrome	Complex cyanotic heart lesions, anomalous pulmonary venous return, dextrocardia, single ventricle, single AV valve
Polysplenia syndrome	Azygos continuation of inferior vena cava, pulmonary atresia, dextrocardia, single ventricle
Fetal alcohol syndrome	VSD, ASD
Fetal hydantoin syndrome (caused by prenatal phenytoin exposure)	TGA, VSD, TOF

**Conotruncal—tetralogy of Fallot, pulmonary atresia, truncus arteriosus, transposition of great arteries.*
†VACTERL association is also known as VATER association, in which the limb anomalies are not included.
ASD, Atrial septal defect; *AV*, atrioventricular; *PDA*, patent ductus arteriosus; *PS*, pulmonic stenosis; *TGA*, transposition of great arteries; *TOF*, tetralogy of Fallot; *VSD*, ventricular septal defect.

coarctation of the aorta. The precordium should be assessed for apical impulse, **point of maximum impulse** (PMI), hyperactivity, and presence of a **thrill**. Abdominal palpation assesses liver and spleen size. The liver size provides an assessment of intravascular volume and is enlarged with systemic venous congestion. The spleen may be enlarged with infective endocarditis.

Auscultation is the most important part of the cardiovascular examination but should supplement what already has been found by inspection and palpation. Systematic listening in a quiet room allows assessment of each portion of the cardiac cycle. In addition to heart rate and regularity, the heart sounds, clicks, and murmurs need to be timed and characterized.

Heart Sounds

S_1 is associated with closure of the mitral and tricuspid valves, is usually single, and is best heard at the left lower sternal border (LLSB) or apex (Fig. 140.1). Although it can normally be split, if a split S_1 is heard, the possibility of an ejection click or, much less commonly, an S_4 should be considered. **S_2** is associated with closure of the aortic and pulmonary valves. It should normally split with inspiration and be single with exhalation. Abnormalities of splitting and intensity of the pulmonary component are associated with significant anatomic and physiologic abnormalities (Table 140.3). **S_3** is heard in early diastole and is related to rapid ventricular filling. It is best heard at the LLSB or apex and may be a normal sound, but a loud S_3 is abnormal and heard in conditions with dilated ventricles. **S_4** occurs late in diastole just before S_1; it is best heard at the LLSB/apex and is associated with decreased ventricular compliance. It is rare and is always abnormal. Differentiation between an S_3 and S_4 can be difficult in children with faster heart rates, and when uncertain consultation is advised.

Clicks

A click implies a valvular abnormality or dilated great artery. It may be ejection or midsystolic in timing and may or may not be associated with a murmur. A midsystolic click is associated

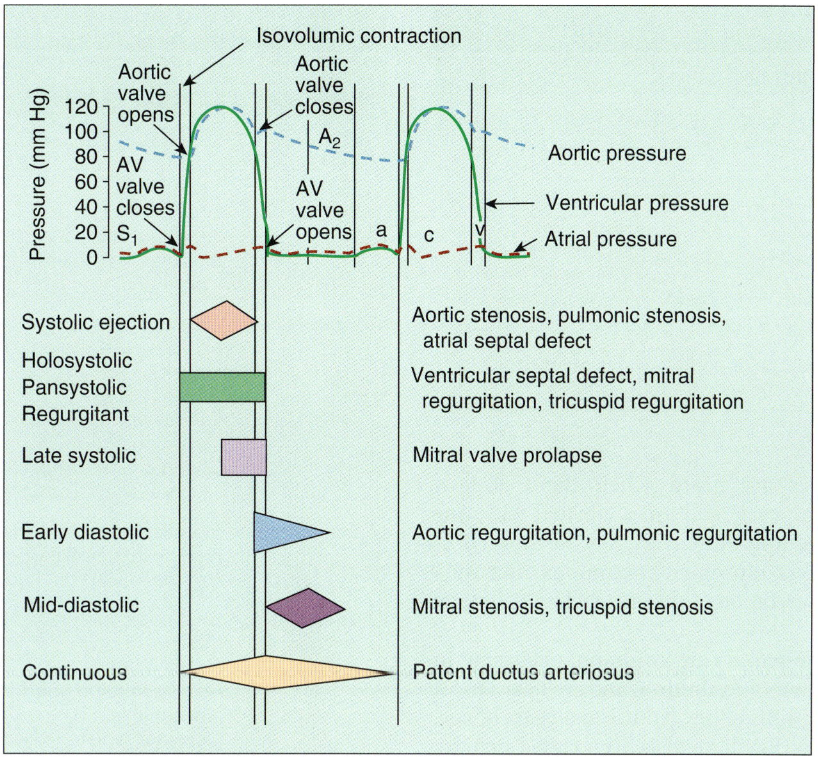

FIGURE 140.1 Timing of heart murmurs. *AV,* Atrioventricular.

TABLE 140.3 Abnormal Second Heart Sound

SINGLE S_2
Pulmonary hypertension (severe) One semilunar valve (aortic atresia, pulmonary atresia, truncus arteriosus) Malposed great arteries (d-TGA, l-TGA) Severe aortic stenosis
WIDELY SPLIT S_2
Increased flow across valve (ASD, PAPVR) Prolonged flow across valve (pulmonary stenosis) Electrical delay (right bundle branch block) Early aortic closure (severe mitral regurgitation)
PARADOXICALLY SPLIT S_2
Severe aortic stenosis
ABNORMAL INTENSITY OF P_2
Increased in pulmonary hypertension Decreased in severe pulmonary stenosis, tetralogy of Fallot

ASD, Atrial septal defect; *d-TGA,* dextro-transposition of the great arteries; *l-TGA,* levo-transposition of the great arteries; *PAPVR,* partial anomalous pulmonary venous return.

with mitral valve prolapse. **Ejection clicks** occur early in systole. Pulmonary ejection clicks are best heard at the left upper sternal border and vary in intensity with respiration. Aortic clicks are often louder at the apex, left midsternal border, or right upper sternal border and do not vary with respiration.

Murmurs

Murmur evaluation should determine timing, duration, location, intensity, radiation, and frequency or pitch of the murmur. The timing determines a murmur's significance and can be used to develop a differential diagnosis (see Fig. 140.1). Murmurs should be classified as **systolic, diastolic,** or **continuous.** Most murmurs are systolic and can be divided further into systolic ejection murmurs or holosystolic (also called pansystolic or regurgitant) murmurs. **Ejection murmurs** are crescendo-decrescendo with a short time between S_1 and the onset of the murmur (isovolumic contraction). Systolic ejection murmurs require the ejection of blood from the ventricle and may occur with aortic stenosis, pulmonary stenosis, atrial septal defects (ASDs), and coarctation of the aorta. **Holosystolic murmurs** have their onset with S_1. The murmur has a plateau quality and may be heard with ventricular septal defects (VSDs) and mitral or tricuspid regurgitation. A late regurgitant murmur may be heard after a midsystolic click in mitral valve prolapse.

Murmurs are often heard along the path of blood flow. This can be reflected in both the location and radiation pattern of the murmur. Ejection murmurs usually are best heard at the base of the heart, whereas holosystolic murmurs are louder at the LLSB and apex. Pulmonary ejection murmurs radiate to the back and axilla. Aortic ejection murmurs radiate to the neck. The **intensity** or loudness of a heart murmur is assessed as grade I through VI (Table 140.4). The **frequency** or pitch of a murmur provides information regarding the pressure gradient. The higher the pressure gradient across a narrowed area (valve, vessel, or defect), the faster the flow and higher the frequency of the murmur. Low-frequency murmurs imply low-pressure gradients and mild obstruction or less restriction to flow.

Diastolic murmurs are much less common than systolic murmurs and should be considered abnormal. Early diastolic murmurs occur when there is regurgitation through the aortic or pulmonary valve. Mid-diastolic murmurs are caused by increased flow (ASD, VSD) or anatomic stenosis across the mitral or tricuspid valves.

TABLE 140.4 Heart Murmur Intensity

GRADE	DESCRIPTION
Grade I	Very soft, heard in quiet room with cooperative patient
Grade II	Easily heard but not loud
Grade III	Loud but no thrill
Grade IV	Loud with palpable thrill
Grade V	Loud with thrill, audible with stethoscope at 45-degree angle
Grade VI	Loud with thrill, audible with stethoscope off chest 1 cm

Continuous murmurs are heard when there is flow through the entire cardiac cycle and are abnormal with one common exception, the **venous hum**. A PDA is the most common abnormal continuous murmur. Continuous murmurs can also be heard with coarctation of the aorta when collateral vessels are present.

Normal or **innocent murmurs** are common, occurring in at least 80% of healthy infants and children and are heard most often during the first 6 months of life, from 3 to 6 years of age, and in early adolescence. They have also been called benign, functional, vibratory, and flow murmurs. Characteristic findings of innocent murmurs include an intermittent nature, having a musical or vibratory quality, a lack of significant radiation, and a significant alteration in the intensity of the murmur with positional changes (Table 140.5). Most important, the cardiovascular history and examination are otherwise normal. The presence of symptoms, including growth faltering or dysmorphic features, should make one cautious about diagnosing a *normal* murmur. Diastolic, holosystolic, late systolic, and continuous (except for the venous hum) murmurs and the presence of a thrill are not normal.

TABLE 140.5 Normal or Innocent Heart Murmurs

MURMUR	CLINICAL FEATURES	USUAL AGE WHEN HEARD
Still's murmur/ vibratory murmur	Systolic ejection murmur LLSB or between LLSB and apex Grades I–III/VI Vibratory, musical quality Intensity decreases in upright position	3–6 yr
Venous hum	Continuous murmur Infraclavicular region (right > left) Grades I–III/VI Louder with patient in upright position Changes with compression of jugular vein or turning head	3–6 yr
Carotid bruit	Systolic ejection murmur Neck, over carotid artery Grades I–III/VI	Any age
Adolescent ejection murmur	Systolic ejection murmur LUSB Grades I–III/VI Usually softer in upright position Does not radiate to back	8–14 yr
Innocent peripheral pulmonary stenosis murmur	Systolic ejection murmur Axilla and back, LUSB/RUSB Grades I–III/VI High frequency	Newborn–6 mo

LLSB, Left lower sternal border; *LUSB*, left upper sternal border; *RUSB*, right upper sternal border.

LABORATORY AND IMAGING TESTS

Pulse Oximetry

Mild desaturation that is not clinically apparent may be the only early finding in complex congenital heart defects. Measurement of pulse oximetry in the right arm and a lower extremity may allow diagnosis of complex congenital heart disease including a ductal-dependent lesion in which desaturated blood flows right to left across a PDA to perfuse the lower body. By improving early diagnosis and management, the routine pulse oximetry screening of newborns between 24 and 48 hours of life has resulted in decreased morbidity and mortality from critical congenital heart disease.

Blood Gas

When a patient demonstrates **hypoxemia**, or an abnormally low oxygen saturation, the next step should be to apply supplemental oxygen. The **hyperoxia test** describes applying 10 minutes of 100% FiO_2 to a patient (usually an infant) with an abnormally low oxygen saturation to assess the response; arterial blood gases are collected before initiation of supplemental oxygen and after 10 minutes of supplemental oxygen. If the patient's partial pressure of oxygen improves with supplemental oxygen, the cause of the hypoxia is likely respiratory. If the patient's oxygen saturation does not significantly improve, the cause of the hypoxia may be cardiac (suggestive of a left-to-right shunt).

Electrocardiography

The 12-lead electrocardiogram (ECG) provides information about the **rate**, **rhythm**, **depolarization**, and **repolarization** of the cardiac cells and the size and wall thickness of the chambers. It should be assessed for rate, rhythm, axis (P wave, QRS, and T wave), intervals (PR, QRS, QTc) (Fig. 140.2), and voltages (left atrial, right atrial, left ventricular, right ventricular) adjusted for the child's age.

The **P wave** represents atrial depolarization. A criterion for right atrial enlargement is an increase of the amplitude of the P wave, reflected best in lead II. The diagnosis of left atrial enlargement is made by prolongation of the second portion of the P wave, exhibited best in the chest leads.

The **PR interval**, measured from the beginning of the P wave to the beginning of the QRS complex, increases with age. Conduction time is shortened when the conduction velocity is increased (as in glycogen storage disease) or when the atrioventricular node is bypassed (as in Wolff-Parkinson-White syndrome). A prolonged PR interval usually indicates slow conduction through the atrioventricular node. Diseases in the atrial myocardium, the bundle of His, or the Purkinje system may also contribute to prolonged PR intervals.

The **QRS complex** represents ventricular depolarization. A greater ventricular volume or mass causes a greater magnitude of the complex, though this is a nonspecific finding. The proximity of the right ventricle to the chest surface accentuates that ventricle's contribution to the complex. Changes in the QRS axis and duration occur with age. Normative data for each age group must be known to make a diagnosis from the ECG.

The **QT interval** is measured from the beginning of the QRS complex to the end of the T wave. The corrected QT interval (corrected for rate) should be less than 0.45 second ($QTc = QT\sqrt{\text{preceding R to R interval}}$). The interval may be prolonged in children with hypocalcemia or severe hypokalemia. It is also prolonged in a group of children at risk for severe ventricular arrhythmias and sudden death **(prolonged QT syndrome)**. Drugs can also prolong the QT interval. Common examples include macrolide or quinolone antibiotics, tricyclic antidepressants, selective serotonin reuptake inhibitors, or antiemetics such as ondansetron. ECG measurement prior to initiating these medications may be indicated.

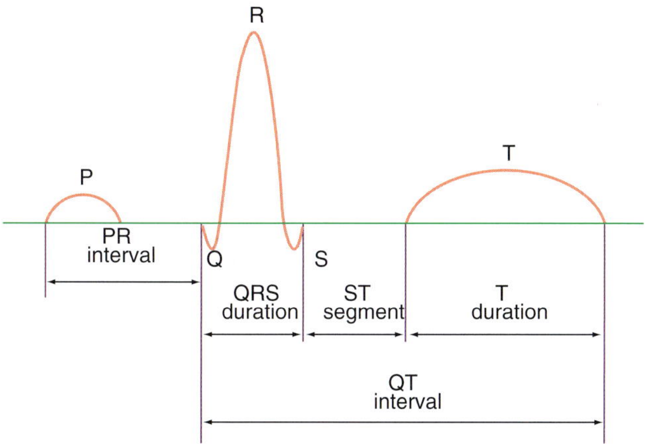

FIGURE 140.2 Nomenclature of electrocardiogram waves and intervals.

Chest Radiography

A systematic approach to reading a chest radiograph includes assessment of extracardiac structures, the shape and size of the heart, and the size and position of the pulmonary artery and aorta (Fig. 140.3). Assessment of the location and size of the heart and **cardiac silhouette** may suggest a cardiac defect. On a good inspiratory film, the cardiothoracic ratio should be less than 55% in infants under 1 year of age and less than 50% in older children and adolescents. An enlarged heart may be due to an increased volume load (left-right shunt) or due to myocardial dysfunction (dilated cardiomyopathy). The shape of the heart may suggest specific congenital heart defects. The most common examples are the boot-shaped heart seen with tetralogy of Fallot, the egg on a string seen with dextro-transposition of the great arteries, and the "snowman" seen with supracardiac total anomalous pulmonary venous return. The chest x-ray can aid in the assessment of **pulmonary blood flow.** Defects associated with left-to-right shunting have increased pulmonary blood flow (shunt vascularity) on x-ray. Right-to-left shunts have decreased pulmonary blood flow.

Echocardiography

Echocardiography has become the most important noninvasive tool in the diagnosis and management of cardiac disease, providing a full anatomic evaluation in most congenital heart defects (Fig. 140.4). Physiologic data on the direction and velocity of blood flow can be obtained with the use of pulsed, continuous-wave, and color flow Doppler. Imaging from multiple views provides an assessment of spatial relationships.

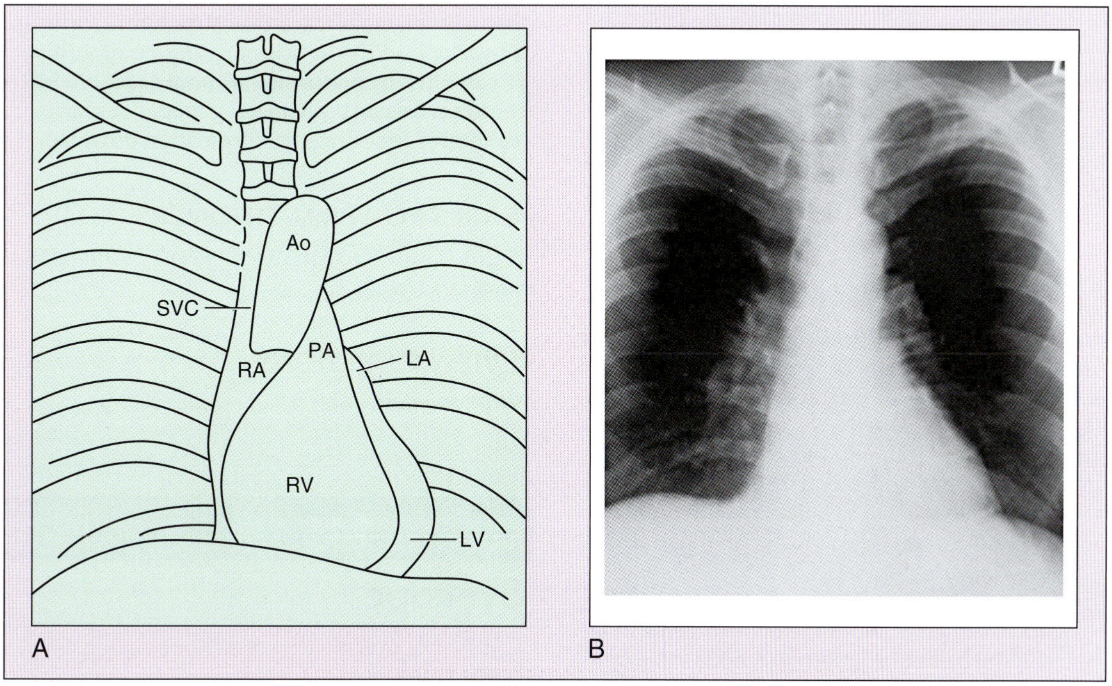

FIGURE 140.3 **(A)** Parts of the heart whose outlines can be identified on a routine chest x-ray. **(B)** Routine posteroanterior x-ray of the normal cardiac silhouette. *Ao*, Aorta; *LA*, left atrium; *LV*, left ventricle; *PA*, pulmonary artery; *RA*, right atrium; *RV*, right ventricle; *SVC*, superior vena cava. (From Andreoli TE, Carpenter CCJ, Plum F, et al., eds. *Cecil Essentials of Medicine*. 2nd ed. Philadelphia: WB Saunders; 1990.)

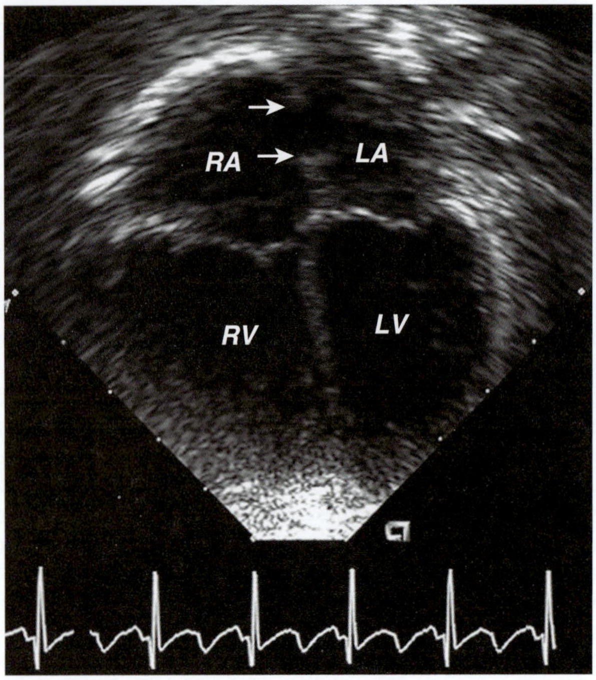

FIGURE 140.4 Four-chamber echocardiogram of an atrial septal defect. The defect margins are identified by the two arrows. *LA*, Left atrium; *LV*, left ventricle; *RA*, right atrium; *RV*, right ventricle.

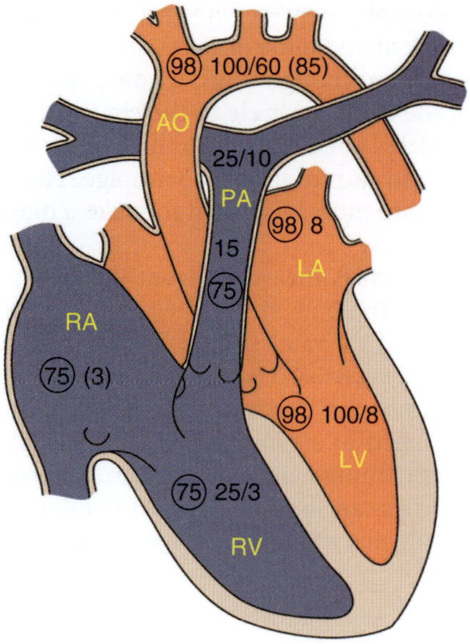

FIGURE 140.5 The normal heart. Circled values are oxygen saturations. *Ao*, Aorta; *LA*, left atrium; *LV*, left ventricle; *PA*, pulmonary artery; *RA*, right atrium; *RV*, right ventricle.

Three-dimensional (3D) and four-dimensional (4D) imaging now allows reconstruction of the heart and manipulation of the images to provide more detail, especially with regard to valve structure and function. Prenatal or fetal echocardiography can diagnose congenital heart disease by 18 weeks of gestation and allows for delivery of the infant at a tertiary care hospital, improving the timeliness of therapy. Most congenital heart defects now are surgically repaired based on the echocardiogram without need for cardiac catheterization.

Though transthoracic echocardiography in pediatrics usually provides diagnostic quality images, transesophageal echocardiography (TEE) can provide higher quality images when transthoracic imaging is inadequate. It is used intraoperatively to assess results and cardiac function after surgery. TEE and intracardiac echocardiography are used to guide interventional catheterization and radiofrequency ablation of dysrhythmias.

Cardiac Catheterization

Cardiac catheterization is performed in patients who need additional anatomic information or precise hemodynamic information before operating or establishing a management plan, or in cases where a catheter-based intervention is possible. Pressures, oxygen saturations, and oxygen content are measured in each chamber and blood vessel entered (Fig. 140.5). This information is used to calculate systemic and pulmonary blood flow and resistance. Angiography is performed by injecting contrast material into selected sites to define anatomy and supplement noninvasive information. An increasing percentage of cardiac catheterizations are done to perform an intervention, including balloon dilation of stenotic valves and vessels, ballooning and stenting of stenotic lesions, closure of collateral vessels by coil embolization, and device closure of PDAs, secundum ASDs, and muscular VSDs. Catheterization with electrophysiologic studies allows for precise mapping of the electrical activity, can assess the risk of abnormal heart rhythms, and is often done in anticipation of radiofrequency ablation of the site of a dysrhythmia.

Cardiac Computed Tomography/Magnetic Resonance Imaging

Computed tomography (CT) and magnetic resonance imaging (MRI) are often used to provide additional structural and functional information in congenital and acquired heart disease. They are especially helpful in providing 3D anatomy and when visualizing extracardiac structures (aortic arch, pulmonary artery and vein anatomy and relationships). Although CT can often be performed without sedation, MRI frequently requires sedation; both imaging modalities have strengths and weaknesses regarding the information provided.

PEARLS FOR PRACTITIONERS

See The Cardiovascular System: Pearls for Practitioners at the end of this section.

REVIEW QUESTIONS

Available online.

CHAPTER 141

Syncope

ETIOLOGY

Syncope is the transient loss of consciousness and muscle tone that, by history, does not suggest other altered states of consciousness. Presyncope or near-syncope has prodromal symptoms without loss of consciousness. Syncope is relatively common and is most commonly due to autonomic dysfunction. The frequency of episodes, amount of stress, and functional impairment caused by syncope vary. Most syncopal events are relatively benign but can represent a serious cardiac condition that may lead to death (see Table 141.1). The differential diagnosis for typical syncope includes vasovagal or orthostatic responses, seizure, hypoglycemia, hyperventilation, atypical migraine, breath holding, and cardiac causes/arrhythmia.

CLINICAL MANIFESTATIONS

Typical syncopal events usually occur in the upright position or are related to changing position. Syncope may be associated with anxiety, pain, phlebotomy or the sight of blood, fasting, a hot environment, or crowded places. The patient often appears pale. A prodrome, consisting of dizziness, lightheadedness, nausea, diaphoresis, visual changes (blacking out), or possibly palpitations, warns the patient and often prevents injury. Unconsciousness lasts for less than 1 minute. A return to normal consciousness occurs relatively quickly. Most of these syncopal episodes are vasovagal or neurocardiogenic in origin. The physical examination is normal. Atypical characteristics that warrant further evaluation include a lack of prodrome, syncope with exercise, and family history of sudden cardiac death. A postictal state or convulsions would increase concern for seizures; however, some episodes of syncope also have rhythmic movement of extremities.

DIAGNOSTIC STUDIES

Syncopal episodes may require no more than reassurance to the patient and family. If the episodes have a significant impact on daily activities, further evaluation may be indicated. An

TABLE 141.1 Etiologies of Syncope and Dizziness

DIAGNOSIS	HISTORY	SIGNS/ SYMPTOMS	DESCRIPTION	HEART RATE/ BLOOD PRESSURE	DURATION	POSTSYNCOPE	RECURRENCE
Neurocardiogenic (vasodepressor)	At rest	Pallor, nausea, visual changes	Brief ± convulsion	↓/↓	<1 min	Residual pallor, sweaty, hot; recurs if child stands	Common
OTHER VAGAL							
Micturition	Postvoiding	Pallor, nausea	Brief; convulsions rare	↓/↓	<1 min		(+)
Hair grooming	Standing getting hair done or ears touched	Pallor, nausea, visual changes, lightheaded	Brief		<1 min	Residual pallor, sweaty, hot, can recur if stands too soon	(+)
Cough (deglutition)	Paroxysmal cough	Cough	Abrupt onset	May not change	<5 min	Fatigue or baseline	(+)
Carotid sinus	Tight collar, turned head	Vague, visual changes	Sudden onset, pallor	Usually ↓/↓	<5 min	Fatigue or baseline	(+)
CARDIAC SYNCOPE							
LVOT obstruction	Exercise	±Chest pain, SOB	Abrupt during or after exertion, pallor	↑/↓	Any duration	Fatigue, residual pallor, and sweating	(+)
Pulmonary hypertension	Any time, especially exercise	SOB	Cyanosis and pallor	↑/↓	Any duration	Fatigue, residual cyanosis	(+)
Myocarditis	Post–viral infection exercise	SOB, chest pain, palpitations	Pallor	↑/↓	Any duration	Fatigue	(+)
Tumor or mass	Recumbent, paroxysmal	SOB ± chest pain	Pallor	↑/↓	Any duration	Baseline	(+)
Coronary artery disease	Exercise	SOB ± chest pain	Pallor	↑/↓	Any duration	Fatigue, chest pain	(+)
Dysrhythmia	Any time	Palpitations ± chest pain	Pallor	↑ or ↑/↓	Usually <10 min	Fatigue or baseline	(+)

±, With or without; (+), yes but not consistent or predictable; *LVOT*, left ventricular outflow tract; *SOB*, shortness of breath.
From Lewis DA. Syncope and dizziness. In Kliegman RM, ed. Practical Strategies in Pediatric Diagnosis and Therapy. *Philadelphia: WB Saunders; 1996.*

electrocardiogram (ECG) should be obtained with attention to the QTc and PR intervals (see Chapter 140). Although reassurance and increasing fluid and salt intake may be adequate to treat most cases of syncope, medical management is sometimes indicated.

PEARLS FOR PRACTITIONERS

See The Cardiovascular System: Pearls for Practitioners at the end of this section.

REVIEW QUESTION

Available online

CHAPTER 142

Chest Pain

ETIOLOGY

Chest pain in the pediatric patient often generates a significant amount of patient and parental concern. Although chest pain is rarely cardiac in origin in children, common knowledge about atherosclerotic heart disease raises concerns about a child experiencing chest pain. Most diagnosable chest pain in childhood is musculoskeletal in origin. However, a significant amount remains idiopathic. Knowledge of the complete differential diagnosis is necessary to make an accurate assessment (Table 142.1).

CLINICAL MANIFESTATIONS

Assessment of a patient with chest pain includes a thorough history to determine activity at the onset; the location, radiation, quality, and duration of the pain; what makes the pain better and worse during the time that it is present; and any associated symptoms. A family history and assessment of how much anxiety the symptom is causing are important and often revealing. A careful general physical examination should focus on the chest wall, heart, lungs, and abdomen. Pain that is reproducible with palpation of the precordium supports a musculoskeletal cause. A history of chest pain associated with exertion, syncope, or palpitations or acute onset associated with fever suggests a cardiac etiology. Cardiac causes of chest pain are generally ischemic, inflammatory, or arrhythmic in origin.

DIAGNOSTIC STUDIES

Tests rarely are indicated based on the history. A chest x-ray, electrocardiogram (ECG), 24-hour Holter monitoring, echocardiogram, and exercise stress testing may be obtained based on history and examination. Referral to a pediatric cardiologist is based on the history, physical examination findings, family history, and, frequently, the level of anxiety in the patient or family members regarding the pain.

TABLE 142.1 Differential Diagnosis of Pediatric Chest Pain

COMMON
Musculoskeletal
Costochondritis Trauma or muscle overuse/strain
Pulmonary
Asthma (often exercise-induced) Severe cough Pneumonia
Gastrointestinal
Reflux esophagitis
Psychogenic
Anxiety, hyperventilation
Miscellaneous
Precordial catch syndrome (Texidor's twinge) Sickle cell vaso-occlusive crisis Idiopathic
UNCOMMON/RARE
Cardiac
Ischemia (coronary artery abnormalities, severe AS or PS, HOCM, cocaine) Infection/inflammation (myocarditis, pericarditis, Kawasaki disease) Dysrhythmia
Musculoskeletal
Abnormalities of rib cage/thoracic spine Tietze syndrome Slipping rib Tumor
Pulmonary
Pleurisy Pneumothorax, pneumomediastinum Pleural effusion Pulmonary embolism
Gastrointestinal
Esophageal foreign body Esophageal spasm
Psychogenic
Functional neurologic disorders Somatization disorders Depression

AS, Aortic stenosis; *HOCM*, hypertrophic obstructive cardiomyopathy; *PS*, pulmonary stenosis.

PEARLS FOR PRACTITIONERS

See The Cardiovascular System: Pearls for Practitioners at the end of this section.

REVIEW QUESTION

Available online.

CHAPTER 143

Dysrhythmias

ETIOLOGY AND DIFFERENTIAL DIAGNOSIS

Cardiac dysrhythmias or abnormal heart rhythms are uncommon in pediatrics but may be caused by infection and inflammation, structural lesions, metabolic abnormalities, and intrinsic conduction abnormalities (Table 143.1). Many pediatric dysrhythmias are normal variants that do not require treatment or even further evaluation.

Sinus rhythm originates in the sinus node and has a normal axis P wave (upright in leads I and aVF) preceding each QRS complex. Because normal rates vary with age, sinus bradycardia and sinus tachycardia are defined based on age. **Sinus arrhythmia** is a common finding in children and represents a normal variation in the heart rate associated with breathing. The heart rate increases with inspiration and decreases with expiration, producing a recurring pattern on the ECG tracing of variation in the R-R interval with no change in P-wave morphology. Sinus arrhythmia is normal and does not require further evaluation or treatment.

TABLE 143.1 Etiology of Dysrhythmias

DRUGS
Intoxication (cocaine, tricyclic antidepressants, and others) Antiarrhythmic agents (proarrhythmic agents [quinidine]) Sympathomimetic agents (caffeine, theophylline, ephedrine, and others) Digoxin
INFECTION AND POSTINFECTION
Myocarditis Lyme disease Endocarditis Diphtheria Guillain-Barré syndrome Rheumatic fever
METABOLIC-ENDOCRINE
Electrolyte disturbances (↓↑K^+, ↓↑Ca^{2+}, ↓Mg^{2+}) Cardiomyopathy Thyrotoxicosis Uremia Pheochromocytoma Porphyria Mitochondrial myopathies
STRUCTURAL LESIONS
Congenital heart defects Ventricular tumor Ventriculotomy Arrhythmogenic right ventricle (dysplasia)
OTHER CAUSES
Adrenergic-induced Prolonged QT interval Maternal collagen vascular disease (+SSA and/or SSB) Idiopathic Central venous catheter

Ca, Calcium; *K*, potassium; *Mg*, magnesium; *SSA*, anti-Ro/SSA antibody; *SSB*, anti-La antibody.

Atrial Dysrhythmias

A **wandering atrial pacemaker** is a change in the morphology of the P waves with variable PR interval and normal QRS complex. This is a benign finding, requiring no further evaluation or treatment.

Premature atrial contractions (PACs) are relatively common prenatally and in infants. A premature P wave, usually with an abnormal axis consistent with its ectopic origin, is present. The premature atrial activity may be blocked (no QRS following it), conducted normally (normal QRS present), or conducted aberrantly (a widened, altered QRS complex). Premature atrial contractions are usually benign and, if present around the time of birth, usually disappear during the first few weeks of life.

Atrial flutter and **atrial fibrillation** are uncommon dysrhythmias in pediatrics and usually present after surgical repair of complex congenital heart disease. They may also be seen in patients with myocarditis or in association with drug toxicity. Neonatal atrial flutter can be a relatively common entity and usually does not recur after cardioversion.

Supraventricular tachycardia (SVT) is the most common symptomatic dysrhythmia in pediatric patients. The rhythm has a rapid, regular rate with a narrow QRS complex. SVT in infants is often 220–300 beats per minute with slower rates for older children and adolescents. The tachycardia has an abrupt onset and termination. In a child with a structurally normal heart, most episodes are relatively asymptomatic other than a pounding heartbeat. If there is structural heart disease or the episode is prolonged (>12 hours), there may be an alteration in the cardiac output and development of symptoms of heart failure. Although most patients with SVT have structurally normal hearts and normal baseline ECGs, some children have Wolff-Parkinson-White syndrome or preexcitation as the cause of the dysrhythmia.

Ventricular Dysrhythmias

Premature ventricular contractions (PVCs) are less common than premature atrial contractions in infancy but more common in older children and adolescents (Table 143.2). The premature beat is not preceded by a P wave, and the QRS complex is abnormal. If the heart is structurally normal and the PVCs are infrequent, singleton, uniform in focus, and disappear with increased heart rate, they are usually benign and require no treatment. Any deviation from the presentation (history of syncope or a family history of sudden death) requires further investigation and possibly treatment with antiarrhythmic medications.

Ventricular tachycardia, defined as three or more consecutive PVCs, is also relatively rare in pediatric patients. Although there are multiple causes of ventricular tachycardia, it can be a sign of serious cardiac dysfunction or disease. Rapid-rate ventricular tachycardia results in decreased cardiac output and cardiovascular instability. Treatment in symptomatic patients is synchronized cardioversion. Medical management with lidocaine or amiodarone may be appropriate in a conscious asymptomatic patient. Complete evaluation of the etiologic picture is necessary, including electrophysiologic study.

TABLE 143.2 Dysrhythmias in Children

TYPE	ELECTROCARDIOGRAM CHARACTERISTICS	TREATMENT
Supraventricular tachycardia	Rate usually >220 beats/min (range, 180–320 beats/min); abnormal atrial rate for age; P waves may be present and are related to QRS complex; normal, narrow QRS complexes unless aberrant conduction is present	Increase vagal tone (bag of ice water to face, Valsalva maneuver), adenosine, digoxin, sotalol, electrical cardioversion if acutely ill, catheter ablation
Atrial flutter	Atrial rate usually 300 beats/min, with varying degrees of block; sawtooth flutter waves	Digoxin, sotalol, cardioversion
Premature ventricular contraction	Premature, wide, unusually shaped QRS complex, with large inverted T wave	None if normal heart and if premature ventricular contractions disappear with exercise; beta blockade, lidocaine, procainamide
Ventricular tachycardia	>3 premature ventricular beats; AV dissociation; fusion beats, blocked retrograde AV conduction; sustained if >30 sec; rate 120–240 beats/min	Lidocaine, amiodarone, procainamide, propranolol, cardioversion
Ventricular fibrillation	No distinct QRS complex or T waves; irregular undulations with varied amplitude and contour, no conducted pulse	Nonsynchronized cardioversion
Complete heart block	Atria and ventricles have independent pacemakers; AV dissociation; escape-pacemaker is at atrioventricular junction if congenital	Awake rate <55 beats/min in neonate or <40 beats/min in adolescent, or hemodynamic instability; requires permanent pacemaker
First-degree heart block	Prolonged PR interval for age	Observe, obtain digoxin level if on therapy
Mobitz type I (Wenckebach) second-degree heart block	Progressive lengthening of PR interval until P wave is not followed by conducted QRS complex	Observe, correct underlying electrolyte or other abnormalities
Mobitz type II second-degree heart block	Sudden nonconduction of P wave with loss of QRS complex without progressive PR interval lengthening	Consider pacemaker
Sinus tachycardia	Rate >100 beats/min in adults or above the normal range for age in children; P waves with constant morphology precede every QRS complex	Treat cause (fever), remove sympathomimetic drugs

AV, Atrioventricular.

Heart Block

First-degree heart block is the presence of a prolonged PR interval. It is asymptomatic and, when present in otherwise healthy children, requires no evaluation or treatment. **Second-degree heart block** is when some, but not all, of the P waves are followed by a QRS complex. Mobitz type I (also known as Wenckebach) is characterized by a progressive prolongation of the PR interval until a QRS complex is dropped. It is often seen during sleep, usually does not progress to other forms of heart block, and does not require further evaluation or treatment in otherwise normal children. Mobitz type II is present when the PR interval does not change, but a QRS is intermittently dropped. This form may progress to complete heart block and may require pacemaker placement. **Third-degree heart block**, whether congenital or acquired, is present when there is no relationship between atrial and ventricular activity. The ventricular rate is much slower than the atrial rate. **Congenital complete heart block** is associated with maternal collagen vascular disease (such as systemic lupus erythematosus or Sjögren syndrome with positive SSA and/or SSB antibodies) or congenital heart disease. The acquired form most often occurs after cardiac surgery but may be secondary to infection, inflammation, or drugs.

TREATMENT

Most atrial dysrhythmias require no intervention. Treatment of SVT depends on presentation and symptoms. Acute treatment of SVT in infants usually consists of **vagal maneuvers**, such as Valsalva or the sudden application of a cold stimulus (ice bag, washcloth, etc.) to the face. Intravenous (IV) **adenosine** usually converts the dysrhythmia by blocking conduction through the atrioventricular node, which forms part of the re-entry circuit in most patients with SVT. In patients with cardiovascular compromise at the time of presentation, **synchronized cardioversion** is indicated using 1–2 J/kg. In patients with palpitations, it is important to document heart rate and rhythm during their symptoms before considering therapeutic options. The frequency, length, and associated symptoms during the episodes, as well as what is required to convert the rhythm, determine the need for ongoing treatment. Some patients require only education regarding the dysrhythmia and follow-up. If pharmacologic treatment is utilized, a β blocker is usually the first choice. Some practitioners still use digoxin for management of SVT, but it is contraindicated in patients with Wolff-Parkinson-White syndrome. Additional antiarrhythmic medications are sometimes needed depending on the mechanism of the SVT. In patients who are

TABLE 143.3 Classification of Drugs for Antiarrhythmia

CLASS	ACTION	EXAMPLE(S)
I	Depression of phase of depolarization (velocity of upstroke of action potential); sodium channel blockade	
Ia	Prolongation of QRS complex and QT interval	Quinidine, procainamide, disopyramide
Ib	Significant effect on abnormal conduction	Lidocaine, mexiletine, phenytoin, tocainide
Ic	Prolongation of QRS complex and PR interval	Flecainide, propafenone, moricizine
II	β Blockade; slowing of sinus rate; prolongation of PR interval	Propranolol, atenolol, acebutolol
III	Prolongation of action potential; prolongation of PR, QT intervals, QRS complex; sodium and calcium channel blockade	Bretylium, amiodarone, sotalol
IV	Calcium channel blockade; reduction in sinus and AV node pacemaker activity and conduction; prolongation of PR interval	Verapamil and other calcium channel blocking agents

AV, Atrioventricular.

symptomatic or for those not wanting to take daily medications, **radiofrequency ablation** may be performed, typically with good outcomes.

A variety of antiarrhythmic agents are used to treat ventricular dysrhythmias that require intervention (Table 143.3). Management of third-degree heart block depends on the ventricular rate and presence of symptoms. Treatment, if needed, often requires placement of a pacemaker.

PEARLS FOR PRACTITIONERS

See The Cardiovascular System: Pearls for Practitioners at the end of this section.

REVIEW QUESTION

Available online.

CHAPTER 144

Acyanotic Congenital Heart Disease

ETIOLOGY AND EPIDEMIOLOGY

Congenital heart disease (CHD) is the most common congenital disorder in newborns and occurs in more than 8 per 1,000 births worldwide. The spectrum of lesions ranges from asymptomatic to fatal. Of newborns born with CHD, 25% have critical CHD requiring surgical or catheter-based intervention in the first year of life. Although most cases of CHD are multifactorial, some lesions are associated with chromosomal disorders, single gene defects, teratogens, or maternal metabolic disease (see Table 140.2).

CHDs can be divided into three pathophysiologic groups (Table 144.1):

1. Left-to-right shunts
2. Right-to-left shunts
3. Obstructive, stenotic lesions

TABLE 144.1 Classification of Congenital Cardiac Defects

	SHUNTING		
STENOTIC	RIGHT→LEFT	LEFT→RIGHT	MIXING
Aortic stenosis	Tetralogy of Fallot	Patent ductus arteriosus	Truncus
Pulmonary stenosis	Transposition	Ventricular septal defect	TAPVR
Coarctation of the aorta	Tricuspid atresia	Atrial septal defect	HLHS

HLHS, Hypoplastic left heart syndrome; *TAPVR,* total anomalous pulmonary venous return.

Acyanotic CHD includes left-to-right shunts resulting in an increase in pulmonary blood flow (e.g., patent ductus arteriosus [PDA], ventricular septal defect [VSD], atrial septal defect [ASD]) and obstructive lesions (e.g., aortic stenosis, pulmonary stenosis, coarctation of the aorta), which usually have normal pulmonary blood flow.

VENTRICULAR SEPTAL DEFECT

Etiology and Epidemiology

VSDs, the most common congenital heart defect, accounts for 25% of all CHD. The ventricular septum is a complex structure that can be divided into four components. The largest component is the **muscular septum**. The inlet or posterior septum comprises **endocardial cushion tissue**. The subarterial or **supracristal septum** comprises conotruncal tissue. The **membranous septum** is below the aortic valve and is relatively small. VSDs occur when any of these components fails to develop normally. **Perimembranous VSDs** are the most common of all VSDs (67%) (Fig. 144.1).

The location of the VSD is important prognostically and in approach to repair; the amount of flow crossing a VSD determines the clinical presentation and depends on the size of the defect and the pulmonary vascular resistance. Large VSDs are not symptomatic at birth because the pulmonary vascular resistance is normally elevated at this time. As the pulmonary vascular resistance decreases over the first 6–8 weeks of life,

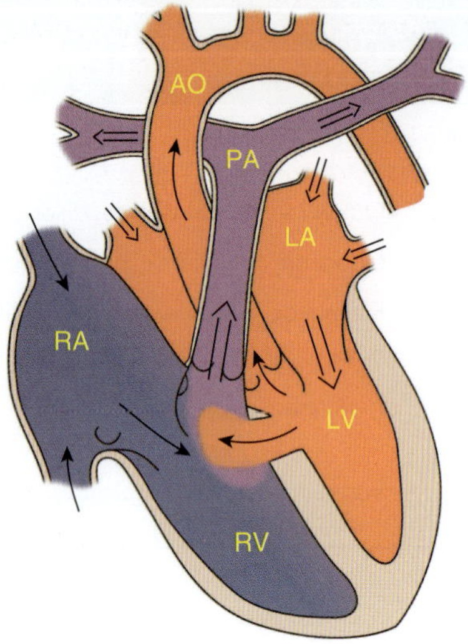

FIGURE 144.1 Ventricular septal defect. *AO*, Aorta; *LA*, left atrium; *LV*, left ventricle; *PA*, pulmonary artery; *RA*, right atrium; *RV*, right ventricle.

shunting of blood across the defect increases, and symptoms may develop.

Clinical Manifestations

Small VSDs with little shunt are often asymptomatic but have a high-frequency, loud murmur. Moderate to large VSDs result in pulmonary overcirculation and heart failure with symptoms of tachypnea and increased work of breathing, poor feeding, and poor weight gain. The typical physical finding with a VSD is a **pansystolic murmur**, usually heard best at the lower left sternal border. There may be a thrill. Large shunts increase flow across the mitral valve causing a **mid-diastolic murmur** at the apex. The splitting of S_2 and intensity of P_2 depend on the pulmonary artery pressure.

Imaging Studies

ECG and chest x-ray findings depend on the size of the VSD. Small VSDs usually have normal studies. Larger VSDs cause volume overload to the left side of the heart, resulting in ECG findings of left atrial and ventricular enlargement and hypertrophy. A chest x-ray may reveal cardiomegaly, enlargement of the left ventricle, an increase in the pulmonary artery silhouette, and increased pulmonary blood flow. Pulmonary hypertension due to either increased flow or increased pulmonary vascular resistance may lead to right ventricular enlargement and hypertrophy. Echocardiography provides the location and size of the defect as well as hemodynamic information regarding the magnitude of the shunt (left heart enlargement) and right heart/pulmonary artery pressure (flow velocity across the defect).

Treatment

Approximately one-third of all VSDs close spontaneously. Small VSDs usually close spontaneously and, if they do not close, surgical closure may not be required. Initial treatment for moderate to large VSDs includes **diuretics** and increasing the caloric density of feeds, with some practitioners also considering **digoxin** and/or **afterload reduction**. Continued poor growth or pulmonary hypertension despite therapy requires closure of the defect, usually between 4 and 6 months of age, though smaller defects can sometimes be followed longer. Most VSDs are closed surgically, but some VSDs, especially muscular defects, can be closed with devices placed via cardiac catheterization.

ATRIAL SEPTAL DEFECT

Etiology and Epidemiology

During the embryologic development of the heart, a septum grows toward the endocardial cushions to divide the atria. Failure of septal growth or excessive reabsorption of tissue leads to ASDs (Fig. 144.2). ASDs represent approximately 10% of all CHD. A secundum defect, with the hole in the region of the foramen ovale, is the most common ASD. A **primum ASD**, located inferiorly in the septum near the crux of the heart, may be part of a complete atrioventricular canal defect or may be present with an intact ventricular septum. The least common ASD is the **sinus venosus defect**, which may be associated with anomalous pulmonary venous return.

Clinical Manifestations

The pathophysiology and amount of shunting depend on the size of the defect and the relative compliance of the ventricles. Even with large ASDs and significant shunts, infants and children are rarely symptomatic. A prominent **right ventricular impulse** at the left lower sternal border (LLSB) often can be palpated. A soft (grade I or II) **systolic ejection murmur** in the region of the right ventricular outflow tract and a **fixed split S_2** (due to overload of the right ventricle with prolonged ejection into the pulmonary circuit) are often audible. A larger shunt may result in a mid-diastolic murmur at the LLSB as a result of the increased volume passing across the tricuspid valve.

Imaging Studies

ECG and chest x-ray findings reflect the **increased blood flow** through the right atrium, right ventricle, pulmonary arteries,

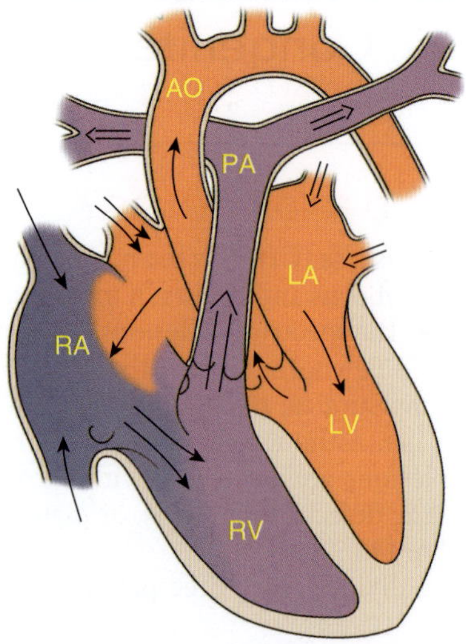

FIGURE 144.2 Atrial septal defect. *AO*, Aorta; *LA*, left atrium; *LV*, left ventricle; *PA*, pulmonary artery; *RA*, right atrium; *RV*, right ventricle.

and lungs. The ECG may show **right axis deviation** and **right ventricular enlargement**. A chest radiograph may show cardiomegaly, right atrial enlargement, and a prominent pulmonary artery. Echocardiography demonstrates the location and size of the defect as well as the magnitude of the shunt (right heart size).

Treatment

Medical management is rarely indicated. If a significant shunt is still present at around 3–5 years of age, usually determined by the presence of right heart dilation, closure is often recommended. Most secundum ASDs can be closed with an ASD **closure device** in the catheterization laboratory. Primum and sinus venosus defects usually require surgical closure.

PATENT DUCTUS ARTERIOSUS

Etiology and Epidemiology

The ductus arteriosus allows blood to flow from the pulmonary artery to the aorta during fetal life. Failure of the normal closure of this vessel results in a PDA (Fig. 144.3). With falling pulmonary vascular resistance after birth, left-to-right shunting of blood and increased pulmonary blood flow occur. Excluding premature infants, PDAs represent approximately 5–10% of CHD.

Clinical Manifestations

Symptoms depend on the amount of pulmonary blood flow. The magnitude of the shunt depends on the size of the PDA (diameter, length, and tortuosity) and the pulmonary vascular resistance. Small PDAs are asymptomatic; moderate to large shunts can produce the symptoms of heart failure, particularly as the pulmonary vascular resistance decreases.

The physical examination findings depend on the size of the shunt. A **widened pulse pressure** is often present as a result of the runoff of blood into the pulmonary circulation during diastole. A **continuous, machine-like murmur** can be heard at the left infraclavicular area, radiating along the pulmonary arteries and often well heard over the left side of the back. Larger shunts with increased flow across the mitral valve may result in a mid-diastolic murmur at the apex and a **hyperdynamic precordium**. Splitting of S_2 and intensity of P_2 depend on the pulmonary artery pressure.

Imaging Studies

ECG and chest x-ray findings are normal with small PDAs. Moderate to large shunts may result in a **full pulmonary artery silhouette** and **increased pulmonary vascularity**. If left heart dilation is present, there may be an **enlarged cardiac silhouette**. ECG findings vary from normal to evidence of left ventricular hypertrophy. If pulmonary hypertension is present, there is also right ventricular hypertrophy. Echocardiography demonstrates the size and anatomy of the PDA as well as hemodynamic information regarding the magnitude of the shunt (left heart size) and pulmonary artery pressure (flow velocity across the PDA).

Treatment

Spontaneous closure of a PDA after a few weeks of age is uncommon in full-term infants. Moderate and large PDAs may be managed initially with **diuretics**, but they eventually require closure. Elective closure of small, hemodynamically insignificant PDAs is controversial. Most PDAs can be closed in the catheterization laboratory by either **coil embolization** or a PDA **closure device**.

ENDOCARDIAL CUSHION DEFECT

Etiology and Epidemiology

Endocardial cushion defects, also referred to as **atrioventricular canal defects** or atrioventricular septal defects, may be complete (Fig. 144.4), partial, or transitional. Abnormal development of the endocardial cushion tissue results in failure of the septum to fuse with the endocardial cushion; this results

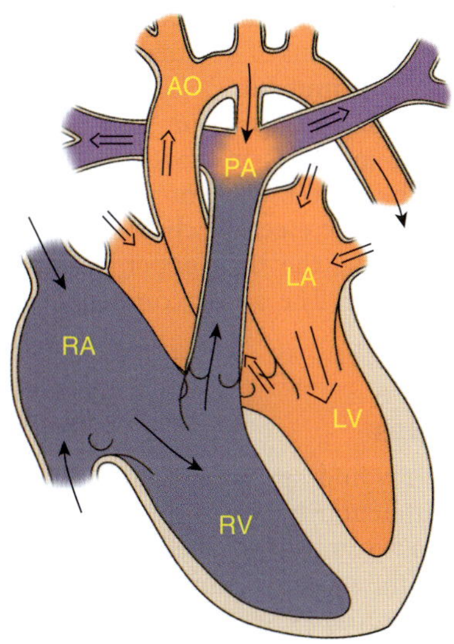

FIGURE 144.3 Patent ductus arteriosus. *AO*, Aorta; *LA*, left atrium; *LV*, left ventricle; *PA*, pulmonary artery; *RA*, right atrium; *RV*, right ventricle.

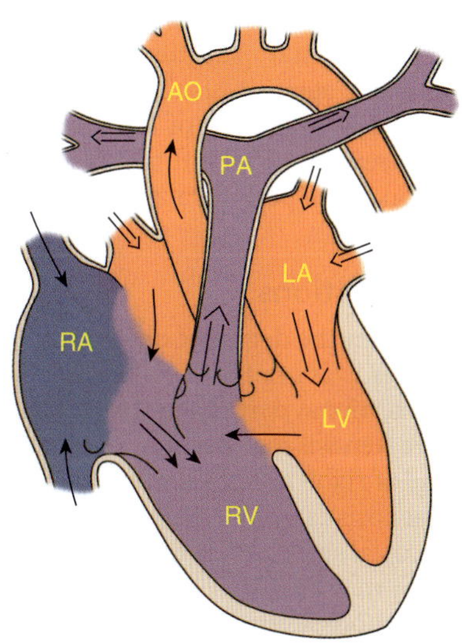

FIGURE 144.4 Atrioventricular canal defects. *AO*, Aorta; *LA*, left atrium; *LV*, left ventricle; *PA*, pulmonary artery; *RA*, right atrium; *RV*, right ventricle.

in **abnormal atrioventricular valves** as well. The complete defect results in a primum ASD, a posterior or inlet VSD, and a common atrioventricular valve with anterior and posterior bridging leaflets. Partial and transitional defects have two separate atrioventricular valves, usually with a "cleft" in the anterior leaflet of the left-sided valve. In addition to left-to-right shunting at both levels, there may be **atrioventricular valve insufficiency**. This is the most common congenital heart defect in children with trisomy 21.

Clinical Manifestations

The symptoms of heart failure usually develop as the pulmonary vascular resistance decreases over the first 6–8 weeks of life. Symptoms may be earlier and more severe with significant atrioventricular valve insufficiency. Pulmonary hypertension can be present due to the increased pulmonary blood flow, and pulmonary vascular obstructive disease may develop early, especially in patients with trisomy 21. The presence of murmurs varies depending on the amount of shunting at both atrial and ventricular levels. If there is a large VSD component, S_2 will be single. Growth is usually poor.

Imaging Tests

The diagnosis usually is made with echocardiography. A chest radiograph reveals cardiomegaly with enlargement of all chambers and the presence of **increased vascularity**. An ECG reveals **left axis deviation** and **combined ventricular hypertrophy** and may show combined atrial enlargement.

Treatment

Initial management can be similar to management of VSDs and includes diuretics. Some practitioners use afterload reduction for treatment of heart failure but, ultimately, surgical repair of the defect is required.

PULMONARY STENOSIS

Etiology

Pulmonary stenosis accounts for approximately 10% of all CHD and can be **valvular**, **subvalvular**, or **supravalvular** in nature. Pulmonary stenosis results from the failure of the development, in early gestation, of the three leaflets of the valve, insufficient resorption of infundibular tissue, or insufficient canalization of the peripheral pulmonary arteries.

Clinical Manifestations

Symptoms depend on the degree of obstruction present. Mild pulmonary stenosis is asymptomatic. Moderate to severe stenosis results in exertional dyspnea and easy fatigability. Newborns with severe stenosis may be more symptomatic and even cyanotic because of right-to-left shunting at the atrial level.

Pulmonary stenosis causes a systolic ejection murmur at the second left intercostal space, which radiates to the back. A thrill may be present. S_2 may be widely split with a quiet pulmonary component. With more severe pulmonary stenosis, an impulse at the lower left sternal border results from **right ventricular hypertrophy**. Valvular stenosis may result in a **click** that varies with respiration. Worsening stenosis causes an increase in the duration of the murmur and a higher frequency of the sound. The systolic ejection murmurs of **peripheral pulmonary stenosis** are heard distal to the site of obstruction in the pulmonary circulation, including radiation to the axillae and back. Benign or innocent peripheral pulmonary stenosis causes a "blowing" systolic murmur in infants in the first week of life and reflects the normal physiologic transition from intrauterine to extrauterine circulation occurring in the pulmonary vasculature. Persistence beyond the first weeks of life is pathologic.

Imaging Tests

ECG and chest x-ray findings are normal in mild stenosis. Moderate to severe stenosis results in **right axis deviation** and **right ventricular hypertrophy**. The heart size is usually normal on chest x-ray, although **dilation of the main pulmonary artery** may be seen. Echocardiography provides assessment of the site of stenosis, degree of hypertrophy, valve morphology, as well as an estimate of the pressure gradient.

Treatment

Valvular pulmonary stenosis usually does not progress after the first few months of life, especially if it is mild. **Balloon valvuloplasty** is often successful in reducing the gradient to acceptable levels for more significant or symptomatic stenosis. **Surgical repair** is required if balloon valvuloplasty is unsuccessful or when subvalvular (muscular) stenosis is present.

AORTIC STENOSIS

Etiology and Epidemiology

Valvular, **subvalvular**, or **supravalvular** aortic stenosis represents approximately 5% of all CHD. Lesions result from failure of development of the three leaflets or failure of resorption of tissue around the valve.

Clinical Manifestations

Mild to moderate obstructions often cause no symptoms. More severe stenosis results in easy fatigability, exertional chest pain, and syncope. Infants with critical aortic stenosis may present with symptoms of heart failure.

A **systolic ejection murmur** is heard at the right second intercostal space along the sternum and radiating into the neck. The murmur increases in length and becomes higher in frequency as the degree of stenosis increases. With valvular stenosis, a **systolic ejection click** often is heard, and a thrill may be present at the right upper sternal border or in the suprasternal notch. The aortic component of S_2 may be decreased in intensity.

Imaging Studies

ECG and chest x-ray findings are normal with mild degrees of stenosis. **Left ventricular hypertrophy** develops with moderate to severe stenosis and is detected on the ECG and chest x-ray. **Dilation** of the ascending aorta or aortic knob due to an intrinsic aortopathy may be seen on chest radiographs. Echocardiography shows the site of stenosis, valve morphology, and the presence of left ventricular hypertrophy, and it allows an estimate of the pressure gradient.

Treatment

The degree of aortic stenosis frequently progresses with growth and age. Aortic insufficiency often develops or progresses. Serial follow-up with echocardiography is indicated. **Balloon valvuloplasty** is usually the first interventional procedure for significant stenosis. It is not as successful as pulmonary balloon valvuloplasty and has a higher risk of significant valvular insufficiency. **Surgical management** is necessary when balloon valvuloplasty is unsuccessful or significant valve insufficiency develops.

COARCTATION OF THE AORTA

Etiology and Epidemiology

Coarctation of the aorta occurs in approximately 10% of all CHD. It is almost always **juxtaductal** in position. During development of the aortic arch, the area near the insertion of the ductus arteriosus fails to develop correctly, resulting in a narrowing of the aortic lumen.

Clinical Manifestations

Timing of presentation depends on the severity of obstruction and associated cardiac defects. Infants presenting with coarctation of the aorta frequently have a hypoplastic aortic arch, abnormal aortic valves, and VSDs. They may be dependent on a PDA to provide descending aortic flow and may present with a differential oxygen saturation between the right arm and leg on newborn screening. Symptoms develop when the aortic ampulla of the ductus closes with classic age of presentation at approximately 2 weeks of age. Less severe obstruction causes no symptoms in infancy.

Symptoms, including poor feeding, respiratory distress, and shock, may develop before 2 weeks of age. Classically, the **femoral pulses** are weaker and delayed compared with the right radial pulse. The blood pressure in the lower extremities is lower than that in the upper extremities. However, if cardiac function is poor, these differences may not be as apparent until appropriate resuscitation is accomplished. In this situation, there may be no murmur, but an S_3 is often present.

Older children presenting with coarctation of the aorta are usually asymptomatic. There may be a history of **leg discomfort** with exercise, headache, or epistaxis. Decreased or absent lower extremity pulses, **hypertension** (upper extremity), or a murmur may be present. The murmur is typically best heard in the left interscapular area of the back. If significant collaterals have developed, continuous murmurs may be heard throughout the chest. An abnormal aortic valve is present approximately 50% of the time, causing a systolic ejection click and systolic ejection murmur of aortic stenosis.

Imaging Studies

The ECG and chest x-ray show evidence of right ventricular enlargement and hypertrophy in infantile coarctation with marked **cardiomegaly** and **pulmonary edema**. In older children, the ECG and chest x-ray usually show left ventricular hypertrophy and a mildly enlarged heart. **Rib notching** may also be seen in older children (>8 years of age) with large collaterals. Echocardiography shows the site and degree of coarctation, the presence of left ventricular hypertrophy, and the aortic valve morphology and function.

Treatment

Management of an infant presenting with cardiac decompensation includes intravenous infusion of **prostaglandin** E_1 (which chemically opens the ductus arteriosus), inotropic agents, diuretics, and other supportive care. **Balloon angioplasty** has been done, especially in critically ill infants, but **surgical repair** of the coarctation is most commonly performed. Ballooning and stenting of older patients with coarctation has become more accepted as primary therapy, but surgical repair remains an option.

PEARLS FOR PRACTITIONERS

See The Cardiovascular System: Pearls for Practitioners at the end of this section.

REVIEW QUESTION

Available online.

CHAPTER 145

Cyanotic Congenital Heart Disease

Cyanotic congenital heart disease (CHD) occurs when some of the systemic venous return crosses from the right side of the heart to the left and returns to the body without going through the lungs **(right-to-left shunt)**. **Cyanosis**, the visible sign of this shunt, occurs when at least 5 g/100 mL of deoxy-hemoglobin is present in systemic blood. Thus a polycythemic patient appears cyanotic with a higher oxygen saturation than a normocythemic patient. A patient with anemia requires a higher percentage of reduced hemoglobin (lower saturation) for the recognition of cyanosis. Oxygen desaturation between 80 and 90% may occur with mixing lesions but does not cause clinically apparent cyanosis (referred to as the **cyanotic blind spot**).

The most common cyanotic congenital heart defects are the five *T*s:

1. Tetralogy of Fallot
2. Transposition of the great arteries
3. Tricuspid atresia
4. Truncus arteriosus
5. Total anomalous pulmonary venous return

Other congenital heart defects that allow complete mixing of systemic and pulmonary venous return can present with cyanosis depending on the amount of pulmonary blood flow that is present. Many cyanotic heart lesions present in the neonatal period (Table 145.1). All cyanotic heart lesions require surgical intervention. Common interventions are summarized in Table 145.2.

TETRALOGY OF FALLOT

Etiology and Epidemiology

Tetralogy of Fallot is the most common cyanotic congenital heart defect, representing about 10% of all CHD (Fig. 145.1). There are four structural defects: **ventricular septal defect (VSD)**, **pulmonary stenosis**, **overriding aorta**, and **right**

TABLE 145.1 Presenting Symptoms and Signs of Congenital Heart Disease in the Neonate*

SYMPTOM/SIGN	PHYSIOLOGIC CATEGORY	ANATOMIC CAUSE	LESION
Cyanosis with respiratory distress	Increased pulmonary blood flow	Transposition	d-Transposition with or without associated lesions
Cyanosis without respiratory distress	Decreased pulmonary blood flow	Right heart obstruction	Tricuspid atresia Ebstein anomaly Pulmonary atresia Pulmonary stenosis Tetralogy of Fallot
Hypoperfusion	Poor cardiac output	Left heart obstruction	Total anomalous pulmonary venous return with obstruction Aortic stenosis Hypoplastic left heart syndrome
	Poor cardiac function	Normal anatomy	Cardiomyopathy Myocarditis
Respiratory distress with desaturation (not visible cyanosis)	Bidirectional shunting	Complete mixing	Truncus arteriosus AV canal Complex single ventricle (including heterotaxias) without pulmonary stenosis
Respiratory distress with normal saturation	Left-to-right shunting	Simple intracardiac shunt	ASD VSD PDA Aortopulmonary window AVM

*Symptoms develop after physiologic transition from high to low pulmonary vascular resistance, which occurs in the first 24–48 hours of life.
ASD, Atrial septal defect; *AV*, atrioventricular; *AVM*, arteriovenous malformation; *PDA*, patent ductus arteriosus; *VSD*, ventricular septal defect.

ventricular hypertrophy. Tetralogy of Fallot is due to abnormal septation of the truncus arteriosus into the aorta and pulmonary artery that occurs early in gestation (3–4 weeks). The VSD is large, and the pulmonary stenosis is most commonly subvalvular or infundibular. It may also be valvular, supravalvular, or, frequently, a combination of levels of obstruction.

Clinical Manifestations

Infants initially may be acyanotic. A **pulmonary stenosis murmur** is the usual initial abnormal finding. The amount of right-to-left shunting at the VSD (and the degree of cyanosis) increases as the degree of pulmonary stenosis increases. With increasing severity of pulmonary stenosis, the murmur becomes shorter and softer due to decreasing flow across the pulmonary valve. In addition to varying degrees of cyanosis and a murmur, a **single S_2** and **right ventricular impulse** at the left sternal border are typical findings.

Hypercyanotic (Tet) spells are less commonly seen than in the past because of early surgical repair but do still occur. During a spell, the child typically becomes restless and agitated and may cry inconsolably. An ambulatory toddler may squat. Hyperpnea occurs with gradually increasing cyanosis and loss of the murmur. In severe spells, prolonged unconsciousness and convulsions, hemiparesis, or death may occur. Independent of hypoxic spells, patients with unrepaired tetralogy of Fallot are at increased risk for cerebral thromboembolism and cerebral abscesses resulting, in part, from their right-to-left intracardiac shunt.

Imaging Studies

The ECG usually has **right axis deviation** and **right ventricular hypertrophy**. The classic chest x-ray finding is a **boot-shaped heart** created by the small main pulmonary artery and upturned apex secondary to right ventricular hypertrophy. Echocardiography shows the anatomic features, including the anatomic level and quantification of pulmonary stenosis. **Anomalous coronary arteries**, most commonly a left anterior descending coronary artery arising from the right coronary artery and crossing the anterior surface of the right ventricular outflow tract, are present in 5% of patients with tetralogy of Fallot.

Treatment

The natural history of tetralogy of Fallot is progression of pulmonary stenosis and cyanosis. Treatment of hypoxic spells consists of oxygen administration (although of minimal value given that worsening cyanosis is due to lack of pulmonary blood flow) and placing the child in the knee-chest position (to increase venous return and systemic vascular resistance [SVR]). Traditionally, morphine sulfate was given (to relax the pulmonary infundibulum and for sedation). The use of ketamine is often beneficial (sedation, increases SVR, and can be given intramuscularly). If necessary, the SVR can be increased acutely through the administration of an α-adrenergic agonist (phenylephrine). The occurrence of a cyanotic spell is an indication to proceed with surgical repair.

Complete surgical repair with VSD closure and removal or patching of the pulmonary stenosis can be performed in infancy. Occasionally, **palliative shunt surgery** between the subclavian artery and pulmonary artery is performed for complex forms of tetralogy of Fallot and more complete repair is done at a later time. **Subacute bacterial endocarditis prophylaxis** is indicated until 6 months after complete repair unless there is a residual VSD. Prophylaxis is then continued as long as there is a residual VSD.

TABLE 145.2 Surgical Approaches to Congenital Heart Disease

SURGICAL METHOD	PATH OF BLOOD FLOW	RELEVANT CLINICAL CONDITIONS
Modified Blalock-Taussig-Thomas shunt (mBTT shunt)	Pulmonary artery to aorta (or one of its branches, such as the subclavian artery)	Single ventricle lesions (HLHS, unbalanced AV canal, some tricuspid atresias), or any other lesions with ductal dependent circulation
Norwood procedure	Atrial septectomy, construction of neoaorta from main pulmonary artery, establishment of pulmonary blood flow, usually with a mBTT shunt or Sano shunt (RV-PA shunt)	Single ventricle*, optimally in newborn period
Bidirectional cavopulmonary shunt (bidirectional Glenn)	Superior vena cava to right and/or left pulmonary artery	Single ventricle*, optimally at 3–6 months
Fontan procedure	Creates Fontan circulation: systemic venous return to pulmonary arteries without intervening ventricular pump, and single ventricle pumps to body	Single ventricle*, optimally at 3 years
Balloon septostomy	Create atrial or ventricular mixing lesion	Complex congenital heart disease which requires mixing lesion to be compatible with life, such as transposition of the great arteries
Arterial switch (Jatene switch)	Connects aorta to the left ventricle and the pulmonary artery to the right ventricle	d-TGA
Atrial switch (Mustard, Senning)	Atrial baffle (structure directing blood flow) created to allow systemic venous blood to flow to the subpulmonary ventricle, and pulmonary venous blood to flow to the subsystemic ventricle	Primarily used in d-TGA prior to the standardization of the arterial switch; most commonly used in the double switch procedure (atrial and arterial switches) in patients with cc-TGA or as an option in patients with d-TGA who are not arterial switch candidates
Rastelli operation	Synthetic patch routes blood from left ventricle through VSD to aorta "ventricular-level switch", pulmonary artery connected to right ventricle	TGA with large VSD and pulmonary stenosis
Nikaidoh procedure	Pulmonary root excised to allow anterior aorta moved posterior, allowing left ventricle to aortic flow and right ventricle to pulmonary artery flow	d-TGA with specific anatomic considerations making other procedures less preferred
PDA stent	Preserves PDA connection between pulmonary artery and aorta	Useful in stabilization of ductal dependent lesions which require patency before more definitive surgical repair
PDA closure	Medical therapies (indomethacin, ibuprofen, acetaminophen) may be trialed first in infants with otherwise normal intracardiac anatomy; catheter-based intervention by coils, device, or surgical ligation of the PDA removes connection between pulmonary artery and aorta	Persistent and clinically significant PDA

**Single ventricle pathology includes tricuspid atresia, severely unbalanced atrioventricular canal defects, and other causes of functional hypoplastic right heart and hypoplastic left heart*

AV, Atrioventricular; *cc-TGA*, congenitally corrected transposition of the great arteries; *d-TGA*, dextro-transposition of the great arteries; *HLHS*, hypoplastic left heart syndrome; *PA*, pulmonary artery; *PDA*, patent ductus arteriosus; *RV*, right ventricle; *VSD*, ventricular septal defect.

TRANSPOSITION OF THE GREAT ARTERIES

Etiology and Epidemiology

Although dextro-transposition of the great arteries (d-TGA) represents only about 5% of CHD, it is the most common cyanotic lesion to present in the newborn period (Fig. 145.2). TGA is ventriculoarterial discordance secondary to abnormalities of septation of the truncus arteriosus. In d-TGA, the aorta arises from the right ventricle, anterior and to the right of the pulmonary artery, which arises from the left ventricle. This results in two separate circulations, with desaturated blood returning to the right side of the heart and being pumped back out to the body, while well-oxygenated blood returning from the lungs enters the left side of the heart and is pumped back to the lungs. Without mixing of the two circulations, death occurs quickly. Mixing can occur at the atrial (patent foramen ovale/atrial septal defect [ASD]) or less commonly at the ventricular (VSD) level. The presence of a patent ductus arteriosus (PDA) increases pulmonary blood flow and will improve mixing if adequate intracardiac communication is present.

Clinical Manifestations

A history of **cyanosis** is always present, although it depends on the amount of mixing. **Quiet tachypnea** (tachypnea without increased work of breathing) and a **single S_2** are typically present. If the ventricular septum is intact, there may be no murmur.

Children with transposition and a large VSD have improved intracardiac mixing and less cyanosis. They may present with signs of heart failure. The heart is hyperdynamic, with palpable left and right ventricular impulses. A loud VSD murmur is heard. S_2 is single.

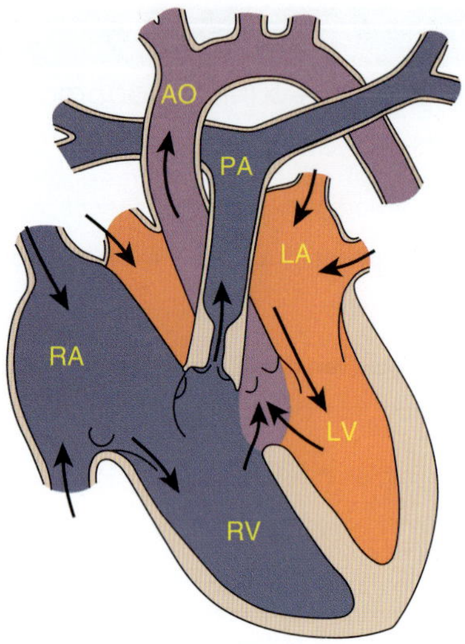

FIGURE 145.1 Tetralogy of Fallot. *AO*, Aorta; *LA*, left atrium; *LV*, left ventricle; *PA*, pulmonary artery; *RA*, right atrium; *RV*, right ventricle.

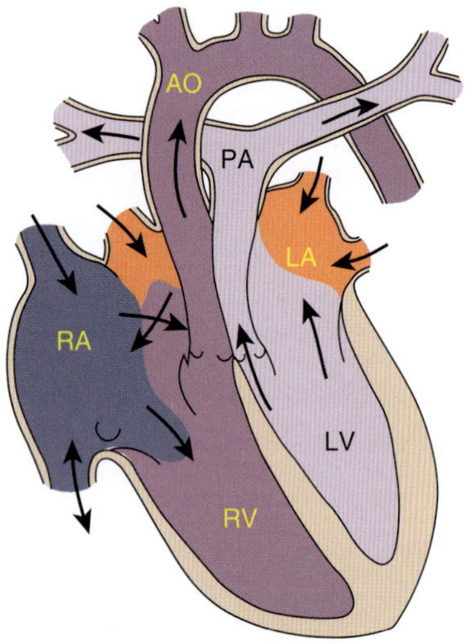

FIGURE 145.2 Transposition of the great arteries. *AO*, Aorta; *LA*, left atrium; *LV*, left ventricle; *PA*, pulmonary artery; *RA*, right atrium; *RV*, right ventricle.

Imaging Studies

ECG findings typically include **right axis deviation** and **right ventricular hypertrophy**. The chest x-ray reveals **increased pulmonary vascularity**, and the cardiac shadow is classically an **egg on a string** created by the narrow superior mediastinum. Echocardiography shows the transposition of the great arteries, the sites and amount of mixing, and any associated lesions.

Treatment

Initial medical management includes **prostaglandin E_1** to maintain ductal patency and increase pulmonary blood flow and return. If significant hypoxia persists on prostaglandin therapy, a **balloon atrial septostomy** improves mixing between the two circulations. Complete surgical repair is most often an **arterial switch**. The arterial switch usually is performed within the first 2 weeks of life, when the left ventricle can still maintain systemic pressure. If there are other cardiac anomalies present, such as significant pulmonary stenosis, then other procedures such as a Rastelli, Nikaidoh, or aortic root translocation may be indicated instead of an arterial switch.

TRICUSPID ATRESIA

Etiology and Epidemiology

Tricuspid atresia accounts for approximately 2% of all CHD (Fig. 145.3). The absence of the tricuspid valve results in a **hypoplastic right ventricle**. All systemic venous return must cross the atrial septum into the left atrium. A PDA or VSD is necessary for pulmonary blood flow and survival.

Clinical Manifestations

Infants with tricuspid atresia are usually **severely cyanotic** and have a **single S_2**. If a VSD is present, there may be a murmur. A diastolic murmur across the mitral valve may be audible. Frequently there is no significant murmur.

Imaging Studies

The ECG shows **left ventricular hypertrophy** and a **superior QRS axis** (between 0 and −90 degrees). The chest x-ray reveals a normal or mildly enlarged cardiac silhouette with **decreased pulmonary blood flow**. Echocardiography shows the anatomy, associated lesions, and source of pulmonary blood flow.

Treatment

Management initially depends on the presence of a VSD and the amount of antegrade blood flow to the lungs. If there is no VSD, or it is small, prostaglandin E_1 maintains pulmonary blood flow until surgery. Surgery is staged with an initial subclavian artery-to-pulmonary shunt (usually a **modified Blalock-Taussig-Thomas shunt)** typically followed by a two-stage procedure: **bidirectional cavopulmonary shunt (bidirectional Glenn)** and **Fontan procedure**. These surgeries direct systemic venous return directly to the pulmonary arteries, creating **Fontan circulation** where there is no ventricle pumping to the lungs, and a systemic ventricle pumping to the body. This surgical pathway is also utilized in other "single ventricle" lesions such as hypoplastic left heart syndrome (see below) or severely unbalanced atrioventricular canal defects.

TRUNCUS ARTERIOSUS

Etiology and Epidemiology

Truncus arteriosus occurs in less than 1% of all cases of CHD (Fig. 145.4). It results from the failure of septation of the truncus during the first 3–4 weeks of gestation. A single arterial trunk arises from the heart with a large VSD. The pulmonary arteries arise from the single arterial trunk either as a single vessel that then divides or individually from the arterial trunk to the lungs.

Clinical Manifestations

Varying degrees of cyanosis depend on the amount of pulmonary blood flow. If not diagnosed at birth, the infant may develop signs of heart failure as pulmonary vascular resistance decreases. The signs include tachypnea, difficulty feeding, and poor growth. Peripheral pulses are usually bounding as a result

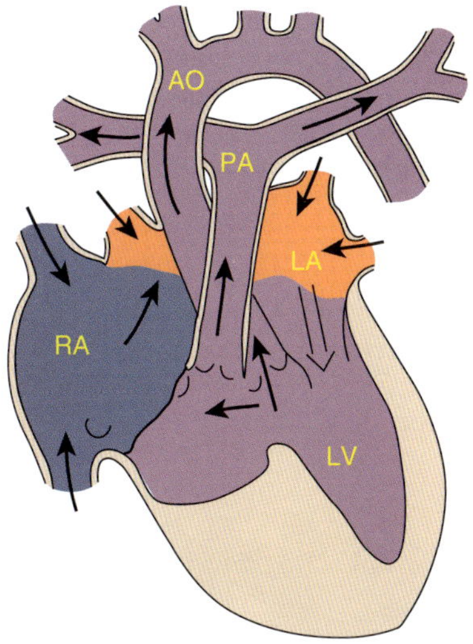

FIGURE 145.3 Tricuspid atresia with ventricular septal defect. *AO*, Aorta; *LA*, left atrium; *LV*, left ventricle; *PA*, pulmonary artery; *RA*, right atrium.

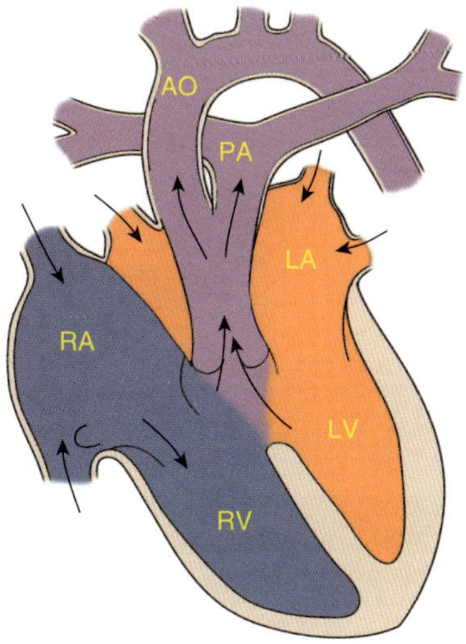

FIGURE 145.4 Truncus arteriosus. *AO*, Aorta; *LA*, left atrium; *LV*, left ventricle; *PA*, pulmonary artery; *RA*, right atrium; *RV*, right ventricle.

of the diastolic runoff into the pulmonary arteries. If there is significant truncal valve dysfunction, then poor systemic output and decreased ventricular function can occur. A single $\mathbf{S_2}$ is due to the single valve. There may be a systolic ejection click, and there is often a **systolic murmur** at the left sternal border.

Imaging Studies

ECG findings include **combined ventricular hypertrophy** and **cardiomegaly**. A chest x-ray usually reveals **increased pulmonary blood** and may show displaced pulmonary arteries. Echocardiography defines the anatomy, including the VSD, truncal valve function, and origin of the pulmonary arteries.

Treatment

Medical management is usually needed and includes anticongestive medications such as **diuretics**. **Surgical repair** includes VSD closure, separation of the pulmonary arteries from the common arterial trunk, and placement of a conduit between the right ventricle and pulmonary arteries.

TOTAL ANOMALOUS PULMONARY VENOUS RETURN

Etiology and Epidemiology

Total anomalous pulmonary venous return accounts for about 1% of CHD (Fig. 145.5). Disruption of the development of normal pulmonary venous drainage during the third week of gestation results in the pulmonary veins failing to connect to the left atrium and returning abnormally to the right side of the heart. They may have **supracardiac**, **infracardiac**, **cardiac**, or **mixed drainage**. An atrial-level communication is required for systemic cardiac output and survival.

Clinical Manifestations

The most important determinant of presentation is the presence or absence of **obstruction** to the pulmonary venous drainage. Infants without obstruction have minimal cyanosis and may be asymptomatic. There is a hyperactive **right ventricular impulse** with a **widely split $\mathbf{S_2}$** (owing to increased right ventricular volume) and a **systolic ejection murmur** at the left upper sternal border. There is usually a mid-diastolic murmur at the lower left sternal border from the increased flow across the tricuspid valve. Growth is relatively poor. Infants with **obstruction** present with cyanosis, marked tachypnea and dyspnea, and signs of right-sided heart failure including hepatomegaly. The obstruction results in pulmonary edema and backup of fluid to the lungs, and little, if any, increase in right ventricular volume, so there may be no murmur or changes in S_2.

Imaging Studies

For infants without obstruction, the ECG is consistent with right ventricular volume overload. Cardiomegaly with increased pulmonary blood flow is seen on chest x-ray. Infants with obstructed veins have right axis deviation and

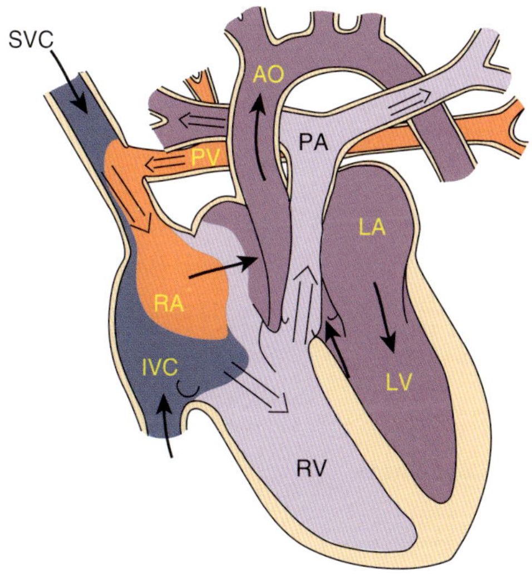

FIGURE 145.5 Total anomalous pulmonary venous return. *AO*, Aorta; *IVC*, inferior vena cava; *LA*, left atrium; *LV*, left ventricle; *PA*, pulmonary artery; *PV*, pulmonary vein; *RA*, right atrium; *RV*, right ventricle; *SVC*, superior vena cava.

right ventricular hypertrophy on ECG. On chest x-ray, the heart is normal or mildly enlarged with varying degrees of pulmonary edema that can appear similar to respiratory distress syndrome or pneumonia. Echocardiography shows the volume-overloaded right side of the heart, right-to-left atrial level shunting, and common pulmonary vein site of drainage and degree of obstruction.

Treatment

At surgery, the common pulmonary vein is opened into the left atrium, and there is ligation of any vein or channel that had been draining the common vein. Obstructed total anomalous pulmonary venous return requires prompt surgical intervention.

HYPOPLASTIC LEFT HEART SYNDROME

Etiology and Epidemiology

Hypoplastic left heart syndrome accounts for 1% of all CHD (Fig. 145.6) but is the most common cause of death from cardiac defects in the first month of life. Hypoplastic left heart syndrome occurs when there is failure of normal development of the mitral or aortic valve. A small left ventricle that is unable to support normal systemic circulation is a central finding, regardless of etiology. Associated degrees of hypoplasia of the ascending aorta and aortic arch are present. Left-to-right shunting occurs at the atrial level pre- and postnatally.

Clinical Manifestations

The newborn is dependent on right-to-left shunting at the ductus arteriosus for systemic blood flow. As the ductus arteriosus constricts, the infant becomes critically ill with signs and symptoms of heart failure from excessive pulmonary blood flow and obstruction of systemic blood flow. Pulses are diffusely weak or absent. S_2 is single and loud. There is usually no heart murmur. Cyanosis may be minimal, but **low cardiac output** gives a grayish color to the cool, mottled skin.

Imaging Studies

ECG findings include **right ventricular hypertrophy** with **decreased left ventricular forces**. The chest x-ray reveals **cardiomegaly** (with right-sided enlargement) and pulmonary venous congestion or pulmonary edema. Echocardiography

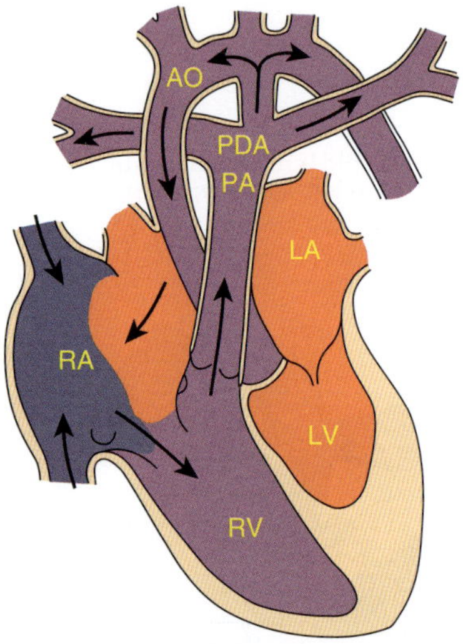

FIGURE 145.6 Hypoplastic left side of the heart. *AO,* Aorta; *LA,* left atrium; *LV,* left ventricle; *PA,* pulmonary artery; *PDA,* patent ductus arteriosus; *RA,* right atrium; *RV,* right ventricle.

TABLE **145.3** Extracardiac Complications of Cyanotic Congenital Heart Disease

PROBLEM	ETIOLOGY	THERAPY
Polycythemia	Persistent hypoxia	Phlebotomy
Relative anemia	Nutritional deficiency	Iron replacement
CNS abscess	Right-to-left shunting	Antibiotics, drainage
CNS thromboembolic stroke	Right-to-left shunting or polycythemia	Phlebotomy
Gingival disease	Polycythemia, gingivitis, bleeding	Dental hygiene
Gout	Polycythemia, diuretic agents	Allopurinol
Arthritis, clubbing	Hypoxic arthropathy	None
Pregnancy	Poor placental perfusion, poor ability to increase cardiac output	Bed rest
Infectious disease	Associated asplenia, DiGeorge syndrome	Antibiotics
	Fatal RSV pneumonia with pulmonary hypertension	Ribavirin, RSV immune globulin
Growth	Growth faltering, increased oxygen consumption, decreased nutrient intake	Treat heart failure; correct defect early
Psychosocial adjustment	Limited activity, peer pressure; chronic disease, multiple hospitalizations, cardiac surgical techniques	Counseling
Eisenmenger Syndrome	Secondary pulmonary arterial hypertension due to undertreated congenital heart defect results in reversal of left-to-right shunt (to right-to-left), causing hypoxemia that is resistant to supplemental oxygen	Diuretics, antiarrhythmics, anticoagulation, vasodilator therapies; Heart and lung transplant

CNS, Central nervous system; *RSV,* respiratory syncytial virus.

shows the small left side of the heart, the degree of stenosis of the aortic and mitral valves, the hypoplastic ascending aorta, and the adequacy of left-to-right atrial flow and right-to-left ductal flow.

Treatment

Medical management includes **prostaglandin E_1** to open the ductus arteriosus, correction of acidosis, and ventilatory and blood pressure support as needed. **Surgical repair** is staged with the first surgery (Norwood procedure) done during the newborn period. Subsequent procedures create a systemic source for the pulmonary circulation (bidirectional Glenn and Fontan procedures), leaving the right ventricle to supply systemic circulation. There have been many modifications to all three stages of the repair. Prognosis for survival has improved significantly over the past 2 decades; however, many long-term complications remain including liver fibrosis and hepatic carcinoma, protein losing enteropathy, plastic bronchitis, and systemic right ventricular failure. Many patients will ultimately require heart transplantation.

COMPLICATIONS OF CONGENITAL HEART DISEASE

Extracardiac complications are summarized in Table 145.3.

PEARLS FOR PRACTITIONERS

See The Cardiovascular System: Pearls for Practitioners at the end of this section.

REVIEW QUESTIONS

Available online.

CHAPTER 146
Heart Failure

ETIOLOGY AND EPIDEMIOLOGY

The force generated by the cardiac muscle fiber depends on its contractile status and basal length. Basal length of the muscle fibers can also be conceptualized as preload. As the preload (fiber length, left ventricular filling pressure, or volume) increases, myocardial performance (stroke volume and wall tension) increases up to a point (the normal Starling curve). The relationship is the **ventricular function curve** (Fig. 146.1). Alterations in the contractile state of the muscle lower the relative position of the curve but retain the relationship of fiber length to muscle work. The cardiac output equals stroke volume times the heart rate; thus heart rate is another important determinant of cardiac work. Additional factors also affect cardiac performance (Table 146.1).

Heart failure occurs when the heart is unable to pump blood at a rate commensurate with metabolic needs (inadequate oxygen delivery). It may be due to a change in **myocardial contractility** that results in low cardiac output or to

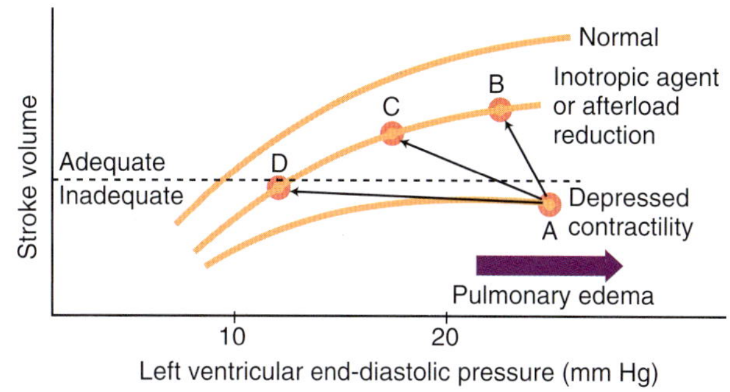

FIGURE 146.1 Ventricular function curve illustrating the effect of inotropic agents or arterial vasodilators. In contrast to diuretics, the effect of digitalis or arterial vasodilator therapy in a patient with heart failure is movement onto another ventricular function curve, which is intermediate between the normal and the depressed curves. When the patient's ventricular function moves from *A* to *B* by the administration of one of these agents, the left ventricular end-diastolic pressure may also decrease because of improved cardiac function; further administration of diuretics or venodilators may shift the function further to the left along the same curve from *B* to *C* and eliminate the risk of pulmonary edema. A vasodilating agent that has arteriolar and venous dilating properties (e.g., nitroprusside) would shift this function directly from *A* to *C*. If this agent shifts the function from *A* to *D* because of excessive venodilation or the administration of diuretics, the cardiac output may decrease too much, even though the left ventricular end-diastolic pressure would be normal (10 mm Hg) for a normal heart. Left ventricular end-diastolic pressures of 15–18 mm Hg are usually optimal in the failing heart to maximize cardiac output but to avoid pulmonary edema. (From Andreoli TE, Carpenter CCJ, Griggs RC, et al., eds. *Cecil Essentials of Medicine*. 5th ed. Philadelphia: Saunders; 2001.)

TABLE 146.1 Factors Affecting Cardiac Performance

PRELOAD (LEFT VENTRICULAR DIASTOLIC VOLUME)
Total blood volume Venous tone (sympathetic tone) Body position Intrathoracic and intrapericardial pressure Atrial contraction Pumping action of skeletal muscle
AFTERLOAD (IMPEDANCE AGAINST WHICH THE LEFT VENTRICLE MUST EJECT BLOOD)
Peripheral vascular resistance Left ventricular volume (preload, wall tension) Physical characteristics of the arterial tree (elasticity of vessels or presence of outflow obstruction)
CONTRACTILITY (CARDIAC PERFORMANCE INDEPENDENT OF PRELOAD OR AFTERLOAD)
Sympathetic nerve impulses* Circulating catecholamines* Digitalis, calcium, other inotropic agents* Increased heart rate or postextrasystolic augmentation* Anoxia, acidosis† Pharmacologic depression† Loss of myocardium† Intrinsic depression†
HEART RATE
Autonomic nervous system Temperature, metabolic rate Medications, drugs

**Increases contractility.*
†Decreases contractility.
Modified from Lohr NL, Benjamin IJ. Structure and function of the normal heart and blood vessels. In Wing EJ, Schiffman FJ, eds. Cecil Essentials of Medicine. *10th ed. Philadelphia: Saunders; 2022:table 2.2.*

abnormal loading conditions being placed on the myocardium. The abnormal loading conditions may be **afterload** (pressure overload, such as with aortic stenosis, pulmonary stenosis, or coarctation of the aorta) or **preload** (volume overload, such as in ventricular septal defect [VSD], patent ductus arteriosus [PDA], or valvular insufficiency). Volume overload is the most common cause of heart failure in children.

The age of presentation is helpful in creating the differential diagnosis (Table 146.2). In the first weeks of life, excessive afterload being placed on the myocardium is most common. Heart failure presenting around 2 months of age is usually due to increasing left-to-right shunts that become apparent as the pulmonary vascular resistance decreases. Acquired heart disease, such as myocarditis and cardiomyopathy, can present at any age.

TABLE **146.2** Etiology of Heart Failure by Age Group

FETUS
Severe anemia (hemolysis, fetal-maternal transfusion, hypoplastic anemia) Supraventricular tachycardia Ventricular tachycardia Complete heart block Atrioventricular valve insufficiency High-output cardiac failure (arteriovenous malformation, teratoma)
PREMATURE NEONATE
Fluid overload PDA VSD Cor pulmonale (BPD)
FULL-TERM NEONATE
Asphyxial cardiomyopathy (e.g., after perinatal hypoxemic event) Arteriovenous malformation (vein of Galen, hepatic) Left-sided obstructive lesions (coarctation of aorta, hypoplastic left heart, critical aortic stenosis) Transposition of great arteries Large mixing cardiac defects (single ventricle, truncus arteriosus) Viral myocarditis Anemia Supraventricular tachycardia Complete heart block
INFANT/TODDLER
Left-to-right cardiac shunts (VSD) Hemangioma (arteriovenous malformation) Anomalous left coronary artery Metabolic cardiomyopathy Acute hypertension (hemolytic uremic syndrome) Supraventricular tachycardia Kawasaki disease Postoperative repair of congenital heart disease
CHILD/ADOLESCENT
Rheumatic fever Acute hypertension (glomerulonephritis) Viral myocarditis Thyrotoxicosis Hemochromatosis/hemosiderosis Cancer therapy (radiation, doxorubicin) Sickle cell anemia Endocarditis Cor pulmonale (cystic fibrosis) Arrhythmias Chronic upper airway obstruction (cor pulmonale) Unrepaired or palliated congenital heart disease Eisenmenger Syndrome Cardiomyopathy

BPD, Bronchopulmonary dysplasia; *PDA*, patent ductus arteriosus; *VSD*, ventricular septal defect.

TABLE **146.3** Treatment of Heart Failure

THERAPY	MECHANISM
GENERAL CARE	
Rest	Reduces cardiac output
Oxygen	Improves oxygenation in the presence of pulmonary edema
Sodium, fluid restrictions	Decreases vascular congestion; decreases preload
DIURETICS	
Furosemide	Salt excretion at ascending loop of Henle; reduces preload; afterload reduces with control of hypertension; may also cause venodilation
Combination of distal tubule and loop diuretics	Greater sodium excretion
INOTROPIC AGENTS	
Digitalis	Inhibits membrane Na^+, K^+-ATPase and increases intracellular Ca^{2+}, improves cardiac contractility, increases myocardial oxygen consumption
Dopamine	Releases myocardial norepinephrine plus a direct effect on β-receptor, may increase systemic blood pressure; at low infusion rates, dilates renal artery, facilitating diuresis
Dobutamine	β1-receptor agent; often combined with dopamine
Milrinone	Phosphodiesterase 3 inhibitor with positive inotropic properties and decreases vascular resistance/ afterload
AFTERLOAD REDUCTION	
Hydralazine	Arteriolar vasodilator
Nitroprusside	Arterial and venous relaxation; venodilation reduces preload
Captopril/enalapril	Inhibition of angiotensin-converting enzyme; reduces angiotensin II production
OTHER MEASURES	
Mechanical counterpulsation	Improves coronary flow, afterload
Transplantation	Removes diseased heart
Extracorporeal membrane oxygenation	Bypasses heart
Carvedilol	β-Blocking agent

CLINICAL MANIFESTATIONS

Heart failure presents in infants as poor feeding, growth faltering, tachypnea, and diaphoresis with feeding. Older children may present with shortness of breath, easy fatigability, and edema. The physical examination findings depend on whether pulmonary venous congestion, systemic venous congestion, or both are present. Tachycardia, a gallop rhythm, and thready pulses may be present with either cause. If left-sided failure is predominant, tachypnea, orthopnea, wheezing, and pulmonary edema are seen. Hepatomegaly, edema, and distended neck veins are signs of right-sided failure.

IMAGING STUDIES

The absence of cardiomegaly on a chest x-ray usually rules out the diagnosis of heart failure. An echocardiogram assesses the heart chamber sizes, measures myocardial function, and diagnoses congenital heart defects when present.

TREATMENT

Initial treatment is directed at improving myocardial function and optimizing preload and afterload. Diuretics, inotropic support, and, often, **afterload reduction** are employed (Table 146.3). Long-term therapy usually consists of diuretics followed by afterload reduction. Long-term therapy with β blockers or angiotensin-converting enzyme inhibitors also may be beneficial. Spironolactone is usually added to the medical regimen because of its effect on cardiac remodeling.

PEARLS FOR PRACTITIONERS

See The Cardiovascular System: Pearls for Practitioners at the end of this section.

REVIEW QUESTIONS

Available online.

CHAPTER 147

Rheumatic Fever

ETIOLOGY AND EPIDEMIOLOGY

Although uncommon in the United States, *acute* rheumatic fever remains an important preventable cause of cardiac disease worldwide. It is most common in children 6–15 years of age. It is due to an immunologic reaction that is a delayed sequela of group A β-hemolytic streptococcal infections of the pharynx. A family history of rheumatic fever and lower socioeconomic status are additional risk factors.

CLINICAL MANIFESTATIONS

Acute rheumatic fever is diagnosed using the clinical and laboratory findings of the **revised Jones criteria** (Table 147.1). The presence of either two **major criteria** or one major and two **minor criteria**, along with evidence of an antecedent **streptococcal infection**, confirms a diagnosis of acute rheumatic fever. The infection often precedes the presentation of rheumatic fever by 2–6 weeks. Streptococcal antibody tests, such as the antistreptolysin O titer, are the most reliable laboratory evidence of prior infection.

Arthritis is the most common major manifestation. It usually involves the large joints and is migratory. Arthralgia cannot be used as a minor manifestation if arthritis is used as a major manifestation. **Carditis** occurs in about 50% of patients. Tachycardia, a new murmur (mitral or aortic regurgitation), pericarditis, cardiomegaly, and signs of heart failure are evidence of carditis. **Erythema marginatum**, a serpiginous, nonpruritic, and evanescent rash, is uncommon, occurs on the trunk, and is brought out by warmth. **Subcutaneous nodules** are seen predominantly with chronic or recurrent disease. They are firm, painless, nonpruritic, mobile nodules found on the extensor surfaces of the large and small joints, the scalp, and the spine. **Chorea** (Sydenham chorea) consists of neurologic and psychiatric signs. It also is uncommon and often presents long after the infection.

TABLE 147.1 Major Jones Criteria for Diagnosis of Acute Rheumatic Fever[*,†]

SIGN	COMMENTS
Arthritis	Common; swelling, limited motion, tender, erythema
	Must be polyarthritis in low-risk populations[‡] but can be monoarthritis or polyarthralgia in moderate- and high-risk groups
	Migratory; involves large joints but rarely small or unusual joints, such as vertebrae
Carditis	Common; pancarditis, valves, pericardium, myocardium
	Tachycardia greater than explained by fever; new murmur of mitral or aortic insufficiency; Carey-Coombs mid-diastolic murmur; heart failure
	Subclinical carditis seen on echocardiography may be used as a major criteria
Chorea (Sydenham chorea)	Uncommon; manifests long after infection has resolved; more common in females; antineuronal antibody positive
Erythema marginatum	Uncommon; pink macules on trunk and proximal extremities, evolving to serpiginous border with central clearing; evanescent, elicited by application of local heat; nonpruritic
Subcutaneous nodules	Uncommon; associated with repeated episodes and severe carditis; located over extensor surface of elbows, knees, knuckles, and ankles, or scalp and spine; firm, nontender

Minor criteria include fever (temperatures of >38.5°C in low-risk populations and >38°C in moderate- and high-risk populations), arthralgias (must be polyarthralgias in low-risk population but mono- or polyarthralgias in moderate- and high-risk populations), elevated erythrocyte sedimentation rate/C-reactive protein, and prolonged PR interval.

†One major and two minor or two major criteria with evidence of recent group A streptococcal disease (e.g., scarlet fever, positive throat culture, or elevated antistreptolysin O or other antistreptococcal antibodies) strongly suggest the diagnosis of acute rheumatic fever.

‡Low-risk populations are those with acute rheumatic fever incidence of <2 per 100,000 school-age children or all-age rheumatic heart disease prevalence <1 per 1000 population per year.

TREATMENT AND PREVENTION

Management of acute rheumatic fever consists of **benzathine penicillin** to eradicate the β-hemolytic streptococcus, antiinflammatory therapy with **salicylates**, and **bed rest**. Additional supportive therapy for heart failure or chorea may be necessary. **Long-term penicillin prophylaxis**, preferably with intramuscular benzathine penicillin G, 1.2 million U every 28 days, is required. Oral regimens for prophylaxis generally are not as effective. The prognosis of acute rheumatic fever depends on the degree of permanent cardiac damage. Cardiac involvement may resolve completely, especially if it is the first episode and the prophylactic regimen is followed. The severity of cardiac involvement worsens with each recurrence of rheumatic fever.

PEARLS FOR PRACTITIONERS

See The Cardiovascular System: Pearls for Practitioners at the end of this section.

REVIEW QUESTION

Available online.

CHAPTER 148

Cardiomyopathies

ETIOLOGY

A cardiomyopathy is an intrinsic disease of the heart muscle and is not associated with other forms of heart disease (Table 148.1). Cardiomyopathies can be generally categorized into three phenotypes based on anatomic and functional features:

1. Dilated
2. Hypertrophic
3. Restrictive

Dilated cardiomyopathies are the most common. They are often idiopathic, but they may be due to infection (echovirus or coxsackie B virus) or be postinfectious, familial, or secondary to systemic disease or to cardiotoxic drugs. **Hypertrophic cardiomyopathies** are usually familial with autosomal dominant inheritance but may occur sporadically. They can also be associated with genetic syndromes or metabolic disorders. **Restrictive cardiomyopathies** are rare; they may be idiopathic or associated with systemic disease (Table 148.2). There are also less common cardiomyopathies such as left ventricular (LV) noncompaction cardiomyopathy and arrhythmogenic cardiomyopathy that do not fit cleanly into the above phenotypes.

TABLE 148.1 Etiology of Myocardial Disease

FAMILIAL/HEREDITARY
Duchenne muscular dystrophy
Other muscular dystrophies (Becker, limb-girdle)
Myotonic dystrophy
Kearns-Sayre syndrome (progressive external ophthalmoplegia)
Carnitine deficiency syndromes
Endocardial fibroelastosis
Mitochondrial myopathy syndromes
Familial dilated cardiomyopathy (dominant, recessive, X-linked with many genes implicated, including *TTN*)
Familial hypertrophic cardiomyopathy (autosomal dominant inheritance, most commonly involved genes are *MYH7, MYBPC3, TNNT2, TNNI3*)
Familial restrictive cardiomyopathy (autosomal dominant inheritance, *TNNI3* and other variants)
Pompe disease (glycogen storage)
INFECTIOUS (MYOCARDITIS)
Viral (e.g., coxsackievirus infection, mumps, Epstein-Barr virus infection, influenza, parainfluenza infection, measles, varicella, HIV infection)
Bacterial (e.g., diphtheria, *Mycoplasma* infection, meningococcal disease, leptospirosis, Lyme disease, psittacosis, *Coxiella* infection, Rocky Mountain spotted fever)
Parasitic (e.g., Chagas disease, toxoplasmosis)
METABOLIC/NUTRITIONAL/ENDOCRINE
Hypothyroidism
Hyperthyroidism
Pheochromocytoma
Mitochondrial myopathies and oxidative respiratory chain defects
Type II, X-linked 3-methylglutaconic aciduria
CONNECTIVE TISSUE/GRANULOMATOUS DISEASE
Systemic lupus erythematosus
Scleroderma
Amyloidosis
Rheumatic fever
Sarcoidosis
Dermatomyositis
DRUGS/TOXINS
Doxorubicin (Adriamycin)
Ipecac
Iron overload (hemosiderosis)
Irradiation
Cocaine
Amphetamines
CORONARY ARTERIES
Anomalous left coronary artery
Kawasaki disease
OTHER DISORDERS/CONDITIONS
Idiopathic
Sickle cell anemia
Endomyocardial fibrosis
Right ventricular dysplasia

CLINICAL MANIFESTATIONS

Dilated cardiomyopathies result in enlargement of the left ventricle only or of both ventricles. Myocardial contractility is variably decreased. Children with dilated cardiomyopathy present with signs and symptoms of inadequate cardiac output and **heart failure**. Tachypnea and tachycardia are present on examination. Peripheral pulses are often weak because of a **narrow pulse pressure**. Rales may be audible on auscultation. The heart sounds may be muffled, and an S_3 is often present. Concurrent infectious illness may result in circulatory collapse and shock in children with dilated cardiomyopathies.

Hypertrophic cardiomyopathy is initially difficult to diagnose. Infants, but not older children, frequently present with signs of heart failure. Sudden death may be the initial presentation in older children. Dyspnea, fatigue, chest pain,

TABLE 148.2 Anatomic and Functional Features of Cardiomyopathies

FEATURE	DILATED	HYPERTROPHIC	RESTRICTIVE
Etiology	Infectious Metabolic Toxic Familial (dominant, recessive, and X-linked inheritance with many genes implicated, including *TTN*) Idiopathic	Sporadic Inherited (autosomal dominant, most commonly involved genes are *MYH7, MYBPC3, TNNT2, TNNI3*)	Infiltrative (amyloidosis, sarcoidosis) Noninfiltrative (idiopathic; familial, including autosomal dominant inheritance of *TNNI3* variants) Storage disease (hemochromatosis, Fabry disease) Endomyocardial disease
Hemodynamics	Decreased systolic function	Diastolic dysfunction (impaired ventricular filling)	Diastolic dysfunction (impaired ventricular filling)
Treatment	Positive inotropes Diuretics Afterload reduction β Blockers Antiarrhythmics Anticoagulants Cardiac transplantation	β Blockers Calcium channel blockers Cardiac transplantation	Diuretics Anticoagulants Cardiac transplantation

syncope or near-syncope, and palpitations may be present. A murmur is heard in more than 50% of children referred after identification of an affected family member. Restrictive cardiomyopathies are relatively rare in pediatrics. Presenting symptoms usually include dyspnea exacerbated by a respiratory illness, syncope, hepatomegaly, and an S_4 heart sound on examination.

IMAGING STUDIES

Cardiomegaly usually is seen on chest radiographs for all three types of cardiomyopathies. The ECG in dilated cardiomyopathy may have nonspecific ST-T-wave changes and left ventricular hypertrophy. ECG evidence of right ventricular hypertrophy is present in 25% of children with cardiomyopathy. The ECG with hypertrophic cardiomyopathy is almost universally abnormal, but changes can be nonspecific. Primary hypertrophic cardiomyopathy is associated with a prolonged QT interval. Children with restrictive cardiomyopathies may show atrial enlargement on the ECG. Echocardiography features vary by type of cardiomyopathy. Dilated cardiomyopathies result in left atrial and ventricular dilation and depressed contractility. Asymmetric septal hypertrophy and left ventricular outflow tract obstruction are seen in hypertrophic cardiomyopathies. Massive atrial dilation is seen in restrictive cardiomyopathies. LV noncompaction cardiomyopathy will show an increase in the ratio of trabeculated to compact LV myocardium. Endomyocardial biopsy specimens, obtained while the patient is hemodynamically stable, identify histologic type and allow tests for mitochondrial or infiltrative diseases.

TREATMENT

Supportive therapy, including **diuretics**, **inotropic medications**, and **afterload reduction**, is provided for all three types of cardiomyopathy. If a specific etiology can be identified, treatment is directed at the etiology. Symptomatic therapy with close monitoring and follow-up is crucial. Because of the high mortality rate associated with all forms of cardiomyopathy, **cardiac transplantation** must be considered.

PEARLS FOR PRACTITIONERS

See The Cardiovascular System: Pearls for Practitioners at the end of this section.

REVIEW QUESTION

Available online.

CHAPTER 149
Pericarditis

ETIOLOGY AND EPIDEMIOLOGY

Pericarditis is inflammation of the parietal and visceral surfaces of the pericardium. It is most often viral in origin, with many viruses identified as causative agents. A bacterial etiology is rare but causes a much more serious and symptomatic pericarditis. *Staphylococcus aureus* and *Streptococcus pneumoniae* are the most likely bacterial causes. Pericarditis is associated with collagen vascular diseases, such as rheumatoid arthritis, and is seen with uremia (Table 149.1). **Postpericardiotomy syndrome** is a relatively common form of pericarditis that follows heart surgery.

CLINICAL MANIFESTATIONS

The symptoms of pericarditis (Table 149.2) depend on the amount of fluid in the pericardial space and how fast it accumulates. Classically, symptoms include chest pain worsened with supine positioning or deep inspiration. A small effusion usually is well tolerated. A large effusion may be well tolerated if it accumulates slowly. The faster the fluid accumulates, the sooner the patient is hemodynamically compromised and develops symptoms, which can include dyspnea, tachypnea, jugular venous distension, edema, and symptoms of poor systemic perfusion including fatigue, hypotension, and ultimately cardiogenic shock.

TABLE 149.1 Etiology of Pericarditis and Pericardial Effusion

IDIOPATHIC (PRESUMED VIRAL) INFECTIOUS AGENTS
Bacterial
Group A streptococci *Staphylococcus aureus* Pneumococcus, meningococcus* *Haemophilus influenzae** *Mycobacterium tuberculosis*
Viral[†]
Coxsackievirus (group A, B) Echovirus Mumps Influenza Epstein-Barr Cytomegalovirus
Fungal
Histoplasma capsulatum *Coccidioides immitis* *Blastomyces dermatitidis* *Candida*
COLLAGEN VASCULAR, INFLAMMATORY, AND GRANULOMATOUS DISEASES
Rheumatic fever Systemic lupus erythematosus (idiopathic and drug-induced) Rheumatoid arthritis Kawasaki disease Scleroderma Mixed connective tissue disease Inflammatory bowel disease Sarcoidosis Vasculitis
TRAUMATIC
Cardiac contusion (blunt trauma) Penetrating trauma Postpericardiotomy syndrome Radiation
CONTIGUOUS SPREAD
Pleural disease Pneumonia Aortic aneurysm (dissecting)
METABOLIC
Hypothyroidism Uremia Chylopericardium
NEOPLASTIC
Primary Contiguous (lymphoma) Metastatic Infiltrative (leukemia)
OTHER ETIOLOGIC DISORDERS/FACTORS
Drug reaction Pancreatitis After myocardial infarction Thalassemia Central venous catheter perforation Heart failure Hemorrhage (coagulopathy)

*Infectious or immune complex.
[†]Common (viral pericarditis or myopericarditis is probably the most common cause of acute pericarditis in a previously normal host).
Modified from Sigman G. Chest pain. In Kliegman RM, Greenbaum LA, Lye PS, eds. Practical Strategies in Pediatric Diagnosis and Therapy. 2nd ed. Philadelphia: Saunders; 2004. Table 9-9.

TABLE 149.2 Manifestations of Pericarditis

SYMPTOMS
Chest pain (worsened if lying down or with inspiration) Dyspnea Malaise Patient assumes sitting position
SIGNS
Nonconstrictive
Fever Tachycardia Friction rub (accentuated by inspiration, body position) Enlarged heart by percussion and x-ray examination Distant heart sounds
Tamponade
Beck's triad: hypotension, jugular venous distension, and muffled heart sounds* Hepatomegaly Pulsus paradoxus (>10 mm Hg with inspiration) Narrow pulse pressure Weak pulse, poor peripheral perfusion
Constrictive
Distended neck veins Kussmaul sign (inspiratory increase in jugular venous pressure) Distant heart sounds Pericardial knock Hepatomegaly Ascites Edema Tachycardia

Beck's triad is not always present in cases of cardiac tamponade.

IMAGING AND LABORATORY STUDIES

Echocardiography is the most specific and useful diagnostic test for detection of pericardial effusions. A chest x-ray may reveal cardiomegaly. A large effusion creates a rounded, globular cardiac silhouette. The ECG may show tachycardia, elevated ST segments, reduced QRS voltage, depressed PR segment, or electrical alternans (variable QRS amplitude). The causative organism may be identified through viral titers, antistreptolysin O (ASO) titers, or diagnostic testing of the pericardial fluid.

TREATMENT

Pericardiocentesis is indicated for the treatment of hemodynamically significant effusions and to determine the etiology of the pericarditis. Additional treatment is directed at the specific etiology. There is no specific treatment for viral pericarditis other than **antiinflammatory medications**.

PEARLS FOR PRACTITIONERS

See The Cardiovascular System: Pearls for Practitioners at the end of this section.

REVIEW QUESTION

Available online.

Suggested Readings

Allen HD, Shaddy RE, Penny DJ, Feltes TF, Cetta F, eds. *Moss and Adams' Heart Disease in Infants, Children, and Adolescents*. 9th ed. Philadelphia: Lippincott Williams & Wilkins; 2016.

Eidem BW, Johnson J, Lopez L, Cetta F, eds. *Echocardiography in Pediatric and Adult Congenital Heart Disease*. 3rd ed. Philadelphia: Lippincott Williams & Wilkins; 2020.

Jefferies JL, Chang AC, Rossano JW, Shaddy RE, Towbin JA, eds. *Heart Failure in the Child and Young Adult, From Bench to Bedside*. London, UK: Academic Press; 2017.

Kliegman RM, St. Geme J, eds. *Nelson Textbook of Pediatrics*. 22nd ed. Philadelphia: Elsevier; 2025.

Park M, Salamat M. *Pediatric Cardiology for Practitioners*. 7th ed. Philadelphia: Elsevier; 2020.

PEARLS FOR PRACTITIONERS

CHAPTER 140

Cardiovascular System Assessment

- Rate of growth is one of the most valuable and objective signs of cardiovascular health.
  - In infants with heart failure, weight gain is more significantly affected than height and head circumference.
- Cardiovascular vital signs vary with age, and one needs to know or have a resource for "normal" for all age groups to be able to recognize/diagnose abnormal.
- Blood pressure should be routinely taken in the right arm and, if elevated, then taken in all four extremities.
  - The presence of a normal right arm blood pressure and normal pedal pulses effectively rules out coarctation of the aorta outside of the newborn period.
- Peripheral cyanosis (hands, feet, perioral), also known as acrocyanosis, is common in infants and needs to be differentiated from central cyanosis (tongue, oral mucosa, trunk).
- Murmurs are "noisy blood flow" and are very common in pediatric patients. They may be normal (innocent) or abnormal.
  - The timing of the murmur is most important in determining the significance of the murmur and developing a differential diagnosis.
  - Diastolic murmurs, holosystolic murmurs, continuous murmurs (with the exception of the venous hum), and murmurs with a palpable thrill are abnormal murmurs.
  - To be a normal (innocent) murmur, the cardiovascular history and remainder of the cardiovascular exam must be normal.
- A normal heart size on chest radiograph virtually rules out heart failure; however, a large heart is not diagnostic of heart failure.
- Echocardiography is the most important noninvasive tool in the diagnosis and management of congenital heart disease with ECG, chest x-ray, cardiac catheterization, and CT/MRI providing additional information.
- Mild desaturation that is not clinically apparent may be the only early finding in complex congenital heart defects. Routine measurement of pulse oximetry in the right arm and a lower extremity between 24 and 48 hours of life may facilitate diagnosis of congenital heart disease.

CHAPTER 141

Syncope

- Syncope is the transient loss of consciousness and muscle tone and is typically associated with an upright position, prodromal symptoms, pale appearance, and brief loss of consciousness with rapid return to normal state of consciousness.
- Syncope occurring during exercise, without any prodrome, or with associated cardiac symptoms should be considered atypical until more extensively evaluated.

CHAPTER 142

Chest Pain

- Chest pain is common in pediatric patients but is rarely cardiac in origin.
- Up to one-third of all pediatric chest pain is idiopathic, with musculoskeletal chest pain being the most common cause of diagnosable chest pain.

CHAPTER 143

Dysrhythmias

- The most common symptomatic dysrhythmia in pediatric patients is supraventricular tachycardia.
- Sinus arrhythmia is common in children and represents a normal variation in heart rate with respiration. It can often mimic an irregular rhythm, ectopy, or heart block on auscultation.

CHAPTER 144

Acyanotic Congenital Heart Disease

- Congenital heart defects occur in about 1% of births and include a wide spectrum of defects from asymptomatic to fatal lesions.
- Ventricular septal defect (VSD) is the most common congenital heart defect.
  - The amount of shunting at a VSD depends on the size of the defect and the pulmonary vascular resistance.

    - Large shunts result in excessive pulmonary blood flow (congestive heart failure), typically presenting with tachypnea, fatigue, and diaphoresis with feeding and poor weight gain.
- Atrial septal defects (ASDs) rarely cause symptoms in childhood.
    - The amount of shunting across an ASD depends on the size of the defect and the relative compliance of the ventricles.
    - In addition to a systolic ejection murmur from increased flow across the pulmonary valve, a widely split S_2 that does not vary with respiration is the classic exam finding associated with an ASD.
- A patent ductus arteriosus (PDA) results in volume overload of the left heart; the shunting is dependent on the size of the PDA and the pulmonary vascular resistance.
- The most common congenital heart defect in children with trisomy 21 is the endocardial cushion defect, which is also called atrioventricular canal defect or atrioventricular septal defect.
- Symptoms and management of pulmonary stenosis and aortic stenosis depend on the severity of the stenosis.
    - Pulmonary valve stenosis is rarely progressive; aortic valve stenosis is usually progressive.
- Coarctation of the aorta usually occurs in the juxtaductal region. Symptoms and presentation depend on the severity of the obstruction and associated congenital heart defects.

CHAPTER 145
Cyanotic Congenital Heart Disease

- Clinical cyanosis occurs when more than 5 g/100 mL of reduced hemoglobin is present in the systemic blood.
- The cyanotic congenital heart defects are the five *Ts*: tetralogy of Fallot, transposition of the great arteries, tricuspid atresia, truncus arteriosus, and total anomalous pulmonary venous return.
- Tetralogy of Fallot is the most common cyanotic congenital heart defect. The degree of cyanosis and the murmur depend on the amount of pulmonary stenosis.
- Transposition of the great arteries is the most common cyanotic lesion to present in the newborn period.
- Congenital heart defects with a functionally single ventricle, such as tricuspid atresia and hypoplastic left heart syndrome (HLHS) require a staged surgical repair. Many will ultimately require heart transplantation.
    - Survival of patients with HLHS—the most common cause of death from a cardiac defect in the first month of life—has improved dramatically with staged surgical and aggressive medical management.

CHAPTER 146
Heart Failure

- Both the most common causes and the clinical manifestations of congestive heart failure vary with age of presentation.
- Diseases/issues that impact preload, afterload, and contractility can all result in worsening cardiac performance and heart failure.
- Treatment of heart failure often includes diuresis, inotropic support, and afterload reduction.

CHAPTER 147
Rheumatic Fever

- Rheumatic fever remains an important, preventable cause of cardiac disease worldwide. Diagnosis of rheumatic fever is made using the clinical and laboratory findings of the revised Jones criteria.
- Antibiotic prophylaxis aimed at decreasing risk of subsequent streptococcal infections is key to the care of patients with a history of rheumatic fever.

CHAPTER 148
Cardiomyopathies

- There are three major types of cardiomyopathy: dilated (most common), hypertrophic, and restrictive.
- Supportive therapy, including diuretics, inotropic medications, and afterload reduction, is used in all three types.
- Cardiac transplantation must be considered due to the high mortality rate seen in all forms of cardiomyopathy.

CHAPTER 149
Pericarditis

- Pericarditis is inflammation of the parietal and visceral surfaces of the pericardium and is most often viral in origin.
    - The severity of symptoms depends on the amount of fluid present in the pericardial space and the rapidity with which the fluid accumulated.

HEMATOLOGY

Melissa Azul | Amanda M. Brandow

CHAPTER 150
Hematology Assessment

HISTORY

A detailed history of the onset, severity, progression, associated symptoms, presence of systemic complaints, and exacerbating factors is crucial to the diagnosis of a blood disorder. In many blood disorders, a **detailed pedigree** identifying a pattern of inheritance can point to the diagnosis.

PHYSICAL EXAMINATION AND COMMON MANIFESTATIONS

The physical examination of patients with blood disorders first focuses on hemodynamic stability. Acute episodes of anemia may be life threatening, presenting with impairment of perfusion and cognitive status. Two common findings of anemia include **pallor** and **jaundice**. The presence of **petechiae**, **purpura**, or deeper sites of **bleeding**, including generalized hemorrhage, indicates abnormalities of platelets, coagulation factors, or both. **Growth parameters** point to whether anemia is an acute or chronic process. Severe types of anemia, thrombocytopenia, and pancytopenia often are associated with congenital anomalies and a pattern of growth delay. Organ system involvement (especially **hepatosplenomegaly** and **lymphadenopathy**) or systemic illness points to a generalized disorder as the cause for hematologic abnormalities (Table 150.1).

INITIAL DIAGNOSTIC EVALUATION

Diagnosis of pediatric blood disorders requires a detailed knowledge of normal hematologic values that vary according to age and, after puberty, according to sex (Table 150.2). Directed by the history, physical examination, and screening laboratory studies, specific diagnostic testing can then confirm the diagnosis.

DEVELOPMENTAL HEMATOLOGY

Hematopoiesis begins by 3 weeks of gestation with **erythropoiesis** in the yolk sac. By 2 months of gestation, the primary site of hematopoiesis migrates to the liver. By 5–6 months of gestation, hematopoiesis shifts from the liver to the bone marrow. An extremely premature infant may have significant **extramedullary hematopoiesis** due to limited bone marrow hematopoiesis. During infancy, virtually all marrow cavities are actively hematopoietic, and the proportion of hematopoietic to stromal elements is elevated. As a child grows, hematopoiesis moves to the central bones of the body (vertebrae, sternum, ribs, and pelvis), and the marrow is gradually replaced with fat. Hemolysis or marrow damage may lead to marrow repopulation of cavities where hematopoiesis

TABLE **150.1** Presentation of Hematologic Disorders

CONDITION	SYMPTOMS AND SIGNS	COMMON EXAMPLES
Anemia	Pallor, fatigue, heart failure, jaundice	Iron deficiency, hemolytic anemia
Polycythemia	Irritability, headache, cyanosis, seizures, jaundice, stroke	Cyanotic heart disease, infant of diabetic mother, cystic fibrosis
Neutropenia	Fever, pharyngitis, oral ulceration, cellulitis, lymphadenopathy, bacteremia, gingivitis, perirectal infections	Viral suppression, congenital or drug-induced agranulocytosis, leukemia
Thrombocytopenia	Petechiae, ecchymosis, epistaxis, gastrointestinal hemorrhage	ITP, leukemia
Coagulopathy	Bruising, hemarthrosis, mucosal bleeding (including menorrhagia)	von Willebrand disease, hemophilia, DIC
Thrombosis	Pulmonary embolism, deep vein thrombosis, cerebral sinus venous thrombosis	Lupus anticoagulant; protein C, protein S, or antithrombin III deficiency; factor V Leiden, prothrombin 20210

DIC, Disseminated intravascular coagulation; *ITP*, immune thrombocytopenia.

TABLE **150.2** Hematologic Values During Infancy and Childhood

AGE	HEMOGLOBIN (g/dL) MEAN	HEMOGLOBIN (g/dL) RANGE	HEMATOCRIT (%) MEAN	HEMATOCRIT (%) RANGE	RETICULOCYTES (%) MEAN	LEUKOCYTES (per mm³) MEAN	LEUKOCYTES (per mm³) RANGE	DIFFERENTIAL COUNTS: NEUTROPHILS (%) MEAN	NEUTROPHILS (%) RANGE	LYMPHOCYTES (%) MEAN	EOSINOPHILS (%) MEAN	MONOCYTES (%) MEAN	NUCLEATED RED CELLS/100 WBCs RANGE
Cord blood	16.8	13.7–20.1	55	45–65	5	18,000	9,000–30,000	61	40–80	31	2	6	7
2 wk	16.5	13–20	50	42–66	1	12,000	5,000–21,000	40		48	3	9	3–10
3 mo	12.0	9.5–14.5	36	31–41	1	12,000	6,000–18,000	30		63	2	5	0
6 mo–6 yr	12.0	10.5–14	37	33–42	1	10,000	6,000–15,000	45		48	2	5	0
7–12 yr	13.0	11–16	38	34–40	1	8,000	4,500–13,500	55		38	2	5	0
POSTPUBERTAL/ADULT													
Female	14.0	12–16	42	37–47	1.6	7,500	5,000–10,000	55	35–70	35	3	7	0
Male	16.0	14–18	47	42–52									

WBCs, White blood cells.
From Behrman RE, ed. Nelson Textbook of Pediatrics. *14th ed. Philadelphia: WB Saunders; 1992.*

previously had ceased or may delay the shift of hematopoiesis. Hepatosplenomegaly in patients with chronic hemolysis may signify extramedullary hematopoiesis. When a patient with cytopenia(s) is being evaluated, a **bone marrow examination** provides valuable information about processes that lead to underproduction of circulating cells. In addition, bone marrow infiltration by neoplastic elements or storage cells often occurs in conjunction with infiltration in the spleen, liver, and lymph nodes.

The hematopoietic cells consist of the following:

1. Small compartment of **pluripotent progenitor stem cells** that resemble small lymphocytes and can form all myeloid elements
2. Large compartment of committed proliferating cells of myeloid, erythroid, and megakaryocytic lineage
3. Large compartment of postmitotic maturing cells (Fig. 150.1)

The bone marrow is the major storage organ for mature neutrophils and contains about seven times the intravascular pool of neutrophils. Bone marrow contains 2.5–5 times as many cells of myeloid lineage as cells of erythroid lineage. Smaller numbers of megakaryocytes, plasma cells, histiocytes, lymphocytes, and stromal cells are also stored in the marrow.

Erythropoiesis (red blood cell [RBC] production) is controlled by **erythropoietin** (EPO), a glycoprotein that stimulates primitive pluripotential stem cells to differentiate along the erythroid line. EPO is made by the juxtaglomerular apparatus of the kidney in response to local tissue hypoxia. The normally high hemoglobin level of the fetus

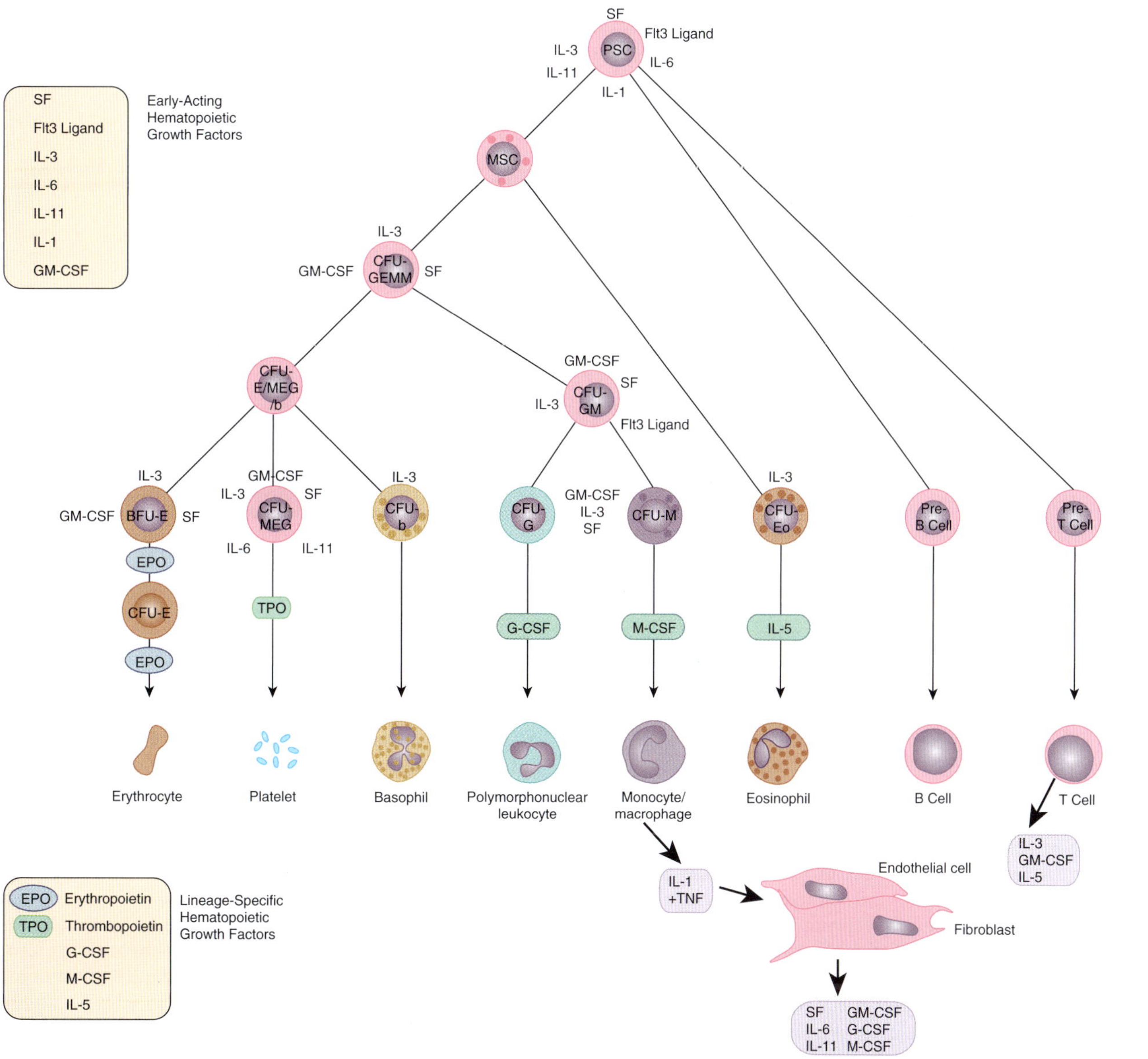

FIGURE 150.1 Major cytokine sources and actions that promote hematopoiesis. Cells of the bone marrow microenvironment, such as macrophages, endothelial cells, and reticular fibroblasts, produce M-CSF, GM-CSF, and G-CSF after stimulation. For all lineages, optimal development requires a combination of early- and late-acting factors. *BFU,* Burst-forming unit; *CFU,* colony-forming unit; *EPO,* erythropoietin; *G-CSF,* granulocyte colony-stimulating factor; *GM-CSF,* granulocyte-macrophage colony-stimulating factor; *IL,* interleukin; *M-CSF,* macrophage colony-stimulating factor; *MSC,* myeloid stem cell; *PSC,* pluripotent stem cell; *TNF,* tumor necrosis factor; *TPO,* thrombopoietin. (From Sieff CA, Nathan DG, Clark SC. The anatomy and physiology of hematopoiesis. In: Orkin SH, Nathan DG, eds. *Hematology of Infancy and Childhood.* 5th ed. Philadelphia: WB Saunders; 1998:168.)

is a result of fetal EPO production in the liver in response to low partial pressure of oxygen (Po_2) in utero. EPO leads to production of the **erythroid colony-forming unit**. The earliest recognizable erythroid cell is the erythroblast, which forms eight or more daughter cells. The RBC nucleus becomes gradually pyknotic and eventually is extruded. The cell is then released from the marrow as a **reticulocyte** that maintains residual mitochondrial and protein synthetic capacity. These relatively large, highly specialized RBC precursors are engaged primarily in the production of **globin chains, glycolytic enzymes**, and **heme**. Iron is taken up via transferrin receptors and incorporated into the heme ring, which combines with globin chains synthesized within the immature RBC. When the messenger RNA and mitochondria are gone from the RBC, heme or protein synthesis is no longer possible; the RBC continues to function for its normal life span of approximately 120 days.

Embryonic hemoglobins are produced during yolk sac erythropoiesis then are replaced by **fetal hemoglobin** (hemoglobin F, $\alpha_2\gamma_2$) during the hepatic phase. During the third trimester, gamma chain production gradually diminishes, replaced by beta chains, resulting in **hemoglobin A** ($\alpha_2\beta_2$). Some fetal factors (e.g., infant of a diabetic mother) delay onset of beta chain production, but premature birth does not. Just after birth, with rapid increases in oxygen saturation, EPO production stops and thus erythropoiesis ceases. Fetal RBCs have a shorter survival time (60 days).

During the first few months of postnatal life, rapid growth, shortened RBC survival, and cessation of erythropoiesis cause a gradual decline in hemoglobin levels, with a nadir at 8–10 weeks of life. This so-called ***physiologic nadir*** is accentuated in premature infants with earlier timing and a lower nadir. EPO is produced in response to the decline in hemoglobin and decreased oxygen delivery. Erythropoiesis subsequently resumes with an increase in the reticulocyte count. The hemoglobin level gradually increases, accompanied by synthesis of increasing amounts of hemoglobin A. By 6 months of age in healthy infants, only trace gamma chain synthesis occurs.

Production of **neutrophil precursors** is controlled predominantly by two different colony-stimulating factors (see Fig. 150.1). The most immature neutrophil precursors are controlled by **granulocyte-macrophage colony-stimulating factor** (GM-CSF), produced by monocytes and lymphocytes. GM-CSF increases the entry of primitive precursor cells into the myeloid line of differentiation. **Granulocyte colony-stimulating factor** (G-CSF) augments the production of more mature granulocyte precursors. GM-CSF and G-CSF, working in concert, can augment production of neutrophils, shorten the usual 10- to 14-day production time from stem cell to mature neutrophil, and stimulate functional activity. The rapid increase in neutrophil count that occurs with infection is caused by release of stored neutrophils from the bone marrow, under the control of GM-CSF. During maturation, a mitotic pool of neutrophil precursors exists—myeloblasts, promyelocytes, and myelocytes possessing primary granules. The postmitotic pool consists of metamyelocytes, bands, and mature polymorphonuclear leukocytes containing secondary or specific granules that define the cell type. Only bands and mature neutrophils are fully functional to perform phagocytosis, chemotaxis, and bacterial killing. Neutrophils migrate from the bone marrow, circulate for 6–7 hours, and then enter the tissues, where they become end-stage cells that do not recirculate. Eosinophil production is under the control of a related glycoprotein hormone, interleukin 3. Eosinophils, which play a role in host defense against parasites, also are capable of living in tissues for prolonged periods.

Megakaryocytes are giant, multinucleated cells derived from the primitive stem cell and are polyploid (16–32 times the normal DNA content) because of nuclear, but not cytoplasmic, cell division. Platelets form by invagination of the megakaryocytic cell membrane and fragment off from these megakaryocyte pseudopods into the blood vessel. **Thrombopoietin** is the primary regulator of platelet production. Platelets adhere to damaged endothelium and subendothelial surfaces via specific receptors for the adhesive proteins, von Willebrand factor, and fibrinogen. Platelets also have dense and alpha granules that readily release their contents after stimulation and trigger the process of platelet aggregation. Platelets circulate for 7–10 days and have no nucleus.

Lymphocytes are particularly abundant in the bone marrow of young children. These are primarily B lymphocytes arising in the spleen and lymph nodes, but T lymphocytes also are present.

PEARLS FOR PRACTITIONERS

See Hematology: Pearls for Practitioners at the end of this section.

REVIEW QUESTIONS

Available online.

CHAPTER 151

Anemia

ETIOLOGY

The diagnosis of anemia is determined by comparison of the patient's **hemoglobin level** with age-specific and sex-specific normal values (see Table 150.2). The production of androgens at the onset of puberty in males results in them maintaining a normal hemoglobin value approximately 1.5–2 g/dL higher than females. The quantitative definition of anemia is any hemoglobin or hematocrit value that is 2 standard deviations (95% confidence limits) below the mean for age and sex. Anemia is often a manifestation of another primary process and may accentuate other organ dysfunction.

Anemias are classified based on the size and hemoglobin content of the cells (Fig. 151.1). **Hypochromic, microcytic anemia** is caused by an inadequate production of hemoglobin. The most common causes of this microcytic anemia are iron deficiency and thalassemia. **Normocytic** anemia is often seen in patients with a systemic illness that impairs adequate marrow synthesis of red blood cells (RBCs). **Macrocytic anemia** is seen in deficiencies of vitamin B_{12} and/or folic acid. **Hemolytic diseases** are mediated either by disorders intrinsic or extrinsic to the RBC that increase RBC destruction. The most common RBC membrane disorders are **hereditary**

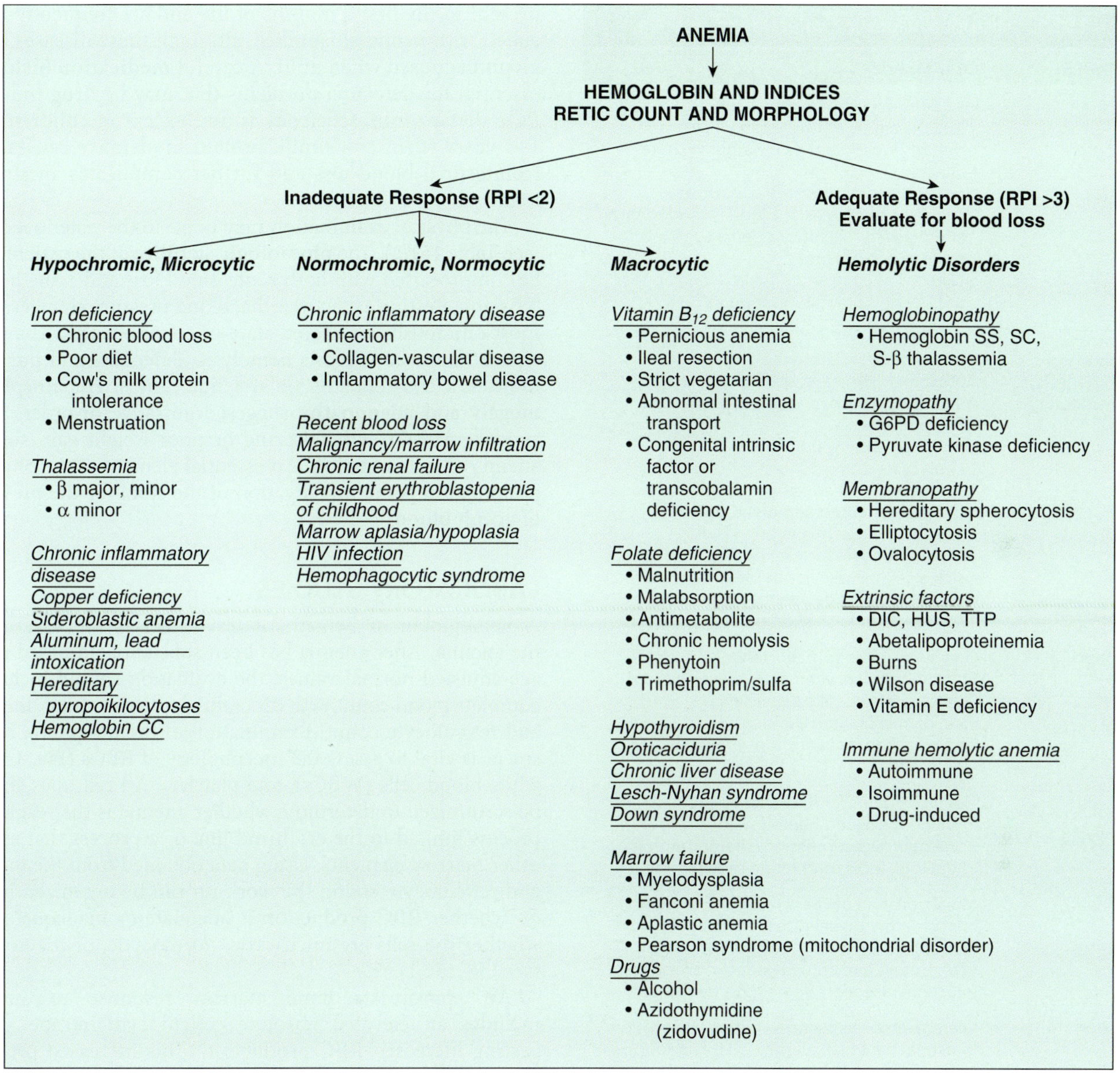

FIGURE 151.1 Use of the complete blood count, reticulocyte count, and blood smear in the diagnosis of anemia. The reticulocyte production index (RPI) is a calculation that measures the rate of red blood cell production. *DIC,* Disseminated intravascular coagulation; *G6PD,* glucose-6-phosphate dehydrogenase; *HUS,* hemolytic uremic syndrome; *TTP,* thrombotic thrombocytopenic purpura.

spherocytosis and **hereditary elliptocytosis**. In both disorders, abnormalities of proteins within the cytoskeleton lead to malformed RBC shape and function. Numerous RBC enzyme deficiencies may lead to hemolysis, including **glucose-6-phosphate dehydrogenase (G6PD) deficiency** (common) and **pyruvate kinase deficiency** (rare). Extravascular hemolysis occurs with immune-mediated hemolysis when RBCs coated with antibodies or complement are phagocytosed by the reticuloendothelial system. Intravascular hemolysis occurs when antibody binding leads to complement fixation and lysis of RBCs or mechanical cleavage secondary to intravascular fibrin stranding.

CLINICAL MANIFESTATIONS

Acute onset of anemia can result in poor compensation, which manifests as tachycardia, systolic flow murmur, dizziness, poor exercise tolerance, headache, fatigue or excessive sleeping (especially in infants), irritability, poor feeding, and syncope. In contrast, chronic anemia often is exceptionally well tolerated in children because of their cardiovascular reserve. Usually, children with chronic anemia will have minimal tachycardia and a systolic flow murmur on examination. The urgency of diagnostic and therapeutic intervention, especially the use of packed RBC transfusion, should be dictated by the extent of cardiovascular or functional impairment more than the absolute level of hemoglobin.

The causes of anemia often can be delineated from a careful history based on the patient's age (Tables 151.1 and 151.2). Anemia at any age demands a search for **blood loss**. A history of jaundice, pallor, previously affected siblings, substance use disorder in mother, or excessive blood loss at the time of birth provides important clues to the diagnosis in newborns. A careful **dietary history** is crucial. A history of **jaundice**, **pallor**, and/or **splenomegaly** are often present

TABLE 151.1 Historical Clues in Evaluation of Anemia

VARIABLE	COMMENTS
Age	Iron deficiency rare in the absence of blood loss before 6 months in term infants or before doubling of birthweight in preterm infants. Neonatal anemia with reticulocytosis suggests hemolysis or blood loss. Neonatal anemia with reticulocytopenia suggests bone marrow failure. Sickle cell anemia and β-thalassemia appear as fetal hemoglobin disappears (4–8 months of age).
Family history and genetic considerations	X-linked: G6PD deficiency Autosomal dominant: spherocytosis Autosomal recessive: sickle cell anemia, Fanconi anemia Family member with history of cholecystectomy (for bilirubin stones) or splenectomy at an early age: spherocytosis or other inherited hemolytic anemias Ethnicity: thalassemia in people of Mediterranean, African, or Asian descent; sickle cell disease in people of African descent; G6PD deficiency in people of African, Greek, or Middle Eastern descent
Nutrition	Cow's milk diet: iron deficiency Strict vegetarian: vitamin B_{12} deficiency Goat's milk diet: folate deficiency Pica: plumbism, iron deficiency Cholestasis, malabsorption: vitamin E deficiency
Medications	G6PD: oxidants (nitrofurantoin, antimalarials) Immune-mediated hemolysis (penicillin) Bone marrow suppression (chemotherapy) Phenytoin, increasing folate requirement
Diarrhea	Malabsorption of vitamin B_{12} or E or iron Inflammatory bowel disease and anemia of inflammation with or without blood loss Milk protein intolerance–induced blood loss Intestinal resection: vitamin B_{12} deficiency
Infection	*Giardia lamblia* infection: iron malabsorption Intestinal bacterial overgrowth (blind loop): vitamin B_{12} deficiency Fish tapeworm: vitamin B_{12} deficiency Epstein-Barr virus, cytomegalovirus infection: bone marrow suppression, hemophagocytic syndromes *Mycoplasma* infection: hemolysis Parvovirus infection: bone marrow suppression HIV infection Chronic infection Endocarditis Malaria: hemolysis Hepatitis: aplastic anemia

G6PD, Glucose-6-phosphate dehydrogenase.

with hemolytic anemia. Due to increased bilirubin production, **gallstones** (bilirubinate) are a common complication of chronic hemolysis. Systemic complaints suggest anemia as part of a larger systemic illness (acute or chronic). In later childhood and adolescence, the presence of constitutional symptoms, unusual diets or supplement use, drug ingestion, or blood loss (often from heavy menstrual bleeding) often points to a diagnosis. **Congenital hemolytic disorders** (e.g., enzyme deficiencies, membrane abnormalities) often present in the first 6 months of life and are frequently associated with neonatal jaundice, although these diseases often go undiagnosed when mild. A careful **medication history** is essential for detecting problems that may be drug induced. Pure dietary iron deficiency is rare except in children ages 1–3 years when cow's milk protein intolerance causes gastrointestinal blood loss and further complicates an already inadequate iron intake.

The physical examination may point to the potential cause (see Table 151.2). The **physiologic stability** of the patient may be compromised with both acute blood loss and acute hemolysis, manifesting as tachycardia, blood pressure changes, and, most ominously, an altered state of consciousness. The presence of jaundice suggests hemolysis. **Petechiae** and **purpura** indicate a coagulopathy or systemic illness. **Hepatosplenomegaly** and **adenopathy** suggest infiltrative disorders such as leukemia. **Growth faltering** or poor weight gain suggest anemia of inflammation. An essential element of the physical examination is the investigation of the stool for the presence of **occult blood**.

LABORATORY STUDIES

A hemoglobin or hematocrit test indicates the severity of the anemia. After anemia has been substantiated based upon age-adjusted normal values, the evaluation should include a complete blood count with differential, platelet count, indices, and reticulocyte count. Examination of the peripheral blood smear is vital to assess the morphology of RBCs (Fig. 151.2), white blood cells (WBCs), and platelets. All cell lines should be scrutinized to determine whether anemia is the result of a process limited to the erythroid line or a process that affects other marrow elements. Using data obtained from the indices and reticulocyte count, the work-up can be organized based on whether RBC production is adequate or inadequate and whether the cells are microcytic, normocytic, or macrocytic (see Fig. 151.1).

An appropriate bone marrow response to anemia includes an elevated absolute reticulocyte number, suggesting increased RBC production. This increased production is frequently a response to either hemolysis or blood loss. Anemia with a normal reticulocyte number suggests decreased or ineffective RBC production for the degree of anemia. Reticulocytopenia signifies either an acute onset of anemia such that the marrow has not had adequate time to respond, nutritional deficiencies leading to decreased RBC production, reticulocytes being destroyed in the marrow (antibody mediated), or that intrinsic bone marrow disease is present. The best indicators of the severity of hemolysis are the hemoglobin level and the elevation of the **reticulocyte count**. Biochemical evidence of hemolysis includes levels of bilirubin and lactate dehydrogenase, as well as a decrease in haptoglobin.

DIFFERENTIAL DIAGNOSIS

Microcytic Anemia

Iron-Deficiency Anemia

Etiology

Infants fed cow's milk when younger than 1 year of age, toddlers fed large volumes of cow's milk, and menstruating adolescent females who are not receiving supplemental iron are at

TABLE **151.2** Physical Findings in the Evaluation of Anemia

SYSTEM/STRUCTURE	OBSERVATION	SIGNIFICANCE
Skin	Hyperpigmentation	Fanconi anemia, dyskeratosis congenita
	Café-au-lait spots	Fanconi anemia
	Vitiligo	Vitamin B_{12} deficiency
	Partial oculocutaneous albinism	Chediak-Higashi syndrome
	Jaundice	Hemolysis
	Petechiae, purpura	Bone marrow infiltration, autoimmune hemolysis with autoimmune thrombocytopenia, hemolytic uremic syndrome, hemophagocytic syndromes
	Erythematous rash	Parvovirus or Epstein-Barr virus infection
	Butterfly rash	SLE antibodies
	Bruising	Bleeding disorder, nonaccidental trauma, scurvy (vitamin C deficiency)
Head	Frontal bossing	Thalassemia major, severe iron deficiency, chronic subdural hematoma
	Microcephaly	Fanconi anemia
Eyes	Microphthalmia	Fanconi anemia
	Retinopathy	Hemoglobin SS, SC disease (see Table 151.7)
	Optic atrophy	Osteopetrosis
	Blocked lacrimal gland	Dyskeratosis congenital
	Kayser-Fleischer ring	Wilson disease
	Blue sclera	Iron deficiency, osteopetrosis
Mouth	Glossitis	Vitamin B_{12} deficiency, iron deficiency
	Angular stomatitis	Iron deficiency
	Cleft lip	Diamond-Blackfan syndrome
	Pigmentation	Peutz-Jeghers syndrome (intestinal blood loss)
	Telangiectasia	Osler-Weber-Rendu syndrome (blood loss)
	Leukoplakia	Dyskeratosis congenital
Chest	Shield chest or widespread nipples	Diamond-Blackfan syndrome
	Murmur	Endocarditis: prosthetic valve hemolysis; severe anemia
Abdomen	Hepatomegaly	Hemolysis, infiltrative tumor, chronic disease, hemangioma, cholecystitis, extramedullary hematopoiesis
	Splenomegaly	Hemolysis, sickle cell disease, (early) thalassemia, malaria, leukemia/lymphoma, Epstein-Barr virus, portal hypertension
	Enlarged kidney	Fanconi anemia
	Absent kidney	Fanconi anemia
Extremities	Absent thumbs	Fanconi anemia
	Triphalangeal thumb	Diamond-Blackfan syndrome
	Spoon nails	Iron deficiency
	Beau line (nails)	Heavy metal intoxication, severe illness
	Mees line (nails)	Heavy metals, severe illness, sickle cell anemia
	Dystrophic nails	Dyskeratosis congenita
Rectal	Hemorrhoids	Portal hypertension
	Heme-positive stool	Gastrointestinal bleeding
Nerves	Irritable, apathy	Iron deficiency
	Peripheral neuropathy	Deficiency of vitamins B_1, B_{12}, and E; lead poisoning
	Dementia	Deficiency of vitamins B_{12} and E
	Ataxia, posterior column signs	Vitamin B_{12} deficiency
	Stroke	Hemoglobin SS or $S\beta^0$-thalassemia, paroxysmal nocturnal hemoglobinuria
General	Small stature	Fanconi anemia, HIV infection, malnutrition

SLE, Systemic lupus erythematosus.

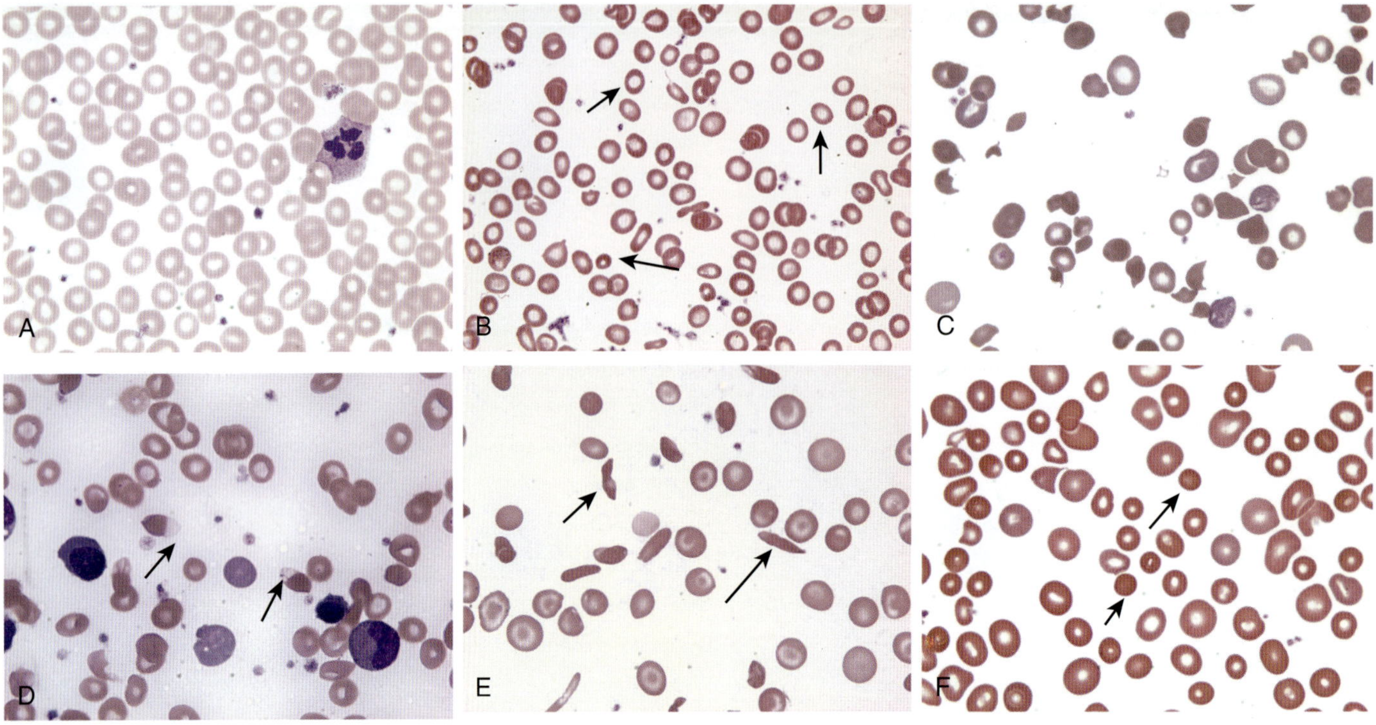

FIGURE 151.2 Morphologic abnormalities of the red blood cell. **(A)** Normal. **(B)** Hypochromic microcytes (iron deficiency). **(C)** Schistocytes (hemolytic uremic syndrome). **(D)** Blister cells (glucose-6-phosphate dehydrogenase deficiency). **(E)** Sickle cells (hemoglobin SS disease). **(F)** Spherocytes (autoimmune hemolytic anemia). *Arrows* represent the cell discussed. (Courtesy B. Trost and J.P. Scott.)

high risk for iron deficiency. **Dietary** iron-deficiency anemia is most common in toddlers who are receiving large volumes of cow's milk and eat minimal amounts of food high in iron content (see Chapters 26 and 29). Gastrointestinal blood loss can lead to iron-deficiency anemia and should be considered, especially in adolescent males. Iron-deficiency anemia also may be found in children with chronic inflammatory diseases, even without **chronic blood loss**.

Epidemiology

The prevalence of iron deficiency, the most common cause of anemia in the world, is approximately 9% in toddlers, 9–11% in adolescent females, and less than 1% in adolescent males. Iron-deficiency anemia occurs in approximately one-third of children who are iron deficient (Table 151.3). Children from low socioeconomic status in the United States may be at increased risk for iron deficiency because of poor dietary intake (see Chapter 29). Breast-fed infants are less likely to have iron deficiency than bottle-fed infants because, although there is less iron in breast milk, this iron is more efficiently absorbed. Infants who continue to be exclusively breast-fed in the second half of the first year of life are at risk for iron deficiency.

Clinical Manifestations

In addition to cardiovascular manifestations of anemia, central nervous system abnormalities **(apathy, irritability, poor concentration)** have been linked to iron deficiency, resulting from alterations of iron-containing enzymes (monoamine oxidase) and cytochromes. Poor muscle endurance, gastrointestinal dysfunction, and impaired WBC and T-cell function have been associated with iron deficiency. Iron deficiency in infancy is associated with later **cognitive deficits** and poor school performance. The gradually developing nature of anemia associated with iron deficiency allows for physiologic compensation so that some children are minimally symptomatic even with severe anemia.

Treatment

In an otherwise healthy child, a **therapeutic trial of oral iron** is the best diagnostic study for iron deficiency as long as the child is re-examined and a response is documented. The response to oral iron includes rapid subjective improvement, especially in neurologic function (within 24–48 hours) and reticulocytosis (48–72 hours); increase in hemoglobin levels (4–30 days); and repletion of iron stores (1–3 months). The usual therapeutic dose of 3–6 mg/day of elemental iron induces an increase in hemoglobin of 0.25–0.4 g/dL per day (a 1%/day increase in hematocrit). If the hemoglobin level fails to increase within 2 weeks after institution of iron treatment, careful re-evaluation for ongoing blood loss, development of infection, poor compliance, malabsorption, or other causes of microcytic anemia is required (Table 151.4; see Fig. 151.1).

Prevention

Bottle-fed infants should receive an iron-containing formula until 12 months of age. Exclusively breast-fed infants older than 6 months of age should receive an iron supplement. The introduction of iron-enriched solid foods at 6 months of age, followed by a transition to a limited amount of cow's milk and increased solid foods at 1 year, will help prevent iron-deficiency anemia. Adolescent females who are menstruating

TABLE 151.3 Stages in Development of Iron Deficiency Anemia

HEMOGLOBIN (g/dL)	PERIPHERAL SMEAR	SERUM IRON (mcg/dL)	BONE MARROW IRON	SERUM FERRITIN (ng/mL)
13+ (normal)	nc/nc	50–150	Fe^{2+}	*Male:* 40–340 *Female:* 40–150
10–12	nc/nc	↓	Fe^{2+} absent, erythroid hyperplasia	<12
8–10	hypo/nc	↓	Fe^{2+} absent, erythroid hyperplasia	<12
<8	hypo/micro*	↓	Fe^{2+} absent, erythroid hyperplasia	<12

Microcytosis, determined by a mean corpuscular volume (in fL) <2 SD below the mean, must be adjusted for age (e.g., −2 SD at 3–6 mo = 74; at 0.5–2 yr = 70; at 2–6 yr = 75; at 6–12 yr = 77; and at 12–18 yr = 78).
Fe^{2+}, Ferrous iron; *hypo/micro*, hypochromic, microcytic; *hypo/nc*, hypochromic, normocytic; *nc/nc*, normochromic, normocytic; *SD*, standard deviations.
From Andreoli TE, Bennett JC, Carpenter CC, et al. Cecil Essentials of Medicine. 4th ed. Philadelphia: WB Saunders; 1997.

TABLE 151.4 Differentiating Features of Microcytic Anemias*

TEST	IRON-DEFICIENCY ANEMIA	THALASSEMIA MINOR†	ANEMIA OF INFLAMMATION‡
Serum iron	Low	Normal	Low
Serum iron-binding capacity	High	Normal	Low or normal
Serum ferritin	Low	Normal or high	Normal or high
Marrow iron stores	Low or absent	Normal or high	Normal or high
Marrow sideroblasts	Decreased or absent	Normal or increased	Normal or increased
Free erythrocyte protoporphyrin	High	Normal or slightly increased	High
Hemoglobin A_2 or F	Normal	High β-thalassemia; normal α-thalassemia	Normal
Red blood cell distribution width§	High	Normal	Normal or high

**See Table 151.3 for definition of microcytosis.*
†α-Thalassemia minor can be diagnosed by the presence of Bart hemoglobin on newborn screening.
‡Usually normochromic; 25% of cases are microcytic.
§Red blood cell distribution width quantitates the degree of anisocytosis (different sizes) of red blood cells.

should have a diet enriched with iron-containing foods. A vitamin with iron may also be used.

Thalassemia Minor

Etiology and Epidemiology

α-Thalassemia and β-thalassemia minor are common causes of microcytosis, either with or without a mild hypochromic, microcytic anemia. They are prevalent in certain ethnic groups (e.g., Mediterranean, Southeast Asian, African). Individuals of Asian descent are at risk of having three or four α genes deleted, resulting in hemoglobin H disease (β_4 tetramers) or hydrops fetalis. Bart (γ_4 tetramers) hemoglobin may present on the newborn screen with either α-thalassemia state (Table 151.5 and Fig. 151.3).

Laboratory Testing

The thalassemia minor syndromes (i.e., α-thalassemia trait, β-thalassemia trait) are characterized by a mild hypochromic, microcytic anemia with a low absolute reticulocyte count (see Table 151.5), due at least in part to ineffective erythropoiesis. The RBC count is usually elevated. As a result, if the mean corpuscular volume (MCV) divided by the RBC count is less than 12.5 **(Mentzer index)**, the diagnosis is suggestive of thalassemia trait. The blood smear reveals only microcytosis with α-thalassemia minor. Outside the neonatal period, when Bart hemoglobin is no longer detectable, the hemoglobin electrophoresis is usually normal in α-thalassemia minor (see Fig. 151.3). Blood smears of patients with β-thalassemia minor also reveal microcytic RBCs. In addition, target cells and basophilic stippled RBCs, caused by precipitation of alpha chain tetramers, may also be present. The diagnosis of β-thalassemia minor is based on an elevation of hemoglobin A_2 and F levels. Molecular testing is indicated for identification of more severe or unusual variants.

Treatment

No treatment is required for children with thalassemia minor. Children with more severe forms of thalassemia, such as β-thalassemia intermedia or major, or children with hemoglobin H disease (β_4 tetramers) with the Constant Spring variant, may require chronic transfusion therapy (see Table 151.5).

Lead Poisoning

Lead poisoning is associated with a hypochromic, microcytic anemia because most patients have concomitant iron deficiency due to competition for uptake between these two divalent cations. The history of living in an older home (built before 1980) with chipped paint or lead dust should raise suspicion of lead poisoning, especially in a child with **pica**. The lead content of water should also be assessed due to the potential for lead-containing pipes. **Basophilic stippling** on the blood smear is common. Lead intoxication rarely causes hemolytic anemia. Detection by routine screening at health

TABLE 151.5 Thalassemia Syndromes

DISORDER	GENOTYPIC ABNORMALITY	CLINICAL PHENOTYPE
β-THALASSEMIA		
Thalassemia major (Cooley anemia)	Homozygous β^0-thalassemia	Severe hemolysis, ineffective erythropoiesis, transfusion dependency, hepatosplenomegaly, iron overload
Thalassemia intermedia	Compound heterozygous β^0- and β^+-thalassemia	Moderate hemolysis, splenomegaly, moderately severe anemia, but not transfusion-dependent; main life-threatening complication is iron overload
Thalassemia minor	Heterozygous β^0- or β^+-thalassemia	Microcytosis, mild anemia
α-THALASSEMIA		
Hydrops fetalis	– –/– –	Severe anemia, intrauterine anasarca from congestive heart failure; death in utero or at birth
Hemoglobin H	α –/– –	Microcytic anemia and mild hemolysis; not transfusion-dependent*
α-Thalassemia trait	αα/– – (α-thalassemia 1, *cis* deletion) *or* α –/α – (α-thalassemia 2, *trans* deletion)	Mild microcytic anemia
Silent carrier	α–/αα	Normal complete blood count

**The Constant Spring variant may require chronic transfusion.*
Modified from Wing E, Schiffman F, et al. Cecil Essentials of Medicine. *10th ed. Philadelphia: Saunders; 2022.*

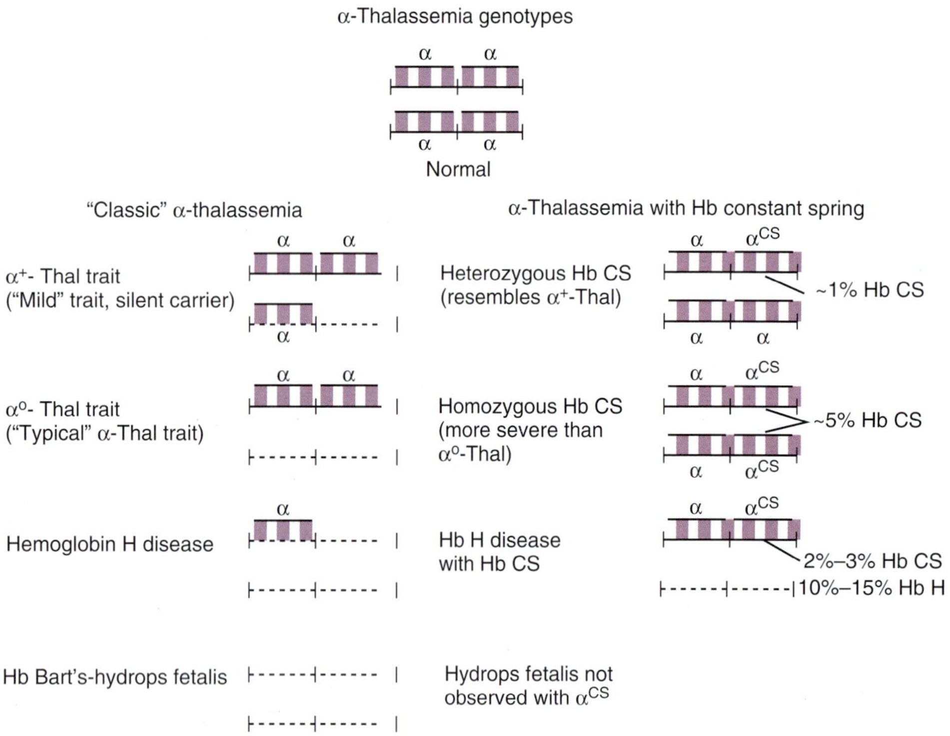

FIGURE 151.3 Genetic origins of the classic α-thalassemia syndromes due to gene deletions in the α-globin gene cluster. Hb CS is an α-globin chain variant synthesized in such small amounts (1–2% of normal) that it has the phenotypic impact of a severe nondeletion α-thalassemia allele; the α^{CS} allele is always linked to a functioning α-globin gene, so it has never been associated with hydrops fetalis. *Hb CS*, Hemoglobin Hb Constant Spring. (From Hoffman R, Benz EJ, Shattil SS, et al., eds. *Hematology: Basic Principles and Practice.* 5th ed. Philadelphia: Churchill Livingstone; 2008.)

care maintenance visits, removal from exposure, chelation therapy, and correction of iron deficiency are crucial to the neurologic development of affected children.

Normocytic Anemia

Etiology and Treatment

Anemia is commonly seen in chronic inflammatory disease. Hepcidin, a protein made in the liver, plays a key role in iron homeostasis. Inflammation causes an increase in the production of hepcidin, interrupting the process of iron release by macrophages and the absorption of iron from the intestines, leading to anemia. **Anemia of inflammation** may be normocytic or, less frequently, microcytic. This may pose a clinical challenge, when children with inflammatory disorders associated with blood loss (e.g., inflammatory bowel disease) exhibit a microcytic anemia. In these circumstances, only a bone marrow aspiration with staining of the sample for iron can differentiate the two entities definitively (see Table 151.4). Low ferritin levels indicate concurrent iron deficiency. A trial of iron therapy is not indicated without a specific diagnosis in children who appear to be systemically ill.

Bone marrow **infiltration by malignant cells** commonly leads to a normochromic, normocytic anemia. The mechanism by which neoplastic cells interfere with RBC and other marrow cell synthesis is multifactorial. The reticulocyte count is often low. Immature myeloid elements may be released into the peripheral blood because of the presence of the infiltrating tumor cells. An examination of the peripheral blood may reveal myelo- or lymphoblasts; when solid tumors metastasize to the marrow, these cells are seldom seen in the peripheral blood. Teardrop cells may be seen in the peripheral blood. A bone marrow examination is often necessary for further evaluation in the face of normochromic, normocytic anemia.

Congenital hypoplastic anemia (Diamond-Blackfan anemia [DBA]), a lifelong disorder, usually presents in the first few months of life or at birth with severe anemia and mild macrocytosis or normocytic anemia. DBA is due to a deficiency of bone marrow RBC precursors (Table 151.6). More than a third of patients have short stature. Many patients (50–66%) respond to corticosteroid treatment but must receive therapy indefinitely. Patients who do not respond to corticosteroid treatment are transfusion-dependent; they are at risk of multiple potential complications of long-term transfusion therapy, especially iron overload. These patients have a higher rate of developing leukemia or other hematologic malignancies than the general population.

In contrast to the congenital hypoplastic anemias, **transient erythroblastopenia of childhood (TEC)**, a normocytic anemia caused by suppression of RBC synthesis, appears between 6 months and 5 years of age in an otherwise well-appearing child (see Table 151.6). Viral infections are a presumed trigger, although the mechanism leading to RBC aplasia is poorly understood. The onset is gradual, but anemia may become severe. Transfusion of packed RBCs may be necessary if the anemia becomes symptomatic before recovery. Recovery is usually spontaneous. Mild neutropenia can be seen in patients with TEC; the well-appearing child with an otherwise normal physical exam helps differentiate from an underlying marrow infiltrative process. Differentiation from Diamond-Blackfan syndrome, in which erythroid precursors also are absent or diminished in the bone marrow, may be challenging.

Aplastic crises may complicate any chronic hemolytic anemia. Human parvovirus B19 (the cause of fifth disease) infects erythroid precursors and shuts down erythropoiesis. In children with chronic hemolytic anemia, these periods of severe reticulocytopenia can lead to an acute exacerbation of the anemia that may precipitate cardiovascular decompensation. Transient erythroid aplasia is without consequence in individuals with normal RBC survival. Recovery from parvovirus infection in hemolytic disease is spontaneous, but patients may need transfusion if the anemia is severe.

Macrocytic Anemia

See Figure 151.1.

Marrow Failure/Pancytopenia

Etiology

Pancytopenia is a simultaneous quantitative decrease in formed elements of the blood—erythrocytes, leukocytes, and platelets. Patients more often exhibit symptoms of infection or bleeding than anemia because of the relatively short life span of WBCs and platelets compared with the life span of RBCs. Causes of pancytopenia include failure of production (intrinsic bone marrow disease), sequestration (hypersplenism), and increased peripheral destruction.

Differential Diagnosis

Features that suggest **bone marrow failure** and mandate an examination of the bone marrow include a low reticulocyte count, teardrop forms of RBCs (implying marrow replacement, not just failure), presence of abnormal forms of leukocytes or myeloid elements more immature than band forms, small platelets, and an elevated MCV in the face of a low reticulocyte count. Pancytopenia resulting from bone marrow failure is usually a gradual process, starting with one or two cell lines but later involving all three cell lines. Features suggesting **increased destruction** include reticulocytosis, jaundice, immature erythroid or myeloid elements on the blood smear, large platelets, and increased serum bilirubin and lactate dehydrogenase.

Aplastic Anemia

Etiology and Epidemiology

In a child with aplastic anemia, pancytopenia evolves as the hematopoietic elements of the bone marrow disappear and the marrow is replaced by fat. Aplastic anemia is often idiopathic although the disorder may be induced by drugs (i.e., chloramphenicol, felbamate) or by toxins (i.e., benzene and pesticides). Infectious processes may also trigger aplastic anemia, particularly hepatitis and infectious mononucleosis (see Table 151.6). Immunosuppression of hematopoiesis is an important mechanism in patients with postinfectious and idiopathic aplastic anemia.

Laboratory Studies

A **bone marrow aspirate and biopsy** are crucial to determine cellularity or the extent of depletion of the hematopoietic elements.

Treatment

For severe aplastic anemia, the survival rate is 20% with supportive care alone; the duration of survival may be years when vigorous blood product and antibiotic support are provided. For children with severe aplastic anemia—defined by an absolute reticulocyte count less than 50,000/μL, absolute neutrophil count less than 500/mm^3, platelet count less than 20,000/mm^3, and bone marrow cellularity on biopsy specimen less than 25% of normal—the treatment of choice is **hematopoietic stem cell transplantation (HSCT)** from a sibling with identical human leukocyte antigen (HLA) and compatible mixed lymphocytes. When HSCT occurs before the recipient is sensitized to blood products, survival rate is greater than 80%. There are two major options for the treatment of aplastic anemia without an HLA-matched donor for HSCT: potent immunosuppressive therapy or unrelated or partially matched HSCT. Data regarding immunosuppressive therapy with antithymocyte globulin, cyclosporine or tacrolimus, and corticosteroids in combination with hematopoietic growth factors have been encouraging. Such therapy is often toxic, and relapses often occur when therapy is stopped.

Fanconi Anemia

Etiology and Epidemiology

Fanconi anemia is a constitutional form of aplastic anemia that usually presents in the latter half of the first decade of life and may evolve over years. A group of pathogenic variants (>20 genes recognized) in proteins involved in **DNA repair** have been identified in Fanconi anemia, which is inherited in an autosomal recessive manner. The diagnosis is based on demonstration of increased chromosomal breakage after exposure to agents that damage DNA. The repair mechanism for DNA damage is abnormal in all cells in Fanconi anemia, which may contribute to the increased risk of malignancies. Acute leukemia develops in 10% of cases. Other malignancies that can occur include solid tumors of the head and neck, gastrointestinal tumors, and gynecologic tumors.

Clinical Manifestations

Patients with Fanconi anemia have numerous characteristic clinical findings (see Table 151.6).

Treatment

HSCT can cure the pancytopenia caused by bone marrow aplasia. Many patients with Fanconi anemia and approximately 20% of children with aplastic anemia may respond for a time to **androgenic therapy**, which induces masculinization and may cause liver injury and liver tumors. Androgenic therapy increases RBC synthesis and can diminish transfusion requirements. The effect on granulocytes, and especially the platelet count, is less impressive.

Other less common etiologies of familial bone marrow failure resulting in pancytopenia are outlined in Table 151.6. These include dyskeratosis congenita and familial hemophagocytic lymphohistiocytosis.

TABLE **151.6** Differentiation of Red Blood Cell Aplasias and Pancytopenia

DISORDER	AGE AT ONSET	CHARACTERISTICS	TREATMENT
CONGENITAL			
Diamond-Blackfan syndrome (congenital hypoplastic anemia)	Newborn–1 mo; 90% of patients are <1 yr of age	Pure red blood cell aplasia, autosomal recessive trait, elevated fetal hemoglobin, fetal i antigen present, macrocytic, short stature, webbed neck, cleft lip, triphalangeal thumb; late-onset leukemia, pathogenic variant analysis	Prednisone, transfusion, hematopoietic stem cell transplant
ACQUIRED			
TEC	6 mo–5 yr of age; 85% of patients are >1 yr of age	Pure red blood cell defect; no anomalies, fetal hemoglobin, or i antigen; spontaneous recovery, normal MCV	Expectant transfusion for symptomatic anemia
Idiopathic aplastic anemia (status posthepatitis, drugs, unknown)	All ages	All cell lines involved; exposure to felbamate, chloramphenicol, radiation	Hematopoietic stem cell transplantation, antithymocyte globulin, cyclosporine, androgens
FAMILIAL			
Fanconi anemia	Usually before 10 yr of age; mean is 8 yr	All cell lines; microcephaly, absent thumbs, café-au-lait spots, cutaneous hyperpigmentation, short stature; chromosomal breaks, high MCV and hemoglobin F; horseshoe or absent kidney; leukemic transformation; autosomal recessive trait	Androgens, corticosteroids, hematopoietic stem cell transplantation
Paroxysmal nocturnal hemoglobinuria	After 5 yr	Initial hemolysis followed by aplastic anemia; increased complement-mediated hemolysis; thrombosis; iron deficiency; CD59 low	Iron, hematopoietic stem cell transplantation, androgens, steroids, eculizumab
Dyskeratosis congenita	Mean is 10 yr for skin; mean is 17 yr for anemia	Pancytopenia; hyperpigmentation, dystrophic nails, leukoplakia; X-linked recessive; lacrimal duct stenosis; high MCV and fetal hemoglobin	Androgens, splenectomy, hematopoietic stem cell transplantation
Familial hemophagocytic lymphohistiocytosis	Before 2 yr	Pancytopenia; fever, hepatosplenomegaly, hypertriglyceridemia, CSF pleocytosis	Transfusion; often lethal; etoposide, dexamethasone, emapalumab, hematopoietic stem cell transplantation, IVIG, cyclosporine
INFECTIOUS			
Parvovirus	Any age	Any chronic hemolytic anemia (i.e., sickle cell); new-onset reticulocytopenia and severe anemia	Red blood cell transfusion
EBV	Any age; usually <5 yr of age	X-linked immunodeficiency syndrome, pancytopenia	Transfusion, bone marrow transplantation
Virus-associated hemophagocytic syndrome (CMV, HHV-6, EBV)	Any age	Pancytopenia; hemophagocytosis in marrow, fever, hepatosplenomegaly	Transfusion, antiviral therapy, IVIG

CMV, Cytomegalovirus; *CSF*, cerebrospinal fluid; *EBV*, Epstein-Barr virus; *HHV-6*, human herpesvirus 6; *IVIG*, intravenous immunoglobulin; *MCV*, mean corpuscular volume; *TEC*, transient erythroblastopenia of childhood.

Marrow Replacement

Marrow replacement may occur because of **leukemia**, **solid tumors** (especially neuroblastoma), **storage diseases**, **osteopetrosis** in infants, and **myelofibrosis**, which is rare in childhood. The mechanisms by which malignant cells impair marrow synthesis of normal hematopoietic elements are complex. Bone marrow aspirate and biopsy are needed for precise diagnosis of the etiology of marrow synthetic failure.

Pancytopenia Resulting From Destruction of Cells

Pancytopenia resulting from destruction of cells may be caused by **intramedullary destruction** of hematopoietic elements (e.g., myeloproliferative disorders, deficiencies of folic acid and vitamin B_{12}) or by the **peripheral destruction** of mature cells. The most common site of peripheral destruction of blood cells is the spleen; the liver and other parts of the reticuloendothelial system may contribute. **Hypersplenism** may be the result of anatomic causes (portal hypertension or splenic hypertrophy from thalassemia), infections (including malaria or Epstein-Barr virus [EBV]), storage diseases (Gaucher disease), or malignancy (lymphomas, histiocytosis). Splenectomy is indicated only when the pancytopenia is of clinical significance.

Hemolytic Anemias

Major Hemoglobinopathies

Alpha Chain Hemoglobinopathies

Etiology. Alpha chains are needed for fetal erythropoiesis and production of hemoglobin F ($\alpha_2\gamma_2$), which results in **alpha chain hemoglobinopathies** being present in utero. Four alpha genes are present on the two number 16 chromosomes (see Fig. 151.3 and Table 151.5). Single gene deletions produce no disorder (silent carrier state) but can be detected by measuring the rates of α and β synthesis or by using molecular biologic techniques. Deletion of two genes produces **α-thalassemia minor** with mild or no anemia and microcytosis. In individuals of African origin, the gene deletions occur on different chromosomes *(trans)*. Thus, infants born to parents that both have α-thalassemia gene deletions in *trans* have a benign disorder. In the Asian population, deletions may occur on the same chromosome *(cis)*. Thus, infants born to parents who both have α-thalassemia gene deletions in *cis* may inherit two number 16 chromosomes lacking three or even four genes, resulting in severe disease. Deletion of three genes produces moderate hemolytic anemia with γ_4 tetramers **(Bart hemoglobin)** in the fetus and β_4 tetramers **(hemoglobin H)** in older children and adults (see Table 151.5). Deletion of all four α genes leads to hydrops fetalis, severe intrauterine anemia, and death, unless intrauterine transfusions are administered.

Beta Chain Hemoglobinopathies

Beta chain hemoglobinopathies are more prevalent in the United States than alpha chain disorders. The major beta hemoglobinopathies include those that alter hemoglobin function (e.g., **hemoglobin S, C, E, and D**) and those that alter beta chain production (e.g., **β-thalassemias**). As each RBC has two copies of chromosome 11 and they express both β-globin genes, most disorders of beta chains are not clinically severe, unless both beta chains are abnormal. By convention, when describing β-thalassemia genes, β^0 indicates a thalassemic gene resulting in absent beta chain synthesis; β^+ indicates a thalassemic gene that permits reduced but not absent synthesis of normal β chains. Disorders of the beta chain usually manifest themselves clinically between 4–12 months of age when fetal hemoglobin nadirs, unless they have been detected prenatally or by cord blood screening.

β-Thalassemia Major (Cooley Anemia)

Etiology and Epidemiology

β-Thalassemia major is caused by pathogenic variants in the *HBB* gene that impair **beta chain synthesis**. Due to the unbalanced synthesis of alpha and beta chains, alpha chains precipitate within the cells, resulting in RBC destruction either in the bone marrow or in the spleen. β-Thalassemia major is most commonly seen in individuals of Mediterranean or Asian descent. The clinical severity of the illness varies based on the specific molecular variant (see Table 151.5).

Clinical Manifestations

Signs and symptoms of β-thalassemia major result from the combination of chronic hemolytic anemia, decreased or absent production of normal hemoglobin A, and ineffective erythropoiesis. The anemia is severe and leads to growth failure and high-output heart failure. **Ineffective erythropoiesis** causes increased expenditure of energy and expansion of the bone marrow cavities of all bones, leading to osteopenia, pathologic fractures, extramedullary erythropoiesis with resultant hepatosplenomegaly, and an increase in the rate of iron absorption.

Treatment

Treatment of β-thalassemia major is based on a **hypertransfusion program** that corrects the anemia and suppresses the patient's own ineffective erythropoiesis, limiting the stimulus for increased iron absorption. This suppression permits the bones to heal, decreases metabolic expenditures, increases growth, and limits dietary iron absorption. Splenectomy may reduce the transfusion volume but adds to the risk of serious infection. **Chelation therapy** with deferasirox or deferoxamine should start when laboratory evidence of iron overload **(hemochromatosis)** is present and before there are clinical signs of iron overload (nonimmune diabetes mellitus, cirrhosis, heart failure, bronzing of the skin, and multiple endocrine abnormalities). HSCT in childhood, before organ dysfunction is induced by iron overload, has good success in β-thalassemia major and is the treatment of choice. There are also Food and Drug Administration–approved gene therapies for transfusion-dependent β-thalassemia. Beti-cel utilizes a lentiviral vector to carry a modified β-globin gene and is approved for age 4 years and older. Exagamglogene autotemcel utilizes genome editing technology, CRISPR/Cas9, to modify patients' stem cells to cut DNA in targeted areas and is approved in patients aged 12 years and older. In clinical trials, both products have resulted in transfusion-independence post-treatment.

Sickle Cell Disease

Etiology and Epidemiology

Sickle cell syndromes include **hemoglobin SS disease**, **hemoglobin SC disease**, **hemoglobin S-β^0-thalassemia**, **hemoglobin S-β^+-thalassemia**, and other rare variants (Table 151.7). The specific hemoglobin genotype must be identified because the clinical complications differ in frequency, type, and severity. As a result of a single **amino acid substitution** (valine for

TABLE 151.7 Comparison of Sickle Cell Syndromes

		PERCENT HEMOGLOBIN					
GENOTYPE	CLINICAL CONDITION	HB A	HB S	HB A_2	HB F	HB C	OTHER FINDING(S)
SA	Sickle cell trait	55–60	40–45	2–3	–	–	Usually asymptomatic
SS	Sickle cell anemia	0	85–95	2–3	5–15	–	Clinically severe anemia; Hb F heterogeneous in distribution
S-β^0 thalassemia	Sickle cell β^0-thalassemia	0	70–80	3–5	10–20	–	Moderately severe anemia; splenomegaly in 50%; smear: hypochromic, microcytic anemia
S-β^+ thalassemia	Sickle cell β^+-thalassemia	10–20	60–75	3–5	10–20	–	Hb F distributed heterogeneously; mild microcytic anemia
SC	Hb SC disease	0	45–50	–	–	45–50	Moderately severe anemia; splenomegaly; retinopathy; target cells
S-HPFH	Sickle-hereditary persistence of Hb F	0	70–80	1–2	20–30	–	Often asymptomatic; Hb F is uniformly distributed

From Andreoli T, Carpenter C, Griggs R, et al. Cecil Essentials of Medicine. *7th ed. Philadelphia: Saunders; 2007.*

glutamic acid at the β6 position), sickle hemoglobin crystallizes and forms a gel in the deoxygenated state. When reoxygenated, the sickle hemoglobin is normally soluble. The so-called *reversible sickle cell* can enter the microcirculation. As the oxygen is extracted and saturation declines, sickling may occur, occluding the microvasculature. The surrounding tissue undergoes infarction, inducing pain and chronic organ dysfunction. This sickling phenomenon is exacerbated by hypoxia, acidosis, fever, hypothermia, and dehydration.

Clinical Manifestations and Treatment

A child with sickle cell disease is vulnerable to **life-threatening infection** by 4 months of age due to splenic dysfunction. **Splenic dysfunction** is caused by sickling of the RBCs within the spleen, resulting in an inability to filter microorganisms from the bloodstream. Splenic dysfunction is followed, eventually, by **splenic infarction**, usually by 2–4 years of age. The loss of normal splenic function makes the patient susceptible to overwhelming infection by encapsulated organisms, especially *Streptococcus pneumoniae* and other pathogens (Table 151.8). The hallmark of infection is fever. A febrile child with sickle cell disease (temperature >38.5°C) must be evaluated immediately (see Chapter 97). Current precautions to prevent infections include prophylactic daily oral penicillin begun at diagnosis and vaccinations against pneumococcus, *Haemophilus influenzae* type b, meningococcus, hepatitis B virus, and influenza virus.

The anemia of hemoglobin SS disease is usually a chronic, moderate-to-severe hemolytic anemia that is not routinely transfusion-dependent. The severity depends in part on the patient's genotype. Manifestations of chronic anemia include jaundice, pallor, variable splenomegaly in infancy, a cardiac flow murmur, and delayed growth and sexual maturation. Decisions about transfusion should be made based on the patient's clinical condition, the hemoglobin level, and the reticulocyte count.

Sickle cell disease is complicated by sudden, sometimes life-threatening events caused by the acute intravascular sickling of the RBCs, with resultant pain or organ dysfunction (i.e., **crisis**). In two different clinical situations, an acute, potentially life-threatening decline in the hemoglobin level may be superimposed on the chronic compensated anemia. **Splenic sequestration crisis** is a life-threatening, hyperacute drop in the hemoglobin level (blood volume) secondary to splenic pooling of the patient's RBCs and sickling within the spleen. The spleen is moderately to markedly enlarged, and the reticulocyte count is elevated. In an **aplastic crisis**, parvovirus B19 infects RBC precursors in the bone marrow and induces transient RBC aplasia with reticulocytopenia and a rapid worsening of anemia because of the very short life span of sickle RBCs. Simple transfusion therapy is indicated for sequestration and aplastic crises when the anemia is symptomatic.

Acute vaso-occlusive events may occur in any organ of the body and manifest as pain and/or significant dysfunction (see Table 151.8). **Acute chest syndrome (ACS)** is a vaso-occlusive event within the lungs with evidence of a new infiltrate on chest radiograph. ACS is often associated with infection and infarction. Patients with ACS may first complain of chest pain but within a few hours develop cough, increasing respiratory and heart rates, hypoxia, and progressive respiratory distress. Physical examination reveals areas of decreased breath sounds and dullness on chest percussion. Treatment involves early recognition and prevention of arterial hypoxemia. Oxygen, fluids, judicious use of analgesic medications, antibiotics, bronchodilators, and RBC transfusion (rarely exchange transfusion) are indicated as treatment. *Incentive spirometry* may help reduce the incidence of ACS in patients presenting with pain in the chest or abdomen.

Acute painful events are the most common type of vaso-occlusive events. Pain usually localizes to the long bones of the arms or legs but may occur in smaller bones of the hands or feet in infancy **(dactylitis)**, ribs, or in the abdomen. Painful events usually last 2–7 days. Repeated painful events within the femur may lead to *avascular necrosis of the femoral head* and chronic hip disease. Treatment of painful events includes analgesia (usually opioids and nonsteroidal antiinflammatory drugs) and supplemental oxygen if the patient is hypoxic. Appropriate use of analgesics is imperative to control pain. Patients with sickle cell disease often require high doses of opioids due to tolerance to provide adequate pain control. The frequency of acute painful events increases with age. In addition, chronic daily pain irrespective of an acute vaso-occlusive event is associated with increasing age, occurring in 30–40% of patients. Chronic nervous system sensitization is likely a

TABLE 151.8 Clinical Manifestations of Sickle Cell Disease*

MANIFESTATION	COMMENTS
Anemia	Chronic, onset 3–4 mo of age; hemoglobin usually 6–10 g/dL
Aplastic crisis	Parvovirus infection, reticulocytopenia; acute and reversible; may need transfusion
Sequestration crisis	Massive splenomegaly (may involve liver), shock; treat with transfusion
Hemolytic crisis	May be associated with G6PD deficiency
Dactylitis	Hand-foot swelling in early infancy
Pain	Microvascular painful vaso-occlusive infarcts of muscle, bone, bone marrow, lung, intestines; chronic pain (nervous system sensitization)
Cerebrovascular accidents (overt and silent)	Large and small vessel occlusion leading to thrombosis (stroke); secondary prevention with chronic transfusions; at risk of neurocognitive deficits
Acute chest syndrome	Infection, asthma, atelectasis, infarction, fat emboli, severe hypoxemia, infiltrate, dyspnea, absent breath sounds; treated with transfusions, antibiotics, oxygen, bronchodilators
Chronic lung disease	Pulmonary fibrosis, restrictive lung disease, cor pulmonale, pulmonary hypertension
Priapism	Causes eventual erectile dysfunction; treated with transfusion, oxygen, or corpora cavernosa-to-spongiosa shunt
Ocular	Retinopathy
Gallbladder disease	Bilirubin stones; cholecystitis
Kidney	Hematuria, papillary necrosis, hyposthenuria; nephropathy
Cardiomyopathy	Heart failure
Skeletal	Osteonecrosis (avascular) most commonly of the femoral or humeral head
Infections	Functional asplenia, defects in properdin system; pneumococcal bacteremia, meningitis, and arthritis; deafness from meningitis; *Salmonella* and *Staphylococcus aureus* osteomyelitis; severe *Mycoplasma* pneumonia
Growth failure, delayed puberty	May respond to nutritional supplements
Mental health conditions	Depression, anxiety

**Clinical manifestations with sickle cell trait are unusual but include renal papillary necrosis (hematuria), sudden death on exertion, intraocular hyphema extension, and sickling in unpressurized airplanes.*
G6PD, Glucose-6-phosphate dehydrogenase.

key driver of the chronic pain seen in patients with sickle cell disease.

Priapism occurs in males, usually when they are older than 6 years of age. The child experiences a sudden, painful onset of a tumescent penis that will not relax. Therapeutic steps for priapism include the administration of oxygen, fluids, analgesia, and transfusion when appropriate to achieve a hemoglobin S less than 30%. Urgent partial exchange transfusion is often required to lower the hemoglobin S. Prompt consultation with urology is recommended.

Stroke occurs in approximately 8–10% of patients with hemoglobin SS/hemoglobin S-β^0-thalassemia disease. Stroke events can present with the sudden onset of an altered state of consciousness, seizures, or focal paralysis. **Silent stroke**, which is defined as evidence of cerebral infarction on imaging studies but a normal neurologic examination, occurs in approximately 20% of patients with hemoglobin SS/hemoglobin S-β^0-thalassemia disease. Neurocognitive changes, such as a significant change in school performance or behavior, are associated with silent stroke, and those with silent stroke are at increased risk for development of overt stroke. Children with hemoglobin SS/hemoglobin S-β^0-thalassemia disease ages 2–16 years should be screened for increased risk of stroke using transcranial Doppler (TCD). Chronic monthly transfusions are indicated in those with overt stroke, silent stroke, and/or abnormal TCDs.

Laboratory Diagnosis

The diagnosis of hemoglobinopathies is made by identifying the precise amount and type of hemoglobin using **hemoglobin electrophoresis**, **isoelectric focusing**, or **high-performance liquid chromatography**. Every member of an at-risk population should have a precise hemoglobin phenotype performed at birth (preferably) or during early infancy. All U.S. states perform newborn screening for sickle cell disease.

Treatment

Disease-modifying therapy for sickle cell disease is evolving. Data support the use of chronic RBC transfusions in children who have had an overt or silent stroke or abnormal TCD. Chronic RBC transfusions can also be used successfully for short time periods to prevent recurrent vaso-occlusive events, including pain, acute chest syndrome, and priapism. **Hydroxyurea**, which increases hemoglobin F, decreases the number and severity of painful events, frequency of ACS, and need for transfusions in children as young as 1 year of age. Clinical care guidelines from the National Institutes of Health/National Heart, Lung, and Blood Institute for patients with sickle cell disease recommend hydroxyurea should be initiated in asymptomatic children with severe sickle cell disease (HbSS or HbS-β^0-thalassemia). Disease-modifying drugs approved by the Food and Drug Administration for the treatment of sickle cell disease include crizanlizumab and L-glutamine. HSCT using a matched sibling donor can be curative for children with sickle cell disease. HSCT using alternative donors for children, without a suitable sibling match, is also available as a curative therapy for patients with severe sickle cell disease. Two gene therapies have been approved by the Food and Drug Administration to treat sickle cell disease. Exagamglogene autotemcel utilizes genome editing technology, and CRISPR/Cas9 modifies patients' stem cells to cut DNA in targeted areas. Lovotibeglogene autotemcel utilizes a lentiviral vector to deliver genetic modification. Both products are made from the patient's own stem cells, eliminating the need for a donor as with HSCT, and they are considered transformative therapies for sickle cell disease. Supportive care for the treatment of end-organ complications (e.g., cardiopulmonary, kidney) is vital to decrease morbidity.

Enzymopathies

Etiology

G6PD deficiency is an abnormality in the **hexose monophosphate shunt pathway** of glycolysis that results in the depletion of reduced nicotinamide adenine dinucleotide phosphate (NADPH) and the inability to regenerate reduced glutathione. When a patient with G6PD deficiency is exposed to significant oxidant stress, hemoglobin is oxidized, forming precipitates of sulfhemoglobin **(Heinz bodies)**, which are visible on specially stained preparations.

The severity of hemolysis depends on the enzyme variant. In many G6PD deficiencies, the enzymes become unstable with aging of the RBC and cannot be replaced because the cell is anucleated. Older cells are most susceptible to oxidant-induced hemolysis. In other variants, the enzyme is kinetically abnormal.

Epidemiology

The most common variants of G6PD deficiency have been found in areas where malaria is endemic. G6PD deficiency protects against parasitism of the erythrocyte. The most common variant with normal activity is **type B**, which is defined by its electrophoretic mobility. The approximate gene frequencies in Black patients are 70% type B, 20% type A, and 10% type A−. Only the **A− variant**, termed the *African variant*, is unstable. Ten percent of Black males are affected. A group of variants found in people of Sardinian, Sicilian, Greek, Sephardic and Oriental Jewish, and Arab descent is termed the **Mediterranean variant** and is associated with chronic hemolysis and potentially life-threatening hemolytic disease. Because the gene for G6PD deficiency is carried on the X chromosome, clinical hemolysis is most common in males. Heterozygous females who have randomly inactivated a higher percentage of X chromosomes with the normal gene may become symptomatic, as may homozygous females with the A− variant (0.5–1% of females of African descent).

Clinical Manifestations

G6PD deficiency has two common presentations. Individuals with the A− variant have normal hemoglobin values when well but develop an **acute episode of hemolysis** triggered by serious (bacterial) infection or ingestion of an oxidant drug. The RBC morphology during episodes of acute hemolysis is striking, appearing to have "bites" taken out of them *(cookie cells)*. These are areas of absent hemoglobin that are produced by phagocytosis of Heinz bodies by splenic macrophages; as a result, the RBCs appear blistered. Clinically evident jaundice, dark urine resulting from bilirubin pigments, hemoglobinuria when hemolysis is intravascular, and decreased haptoglobin levels are common during hemolytic episodes. Early on, the hemolysis usually exceeds the ability of the bone marrow to compensate, so the reticulocyte count may be low for 3–4 days.

Laboratory Studies

The diagnosis of G6PD deficiency is based on decreased NADPH formation. G6PD levels during an acute, severe hemolytic episode may be normal because the most deficient cells have been destroyed and reticulocytes are enriched with G6PD. Repeating testing at a later time when the patient is in a steady-state condition, testing the mothers of males with suspected G6PD deficiency, or performing electrophoresis to identify the precise variant present aids in diagnosis.

Treatment and Prevention

The treatment of G6PD deficiency is supportive. Transfusions are indicated when significant anemia associated with cardiovascular compromise is present. Maintaining hydration and urine alkalization protects the kidneys against damage from precipitated free hemoglobin. Hemolysis is prevented by avoidance of known oxidants, particularly long-acting sulfonamides, nitrofurantoin, primaquine, dimercaprol, and moth balls (naphthalene). Fava beans (favism) have triggered hemolysis, particularly in patients with the Mediterranean variant. Serious infection also is a potential precipitant of hemolysis in G6PD-deficient young children.

Pyruvate kinase deficiency is much less common than G6PD deficiency and represents a clinical spectrum of disorders caused by the functional deficiency of pyruvate kinase. Some individuals have a true deficiency state, and others have abnormal enzyme kinetics. The metabolic consequence of pyruvate kinase deficiency is adenosine triphosphate depletion, impairing RBC survival. Pyruvate kinase deficiency is usually an autosomal disorder due to a pathogenic variant in the *PKLR* gene, and most children who are affected are double heterozygotes for two abnormal enzymes. Hemolysis is not aggravated by oxidant stress due to the profound reticulocytosis in this condition. Aplastic crises can be life threatening. The spleen is the site for RBC removal in pyruvate kinase deficiency. Most patients have amelioration of the anemia and a reduction of transfusion requirements after splenectomy.

Membrane Disorders

Etiology

The biochemical basis of **hereditary spherocytosis** and **hereditary elliptocytosis** is similar. Both conditions have a defect in the protein lattice (spectrin, ankyrin, protein 4.2, band 3) that underlies the RBC lipid bilayer and provides stability for the membrane shape. In hereditary spherocytosis, pieces of membrane bud off as microvesicles because of abnormal vertical interaction of the cytoskeletal proteins and uncoupling of the lipid bilayer from the cytoskeleton. When the RBC loses membrane, cell shape changes from a biconcave disk to a spherocyte. This shape is less deformable when passing through narrow passages in the spleen. Hereditary elliptocytosis is a disorder of spectrin dimer interactions that occurs primarily in individuals of African descent. The transmission of hereditary spherocytosis can be autosomal dominant, autosomal recessive, or occur through a spontaneous pathogenic variant. **Hereditary pyropoikilocytosis** (unusual instability of the erythrocytes when they are exposed to heat at 45°C) is the result of a structural abnormality of spectrin.

Clinical Manifestations

Hereditary spherocytosis varies greatly in clinical severity, ranging from an asymptomatic, well-compensated, mild hemolytic anemia that may be discovered incidentally to a severe hemolytic anemia with growth failure, splenomegaly, and chronic transfusion requirements in infancy necessitating early splenectomy. The most common variant of hereditary elliptocytosis is a clinically insignificant morphologic abnormality without shortened RBC survival. The less common variant is associated with spherocytes, ovalocytes, and elliptocytes with a moderate, usually compensated, hemolysis. Far more significant hemolysis occurs in hereditary pyropoikilocytosis. The peripheral blood smear in hereditary pyropoikilocytosis often includes elliptocytes, spherocytes, fragmented RBCs, and striking microcytosis. Such patients may have unique blood smears in the newborn period with small, fragmented RBCs.

Laboratory Diagnosis

The clinical diagnosis of hereditary spherocytosis should be suspected in patients with even a few spherocytes found on the blood smear because the spleen preferentially removes spherocytes. An incubated **osmotic fragility test** confirms the presence of spherocytes and increases the likelihood of the diagnosis. The osmotic fragility test result is abnormal in any hemolytic disease in which spherocytes are present (e.g., in antibody-mediated hemolysis). Further genetic testing (band 3 gene pathogenic variant) can confirm the diagnosis of hereditary spherocytosis.

Treatment

Splenectomy corrects the anemia and normalizes the RBC survival in patients with hereditary spherocytosis, but the morphologic abnormalities persist. Splenectomy should be reserved for children with severe hereditary spherocytosis causing chronic anemia or growth failure. Splenectomy should be deferred until age 5 years, if possible, to minimize the risk of overwhelming postsplenectomy sepsis and to maximize the antibody response to the polyvalent pneumococcal and meningococcal vaccine. Partial splenectomy should be considered to improve the hemolytic anemia and maintain splenic function in host defense.

Hemolytic Anemia Caused by Disorders Extrinsic to the Red Blood Cell

Etiology and Clinical Manifestations

Isoimmune hemolysis is caused by active maternal immunization against fetal antigens that the mother's erythrocytes do not express (see Chapter 61). Examples are antibodies to the A, B, and Rh D antigens; other Rh antigens; and the Kell, Duffy, and other blood groups. Anti-A and anti-B hemolysis are caused by the placental transfer of naturally occurring maternal antibodies from mothers who lack A or B antigen (usually blood type O). Positive results of the direct antiglobulin **(Coombs)** test on the infant's RBCs (Fig. 151.4), the indirect antiglobulin test on the mother's serum, and the presence of spherocytes and immature erythroid precursors (erythroblastosis) on the infant's blood smear confirm this diagnosis. Isoimmune hemolytic disease varies in clinical severity, ranging from infants being asymptomatic to having jaundice, severe anemia, and/or hydrops fetalis.

Autoimmune hemolytic anemia is usually an acute, self-limited Coombs-positive process that develops after an infection (e.g., *Mycoplasma*, EBV, or other viral infections) due to the production of autoantibodies that cause red cell destruction. Autoimmune hemolytic anemia may also be the presenting symptom of a chronic autoimmune disease (e.g., systemic lupus erythematosus, lymphoproliferative disorders, or immunodeficiency). Drugs may induce a Coombs-positive hemolytic anemia by forming a hapten on the RBC membrane (penicillin) or by forming immune complexes (quinidine) that attach to the RBC membrane. Antibodies then activate complement-induced intravascular hemolysis. The third type of drug-induced immune hemolysis occurs during treatment with α-methyldopa and a few other drugs. In this type, prolonged drug exposure alters the RBC membrane, inducing neoantigen formation. Antibodies are produced that bind to the neoantigen; this produces a positive antiglobulin test result far more commonly than it induces hemolysis. In each of these conditions, the erythrocyte is an *innocent bystander*.

A second form of acquired hemolytic disease is caused by mechanical damage to the RBC membrane during circulation. In **thrombotic microangiopathy**, the RBCs are trapped by fibrin strands in the circulation and physically broken by shear stress as they pass through these strands. Hemolytic uremic syndrome, disseminated intravascular coagulation (DIC), thrombotic thrombocytopenic purpura, malignant hypertension, toxemia, and hyperacute kidney graft rejection can produce thrombotic microangiopathy. The platelets are usually large, indicating that they are young, but have a decreased survival, even if the numbers are normal. Consumption of clotting factors is more prominent in DIC than in the other forms of thrombotic microangiopathy. The smear shows RBC fragments (schistocytes), microspherocytes, teardrop forms, and polychromasia. Other examples of mechanical injury to RBCs include damage by exposure to nonendothelialized surfaces (as in artificial heart valves) and damage because of high flow and shear rates in giant hemangiomas **(Kasabach-Merritt syndrome)**.

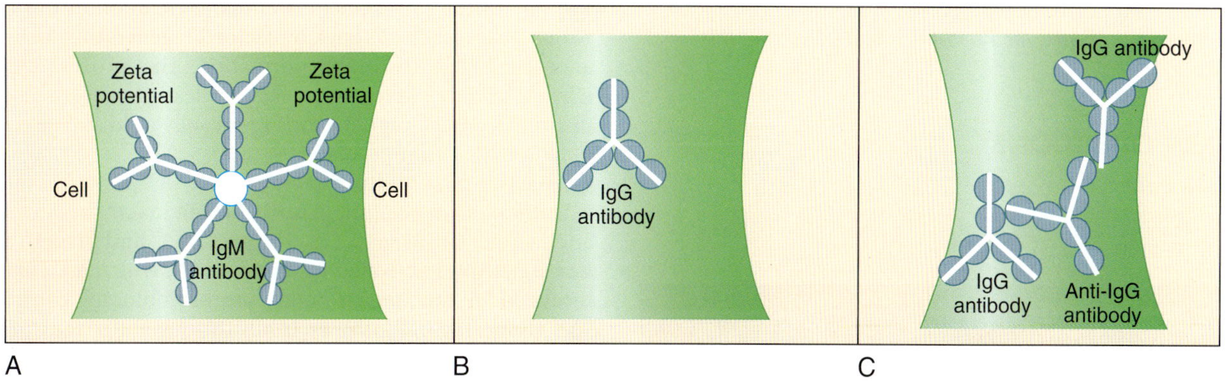

FIGURE 151.4 Coombs or DAT. In the DAT, so-called *Coombs serum* that recognizes human Ig or C is used to detect the presence of antibody or C on the surface of the RBCs by agglutination. **(A)** An IgM antibody can bind two RBCs simultaneously because of its multiple antigen-binding sites. The great size of the IgM allows it to bridge the surface repulsive forces (zeta potential) between RBCs and cause agglutination. **(B)** An IgG antibody is too small to bridge the zeta potential and cause agglutination. **(C)** On the addition of Coombs serum, the zeta potential is bridged successfully, and RBCs agglutinate. *C*, Complement; *DAT*, direct antiglobulin test; *Ig*, immunoglobulin; *RBCs*, red blood cells. (Modified from Ware RE, Rosse WF. Autoimmune hemolytic anemia. In: Orkin SH, Nathan DG, Look AT, et al., eds. *Hematology of Infancy and Childhood*. 6th ed. Philadelphia: Saunders; 2003:530.)

Alterations in plasma lipids, especially cholesterol, may lead to damage to the RBC membrane and a shortened RBC survival. Lipids in the plasma are in equilibrium with lipids in the RBC membrane. High cholesterol levels increase the membrane cholesterol and the total membrane surface without affecting the volume of the cell. This condition produces **spur cells** that may be seen in abetalipoproteinemia and liver diseases. Hemolysis occurs in the spleen where poor RBC deformability results in erythrocyte destruction. **Circulating toxins** (e.g., snake venoms and heavy metals) that bind sulfhydryl groups may damage the RBC membrane and induce hemolysis. Irregularly spiculated RBCs (burr cells) are seen in kidney failure. **Vitamin E deficiency** can also cause an acquired hemolytic anemia because of abnormal sensitivity of membrane lipids to oxidant stress. Vitamin E deficiency may occur in premature infants who are not being supplemented with vitamin E or who have insufficient nutrition, in infants with severe malabsorption syndromes (including cystic fibrosis), and in infants with transfusional iron overload, which can lead to severe oxidant exposure.

Laboratory Diagnosis

The peripheral blood smear in autoimmune hemolytic anemia usually reveals spherocytes and occasionally nucleated RBCs. The reticulocyte count varies because some patients have relatively low reticulocyte counts due to autoantibodies that cross react with RBC precursors.

Treatment and Prognosis

Transfusion may be lifesaving in the management of autoimmune hemolytic anemia. Cross matching of RBCs in preparation for transfusion can be difficult because autoantibodies react with virtually all RBCs. In addition to **transfusion**, further management of autoimmune hemolytic anemia depends on antibody type. Acute management may involve administration of **corticosteroids** and, at times, **intravenous immunoglobulin**. Corticosteroids reduce the clearance of sensitized RBCs in the spleen. More than 80% of children with autoimmune hemolytic anemia recover spontaneously. In drug-induced hemolysis, withdrawal of the drug usually leads to resolution of the hemolytic process.

PEARLS FOR PRACTITIONERS

See Hematology: Pearls for Practitioners at the end of this section.

REVIEW QUESTIONS

Available online.

CHAPTER 152

Hemostatic Disorders

NORMAL HEMOSTASIS

Hemostasis is the dynamic process of **coagulation** as it occurs in areas of vascular injury, involving the carefully modulated interaction of platelets, the vascular wall, and procoagulant and anticoagulant proteins. After an injury to the vascular endothelium, subendothelial collagen induces a conformational change in **von Willebrand factor** (VWF), an adhesive protein to which platelets bind via their glycoprotein Ib receptor. After adhesion, platelets undergo activation and release various molecular contents, including adenosine diphosphate, from intracellular granules. These **activated platelets** subsequently induce aggregation of additional platelets. Simultaneously, tissue factor, collagen, and other matrix proteins in tissue activate the coagulation cascade, leading to the formation of the enzyme **thrombin** (Fig. 152.1). Thrombin causes further aggregation of platelets, a positive feedback activation of factors 5 and 8, the conversion of fibrinogen to fibrin, and the activation of factor 11. A **platelet plug** forms and bleeding ceases, usually within 3–7 minutes. This process of platelet plug formation is referred to as *primary hemostasis.* The generation of thrombin leads to formation of a more stable clot by the activation of factor 13, which cross-links fibrin, forming a stable thrombus. Finally, contractile elements within the platelet mediate **clot retraction**. The production and retraction of a thrombin clot is known as *secondary hemostasis.* Thrombin also contributes to the eventual limitation of clot size by binding to the protein thrombomodulin on intact endothelial cells, converting protein C into activated protein C, which binds to protein S to downregulate the activation of factors 5 and 8. Thrombin also contributes to the eventual lysis of the thrombus by activating plasminogen to plasmin. All the hemostatic processes are closely interwoven and occur on biologic surfaces that mediate coagulation by bringing the critical players (platelets, endothelial cells, and subendothelium) into close proximity with pro- and anticoagulant proteins.

Despite coagulation often being labeled as having **intrinsic and extrinsic pathways**, in reality these pathways are closely interactive and do not react independently (Fig. 152.2). For ease of use, all coagulation factors are denoted herein using Arabic rather than Roman numerals to prevent misreading factor VII (7) as factor VIII (8), and so forth. In vivo, factor 7 autocatalyzes to form small amounts of factor 7a. When tissue is injured, **tissue factor** is released and causes a burst of factor 7a generation. Tissue factor, in combination with calcium and factor 7a, activates factor 9 and factor 10. The activation of factor 9 by factor 7a results in eventual generation of thrombin, which positively feeds back on factor 11, generating factor 11a and accelerating thrombin formation. This process explains why deficiency of factor 8 or factor 9 leads to severe bleeding disorders; deficiency of factor 11 is usually mild and deficiency of factor 12 is asymptomatic.

A series of **inhibitory factors** serve to tightly regulate the activation of coagulation. **Antithrombin** inactivates thrombin and factors 9a, 10a, and 11a. The **protein C and protein S** system inactivates activated factors 5 and 8, which are cofactors localized in the "tenase" and "prothrombinase" complexes. The **tissue factor pathway inhibitor**, an anticoagulant protein, limits activation of the coagulation cascade by factor 7a and factor 10a. **Fibrinolysis** is initiated by the action of tissue plasminogen activator on plasminogen, producing plasmin, the active enzyme that degrades fibrin into split products. Fibrinolysis eventually dissolves the clot and allows normal flow to resume. Acquired or inherited deficiencies of anticoagulant proteins may predispose to thrombosis.

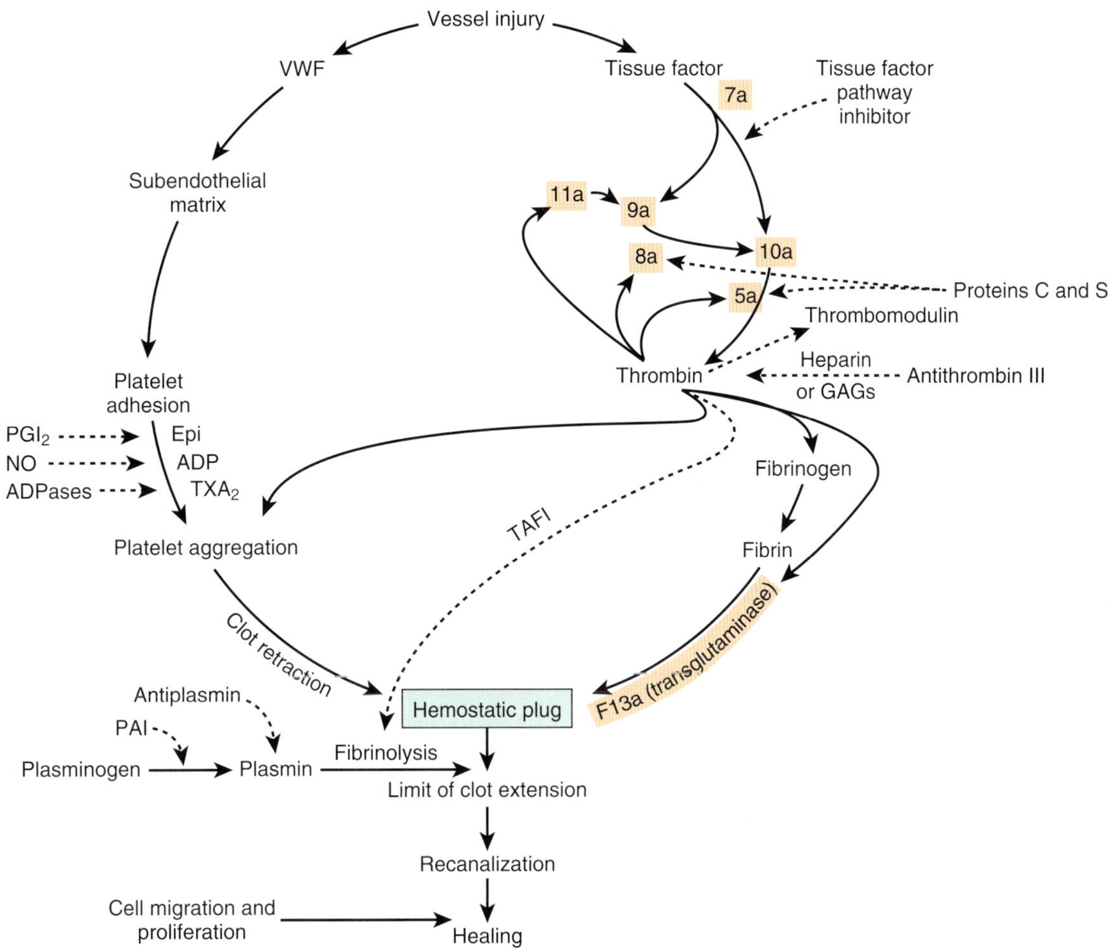

FIGURE 152.1 Diagram of the multiple interactions of the hemostatic mechanism. *Solid lines* indicate reactions that favor coagulation, and *dashed lines* indicate reactions that inhibit clotting. *Epi*, Epinephrine; *GAGs*, glycosaminoglycans; *NO*, nitric oxide; *PAI*, plasminogen activator inhibitor; *PGI2*, prostaglandin I_2 (prostacyclin); *TAFI*, thrombin-activated fibrinolytic inhibitor; *TXA2*, thromboxane A_2; *VWF*, von Willebrand factor. (Modified from Branchford BR, Samelson-Jones BJ, Raffini LJ, Flood VH. Hemostasis. In: Kliegman RM, St. Geme J, eds. *Nelson Textbook of Pediatrics*. 22nd ed. Philadelphia: Elsevier; 2024:Fig 524.2.)

DEVELOPMENTAL HEMOSTASIS

In the fetus, procoagulant factors such as fibrinogen, factor 5, factor 8, and platelets approach normal levels during the second trimester. Levels of other clotting factors and anticoagulant proteins increase gradually throughout gestation. The premature infant is simultaneously at increased risk of bleeding and clotting complications that are exacerbated by many of the medical interventions needed for care and monitoring, especially indwelling arterial or venous catheters. Children attain normal levels of procoagulant and anticoagulant proteins by 1 year of age, although levels of protein C may lag and normalize in adolescence.

HEMOSTATIC DISORDERS

Etiology and Epidemiology

A detailed **family history** is crucial to the diagnosis of bleeding and thrombotic disorders. **Hemophilia** is X linked, and most affected children are male. **von Willebrand disease** (VWD) usually is inherited in an autosomal dominant fashion. The causes of bleeding may be hematologic in origin or due to vascular, nonhematologic causes (Fig. 152.3). In the evaluation of thrombotic disorders, a personal or family history of blood clots in the legs or lungs, early-onset stroke, or myocardial infarction suggests a hereditary predisposition to thrombosis. Thrombotic disorders can be congenital or acquired (Table 152.1) and frequently present after an initial event (e.g., indwelling catheter, trauma, malignancy, infection, pregnancy, or treatment with estrogens) provides a nidus for clot formation or creates a procoagulant stimulus.

Clinical Manifestations

Patients with hemostatic disorders may have complaints of either bleeding or clotting. Age at onset of bleeding can provide clues to whether the problem is congenital or acquired. The **sites of bleeding** (mucocutaneous or muscle/joint) and **degree of trauma** (spontaneous or significant) required to induce injury can suggest the type and severity of the disorder. Certain medications (e.g., aspirin, valproic acid) are known to exacerbate preexisting bleeding disorders by interfering with platelet function.

The **physical examination** should characterize the presence of skin or mucous membrane bleeding and deeper sites of hemorrhage into the muscles and joints or internal bleeding sites. The term ***petechia*** refers to a nonblanching lesion less

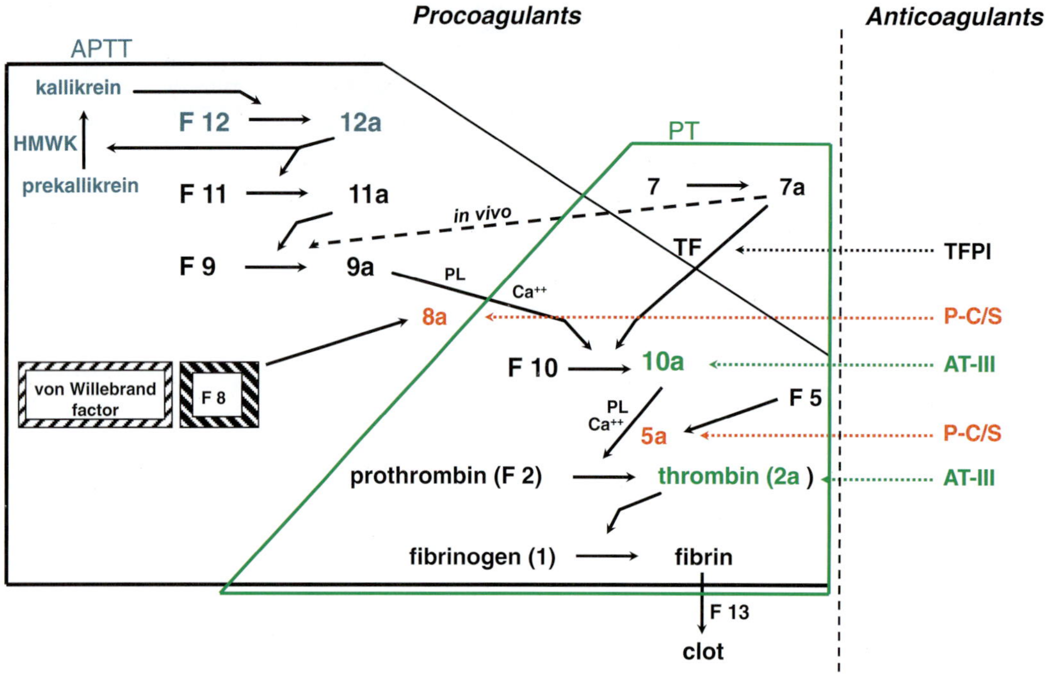

FIGURE 152.2 Simplified pathways of blood coagulation. The area inside the *solid black line* is the intrinsic pathway measured by the APTT. The area inside the *green line* is the extrinsic pathway, measured by the PT. The area encompassed by *both lines* is the common pathway. *APTT,* Activated partial thromboplastin time; *AT-III,* antithrombin III; *F,* factor; *HMWK,* high molecular weight kininogen; *P-C/S,* protein C/S; *PL,* phospholipid; *PT,* prothrombin time; *TFPI,* tissue factor pathway inhibitor. (Modified from Branchford BR, Samelson-Jones BJ, Raffini LJ, Flood VH. Hemostasis. In: Kliegman RM, St. Geme J, eds. *Nelson Textbook of Pediatrics.* 22nd ed. Philadelphia: Elsevier; 2024;Fig 524.1.)

than 2 mm in size. **Purpura** is a group of adjoining petechiae; **ecchymoses** (bruises) are isolated lesions larger than petechiae; and **hematomas** are raised, palpable ecchymoses.

The physical examination should also search for manifestations of an underlying disease such as lymphadenopathy, hepatosplenomegaly, vasculitic rash, edema, or jaundice. **Superficial venous thrombi (thrombophlebitis)** can manifest as erythematous, painful "cord" type swelling along the track of a superficial vein, often following localized trauma such as venipuncture or peripheral intravenous (IV) line insertion. **Deep venous thrombi** may cause warm, swollen (distended), painful, purplish discolored extremities or no findings. **Pulmonary emboli** can be asymptomatic or cause symptoms such as chest pain, shortness of breath, hypoxia, respiratory distress, and tachycardia (see Chapter 137). **Cerebral sinus venous thrombosis** can be associated with headache, seizure, or visual disturbance. **Arterial clots** may cause acutely painful, pale, and poorly perfused extremities. Arterial thrombi of the internal organs present with signs and symptoms of infarction.

Laboratory Testing

Screening laboratory studies for bleeding patients include a **platelet count, prothrombin time, partial thromboplastin time, thrombin time, fibrinogen,** and screening test of platelet function. The platelet function analyzer (PFA) screens for platelet function abnormalities and VWD and is particularly useful when blood volume is limited, as with infants. The PFA has variable sensitivity and specificity for common bleeding disorders. No single laboratory test can screen for all bleeding disorders. The findings on screening tests for bleeding vary with the specific disorder (Table 152.2).

Differential Diagnosis

Disorders of Platelets

Platelet counts less than 150,000/mm^3 constitute **thrombocytopenia**. Mucocutaneous bleeding and/or petechiae are the hallmarks of platelet disorders, including thrombocytopenia. The risk of bleeding correlates imperfectly with the platelet count. Children with platelet counts greater than 80,000/mm^3 can withstand all but the most extreme hemostatic challenges, such as surgery or major trauma. Children with platelet counts less than 20,000/mm^3 are at risk for spontaneous bleeding. These generalizations are modified by factors such as the age of the platelets (young, large platelets usually function better than older ones) and the presence of inhibitors of platelet function, such as antibodies, drugs (especially aspirin), fibrin degradation products, and toxins formed in the presence of hepatic or kidney disease. The size of platelets is routinely measured as the mean platelet volume. The etiology of thrombocytopenia (Fig. 152.4) may be organized into three mechanisms:

1. Decreased platelet production
2. Increased destruction
3. Sequestration

Thrombocytopenia Resulting From Decreased Platelet Production

Primary disorders of megakaryopoiesis (platelet production) are rare in childhood, other than as part of an aplastic syndrome. **Thrombocytopenia with absent radii syndrome** in newborns is characterized by severe thrombocytopenia in association with orthopedic abnormalities, especially of the upper extremities. The thrombocytopenia usually improves spontaneously over time. **Congenital amegakaryocytic thrombocytopenia** presents at birth or shortly thereafter with findings of severe

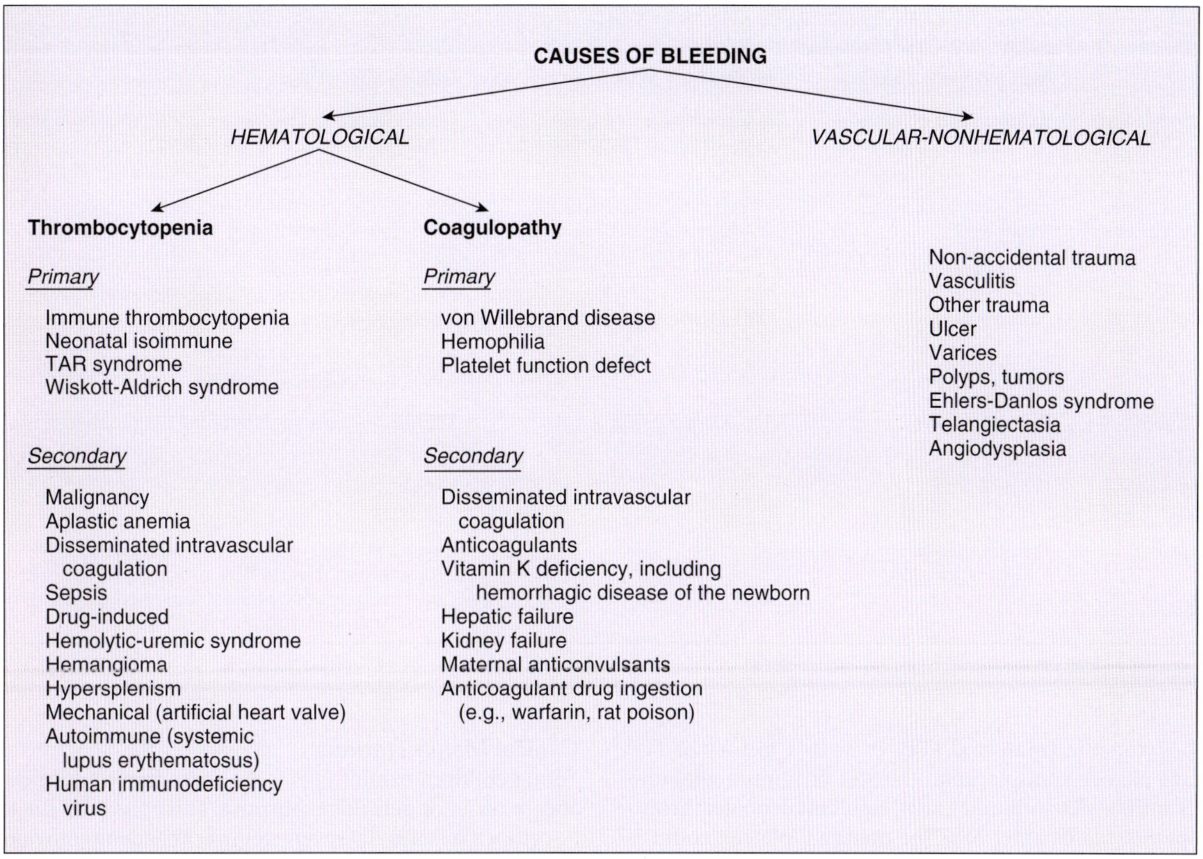

FIGURE 152.3 Common causes of bleeding. *TAR,* Thrombocytopenia with absence of radius (syndrome).

TABLE **152.1** Common Hypercoagulable States

CONGENITAL DISORDERS
Factor V Leiden (activated protein C resistance) Prothrombin 20210 Protein C deficiency Protein S deficiency Antithrombin deficiency Plasminogen deficiency Dysfibrinogenemia Homocystinuria
ACQUIRED DISORDERS
Indwelling catheters Lupus anticoagulant/antiphospholipid syndrome Nephrotic syndrome Malignancy Pregnancy Oral contraceptives (estrogen containing) Autoimmune disease Immobilization/surgery Trauma Infection Inflammatory bowel disease

From Scott JP. Bleeding and thrombosis. In: Kliegman RM, ed. Practical Strategies in Pediatric Diagnosis and Therapy. *Philadelphia: WB Saunders; 1996.*

thrombocytopenia but no other congenital anomalies. The marrow is devoid of megakaryocytes and usually progresses to aplasia of all hematopoietic cell lines. This disorder results from pathogenic variants in *c-mpl*, resulting in abnormal thrombopoietin (TPO) receptors that do not respond to stimulation by TPO.

Acquired thrombocytopenia due to decreased production is rarely an isolated finding; it is seen more often in the context of **pancytopenia resulting from bone marrow failure** caused by infiltrative or aplastic processes. Certain chemotherapeutic agents may affect megakaryocytes selectively more than other marrow elements. **Cyanotic congenital heart disease with polycythemia** often is associated with thrombocytopenia, but this is rarely associated with significant clinical bleeding. **Congenital** (TORCH [toxoplasmosis, other agents, rubella, cytomegalovirus, herpes simplex]) and **acquired viral infections** (HIV, Epstein-Barr virus, and measles) and some **drugs** (anticonvulsants, antibiotics, cytotoxic agents, heparin, and quinidine) may induce thrombocytopenia. Postnatal infections and drug reactions usually cause transient thrombocytopenia; congenital infections may produce prolonged suppression of bone marrow function.

Thrombocytopenia Resulting From Peripheral Destruction

Etiology

In a child who appears well, **immune-mediated mechanisms** are the most common cause of thrombocytopenia, resulting from rapid peripheral destruction of antibody-coated platelets by reticuloendothelial cells. **Neonatal alloimmune thrombocytopenia** (NAIT) occurs because of sensitization of the mother to antigens present on fetal platelets (most commonly HPA-1a). Antibodies cross the placenta and attack the fetal platelets (see Chapter 58). Many platelet alloantigens have been identified and sequenced, permitting prenatal diagnosis of the condition in an at-risk fetus. Mothers with immune

TABLE 152.2 Screening Tests for Bleeding Disorders

TEST	MECHANISM TESTED	NORMAL VALUES	DISORDER
Prothrombin time	Extrinsic and common pathway	<12 sec beyond neonate; 12–18 sec in term neonate	Defect in vitamin K–dependent factors; hemorrhagic disease of newborn, malabsorption, liver disease, DIC, oral anticoagulants, ingestion of rat poison
Activated partial thromboplastin time	Intrinsic and common pathway	70 sec in term neonate 25–40 sec beyond neonate	Hemophilia; von Willebrand disease, heparin; DIC; deficient factors 12 and 11; lupus anticoagulant
Thrombin time	Fibrinogen to fibrin conversion	12–17 sec in term neonate; 10–15 sec beyond neonate	Fibrin split products, DIC, hypofibrinogenemia, heparin, uremia
Bleeding time	Hemostasis, capillary and platelet function	3–7 min beyond neonate	Platelet dysfunction, thrombocytopenia, von Willebrand disease, aspirin
Platelet count	Platelet number	150,000–450,000/mL	Thrombocytopenia differential diagnosis (see Fig. 152.4)
Platelet function analyzer-100	Closure time		Platelet function disorders
Blood smear	Platelet number and size; RBC morphology	–	Large platelets suggest peripheral destruction; fragmented, bizarre RBC morphology suggests microangiopathic process (e.g., hemolytic uremic syndrome, hemangioma, DIC)

DIC, Disseminated intravascular coagulation; *RBC*, red blood cell.

thrombocytopenia **(maternal ITP)** or with a history of ITP may have passive transplacental transfer of immunoglobulin G (IgG) antiplatelet antibodies, with resultant neonatal thrombocytopenia (see Chapter 58). The maternal platelet count is sometimes a useful indicator of the probability that the infant will be affected.

Clinical Manifestations

The infant with NAIT is at risk for **intracranial hemorrhage** in utero and during the immediate delivery process. In ITP, the greatest risk seems to be present during passage through the birth canal, during which molding of the head may induce intracranial hemorrhage. Fetal scalp sampling or percutaneous umbilical blood sampling may be performed to measure the fetal platelet count.

Treatment

Administration of intravenous immunoglobulin (IVIG) before delivery increases fetal platelet counts and may alleviate thrombocytopenia in infants with NAIT and ITP. Delivery by cesarean section is recommended to prevent central nervous system bleeding (see Chapter 58). Neonates with severe thrombocytopenia (platelet counts <20,000/mm^3) can be treated with IVIG or corticosteroids or both until thrombocytopenia remits. If necessary, infants with NAIT may receive washed maternal platelets.

Immune Thrombocytopenia

Etiology

Immune thrombocytopenia of childhood (childhood ITP) is a common disorder that usually follows an acute viral infection. Childhood ITP is caused by an antibody (IgG or IgM) that binds to the platelet membrane. The condition results in Fc receptor–mediated splenic destruction of antibody-coated platelets. Rarely, ITP may be the presenting symptom of an autoimmune disease, such as systemic lupus erythematosus (SLE).

Clinical Manifestations

Young children exhibit ITP 1–4 weeks after viral illness, with abrupt onset of petechiae, purpura, and epistaxis. The thrombocytopenia is usually severe. Significant adenopathy or hepatosplenomegaly is unusual, and the red blood cell (RBC) and white blood cell (WBC) counts are normal.

Diagnosis

The diagnosis of ITP usually is based on clinical presentation and the platelet count; bone marrow examination is usually not necessary. Peripheral blood smear reveals severe thrombocytopenia with increased platelet size and normal RBC and WBC morphology. If atypical findings are noted, marrow examination is indicated to evaluate for an infiltrative disorder (leukemia) or an aplastic process (aplastic anemia). With ITP, an examination of the bone marrow reveals increased megakaryocytes and normal erythroid and myeloid elements.

Treatment and Prognosis

Treatment for ITP is seldom indicated for platelet counts greater than 20,000/mm^3. Treatment does not affect the long-term outcome of ITP but is intended to increase the platelet count acutely. For moderate and severe clinical bleeding with severe thrombocytopenia (platelet count <10,000/mm^3), therapeutic options include **prednisone** (starting dose of 2–4 mg/kg/day for 5–7 days) or IVIG (1 g/kg once). These approaches decrease the rate of clearance of sensitized platelets, rather than decreasing production of antibody. Splenectomy is indicated in acute ITP only for life-threatening bleeding. Spontaneous resolution of ITP occurs in 80% of children within 6 months of diagnosis. Serious bleeding, especially intracranial bleeding, occurs in fewer than 1% of patients with ITP. There is no evidence that early treatment prevents intracranial bleeding.

ITP that persists for 6–12 months is classified as **chronic ITP**. In children who do not respond to first-line treatment

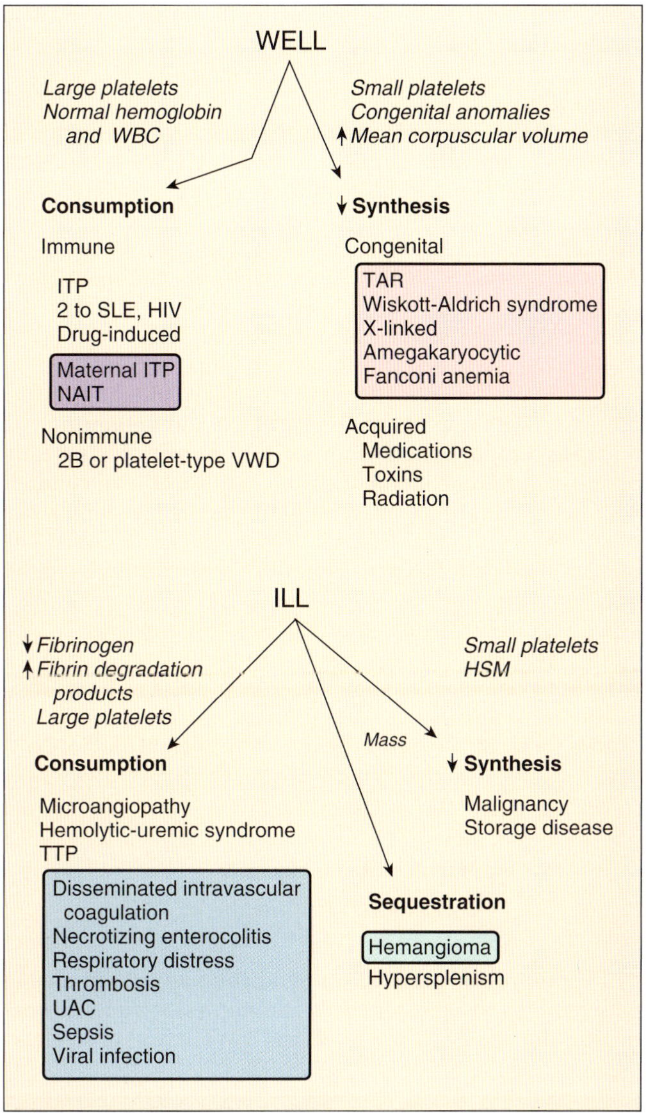

FIGURE 152.4 Differential diagnoses of childhood thrombocytopenic syndromes. The syndromes initially are separated by their clinical appearances. Clues leading to the diagnosis are presented in *italics.* The mechanisms and common disorders leading to these findings are shown in the *lower part* of the figure. Disorders that commonly affect neonates are listed in the *shaded boxes. HSM,* Hepatosplenomegaly; *ITP,* immune thrombocytopenia; *NAIT,* neonatal alloimmune thrombocytopenia; *SLE,* systemic lupus erythematosus; *TAR,* thrombocytopenia with absence of radius (syndrome); *TTP,* thrombotic thrombocytopenic purpura; *UAC,* umbilical artery catheter; *VWD,* von Willebrand disease; *WBC,* white blood cell. (From Scott JP. Bleeding and thrombosis. In: Kliegman RM, Greenbaum LA, Lye PS, eds. *Practical Strategies in Pediatric Diagnosis and Therapy.* Philadelphia: Saunders; 2004:920.)

with high-dose steroids or IVIG, thrombopoietin receptor agonists (i.e., eltrombopag, romiplostim) or rituximab is suggested as a second-line therapy. If persistent, splenectomy can be considered in the management of children with moderate-severe chronic ITP.

Secondary causes of chronic ITP, especially SLE or immunologic abnormalities, should be ruled out. Splenectomy induces a remission in 70–80% of childhood chronic ITP cases. The risks of splenectomy (surgery, sepsis from encapsulated bacteria, pulmonary hypertension) must be weighed against the risk of severe bleeding.

Other Disorders

Wiskott-Aldrich syndrome is an X-linked disorder characterized by hypogammaglobulinemia, eczema, and microthrombocytopenia caused by a molecular defect in a cytoskeletal protein common to lymphocytes and platelets (see Chapter 73). Small platelets are seen on a peripheral blood smear. Nevertheless, thrombocytopenia often is improved by splenectomy. Hematopoietic stem cell transplantation cures the immunodeficiency and thrombocytopenia. Familial X-linked thrombocytopenia can be seen as a variant of Wiskott-Aldrich syndrome or a pathogenic variant in the *GATA1* gene. Autosomal macrothrombocytopenia is due to deletions in chromosome 22q11 or pathogenic variants in 22q12.

Thrombotic microangiopathy causes thrombocytopenia, anemia secondary to intravascular RBC destruction, and, in some cases, depletion of clotting factors. Children with thrombotic microangiopathy usually are quite ill. In a child with **disseminated intravascular coagulation (DIC)**, the deposition of fibrin strands within the vasculature and activation of thrombin and plasmin result in a wide-ranging hemostatic disorder with activation and clearance of platelets. **Hemolytic uremic syndrome** occurs because of exposure to a toxin that induces endothelial injury, fibrin deposition, and platelet activation and clearance (see Chapter 165). In **thrombotic thrombocytopenic purpura**, platelet consumption, precipitated by a congenital or acquired (antibody-mediated) deficiency of a metalloproteinase that cleaves VWF, seems to be the primary process, with a modest deposition of fibrin and RBC destruction.

Disorders of Platelet Function

Etiology

Primary disorders of platelet function involve receptors on platelet membranes for adhesive proteins. Deficiency of glycoprotein Ib complex (VWF receptor) causes **Bernard-Soulier syndrome**. A deficiency of glycoprotein IIb-IIIa (the fibrinogen receptor) causes **Glanzmann thrombasthenia**. Mild abnormalities of platelet aggregation and granule release, detectable by platelet aggregometry, are far more common. Secondary disorders caused by toxins and drugs (uremia, valproic acid, aspirin, nonsteroidal antiinflammatory drugs, and infections) cause a broad spectrum of platelet dysfunction.

Clinical Manifestations

Disorders of platelet function present with mucocutaneous bleeding and a prolonged bleeding time or delayed PFA closure time; they may be primary or secondary. The bleeding time is an insensitive screen for mild and moderate platelet function disorders but is usually prolonged in severe platelet function disorders, such as Bernard-Soulier syndrome or Glanzmann thrombasthenia.

Disorders of Clotting Factors

Etiology

Hereditary deficiencies of most procoagulant proteins lead to bleeding. The genes for factor 8 and factor 9 are on the X chromosome; virtually all the other clotting factors are coded on autosomal chromosomes. **Factor 8 and factor 9 deficiencies** are the most common severe inherited bleeding disorders. **von Willebrand disease (VWD)** is the most common inherited bleeding disorder. Of the procoagulant proteins, low levels of the contact factors (prekallikrein, high molecular weight kininogen, and Hageman factor [factor 12]) cause a prolonged activated partial thromboplastin time (aPTT) but are not associated with a predisposition to bleeding.

Hemophilia

Etiology

Hemophilia A (factor 8 deficiency) occurs in 1 in 5,000 males. **Hemophilia B** (factor 9 deficiency) occurs in approximately 1 in 25,000 males. Clinically, the two disorders are indistinguishable other than by their therapy (Table 152.3). The lack of factor 8 or factor 9 delays the generation of thrombin, which is crucial to forming a normal, functional fibrin clot and solidifying the platelet plug that has formed in areas of vascular injury. The severity of the disorder is determined by the degree of clotting factor deficiency.

Clinical Manifestations

Patients with less than 1% (severe hemophilia) factor 8 or factor 9 may have **spontaneous bleeding** (often in joints or muscles [**hemarthroses**]) or bleeding with minor trauma. Patients with 1–5% (moderate hemophilia) factor 8 or factor 9 usually require moderate trauma to induce bleeding episodes. In mild hemophilia (5–40% factor 8 or factor 9), significant trauma is necessary to induce bleeding; spontaneous bleeding does not occur. Mild hemophilia may go undiagnosed for many years; severe hemophilia manifests in infancy.

Laboratory Studies

The diagnosis of hemophilia is based on a **prolonged aPTT**. In the aPTT, a surface-active agent activates the intrinsic system of coagulation, of which factors 8 and 9 are crucial components. In factor 8 or factor 9 deficiency, the aPTT is prolonged but should correct to normal when the patient's plasma is mixed 1:1 with normal plasma. When an abnormal aPTT is obtained and corrects upon mixing with normal plasma, **specific factor assays** are needed to make a precise diagnosis (see Table 152.2) to determine the appropriate factor replacement therapy. Prenatal diagnosis and carrier diagnosis can be made with molecular testing.

Treatment

Early, appropriate **replacement therapy** is the hallmark of excellent hemophilia care. Acute bleeding episodes are best treated in the home with IV infusion assuming patient cooperation, caregiver comfort, and available IV access (whether through peripheral venipuncture or central venous catheter). Early institution of factor replacement and continuous prophylaxis beginning in early childhood are likely to reduce the chronic joint disease associated with hemophilia.

Bleeding associated with surgery, trauma, or dental extraction often can be anticipated, and excessive bleeding can be prevented with appropriate replacement and antifibrinolytic therapies. Prophylactic therapy starting in infancy has greatly diminished the likelihood of chronic arthropathy in children with hemophilia. To manage life-threatening bleeding, levels of 80–100% of normal factor 8 or factor 9 are necessary. For mild-to-moderate bleeding episodes (hemarthroses), a 40% level for factor 8 or a 30–40% level for factor 9 is appropriate. The dose can be calculated using the knowledge that 1 U/kg body weight of factor 8 increases the plasma level 2% and 1.5 U/kg of recombinant factor 9 increases the plasma level 1%:

$$\text{Dose for factor 8} = \text{desired level } (\%) \times \text{weight (kg)} \times 0.5$$

or

$$\text{Dose for recombinant factor 9} = \text{desired level}(\%) \times \text{weight (kg)} \times 1.5$$

Desmopressin acetate is a synthetic vasopressin analog with minimal vasopressor effect. Desmopressin triples or quadruples the initial factor 8 level (and VWF levels) of a patient

TABLE **152.3** Comparison of Hemophilia A, Hemophilia B, and von Willebrand Disease

FEATURE	HEMOPHILIA A	HEMOPHILIA B	VON WILLEBRAND DISEASE
Inheritance	X linked	X linked	Autosomal dominant
Factor deficiency	Factor 8	Factor 9	VWF, factor 8
Bleeding site(s)	Muscle, joint, surgical	Muscle, joint, surgical	Mucous membranes, skin, surgical, menstrual
Prothrombin time	Normal	Normal	Normal
Activated partial thromboplastin time	Prolonged	Prolonged	Prolonged or normal
Bleeding time/PFA-100	Normal	Normal	Prolonged or normal
Factor 8 coagulant activity	Low	Normal	Low or normal
VWF antigen	Normal	Normal	Low
VWF activity	Normal	Normal	Low
Factor 9	Normal	Low	Normal
Ristocetin-induced platelet agglutination	Normal	Normal	Normal, low, or increased at low-dose ristocetin
Platelet aggregation	Normal	Normal	Normal
Treatment	DDAVP* or recombinant factor 8	Recombinant factor 9	DDAVP* or VWF concentrate

**DDAVP may be used to treat mild-to-moderate hemophilia A or type 1 von Willebrand disease.*
DDAVP, Desmopressin; *PFA*, platelet function analyzer-100; *VWF*, von Willebrand factor.

with mild or moderate (not severe) hemophilia A but has no effect on factor 9 levels. When adequate hemostatic levels can be attained, desmopressin is the treatment of choice for individuals with mild and moderate hemophilia A. Aminocaproic acid is an inhibitor of fibrinolysis with systemic (and topical, in the liquid form) activity that may be useful for oral/nasal mucosal bleeding. Patients treated with older factor 8 or 9 concentrates derived from large pools of plasma donors were at risk for hepatitis B, C, and D and HIV. Recombinant factor 8 and factor 9 concentrates are safe from virally transmitted illnesses.

Factor inhibitors are IgG antibodies directed against transfused factor 8 or factor 9 in congenitally deficient patients, whose immune systems recognize the transfused factors as foreign proteins. Inhibitors arise in 15–30% of patients with severe factor 8 deficiency but are less common (1–5%) in patients with severe factor 9 deficiency. They may be high or low titer and show an anamnestic response to treatment. The treatment of bleeding patients with an inhibitor is difficult. For low titer inhibitors, options include high-dose or continuous factor 8 infusions. For high titer inhibitors, it is usually necessary to administer a product that bypasses the inhibitor, such as recombinant factor 7a. Activated prothrombin complex concentrates, used in the past to treat inhibitor patients, paradoxically increased the risks of thrombosis, resulting in fatal complications, such as myocardial infarction. For long-term treatment of inhibitor patients, induction of immune tolerance by repeated infusion of the deficient factor with or without immunosuppression may be beneficial.

Emicizumab is a bispecific antibody that mimics the activity of factor 8 to bridge factors 9a and 10, catalyzing the activation of factor 10 and leading to downstream thrombin production. Emicizumab promotes effective hemostasis in individuals with hemophilia A without inhibitors; the pharmacokinetics allows for subcutaneous injection with infrequent dosing, thus making it a popular treatment option. Additionally, multiple gene therapy strategies are available for adults with hemophilia A or B; these remain in clinical trial for pediatric patients.

von Willebrand Disease

Etiology

VWD is a common disorder (1% of the general population) caused by a deficiency of **VWF**, an adhesive protein that serves two functions: it acts as a bridge between subendothelial collagen and platelets and binding circulating factor 8 and protects factor 8 from rapid clearance from the circulation. VWD usually is inherited as an autosomal dominant trait and, rarely, as an autosomal recessive trait. VWF may be either quantitatively deficient (partial = type 1 or absolute = type 3) or qualitatively abnormal (type 2 = dysproteinemia). Approximately 80% of patients with VWD have classic (type 1) disease (i.e., a mild-to-moderate deficiency of VWF). Several other subtypes are clinically important, each requiring different therapy.

Clinical Manifestations

Mucocutaneous bleeding, epistaxis, gingival bleeding, cutaneous bruising, and menorrhagia may occur in patients with VWD. In severe disease, factor 8 deficiency may be profound, and the patient may also have manifestations similar to hemophilia A (hemarthrosis). Findings in classic VWD differ from findings in hemophilia A and B (see Table 152.3).

Laboratory Testing

VWF testing involves measurement of the amount of protein, usually measured immunologically as the **VWF antigen** (VWF:Ag). VWF activity (VWF:Act) is measured functionally in the **ristocetin cofactor assay** (VWFR:Co), which uses the antibiotic ristocetin to induce VWF to bind to platelets. Alternatively, VWF activity may be evaluated using a gain-of-function variant of GPIb (GPIbM) instead of ristocetin. VWF multimer testing assesses the protein structure and assists in the diagnosis of the qualitative disorders (type 2 = dysproteinemia).

Treatment

The treatment of VWD depends on the severity of bleeding. **Desmopressin** is the treatment of choice for most bleeding episodes in patients with type 1 disease and some patients with type 2 disease. When high levels of VWF are needed but cannot be achieved with desmopressin, treatment with a virally attenuated, **VWF-containing plasma-derived concentrate or recombinant VWF concentrate** may be appropriate. Cryoprecipitate should not be used because it is not virally attenuated. Hepatitis B vaccine should be given before the patient is exposed to plasma-derived products. As in all bleeding disorders, aspirin and nonsteroidal antiinflammatory drugs should be avoided.

Vitamin K Deficiency

For discussion of vitamin K deficiency, see Chapters 25 and 29.

Disseminated Intravascular Coagulation

Etiology

DIC is a disorder with widespread activation of the coagulation mechanism and is usually associated with decreased organ perfusion, seen in shock. Normal hemostasis is a balance between hemorrhage and thrombosis. In DIC, this balance is altered by the severe illness, so the patient has activation of coagulation (thrombosis) mediated by thrombin and fibrinolysis mediated by plasmin (bleeding). Coagulation factors—especially platelets, fibrinogen, and factors 2, 5, and 8—are consumed, as are the anticoagulant proteins, especially antithrombin, protein C, and plasminogen. Endothelial injury (crush injuries, burns), tissue release of thromboplastic procoagulant factors, or, rarely, exogenous factors (snake venoms, severe infections) directly activate the coagulation mechanism (Table 152.4).

Clinical Manifestations

The diagnosis of DIC usually is suspected clinically and is confirmed by laboratory findings of a **decrease in platelets and fibrinogen** associated with elevated PTT, aPTT, and elevated levels of D-dimer, formed when fibrinogen is clotted and then degraded by plasmin (Table 152.5). In some patients, DIC may evolve more slowly, and there may be a degree of compensation. In a severely ill patient, the new onset of bleeding from a venipuncture or incision site, gastrointestinal or pulmonary hemorrhage, petechiae, ecchymosis, or evidence of peripheral gangrene or thrombosis suggests the diagnosis of DIC.

TABLE 152.4 Causes of Disseminated Intravascular Coagulation
INFECTIOUS
Meningococcemia (purpura fulminans) Other gram-negative bacteria *(Haemophilus, Salmonella, Escherichia coli)* Rickettsiae (Rocky Mountain spotted fever) Virus (cytomegalovirus, herpes, hemorrhagic fevers) Malaria Fungus
TISSUE INJURY
Central nervous system trauma (massive head injury) Multiple fractures with fat emboli Crush injury Profound shock or asphyxia Hypothermia or hyperthermia Massive burns
MALIGNANCY
Acute promyelocytic leukemia Acute monoblastic or myelocytic leukemia Widespread malignancies (neuroblastoma)
VENOM OR TOXIN
Snake bites Insect bites
MICROANGIOPATHIC DISORDERS
"Severe" thrombotic thrombocytopenic purpura Hemolytic uremic syndrome Giant hemangioma (Kasabach-Merritt syndrome)
GASTROINTESTINAL DISORDERS
Fulminant hepatitis Severe inflammatory bowel disease Reye syndrome
HEREDITARY THROMBOTIC DISORDERS
Antithrombin deficiency Homozygous protein C deficiency
NEONATAL PERIOD
Maternal toxemia Group B streptococcal infections Abruptio placentae Severe respiratory distress syndrome Necrotizing enterocolitis Congenital viral disease (e.g., cytomegalovirus infection or herpes) Erythroblastosis fetalis
MISCELLANEOUS CONDITIONS/DISORDERS
Severe acute graft rejection Acute hemolytic transfusion reaction Severe collagen vascular disease Kawasaki disease Heparin-induced thrombosis Infusion of "activated" prothrombin complex concentrates Hyperpyrexia/encephalopathy, hemorrhagic shock syndrome

From Scott JP. Bleeding and thrombosis. In: Kliegman RM, ed. Practical Strategies in Pediatric Diagnosis and Therapy. *Philadelphia: WB Saunders; 1996.*

Treatment

The treatment of DIC is challenging. General guidelines include: treat the underlying disorder inducing the DIC first; support the patient by correcting hypoxia, acidosis, and poor perfusion; and consider replacing depleted blood-clotting factors, platelets, and anticoagulant proteins by transfusion, especially in the bleeding patient.

Heparin may be used to treat significant arterial or venous thrombotic disease unless sites of life-threatening bleeding coexist.

Thrombosis

Etiology

A hereditary predisposition to **thrombosis** (see Table 152.1) may be caused by a deficiency of an anticoagulant protein (**protein C or S, antithrombin**, or **plasminogen**) (Fig. 152.5), by an abnormality of a procoagulant protein making it resistant to proteolysis by its respective inhibitor **(factor 5 Leiden)**, by a pathogenic variant resulting in an increased level of a procoagulant protein (prothrombin 20210), or by damage to endothelial cells **(homocysteinemia)**. Neonates with deficiency syndromes may be particularly vulnerable to thrombosis. Neonates with homozygous protein C deficiency present with purpura fulminans or thrombosis of the major arteries and veins or both. Some individuals with an inherited predisposition to thrombosis do not exhibit symptoms until adolescence or early adulthood. Protein C deficiency due to a pathogenic variant in *PROC* can present in young adulthood (autosomal dominant trait); the homozygous form usually is autosomal recessive and may present in younger children. Protein S and antithrombin deficiencies are inherited as autosomal dominant traits. Factor 5 Leiden is the most common hereditary cause of a predisposition to thrombosis, appearing in 3–5% of White people. **Acquired antiphospholipid antibodies** (anticardiolipin and anti-β_2-glycoprotein antibodies and lupus anticoagulant) also predispose to thrombosis.

Clinical Manifestations

Neonates and adolescents are the most likely pediatric patients to present with thromboembolic disease. Indwelling catheters (with unfavorable catheter:vein size ratio), vasculitis, sepsis, immobilization, nephrotic syndrome, coagulopathy, trauma, infection, surgery, inflammatory bowel disease, oral contraceptive agents, and pregnancy all predispose to thrombosis. The manifestations of pulmonary emboli vary from no findings to chest pain, diminished breath sounds, a loud S2, cyanosis, tachypnea, and hypoxemia.

Diagnostic and Imaging Studies

Venous thrombosis can be detected noninvasively by ultrasound Doppler flow compression studies. The gold standard for diagnosis is the venogram. An abnormal *(high probability)* ventilation-perfusion scan or detection of an intravascular thrombus on helical computed tomography is diagnostic of pulmonary emboli in young adults. Cerebral sinus venous thrombosis is often diagnosed by magnetic resonance venography. There are no appropriate screening studies for thrombotic disorders. Diagnosis of a congenital or acquired predisposition to thrombosis requires a battery of specific assays.

Treatment

Therapy of thrombotic disorders depends on the underlying condition and usually initially involves unfractionated or low molecular weight **heparin** or a **direct oral anticoagulant (DOAC)**. In some clinical scenarios, long-term anticoagulation is needed with a DOAC or **warfarin**. Direct thrombin inhibitors may also be used in children and may be favored depending on the clinical circumstance. Major vessel thrombosis, life-threatening

TABLE 152.5 Differential Diagnoses of Coagulopathies That Can Be Confused With DIC

	PROTHROMBIN TIME	PARTIAL THROMBOPLASTIN TIME	FIBRINOGEN	PLATELETS	D-DIMER	CLINICAL KEY(S)
DIC	↑	↑	↓	↓	↑	Shock
Liver failure	↑	↑	↓	Normal or ↓	↑	Jaundice
Vitamin K deficiency	↑	↑	Normal	Normal	Normal	Malabsorption, liver disease
Sepsis without shock	↑	↑	Normal	Normal	↑ or normal	Fever

DIC, Disseminated intravascular coagulation.
From Scott JP. Bleeding and thrombosis. In: Kliegman RM, ed. Practical Strategies in Pediatric Diagnosis and Therapy. *Philadelphia: WB Saunders; 1996.*

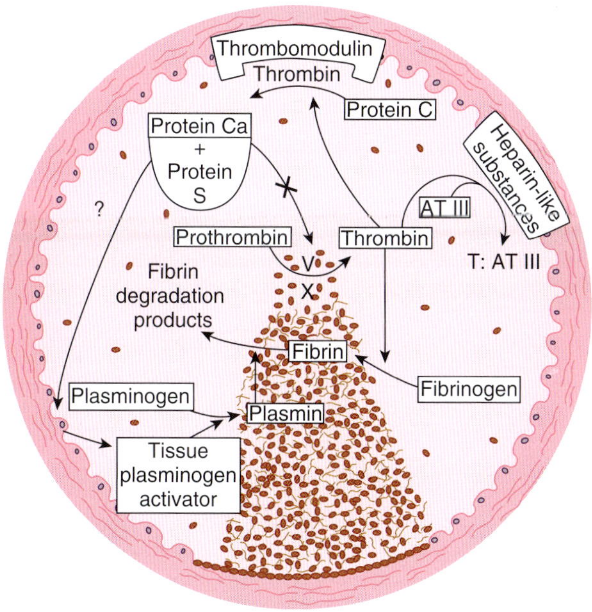

FIGURE 152.5 Formation of the hemostatic plug at the site of vascular injury. Three major physiologic anticoagulant mechanisms—AT, protein C, and the fibrinolytic system—are activated to limit clot formation to the site of damage and to prevent generalized thrombosis. *AT*, Antithrombin; *T*, thrombin. (From Schafer A. The hypercoagulable state. *Ann Intern Med.* 1985;102:814–828.)

thrombosis, or arterial thrombosis may necessitate treatment with **fibrinolytic agents** (recombinant tissue plasminogen activator). In newborns, inherited deficiency syndromes may present as emergencies and necessitate **replacement** with plasma, antithrombin concentrates, or protein C concentrates.

PEARLS FOR PRACTITIONERS

See Hematology: Pearls for Practitioners at the end of this section.

REVIEW QUESTIONS

Available online.

CHAPTER 153

Blood Component Therapy

Transfusion of red blood cells (RBCs), platelets, plasma, cryoprecipitate, and granulocytes can be lifesaving or life sustaining (Table 153.1). **Whole blood** is rarely indicated and is most useful to provide both oxygen-carrying capacity and functional procoagulant and anticoagulant factors. **Packed RBCs** are used to treat anemia to increase oxygen-carrying capacity. RBC transfusions should not be used to treat asymptomatic nutritional deficiencies that can be corrected by administering the appropriate deficient nutrient (e.g., iron or folic acid).

Blood component therapy requires proper anticoagulation of the component unit, screening for infectious agents, and blood group compatibility testing before administration. Typical **transfusion reactions** are listed in Table 153.2. Transfusion may also result in circulatory overload, especially in the presence of cardiopulmonary deficiency. Filtering of blood products to remove white blood cells may prevent febrile reactions. Long-term complications of transfusions include graft versus host disease and **infectious diseases** such as **hepatitis B** (<1:1,000,000 units) and **C** (1:2,000,000 units), **HIV** (<1:2,000,000 units), malaria, syphilis, babesiosis, brucellosis, and Chagas disease. Patients who are chronically transfused are more prone to iron overload and alloimmunization to RBCs and platelets. Iron overload may be treated with chelation therapy to prevent organ damage and further iron overload. Patients with alloimmunization who require future transfusions should be matched for RBC antigens to minimize further alloimmunization.

TABLE 153.1 Commonly Used Transfusion Products

COMPONENT	CONTENT	INDICATION	DOSE	EXPECTED OUTCOME
Packed RBCs	250–300 mL/unit	↓ Oxygen-carrying RBCs	10–15 mL/kg	↑ Hgb by 2–3 g/dL
Platelet concentrate from whole blood donation	$5–7 \times 10^{10}$ platelets/unit	Severe thrombocytopenia ± bleeding	1 unit/10 kg	↑ Platelet count by 50,000/μL
Platelet concentrate	3×10^{11} platelets/unit	Severe thrombocytopenia ± bleeding	1 unit/70 kg	↑ Platelet count by 30,000–50,000/μL
Fresh frozen plasma	1 unit of each clotting factor/mL	Multiple clotting factor deficiency	10–20 mL/kg	Improvement in significantly prolonged prothrombin and partial thromboplastin times
Cryoprecipitate	Fibrinogen, factor 8, VWF, factor 13	Hypofibrinogenemia, factor 13 deficiency	1 unit/5–10 kg	↑ Fibrinogen by 50–100 mg/dL
Recombinant factor concentrates	Units as labeled	Hemophilic bleeding or prophylaxis	F8: 20–50 units/kg F9: 40–120 units/kg	F8: ↑ 2%/unit/kg F9: ↑ 0.7 unit/kg
Recombinant factor VIIa (NovoSeven)	Micrograms (mcg)	Hemophilic bleeding in patient with inhibitor; also used for uncontrolled postoperative hemorrhage	30–90 mcg/kg/dose	Cessation of bleeding

Hgb, Hemoglobin; *RBCs*, red blood cells; *VWF*, von Willebrand factor.

TABLE 153.2 Evaluation of Transfusion Reactions

TYPE OF REACTION	CLINICAL SIGNS	MANAGEMENT
Acute hemolytic transfusion reaction (incidence of 1:250,000–1:1,000,000)	Acute shock, back pain, flushing, early fever, intravascular hemolysis, hemoglobinemia, hemoglobinuria (may be delayed 5–10 days and less severe if anamnestic response is present)	Stop transfusion; return blood to bank with fresh sample of patient's blood Hydrate intravenously; support blood pressure, maintain high urine flow, alkalinize urine Check for and correct electrolyte abnormalities (hyperkalemia)
Delayed hemolytic transfusion reaction (incidence of 1:100,000)	Onset 7–14 days after transfusion: pain, fever, jaundice, hemoglobinuria; fall in hemoglobin; reticulocytopenia	Transfuse only antigen-negative RBCs if needed
Febrile nonhemolytic transfusion reaction (incidence of 1:100)	Fever during or within 4 hr after end of transfusion, chills, usually from passively transfused cytokines or recipient reaction to leukocytes Bacterial contamination can occur in 1:100,000 platelet transfusions	Antipyretics for symptomatic treatment or pretreatment for future transfusions; leukocyte reduction has decreased incidence of febrile reactions Blood culture if high suspicion for bacterial infection
Allergic transfusion reaction (incidence of 1:100)	Urticaria, pruritus, maculopapular rash, edema, respiratory distress, hypotension during or within 4 hr of transfusion; often because recipient has preformed antibodies against donor antigens, occasionally from passive infusion of antibodies from atopic donor	Diphenhydramine ± hydrocortisone for acute management For future transfusions consider: Pretreatment with diphenhydramine ± hydrocortisone Volume reduction to reduce donor plasma Washing cellular products to remove all donor plasma (for severe reactions)

RBCs, Red blood cells.
Modified from Andreoli TE, Bennett JC, Carpenter CC, et al. *Cecil Essentials of Medicine*. 4th ed. Philadelphia: WB Saunders; 1997.

PEARLS FOR PRACTITIONERS

See Hematology: Pearls for Practitioners at the end of this section.

REVIEW QUESTIONS

Available online.

Suggested Readings

Alter BP. Bone marrow failure syndromes in children. *Pediatr Clin North Am*. 2002;49(5):973–988.

Chou ST, Alsawas M, Fasano RM, et al. American Society of Hematology 2020 guidelines for sickle cell disease: transfusion support. *Blood Adv*. 2020;4(2):327–355.

Hartung HD, Olson TS, Bessler M. Acquired aplastic anemia in children. *Pediatr Clin North Am*. 2013;60(6):1311–1336.

Key NS, Negrier C. Coagulation factor concentrates: past, present, and future. *Lancet*. 2007;370(9585):439–448.

Klein HG, Spahn DR, Carson JL. Red blood cell transfusion in clinical practice. *Lancet*. 2007;370(9585):415–426.

Lavin M, O'Donnell JS. New treatment approaches to von Willebrand disease. *Hematology Am Soc Hematol Educ Program*. 2016;2016(1):683–689.

Meeks SL, Batsuli G. Hemophilia and inhibitors: current treatment options and potential new therapeutic approaches. *Hematology Am Soc Hematol Educ Program*. 2016;2016(1):657–662.

Monagle P, Chan AKC, Goldenberg NA, et al. Antithrombotic therapy in neonates and children: Antithrombotic Therapy and Prevention of Thrombosis, 9th ed: American College of Chest Physicians Evidence-Based Clinical Practice Guidelines. [published correction appears in Chest. 2014 Dec;146(6):1694. Dosage error in article text] [published correction appears in Chest. 2014 Nov;146(5):1422]. *Chest*. 2012; 141(2 suppl):e737S–e801S.

National Heart, Lung, and Blood Institute. Evidence-Based Management of Sickle Cell Disease. *Expert Panel Report, 2014. NHLBI*, National Institutes of Health, Bethesda, Maryland.
Neunert C, Lim W, Crowther M, et al. The American Society of Hematology 2011 evidence-based practice guideline for immune thrombocytopenia. *Blood*. 2011;117(16):4190–4207.
Stroncek DF, Rebulla P. Platelet transfusions. *Lancet*. 2007;370(9585):427–438.
Tolar J, Mehta PA, Walters MC. Hematopoietic cell transplantation for nonmalignant disorders. *Biol Blood Marrow Transplant*. 2012;18(1 suppl):S166–S171.
Tsai SF, Chen SJ, Yen HJ, et al. Iron deficiency anemia in predominantly breastfed young children. *Pediatr Neonatol*. 2014;55(6):466–469.

PEARLS FOR PRACTITIONERS

CHAPTER 150

Hematology Assessment

- Normal hematologic values vary according to age and, after puberty, also vary according to sex.
- The physiologic nadir occurs at 8–10 weeks of life; this nadir is accentuated in premature infants.
- The presence of petechiae, purpura, or deeper sites of bleeding, including generalized hemorrhage, indicates abnormalities of platelets, coagulation factors, or both.
- Organ system involvement or systemic symptoms point to a generalized illness as the cause of hematologic abnormalities.

CHAPTER 151

Anemia

- Anemia is defined as any hemoglobin or hematocrit value that is 2 standard deviations (SDs) below the mean for age and sex.
- Androgens at the onset of puberty result in hemoglobin values in males that are about 1.5–2 g/dL higher than females.
- Anemia is classified based on red blood cell (RBC) size: microcytic, normocytic, or macrocytic.
- Key clinical findings in patients with hemolytic anemias are jaundice, pallor, and splenomegaly.
- An elevated reticulocyte count suggests increased RBC production.
- Anemia with a normal reticulocyte count suggests decreased or ineffective production.

Microcytic Anemia

Iron-Deficiency Anemia

- Pure dietary iron deficiency is rare except in children 1–3 years of age; it is most common in toddlers receiving large amounts of cow's milk and lacking food high in iron.
- Menstruating adolescent females who are not receiving supplemental iron are at risk for iron deficiency.
- Iron deficiency in adolescent males is rare and should prompt evaluation for chronic gastrointestinal blood loss.
- In an otherwise healthy child, a therapeutic trial of oral iron is the best diagnostic study for iron deficiency as long as the child is re-examined and a response is documented, including reticulocytosis (48–72 hours), increase in hemoglobin levels (4–30 days), and repletion of iron stores (in 1–3 months).

Thalassemias

- α-Thalassemia minor and β-thalassemia minor are common causes of microcytic anemia in otherwise healthy children of Mediterranean, Southeast Asian, or African descent.

Lead Poisoning

- Lead poisoning is associated with hypochromic, microcytic anemia because most patients have concomitant iron deficiency.

Normocytic Anemia

- Chronic inflammation can lead to normocytic anemia that is likely mediated through hepcidin.
- Malignancy can result in normocytic anemia; RBC aplasia (congenital and acquired) results in normocytic anemia.

Macrocytic Anemia

- Macrocytic anemia should prompt an evaluation for vitamin B_{12} and folate deficiency, as well as careful evaluation for bone marrow failure, dysplasia, or infiltrative process.

Pancytopenia

- Pancytopenia is a simultaneous quantitative decrease in all formed elements of the blood.
- A low reticulocyte count, presence of abnormal forms of leukocytes or myeloid elements less mature than band forms, small platelets, and an elevated mean corpuscular volume in the face of a low reticulocyte count suggest bone marrow failure and require bone marrow examination.
- The etiology of aplastic anemia can be idiopathic, drug induced, or postinfectious.
- Fanconi anemia, an autosomal recessive defect in DNA repair that leads to bone marrow failure, presents with multiple congenital anomalies and can evolve into acute leukemia.

Hemoglobinopathies

- Alpha chain hemoglobinopathies present in utero because alpha chains are needed for fetal erythropoiesis.
- Four alpha genes are present on chromosome 16. A single-gene deletion is a silent carrier, two-gene deletion results in α-thalassemia minor (trait), three-gene deletion results in hemoglobin H disease (moderate hemolytic anemia), and four-gene deletion results in hydrops fetalis with severe intrauterine anemia.
- Beta chain hemoglobinopathies present between 4–12 months of age when fetal hemoglobin nadirs.

Sickle Cell Disease

- Sickle cell syndromes include hemoglobin SS disease, hemoglobin SC disease, hemoglobin S-β^0-thalassemia, and hemoglobin S-β^+-thalassemia.
- A child with sickle cell disease is vulnerable to:
  - Life-threatening infection by 4 months of age due to splenic dysfunction. A febrile patient with sickle cell disease must be evaluated immediately and empirically treated with antibiotics.
  - Sudden, severe, and sometimes life-threatening events, which are caused by the acute intravascular sickling of the RBCs, with resultant pain or organ dysfunction.
  - Acute painful events, which are usually localized to the long bones of the arms or legs but may occur in smaller bones of the hands or feet in infancy (dactylitis), ribs, or in the abdomen.
  - Overt stroke, which occurs in approximately 8–10% of patients with hemoglobin SS or hemoglobin S-β^0-thalassemia and is an indication for chronic transfusion.
- Hydroxyurea should be initiated in asymptomatic children with severe sickle cell disease (HbSS or HbSβ^0-thalassemia).

Enzymopathies

- RBC enzyme disorders include glucose-6-phosphate dehydrogenase (G6PD) deficiency (common) and pyruvate kinase deficiency (rare).
- The gene for G6PD is on the X chromosome.
- Patients with pyruvate kinase deficiency have depletion of adenosine triphosphate, which impairs RBC survival.

Membrane Disorders

- The most common RBC membrane hemolytic disorders are hereditary spherocytosis and hereditary elliptocytosis.
- A positive osmotic fragility test supports the diagnosis of hereditary spherocytosis.

Hemolytic Anemia Caused by Disorders Extrinsic to the Red Blood Cell

- Isoimmune hemolysis is caused by active maternal immunization against fetal antigens (i.e., A, B, and Rh D antigens).
- Autoimmune hemolytic anemia is Coombs positive due to the production of autoantibodies that cause RBC destruction, often following an infection.
- Treatment of autoimmune hemolytic anemia often requires RBC transfusion in addition to corticosteroids for some types.

CHAPTER 152

Hemostatic Disorders

Normal Hemostasis

- All the hemostatic processes are closely interwoven and occur on biologic surfaces that mediate coagulation by bringing platelets, endothelial cells, and subendothelium into close proximity with pro- and anticoagulant proteins.
- Deficiency of factor 8 or factor 9 leads to severe bleeding disorders, deficiency of factor 11 can be associated with mild bleeding, and deficiency of factor 12 is asymptomatic.
- Fibrinolysis is initiated by the action of tissue plasminogen activator on plasminogen, producing plasmin, the active enzyme that degrades fibrin into split products.

Developmental Hemostasis

- Children attain normal levels of procoagulant and anticoagulant proteins by 1 year of age; levels of protein C lag and normalize in adolescence.

Hemostatic Disorders

- A detailed family history is crucial to the diagnosis of bleeding and thrombotic disorders.
- No single laboratory test can screen for all bleeding disorders.

Platelet Disorders

- Platelet counts less than 150,000/mm^3 constitute thrombocytopenia. Mucocutaneous bleeding is the hallmark of platelet disorders. The risk of bleeding correlates imperfectly with the platelet count.
- The etiology of thrombocytopenia is organized into three mechanisms:
  - Decreased platelet production
  - Increased platelet destruction, as found in neonatal autoimmune thrombocytopenia, acute idiopathic thrombocytopenia purpura, and thrombotic microangiopathy
  - Platelet sequestration/consumption
- Disorders of platelet function present with mucocutaneous bleeding, prolonged bleeding time, or long PFA closure time and can be primary or secondary disorders.

Disorders of Clotting Factors

- Hemophilia A (factor 8 deficiency) and hemophilia B (factor 9 deficiency) are X-linked, potentially severe bleeding disorders.
  - Clinical bleeding often occurs in the muscles and joints; the severity of bleeding is proportional to the patient's baseline level of factor 8 or 9.
  - Factor 8 or factor 9 recombinant replacement therapy is used to treat acute bleeds, for hemostasis for surgical procedures, and as prophylaxis in patients with severe hemophilia.
  - Other treatment options, such as a bispecific antibody that mimics factor 8 activity and gene therapy, are shifting the paradigm in hemophilia management.
- von Willebrand disease is an inherited bleeding disorder that affects about 1% of the general population.
  - It is associated with mucocutaneous bleeding such as epistaxis, gingival bleeding, cutaneous bruising, and menorrhagia.

- The treatment depends on the type and the severity of bleeding; it commonly includes desmopressin (DDAVP).

Disseminated Intravascular Coagulation

- Disseminated intravascular coagulation (DIC) is a disorder with widespread activation of coagulation (thrombosis) and fibrinolysis (bleeding).
  - Diagnosis usually is suspected clinically and is confirmed by laboratory findings.
  - General treatment guidelines include:
    - Treat the underlying disorder inducing DIC first.
    - Support the patient by correcting hypoxia, acidosis, and poor perfusion.
    - Replace depleted blood-clotting factors, platelets, and anticoagulant proteins by transfusion, especially in a bleeding patient.

Thrombosis

- Hereditary predisposition to thrombosis:
  - Protein C or S, antithrombin, or plasminogen deficiency
  - Abnormality of a procoagulant protein (factor 5 Leiden)
  - Increased level of a procoagulant protein (prothrombin 20210)
  - Damage to endothelial cells (homocysteinemia)
- Acquired thrombosis may be due to indwelling catheters, vasculitis, sepsis, immobilization, nephrotic syndrome, coagulopathy, trauma, infection, surgery, inflammatory bowel disease, oral contraceptive agents, and pregnancy.
- Venous thromboses cause warm, swollen, tender, or purplish discolored extremities; arterial thromboses cause painful, pale, and poorly perfused extremities.
  - Venous thrombosis can be detected noninvasively by ultrasound Doppler flow compression studies. The gold standard for diagnosis is venogram. Pulmonary embolism is detected by spiral computed tomography scan of the chest. Cerebral sinus venous thrombosis is often diagnosed by magnetic resonance venography.
- Therapy of thrombotic disorders usually initially involves unfractionated or low molecular weight heparin followed by longer term anticoagulation with warfarin or other oral anticoagulants.

CHAPTER 153

Blood Component Therapy

- Transfusion of RBCs, platelets, plasma, cryoprecipitate, and granulocytes can be lifesaving or life sustaining.
- Packed RBCs are used to treat anemia to increase oxygen-carrying capacity.
- Long-term complications of transfusions include:
  - Graft versus host disease
  - Infectious diseases such as hepatitis B (<1:1,000,000 units) and C (1:2,000,000 units), HIV (<1:2,000,000 units), malaria, syphilis, babesiosis, brucellosis, and Chagas disease.
- Patients who are chronically transfused are prone to developing iron overload and alloimmunization to RBCs and platelets.

SECTION 21

ONCOLOGY

Sarah P. Supples | Thomas W. McLean

CHAPTER 154

Oncology Assessment

Childhood cancer is rare; only about 1% of new cancer cases in the United States occur among children younger than 19 years of age, yet cancer is the leading cause of disease-related death in children aged 1–14 years. Acute leukemia is the most common childhood cancer, followed by central nervous system (CNS) tumors, lymphomas, sarcomas of soft tissue and bone, and germ cell and gonadal tumors (Fig. 154.1). There is wide variability in the age-specific incidence of childhood cancers. Embryonal tumors, such as neuroblastoma and retinoblastoma, peak during the first 2 years of life; acute lymphoblastic leukemia peaks during early childhood (ages 2–4 years); osteosarcoma peaks during adolescence; and Hodgkin lymphoma peaks during late adolescence and young adulthood (Fig. 154.2). The overall incidence of cancer among White children is higher than in other ethnic groups and is approximately 40% higher than in Black children in the United States.

HISTORY

Signs and symptoms of childhood cancer are often nonspecific. Most children with fever, fatigue, weight loss, or limp do not have cancer, yet each of these symptoms may be a manifestation of an underlying malignancy. Uncommonly, a child with cancer will have no symptoms at all. An abdominal mass may be palpated on routine examination, or a complete blood count (CBC) may be unexpectedly abnormal.

It is important to explore quality, duration, location, severity, and precipitating events of the chief complaint. A prominent lymph node that does not resolve (with or without antibiotics) may warrant further evaluation with imaging and/or a biopsy. A limp that does not improve within 1–2 weeks should prompt a CBC and a radiograph. Fever, night sweats, or weight loss should raise the concern for malignancy. In addition, it is important to obtain the birth history, medical and surgical history, growth history, developmental history, family history, and social history. Variants in cancer-predisposing genes (such as *TP53*) are found in approximately 9% of children and adolescents with cancer, even though family history in most patients does not predict an underlying predisposition syndrome. If known to have a genetic susceptibility to cancer, the child should be screened appropriately (Table 154.1).

PHYSICAL EXAMINATION

Growth parameters and vital signs are important to obtain in all patients. Pulse oximetry should be obtained if respiratory symptoms are present. The general appearance of the patient should be noted, along with signs of pain, cachexia, pallor, and respiratory distress. Palpable masses should be measured, if possible. Lymphadenopathy and organomegaly, if present, should be quantified. A thorough examination of the skin may reveal rashes, bruises, and petechiae. A genitourinary exam is important in any patient with unexplained findings. Careful neurologic and ophthalmologic examinations are crucial if headache or vomiting is present as most patients with CNS tumors have abnormal neurologic examinations.

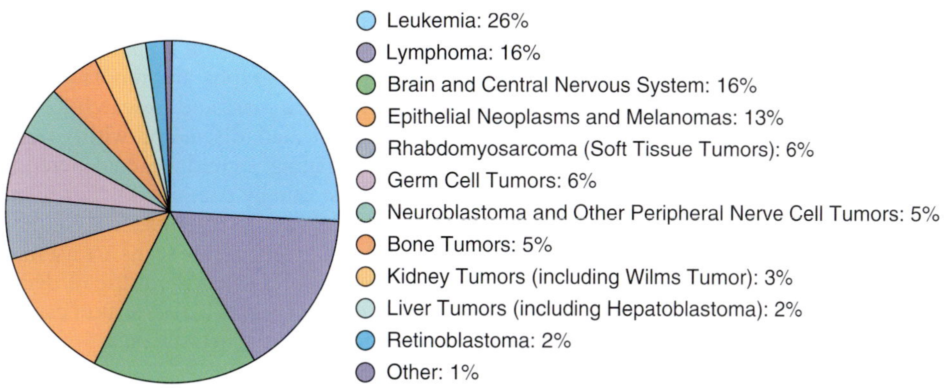

FIGURE 154.1 Number of childhood cancer diagnoses per year, ages 0–19. (Source: NCCR Explorer: An interactive website for NCCR cancer statistics. National Cancer Institute. Accessed at nccrexplorer.ccdi.cancer.gov. Years 2015–2019, by cancer site, both sexes, all backgrounds, ages <20.)

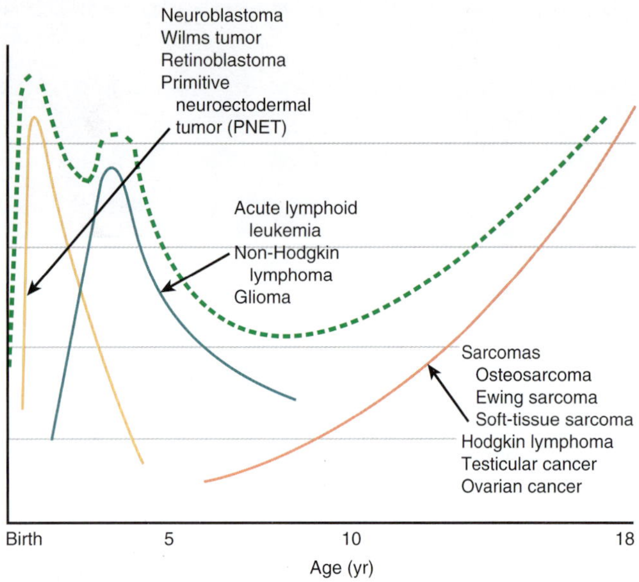

FIGURE 154.2 Incidence of the most common types of cancer in children by age. The cumulative incidence is shown as a *dashed line*. (Courtesy Archie Bleyer, MD.)

COMMON MANIFESTATIONS

The most common manifestations of childhood cancer are fatigue, anorexia, malaise, pain, fever, abnormal lump or mass, pallor, bruising, petechiae, bleeding, headache, vomiting, visual changes, weight loss, and night sweats (Table 154.2). Lymphadenopathy and organomegaly are common in leukemia, particularly with T-cell acute lymphoblastic leukemia or lymphoma. Patients with solid tumors often have a palpable mass. Children with retinoblastoma may have leukocoria or absence of the red reflex (which may be seen on a photograph). Other signs and symptoms of malignancy include limp, cough, dyspnea, cranial nerve palsies, and papilledema. In general, malignant masses are large/growing, firm, fixed, and nontender; masses that are infectious or inflammatory are relatively smaller/stable in size, softer, mobile, and tender to palpation.

DIFFERENTIAL DIAGNOSIS

Distinguishing a malignant process from another disease can be difficult. Ultimately, a tissue diagnosis (from bone marrow or solid tumor biopsy) with pathologic confirmation is required to confirm a diagnosis of cancer. Infection commonly masquerades as a potential malignancy. Epstein-Barr virus, cytomegalovirus, HIV, and mycobacterial infections can mimic leukemia or lymphoma by causing fever, night sweats, lymphadenopathy, organomegaly, weight loss, and abnormal blood counts. Trauma may produce swelling that can mimic solid tumors. Immune thrombocytopenia and iron deficiency can produce thrombocytopenia and anemia, respectively. Immune deficiencies or irregularities (such as autoimmune hemolytic anemia, autoimmune neutropenia, or transient erythroblastopenia of childhood) can also produce cytopenias. Juvenile idiopathic arthritis, systemic lupus erythematosus, and other collagen vascular disease can cause musculoskeletal pain, anemia, or thrombocytopenia, mimicking leukemia. Benign masses are relatively common in children, including reactive adenopathy, mature germ cell tumors/hamartomas, hemangiomas or other vascular tumors, mesoblastic nephromas, and bone cysts.

INITIAL DIAGNOSTIC EVALUATION

Screening Tests

A CBC with differential and review of the peripheral blood smear is the best screening test for many pediatric malignancies. Leukopenia (with or without neutropenia), anemia, or thrombocytopenia may be present in leukemia or any cancer that invades the bone marrow (e.g., neuroblastoma, rhabdomyosarcoma, and Ewing sarcoma). Leukemia may also produce leukocytosis, usually with blasts present on the peripheral blood smear. An isolated cytopenia (neutropenia, anemia, or thrombocytopenia) widens the differential diagnosis but still could be the only abnormal laboratory finding. Of note, a patient with leukemia may also have a normal CBC. Lactate dehydrogenase and uric acid are often elevated in fast-growing tumors (leukemia or lymphoma) and occasionally in sarcomas or neuroblastoma. It is appropriate to assess electrolytes as well as kidney and liver function in the screening process. Elevated blood pressure, if confirmed by repeat measurements, should prompt a urinalysis, as should the palpation of an abdominal mass. Serum (and/or cerebrospinal fluid) α-fetoprotein (AFP) and β-human chorionic gonadotropin are screening tests (and tumor markers) for germ cell tumors. Serum AFP is also a tumor marker for hepatoblastoma. Urine homovanillic acid and vanillylmandelic acid are tumor markers for neuroblastoma.

Diagnostic Imaging

A chest x-ray (CXR) (posteroanterior and lateral) is the best screening radiographic study for a patient with suspicious lymphadenopathy, fever, and weight loss. Mediastinal masses and pleural effusions can be detected on CXR. Concerning abdominal signs or symptoms usually warrant an ultrasound or computed tomography (CT) scan. Persistent headaches or morning vomiting should prompt a CT scan or magnetic resonance imaging (MRI) of the head. For suspected bone tumors, plain radiographs are indicated and will usually reveal the lesion(s), if present, although radiographs may be normal when a bony pelvic lesion is suspected. CT or MRI should be obtained if radiographs are abnormal. Other imaging studies to delineate a mass and to search for suspected metastases are often indicated; discussion with a radiologist to ascertain the best imaging should be considered. Positron emission tomography, usually combined with CT or MRI, is useful for staging and assessing response for lymphomas and sarcomas. Metaiodobenzylguanidine scans are useful for neuroblastoma. Table 154.3 shows the general use of diagnostic imaging following confirmation of a diagnosis of cancer, assessing the primary tumor and for metastases.

TABLE 154.1 Known Risk Factors for Selected Childhood Cancers

CANCER TYPE	RISK FACTOR	COMMENTS
ALL	Ionizing radiation	Prenatal diagnostic x-ray exposure and therapeutic irradiation for cancer treatment increases risk.
	Race and ethnicity	White children have a twofold higher rate than Black children in the United States.
	Genetic conditions	Down syndrome is associated with an estimated 10- to 20-fold increased risk. Neurofibromatosis 1, Bloom syndrome, and ataxia-telangiectasia, among others, are associated with an elevated risk.
	Other	Air pollution, ancestry, increased maternal age, pesticides, and structural birth defects increase the risk of ALL.
AML	Chemotherapy and radiation therapy	Alkylating agents and epipodophyllotoxins increase risk, as does radiation therapy for other cancers.
	Genetic factors	Down syndrome and neurofibromatosis 1 are strongly associated. Familial monosomy 7 and several other genetic syndromes are also associated with increased risk of AML.
CNS tumors	Ionizing radiation to the head	Radiation therapy for one brain tumor can lead to a secondary brain tumor.
	Genetic factors	Neurofibromatosis 1 is strongly associated with optic gliomas and, to a lesser extent, with other CNS tumors. Tuberous sclerosis and several other genetic syndromes are associated with increased risk.
	Other	Air pollution, positive family history, higher birth weight, increased maternal age, and structural defects increase the risk of CNS tumors.
Hodgkin lymphoma	Family history	Monozygotic twins and siblings are at increased risk.
	Infections	Epstein-Barr virus and papillomaviruses are associated with increased risk.
Non-Hodgkin lymphoma	Immunodeficiency	Acquired and congenital immunodeficiency disorders and immunosuppressive therapy increase risk.
	Infections	Epstein-Barr virus is associated with increased risk in African countries.
Osteosarcoma	Ionizing radiation	Cancer radiation therapy and high radium exposure increase risk.
	Chemotherapy	Alkylating agents increase risk.
	Genetic factors	Increased risk is apparent with Li-Fraumeni syndrome and hereditary retinoblastoma.
Ewing sarcoma	Race and ethnicity	Incidence is about nine times higher in White children than in Black children in the U.S.
Neuroblastoma	Genetic factors	Chromosome 6p22 variants and pathogenic variants in the *ALK* and *PHOX* genes are associated with increased risk.
Retinoblastoma	Genetic factors	Pathogenic variants in the *Rb* gene on chromosome 14
Wilms tumor	Congenital anomalies	Aniridia, Beckwith-Wiedemann syndrome, and other congenital and genetic conditions are associated with increased risk.
Renal medullary carcinoma	Sickle cell trait	Etiology is unknown.
Rhabdomyosarcoma	Congenital anomalies and genetic conditions	Li-Fraumeni syndrome and neurofibromatosis 1 are associated with increased risk.
Hepatoblastoma	Prematurity	Etiology is unknown.
	Genetic factors	Beckwith-Wiedemann syndrome, hemihypertrophy, Gardner syndrome, and familial adenomatous polyposis are associated with increased risk.
Hepatocellular carcinoma	Infections	Hepatitis B virus infection increases risk.
Malignant germ cell tumors	Cryptorchidism	Cryptorchidism is a risk factor for testicular germ cell tumors.

ALL, Acute lymphoid leukemia; *AML*, acute myeloid leukemia; *CNS*, central nervous system.
Modified from Scheurer ME, Lupo PL, Schuz J, Spector LG. Epidemiology of childhood cancer. In: Pizzo and Poplack's Pediatric Oncology. *8th ed. Philadelphia: Wolters Kluwer; 2021:11.*

TABLE 154.2 Common Manifestations of Childhood Malignancies

SIGN/SYMPTOM	SIGNIFICANCE	EXAMPLE
HEMATOLOGIC		
Pallor, anemia	Bone marrow infiltration	Leukemia, neuroblastoma
Petechiae, thrombocytopenia	Bone marrow infiltration	Leukemia, neuroblastoma
Fever, neutropenia	Bone marrow infiltration	Leukemia, neuroblastoma
SYSTEMIC		
Bone pain, limp, arthralgia	Primary bone tumor, metastasis to bone	Osteosarcoma, Ewing sarcoma, rhabdomyosarcoma, leukemia, neuroblastoma
Fever of unknown origin, weight loss, night sweats	Lymphoreticular malignancy	Hodgkin or non-Hodgkin lymphoma
Painless lymphadenopathy (especially in the cervical region)	Lymphoreticular malignancy, metastatic solid tumor	Leukemia, Hodgkin and non-Hodgkin lymphoma, Burkitt lymphoma, nasopharyngeal carcinoma, thyroid carcinoma
Cutaneous lesion	Primary or metastatic disease	Neuroblastoma, leukemia, lymphoma, Langerhans cell histiocytosis, melanoma
Abdominal mass	Abdominal/pelvic organ	Neuroblastoma, Wilms tumor, Burkitt lymphoma, hepatoblastoma, germ cell tumor
Hypertension	Sympathetic nervous system tumor	Wilms tumor, neuroblastoma, pheochromocytoma
Diarrhea	Vasoactive intestinal polypeptide	Neuroblastoma
Soft tissue mass	Local or metastatic tumor	Ewing sarcoma, osteosarcoma, neuroblastoma, rhabdomyosarcoma, germ cell tumor, thyroid carcinoma
Diabetes insipidus, galactorrhea, poor growth	Neuroendocrine involvement of hypothalamus or pituitary gland	Germ cell tumor, adenoma, craniopharyngioma, prolactinoma, Langerhans cell histiocytosis
Emesis, visual disturbances, ataxia, headache, papilledema, cranial nerve palsies	Increased intracranial pressure	Primary brain tumor; metastasis
OPHTHALMOLOGIC		
Leukocoria	White pupil	Retinoblastoma
Periorbital ecchymosis	Metastasis	Neuroblastoma
Miosis, ptosis, heterochromia	Horner syndrome: compression of cervical sympathetic nerves	Neuroblastoma
Opsomyoclonus, ataxia	Paraneoplastic/immune	Neuroblastoma
Exophthalmos, proptosis	Orbital tumor	Rhabdomyosarcoma, neuroblastoma, lymphoma
THORACIC		
Anterior mediastinal mass	Cough, stridor, shortness of breath, pneumonia, tracheal-bronchial compression	Germ cell tumor, T-cell lymphoma/leukemia, Hodgkin disease, primary mediastinal large B-cell lymphoma
Posterior mediastinal mass	Vertebral or nerve root compression; dysphagia	Neuroblastoma, ganglioneuroblastoma, ganglioneuroma

TABLE 154.3 Baseline Work-Up for Common Pediatric Malignancies to Assess Primary Tumor and Potential Metastases*

MALIGNANCY	BMA/BX	CXR	CT SCAN	MRI	BONE SCAN, OR PET-CT SCAN	CSF ANALYSIS	MARKER(S)	OTHER
Leukemia	Yes	Yes	—	—	—	Yes	—	—
Non-Hodgkin lymphoma	Yes	Yes	Yes	—	Yes	Yes	—	—
Hodgkin lymphoma	Yes	Yes	Yes	—	Yes	—	—	—
CNS tumors	—	—	—	Yes	—	Yes	—	—
Neuroblastoma	Yes	—	Yes	—	—	—	VMA, HVA	mIBG scan
Wilms tumor	—	Yes	Yes	—	—	—	—	—
Rhabdomyosarcoma	Yes	Yes	Yes	—	Yes	Yes, for parameningeal tumors only	—	—

(Continued)

TABLE 154.3 Baseline Work-Up for Common Pediatric Malignancies to Assess Primary Tumor and Potential Metastases*—cont'd

MALIGNANCY	BMA/BX	CXR	CT SCAN	MRI	BONE SCAN, OR PET-CT SCAN	CSF ANALYSIS	MARKER(S)	OTHER
Osteosarcoma	—	Yes	Yes (chest)	Yes (primary)	Yes	—	—	—
Ewing sarcoma	Yes	Yes	Yes (chest)	Yes (primary)	Yes	—	—	—
Germ cell tumors	—	Yes	Yes	—	—	—	AFP, β-hCG	Consider brain MRI
Liver tumors	—	Yes	Yes	—	—	—	AFP	
Retinoblastoma	±	—	Yes, if MRI not available	Yes (brain)	±	Yes	—	Rb gene analysis

*Individual cases may require additional studies.
AFP, α-fetoprotein; *β-HCG*, β-human chorionic gonadotropin; *BMA/bx*, bone marrow aspirate/biopsy; *CNS*, central nervous system; *CSF*, cerebrospinal fluid; *CT*, computed tomography; *CXR*, chest x-ray; *HVA*, homovanillic acid; *mIBG*, metaiodobenzylguanidine; *MRI*, magnetic resonance imaging; *PET*, positron emission tomography; *Rb*, retinoblastoma; *VMA*, vanillylmandelic acid.

PEARLS FOR PRACTITIONERS

See Oncology: Pearls for Practitioners at the end of this section.

REVIEW QUESTIONS

Available online.

CHAPTER 155

Principles of Cancer Treatment

The overarching goal of pediatric oncology is to cure all patients with minimal toxicity. The prognosis for children with cancer has improved dramatically in the past 60 years, with long-term survival improving from about 20% to greater than 80%. Treatment for children with cancer is often multimodal and may involve surgery, radiation therapy, chemotherapy, and immunotherapy. Surgery and radiation are generally local treatment modalities (an exception is total body irradiation as part of a bone marrow or stem cell transplant); chemotherapy and immunotherapy have both local and systemic effects.

Primary prevention strategies for most pediatric malignancies are unknown. Two exceptions are the use of hepatitis B vaccine to lower the rates of hepatocellular carcinoma and the use of human papillomavirus vaccine to reduce the risk of genitourinary and oropharyngeal cancers. Unlike adult malignancies, childhood malignancies are not associated with tobacco or alcohol use, dietary factors, or sun exposure. Treatment with certain chemotherapy agents and radiation therapy increases the rate of secondary malignancies. Secondary prevention may be accomplished by screening the at-risk child (e.g., a child with Beckwith-Wiedemann syndrome or the twin of a patient with leukemia), but these opportunities are rare.

ONCOLOGIC EMERGENCIES

Adverse effects of tumors and treatments may result in oncologic emergencies in pediatric patients (Table 155.1). Mediastinal masses from lymphoma can cause life-threatening airway obstruction. Cancers with a large tumor burden (e.g., lymphoma, leukemia) may adversely affect kidney function from tubular deposition of uric acid crystals. Allopurinol or rasburicase can be administered before chemotherapy to minimize this effect.

A common metabolic emergency is **tumor lysis syndrome**, often seen in treatment of leukemia and lymphoma. Large amounts of phosphate, potassium, and uric acid are released into the circulation from lysed cells. Other oncologic emergencies include bleeding, acute infections, and spinal cord compression with neurologic compromise.

SURGERY

Appropriate imaging (usually CT or MRI) for solid tumors presenting as a palpable mass or mass-related symptoms (pain, respiratory distress, intestinal obstruction) should be obtained and followed by resection (when possible) or biopsy (if complete resection is not feasible or indicated). Pediatric lymphomas are chemosensitive and rarely require complete surgical resection.

It is crucial to determine the amount of tissue required and the appropriate distribution of the tissue for testing so that all necessary studies are performed. As targeted therapies become more available, genetic testing of tumor tissue (i.e., next-generation sequencing of specific genes) is becoming standard practice. A general oncologic surgery principle is to resect not just the tumor but also, in most cases, a surrounding margin of normal tissue to ensure the entire tumor has been resected. A central line (usually a port-a-cath) is often inserted at the time of tumor biopsy.

CHEMOTHERAPY

As most pediatric solid tumors have a high risk for micrometastatic disease at the time of diagnosis, chemotherapy is used in almost all cases (Table 155.2). Exceptions include low-stage neuroblastoma and Wilms tumor (particularly in infants), low-grade central nervous system (CNS) tumors that have been completely excised, and small (≤5 cm) nonrhabdomyosarcoma soft tissue sarcomas that have been completely

TABLE 155.1 Oncologic Emergencies

CONDITION	MANIFESTATIONS	ETIOLOGY	MALIGNANCY	TREATMENT
METABOLIC				
Hyperuricemia	Uric acid nephropathy, kidney insufficiency or failure	Tumor lysis syndrome	Lymphoma, leukemia	Allopurinol, hydration, rasburicase
Hyperkalemia	Arrhythmias	Tumor lysis syndrome	Lymphoma, leukemia	Kayexalate; sodium bicarbonate, glucose plus insulin
Hyperphosphatemia	Kidney insufficiency, hypocalcemic tetany; metastatic calcification, photophobia, pruritus	Tumor lysis syndrome	Lymphoma, leukemia	Hydration, diuresis; oral aluminum hydroxide to bind phosphate
Hypercalcemia	Anorexia, nausea, polyuria, pancreatitis, gastric ulcers; prolonged PR/shortened QT interval	Bone resorption; ectopic parathyroid-hormone related protein, vitamin D, or prostaglandins	Metastasis to bone, rhabdomyosarcoma	Hydration and furosemide diuresis; corticosteroids; mithramycin; calcitonin, bisphosphonates
HEMATOLOGIC				
Anemia	Pallor, weakness, heart failure	Bone marrow suppression or infiltration; blood loss	Any with chemotherapy	Packed red blood cell transfusion
Thrombocytopenia	Petechiae, hemorrhage	Bone marrow suppression or infiltration	Any with chemotherapy	Platelet transfusion
Disseminated intravascular coagulation	Shock, hemorrhage	Sepsis, hypotension, tumor factors	Promyelocytic leukemia, others	Fresh frozen plasma, cryoprecipitate, platelets, treat underlying cause
Neutropenia	Infection	Bone marrow suppression or infiltration	Any with chemotherapy	If patient is febrile, administer broad-spectrum antibiotics, consider filgrastim (G-CSF)
Hyperleukocytosis (WBC ≥100,000/mm^3)	Hemorrhage, thrombosis; pulmonary infiltrates, hypoxia; tumor lysis syndrome	Leukostasis; vascular occlusion	Leukemia	Hydration; chemotherapy; possibly leukapheresis
Graft versus host disease	Dermatitis, diarrhea, hepatitis	Immunosuppression and nonirradiated blood products; bone marrow transplantation	Any with immunosuppression	Corticosteroids; cyclosporine; methotrexate; tacrolimus; mycophenolate mofetil; antithymocyte globulin
SPACE-OCCUPYING LESIONS				
Spinal cord compression	Back pain, motor and sensory deficits	Invasion of spinal canal by primary tumor or metastases	Neuroblastoma, medulloblastoma	MRI for diagnosis; corticosteroids; radiation therapy; laminectomy; chemotherapy
Increased intracranial pressure	Headache, confusion, coma, emesis, headache, hypertension, bradycardia, seizures, papilledema, hydrocephalus; cranial nerve III and VI palsies	Primary or metastatic brain tumor	Astrocytoma, medulloblastoma, others; neuroblastoma	CT or MRI for diagnosis; corticosteroids; ventriculoperitoneal shunt; radiation therapy; chemotherapy
Superior vena cava syndrome	Distended neck veins, plethora, edema of head and neck, cyanosis, proptosis; Horner syndrome	Superior mediastinal mass	Lymphoma	Chemotherapy; radiation therapy
Tracheal compression	Respiratory distress	Mediastinal mass compressing trachea	Lymphoma	Radiation therapy, corticosteroids, chemotherapy

CT, Computed tomography; *G-CSF*, granulocyte colony–stimulating factor; *MRI*, magnetic resonance imaging; *WBC*, white blood cell.

TABLE 155.2 Cancer Chemotherapy

DRUG	ACTION	INDICATION	ACUTE TOXICITY*
Methotrexate	Folic acid antagonist; inhibits dihydrofolate reductase	ALL, lymphoma, medulloblastoma, osteosarcoma	Myelosuppression (nadir 7–10 days), mucositis, dermatitis, hepatitis, kidney and CNS effects with high-dose administration; prevent with hydration and leucovorin, monitor levels
6-Mercaptopurine	Purine analog	ALL	Myelosuppression; hepatitis; mucositis; allopurinol increases toxicity
Ara-C	Pyrimidine analog; inhibits DNA polymerase	ALL, AML, lymphoma	Myelosuppression, conjunctivitis, mucositis, neurotoxicity
Cyclophosphamide	Alkylates guanine; inhibits DNA synthesis	ALL, lymphoma, sarcoma, brain tumors	Myelosuppression; hemorrhagic cystitis
Ifosfamide	Similar to cyclophosphamide	Lymphoma, Wilms tumor, sarcoma, germ cell and testicular tumors	Similar to cyclophosphamide; neurotoxicity, cardiac toxicity
Carmustine (BCNU), lomustine (CCNU)	Carbamylation of DNA; inhibits DNA synthesis	CNS tumors, lymphoma, Hodgkin lymphoma	Delayed myelosuppression (4–6 wk); pulmonary fibrosis, carcinogenic, stomatitis
Cisplatin	Inhibits DNA synthesis	Osteosarcoma, neuroblastoma, CNS tumors, germ cell tumors	Nephrotoxic; myelosuppression, ototoxicity, neurotoxicity, hemolytic uremic syndrome
Carboplatin	Inhibits DNA synthesis	Same as for cisplatin	Myelosuppression
Doxorubicin and daunorubicin	Intercalation, DNA strand breaks	ALL, AML, osteosarcoma, Ewing sarcoma, lymphoma, neuroblastoma	Cardiomyopathy, red urine, tissue necrosis on extravasation, myelosuppression, conjunctivitis, radiation dermatitis, arrhythmia
Dactinomycin	Intercalation, DNA strand breaks	Wilms tumor, rhabdomyosarcoma, Ewing sarcoma	Tissue necrosis on extravasation, myelosuppression, hepatopathy with thrombocytopenia, stomatitis
Etoposide (VP-16)	DNA strand breaks	ALL, AML, lymphoma, germ cell tumor, sarcoma	Myelosuppression, secondary leukemia, allergic reaction
Topotecan	DNA strand breaks	Neuroblastoma, rhabdomyosarcoma	Myelosuppression, diarrhea, mucositis
Vincristine	Inhibits microtubule formation	ALL, lymphoma, Wilms tumor, Hodgkin lymphoma, Ewing sarcoma, neuroblastoma, rhabdomyosarcoma, brain tumors	Local cellulitis, peripheral neuropathy, constipation, ileus, jaw pain, inappropriate ADH secretion, seizures, ptosis, minimal myelosuppression
Vinblastine	Inhibits microtubule formation	Hodgkin lymphoma, Langerhans cell histiocytosis	Local cellulitis, myelosuppression
Asparaginase	Depletion of asparagine	ALL, AML	Allergic reaction; pancreatitis, hyperglycemia, platelet dysfunction and coagulopathy, encephalopathy, stroke, thrombosis
Prednisone, dexamethasone	Direct lymphocyte cytotoxicity	ALL; Hodgkin lymphoma, lymphoma	Cushing syndrome, cataracts, diabetes, hypertension, myopathy, osteoporosis, infection, peptic ulceration, irritability, psychosis, hunger, fluid retention
Rituximab	Anti-CD20	CD20+ B-cell leukemia, lymphoma	Fever, chills, allergy
Brentuximab	Anti-CD30	CD30+ lymphomas	Myelosuppression, peripheral neuropathy, fatigue, fever
Blinatumomab	Anti-CD19 and anti-CD3	CD19+ B-lymphoblastic leukemia	Cytokine release syndrome, neurotoxicity
Dinutuximab	Anti-GD2	High-risk neuroblastoma	Neuropathic pain, hypotension, hypoxia, fever, capillary leak syndrome, hypersensitivity reactions
Imatinib	Inhibits BCR-ABL, VEGF, c-KIT kinases	Ph+ CML, ALL	Nausea, vomiting, fatigue, headache
Dasatinib	Inhibits BCR-ABL, c-KIT, and other kinases	Ph+ CML, ALL	Fluid retention, rash, nausea
Tretinoin (ATRA) and isotretinoin (CRA)	Promotes differentiation	Acute promyelocytic leukemia (ATRA); neuroblastoma (CRA)	Fever, respiratory distress, leukocytosis (ATRA); dry mouth, hair loss, pseudotumor cerebri (CRA)
Arsenic	Promotes differentiation, apoptosis	Acute promyelocytic leukemia	Transaminitis, nausea, vomiting, abdominal pain, QTc prolongation
Tisagenlecleucel	Anti-CD19 CART therapy	CD19+ refractory B-lymphoblastic leukemia	Cytokine release syndrome, hypogammaglobulinemia

*Many drugs produce nausea and vomiting during administration, and many cause alopecia with repeated doses.

ADH, Antidiuretic hormone; *ALL*, acute lymphoblastic leukemia; *AML*, acute myeloid leukemia; *Ara-C*, cytosine arabinoside; *ATRA*, all-*trans* retinoic acid; *CART*, chimeric antigen receptor T cell; *CML*, chronic myeloid leukemia; *CNS*, central nervous system; *CRA*, *cis*-retinoic acid; *Ph*, Philadelphia chromosome; *VEGF*, vascular endothelial growth factor.

excised. For patients with localized solid tumors, chemotherapy administered after removal of the primary tumor is referred to as ***adjuvant therapy*** (often called *consolidation*). Chemotherapy administered while the primary tumor is still present is referred to as ***neoadjuvant chemotherapy***, often called *induction*. Neoadjuvant chemotherapy has numerous potential benefits, including an early attack on presumed micrometastatic disease, shrinkage of the primary tumor to facilitate local control, and additional time to plan for definitive surgery.

Resistance to chemotherapeutic agents can develop quickly; combinations of chemotherapy drugs are used (as opposed to sequential single agents) to treat childhood cancer. The blood-brain barrier prevents the penetration of many chemotherapeutic drugs into the CNS; administration of chemotherapy directly into the cerebrospinal fluid (by lumbar puncture) is used for leukemia and lymphoma. Radiation therapy also circumvents the blood-brain barrier and may be used in selected cases.

RADIATION THERAPY

Radiation therapy delivers ionizing radiation to malignant cells to kill them directly or, more commonly, prevent them from dividing by interfering with DNA replication. Conventional radiation therapy uses photons, but atomic particles such as electrons, protons, and neutrons can also be used. Not all tumors are radiosensitive, and radiation therapy is not necessary in all tumors that are radiosensitive. Radiation is known to adversely affect growing children, and it is only used after careful consideration of the risks and benefits.

OTHER THERAPIES

Certain cancers can be treated with biologic response modifiers, tyrosine kinase inhibitors, or monoclonal antibodies in addition to standard treatments. **Targeted therapies** specifically target tumor cells, sparing normal host cells. Imatinib, the first tyrosine kinase inhibitor (TKI) approved by the United States Food and Drug Administration, targets the effects of the t(9;22) translocation *(BCR-ABL)* of chronic myeloid leukemia and acute lymphoblastic leukemia. Other TKIs have since been developed and approved to treat a variety of malignancies. Rituximab is a monoclonal antibody directed against the cell surface antigen CD20 expressed in some lymphomas and leukemias. Dinutuximab is an anti-GD2 monoclonal antibody used for neuroblastoma. Chimeric antigen receptor T-cell therapy (tisagenlecleucel) and bi-specific T-cell engager therapy (blinatumomab) are immunotherapies that leverage the patient's own T cells to kill CD19-positive leukemia cells.

Supportive care also plays an important role in pediatric oncology, including the use of appropriate antiemetics, antimicrobial agents, blood products, nutritional support, intensive care, pain control, psychosocial support, and integrative therapies.

ADVERSE EFFECTS

Chemotherapy is well known to cause side effects. Bone marrow suppression, immunosuppression, nausea, vomiting, and alopecia are general adverse effects of commonly used chemotherapy drugs. Each chemotherapy drug also has specific toxicities. Doxorubicin can cause cardiac damage; cisplatin can cause kidney damage and ototoxicity; cyclophosphamide and ifosfamide can cause hemorrhagic cystitis; and vincristine can cause peripheral neuropathy. Radiation therapy produces adverse effects such as mucositis, growth retardation, organ dysfunction, and the later development of secondary cancers. Significant therapy-related **late side effects** may develop in patients with pediatric cancer (Table 155.3).

TABLE 155.3 Long-Term Sequelae of Cancer Therapy

PROBLEM	ETIOLOGIC AGENT(S)
Infertility	Alkylating agents; radiation
Secondary cancers	Genetic predisposition; radiation; alkylating agents, etoposide, topoisomerase II inhibitors
Sepsis	Splenectomy
Hepatotoxicity	Methotrexate, 6-mercaptopurine; radiation
Scoliosis	Radiation
Pulmonary (fibrosis)	Radiation; bleomycin, busulfan
Cardiomyopathy	Doxorubicin, daunorubicin; radiation
Leukoencephalopathy	Cranial radiation, methotrexate
Cognition/intelligence	Cranial radiation, methotrexate
Pituitary dysfunction (growth hormone deficiency, panhypopituitarism)	Cranial radiation
Psychosocial	Stress, anxiety, death of peers; conditioned responses to chemotherapy
Thyroid dysfunction	Radiation
Osteonecrosis	Corticosteroids

PEARLS FOR PRACTITIONERS

See Oncology: Pearls for Practitioners at the end of this section.

REVIEW QUESTIONS

Available online.

CHAPTER 156

Leukemia

ETIOLOGY

The etiology of childhood leukemia is unknown and is thought to be multifactorial, with both genetics and environmental factors contributing to malignant transformation. A variety of genetic syndromes and diseases, including Down syndrome (trisomy 21), Fanconi anemia, Bloom syndrome, ataxia-telangiectasia, Wiskott-Aldrich syndrome, neurofibromatosis type 1, and rare familial leukemia syndromes can predispose children to the development of acute leukemia. Siblings of children with leukemia are also at an increased risk of developing leukemia compared to the general pediatric population. Other factors that may increase the risk of leukemia include ionizing radiation, certain chemotherapy agents (i.e., etoposide), air pollution, pesticides, increased maternal age, and some structural birth defects. Certain leukemias are associated with specific somatic pathogenic variants. For example, **chronic myeloid leukemia (CML)** and less commonly in **acute lymphoblastic leukemia (ALL)**, a translocation involving chromosomes 9 and 22 (Philadelphia [Ph] chromosome) results in a fusion gene called *BCR-ABL*, which leads to a constitutively activated tyrosine kinase that drives development of CML and Ph-positive ALL.

EPIDEMIOLOGY

ALL accounts for approximately 75% of leukemia cases in the pediatric population, followed by **acute myeloid leukemia (AML)** at approximately 20% and CML at less than 5%. Other chronic leukemias, including juvenile myelomonocytic leukemia, chronic myelomonocytic leukemia, and chronic lymphocytic leukemia, are rare in childhood. ALL is the most common childhood cancer overall, comprising 25% of cancer prior to the age of 15 years (40 per 1 million children age <15 years) and approximately 20% of cancer prior to the age of 20 years.

ALL is classified according to lymphoid lineage as either B cell or T cell. The incidence of B-lineage ALL peaks at 2–4 years of age and is slightly more common in males than in females. T-cell ALL is associated with male predominance as well as an older age of onset. In the United States, ALL is more common in White than in Black children. The incidence of AML is relatively higher in the first year of life, then drops and stabilizes until adolescence when there is a slight increase, which continues into adulthood. Males and females are equally affected by AML. Hispanic and Black children have a slightly higher incidence of AML than White children.

CLINICAL MANIFESTATIONS

Signs and symptoms of acute leukemia are related to the infiltration of leukemic cells into normal tissues, resulting in bone marrow failure (anemia, neutropenia, thrombocytopenia), leukocytosis, and/or specific tissue infiltration (lymph nodes, liver, spleen, brain, bone, skin, gingiva, testes). Common presenting symptoms are fever, pallor, petechiae and/or ecchymoses, malaise, anorexia, and musculoskeletal pain. Physical examination frequently reveals lymphadenopathy and hepatosplenomegaly. The testes and central nervous system (CNS) are common extramedullary sites for ALL involvement; neurologic symptoms or a painless enlargement of one or both testes may be seen. Patients with T-cell ALL often have high white blood cell (WBC) counts, an anterior mediastinal mass (mediastinal adenopathy and/or thymic infiltration), cervical lymphadenopathy, hepatosplenomegaly, and CNS involvement. In patients with AML, extramedullary soft tissue tumors may be found in various sites.

LABORATORY AND IMAGING STUDIES

The diagnosis of acute leukemia is confirmed by finding immature blast cells on either the peripheral blood smear, bone marrow aspirate, or both. Most patients have abnormal blood counts; anemia and thrombocytopenia are common. The WBC count may be low, normal, or high; 10% to 20% of patients have a WBC count of 100,000/mm^3 or higher (hyperleukocytosis) at presentation. Definitive diagnosis requires the evaluation of cell surface markers (immunophenotype) by flow cytometry. Cytogenetic analysis should be done in all cases of acute leukemia because recurring cytogenetic abnormalities have prognostic implications and are used in combination with other risk factors to assign therapy to optimize outcome. In B-lineage ALL, the t(12;21) translocation (*ETV6/RUNX1* fusion) is the most common (approximately 20% of all cases) and is associated with a favorable prognosis when combined with other low-risk features. The t(9;22) translocation (Ph chromosome) occurs in 3% of cases and has a worse prognosis. Much like in CML, the use of tyrosine kinase inhibitors (TKIs) in Ph-positive ALL has resulted in significant improvement in outcomes. Ph-like ALL exhibits a similar genotype (by gene expression profiling) to Ph+ ALL but lacks the t(9;22) translocation. The use of TKIs in Ph-like ALL is under investigation. The t(4;11) translocation (and other translocations involving the *KMT2A* gene on chromosome 11) often occurs in infant ALL and patients with secondary AML (often in patients that have been exposed to etoposide) and is associated with a poor prognosis. Fluorescent in situ hybridization, polymerase chain reaction, DNA microarray techniques, and/or next-generation sequencing are utilized in most cases of leukemia because some DNA abnormalities may not be apparent on routine karyotypes. A lumbar puncture should always be performed at the time of diagnosis to evaluate the possibility of CNS involvement. A chest x-ray should be obtained in all patients to assess for an anterior mediastinal mass. Electrolytes (particularly potassium, phosphorus, and calcium), uric acid, and kidney function should be monitored in all patients to assess and treat patients at risk for tumor lysis syndrome.

DIFFERENTIAL DIAGNOSIS

The differential diagnoses of acute leukemia include nonmalignant and malignant diseases. Acute infection is probably the most common mimicker of acute leukemia, particularly Epstein-Barr virus. Other infections (cytomegalovirus, other viruses, mycobacteria) also can produce signs and symptoms common to leukemia. Noninfectious considerations include aplastic anemia, histiocytosis, juvenile idiopathic arthritis, systemic lupus erythematosus, immune thrombocytopenia, and congenital or acquired conditions that result in neutropenia or anemia. Several malignant diagnoses also can mimic leukemia, including neuroblastoma, rhabdomyosarcoma, and Ewing sarcoma. Newborns with trisomy 21 may have a condition known as *transient myeloproliferative disorder*, which produces elevated WBC counts with peripheral blasts, anemia, and thrombocytopenia. It usually resolves with supportive care only, but these children have a significantly increased risk (30%) of developing acute leukemia (ALL or AML) within the next few months to years of life.

TREATMENT

Patients with B-lineage ALL generally receive three- or four-agent induction chemotherapy based on their age at diagnosis (1–9 years is favorable) and highest pretreatment WBC count (<50,000/mm^3 is favorable). All patients with T-cell ALL receive a four-agent induction. Standard-risk patients receive vincristine, corticosteroids, and pegylated asparaginase over 4 weeks; high-risk patients also receive an anthracycline like daunorubicin. Intrathecal therapy with cytarabine or methotrexate is given to prophylax against or treat existing CNS leukemia. Following induction therapy, patients undergo an end-of-induction bone marrow evaluation to assess for remission (nearly all patients with ALL achieve a morphologic remission). The intensity of postinduction therapy relies on risk adaptation, utilizing a variety of prognostic tools including genetic evaluation of the leukemia cells and minimal residual disease assessment. Patients with ALL and CNS involvement detected at diagnosis require more intensive CNS-directed treatment including intrathecal therapy and, in rare cases, cranial radiation therapy. After a 1-month induction, the typical phases of therapy include consolidation (2 months), delayed intensification (2 months), and maintenance (2+ years), for a total duration of therapy of about 2.5 years. The treatment of AML is divided into three general types including (1) acute promyelocytic leukemia with a t(15;17) translocation *(PML-RARA)* that relies heavily on all-trans retinoic acid and arsenic trioxide, (2) myeloid leukemias of Down syndrome in which less intensive therapy is administered, and (3) AML that parallels the risk and biologic features most commonly seen in adult AML resulting in the need for intensive therapy and, in select high-risk patients, the use of stem cell transplantation after receiving upfront intensive chemotherapy. Most pediatric patients with AML have the latter form requiring four or five cycles of intensive cytarabine-based chemotherapy. Much like ALL, risk adaptive therapy is based on cytogenetics and response to therapy. Additionally, the availability of an HLA-matched donor (ideally an HLA-matched sibling) may determine the use of stem cell transplantation in first remission. Unlike ALL, there is little evidence that low-dose continuation therapy is helpful in AML (with the exception of acute promyelocytic leukemia).

COMPLICATIONS

Major short-term complications associated with the treatment of leukemia result from bone marrow suppression caused by chemotherapy. Patients may have bleeding and significant anemia that necessitates transfusion of platelets and red blood cells. The development of neutropenia predisposes patients to a significant risk of both bacterial and fungal infections. Cell-mediated immunosuppression increases the risk of *Pneumocystis jirovecii* pneumonia; prophylaxis is recommended with oral trimethoprim-sulfamethoxazole. Prophylaxis with antibiotics and antifungal agents has become standard practice in patients with AML and high-risk ALL. Long-term sequelae of therapy are less common than in previous treatment eras but continue to be a priority for prevention, recognition, and treatment. These sequelae include neurocognitive impairment, cardiac dysfunction, osteonecrosis, infertility, secondary malignant neoplasms, and psychosocial problems (see Table 155.3).

TABLE 156.1 General Prognostic Factors in Acute Lymphoblastic Leukemia

FACTOR	FAVORABLE (LOWER RISK)	UNFAVORABLE (HIGHER RISK)
Age	1–9.99 yr	<1 or ≥10 yr
Background and ethnicity	White, Asian/ Pacific Islanders	Black, Hispanic, Native American
Initial WBC count	<50,000/mm^3	≥50,000/mm^3
CNS disease at diagnosis	Absent	Present
Immunophenotype	B lineage	T cell
Ploidy (number of chromosomes)	Hyperdiploidy (>50)	Hypodiploidy (<44)
Genetics	t(12;21), trisomies of chromosomes 4, 10, and 17	t(4;11), t(9;22), Ph-like, iamp21, *IKZF1* pathogenic variants
Minimal residual disease after induction therapy	Negative	Positive

CNS, Central nervous system; *WBC*, white blood cell.

PROGNOSIS

Patients with ALL are classified into prognostic risk groups based on age, initial WBC count, genetic characteristics, extramedullary involvement at diagnosis (testicular and/or CNS involvement), and response to induction therapy using minimal residual disease techniques. Risk stratification factors can be seen in Table 156.1; the general categories are low, average, high, and very high risk. The overall cure rate for childhood B-lineage ALL is approximately 90%. Relapse of ALL occurs most commonly in the bone marrow but can involve other extramedullary sites, such as the CNS or testicles. Relapse therapy relies on treatment options based on the timing and location of relapse as well as response to initial reinduction with chemotherapy. Thereafter, treatment options include additional chemotherapy combined with immunotherapy (blinatumomab), stem cell transplantation, and chimeric antigen receptor T-cell therapy (tisagenlecleucel). The current overall cure rate for childhood AML is approximately 65%. The prognosis for relapsed AML is poor, particularly in patients who have already received a stem cell transplant.

PEARLS FOR PRACTITIONERS

See Oncology: Pearls for Practitioners at the end of this section.

REVIEW QUESTIONS

Available online.

CHAPTER 157 Lymphoma

ETIOLOGY

Lymphomas are malignancies of lymphoid tissues and are the third most common malignancy in childhood, behind leukemias and central nervous system (CNS) tumors. There are two major types of lymphoma: **Hodgkin lymphoma (HL)** and **non-Hodgkin lymphoma (NHL)**. The etiology of lymphoma is multifactorial. Both congenital and acquired immunodeficiencies are more commonly associated with NHL; the Epstein-Barr virus (EBV) has been associated with both HL and NHL.

Almost all cases of NHL in childhood are diffuse, highly malignant, and show little differentiation. NHL has three main histologic subtypes: small noncleaved cell (Burkitt lymphoma [BL]), lymphoblastic, and large cell. For simplicity, these may be regarded as *B cell*, *T cell*, and *large cell* (which may be of B-cell or T-cell origin) (Table 157.1). Chromosomal translocations can result in unregulated/increased expression of an oncogene that drives malignant transformation. In BL, translocations occurring between chromosome 8 (*c-myc* oncogene) and the immunoglobulin gene locus (found on chromosome 2, 14, or 22) lead to overexpression of *c-myc*, causing malignant transformation.

EPIDEMIOLOGY

The incidence of HL has a bimodal distribution with peaks in the adolescent/young adult years and again after age 50; it is rarely seen in children younger than 5 years of age. In children, males are affected more commonly than females; in adolescents, the gender ratio is approximately equal. The incidence of NHL increases with age. It is twice as common in White children as in Black children and has a male predominance. NHL has been described in association with congenital or acquired immunodeficiency states and after transplantation (organ or stem cell). BL commonly is divided into two forms: a sporadic form commonly seen in North America and an endemic form commonly seen in Africa, which has a strong association with EBV.

CLINICAL MANIFESTATIONS

The most common clinical presentation of HL is painless, firm lymphadenopathy often confined to one or two contiguous lymph node areas (most commonly the cervical and supraclavicular nodes). Mediastinal lymphadenopathy producing cough or shortness of breath is a frequent presenting symptom. The presence of one of three **B symptoms** has adverse prognostic value: fever (>38°C for 3 consecutive days), drenching night sweats, and unintentional weight loss of 10% or more within 6 months of diagnosis.

The sporadic (North American) form of BL more commonly has an abdominal presentation (usually with pain); the endemic (African) form frequently presents with tumors of the head and neck. The anterior mediastinum and cervical nodes are the usual primary sites for T-cell lymphomas. These lymphomas may cause airway or superior vena cava obstruction, pleural effusion, or both.

The diagnosis of lymphoma is established through biopsy of an involved lymph node. Systemic symptoms such as fever and weight loss may be present, particularly in patients with anaplastic large cell lymphoma, which can be insidious in onset. If the bone marrow contains 20% or greater blasts, the disease is classified as acute lymphoblastic leukemia (ALL; either B-lineage ALL, T-cell ALL, or Burkitt leukemia). This distinction makes little prognostic or therapeutic difference because they all require aggressive, systemic therapy in addition to CNS-directed therapy.

LABORATORY/IMAGING STUDIES

Patients suspected to have lymphoma should have a CBC, erythrocyte sedimentation rate, and measurement of serum electrolytes (particularly potassium, phosphorus, and calcium), lactate dehydrogenase, and uric acid as well as a chest x-ray to assess for a mediastinal mass (Fig. 157.1). The diagnosis ultimately requires a pathologic confirmation from tissue or fluid sampling (pleural or peritoneal fluid). For staging purposes, a bone marrow evaluation, lumbar puncture, and positron emission tomography-computed tomography (PET-CT) scan are indicated to assess extent of disease. The pathologic hallmark of classic HL is the identification of **Reed-Sternberg cells**. Histopathologic subtypes in childhood HL are the same as those reported in adults. Nodular sclerosis is the most common subtype in adolescents/young adults; mixed cellularity subtypes and nodular lymphocyte predominant are more common in younger children. Staging of HL is according to the Ann Arbor system; classification is based on where lymph node involvement is located. About half of pediatric patients will have stage II involvement at presentation (I, 19%; II, 49%; III, 19%; IV, 13%), and about 39% will have B symptoms.

DIFFERENTIAL DIAGNOSIS

The differential diagnoses for lymphomas in children include leukemia, rhabdomyosarcoma, nasopharyngeal carcinoma,

TABLE 157.1 Subtypes of Non-Hodgkin Lymphoma in Children

HISTOLOGIC CATEGORY	IMMUNOPHENOTYPE	USUAL PRIMARY SITE	MOST COMMON TRANSLOCATION(S)
Small noncleaved (Burkitt lymphoma)	Mature B cell (surface immunoglobulin present)	Abdomen (sporadic form) Head and neck (endemic form)	t(8;14)(q24;q32) t(2;8)(p11;q24) t(8;22)(q24;q11)
Lymphoblastic	T cell (rarely pre–B cell)	Neck and/or anterior mediastinum	Many
Large cell	T cell, B cell, or indeterminate	Lymph nodes, skin, soft tissue, bone	t(2;5)(p23;q35)

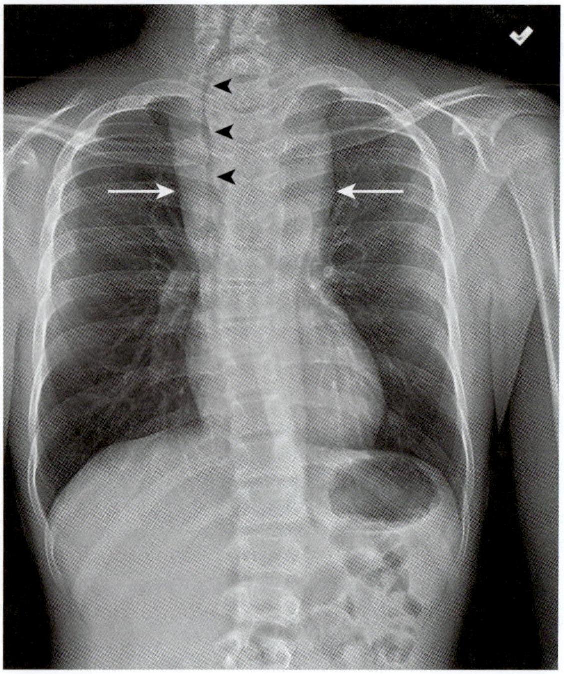

FIGURE 157.1 Chest x-ray of a 15-year-old male demonstrating a large superior anterior mediastinal mass *(large white arrows)* compressing the trachea and deviating it rightward *(black arrowheads)*. Biopsy revealed non-Hodgkin lymphoma.

germ cell tumors, and thymomas. Nonmalignant diagnoses include infectious mononucleosis (EBV infection), branchial cleft and thyroglossal duct cysts, cat scratch disease *(Bartonella henselae)*, bacterial or viral lymphadenitis, mycobacterial infection, toxoplasmosis, and even tinea capitis, all of which can produce significant lymphadenopathy that can mimic lymphoma. Patients with acute abdominal pain from BL may be misdiagnosed as having appendicitis.

TREATMENT

Pediatric HL is highly curable even with advanced disease, with overall survival rates exceeding 90%. Risk adaptive therapy using stage, the presence of bulky disease, the presence or absence of B symptoms, serum albumin, and response to upfront chemotherapy has been employed to reduce the need for radiation therapy and excess chemotherapy. Multiagent chemotherapy usually consists of drugs such as doxorubicin, vincristine, vinblastine, etoposide, prednisone, cyclophosphamide, and brentuximab (a monoclonal antibody directed against CD30). The checkpoint inhibitor antibodies nivolumab and pembrolizumab are also safe and effective in treating pediatric classic HL and are becoming first-line therapies for selected patients. In general, four to six courses of chemotherapy are given. Response to therapy is usually assessed after two courses of chemotherapy, relying on a PET-CT scan to determine the need for subsequent chemotherapy (slow response obligates more aggressive chemotherapy) as well as the need for radiation therapy. Of interest, patients with stage I (single node with complete resection) nodular lymphocyte predominant HL will be cured with surgery alone 80% of the time.

Distant, noncontiguous metastases are common in childhood NHL. Systemic chemotherapy should be administered to virtually all children with NHL, although patients with stage I pediatric-type follicular lymphoma can be cured with surgery alone. B-cell and T-cell lymphoblastic lymphoma and anaplastic large cell lymphoma generally are treated with aggressive multidrug regimens similar to the regimens used in ALL. Surgery and radiation therapy are not commonly used because NHL is rarely localized and is highly sensitive to chemotherapy. BL and diffuse large B-cell lymphomas (even high stage) are highly curable with rituximab, cyclophosphamide, vincristine, prednisolone, doxorubicin, and methotrexate.

COMPLICATIONS

The short-term complications from the treatment of lymphoma are similar to other pediatric malignancies, including immunosuppression, related sequelae from myelosuppression, nausea, vomiting, and alopecia. Late adverse effects include second malignant neoplasms (acute myeloid leukemia or myelodysplasia, thyroid malignancies, and breast cancer), hypothyroidism, impaired soft tissue and bone growth, and cardiac dysfunction.

PROGNOSIS

Children and adolescents with HL are classified as low, intermediate, or high risk according to stage, nodal bulk, the presence of B symptoms, and the serum albumin at presentation. The prognosis is generally excellent, with overall survival exceeding 90% for most patients (approaching 100% for low-risk patients). The overall 3-year survival rates for B-cell, T-cell, and large cell NHL are 70% to 90%.

PEARLS FOR PRACTITIONERS

See Oncology: Pearls for Practitioners at the end of this section.

REVIEW QUESTIONS

Available online.

CHAPTER 158

Central Nervous System Tumors

ETIOLOGY

Most central nervous system (CNS) tumors in pediatric patients are **primary tumors** that originate in the CNS and include gliomas (especially low-grade gliomas) and embryonal neoplasms (i.e., medulloblastoma). In contrast, CNS tumors in adults are often high-grade gliomas or **secondary tumors** that are metastatic from another site. Radiation previously directed at the CNS can result in secondary malignancy of the CNS. The classification of CNS tumors is complex and evolving, with the World Health Organization classification being the most complete and accurate system. Tumors continue to be renamed and reclassified as new molecular data emerge.

EPIDEMIOLOGY

CNS tumors are the most common solid tumors in children, second to leukemia in overall cancer incidence during childhood. Due primarily to improved outcomes for leukemia, CNS tumors are now the leading cause of childhood cancer deaths. About 3,400 new cases occur each year in the United States; the rate is approximately 6 cases per 100,000 children under 15 years of age. The incidence peaks before age 10 years and then decreases until a second peak after age 70. For medulloblastoma and ependymoma, males are more affected than females; for other tumor types, no gender differences exist. In the first 2–3 years of life, White children are affected more than non-White children; after age 3 incidence rates are essentially equal for White and non-White children.

Children with certain inherited syndromes, such as neurofibromatosis (types 1 and 2), Li-Fraumeni syndrome, tuberous sclerosis, Turcot syndrome, and von Hippel-Lindau syndrome, have an increased risk for developing a CNS tumor. The majority of CNS tumors arise in children with no known underlying disorder or risk factor.

CLINICAL MANIFESTATIONS

CNS tumors can cause symptoms by impingement on normal tissue (usually cranial nerves) or by an increase in intracranial pressure caused either by obstruction of cerebrospinal fluid (CSF) flow or by a direct mass effect. Tumors that obstruct the flow of CSF quickly become symptomatic. Symptoms of **increased intracranial pressure** include lethargy, headache, and vomiting (particularly in the morning upon awakening). Irritability, anorexia, poor school performance, and loss of developmental milestones all may be signs of slow-growing CNS tumors. In young children with open cranial sutures, an increase in head circumference may occur. Optic pathway tumors may lead to visual defects. Inability to abduct the eye as the result of sixth cranial nerve palsy is a common sign of increased intracranial pressure. Other cranial nerve deficits suggest involvement of the brainstem. Seizures occur in 20–50% of patients with supratentorial tumors; focal weakness or sensory changes also may be seen. Pituitary involvement can produce neuroendocrine effects such as precocious puberty or diabetes insipidus. Cerebellar tumors are associated with ataxia and diminished coordination. A history and physical examination are fundamental for evaluation and should include a thorough neurologic assessment with assessment of visual fields and a funduscopic examination.

LABORATORY/IMAGING STUDIES

If an intracranial lesion is suspected, imaging (MRI or CT) should be obtained (Fig. 158.1). Examination of CSF by cytocentrifuge histologic testing is indicated to determine the presence of metastatic disease in embryonal tumors, germ cell tumors, and pineal region tumors. A lumbar puncture should not be performed before imaging has been obtained to evaluate for evidence of increased intracranial pressure. If a tumor is suspected to have metastatic potential (e.g., medulloblastoma), MRI of the entire spine should be obtained before surgery to assess for neuraxial dissemination. A postoperative MRI study of the brain should be obtained within 24–48 hours of surgery to assess the extent of resection.

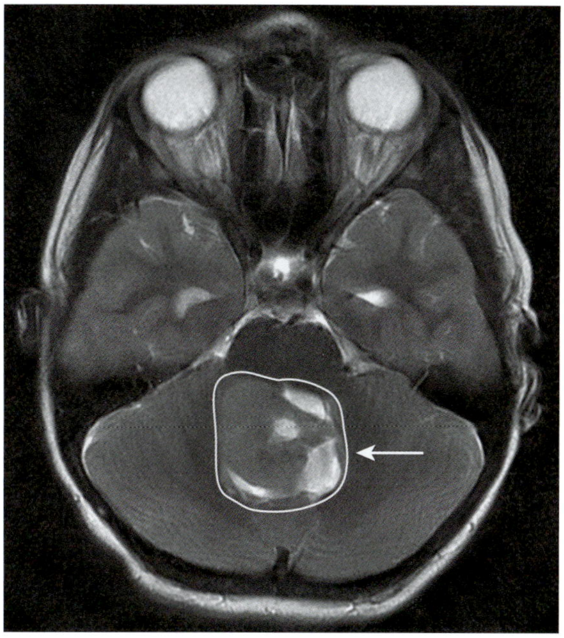

FIGURE 158.1 Magnetic resonance imaging of a 9-year-old male showing a heterogeneously enhancing fourth ventricular mass *(arrow)*. The mass was resected; pathology revealed medulloblastoma.

DIFFERENTIAL DIAGNOSIS

The differential diagnoses of a CNS mass lesion include malignant tumor, benign tumor, arteriovenous malformation, aneurysm, abscess, cysticercosis, granulomatous disease (tuberculosis, sarcoid), Langerhans cell histiocytosis, intracranial hemorrhage, pseudotumor cerebri, vasculitis, and, rarely, metastatic tumor.

TREATMENT

The therapy for children with CNS tumors is individualized and depends on the tumor type, location, size, and associated symptoms. High-dose **dexamethasone** is often administered immediately to reduce tumor-associated edema. Surgical objectives are complete excision, if possible, and maximal debulking if a complete excision is not possible. In children, radiation therapy is often combined with chemotherapy; in young children, radiation therapy may be delayed or avoided altogether to limit late side effects. Medulloblastoma and germ cell tumors are sensitive to chemotherapy; gliomas are less sensitive to chemotherapy. Chemotherapy plays an especially important role in infants, in whom radiation therapy may have devastating effects on growth and neurocognitive development. High-dose chemotherapy with autologous stem cell rescue is sometimes used to help avoid radiation therapy. As knowledge of the molecular drivers of tumorigenesis evolves, targeted therapies are gaining approval as frontline treatment (e.g., dabrafenib [a *BRAF* inhibitor] plus trametinib [a *MEK* inhibitor] for certain low-grade gliomas), and others are under investigation in clinic trials.

COMPLICATIONS

Short-term adverse effects of therapy include nausea, vomiting, anorexia, fatigue, immunosuppression, and cushingoid features. Long-term adverse effects include neurocognitive deficits, endocrinologic sequelae, decreased bone growth, ototoxicity, kidney insufficiency, cataracts, infertility, and secondary malignant neoplasms. The neurocognitive deficits can be significant, particularly in infants and young children, and are the primary reason for the continued search for the lowest efficacious radiation therapy dose and the most conformal delivery methods. **Posterior fossa syndrome** (also known as *cerebellar mutism*) occurs in up to 25% of patients after resection of a posterior fossa tumor and is characterized by an acute decrease in speech, behavioral changes (e.g., irritability, apathy, or both), diffuse cerebellar dysfunction, and other neurologic abnormalities. Posterior fossa syndrome may begin within hours to days of surgery and is usually self-resolving within weeks to months, although some neurologic complications may persist. **Somnolence syndrome**, which is characterized by excessive fatigue and sleepiness, may occur in the months after completion of radiation therapy and is self-limited.

PROGNOSIS

Improvements in diagnosis, neurosurgical techniques, chemotherapy regimens, and radiation therapy techniques have improved overall outcome. The 5-year overall survival rate associated with all childhood CNS tumors is approximately 50–60% (Table 158.1). Patients with low-grade gliomas that are completely resected have an excellent prognosis. Patients with diffuse intrinsic pontine gliomas and glioblastoma multiforme have poor prognoses.

TABLE 158.1 Location, Incidence, and Prognosis of Central Nervous System Tumors in Children

LOCATION	INCIDENCE (%)	5-YR SURVIVAL (%)
Infratentorial (posterior fossa)	50–60	—
Astrocytoma (cerebellum)	15	90
Medulloblastoma	15	50–80
Glioma (brainstem)	15	High grade: 0–5; low grade: 30
Ependymoma	5	50–60
Supratentorial (cerebral hemispheres)	35–45	—
Astrocytoma	20	50–75
Glioblastoma multiforme	10	0–5
Ependymoma	5	50–75
Choroid plexus papilloma	2	95
Midline	10–15	—
Craniopharyngioma	6	70–90
Germ cell tumors	3	65–95
Pineal	1	65–75
Optic nerve glioma	3	90

PEARLS FOR PRACTITIONERS

See Oncology: Pearls for Practitioners at the end of this section.

REVIEW QUESTIONS

Available online.

CHAPTER 159 Neuroblastoma

ETIOLOGY

Neuroblastoma is derived from **neural crest cells** that form the adrenal medulla and the sympathetic nervous system. Most cases occur in young children; the cause is most often unknown. Neuroblastoma may rarely (1–2% of cases) be hereditary. Germline genetic variants in the *ALK*, *PHOX2B*, and *TP53* genes have been associated with familial cases. In sporadic cases, several somatic genetic variants have been identified, with *MYCN* amplification being the most common.

EPIDEMIOLOGY

Neuroblastoma is the most common extracranial solid tumor of childhood and the most common malignancy in infancy. The median age at diagnosis is 17 months. There are approximately 800 new cases of neuroblastoma in the United States each year. The prevalence is estimated to be 1 in 7,000 live births.

CLINICAL MANIFESTATIONS

Neuroblastoma is remarkable for its broad spectrum of clinical behavior, ranging from spontaneous regression to rapid progression with metastases resulting in death. Children with localized disease are often asymptomatic at diagnosis; children with metastases often appear ill and have systemic symptoms such as fever, weight loss, bruising, and pain. The most common presentation is abdominal pain or mass. The mass is often palpated in the abdomen or flank and is hard and nontender. Approximately 45% of tumors arise in the adrenal gland, and 25% arise in the retroperitoneal sympathetic ganglia. Other sites of origin are the paravertebral ganglia of the chest and neck. Paraspinal tumors may invade through the neural foramina and cause spinal cord compression. *Horner syndrome* is sometimes seen with neck or apical masses. Several **paraneoplastic syndromes**, including secretory diarrhea, profuse sweating, and **opsoclonus-myoclonus-ataxia syndrome**, are associated with neuroblastoma.

Neuroblastoma can metastasize to multiple organs, including the liver, bone, bone marrow, and lymph nodes. Periorbital ecchymoses ("raccoon eyes") are a sign of orbital bone metastases in the presence of thrombocytopenia. A unique category of neuroblastoma, **stage MS**, is defined in infants (<18 months old) with metastases limited to skin, liver, or bone marrow. It is associated with a favorable outcome. Some cases of stage MS neuroblastoma can regress spontaneously; others may require chemotherapy to achieve a cure.

LABORATORY/IMAGING STUDIES

A CBC and plain radiographs may help identify patients with neuroblastoma. Calcification within abdominal neuroblastoma tumors is often observed on plain radiographs of the abdomen. About 90% of neuroblastomas produce **catecholamines (vanillylmandelic acid; homovanillic acid)** that can be detected in the urine. Definitive diagnosis of neuroblastoma requires tissue biopsy for microscopic examination and genetic testing. A CT scan of the chest, abdomen, and pelvis (Fig. 159.1); an iodine-123-metaiodobenzylguanidine (^{123}I-MIBG) scan; and bilateral bone marrow aspirations/biopsies complete the evaluation.

DIFFERENTIAL DIAGNOSIS

The abdominal presentation of neuroblastoma must be differentiated from Wilms tumor and hepatoblastoma, which can also present as an abdominal or flank mass. Ultrasound or CT examination usually distinguishes the tumors prior to surgery. Periorbital ecchymoses from orbital metastases can be mistaken for child abuse. Because children with bone marrow involvement may have anemia, thrombocytopenia, or neutropenia, leukemia and metastatic sarcomas are often considered in the differential.

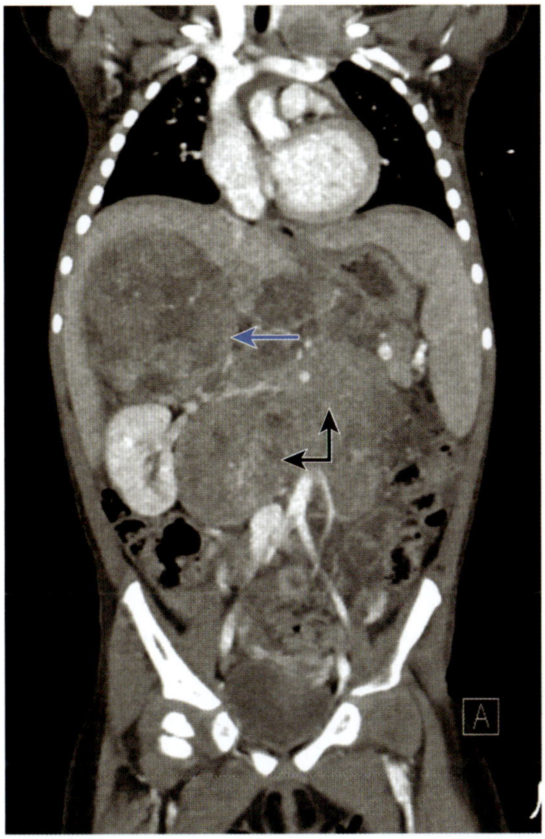

FIGURE 159.1 Neuroblastoma. Computed tomography (CT) scan of a 2-year-old who presented with bilateral periorbital ecchymoses, fatigue, pallor, and pancytopenia. CT shows a large right suprarenal mass *(blue arrow)* and large retroperitoneal abdominal lymph nodes *(black arrows)*. An iodine-123-metaiodobenzylguanidine (^{123}I-MIBG) scan and bone marrow biopsies revealed widespread metastatic disease.

TREATMENT

Treatment of neuroblastoma is based on risk classification, which is determined by factors including age, presence or absence of image-defined risk factors and metastatic disease, histopathology (favorable or unfavorable histology), and cytogenetic features such as presence or absence of *MYCN* amplification and segmental chromosomal aberrations. Complete surgical excision is the treatment of choice for localized neuroblastoma. Children with very low or low-risk tumors who undergo a gross total resection require no further therapy. Patients with intermediate-risk disease are usually treated with surgery and four to eight cycles of chemotherapy. In patients with high-risk disease, combination chemotherapy is given after confirmation of the diagnosis. The most commonly used agents are vincristine, cyclophosphamide, topotecan, doxorubicin, cisplatin, and etoposide. Resection of the primary tumor is undertaken after several courses of chemotherapy. Patients then undergo two courses of **high-dose chemotherapy with autologous stem cell rescue**. Radiation therapy is administered to the primary tumor bed and major areas of metastatic disease. Finally, **cis-retinoic acid** (isotretinoin) and **dinutuximab** (a monoclonal antibody directed against the GD2 antigen) are administered to treat minimal residual disease. *ALK* aberrations (pathogenic variants and amplifications) have been identified in approximately 14% of high-risk neuroblastoma tumors and are associated with inferior outcomes. This has led to the investigation of small molecule *ALK* inhibitors. Therapeutic ^{131}I-MIBG has shown promising results and is currently under investigation in high-risk neuroblastoma. In addition, some patients with high-risk neuroblastoma may receive eflornithine as maintenance therapy.

COMPLICATIONS

Spinal cord compression from neuroblastoma may cause an irreversible neurologic deficit and is an oncologic emergency. Children with opsoclonus-myoclonus-ataxia syndrome may suffer from developmental delay. The aggressive chemotherapy and radiation therapies currently used to treat high-risk neuroblastoma may result in complications such as acute infection, bleeding, ototoxicity, cardiotoxicity, nephrotoxicity, growth problems, and secondary malignancies.

PROGNOSIS

The prognosis is affected by age at diagnosis, disease stage (based on presence or absence of metastases and image-defined risk factors), *MYCN* status, and histopathology (grade of tumor differentiation). Similar to leukemias and sarcomas, a favorable response to induction therapy is associated with improved long-term outcomes. Currently, children with neuroblastoma can be divided into four groups: very low, low, intermediate, and high risk. Patients with favorable biology tend to be younger and often have localized disease. Older patients with metastatic disease have unfavorable biology; approximately 50% will ultimately relapse due to drug-resistant residual disease. The continued intensification of high-risk patients with immunotherapy and high-dose chemotherapy with autologous stem cell rescue has provided promising improvements in event-free survival. Although neuroblastoma represents only 8% of cases of childhood cancer, it is responsible for 15% of cancer deaths in children.

PEARLS FOR PRACTITIONERS

See Oncology: Pearls for Practitioners at the end of this section.

REVIEW QUESTIONS

Available online.

CHAPTER 160

Wilms Tumor

ETIOLOGY AND EPIDEMIOLOGY

Wilms tumor is thought to arise from primitive, metanephric blastema, the precursor of a normal kidney. Nephrogenic rests are foci of embryonal cells that are rarely (<1%) found in normal infant kidneys and commonly (25–40%) found in Wilms tumor-bearing kidneys. Although the cause of Wilms tumor is unknown, approximately 15–20% of sporadic tumors have *WT1* variants. Over 70% of Wilms tumors demonstrate loss of imprinting or loss of heterozygosity at 11p15, leading to overexpression of *IGF2*, thought to play a key role in tumorigenesis. Certain syndromes, including Beckwith-Wiedemann and WAGR (Wilms tumor, aniridia, genitourinary anomalies, and range of developmental delays; pathogenic variant involving 11p13 region), are associated with an increased risk of developing the disease.

Wilms tumor is the most common malignant kidney tumor of childhood, with approximately 500 new cases per year in the United States. Unilateral tumors have a median age of diagnosis of 44 months of age versus bilateral tumors, which have a median age of diagnosis of 31 months. Bilateral presentations are commonly associated with hereditary forms of the disease.

CLINICAL MANIFESTATIONS

Most children with Wilms tumor are brought to medical attention because they have an abdominal mass that is discovered by their parents. Although many children do not have complaints at the time that the mass is first noted, associated symptoms and signs may include abdominal pain (often mistaken for constipation), fever, hypertension, and hematuria.

LABORATORY/IMAGING STUDIES

An abdominal ultrasound or CT scan (Fig. 160.1) can usually distinguish an intrarenal mass from a mass arising from the adrenal gland (most commonly neuroblastoma) or other surrounding structures. Evaluation of the inferior vena cava is crucial because the tumor may extend from the kidney into the vena cava. The diagnostic evaluation includes a CBC, urinalysis, liver and kidney function studies, as well as a CT scan of the chest, abdomen, and pelvis to assess for metastatic involvement. Pulmonary involvement is the most common metastatic site, followed by regional lymph nodes. The diagnosis is confirmed by histologic examination of the tumor.

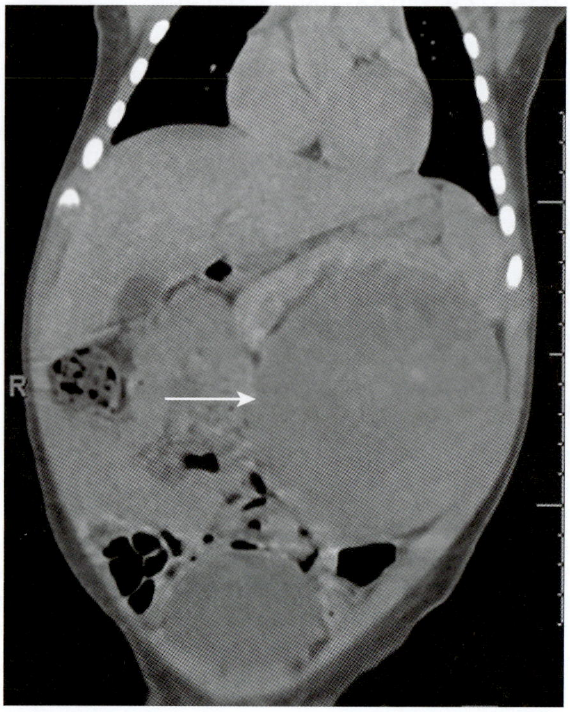

FIGURE 160.1 Wilms tumor. Computed tomography (CT) scan of a 2-year-old with a large heterogenous mass arising from the left kidney *(arrow)*. The child underwent a nephrectomy and pathology revealed Wilms tumor.

DIFFERENTIAL DIAGNOSIS

The differential diagnoses of Wilms tumor include hydronephrosis and polycystic disease of the kidney; benign kidney tumors, such as mesoblastic nephroma and hamartoma; and other malignant tumors, such as neuroblastoma, renal cell carcinoma, lymphoma, and retroperitoneal rhabdomyosarcoma.

TREATMENT

The timing of nephrectomy for unilateral, resectable Wilms tumor remains divided between the North American approach and the European approach. Both approaches have a similar overall survival. The North American approach recommends an upfront nephrectomy if deemed safe and feasible (confirming tissue diagnosis) followed by adjuvant chemotherapy with or without radiation therapy; the European approach is to make a diagnosis relying predominantly on imaging (usually without a biopsy), upfront (neoadjuvant) chemotherapy, then nephrectomy of the involved kidney followed by adjuvant chemotherapy with or without radiation therapy. The Children's Oncology Group (North American approach) relies on stage, histology (favorable vs unfavorable/anaplastic), patient age, tumor weight, loss of heterozygosity of 1p and 16q, and imaging response of pulmonary nodules after initial chemotherapy to risk-stratify patients. Most patients will receive a two- or three-drug chemotherapy regimen (vincristine, actinomycin, with or without doxorubicin); those with high-risk features will also receive radiation therapy. Patients designated with very low-risk unilateral Wilms tumor are often cured with surgery only.

Bilateral Wilms tumor is present in about 5% of children on initial presentation. The treatment goal for patients with bilateral Wilms tumor is to balance the need to achieve a cure while retaining as much normal kidney function as possible.

PROGNOSIS AND COMPLICATIONS

The overall survival rate for Wilms tumor is 90%. Unfortunately, 25% of survivors will experience serious chronic health conditions. Survivors of Wilms tumor are at risk for chronic kidney disease (based on single kidney physiology), cardiomyopathy, hypertension, pulmonary dysfunction, hepatic dysfunction, infertility, and secondary malignancies. Patients with bilateral Wilms tumor are sometimes left with chronic kidney disease or failure, requiring dialysis or a kidney transplant.

PEARLS FOR PRACTITIONERS

See Oncology: Pearls for Practitioners at the end of this section.

REVIEW QUESTIONS

Available online.

CHAPTER 161
Sarcomas

Sarcomas are generally divided into soft tissue and bone cancers. Soft tissue sarcomas arise primarily from the connective tissues of the body, such as muscle. **Rhabdomyosarcoma (RMS)**, the most common soft tissue sarcoma in children, is derived from mesenchymal cells of muscle lineage. Less common soft tissue sarcomas include fibrosarcoma, synovial sarcoma, and extraosseous Ewing sarcoma. The most common malignant bone cancers in children are **osteosarcoma** and **Ewing sarcoma**. Osteosarcomas derive from primitive bone-forming mesenchymal stem cells. Ewing sarcomas are thought to be of neural crest cell origin.

ETIOLOGY

The cause is unknown for most children diagnosed with sarcoma, although there are some known risk factors. Individuals with Li-Fraumeni syndrome (associated with a germline *TP53* pathogenic variant) and neurofibromatosis (associated with *NF1* pathogenic variants) have an increased risk of soft tissue sarcomas. There is a 500-fold increased risk for osteosarcoma for individuals with hereditary retinoblastoma. Prior treatment for childhood cancer with radiation therapy or chemotherapy (specifically alkylating agents) increases the risk for osteosarcoma as a second malignancy.

EPIDEMIOLOGY

In the United States, 850–900 children and adolescents under 20 years of age are diagnosed with soft tissue sarcomas each year; approximately 350 are RMS. The incidence of RMS has a bimodal peak in children 2–6 years old and again in adolescents. The early peak is associated with tumors in the genitourinary region, head, and neck; the later peak is associated with tumors in the extremities, trunk, and male genitourinary tract. Males are affected 1.5 times more often than females. Of the 650–700 U.S. children and adolescents under 20 years of age diagnosed with bone tumors each year, approximately two-thirds have osteosarcoma and one-third have Ewing sarcoma. Osteosarcoma most commonly affects adolescents; the peak incidence occurs during the period of maximum growth velocity. The incidence of Ewing sarcoma peaks between ages 10–20 years but may occur at any age. Ewing sarcoma primarily affects White children; it rarely occurs in Black or Asian children.

CLINICAL MANIFESTATIONS

The clinical presentation of RMS depends on the site of origin, associated mass effect, and presence of metastatic disease. Periorbital swelling, proptosis, and limitation of extraocular motion may be seen with an orbital tumor. Oropharyngeal or nasal mass, dysphagia, neck mass, and cranial nerve involvement may be noted with tumors in other head and neck sites. Urethral or vaginal masses, paratesticular swelling, hematuria, and urinary frequency or retention may be noted with tumors in the genitourinary tract. Trunk or extremity lesions often present as rapidly growing masses that may or may not be painful. If there is metastatic disease to bone or bone marrow, limb pain and cytopenias may be present.

Osteosarcoma is often located at the epiphysis or metaphysis of long bones that are associated with maximum growth velocity (distal femur, proximal tibia, proximal humerus), but any bone may be involved. Osteosarcoma presents with pain and may be associated with a palpable mass. As the pain and swelling often are initially thought to be related to trauma, radiographs of the affected region are frequently obtained; the radiographs usually reveal a lytic lesion, sometimes associated with calcification in the soft tissue surrounding the lesion. Although 75–80% of patients with osteosarcoma have apparently localized disease at diagnosis, most patients are believed to have micrometastatic disease as well.

The femur and pelvis are the most common sites for Ewing sarcoma, although it can occur in almost any bone in the body. In addition to local pain and swelling, clinical manifestations may include constitutional symptoms such as fever, fatigue, and weight loss.

LABORATORY/IMAGING STUDIES

Tissue biopsy is needed for a definitive diagnosis of sarcoma. Selection of the biopsy site is important and has implications for future surgical resection and radiation therapy. Under light microscopy, RMS and Ewing sarcoma appear as small, round, blue cell tumors. Osteosarcomas are distinguishable by the presence of osteoid.

Immunohistochemical staining for muscle-specific proteins, such as actin and myosin, helps confirm the diagnosis of RMS. Two major histologic variants exist for RMS: embryonal and alveolar. The embryonal variant is most common in younger children with head, neck, and genitourinary primary tumors. The alveolar variant occurs in older patients and is seen most commonly in trunk and extremity tumors. Alveolar RMS is usually characterized by the specific translocations t(2;13) or t(1;13), involving the *FOXO1* gene on chromosome 13. The fusion status (*FOXO1* translocation positive or negative) is preferred over the morphologic description (embryonal vs alveolar) to assign risk group and treatment intensity, with fusion positive being unfavorable. Metastatic evaluation for patients with RMS should include positron emission tomography-computed tomography (PET-CT) scan, chest CT, and bilateral bone marrow aspirations/biopsies. A lumbar puncture is required in patients with a parameningeal tumor due to the risk of direct extension into the central nervous system.

The diagnosis of osteosarcoma is established with immunohistochemical analyses of the biopsy material and the presence of osteoid matrix. The extent of the primary tumor should be delineated carefully with MRI before starting chemotherapy to determine surgical resection options. Osteosarcoma metastasizes most commonly to the lungs and, rarely, to other bones. Metastatic evaluation includes a chest CT scan and a bone scan or PET-CT scan.

The diagnosis of Ewing sarcoma is established with immunohistochemical analyses along with cytogenetic and molecular diagnostic studies of the biopsy material. Ewing sarcoma is characterized by a specific chromosomal translocation, t(11;22), which is seen in 95% of tumors. MRI of the primary lesion should be performed to delineate extent of the lesion and any associated soft tissue mass. Metastatic evaluation involves a PET-CT scan, chest CT scan, and bilateral bone marrow aspirations/biopsies.

DIFFERENTIAL DIAGNOSIS

Patients with Ewing sarcoma may be misdiagnosed as having osteomyelitis; children with osteogenic sarcoma are often initially believed to have pain and swelling related to trauma. The differential diagnosis for RMS depends on the location of the tumor. Tumors of the trunk and extremities often present as a painless mass and may initially be thought to be benign tumors. Head and neck RMS may be misdiagnosed as reactive adenopathy, orbital cellulitis, or chronic infection of ears or sinuses. The differential diagnoses for intraabdominal RMS include other abdominal malignancies, such as Wilms tumor and neuroblastoma.

TREATMENT

Treatment of RMS is currently based on a staging system that incorporates numerous diagnostic features including primary site, histologic subtype, *FOXO1* fusion status, stage (local, regional, or metastatic involvement), and surgical grouping (the ability or inability to achieve a gross total resection prior to chemotherapy/radiation). The most common chemotherapy agents used in RMS are vincristine, dactinomycin, and cyclophosphamide. Radiation is administered to the primary tumor when surgical resection is incomplete or would be morbid. Radiation may also be administered to involved regional nodal sites and sometimes to distant metastatic sites.

The current treatment of osteosarcoma involves neoadjuvant chemotherapy and surgical resection of the primary tumor, followed by adjuvant chemotherapy. The most common chemotherapy agents used for osteosarcoma are high-dose methotrexate, doxorubicin, and cisplatin. The ability to surgically resect the primary tumor and sites of metastatic disease is critical for long-term survival. Radiation therapy is relatively ineffective for osteosarcoma, although it is sometimes used for tumors that cannot be resected or with palliative intent to treat pain. The treatment for Ewing sarcoma is similar to osteosarcoma and requires neoadjuvant chemotherapy, local control measures, and adjuvant chemotherapy. The most common chemotherapy agents used for Ewing sarcoma are vincristine, doxorubicin, and cyclophosphamide in combination with ifosfamide and etoposide. In contrast to osteosarcoma, Ewing sarcoma is radiation sensitive, and radiation therapy is administered to patients when the primary tumor cannot be safely resected. Radiation therapy is also administered to metastatic sites.

COMPLICATIONS

In addition to potential late effects from the chemotherapy, children with sarcomas may have complications related to local control of the tumor. If the local disease is controlled with surgery, the long-term sequelae may include loss of limb or limitation of function. If local control is accomplished with radiation therapy, the late effects depend on the dose of radiation given, the extent of the radiated site, and the development of the child at the time of radiation therapy. Irradiating tissues interferes with growth and development, causes organ damage, and increases the risk of secondary malignant neoplasms. Other long-term side effects can include cardiotoxicity and infertility.

PROGNOSIS

For all children with sarcoma, presence or absence of metastatic disease at presentation is the most important prognostic factor. The outlook remains poor for patients who have distant metastases from Ewing sarcoma, RMS, or osteosarcoma. Patients with localized RMS in favorable sites have an excellent prognosis when treated with surgery followed by chemotherapy. In patients with osteosarcoma, the amount of tumor necrosis after preoperative chemotherapy is prognostic. Patients who achieve greater than 90% tumor necrosis after neoadjuvant chemotherapy have an overall survival rate of approximately 80% versus approximately 50% for patients who have less than 90% tumor necrosis. The overall cure rate for patients with localized osteosarcoma and Ewing sarcoma is approximately 70%. Patients who have lung metastasis at diagnosis have a cure rate of approximately 30%. Patients with metastases to other bones have a very poor prognosis (less than 20%).

PEARLS FOR PRACTITIONERS

See Oncology: Pearls for Practitioners at the end of this section.

REVIEW QUESTIONS

Available online.

Suggested Readings

Chung C, Boterberg T, Lucas J, et al. Neuroblastoma. *Pediatr Blood Cancer*. 2021;68(suppl 2):e28473.

Derebas J, Panuciak K, Margas M, Zawitkowska J, Lejman M. The New Treatment Methods for Non-Hodgkin Lymphoma in Pediatric Patients. *Cancers (Basel)*. 2022;14(6):1569.

Eaton BR, Claude L, Indelicato DJ, et al. Ewing sarcoma. *Pediatr Blood Cancer*. 2021;68(suppl 2):e28355.

Eaton BR, Schwarz R, Vatner R, et al. Osteosarcoma. *Pediatr Blood Cancer.* 2021;68(suppl 2):e28352.
Elgarten CW, Aplenc R. Pediatric acute myeloid leukemia: updates on biology, risk stratification, and therapy. *Curr Opin Pediatr.* 2020:32(1): 57–66.
Inaba H, Mulligan CG. Pediatric acute lymphoblastic leukemia. *Haematologica.* 2020;105(11):2524–2539.
Lo AC, Dieckmann K, Pelz T, et al. Pediatric classical Hodgkin lymphoma. *Pediatr Blood Cancer.* 2021;68(suppl 2):e28562.
Malbari F. Pediatric Neuro-Oncology. *Neurol Clin.* 2021;39(3):829–845.
Pater L, Melchior P, Rübe C, et al. Wilms tumor. *Pediatric Blood Cancer.* 2021;68(suppl 2):e28257.
Yechieli RL, Mandeville HC, Hiniker SM, et al. Rhabdomyosarcoma. *Pediatr Blood Cancer.* 2021;68(suppl 2):e28254.

PEARLS FOR PRACTITIONERS

CHAPTER 154
Oncology Assessment

- The most common cancers in children and adolescents are leukemia, brain tumors, and lymphoma, followed by sarcomas of soft tissue and bone and germ cell and gonadal tumors.
- Neuroblastoma, Wilms tumor, retinoblastoma, and hepatoblastoma are seen almost exclusively in children, as opposed to adolescents and adults.
- Signs and symptoms of childhood cancer are often nonspecific. Pain, fatigue, pallor, bruising/petechiae/bleeding, and a growing mass are all common presenting signs and symptoms.
- A careful history and physical exam are crucial in a child with suspected cancer.
- Laboratory and imaging tests are helpful, but cancer ultimately requires a tissue sample (bone marrow aspirate or biopsy) with pathology review to confirm the diagnosis.
    - Urine homovanillic acid (HVA) and vanillylmandelic acid (VMA) are tumor markers for neuroblastoma.
    - Serum (and/or cerebrospinal fluid) α-fetoprotein (AFP) and β-human chorionic gonadotropin (β-HCG) are tumor markers for germ cell tumors.
    - AFP is a tumor marker for hepatoblastoma.

CHAPTER 155
Principles of Cancer Treatment

- The prognosis for children with cancer has improved dramatically in the past 60 years, with long-term survival improving from about 20% to greater than 80%.
- Treatment for children with cancer is usually multimodal and may involve surgery, radiation therapy, chemotherapy, and immunotherapy. Targeted therapies (i.e., rituximab, brentuximab, and tyrosine kinase inhibitors) and immunotherapies (i.e., chimeric antigen receptor [CAR] T-cell therapy) are also used to treat specific pediatric cancers.
- Survivors of childhood cancer may suffer long-term side effects from the treatment. As the prognosis for childhood cancer continues to improve, clinical trials are shifting focus from improving survival to decreasing long-term side effects.
- Prognostic factors for pediatric cancers still incorporate clinical aspects such as age, histology, and the presence or absence of metastases. Genetic factors (of both the cancer and the patient) and response to initial therapy are powerful determinants of survival.
- Tumor lysis syndrome is a life-threatening complication and may be seen in patients with leukemia and lymphoma. Tumor lysis syndrome is best treated with hydration, allopurinol, and/or rasburicase (to treat hyperuricemia) and by treating the underlying cancer.
- Airway compression, spinal cord compression, bleeding, and infection are other oncologic emergencies.

CHAPTER 156
Leukemia

- Children with cytopenias and/or blasts in the peripheral blood should be considered for bone marrow aspiration to assess for acute leukemia.
- Children with acute lymphoblastic leukemia generally have an excellent prognosis (cure rate of 90%); children with acute myeloid leukemia have a more guarded prognosis (cure rate of 65%).

CHAPTER 157
Lymphoma

- Malignant lymph nodes tend to be large, firm, fixed, and nontender; reactive lymph nodes tend to be small, soft, mobile, and tender.
- There are two major types of lymphoma: Hodgkin lymphoma (HL) and non-Hodgkin lymphoma (NHL).
- Children and adolescents with HL are classified as low, intermediate, or high risk according to stage, nodal bulk, the presence of B symptoms, and the serum albumin at presentation.
- The prognosis for lymphoma is generally excellent, with overall survival exceeding 90% for most patients (approaching 100% for low-risk patients). The overall 3-year survival rates for B-cell, T-cell, and large cell NHL are 70% to 90%.

CHAPTER 158

Central Nervous System Tumors

- Most central nervous system (CNS) tumors in pediatric patients are primary tumors that originate in the CNS and include astrocytomas/gliomas or embryonal neoplasms (i.e., medulloblastoma).
- Lethargy, headache, ataxia, and morning vomiting are common presenting symptoms of brain tumors; these symptoms should prompt consideration for imaging the brain (computed tomography and/or magnetic resonance imaging).

CHAPTER 159

Neuroblastoma

- A child with an abdominal mass should prompt consideration for neuroblastoma, Wilms tumor, and hepatoblastoma.
- Compared with toddlers and older children, infants with neuroblastoma are generally well, have less aggressive disease, and have an excellent prognosis.
- About 90% of neuroblastomas produce catecholamines (specifically vanillylmandelic acid [VMA] and homovanillic acid [HMA]), which can be detected in urine.
- Children with high-risk neuroblastoma have a guarded prognosis, even with aggressive treatment including chemotherapy, surgery, radiation therapy, retinoic acid, and immunotherapy.

CHAPTER 160

Wilms Tumor

- Wilms tumor usually presents with an abdominal mass in a relatively well-appearing child.
- Wilms tumor may be unilateral or bilateral; lungs and lymph nodes are the most common sites of metastases.
- The prognosis for patients with Wilms tumor is generally very good with multimodal therapy.

CHAPTER 161

Sarcomas

- Sarcomas originating in the bone, such as osteosarcoma and Ewing sarcoma, usually present with a mass and/or pain.
- Prognostic factors for patients with sarcomas include the presence or absence of metastases, the extent of surgical resection, and the response to chemotherapy (usually measured by the amount of tumor necrosis).

SECTION 22

NEPHROLOGY AND UROLOGY

Hiren P. Patel | Beth A. Vogt

CHAPTER 162

Nephrology and Urology Assessment

The kidneys preserve homeostasis through (1) maintaining fluid and electrolyte balance, (2) excreting metabolic waste products through glomerular filtration and tubular secretion, and (3) producing important endocrine hormones (e.g., renin, vitamin D metabolites, erythropoietin). There are a wide variety of kidney disorders (Table 162.1), which can manifest in different ways.

KIDNEY PHYSIOLOGY

Normal kidney function depends on intact **glomerular filtration** and **tubular function** (**proximal tubule** [PT], **loop of Henle**, and **distal tubule** [DT]) to produce **urine** (Fig. 162.1). Net glomerular pressure favors movement of fluid out of glomerular capillaries into Bowman's space, which leads to the PT. **Renin** is generated by cells in the juxtaglomerular apparatus, located at the base of each glomerulus near the afferent/efferent arterioles and DT of that nephron. Renin is released in response to decreased kidney perfusion pressure, decreased sodium delivery to the DT, and sympathetic nervous system activity and helps maintain intraglomerular pressure.

The PT reabsorbs (see Fig. 162.1) approximately two-thirds of filtered water, sodium, and chloride. Glucose, amino acids, potassium, and phosphate are almost completely reabsorbed in this segment. Approximately 75% of filtered bicarbonate is reabsorbed in the PT. The PT also secretes compounds such as organic acids, penicillins, and other compounds. The most active form of vitamin D—1,25$(OH)_2$-cholecalciferol **(calcitriol)**—is produced by PT cells in response to parathyroid hormone and intracellular calcium and phosphorus concentrations.

The loop of Henle is the site of reabsorption of 25% of filtered sodium chloride (see Fig. 162.1). Active chloride transport drives the countercurrent multiplier and constructs the medullary interstitial hypertonic gradient required for urinary concentration.

The DT is composed of the **distal convoluted tubule** (DCT) and **collecting duct** (CD). The DCT is water impermeable and contributes to urine dilution by active sodium chloride absorption. The CD is the primary site of **antidiuretic hormone** (vasopressin) response, which leads to urine concentration. Sodium-potassium and sodium-hydrogen exchange

TABLE 162.1 Causes of Kidney and Urinary Tract Disease in Children

GLOMERULAR DISORDERS	
Nephrotic syndrome	Minimal change disease Focal segmental glomerulosclerosis Membranous nephropathy Congenital nephrotic syndrome
Glomerulonephritis	Postinfectious GN Infectious GN Lupus nephritis Membranoproliferative GN (C3GN, DDD) IgA nephropathy IgA vasculitis nephritis Pauci-immune GN (GPA, MPA) Anti-GBM disease
Hereditary disorders	Alport syndrome Thin basement membrane disease
TUBULOINTERSTITIAL DISORDERS	
Acquired	Hypoxic-ischemic injury (ATN) Infection (sepsis, pyelonephritis) Nephrotoxin-induced injury Medication Endogenous (e.g., myoglobin, uric acid) Interstitial nephritis Kidney tumors
Congenital	CAKUT Renal dysplasia Obstructive uropathy Cystic diseases Hereditary tubular disorders
VASCULAR DISORDERS	
	Thrombotic microangiopathies (HUS, TTP) Renal vein thrombosis Sickle cell nephropathy Renal artery stenosis
URINARY TRACT DISORDERS	
	Urinary tract infection Vesicoureteral reflux Voiding dysfunction Urinary tract obstruction Urinary stone disease Urinary tract trauma

ATN, Acute tubular necrosis; *C3GN*, C3 glomerulonephritis; *CAKUT*, congenital anomalies of the kidneys and urinary tract; *DDD*, dense deposit disease; *GBM*, glomerular basement membrane; *GN*, glomerulonephritis; *GPA*, granulomatosis with polyangiitis; *HUS*, hemolytic uremic syndrome; *IgA*, immunoglobulin A; *MPA*, microscopic polyangiitis; *TTP*, thrombotic thrombocytopenic purpura.

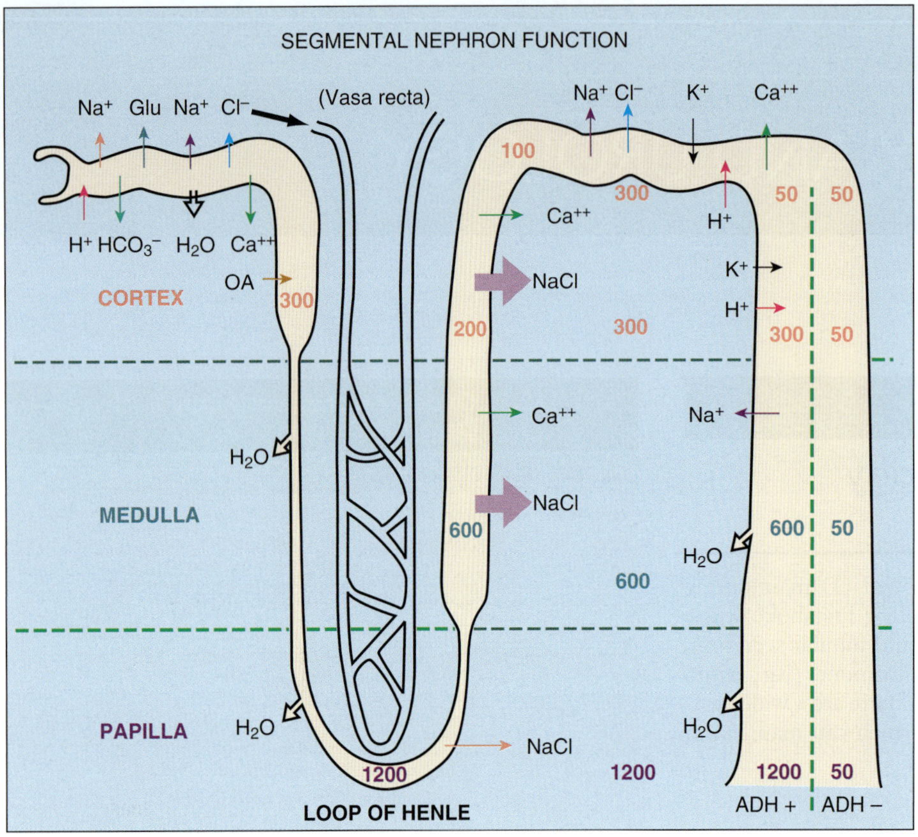

FIGURE 162.1 Illustration of a nephron highlighting major electrolyte transport functions of each nephron segment, including representative osmolalities in the interstitium and the tubular lumen at different levels within the kidney. *ADH*, Antidiuretic hormone; *Glu*, glucose; *OA*, organic acid. (From Andreoli TE, Carpenter CCJ, Plum F, et al., eds. *Cecil Essentials of Medicine*. Philadelphia: WB Saunders; 1986.)

in the CD is regulated by aldosterone. Active hydrogen ion secretion, responsible for final acidification of the urine, also occurs in the CD. Kidney ammonia production and intraluminal generation of ammonium (NH_4^+) facilitate urine hydrogen ion excretion.

Maximum **urinary concentrating capacity** in a preterm newborn (~400 mOsm/L) is less than that of a full-term newborn (600–800 mOsm/L), which is less than that of older children and adults (1,200 mOsm/L). Neonates can dilute urine similar to adults (75–90 mOsm/L), but because their **glomerular filtration rate** (GFR) is lower, their capacity to excrete a water load is limited. Tubular reabsorption of sodium, potassium, and bicarbonate and excretion of hydrogen are all reduced in infants relative to adults. These functions mature independently and at different ages, so a neonate rapidly develops the ability to reabsorb sodium efficiently, but it takes up to 2 years for bicarbonate reabsorption to fully mature. **Erythropoietin** is secreted by interstitial cells in the kidney medulla in response to low oxygen delivery and helps regulate bone marrow red blood cell production.

CLINICAL MANIFESTATIONS

The clinical presentation of kidney and urologic disease will depend on the type of disorder (glomerular, tubulointerstitial, vascular, lower urinary tract) and its severity (Table 162.2). The presentation will also be influenced by whether the disorder is acute or chronic (congenital in some cases) and whether the disorder is a primary intrinsic kidney disease or secondary to a systemic process. Kidney and urologic conditions may present with obvious signs (e.g., hematuria, edema, abnormal urine stream) or with nonspecific findings such as poor growth, fever, or vomiting. In some cases, the child may be asymptomatic and have evidence of kidney or urologic disease discovered by incidental findings on labs or imaging. Presentation of a disorder may also vary by age. For example, neonates and infants with **urinary tract infections** (UTIs) may present with fever, irritability, and vomiting, whereas frequency and dysuria suggest UTI in older children.

HISTORY AND PHYSICAL EXAMINATION

Depending on the clinical suspicion or scenario, attention should be directed to the applicable history and exam elements as listed in Table 162.2. In addition to the present illness, a detailed medical and family history is important. In some cases, a prenatal history is also valuable. Congenital kidney disorders may be associated with reduced (oligohydramnios) or increased amniotic fluid volume (polyhydramnios) as fetal urine production is the primary source of amniotic fluid volume in the second and third trimesters. Pulmonary hypoplasia and fetal maldevelopment of the face and extremities may result from insufficient amniotic fluid (Potter sequence; see Chapters 58 and 60).

Risk factors for kidney and urologic disease (e.g., acute kidney injury, UTI) can often be detected by a careful history. Congenital kidney anomalies may be associated with other extrarenal manifestations including ear, eye, and skin findings or other dysmorphic features. Attention should be paid to the blood pressure because many kidney disorders are associated with hypertension.

TABLE 162.2 Common Manifestations of Kidney and Urinary Tract Disease

TYPE OF DISORDER	COMMON MANIFESTATIONS
Glomerular	**H&P:** Red urine, swelling, oliguria, hypertension, systemic symptoms and signs related to underlying process (e.g., preceding illness, fever, rash, arthralgias, hemoptysis) **Labs:** Hematuria, proteinuria, elevated serum creatinine, hypoalbuminemia, hypercholesterolemia, decreased C3/C4 complement, labs related to underlying process (e.g., positive ANA, ANCA, infectious serologies) **Imaging:** Increased echogenicity and decreased corticomedullary differentiation on ultrasound, enlarged kidneys
Tubulointerstitial	**H&P:** Oliguria, polyuria, dehydration, exposure history to nephrotoxic agents, abdominal/flank mass, fever, poor growth **Labs:** Hematuria, proteinuria, glucosuria, pyuria, dilute urine, elevated serum creatinine, electrolyte abnormalities **Imaging:** Increased echogenicity and decreased corticomedullary differentiation on ultrasound, hydronephrosis, renal cysts, renal mass
Vascular	**H&P:** Hematuria, oliguria, flank pain, malaise, hypertension, petechiae **Labs:** Hematuria, proteinuria, elevated serum creatinine, anemia, thrombocytopenia **Imaging:** Increased echogenicity and decreased corticomedullary differentiation on ultrasound, renal vein thrombosis on Doppler ultrasound, papillary necrosis on CT scan
Urinary tract	**H&P:** Dysuria, urinary urgency, hematuria, fever, enuresis, flank pain, recurrent UTI, vomiting, flank mass, suprapubic mass, urethral anomalies **Labs:** Pyuria, hematuria, positive urine culture, hypercalciuria **Imaging:** Hydronephrosis, urinary tract stones, vesicoureteral reflux on VCUG, thickened bladder wall ± trabeculation, ureterocele, renal scarring, delayed emptying on renal scintigraphy, kidney laceration on CT scan

ANA, Antinuclear antibody; *ANCA,* antineutrophil cytoplasmic antibody; *CT,* computed tomography; *H&P,* history and physical; *UTI,* urinary tract infection; *VCUG,* voiding cystourethrogram.

DIAGNOSTIC STUDIES

Laboratory Studies

Blood urea nitrogen is affected by kidney function but is also affected by hydration, nutrition, catabolism, and tissue breakdown. **Serum creatinine** is a more specific marker of kidney function and is commonly used to approximate GFR. Creatinine is derived from muscle and increases with age as muscle mass increases. The correlation between serum creatinine and GFR can be used to estimate GFR with the revised bedside Schwartz formula:

$$GFR = \frac{0.413 \times Ht}{Cr_{serum}}$$

(height in cm; serum creatinine in mg/dL). This formula is most useful when body habitus and muscle mass are reasonably normal and when kidney function is relatively stable. This formula is most accurate in a GFR range of 15–75 mL/min/1.73 m^2. **Serum cystatin C** is another marker of kidney function that is not affected by muscle mass and can be used to estimate GFR. Serum creatinine and cystatin C can more accurately estimate GFR than the bedside equation above using the Chronic Kidney Disease in Children U25 formulas. GFR can be measured rather than estimated by a 24-hour creatinine clearance; however, this will overestimate GFR to some degree due to creatinine secretion in the PT. This degree of overestimation is greater in children with lower GFR.

By convention, GFR is corrected to body surface area of 1.73 m^2 to allow comparison between different-sized individuals. In a full-term newborn, an uncorrected GFR of 4–5 mL/min corrects to approximately 40 mL/min/1.73 m^2. GFR increases rapidly during the first 2 years of life until it achieves adult values (100–120 mL/min/1.73 m^2). After that, GFR and body size increase proportionately, so GFR/1.73 m^2 remains stable.

Urinalysis is a useful screen for kidney disease. **Macroscopic urinalysis** uses a **urine dipstick** to assess urine concentration, pH, and the presence of blood, protein, glucose, ketones, and leukocytes (via **leukocyte esterase** reaction). Dilute urine may result in a false-negative result for protein; false-positive results may occur with alkaline or concentrated urine. Urine dipsticks are exquisitely sensitive to the presence of heme (whether in red blood cells, free hemoglobin, or myoglobin); there are few false-negative test results but many false-positive results. The **nitrite test** may detect bacteriuria if the bacteria can reduce nitrate to nitrite and have sufficient urine contact time. False-negative results occur with frequent voiding, low urine bacterial count, urinary tract obstruction, and infection with bacteria unable to generate nitrite. Gross hematuria or bacterial colonization of an uncircumcised prepuce may result in a false-positive nitrite test. **Microscopic urinalysis** is used to confirm pyuria and hematuria as well as detect casts and crystals.

Proteinuria can be more accurately assessed by a **spot urine protein/creatinine** ($U_{Pr}/_{Cr}$) ratio in a single urine specimen, preferably from a first-morning void. This value correlates well with 24-hour urine protein excretion. Normal spot $U_{Pr}/_{Cr}$ ratio is less than 0.2 mg/mg; a $U_{Pr}/_{Cr}$ ratio >2 mg/mg is considered nephrotic range in children.

Imaging Studies

Ultrasound is a noninvasive test that reliably assesses kidney size and urinary tract dilation and can detect most cysts, stones, and masses unless very small. Ultrasound examination of the kidneys should also include visualization of the bladder. **Doppler studies** assess arterial and venous blood flow and can provide evidence of renal artery stenosis and renal vein thrombosis.

A **voiding cystourethrogram** involves filling of the bladder with contrast to detect vesicoureteral reflux and to evaluate the urethra. **Computed tomography** (CT) and **magnetic resonance imaging** have replaced the **intravenous pyelogram** to evaluate kidney structure. These two studies provide the most detail on kidney structure but are more expensive, may require sedation in younger children, and involve radiation exposure in the case of CT. Radionuclide studies can identify kidney scars, differential kidney function, and delayed excretion suggestive of obstruction.

PEARLS FOR PRACTITIONERS

See Nephrology and Urology: Pearls for Practitioners at the end of this section.

REVIEW QUESTION

Available online.

CHAPTER 163

Nephrotic Syndrome and Proteinuria

ETIOLOGY AND EPIDEMIOLOGY

Small amounts of protein are found in the urine of healthy children (<4 mg/m^2/hour or urine protein/creatinine [$U_{Pr}/_{Cr}$] <0.2 mg/mg). **Nephrotic proteinuria** in children is defined as protein excretion greater than 40 mg/m^2/hour or $U_{Pr}/_{Cr}$ greater than 2 mg/mg. Proteinuria between these levels is mildly to moderately elevated but not nephrotic. There are three general patterns of proteinuria: transient, orthostatic (postural), and persistent (fixed). Nephrotic syndrome is a clinical subset defined by massive persistent proteinuria and edema.

Transient proteinuria can be seen in children with fever and dehydration or following seizure or vigorous exercise; it resolves within a few days, does not indicate kidney disease, and needs no further evaluation or treatment.

Orthostatic (postural) proteinuria is a benign condition defined by mild to moderate proteinuria ($U_{Pr}/_{Cr}$ typically 0.2–1 mg/mg) on a mid-day sample but normal protein excretion on a first morning sample. Orthostatic proteinuria is more common in adolescents and tall, thin individuals; it is not associated with progressive kidney disease. Many children with orthostatic proteinuria continue this process into adulthood.

Persistent (fixed) proteinuria indicates intrinsic kidney disease. Most persistent proteinuria is **glomerular** in origin and characterized by a combination of large and small molecular weight proteins, variable levels of proteinuria, and, often, other evidence of glomerular disease (hematuria, red blood cell casts, hypertension, and acute kidney injury). **Tubular** proteinuria is characterized by low molecular weight proteinuria and is seen in conditions of tubulointerstitial injury. Patients with tubular proteinuria may have a negative urine dipstick because this test specifically measures urinary albumin. The combination of tubular proteinuria with tubular electrolyte wasting and glycosuria is termed **Fanconi syndrome.**

Nephrotic syndrome (NS) is defined as persistent heavy **proteinuria** (mainly albuminuria; >40 mg/m^2/hour), **hypoalbuminemia** (serum albumin <3.0 g/dL), **hypercholesterolemia** (>250 mg/dL), and **edema**. Urinary protein losses occur due to abnormalities in the glomerular epithelial cell (podocyte) that normally restricts protein filtration. The resultant massive proteinuria leads to decreased serum albumin and reduction in plasma oncotic pressure, leading to fluid shifts from vascular to interstitial compartments with plasma volume contraction. Edema results from decreased oncotic pressure as well as increase in tubular sodium reabsorption from reduced effective circulating blood volume. Hypoalbuminemia stimulates hepatic lipoprotein synthesis and diminishes lipoprotein metabolism, leading to elevated serum lipids (cholesterol, triglycerides) and lipoproteins.

There are three main causes of primary NS in children and a number of less common secondary causes (Table 163.1). **Minimal change nephrotic syndrome** (MCNS) is the most common histologic form of primary NS in children. More than 80% of children <7 years of age with NS have MCNS. Children 7–16 years old with NS have an ~50% chance of having MCNS. Males are affected more frequently than females (2:1), and the peak age of presentation is in the preschool years.

Focal segmental glomerulosclerosis (FSGS) accounts for ~10–20% of children with NS. Children with FSGS present like those with MCNS but may have a less favorable response to treatment. More than 35% of children with FSGS progress to end-stage kidney disease. Most cases are idiopathic, meaning that no secondary or genetic cause is identified.

Membranous nephropathy represents <5% of children with NS. It is seen most commonly in adolescents and children with systemic infections (hepatitis B, syphilis, malaria, and toxoplasmosis), with exposure to specific medications (gold, penicillamine), or with autoimmune disease such as systemic lupus erythematosus.

NS may be a feature of severe cases of any type of glomerulonephritis including immunoglobulin A (IgA) nephropathy, IgA vasculitis nephritis, postinfectious glomerulonephritis, lupus nephritis, and membranoproliferative glomerulonephritis. NS

TABLE 163.1 Primary and Secondary Forms of Nephrotic Syndrome

PRIMARY NEPHROTIC SYNDROME
Minimal change NS Focal segmental glomerulosclerosis Membranous nephropathy Hereditary NS (congenital NS, infantile NS)
SECONDARY NEPHROTIC SYNDROME
Systemic lupus erythematosus and other glomerulonephritides (e.g., MPGN, PIGN) IgA vasculitis, granulomatosis with polyangiitis and other vasculitides Chronic infections (hepatitis B, hepatitis C, malaria, HIV) Allergic interstitial nephritis Diabetic kidney disease Amyloidosis Malignancy (Hodgkin's lymphoma)

HIV, Human immunodeficiency virus; *IgA,* immunoglobulin A; *MPGN,* membranoproliferative glomerulonephritis; *NS,* nephrotic syndrome; *PIGN,* postinfectious glomerulonephritis.

may also occur due to secondary causes including amyloidosis, allergic interstitial nephritis, advanced diabetic kidney disease, and lymphoma (see Table 163.1).

Congenital NS (CNS) presents during the first 3 months of life. Autosomal recessive inheritance of pathogenic variants of *NPHS1* (encoding nephrin, with variants causing Finnish-type CNS) and *NPHS2* (encoding podocin) causes a decrease or absence of key protein components of the podocyte slit diaphragm. A heterogeneous group of other disorders, including diffuse mesangial sclerosis and conditions associated with medications or congenital infections, may also cause CNS. **Infantile NS** presents between 3 and 12 months of age and is usually caused by pathogenic variants encoding other proteins of the glomerular filtration barrier such as podocin.

CLINICAL MANIFESTATIONS

Children with NS initially present with facial and periorbital edema that progresses to more widespread edema including abdominal swelling, lower extremity edema, and even anasarca. The early stages of disease may be mistaken for an allergic reaction. Initial presentation often follows an immune trigger such as an upper respiratory infection. Anorexia, malaise, abdominal pain, diarrhea (due to intestinal wall edema), and respiratory distress (due to presence of ascites and/or pleural effusion) may be present. MCNS is characterized by *absence* of gross hematuria, kidney dysfunction, and hypertension.

DIAGNOSTIC STUDIES

A urine dipstick with trace or negative protein and a $U_{Pr}/_{Cr}$ <0.2 mg/mg on a first morning specimen suggests orthostatic proteinuria, and no further evaluation is needed. Proteinuria of 1+ or higher with a $U_{Pr}/_{Cr}$ >0.2 mg/mg on a first morning urine specimen indicates abnormal proteinuria that should be further evaluated. $U_{Pr}/_{Cr}$ values >2 mg/mg indicate nephrotic range proteinuria.

Children with persistent proteinuria should have kidney function assessed with serum creatinine, electrolyte panel, and albumin level. Routine testing typically includes a serum C3 complement. In children with NS, a low serum C3 implies a lesion other than MCNS. Kidney ultrasound is often useful to rule out structural abnormalities of the urinary tract. Kidney biopsy is recommended in children with persistent proteinuria including NS when MCNS is not suspected (e.g., kidney dysfunction, age >13 years, presence of hematuria, and hypertension).

TREATMENT

Because >80% of children <13 years of age with NS have steroid-responsive forms (chiefly MCNS), empiric steroid therapy may be initiated without a kidney biopsy if a child has typical features of MCNS. Over 90% of children who respond to steroids do so within 4 weeks. A kidney biopsy is indicated for patients who do not respond to steroid therapy in 6 weeks. Relapses of NS are treated with shorter courses of high-dose steroids. Children with frequent relapses, steroid dependence, or steroid resistance may require additional immunosuppressive therapy.

Treatment responses in FSGS are highly variable. Approximately one third of children respond to steroid therapy; others may respond to additional immunosuppressive therapy. Children with membranous nephropathy do not reliably remit with standard NS steroid therapy but often improve with other immunosuppressive therapy. Infants with congenital or infantile NS should not receive immunosuppression and are instead treated with supportive care, aggressive nutritional support, dialysis, and transplantation.

The cornerstone of edema management is dietary salt restriction. Severe edema may require use of loop diuretics or fluid restriction. When these therapies are not successful, cautious parenteral administration of 25% albumin (0.5–1 g/kg intravenously over 2–4 hours) followed by an intravenous loop diuretic may achieve diuresis. Supportive strategies include elevation of the legs or other body parts with severe swelling, careful monitoring of daily weights, and strict documentation of intake and output.

COMPLICATIONS

Side effects of steroids, such as increased appetite, weight gain, hypertension, and irritability, are most common in steroid-dependent and frequently relapsing patients who have greatest exposure to steroids. Hypovolemia and acute kidney injury may result from overaggressive diuresis. Serious infections, including **bacteremia** and **peritonitis** (particularly *Streptococcus pneumoniae, Escherichia coli,* or *Klebsiella*), may occur due to urinary loss of immunoglobulins and complement. **Thrombotic events** including deep vein thrombosis, cerebral venous sinus thrombosis, renal vein thrombosis, and pulmonary embolism may occur due to the hypercoagulable state caused by urinary losses of coagulation inhibitors such as antithrombin 3 as well as increased hepatic production of fibrinogen. Although routine anticoagulation is not recommended in children with NS, it may be considered in those with a history of prior thrombosis or those at particularly high risk. Persistent hyperlipidemia in children with steroid-resistant NS promotes increased risk of atherosclerotic vascular disease.

PROGNOSIS

Nearly 80% of children with steroid-responsive MCNS experience at least one NS relapse, defined as heavy proteinuria that persists for 3 or more consecutive days. Relapse patterns include **infrequently relapsing**, **frequently relapsing** (four or more relapses/year), and **steroid-dependent** (relapse within 2 weeks of steroid discontinuation). Some children do not respond to steroids initially, or despite initial response they become **steroid resistant**. Steroid-responsive patients have little risk of progressive chronic kidney disease. Patients who are steroid resistant, however, are more likely to progress to end-stage kidney disease (see Chapter 166). Recurrence of disease occurs in ~30% of children with steroid-resistant FSGS who undergo kidney transplantation.

PEARLS FOR PRACTITIONERS

See Nephrology and Urology: Pearls for Practitioners at the end of this section.

REVIEW QUESTION

Available online.

CHAPTER 164

Glomerulonephritis and Hematuria

ETIOLOGY AND EPIDEMIOLOGY

Hematuria, defined as five or more red blood cells (RBCs) per high-power field, is a common clinical issue in pediatrics. Hematuria may originate from glomerular, tubulointerstitial, or lower urinary tract disorders (Table 164.1). **Microscopic hematuria** is found in up to 5% of healthy children but in most cases is a transient finding and resolves on repeated testing. Persistent microscopic hematuria raises concern for conditions such as glomerular disease, crystalluria, or inherited disorders such as sickle cell trait/disease or polycystic kidney disease. **Macroscopic (gross) hematuria** is defined as visible blood in the urine and may be seen in conditions such as urolithiasis, urinary tract infection, and acute or chronic glomerulonephritis (GN). **Postinfectious glomerulonephritis (PIGN)** is the most common form of acute GN and **immunoglobulin A (IgA) nephropathy** is the most common form of chronic GN.

CLINICAL MANIFESTATIONS

PIGN occurs most frequently in children 2–12 years of age and is more common in males. Children with PIGN commonly present with hematuria (macro- or microscopic) and other cardinal features of glomerular injury (proteinuria, hypertension, edema, oliguria, and acute kidney injury). Clinical onset of PIGN typically develops on average 10 days after streptococcal pharyngitis, 4–6 weeks after impetigo, or 2 weeks after other bacterial or viral infections. Antibiotic treatment of streptococcal or other infections does not prevent or delay development of GN.

IgA nephropathy has a more variable presentation and may take the form of acute GN, asymptomatic microscopic hematuria, or the classic presentation of recurrent macroscopic hematuria concurrent with an upper respiratory infection. In contrast to PIGN, macroscopic hematuria occurs at the same time as the associated infection in IgA nephropathy. The cause is unknown, although some cases appear to be familial.

There are many other types of secondary GN including IgA vasculitis, systemic lupus erythematosus, and vasculitis. Children with these conditions typically present with systemic features of the respective condition.

Rapidly progressive glomerulonephritis (RPGN) is a severe form of acute GN associated with a rapid loss of kidney function over days to weeks. RPGN may be seen in patients with any form of acute GN. A common feature on kidney biopsy is glomerular epithelial cell proliferation with crescents. Early recognition and treatment of RPGN is crucial to prevent progression to end-stage kidney disease (ESKD).

Several hereditary kidney conditions can cause hematuria. **Alport syndrome** is caused by pathogenic variants encoding type IV collagen (pathogenic variants in *COL4A3, COL4A4,* or *COL4A5*), which leads to construction of abnormal glomerular basement membrane (GBM) in the kidneys, bilateral high-frequency sensorineural hearing loss, and anterior lenticonus and perimacular flecks in the eyes. The most common inheritance pattern is X-linked, but autosomal dominant and recessive forms exist. Males with Alport syndrome present with either painless microscopic or macroscopic hematuria, progressive proteinuria, hypertension, loss of kidney function, and sensorineural hearing loss. Females typically have a more benign course with microscopic hematuria, although some can develop progressive chronic kidney disease. **Thin basement membrane disease** (benign familial hematuria) is also caused by autosomal dominant collagen pathogenic variants *(COL4A3, COL4A4)* that lead to GBM thinning and persistent hematuria. There is often a family history of hematuria in first-degree relatives. As opposed to Alport syndrome, thin basement membrane disease is not associated with hearing loss or ocular symptoms, is typically not progressive, and usually has an excellent prognosis.

Nonglomerular causes of hematuria have a more variable presentation related to the underlying etiology. **Urinary tract infection (UTI)** is typically associated with dysuria and urinary frequency. **Urolithiasis** may be associated with flank or abdominal pain, although some children with stones are asymptomatic. **Hypercalciuria** can cause either macroscopic or microscopic hematuria with classic symptoms of UTI but without pyuria or a positive urine culture. **Strenuous exercise**, **sickle cell trait/disease**, and **Wilms tumor** can cause painless macroscopic hematuria. **Autosomal dominant polycystic kidney disease** or **nutcracker syndrome** (compression of the left renal vein) may be associated with macroscopic hematuria with flank pain. Hematuria following **trauma** may occur with severe kidney or lower urinary tract injury.

TABLE 164.1 Differential Diagnosis of Red Urine/Hematuria

PSEUDOHEMATURIA
Nonpathologic (urate crystals in infants, ingested foods, medications, dyes)
Pathologic (hemoglobinuria from hemolytic anemia, myoglobinuria from rhabdomyolysis)
GLOMERULAR
Immunologic injury (GN; e.g., PIGN, IgA nephropathy, MPGN, lupus nephritis, vasculitis)
Hereditary disorder (Alport syndrome, thin basement membrane disease)
Thrombotic microangiopathy (HUS, TTP)
TUBULOINTERSTITIAL/PARENCHYMAL
Inflammation (interstitial nephritis, pyelonephritis)
Vascular (sickle cell trait/disease, nutcracker syndrome)
Structural (cyst rupture, Wilms tumor, urinary tract obstruction, renal trauma)
LOWER URINARY TRACT
Inflammation (cystitis, hemorrhagic cystitis, urethritis)
Injury (trauma, kidney stone)
Hypercalciuria

GN, Glomerulonephritis; *HUS*, hemolytic uremic syndrome; *IgA*, immunoglobulin A; *MPGN*, membranoproliferative glomerulonephritis; *PIGN*, postinfectious glomerulonephritis; *TTP*, thrombotic thrombocytopenic purpura.

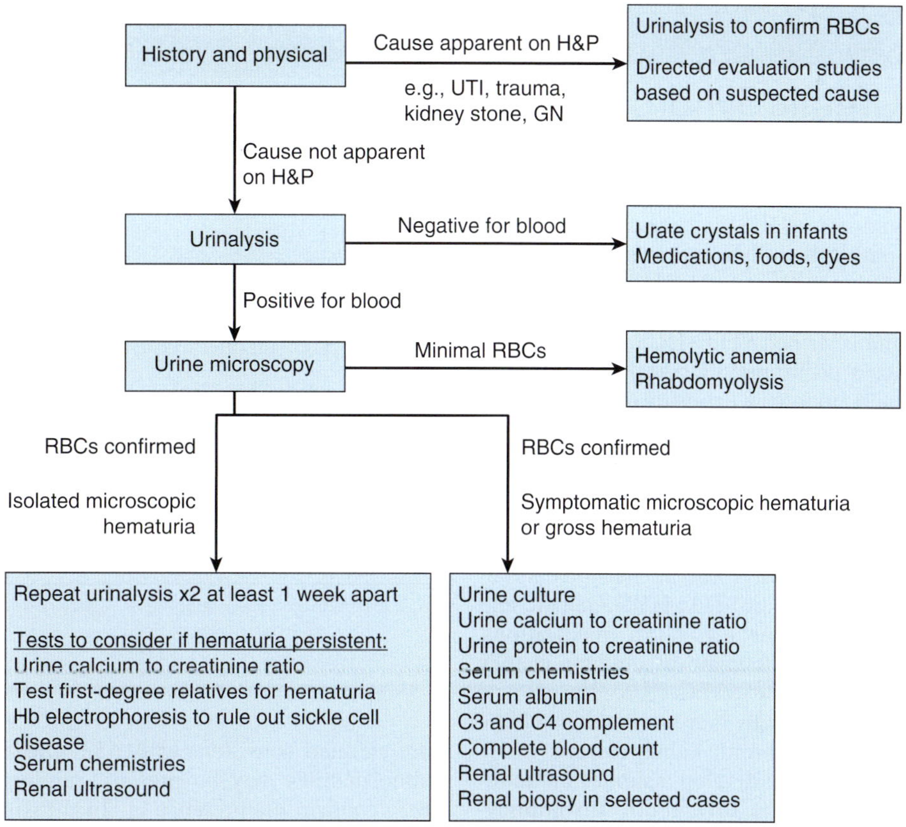

FIGURE 164.1 Suggested diagnostic algorithm for evaluation of red urine/hematuria. *GN*, Glomerulonephritis; *Hb*, hemoglobin; *H&P*, history and physical; *RBCs*, red blood cells; *UTI*, urinary tract infection.

DIAGNOSTIC STUDIES

All patients with hematuria should have a careful history and physical (including blood pressure) along with urinalysis including microscopic examination to identify RBCs. Glomerular hematuria is suggested by red or brown (tea- or cola-colored) urine and presence of RBC casts on urine microscopy. Urine color that is more bright red without RBC casts is more suggestive of a lower urinary tract source.

Children with macroscopic or persistent microscopic hematuria should have additional evaluation. A suggested algorithm for the evaluation of hematuria is given in Fig. 164.1. In patients with suspected GN, complement C3 should be measured as hypocomplementemia narrows the differential diagnosis to PIGN, membranoproliferative GN, and lupus nephritis. Kidney ultrasound is helpful in ruling out tumor, hydronephrosis, cystic disease and urolithiasis. Urine calcium to creatinine ($U_{Ca/Cr}$) ratio screens for hypercalciuria; abnormal findings (>0.2 mg/mg) should be confirmed with a 24-hour urine collection for calcium and creatinine. Children with isolated, asymptomatic microscopic hematuria with negative evaluation may be observed with yearly urinalyses. If the child develops proteinuria, hypertension, or loss of kidney function, nephrology referral is appropriate.

TREATMENT

Treatment of PIGN involves supportive care with dietary sodium restriction, diuretics, and antihypertensive agents. Immunosuppression is not indicated because this condition resolves spontaneously over time. Antibiotics are warranted if there is an active streptococcal or other bacterial infection. Treatment of children with other forms of GN depends on the underlying cause and severity and may include corticosteroids and/or other immunosuppressive agents. Treatment with angiotensin-converting enzyme inhibitors may be helpful in the chronic setting to reduce proteinuria but should be used with caution in the setting of acute kidney injury.

PROGNOSIS AND PREVENTION

PIGN usually has a favorable outcome. In typical cases, the macroscopic hematuria, proteinuria, and edema decline quickly (5–10 days), whereas microscopic hematuria may persist for months or even years; >95% of children recover completely with no long-term sequelae.

Children with IgA nephropathy and other forms of chronic GN have greater risk of progression to ESKD, which is variable and related to the underlying disorder and disease severity. The presence of persistent and heavy proteinuria, hypertension, decreased kidney function, and severe glomerular lesions on kidney biopsy are associated with poor outcomes.

Children with idiopathic isolated, asymptomatic microscopic hematuria, or suspected thin basement membrane disease typically have an excellent prognosis. Long-term follow-up, including yearly urinalysis and blood pressure measurement, is required to exclude progressive forms of kidney disease.

PEARLS FOR PRACTITIONERS

See Nephrology and Urology: Pearls for Practitioners at the end of this section.

REVIEW QUESTIONS

Available online.

CHAPTER 165

Hemolytic Uremic Syndrome

ETIOLOGY AND EPIDEMIOLOGY

Hemolytic uremic syndrome (HUS) is characterized by the triad of **microangiopathic hemolytic anemia**, **thrombocytopenia**, and **acute kidney injury (AKI)**. The most common form of HUS is associated with **Shiga-toxin producing *Escherichia coli* (STEC)** and is termed **STEC-HUS**. Children with STEC-HUS experience a prodromal diarrheal illness due to hemorrhagic enterocolitis following exposure to a pathogenic agent (most commonly ***E. coli* O157:H7**). STEC-HUS outbreaks have been associated with contaminated ground beef, fruit, vegetables, or water. STEC-HUS occurs in ~5–15% of children with STEC infection.

HUS may also occur unrelated to STEC infection **(non-STEC-HUS)**. Infection with *Streptococcus pneumoniae* or HIV has been associated with non-STEC-HUS. Genetic and acquired defects in complement regulation, medications, malignancy, systemic lupus erythematosus, and pregnancy may also be associated with non–STEC-HUS. The clinical course of non–STEC-HUS is usually more severe than STEC-HUS and more likely to lead to chronic kidney disease.

Less commonly, children may develop a similar microangiopathic syndrome, identified as **thrombotic thrombocytopenic purpura** (TTP). Children with TTP typically have predominantly central nervous system symptoms but may also have significant kidney involvement. Because central nervous system involvement is also seen in HUS, TTP can be difficult to distinguish from HUS. Children with TTP have severe deficiency of ADAMTS13, a von Willebrand factor–cleaving protease.

CLINICAL MANIFESTATIONS

STEC-HUS typically occurs in children <5 years of age but can occur in older children. Classic STEC-HUS begins with enterocolitis, often with bloody stools, followed in 7–10 days by weakness, lethargy, and oliguria/anuria. Physical examination reveals irritability, pallor, and petechiae. Volume depletion is common at presentation; however, some children have volume overload. Hypertension may be present due to volume overload and/or kidney injury. Central nervous system involvement, including seizures, occurs in up to 25% of cases. Other organ involvement can include pancreatitis, cardiac dysfunction, and colonic perforation. Children with non–STEC-HUS have similar clinical presentation but usually without a recent history of enterocolitis.

DIAGNOSTIC STUDIES

Common laboratory findings in HUS are listed in Table 165.1. Peripheral blood smear reveals evidence of microangiopathic hemolysis with schistocytes and thrombocytopenia. Coombs test is negative. Serum blood urea nitrogen and creatinine are elevated consistent with AKI, and associated electrolyte abnormalities may be present. Serologic and stool studies may confirm the presence of Shiga toxin, although the toxin may no longer be present by the time of diagnosis of HUS. ADAMTS13 level is normal in all forms of HUS but is severely deficient in TTP.

TABLE 165.1 Common Laboratory Findings With Hemolytic Uremic Syndrome

EVIDENCE OF MICROANGIOPATHIC HEMOLYTIC ANEMIA
Anemia (schistocytes, helmet cells, and burr cells on peripheral blood smear) Thrombocytopenia Increased LDH Decreased haptoglobin Increased indirect bilirubin Increased AST Elevated reticulocyte count
EVIDENCE OF KIDNEY INJURY
Elevated serum creatinine Hematuria, proteinuria, casts on urinalysis
OTHER POTENTIAL FINDINGS
Leukocytosis Positive stool culture for *E. coli* O157:H7 Positive stool test for Shiga toxin Elevated amylase/lipase

AST, Aspartate aminotransferase; *LDH*, lactate dehydrogenase.

TREATMENT AND PROGNOSIS

Therapy for STEC-HUS is supportive and includes volume repletion, treatment of hypertension, and management of complications of AKI, including dialysis when indicated. Early and aggressive intravenous hydration with isotonic saline during the diarrheal phase may lessen the severity of AKI. Red blood cell transfusions are provided as needed. Platelet transfusions should be reserved for active hemorrhage or prior to invasive procedures because they may fuel the thrombotic microangiopathy process. Antibiotics and antidiarrheal agents should be avoided in children with STEC infection as they increase the risk of developing HUS. Most children with STEC-HUS survive the acute phase and recover normal kidney function (>95%), although some may have evidence of chronic kidney disease and other morbidity. Treatment of non–STEC-HUS depends on the underlying etiology.

PEARLS FOR PRACTITIONERS

See Nephrology and Urology: Pearls for Practitioners at the end of this section.

REVIEW QUESTIONS

Available online.

CHAPTER 166

Acute Kidney Injury and Chronic Kidney Disease

ACUTE KIDNEY INJURY

Etiology

Acute kidney injury (AKI), formerly termed *acute renal failure*, refers to an abrupt decrease in glomerular filtration rate (GFR) leading to accumulation of waste products (e.g., urea) and disturbances in fluid, electrolyte, and acid-base balance. AKI may be **oliguric** (<1 mL/kg/hr in neonates and infants, <0.5 mL/kg/hr in children) or **nonoliguric**, which may be more difficult to recognize.

Causes of AKI may be divided into prerenal (renal hypoperfusion), intrinsic (tubular, glomerular, or vascular injury), and postrenal (urinary tract obstruction) categories (Table 166.1). In many cases, the cause of AKI is multifactorial. **Prerenal AKI** is most commonly due to **volume depletion** but may be secondary to other mechanisms of glomerular hypoperfusion such as cardiac dysfunction or sepsis. **Intrinsic AKI** may be due to **acute tubular necrosis** (ATN), which can be caused by a hypoxic-ischemic insult and/or exposure to nephrotoxic agents (medications, contrast, myoglobin). Acute glomerulonephritis, acute tubulointerstitial nephritis, and vascular thromboses are other causes of intrinsic AKI. **Postrenal AKI** occurs due to conditions that result in either structural or functional **urinary tract obstruction**.

Clinical Manifestations

History, physical examination, and basic laboratory studies usually allow proper classification of the child with AKI (Table 166.2). Prerenal AKI is characterized by history of precipitating factors leading to poor renal perfusion, most commonly due to volume depletion. Urine output is low. Intrinsic AKI from ATN is associated with precipitating factors such as prolonged hypotension or exposure to nephrotoxic agents. Urine output in ATN may be low, normal, or high, depending on the severity of the injury; muddy brown casts are often seen in the urine. Children with intrinsic AKI from glomerulonephritis present with hematuria, edema, hypertension, and oliguria. Postrenal AKI is characterized by low or normal urine output and may be associated with flank masses or a distended bladder on examination. Depending on the underlying cause and severity of illness, AKI can be associated with signs of volume depletion or volume overload.

TABLE 166.1 Causes of Acute Kidney Injury

PRERENAL
Dehydration
Hemorrhage
Septic shock
Burns
Heart failure
Cirrhosis
INTRINSIC
Acute tubular necrosis (hypoxic-ischemic insult +/− nephrotoxin exposure)
Infection (sepsis)
Interstitial nephritis (allergic, drug-induced)
Glomerular injury (glomerulonephritis, vasculitis, hemolytic uremic syndrome)
Vascular (renal vein thrombosis, arterial emboli, malignant hypertension)
POSTRENAL (OBSTRUCTION)
Urethral obstruction (stricture, posterior urethral valves)
Ureteral obstruction (stone)
Ureterocele
Bladder outlet obstruction (extrinsic tumor)
Neurogenic bladder (myelomeningocele, spinal cord injury)

Diagnostic Studies

Early recognition and management of AKI is crucial. A **urinalysis** (UA) should be obtained in all children with AKI. In children with prerenal AKI, the UA lacks hematuria or significant proteinuria, but shows a high specific gravity reflecting appropriate urinary concentration. Neonates, children with preexisting kidney disease, and individuals with sickle cell disease may not be able to concentrate urine well despite volume depletion. In children with intrinsic AKI, the UA may show hematuria and proteinuria or casts. Differentiation between prerenal AKI and ATN may be made by determining urine osmolality, fractional excretion of sodium, and urine biomarkers such as neutrophil gelatinase-associated lipocalin (NGAL) (see Table 166.2). **Kidney ultrasound** may show hydronephrosis in patients with postrenal AKI (see Table 166.2). Kidney biopsy is indicated only in select cases of intrinsic AKI.

Common laboratory abnormalities seen in AKI include hyperkalemia, hyponatremia, metabolic acidosis, hypocalcemia, and hyperphosphatemia. Blood work should be trended over time, the frequency of which depends on initial results and the patient's clinical course. A complete blood count should be measured as anemia is frequently observed in children with AKI. Other laboratory studies may be obtained as clinically indicated.

Treatment

In some cases, treating the underlying disorder will improve AKI. Examples include volume repletion in dehydration, stopping an offending nephrotoxic medication, or relieving urinary tract obstruction. In all cases, efforts should be made to limit additional kidney injury (e.g., ensuring adequate kidney perfusion and avoiding nephrotoxic medications). Medication dosages and intervals should be adjusted for decreased GFR as appropriate.

Initial approach to fluid therapy depends on the child's volume status and urine output. If hypovolemia is present, intravascular volume should be expanded using intravenous saline administration. If hypervolemia is present, 1–2 mg/kg of furosemide and fluid restriction may be indicated. If euvolemia is present, total fluid input should be adjusted to match insensible losses and urine output, which may be higher or lower than normal. All children with AKI should have careful measurement of intake and output as well as serial body weight measurements and physical examination with attention to volume status.

TABLE 166.2 Laboratory and Clinical Evaluation of Acute Kidney Injury

LABORATORY/ CLINICAL FEATURE	PRERENAL		RENAL		POSTRENAL
	CHILD	NEONATE	CHILD	NEONATE	
Urine output	Low		Low, normal, or high		Low or normal
Urinalysis	Normal		RBCs, WBCs, protein, casts		Variable
Urine Na^+ (mEq/L)	<15	<20–30	>40	>50	Variable, may be >40
FE_{Na}* (%)	<1	<2.5	>2	>2.5	Variable, may be >2
Urine osmolality (mOsm/L)	>500	>350	~300	~300	Variable, may be <300
Renal ultrasound	Normal		Increased echogenicity, decreased corticomedullary differentiation		Hydronephrosis

*FE_{Na} (%) = [(urine sodium/plasma sodium) ÷ (urine creatinine/plasma creatinine)] × 100.
FE_{Na}, Fractional excretion of sodium; *RBCs*, red blood cells; *WBCs*, white blood cells.

Treatment of AKI involves prevention and management of potential complications, including electrolyte abnormalities. Potassium intake and medications that increase potassium should be restricted. If hyperkalemia occurs, intravenous calcium will lower the risk of arrhythmia while measures are initiated to shift potassium into cells (bicarbonate, β-agonists, insulin/dextrose) and hasten removal (diuretics, sodium-potassium exchange resins, dialysis). Hyperphosphatemia should be treated with phosphorus restriction and administration of phosphate binders. Hypertension may be treated with diuretics, calcium channel blockers, and vasodilators. Angiotensin-converting enzyme (ACE) inhibitors are usually avoided in the setting of AKI.

Indications for **acute dialysis** (kidney support therapy) are listed in Table 166.3. There is no specific blood urea nitrogen or creatinine level at which dialysis is needed in patients with AKI. Kidney support therapy options in children include hemodialysis, peritoneal dialysis, and continuous renal replacement therapy (CRRT). The mode is selected based on individual factors.

Prognosis

Recovery from AKI depends on the etiology and severity of AKI and other patient characteristics. Preterm infants who experience AKI prior to completion of kidney development are at particularly high risk. Even with seemingly good recovery, a history of moderate to severe AKI, especially if kidney support therapy was required, places the child at increased risk for future chronic kidney disease (CKD).

TABLE 166.3 Indications for Kidney Support Therapy

ACUTE AND/OR CHRONIC DIALYSIS
Volume overload Metabolic acidosis Electrolyte abnormalities (hyperkalemia) Uremia
ACUTE DIALYSIS
Certain ingestions Hyperammonemia
CHRONIC DIALYSIS
Poor growth Stage 5 chronic kidney disease (end-stage kidney disease)

CHRONIC KIDNEY DISEASE

Etiology and Epidemiology

Congenital anomalies of the kidney and urinary tract (CAKUT), such as renal dysplasia, are the most common causes of CKD in children. Acquired kidney diseases, such as focal segmental glomerulosclerosis and chronic glomerulonephritis (GN), are more common causes of CKD in older children and teens. The risk of progression to end-stage kidney disease (ESKD) is related to the underlying cause and severity of CKD. Kidney function may deteriorate more rapidly during puberty due to increased demands of growth and maturation.

CKD is staged to facilitate appropriate evaluation and monitoring according to estimated GFR (Table 166.4). GFR can be estimated in children using the Chronic Kidney Disease in Children U25 formula (see Chapter 162). Most metabolic complications of CKD do not begin to manifest until at least stage 3 CKD. In stage 4 CKD, complications become more numerous and severe. Children with stage 5 CKD (ESKD) require treatment with either dialysis or kidney transplantation.

Clinical Manifestations

The clinical presentation of a child with CKD is related to both the underlying etiology and stage of CKD at time of diagnosis. A child with CAKUT may have polyuria, polydipsia, and recurrent urinary tract infections. A child with GN may have hematuria, proteinuria, edema, and hypertension. Common complications of CKD in children are listed in Table 166.5. Most of these complications are multifactorial in etiology. For example, **anemia** results primarily from a failure to produce adequate **erythropoietin** as well as iron deficiency. **Growth failure** may result from poor nutrition, metabolic acidosis, hormonal abnormalities, resistance to growth hormone, and **CKD–mineral bone disorder (CKD-MBD)**. CKD-MBD is usually due to **secondary hyperparathyroidism** as a result of hyperphosphatemia, hypocalcemia, and diminished 1,25-dihydroxyvitamin D production in the kidneys. If prolonged and/or severe, CKD-MBD may lead to rickets and bone

TABLE 166.4 Classification of the Stages of Chronic Kidney Disease

STAGE	GFR (mL/min/1.73 m^2)*	DESCRIPTION
1	>90	Minimal kidney damage
2	60–89	Kidney damage with mild reduction of GFR
3	30–59	Moderate reduction of GFR
4	15–29	Severe reduction of GFR
5	<15 (or dialysis)	End-stage kidney disease

*GFR ranges apply for children age ≥2 yr.
GFR, Glomerular filtration rate.
From National Kidney Foundation Kidney Disease Outcomes Quality Initiative.

TABLE 166.5 Common Complications and Treatments of Chronic Kidney Disease

COMPLICATION	TREATMENT
Poor growth	Increased caloric intake, treat acidosis, treat CKD MBD, recombinant GH
Anemia	Erythropoietin, iron supplementation
CKD-MBD/secondary hyperparathyroidism	1,25-Dihydroxyvitamin D supplementation, dietary phosphorus restriction, phosphate binders
Hypertension ± left ventricular hypertrophy	Antihypertensive medications Sodium/fluid restriction Diuretics
Electrolyte abnormalities	
Hyperkalemia	Low-K diet, furosemide, sodium polystyrene sulfonate
Hyponatremia	Sodium supplementation
Metabolic acidosis	Alkali replacement

CKD-MBD, Chronic kidney disease–mineral bone disorder; *GH*, growth hormone; *K*, potassium.

deformities. **Hypertension** and **left ventricular hypertrophy** are common cardiovascular complications. Delayed puberty results from altered gonadotropin secretion and regulation. Learning and school performance may also be impaired in children with CKD.

Treatment

The management of children with advanced CKD requires a multidisciplinary team, which ideally includes a pediatric nephrologist, nurse, dietitian, social worker, and psychologist. Adequate nutrition should be ensured even if it requires enteral supplements and tube feedings. Some infants and young children with CAKUT require supplemental salt due to urinary sodium wasting. Conversely, children with GN require salt restriction to assist in management of hypertension or edema. Common treatment considerations for CKD complications are listed in Table 166.5.

Several measures can be taken to preserve kidney function or slow progression of CKD. ACE inhibitors or angiotensin receptor blockers should be used to reduce proteinuria and control blood pressure. Potentially nephrotoxic medications such as nonsteroidal antiinflammatory drugs (NSAIDs) should be avoided when feasible. Medication adjustment for reduced kidney function is important. Protein intake is typically not restricted in pediatric CKD due to growth needs.

Children with stage 5 CKD (ESKD) require either kidney transplantation or dialysis support. The optimal treatment of ESKD is **kidney transplantation**. **Maintenance dialysis** is effective as a bridge to kidney transplantation or when kidney transplantation is not possible. **Peritoneal dialysis** is done at home by the family. **Hemodialysis** is performed three times a week at a dialysis facility. Indications for chronic dialysis are listed in Table 166.3.

Prognosis

Children with mild CKD (stages 1 and 2) are usually asymptomatic but need to be monitored for progressive loss of kidney function. Children with stages 3 and 4 CKD have a high likelihood of progressing to ESKD at some point, although the timing can vary. Because children on maintenance dialysis have the highest morbidity and mortality, the goal is to provide a kidney transplant for all children with ESKD. Children with kidney transplants generally do well but must take lifelong immunosuppressive medications associated with a variety of side effects, including infections, nephrotoxicity, cardiovascular complications, and increased risk for certain malignancies. Transplanted kidneys can last for more than 10–20 years but eventually fail, requiring re-transplantation.

PEARLS FOR PRACTITIONERS

See Nephrology and Urology: Pearls for Practitioners at the end of this section.

REVIEW QUESTIONS

Available online.

CHAPTER 167
Hypertension

DEFINITION

In children up to 12 years of age, hypertension (HTN) is defined as blood pressure (BP) >95th percentile for age, gender, and height measured on at least three different occasions. In adolescents ≥13 years of age, a cutoff of ≥130/80 is used to define HTN. The context of BP measurement (e.g., cuff size, pain, anxiety) is important. Staging of HTN is listed in Table 167.1. Severe hypertension (hypertensive crisis) has been traditionally divided into hypertensive emergency and hypertensive urgency. Hypertensive emergency is defined as markedly elevated BP associated with target organ damage (encephalopathy, papilledema, retinal hemorrhages, heart

TABLE 167.1 Classification of Blood Pressure

BP CATEGORY	AGE 1 TO <13 YR	AGE ≥13 YR
Normal	<90th BP percentile	<120/<80
Elevated BP	90th to <95th BP percentile	120/<80 to 129/<80
Stage 1 hypertension	95th BP percentile to <95th BP percentile + 12 mm Hg	130/80 to 139/89
Stage 2 hypertension	≥95th BP percentile + 12 mm Hg	≥140/90

BP, Blood pressure.
Adapted from Flynn JT, Kaelber DC, Baker-Smith CM, et al. Clinical practice guideline for screening and management of high blood pressure in children and adolescents. Pediatrics. *2017;140(3):7,e20171904. Table 3.*

failure, and AKI). Hypertensive urgency is defined as markedly elevated BP without symptoms or target organ damage.

ETIOLOGY

Pediatric HTN has many causes (Table 167.2) that are either **primary** (essential) or **secondary**. **Primary HTN** is the most common cause of HTN in children and adolescents, particularly in those who are obese. Secondary HTN should be suspected in younger and/or non-overweight children with more severely elevated BP. **Kidney disease** is the most common cause of secondary HTN in children.

CLINICAL MANIFESTATIONS

Most children with HTN have no symptoms, although those with hypertensive emergency may have symptoms of encephalopathy, heart failure, stroke, and retinopathy. Neonatal history (prematurity, low birthweight, or use of umbilical artery catheter); family history of HTN, stroke, or heart disease; and dietary history (excessive salt or caffeine, medications, and substance use) are important. Additional findings that may suggest specific causes include abdominal bruit (renal artery stenosis); diminished leg pressure and weak femoral pulse (coarctation of aorta); café-au-lait spots (neurofibromatosis-associated renal artery stenosis); flank mass (hydronephrosis, Wilms tumor); tachycardia with flushing and diaphoresis (pheochromocytoma); truncal obesity, acne, striae, and buffalo hump (Cushing syndrome); and hematuria, proteinuria, and edema (underlying kidney disease).

DIAGNOSTIC STUDIES

Children with suspected HTN should ideally have a 24-hour ambulatory blood pressure monitoring (ABPM) study to confirm the diagnosis and evaluate for **white coat hypertension** (elevated BP in the office setting only). If the ABPM confirms hypertension, the recommended evaluation includes the following:

1. Baseline assessment—urinalysis, electrolytes, blood urea nitrogen, creatinine, and kidney ultrasound (age <6 years)
2. Focused studies based on clinical suspicion (e.g., plasma metanephrines, renin, aldosterone, thyroid studies, vascular imaging)

TABLE 167.2 Causes of Hypertension

PRIMARY HYPERTENSION
Obesity/metabolic syndrome Genetically influenced hypertension
RENAL CAUSES
Congenital anomalies (renal dysplasia, obstructive uropathy) Structural disorders (Wilms tumor, polycystic kidney disease) Glomerulonephritis Acquired injury (kidney scarring, acute tubular necrosis) Obstructive uropathy
ENDOCRINE CAUSES
Catecholamine-secreting tumors (pheochromocytoma, neuroblastoma) Hypercortisolism (Cushing syndrome) Hyperaldosteronism Hyperthyroidism
NEUROLOGIC CAUSES
Increased sympathetic activity (stress, anxiety, pain) Dysautonomia Increased intracranial pressure
VASCULAR CAUSES
Coarctation of the aorta Renal artery embolism (from umbilical artery catheter) Renal vein thrombosis Renal artery stenosis Vasculitis
OTHER CAUSES
Obstructive sleep apnea Medications, substance use

3. Assessment of other cardiovascular risk factors (lipids, fasting glucose, hemoglobin A_{1c}, sleep study)
4. Assessment for target organ damage (echocardiogram for left ventricular hypertrophy when considering initiation of antihypertensive medication)

TREATMENT

Therapeutic lifestyle changes (diet, exercise) should be initiated for asymptomatic stage 1 HTN. Antihypertensive medication should be started for children with stage 2 or symptomatic HTN and stage 1 HTN that fails to respond to lifestyle changes. Calcium channel blockers, angiotensin-converting enzyme inhibitors, angiotensin receptor blockers, and thiazide diuretics are recommended first-line antihypertensive agents. More than one agent may be needed. Hypertensive emergency requires prompt hospitalization and may require parenteral antihypertensive treatment with nicardipine, labetalol, esmolol, or sodium nitroprusside.

PROGNOSIS

Prognosis depends on the underlying etiology and adequacy of BP control. Primary HTN is usually not associated with morbidity at presentation. However, untreated asymptomatic stage 1 HTN may increase risk for cardiovascular, central nervous system, and chronic kidney disease in adulthood.

PEARLS FOR PRACTITIONERS

See Nephrology and Urology: Pearls for Practitioners at the end of this section.

REVIEW QUESTIONS

Available online.

CHAPTER 168

Vesicoureteral Reflux

ETIOLOGY AND EPIDEMIOLOGY

Vesicoureteral reflux (VUR) is retrograde flow of urine from the bladder to the ureter and/or kidney. VUR is the most common anatomic abnormality found in infants and young children with febrile urinary tract infection (UTI). Primary VUR is most common and results from a congenitally short segment of ureter within the bladder wall that does not get fully compressed during bladder contraction. There is a genetic predisposition to primary VUR, with an increased risk in children with affected parents or siblings.

Secondary VUR may be present in children with other urinary tract anomalies. In children with **ureteral duplication**, VUR is commonly seen in the ureter draining the lower pole of the kidney. VUR is seen in up to 50% of children with **neurogenic bladder**. VUR may also be seen in children with increased intravesicular pressure due to **bladder outlet obstruction** (e.g., posterior urethral valves, prune belly syndrome).

CLINICAL MANIFESTATIONS

The most common clinical manifestation of VUR is **febrile UTI** (see Chapter 115). Recurrent febrile UTI is more likely in children with higher grade VUR. **Reflux nephropathy** involves development of kidney scarring in a child with VUR and recurrent febrile UTI; this complication is more likely in children with higher grade VUR and more frequent infections. Kidney scarring is not always visible on ultrasound and is best identified by **nuclear renal scan** (also termed *renal scintigraphy*).

DIAGNOSTIC STUDIES

Kidney ultrasound is typically obtained first to evaluate the kidneys and urinary tract. Although the presence of ultrasound anomalies make VUR more likely, a normal kidney ultrasound does not rule out VUR. Therefore a **voiding cystourethrogram** (VCUG) is required to assess for VUR in a child with recurrent febrile UTI. An international grading system based on VCUG imaging is useful to describe the severity of reflux (Fig. 168.1). For follow-up studies, either VCUG or **radionuclide cystogram** (RNC) may suffice.

The American Academy of Pediatrics recommends obtaining a kidney ultrasound in children 2–24 months of age following an initial febrile UTI. A VCUG is indicated if the kidney ultrasound reveals hydronephrosis, scarring, or findings suggestive of either high-grade VUR or obstructive uropathy and in other atypical or complex clinical circumstances. In children with a normal kidney ultrasound a VCUG is recommended after the second febrile UTI.

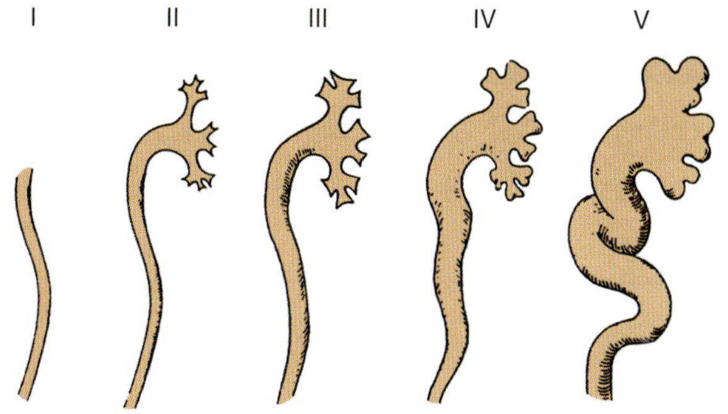

FIGURE 168.1 International classification of vesicoureteral reflux. Grade I: into a nondilated ureter; grade II: into the pelvis and calyces without dilation; grade III: mild to moderate dilation of the ureter, renal pelvis, and calyces with minimal blunting of the fornices; grade IV: moderate ureteral tortuosity and dilation of the pelvis and calyces; grade V: gross dilation of the ureter, pelvis, and calyces; loss of papillary impressions; and ureteral tortuosity. (From Partin A, Dmochowski R, Kavoussi L, et al., eds. *Campbell-Walsh-Wein Urology*. 12th ed. Philadelphia: Elsevier; 2021.)

MANAGEMENT

Grades 1 and 2 primary VUR will likely self-resolve as the intravesical ureteral segment lengthens with growth. Many cases of grades 3 and 4 primary VUR resolve when VUR is diagnosed before 2 years of age and is unilateral. Severe (grade 5) primary VUR and secondary VUR are less likely to resolve spontaneously. Management options for a child with VUR include surveillance, medical therapy, and surgical intervention, but there is lack of consensus on when these options are indicated.

In children with low-grade VUR, a surveillance approach with early evaluation of suspected UTI is often recommended. Antibiotic prophylaxis may benefit children with moderate- to high-grade VUR and/or recurrent UTI. Although there is evidence that antibiotic prophylaxis reduces UTI frequency, it is not clear that antibiotic prophylaxis reduces kidney scarring. Children with VUR should be monitored for bowel and bladder dysfunction because medical treatment of these comorbidities may facilitate resolution of VUR and reduce risk of UTI. Children with high-grade VUR or VUR complicated by recurrent febrile UTI despite antibiotic prophylaxis should be referred to urology because surgical intervention may be indicated. Children with VUR and recurrent UTI should be monitored for evidence of CKD including poor growth, hypertension, and proteinuria.

PEARLS FOR PRACTITIONERS

See Nephrology and Urology: Pearls for Practitioners at the end of this section.

REVIEW QUESTION

Available online.

CHAPTER 169

Congenital and Developmental Abnormalities of the Urinary Tract

ETIOLOGY AND EPIDEMIOLOGY

Congenital anomalies of the kidneys and urinary tract (CAKUT) are a leading cause of pediatric chronic kidney disease (CKD) and occur in up to 4% of infants. CAKUT may be an isolated condition or may be part of a broader syndrome that includes extrarenal manifestations. Both genetic and environmental factors may play a role in development of CAKUT.

Abnormal Kidney Structure

Renal agenesis results from early disruption in embryonal kidney development. In most cases, bilateral renal agenesis is lethal due to severe oligohydramnios and pulmonary hypoplasia since lung development is dependent on fetal urine production. Unilateral renal agenesis can be observed with other CAKUT or extrarenal anomalies such as VACTERL association (vertebral abnormalities, anal atresia, cardiac abnormalities, tracheoesophageal fistula, renal anomalies, and limb defects). Unilateral renal agenesis is usually characterized by normal or minimally reduced renal function at birth. Children with a solitary kidney should have periodic kidney ultrasounds to confirm compensatory hypertrophy of the solitary kidney and be monitored for the development of proteinuria, hypertension, and CKD over time.

Renal hypoplasia/dysplasia refers to kidneys that are congenitally small, malformed, or both. Kidney ultrasonography shows increased echogenicity, decreased corticomedullary differentiation, and in some cases renal cysts. Many affected children will develop progressive CKD due to reduced nephron number, so periodic monitoring of kidney function and surveillance for CKD complications is recommended. Some children have polyuria due to an inability to fully reabsorb sodium and water in which case salt and water supplementation may be indicated.

A **multicystic dysplastic kidney** (MCDK) is a nonfunctioning kidney with many cysts of variable size separated by dysplastic tissue. MCDK is usually identified on prenatal ultrasounds but may also be detected as a flank mass in the neonate. The contralateral kidney is often structurally normal but may be associated with other abnormalities, the most common being vesicoureteral reflux (VUR). In many children, the MCDK spontaneously involutes over time while the contralateral kidney undergoes compensatory hypertrophy. Children with MCDK should be monitored similarly to children with solitary kidney due to renal agenesis.

Polycystic kidney diseases (PKDs) are a group of genetic disorders affecting the kidneys and other tissues. **Autosomal recessive PKD (ARPKD)** is caused by pathogenic variants in the *PKHD1* gene and is clinically characterized by marked bilateral kidney enlargement due to numerous microcysts. In some cases, kidney failure develops in utero resulting in oligohydramnios and pulmonary hypoplasia. Congenital **hepatic fibrosis** is universally present and may lead to bile duct ectasia, biliary dysgenesis, and portal hypertension. Common clinical features include flank masses, hepatosplenomegaly, hypertension, proteinuria, and/or hematuria. End-stage kidney disease often occurs by early childhood.

Autosomal dominant PKD (ADPKD) occurs in 1 in 400–1,000 individuals, making it the most common inherited kidney disease. ADPKD is caused by pathologic variants in *PKD1* or *PKD2*. It is clinically characterized by progressive development of kidney cysts, typically beginning in childhood or young adulthood, but can manifest in a small subset during infancy. Most children and adolescents are asymptomatic, and complications such as hypertension, flank pain, and progressive CKD usually develop in adulthood. Extrarenal manifestations include cysts in other organs (most commonly the liver) and cerebral aneurysms. Cystic kidney disease can be a feature of other inherited disorders such as tuberous sclerosis complex, Bardet-Biedl syndrome, and von Hippel–Lindau syndrome.

Abnormal Kidney Position

Disruption of the normal migration of the kidneys from the pelvis to the renal fossae during embryological development can lead to ectopic kidney or fusion anomalies. The most common form of ectopic kidney is **pelvic kidney**, which is usually unilateral. Fusion anomalies involve congenital fusion of the kidneys, usually at the lower poles, with at least one kidney being ectopic. **Horseshoe kidney** is the most common fusion anomaly in which the renal pelvis of both kidneys remains on its respective side of the midline. In **crossed fused ectopia**, one kidney crosses the midline to fuse with the contralateral kidney.

Children with ectopic kidney or fusion abnormalities have an increased risk of hydronephrosis, VUR, urinary tract infection (UTI), and kidney stones. However, both conditions typically have excellent prognosis for most patients.

Abnormal Urinary Tract

Anomalies of the urinary tract may occur anywhere from the renal pelvis to the urethra (Table 169.1). **Urinary tract obstruction** (UTO) is one of the most concerning conditions

TABLE 169.1 Urinary Tract Anomalies by Site

SITE	URINARY TRACT ANOMALY
Renal pelvis	Duplicated collecting system Hydronephrosis Ureteropelvic junction obstruction
Ureter	Duplicated renal collecting system Megaureter Ectopic ureter Ureterocele
Bladder	Vesicoureteral reflux Bladder diverticulum Bladder/cloacal exstrophy
Urethra	Posterior urethral valves Urethral stricture Hypospadias

because severe obstruction can lead to irreversible kidney injury. UTO is most commonly identified by the presence of urinary tract dilation (hydronephrosis ± hydroureter) on prenatal ultrasound or on imaging obtained following UTI. Severe prenatal obstruction can interfere with normal development resulting in renal dysplasia; obstruction that develops later in childhood can result in kidney scarring. UTO predisposes to UTI due to urinary stasis.

Posterior urethral valves (PUV) are the most common cause of **bladder outlet obstruction** in males. Most affected infants are initially identified by the presence of bilateral urinary tract dilation on prenatal ultrasonography. Prenatal obstruction of the bladder leads to abnormal bladder development. Parents may note a poor urinary stream. PUV commonly results in renal dysplasia, hydronephrosis, VUR, and bladder dysfunction, which can persist after valve ablation.

Hydronephrosis in the absence of UTO is one of the most common forms of CAKUT. Hydronephrosis seen on prenatal ultrasound should be confirmed on postnatal ultrasound done from 48 hours (when urine output is well established) to 4 weeks of life. If clinically indicated due to signs of kidney dysfunction, ultrasound may be obtained sooner than 48 hours. For patients with moderate to severe hydronephrosis, additional imaging with voiding cystourethrogram (to evaluate for VUR and bladder outlet obstruction) and/or diuretic renogram (to evaluate for UTO such as ureteropelvic junction obstruction) may be considered. Diuretic renogram should usually be delayed until 1 month of age when the glomerular filtration rate is higher. Duplicated (or duplex) collecting system is also frequently observed and may involve a complete or more commonly partial duplication. Duplicated collecting systems are commonly benign but may have increased risk for UTO of the upper pole and VUR of the lower pole.

PEARLS FOR PRACTITIONERS

See Nephrology and Urology: Pearls for Practitioners at the end of this section.

REVIEW QUESTIONS

Available online.

CHAPTER 170

Other Urinary Tract and Genital Disorders

URINARY STONE DISEASE

Etiology

Kidney stones have become increasingly common in the pediatric population. An underlying risk factor can be identified in many children with **urolithiasis**. Risk factors for kidney stones include urinary tract structural abnormalities such as hydronephrosis or an underlying metabolic predisposition including hypercalciuria (most common), hypocitraturia, hyperoxaluria, hyperuricosuria, and cystinuria. Risk factors for primary bladder stones include recurrent urinary tract infection (UTI), neurogenic bladder, and intestinal bladder augmentation.

Clinical Manifestations

Acute obstruction of urine flow occurs when a stone becomes lodged in the urinary tract (commonly at the ureteropelvic junction or the ureterovesical junction) and causes renal colic, a severe sharp intermittent pain in the flank or lower abdomen often radiating to the groin and commonly associated with nausea and vomiting. In younger children, fussiness, abdominal pain, and vomiting may be the only symptoms. Hematuria may be gross or microscopic and typically clears rapidly with passage of stone material. Nonobstructing stones in the kidney are typically asymptomatic and may be identified incidentally on imaging done for other purposes.

Diagnostic Studies

Renal ultrasound is usually the initial test of choice for suspected stones in children. Ultrasound can identify hydronephrosis and most stones in the kidney but can miss very small stones and stones distal to the kidney. Noncontrast computed tomography (CT) can identify stones of all sizes throughout the entire urinary tract. Plain abdominal radiography is less sensitive for identifying stones than ultrasound and CT. Chemical analysis of stone material can identify the stone composition and inform the underlying stone etiology. After a child has recovered from an acute stone episode and is back to a typical diet, a 24-hour urine collection (or spot studies if not toilet trained) and blood work can help identify underlying metabolic risk factors for stone formation.

Treatment

Acute treatment of a child with active stone disease consists primarily of hydration and analgesia. Tamsulosin has been used with success in older children to promote passage of distal ureteral stones. Surgical intervention by a pediatric urologist may be required for children with large, infected, or obstructing stones. Long-term management is directed at stone prevention with the most important component being vigorous fluid intake, ideally at a rate greater than the usual maintenance volume. Specific metabolic conditions require specific treatments. For children with hypercalciuria, dietary interventions include increased fluid intake, low sodium and oxalate intake, and normal calcium intake. Children with hypercalciuria and recurrent stones despite dietary management may benefit from treatment with thiazide diuretics or potassium citrate. Children with hypocitraturia may benefit from potassium citrate supplementation.

VOIDING DYSFUNCTION

Etiology and Epidemiology

Voiding difficulties are frequent in preschool-aged children due to immature bladder and micturition pathways. Normal voiding patterns and continence rely on urinary tract structural integrity, neurologic maturation, and coordination between somatic and autonomic nervous system units. Daytime continence is usually achieved before nighttime continence. Most children are dry during both day and night by 5–7 years of age. **Primary nocturnal enuresis** is defined as the involuntary loss of urine during sleep in a child 5 years of age and older who has not had a 6-month span of nighttime continence. Up to 20% of 5-year-old children have primary nocturnal enuresis, with ~15% spontaneous resolution per year. Males are affected more than females, and there is a familial predisposition (40% prevalence at 6 years of age if one affected parent, 70% if two affected parents). **Secondary enuresis** involves loss of nighttime control after an extended period of dryness and generally requires further evaluation.

Clinical Manifestations

Dysfunctional voiding (DV) may manifest as incontinence, frequency, urgency, hesitancy, holding maneuvers, dysuria, lower abdominal pain, or recurrent UTI. Concomitant bowel dysfunction is common including constipation and encopresis. DV symptoms may also be affected by recent UTI or life stressors. Most children with DV are anatomically, neurologically, and psychologically normal. Children with primary nocturnal enuresis typically have no symptoms during the day, but recent life stressors may be associated with more frequent bedwetting.

Diagnostic Studies

Evaluation for DV may be performed at any age, but isolated urinary incontinence in an otherwise normal child is usually not evaluated until 5 years of age. Urinalysis and urine culture should be obtained to exclude occult infection and renal disease. Indications for ultrasound imaging include suspicion of neurologic or urinary tract abnormality, UTI, continuous incontinence, and failure to improve with conservative management. Urodynamic evaluation is typically reserved for children with suspected neurogenic bladder, severe bladder dysfunction with hydronephrosis, urinary tract abnormalities, or DV refractory to treatment. Evaluation of primary nocturnal enuresis is usually limited but should include urinalysis.

Treatment

Timed voiding and anticholinergic medications are used to treat sensory defects and bladder hyperactivity. More complicated treatment regimens include biofeedback, α-blockers, and intermittent catheterization. For children with isolated primary nocturnal enuresis, bed-wetting alarms provide safe and effective resolution of enuresis for >70% of affected children. Oral desmopressin may also be considered in selected children with anticholinergics and imipramine less commonly used.

DISORDERS OF THE PENIS

Etiology

Hypospadias occurs in ~1 in 500 newborn infants. In this condition, the urethral folds fail to fuse completely over the urethral groove, leaving the urethral meatus ventral and proximal to its normal position. The ventral foreskin is also lacking, and the dorsal portion gives the appearance of a hood. It can be associated with **chordee**, a fixed ventral curvature of the penile shaft. Rarely, when the urethra opens onto the perineum, the chordee is extreme, the scrotum is bifid and sometimes extends to the dorsal base of the penis.

Both genetic and environmental factors that interfere with androgenic stimulation have been associated with increased risk for hypospadias. Other urinary tract anomalies are uncommonly associated with hypospadias. Severe hypospadias with undescended testes suggests a disorder of sexual differentiation (see Chapter 178).

In 90% of uncircumcised males, the foreskin should be retractable by adolescence. Before this age, a tight prepuce may be normal and does not need treatment. After this age, the inability to retract the prepuce is termed **phimosis**. The condition may be congenital or the result of inflammation. **Paraphimosis** occurs when the prepuce has been retracted behind the coronal sulcus, cannot resume its normal position, and causes pain and swelling of the glans.

Clinical Manifestations and Treatment

The meatal opening in **hypospadias** may be located anteriorly (on the glans, coronal, or distal third of the shaft), on the middle third of the shaft, or posteriorly (near the scrotum). Undescended testes and inguinal hernias are commonly associated conditions with severe hypospadias. Males with hypospadias should not be circumcised, particularly if the meatus is proximal to the glans, because the foreskin may be necessary for later repair. Most pediatric urologists repair hypospadias before 18 months of age.

Phimosis is rarely symptomatic. Parents should be reassured that loosening of the prepuce usually occurs during puberty. A topical steroid is used for treatment if needed. If the narrowing is severe, gentle stretching may be useful. Circumcision is reserved for the most severe cases. **Paraphimosis** with venous stasis and edema leads to severe pain. When paraphimosis is discovered early, reduction of the foreskin may be possible with lubrication. In some cases, emergent circumcision is needed.

DISORDERS OF THE SCROTUM AND ITS CONTENTS

Epidemiology

Undescended testes (cryptorchidism) describes testes in a position along the path of testicular descent but not in the scrotum and is diagnosed in ~1% of males after 1 year of age. Unilateral or bilateral undescended testes at birth are more common in preterm infants than full-term newborns (30% vs. 3%) and are associated with low birth weight (20% in 2,000- to 2,500-g infants). Cryptorchidism at birth is bilateral in 10% of cases. Spontaneous testicular descent rarely occurs after 6 months of age. Failure to find one or both testes in the scrotum does not necessarily indicate undescended testicles. **Ectopic testes** are testes located outside the path of testicular descent, making this diagnosis distinct from cryptorchidism. Although most cases of cryptorchidism are isolated and do not have an identified cause, cryptorchidism can be a symptom of underlying conditions impacting the hypothalamic-pituitary-gonadal axis.

Clinical Manifestations

A history of whether the testis was ever noted in the scrotum, prenatal exposures (such as tobacco, diethylstilbestrol), and family history are important in the evaluation of a child with apparent cryptorchidism. The true undescended testis is found along the normal embryologic path of descent, usually in the presence of a patent processus vaginalis. An undescended testis is often associated with an inguinal hernia; it is also at risk of **testicular torsion**. There is a high incidence of infertility in adulthood. When bilateral and untreated, infertility is uniform. There is increased malignancy risk (five times the normal rate) with undescended testis, usually presenting between 20 and 30 years of age. The risk is greater in untreated males and those who had surgical correction during or after puberty.

Retractile testes are normal testes that retract into the inguinal canal from an exaggerated cremasteric reflex. The diagnosis of retractile testes is likely if testes are palpable in the newborn period but not at later examination. Parents frequently describe seeing testes in the scrotum when their child is in the bath and seeing one or both "disappear" in other settings.

Complications

Testicular torsion is an emergency requiring prompt diagnosis and treatment to save the affected testis. Torsion accounts for 40% of cases of acute scrotal pain and swelling and is the major cause of acute scrotum in patients less than 6 years of age. It is thought to arise from abnormal fixation of the testis to the scrotum. On examination, the testicle is swollen and tender, and the cremasteric reflex is absent. The absence of blood flow on Doppler ultrasound is consistent with torsion.

The differential diagnosis of testicular pain includes trauma, incarcerated hernia, and torsion of the testicular epididymal appendix. Torsion of the appendix testis is associated with point tenderness over the lesion and minimal swelling. In adolescents, the differential diagnosis of testicular torsion also must include **epididymitis**, the most common cause of acute scrotal pain and swelling in older adolescents. Diagnosis is aided by an antecedent history of sexual activity or UTI. Testicular torsion must still be considered as the principal diagnosis when acute severe testicular pain is present.

Treatment

The undescended testis is usually histologically normal at birth with progressive atrophy and dysplasia occurring over time. Some patients have congenital dysplasia in the contralateral descended testis. Surgical correction at an early age improves adult fertility potential. **Orchidopexy** is usually done between 6 and 12 months of life. Most extraabdominal testes can be brought into the scrotum with correction of the associated hernia. If the testis is not palpable, ultrasound or magnetic resonance imaging may determine its location for surgical planning. The closer the testis is to the internal inguinal ring, the better the chance of successful orchidopexy.

Optimal timing for surgical correction of testicular torsion is within 6 hours of torsion. Torsion of the appendix testis and epididymitis are managed with nonsteroidal antiinflammatory medications, scrotal support, and elevation.

We gratefully acknowledge the invaluable contributions of Rama Jayanthi, MD, Pediatric Urology, Nationwide Children's Hospital, Columbus, Ohio.

PEARLS FOR PRACTITIONERS

See Nephrology and Urology: Pearls for Practitioners at the end of this section.

REVIEW QUESTIONS

Available online.

Suggested Readings

Boyer O, Niaudet P. Hemolytic-Uremic syndrome in children. *Pediatr Clin North Am*. 2022;69:1181–1197.

Flynn JT, Kaelber DC, Baker-Smith CM, et al. Clinical Practice Guideline for Screening and Management of High Blood Pressure in Children and Adolescents [published correction appears in *Pediatrics*. 2017 Dec;140(6):e20173035] [published correction appears in *Pediatrics*. 2018 Sep;142(3):e20181739]. *Pediatrics*. 2017;140(3):e20171904.

Imam AA, Saadeh SA. Evaluation of proteinuria and hematuria in the ambulatory setting. *Pediatr Clin North Am*. 2022;69:1037–1049.

Janjua, Lam SK, Gupta V, et al. Congenital anomalies of the kidneys, collecting system, bladder, and urethra. *Pediatr Rev*. 2019;40:619–626.

Mattoo TK, Mohammad D. Primary vesicoureteral reflux and renal scarring. *Pediatr Clin North Am*. 2022;18:1115–1129.

Mattoo TK, Sanjad S. Current understanding of nephrotic syndrome in children. *Pediatr Clin North Am*. 2022;69:1079–1098.

Menon S, Symons JM, Selewski DT. Acute kidney injury. *Pediatr Rev*. 2023;44:265–279.

National Institute of Diabetes and Digestive and Kidney Diseases. eGFR Calculators for Adults & Pediatrics. United States Health and Human Services National Institutes of Health. Updated May 2024. Accessed Nov 1, 2024. https://www.niddk.nih.gov/health-information/professionals/clinical-tools-patient-management/kidney-disease/laboratory-evaluation/estimated-gfr-calculators/adults-pediatrics.

Panzarino V, Lesser J, Cassani FA. Pediatric chronic kidney disease. *Adv Pediatr*. 2022;69:123–132.

Saadeh SA. Pediatric nephrolithiasis: risk factors, evaluation, and prevention. *Pediatr Ann*. 2020;49:e262–e267.

Subcommittee on Urinary Tract Infection, Steering Committee on Quality Improvement and Management, Roberts KB. Urinary tract infection: clinical practice guideline for the diagnosis and management of the initial UTI in febrile infants and children 2 to 24 months. *Pediatrics*. 2011;128(3):595–610.

PEARLS FOR PRACTITIONERS

CHAPTER 162

Nephrology and Urology Assessment

- The kidneys have many important functions including maintaining fluid and electrolyte balance, excreting metabolic waste products, and producing hormones.
- The clinical presentation of kidney and urologic disease will be affected by many factors including type of disorder, severity, chronicity, and age with characteristic findings on blood, urine, and imaging studies.
- Fetal urine production contributes to amniotic fluid volume, lung maturation, and somatic development; reduced (oligohydramnios) or increased amniotic fluid volume

(polyhydramnios) may be a sign of a congenital kidney disorder.

- Glomerular filtration rate (GFR) is normally low in newborn infants (~40 mL/min/1.73 m^2), and it takes up to 2 years to develop adult levels of GFR (100–120 mL/min/1.73 m^2). The GFR can be estimated using the Chronic Kidney Disease in Children U25 formulas. Free calculators are available online, such as from the United States Health and Human Services National Institutes of Health https://www.niddk.nih.gov/health-information/professionals/clinical-tools-patient-management/kidney-disease/laboratory-evaluation/estimated-gfr-calculators/adults-pediatrics.

CHAPTER 163

Nephrotic Syndrome and Proteinuria

- Urine protein is best quantified by a spot urine protein/creatinine ($U_{Pr}/_{Cr}$) ratio. $U_{Pr}/_{Cr}$ ratio <0.2 mg/mg is normal, between 0.2 and 2 mg/mg indicates mild to moderate proteinuria, and >2 mg/mg indicates severe (nephrotic range) proteinuria.
- Nephrotic syndrome (NS) is characterized by persistent severe proteinuria (mainly albuminuria; $U_{Pr}/_{Cr}$ ratio >2 mg/mg), hypoalbuminemia (serum albumin <3 g/dL), edema, and hypercholesterolemia (>250 mg/dL).
- Primary forms of NS include minimal change nephrotic syndrome (MCNS; most common form of childhood NS), focal segmental glomerulosclerosis, and membranous nephropathy. In addition, nephrotic syndrome may be a feature in patients with many types of glomerulonephritis (e.g., IgA nephropathy, lupus nephritis, vasculitis).
- For the child with likely MCNS (presentation between 2 and 12 years of age, no signs of systemic disorder, minimal hematuria, normal GFR, and normal C3 complement), a corticosteroid trial is warranted.
- Complications of childhood NS include serious bacterial infections, thrombosis, acute kidney injury, poor growth, and progressive chronic kidney disease if steroid resistant.

CHAPTER 164

Glomerulonephritis and Hematuria

- Hematuria may originate from glomerular, tubulointerstitial, or lower urinary tract disorders.
- Cardinal features of glomerulonephritis (GN) include hematuria, proteinuria, decreased renal function, hypertension, oliguria, and/or edema.
- Postinfectious GN is the most common form of acute GN, and immunoglobulin A (IgA) nephropathy is the most common form of chronic GN in children.
- Hypocomplementemia (low C3) characterizes acute postinfectious GN, membranoproliferative GN, and lupus nephritis; all other causes of GN have normal C3 complement.

CHAPTER 165

Hemolytic Uremic Syndrome

- Hemolytic uremic syndrome (HUS) is characterized by the triad of microangiopathic hemolytic anemia, thrombocytopenia, and acute kidney injury.
- The most common type of HUS is associated with Shiga toxin–producing *Escherichia coli* (STEC-HUS) due to contamination of meat, fruit, vegetables, or water (most commonly with *E. coli* O157:H7) and is most common in children <5 years of age.
- Other causes of HUS/thrombotic microangiopathy include other infections, disorders of complement regulation, medications, malignancy, systemic lupus erythematosus, and pregnancy.
- Children with HUS can become critically ill with need for kidney support therapy and red blood cell transfusion.
- TTP and HUS may have similar clinical presentations, but TTP is distinguished by severe deficiency in ADAMTS13.

CHAPTER 166

Acute Kidney Injury and Chronic Kidney Disease

- Acute kidney injury (AKI) may be oliguric or nonoliguric and can be classified as prerenal (renal hypoperfusion), intrinsic (tubular, glomerular, or vascular injury), or postrenal (urinary tract obstruction).
- The most common causes of CKD in children are congenital anomalies of the kidney and urinary tract and glomerular disorders.
- Complications of CKD in children include poor growth, anemia, CKD-MBD, cardiovascular issues (hypertension, left ventricular hypertrophy), metabolic acidosis, and electrolyte disturbances (Na, K, Ca, P).
- Indications for acute dialysis in children include volume overload, metabolic acidosis, electrolyte abnormalities, uremia, certain ingestions, and metabolic disorders (e.g., hyperammonemia); indications for chronic dialysis include all of the above as well as poor growth due to chronic kidney disease (CKD) and stage 5 CKD due to its significant risks of serious complications.

CHAPTER 167

Hypertension

- Hypertension (HTN) in children is most frequently primary (essential) in etiology. Secondary forms are more likely in younger children or with more severe HTN; the most common secondary cause in children is kidney disease.
- Blood pressure (BP) can be classified into categories of normal, elevated BP, stage 1 HTN, and stage 2 HTN.

- Evaluation of children with HTN includes studies to evaluate for underlying secondary causes, co-morbidities (lipids, fasting glucose), and evidence of target organ damage (echocardiogram).
- Treatment of HTN includes therapeutic lifestyle changes ± antihypertensive medications.

CHAPTER 168

Vesicoureteral Reflux

- Primary vesicoureteral reflux (VUR) results from congenital incompetence of the ureterovesical (UV) junction and often resolves with growth.
- VUR secondary to urinary tract anomalies is less likely to self-resolve.
- The most common clinical manifestation of VUR is febrile UTI.
- VUR is identified by a voiding cystourethrogram (VCUG) study.
- VUR may be managed with surveillance, medical therapy, and surgical intervention.
- Reflux nephropathy refers to development and progression of kidney scarring associated with VUR and febrile UTI; the incidence is higher in children with recurrent UTI.

CHAPTER 169

Congenital and Developmental Abnormalities of the Urinary Tract

- Congenital anomalies of the kidneys and urinary tract (CAKUT) occur in up to 4% of infants.
- The two most common forms of CAKUT are hydronephrosis in the absence of urinary tract obstruction and duplicated collecting system of the kidney.
- CAKUT also includes abnormal kidney structure (renal agenesis, renal hypoplasia/dysplasia, multicystic dysplastic kidney, polycystic kidney disease), abnormal kidney location (ectopic kidney, fused kidneys), and abnormal urinary tract (urinary tract obstruction). These disorders often result in abnormal kidney function.

CHAPTER 170

Other Urinary Tract and Genital Disorders

- In childhood urinary stone disease, kidney stones commonly result from a urinary tract structural abnormality or an underlying metabolic predisposition.
- The most common metabolic risk factor for urinary stone disease is hypercalciuria.
- Renal ultrasound is the initial test of choice for diagnosing urinary stone disease.
- Most children are dry during both day and night by 5–7 years of age; primary nocturnal enuresis is common.
- Untreated cryptorchidism is associated with increased risk of infertility and neoplasm later in life. Orchidopexy is usually performed during the first year of life to preserve testicular function.
- Testicular torsion is a urologic emergency and must be identified and treated quickly (ideally within 6 hours) to salvage the testis.

SECTION 23

ENDOCRINOLOGY

Paola Palma Sisto | Mary Kathleen Heneghan

CHAPTER 171

Endocrinology Assessment

Endocrinology is the study of unique chemical messengers known as *hormones* and their impact on normal physiological processes, as well as their effect on morbidity from the pathologic effects of their production, action, and hormone signaling in disease states. Classically, hormones are produced in a regulated fashion in one cell and then travel through the bloodstream, often bound to binding factors, to a target cell. Then, hormones either bind to receptors on the plasma membranes of target cells, or they are transported into cells to bind to intracellular receptors. The target cell has its own influence on its hormonal regulatory response. Hormones generally are regulated in a **feedback loop** so that the production of a hormone is linked to its effect or its circulating concentration.

Hormone action also may be **paracrine** (acting on neighboring cells that are adjacent to the cell of origin of the hormone). The regulation of hormone signaling is tightly controlled and differs between endocrine and paracrine effects (Fig. 171.1). Endocrine disorders generally manifest from one of four ways:

1. By **hormone overproduction:** In Cushing syndrome, there is an excess of glucocorticoid present; the excess is secondary to autonomous glucocorticoid secretion by the adrenal gland.
2. By **hormone underproduction:** In autoimmune hypothyroidism, there is a reduced production of thyroid hormone caused by autoimmune destruction of thyroid cells.
3. By an abnormal **response of end-organ** to hormone: In pseudohypoparathyroidism, pathogenic variants in the gene *(GNAS1)* encoding the alpha subunit of the stimulatory G protein (Gsα) are manifested by elevated parathyroid hormone (PTH) levels in the face of deficient PTH function (PTH resistance).
4. By pathologic **gland enlargement** that may have effects as a result of size rather than function: With a large, nonfunctioning pituitary adenoma, compression of surrounding tissue leads to abnormal visual fields and other neurological signs and symptoms even though no hormone is produced by the tumor.

Peptide hormones act through specific cell membrane receptors; when the hormone is attached to the receptor, the complex triggers various intracellular second messengers that cause the biological effects. Peptide hormone receptor number and avidity may be regulated by hormones. **Steroid hormones** exert their effects by attachment to intranuclear receptors, and the hormone-receptor complex translocates to the nucleus, where it binds with DNA and leads to further gene activation.

The interpretation of serum hormone levels must be related to their regulating factors. For example, a given value of parathyroid hormone may be normal in a eucalcemic patient but inadequate in a hypocalcemic patient with partial hypoparathyroidism or excessive in a hypercalcemic patient with hyperparathyroidism.

HYPOTHALAMIC-PITUITARY AXIS

The hypothalamus' essential role in homeostasis comes from its ability to organize coordinated endocrine, autonomic, and behavioral responses. The **hypothalamus** receives sensory information from both external and internal factors. In turn, the hypothalamus is modulated by a number of factors, including hormones, which can exert both negative and positive feedback. The median eminence is the region that connects the hypothalamus and the anterior pituitary gland. Its location in the center of the tuber cinereum and extensive blood vessels allow direct connections between the hypothalamus and pituitary gland. The **pituitary glands**, composed of anterior and posterior regions, produce a number of hormones that are released and exert effects on their target glands. The pituitary gland is regulated by the hypothalamus through its releasing factors formed in the hypothalamic neurosecretory neurons, through positive and negative feedback of hormones themselves, as well as both paracrine and autocrine factors of the pituitary. The **anterior pituitary** *(adenohypophysis)* houses five different hormone-secreting cell types, which produce adrenocorticotropic hormone (ACTH), growth hormone (GH), thyroid-stimulating hormone (TSH), luteinizing hormone (LH), and prolactin (Fig. 171.2). The **posterior pituitary** *(neurohypophysis)* houses terminal axons of hypothalamic neurons and releases arginine vasopressin (also known as *antidiuretic hormone*) and oxytocin. Alpha-melanocyte stimulating hormone shares the precursor pro-opiomelanocortin (POMC) with ACTH and is secreted by both the hypothalamus and anterior pituitary.

The assessment of pituitary function may be done by measuring some of the specific pituitary hormones in the basal state; other assessments require the measurement after stimulation. Indirect assessment of pituitary function can be obtained by measuring serum concentrations of the target gland hormones (Table 171.1). Several tests of pituitary function are listed in Table 171.2.

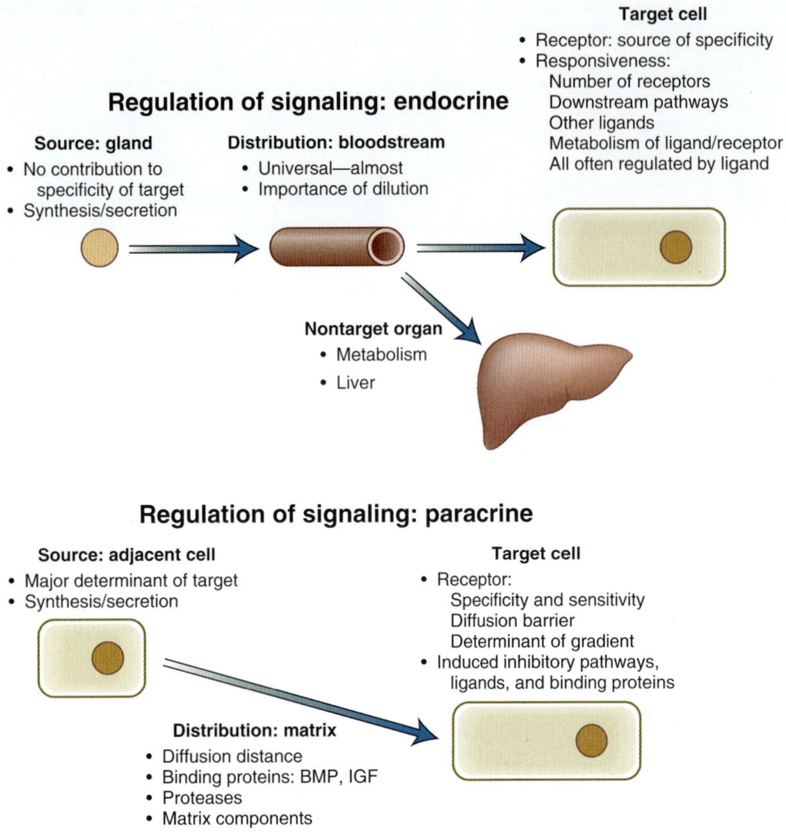

FIGURE 171.1 Comparison of determinants of endocrine and paracrine signaling. *BMP,* Bone morphogenetic protein; *IGF,* insulin-like growth factor. (From Melmed S, Auchus RJ, Goldfine AB, et al. Principles of endocrinology. In: Melmed S, Auchus RJ, Goldine AB, et al., eds. *Williams Textbook of Endocrinology.* 15th ed. Philadelphia: Elsevier; 2025: Fig. 1.1.)

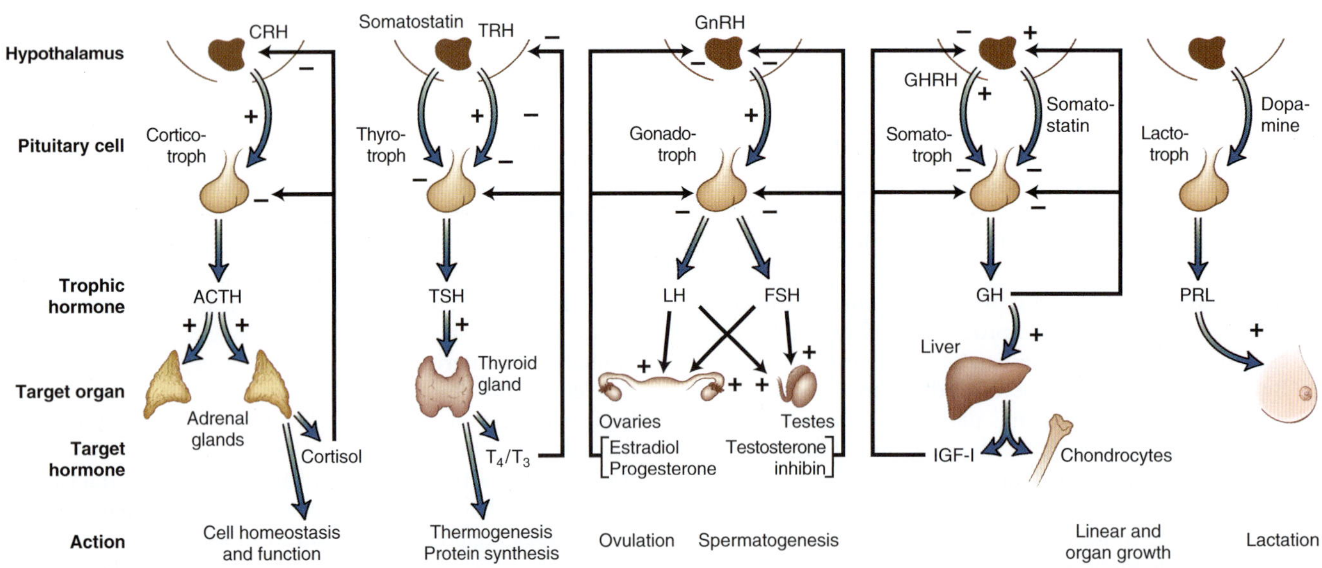

FIGURE 171.2 Control of hypothalamic-pituitary target organ axes. *ACTH,* Adrenocorticotropic hormone; *CRH,* corticotropin-releasing hormone; *FSH,* follicle-stimulating hormone; *GH,* growth hormone; *GHRH,* growth hormone–releasing hormone; *GnRH,* gonadotropin-releasing hormone; *IGF,* insulin-like growth factor; *LH,* luteinizing hormone; *PRL,* prolactin; T_3, triiodothyronine; T_4, thyroxine; *TRH,* thyrotropin-releasing hormone; *TSH,* thyroid-stimulating hormone. (Adapted from Melmed S. Mechanisms for pituitary tumorigenesis: the plastic pituitary. *J Clin Invest.* 2003;112:1603–1618.)

DISORDERS OF THE HYPOTHALAMIC-PITUITARY AXIS

Disorders of pituitary function may arise from a number of causes. *Congenital* hypopituitarism is often caused by genetic variation altering a specific level of pituitary function, including hormones, receptors, and transcription factors that determine anterior pituitary development. In addition, pathogenic variants in specific genes that produce GH, POMC, TSH, LH, and follicle-stimulating hormone can lead to single hormone deficiencies.

TABLE 171.1 Diagnostic Evaluation for Hypopituitarism

MANIFESTATION	CAUSE	TESTS*
Growth failure, hypothyroidism, or both	GH deficiency, TRH/TSH deficiency, or both	Provocative GH tests, free T_4, bone age, IGF-1, IGF-BP3
Hypoglycemia	GH deficiency, ACTH insufficiency, or both	Provocative GH tests, test of ACTH secretion, IGF-1, IGF-BP3
Micropenis, pubertal delay or arrest	Hypogonadotropic hypogonadism with or without GH deficiency	Sex steroids (E_2, testosterone), basal LH and FSH (analyzed by ultrasensitive assays) or after LHRH administration, provocative GH tests, IGF-1, IGF-BP3
Polyuria, polydipsia	ADH deficiency	Urine analysis (specific gravity), serum electrolytes, urine and serum osmolality, water deprivation test

**Each patient with hypopituitarism should have CNS MRI as part of evaluation to determine the etiology of the condition.*
ACTH, Adrenocorticotropic hormone; *ADH,* antidiuretic hormone; *CNS,* central nervous system; *E_2,* estradiol; *FSH,* follicle-stimulating hormone; *GH,* growth hormone; *IGF-1,* insulin-like growth factor 1; *IGF-BP3,* insulin-like growth factor-binding protein 3; *LH,* luteinizing hormone; *LHRH,* luteinizing hormone releasing hormone; *MRI,* magnetic resonance imaging; *T_4,* thyroxine; *TRH,* thyrotropin-releasing hormone; *TSH,* thyroid-stimulating hormone.

TABLE 171.2 Anterior Pituitary Hormone Function Testing

RANDOM HORMONE MEASUREMENTS	PROVOCATIVE OR OTHER TESTS	TARGET HORMONE MEASUREMENT
GH (not useful as a random determination except in newborns and in GH resistance or in pituitary gigantism)	Arginine (a weak stimulus) L-dopa (useful clinically) Insulin-induced hypoglycemia (a dangerous but accurate test)	IGF-1, IGF-BP3 (affected by malnutrition as well as GH excess)
	Clonidine (useful clinically) GHRH	
	12- to 24-hr integrated GH levels (of questionable utility)	
ACTH (early-morning sample useful only if in high-normal range)	Cortisol after insulin-induced hypoglycemia (a dangerous but accurate test)	8 A.M. cortisol 24-hr urinary free cortisol
	ACTH stimulation test (may differentiate ACTH deficiency from primary adrenal insufficiency)	
TSH LH, FSH	LHRH (difficult to interpret in prepubertal subjects)	FT_4 Testosterone/estradiol
Prolactin (elevated in hypothalamic disease and decreased in pituitary disease)		None

ACTH, Adrenocorticotropic hormone; *BP3,* insulin-like growth factor-binding protein 3; *FSH,* follicle-stimulating hormone; *FT_4,* free thyroxine; *GH,* growth hormone; *GHRH,* growth hormone-releasing hormone; *IGF-1,* insulin-like growth factor 1; *IGF-TSH,* thyroid-stimulating hormone; *LH,* luteinizing hormone; *LHRH,* luteinizing hormone releasing hormone.

Structural defects in hypothalamic and/or pituitary regions of the brain, whether present from birth due to developmental malformations of the brain (e.g., optic nerve hypoplasia, holoprosencephaly), or acquired, such as through surgical interventions for tumors, are also causes of hypopituitarism. Each patient with hypopituitarism should have magnetic resonance imaging (MRI) of the brain as part of their evaluation to determine the etiology of the condition. The MRI findings of congenital hypopituitarism may include an ectopic posterior pituitary gland *bright spot*, the appearance of a *pituitary stalk transection*, and/or a small pituitary gland.

Acquired conditions that cause pituitary insufficiency include pituitary tumors such as craniopharyngioma, parasellar masses, hypophysitis, aneurysms, and pituitary apoplexy, in addition to conditions causing infiltration of the pituitary gland (Langerhans cell histiocytosis, lymphoma, and sarcoidosis). Pituitary insufficiency can also be the result of radiation therapy and a consequence of autoimmunity against the pituitary gland.

PEARLS FOR PRACTITIONERS

See Endocrinology: Pearls for Practitioners at the end of this section.

REVIEW QUESTION

Available online.

CHAPTER 172 Diabetes Mellitus

Diabetes mellitus (DM), characterized by hyperglycemia and glycosuria, has multiple etiologies (see Table 172.1). The most common type occurring in childhood is **type 1 DM** (T1D), which is caused by autoimmune destruction of the insulin-producing β cells (islets) of the pancreas, leading to permanent insulin deficiency. **Type 2 DM** (T2D) results from insulin resistance and relative insulin deficiency, usually in the context of exogenous obesity. The incidence of T1D and T2D in the United States is increasing. Less common types of diabetes result from genetic defects of the insulin receptor or inherited abnormalities in sensing of ambient glucose concentration by pancreatic β cells.

DEFINITION

A diagnosis of DM is made based on four glucose abnormalities that may need to be confirmed by repeat testing: (1) fasting serum glucose concentration of 126 mg/dL or above, (2) a random venous plasma glucose of 200 mg/dL or above with symptoms of hyperglycemia, (3) an abnormal oral glucose tolerance test (OGTT) with a 2-hour postprandial serum glucose concentration of 200 mg/dL or above, and (4) a hemoglobin A_{1c} (HbA_{1c}) of 6.5% or above.

A patient is considered to have **impaired fasting glucose** if fasting serum glucose concentration is 100–125 mg/dL or **impaired glucose tolerance** if 2-hour plasma glucose following an OGTT is 140–199 mg/dL. Sporadic hyperglycemia can occur in children, usually in the setting of an intercurrent illness. When the hyperglycemic episode is clearly related to an illness or other physiologic stress, the probability of incipient diabetes is small (<5%).

TYPE 1 DIABETES MELLITUS

Etiology

T1D results from the autoimmune destruction of insulin-producing β cells (islets) of the pancreas. In addition to the presence of diabetes susceptibility genes, an unknown environmental insult presumably triggers the autoimmune process. A variety of studies have produced conflicting data regarding a host of environmental factors. These include cow's milk feeding at an early age, viral infectious agents (coxsackievirus, enterovirus, cytomegalovirus, mumps, rubella), vitamin D deficiency, and perinatal factors. T1D is thought to be primarily a T-cell–mediated disease.

Antibodies to islet cell antigens may be seen months to years before the onset of β cell dysfunction (Fig. 172.1). These include islet cell antibodies; insulin autoantibodies; and antibodies to insulinoma-associated protein 2 (IA-2), glutamic acid decarboxylase (GAD), and Zn transporter 8 (ZnT8), among others. The risk for diabetes increases with the number of antibodies detected in the serum. In individuals with only one detectable antibody, the risk is only 10–15%, while in individuals with three or more antibodies the risk is 55–90%. When 80–90% of the β-cell mass has been destroyed, the remaining β-cell mass is insufficient to maintain euglycemia, and clinical manifestations of diabetes result (see Fig. 172.1).

Epidemiology

The annual incidence of T1D is increasing steadily with significant geographic differences. In the United States, the annual incidence is approximately 20 in 100,000. The annual incidence in children ranges from a high of 40 in 100,000 among Scandinavian populations to less than 1 in 100,000 in China.

No overall gender difference in incidence exists. There is a peak at 4–6 years of age and a second peak at about 10–14 years of age. While genetic determinants play a role in the susceptibility to T1D, the mode of inheritance is complex and multigenic. With no family history of T1D, there is about a 0.4% risk; siblings or offspring of patients with diabetes have a risk of 2–8% for the development of diabetes; an identical twin has a 30–50% risk. The human leukocyte antigen (HLA) region on chromosome 6 provides the strongest determinant of susceptibility, accounting for approximately 40% of familial inheritance of T1D. Specific class II DR and DQ HLA alleles (HLA DR3 and HLA DR4) increase the risk of developing T1D, whereas other specific HLA alleles exert a protective effect. More than 90% of children with T1D possess HLA DR3 alleles, HLA DR4 alleles, or both. The insulin gene region variable number tandem repeat on chromosome 11 is also linked to T1D susceptibility. There is evidence for association, beyond HLA, of more than 100 other loci with T1D. Genetic factors do not fully account for susceptibility to T1D; environmental factors also play a role.

T1D is also associated with celiac disease and other autoimmune or inflammatory polyendocrinopathies such as IPEX (immune dysregulation, polyendocrinopathy, enteropathy X-linked) syndrome.

Screening and Prevention

Early prediction of T1D can help prevent occurrence of diabetic ketoacidosis. Screening and prevention of T1D has seen promising advancements with development of immunotherapies. Screening for number of positive antibodies present in children at risk for development of T1D may help determine those who would benefit from immunologic therapy.

Clinical Manifestations

Hyperglycemia results when insulin secretory capacity becomes inadequate to enhance peripheral glucose uptake and to suppress hepatic and renal glucose production. Insulin deficiency usually first causes postprandial hyperglycemia and then fasting hyperglycemia. Ketogenesis is a sign of more complete insulin deficiency. Lack of suppression of gluconeogenesis and glycogenolysis further exacerbates hyperglycemia, while fatty acid oxidation generates the ketone bodies β-hydroxybutyrate, acetoacetate, and acetone. Protein stores in muscle and fat stores in adipose tissue are metabolized to provide substrates for gluconeogenesis and fatty acid oxidation.

The classic presentation of T1D includes polyuria, polydipsia, polyphagia, and weight loss. Glycosuria occurs when the serum glucose concentration exceeds the renal threshold for glucose reabsorption (from 160–190 mg/dL). Glycosuria causes an osmotic diuresis (including obligate loss of sodium, potassium, and other electrolytes), leading to dehydration. Polydipsia occurs as the patient attempts to compensate for

TABLE 172.1 Classification of Diabetes Mellitus in Children and Adolescents

TYPE	COMMENT
TYPE 1 (INSULIN DEPENDENT)	
Transient neonatal	Intrauterine growth restriction followed by postnatal hyperglycemia, dehydration, and poor growth; spontaneous remission in 1–3 mo with risk of relapse later in life; genetic causes include pathogenic variants in *KCNJ11* and *ABCC8* or abnormal imprinting of 6q24
Permanent neonatal	Postnatal hyperglycemia, dehydration, and poor growth that does not remit; associated with pathogenic variants in *KCNJ11* and *ABCC8*
Classic type 1	Glycosuria, ketonuria, hyperglycemia, islet cell autoimmunity; multifactorial development, but HLA region on chromosome 6 contributes to heritable predisposition
TYPE 2 (NOT INSULIN DEPENDENT)	
Secondary	Cystic fibrosis, hemochromatosis, medications (L-asparaginase, tacrolimus)
Adult type (classic)	Associated with obesity, insulin resistance; heritable predisposition overlaps with heritability of obesity, as well as environmental drivers and epigenetics
OTHER	
Gestational diabetes	Abnormal glucose tolerance during pregnancy only, which reverts to normal postpartum; increased risk for later onset of diabetes
Maturity-onset diabetes of youth	Autosomal dominant, onset before age 25 yr; not associated with obesity or autoimmunity Single-gene pathogenic variants include hepatocyte nuclear factors 1β, 1α, 4α; glucokinase; insulin promoter factor 1
Mitochondrial diabetes	Associated with deafness and other neurologic defects, exclusively maternal transmission of mtDNA point pathogenic variants

HLA, Human leukocyte antigen.

the excess fluid losses. Weight loss results from the persistent catabolic state and the loss of calories through glycosuria and ketonuria.

DIABETIC KETOACIDOSIS

If the clinical features of new-onset T1D are not detected, **diabetic ketoacidosis (DKA)** will occur. DKA may also occur in patients with known T1D if insulin injections are omitted or during an intercurrent illness when greater insulin requirements are unmet in the presence of elevated concentrations of the counter-regulatory and stress hormones (glucagon, growth hormone [GH], cortisol, and catecholamines). DKA can be considered present if (1) the arterial pH is below 7.3, (2) the serum bicarbonate level is below 15 mEq/L, and (3) ketones are elevated in serum or urine.

Pathophysiology

In the absence of adequate insulin secretion, persistent partial hepatic oxidation of fatty acids to ketone bodies occurs. Two of these three ketone bodies are organic acids and lead to metabolic acidosis with an elevated anion gap. Lactic acid may contribute to the acidosis when severe dehydration results in decreased tissue perfusion. Hyperglycemia causes an osmotic diuresis that is initially compensated for by increased fluid intake. As the hyperglycemia and diuresis worsen, most patients are unable to maintain the large fluid intake and thus dehydration occurs. Vomiting and increased insensible water losses caused by tachypnea can worsen the dehydration. Electrolyte abnormalities occur through a loss of electrolytes in the urine and transmembrane alterations resulting from acidosis. As hydrogen ions accumulate because of ketoacidosis, intracellular potassium is exchanged for hydrogen ions. Serum concentrations of potassium increase initially with acidosis then decrease as serum potassium is cleared by the kidney. Depending on the duration of ketoacidosis, serum potassium concentrations at diagnosis may be increased, normal, or decreased, but intracellular potassium concentrations are depleted. A decreased serum potassium concentration is an ominous sign of total body potassium depletion. Phosphate depletion can occur because of the increased renal phosphate excretion required for elimination of excess hydrogen ions. Sodium depletion is also common in ketoacidosis, resulting from renal losses of sodium caused by osmotic diuresis and from gastrointestinal losses from vomiting (Fig. 172.2).

Clinical Presentation

Patients with DKA present initially with polyuria, polydipsia, nausea, and vomiting. Abdominal pain occurs frequently and can mimic an acute abdomen. The abdomen may be tender from vomiting or distended secondary to a paralytic ileus. The presence of polyuria, despite a state of clinical dehydration, indicates osmotic diuresis and differentiates patients with DKA from patients with gastroenteritis or other gastrointestinal disorders. Respiratory compensation for acidosis results in tachypnea with deep **(Kussmaul)** respirations. The *fruity* odor of acetone frequently can be detected on the patient's breath. Altered mental status can occur, ranging from disorientation to coma.

Laboratory studies reveal hyperglycemia (serum glucose concentrations ranging from 200 mg/dL to >1,000 mg/dL). Arterial pH is below 7.30, and serum bicarbonate concentration is less than 15 mEq/L. Serum sodium concentrations may be elevated, normal, or low, depending on the balance of sodium and free water losses. The measured serum sodium concentration is artificially low, however, because of hyperglycemia. The corrected Na can be calculated using the following equation: corrected Na = measured Na + (1.6[glucose − 100]/100). Hyperlipidemia also contributes to the decrease in measured serum sodium. The level of blood urea nitrogen (BUN) can be elevated with prerenal azotemia secondary to dehydration. The white blood cell count is usually elevated and

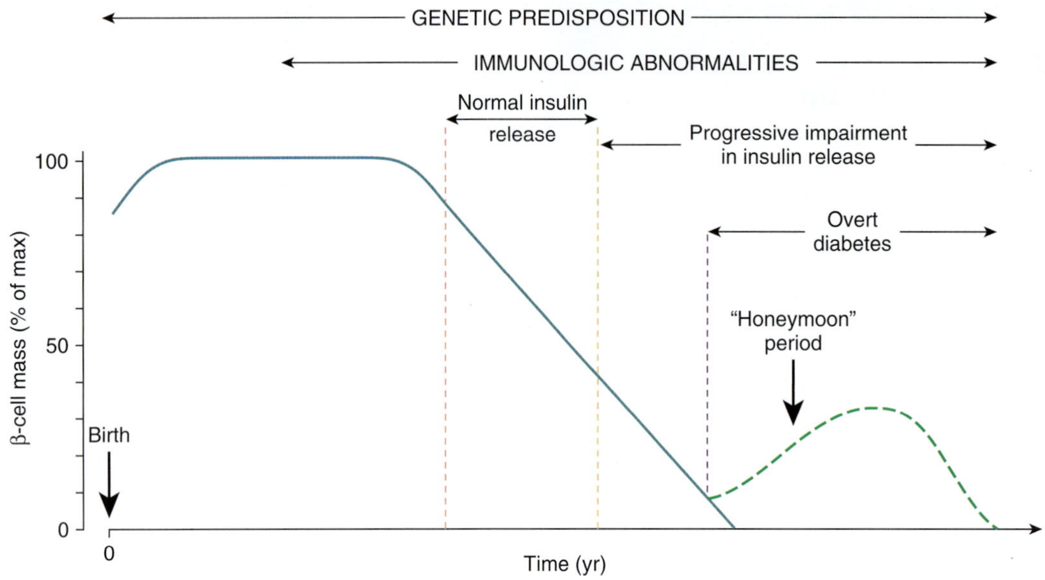

FIGURE 172.1 Schematic representation of the autoimmune evolution of diabetes in genetically predisposed individuals.

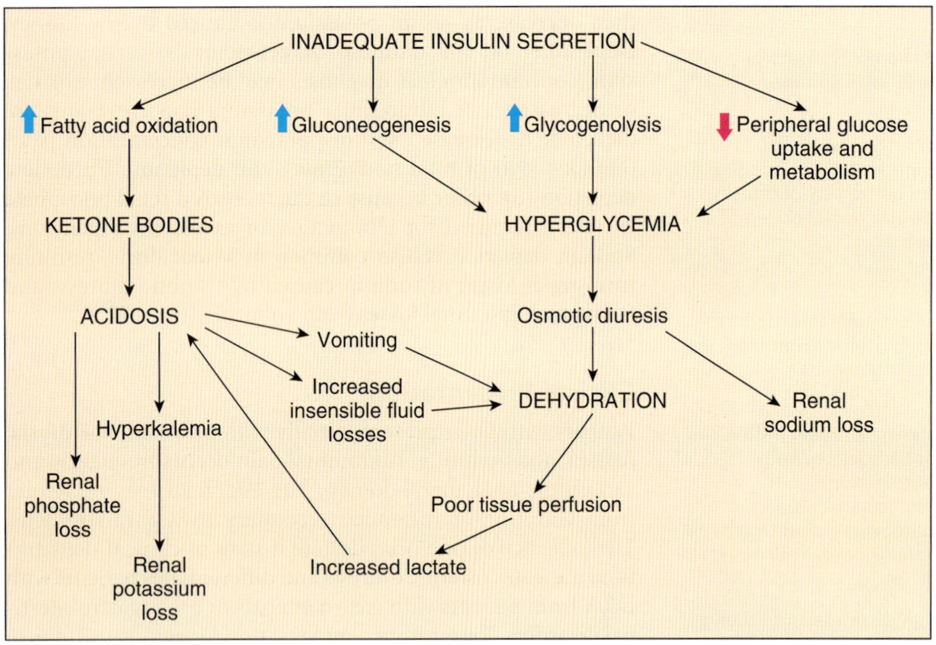

FIGURE 172.2 Pathophysiology of diabetic ketoacidosis.

can be left-shifted without implying the presence of infection. Fever is unusual and should prompt a search for infectious sources that may have triggered the episode of DKA.

Treatment

Therapy for patients with DKA involves careful replacement of fluid deficits, correction of acidosis and hyperglycemia via insulin administration, correction of electrolyte imbalances, and monitoring for complications of treatment. The optimal approach to management of DKA must strike a balance between adequate correction of fluid losses and avoidance of rapid shifts in osmolality and fluid balance. The most serious complications of DKA and its treatment are **cerebral edema** and cerebral herniation.

A patient with severe DKA is assumed to be approximately 10% dehydrated. If a recent weight measurement is available, the precise extent of dehydration can be calculated. An initial intravenous (IV) fluid bolus of a glucose-free isotonic solution (normal saline, lactated Ringer solution) at 10–20 mL/kg should be given to restore intravascular volume and kidney perfusion. The remaining fluid deficit after the initial bolus should be added to maintenance fluid requirements; the total should be replaced slowly over 36–48 hours. Ongoing losses resulting from osmotic diuresis usually do not need to be replaced unless urine output is large or signs of poor perfusion are present. Osmotic diuresis is usually minimal when the serum glucose concentration decreases to less than 300 mg/dL. To avoid rapid shifts in serum osmolality, 0.9% sodium chloride can be used as the replacement fluid for the initial 4–6 hours, followed by 0.45% sodium chloride.

Hyperglycemia

Fast-acting soluble insulin should be administered as a continuous IV infusion (0.1 U/kg/hr). Serum glucose concentrations should decrease at a rate no faster than 100 mg/dL/hr. When serum glucose concentrations decrease to less than 250–300 mg/dL, glucose should be added to the IV fluids. If serum glucose concentrations decrease to less than 200 mg/dL before correction of acidosis, the glucose concentration of the IV fluids should be increased, but the insulin infusion should not be decreased by more than half, and it should never be discontinued before resolution of acidosis.

Acidosis

Insulin therapy decreases the production of free fatty acids and protein catabolism and enhances glucose usage in target tissues. These processes correct acidosis. Bicarbonate therapy should be avoided. Potential adverse effects of bicarbonate administration include paradoxical increases in central nervous system (CNS) acidosis caused by increased diffusion of carbon dioxide across the blood-brain barrier, potential tissue hypoxia caused by shifts in the oxyhemoglobin dissociation curve, abrupt osmotic changes, and increased risk of the development of cerebral edema.

As acidosis is corrected, urine ketone concentrations may appear to rise. β-Hydroxybutyrate, which is not detected in urine ketone assays, is converted with treatment to detectable acetoacetate. Hence, minute-to-minute urine ketone concentrations are not a required index of the adequacy of therapy.

Electrolyte Imbalances

Regardless of the serum potassium concentration at presentation, total body potassium depletion is likely. Serum potassium concentrations can decrease rapidly as insulin and then glucose therapy improve acidosis and potassium is exchanged for intracellular hydrogen ions. When adequate urine output is shown, potassium should be added to the IV fluids. Potassium replacement should be given as 50% potassium chloride and 50% potassium phosphate at a concentration of 20–40 mEq/L. This combination provides phosphate for replacement of deficits but avoids excess phosphate administration, which may precipitate hypocalcemia. If the serum potassium level is greater than 6 mEq/L, potassium should not be added to IV fluids until the potassium level decreases.

Monitoring

Initial laboratory measurements should include serum glucose, sodium, potassium, chloride, bicarbonate, BUN, creatinine, calcium, phosphate, and magnesium concentrations; arterial or venous pH; and a urinalysis. Serum glucose measurement should be repeated every hour during therapy, and electrolyte concentrations should be repeated every 2–3 hours. Calcium, phosphate, and magnesium concentrations should be measured every 4–6 hours during therapy. Neurologic and mental status should be assessed at frequent intervals. Any complaints of headache or deterioration of mental status should prompt rapid evaluation for possible cerebral edema. Symptoms indicative of possible cerebral edema include a decreased sensorium, sudden severe headache, vomiting, change in vital signs (bradycardia, hypertension, apnea), a dilated pupil, ophthalmoplegia, or seizure.

Complications

Clinically apparent cerebral edema occurs in 1–5% of cases of DKA. Cerebral edema is the most serious complication of DKA, with a significant mortality rate. The pathogenesis of cerebral edema likely involves osmolar shift resulting in fluid accumulation in the intracellular compartment and neuronal cell swelling. Subclinical cerebral edema is common in children with DKA, although the factors that exacerbate this process leading to symptomatic brain swelling and possible cerebral herniation are not clearly defined. Cerebral edema typically occurs 6–12 hours after therapy for DKA is begun, often following a period of apparent clinical improvement. Factors that correlate with increased risk for cerebral edema include higher initial BUN concentration, lower initial Pco_2, failure of the serum sodium concentration to increase as glucose concentration decreases during treatment, and treatment with bicarbonate.

Signs of advanced cerebral edema include obtundation, papilledema, pupillary dilation or inequality, hypertension, bradycardia, and apnea. Treatment involves the rapid use of IV hypertonic saline or mannitol, endotracheal intubation, and ventilation and may require the use of a subdural bolt. Other complications of DKA are intracranial thrombosis or infarction, acute kidney injury caused by severe dehydration, pancreatitis, arrhythmias caused by electrolyte abnormalities, pulmonary edema, and bowel ischemia. Peripheral edema may occur 24–48 hours after therapy is initiated and may be related to residual elevations in antidiuretic hormone and aldosterone.

Transition to Outpatient Management

When the acidosis has been corrected and the patient tolerates oral feedings, the IV insulin infusion can be discontinued, and a regimen of subcutaneous (SC) insulin injections can be initiated. The first SC insulin dose should be given 30–45 minutes before discontinuation of the IV insulin infusion. Further adjustment of the insulin dose should be made over the following 2–3 days. A patient previously diagnosed with T1D may be restarted on the prior doses if they were adequate. For a patient with new-onset T1D, typical starting total daily doses are approximately 0.5–0.7 U/kg per 24 hours for prepubertal patients and approximately 0.7–1 U/kg per 24 hours for adolescents, using any number of the available insulin combinations. The best and most common choice for making the transition to SC insulin is to begin by giving injections of fast-acting (bolus) insulin (lispro, aspart, or glulisine insulin) with each meal and long-acting (basal) insulin (glargine, detemir, or degludec) at bedtime. This regimen of multiple daily injections provides the most flexibility but requires the patient to administer many injections per day and to count carbohydrates in food. An alternative is a fixed mixed split dosing regimen (neutral protamine Hagedorn [NPH] and fast-acting insulin) with two daily injections.

Externally worn pumps that provide a continuous SC infusion of fast-acting insulin are available. Insulin pumps provide fast-acting insulin in small basal amounts continuously every hour and will provide bolus insulin when instructed. Insulin pumps may be used by all age groups in patients who are highly motivated to achieve tight control. The absence of SC depot insulin, risk of insulin running out, and pump malfunction can increase the risk of DKA.

Serum glucose concentrations should be assessed before each meal, at bedtime, and periodically at 2–3 A.M. to provide information for adjustment of the regimen. Patients and their families should begin learning the principles of diabetes care as soon as possible. Demonstration of the ability to administer insulin injections and test glucose concentrations using a glucose meter is necessary before discharge, as is knowledge of hypoglycemia management. Meal planning is crucial to control glucose in T1D. Nutrition services must be part of the care delivered to the families from diagnosis.

Honeymoon Period

In some patients with new onset of T1D, the β-cell mass has not been completely destroyed. The remaining functional β cells seem to recover function with insulin treatment. When this occurs, exogenous insulin requirements decrease. This is a period of stable blood glucose control, often with nearly normal glucose concentrations. This phase of the disease, known as the *honeymoon period*, usually starts in the first weeks of therapy, often continues for 3–6 months, and can last 2 years.

Outpatient Type 1 Diabetes Mellitus Management

Management of T1D in children requires a comprehensive approach with attention to medical, nutritional, and psychosocial issues. Therapeutic strategies should be flexible with the individual needs of each patient and the family taken into account. Optimal care involves a team of diabetes professionals, including a physician, a diabetes nurse educator, a dietitian, and a social worker or psychologist.

Goals

The Diabetes Control and Complications Trial established that intensive insulin therapy, with the goal of maintaining blood glucose concentrations as close to normal as possible, can delay the onset and slow the progression of complications of diabetes (retinopathy, nephropathy, neuropathy). Attaining this goal using intensive insulin therapy can increase the risk of hypoglycemia. The adverse effects of hypoglycemia in young children may be significant because the immature CNS may be more susceptible to glycopenia. Although the risk for diabetic complications increases with duration of diabetes, there is controversy as to whether the increase of risk is lower in the prepubertal years than in adolescence and adulthood.

Given the benefits of stable, near normal blood glucose concentrations, a goal of HbA_{1c} below 7.5% is set for children of all ages. Preprandial blood glucose target concentrations are 80–130 mg/dL and concentrations before bedtime and overnight are 80–150 mg/dL. Goals of therapy need to consider other individual characteristics, such as a history of severe hypoglycemia and the abilities of the patient and family.

Insulin Regimens

Many types of insulin differ in duration of action and time to peak effect (Table 172.2). These insulin types can be used in various combinations, depending on the needs and goals of the individual patient. The most commonly used regimen is that of multiple injections of fast-acting insulin given with meals in combination with long-acting basal insulin given at bedtime. This regimen provides flexibility but requires administration of many injections per day and will require assistance for young children. After the total daily dose of insulin is determined, 30–50% is given as long-acting insulin, and the remainder is given as fast-acting insulin, divided according to the need for corrections of high glucose levels and for meals. To correct for hyperglycemia, one can determine the insulin sensitivity using the 1,800/1,500 rule: dividing 1,800 (or 1,500) by the total daily dose of insulin to determine how many milligrams per deciliter of glucose will decrease with one unit of insulin. The insulin:carbohydrate ratio is used to calculate insulin for the carbohydrate content of food; 500 divided by the total daily dose determines the number of grams of carbohydrate that requires one unit of insulin.

Lispro, aspart, and glulisine insulin are synthetic human insulin analogs in which amino acid alterations result in fast

TABLE 172.2 Action Profiles of Insulin Formulations

INSULIN	ONSET	PEAK ACTION	DURATION
VERY SHORT ACTING			
Lispro, aspart, glulisine	5–15 min	30–90 min	3–5 hr
SHORT ACTING			
Regular	30–60 min	2–3 hr	5–8 hr
INTERMEDIATE ACTING			
NPH (isophane)	2–4 hr	4–10 hr	10–16 hr
LONG ACTING			
Glargine	2–4 hr	Minimal	20–24 hr
Detemir	2–4 hr	Minimal	12–24 hr
Degludec	2–4 hr	Minimal	24+ hr

NPH, Neutral protamine Hagedorn.

absorption and onset of action (see Table 172.2). Because of the short duration of action, these are used in combination with long-acting insulin. Glargine and detemir are insulin analogs with increased solubility at acidic pH and decreased solubility at physiologic pH. They can have a duration of up to 24 hours and act as a basal insulin.

Newly diagnosed patients in the honeymoon period may require 0.4–0.6 U/kg per 24 hours. Prepubertal patients with diabetes longer than 1–2 years typically require 0.5–1 U/kg per 24 hours. During middle adolescence when elevated GH concentrations produce relative insulin resistance, insulin requirements increase by 40–50%, and doses of 1–2 U/kg per 24 hours are typical.

Blood Glucose Testing

Blood glucose should be routinely monitored before each meal and at bedtime. Hypoglycemia during the night or excessive variability in the morning glucose concentrations should prompt additional testing at 2 or 3 A.M. to ensure that there is no consistent hypoglycemia or hyperglycemia. During periods of illness or when blood glucose concentrations are higher than 300 mg/dL, urine ketones also should be tested. **Continuous glucose monitors (CGM)**, which provide minute-to-minute blood glucose concentration information, can be useful in following trends of blood glucose concentrations and have been approved to replace fingerstick blood glucose testing.

Insulin Pumps, Continuous Glucose Monitors, and Closed-Loop Systems

Insulin pumps that provide a continuous SC infusion of short-acting insulin also are available and are being used by children and adolescents who are highly motivated to achieve tight control. Sensor augmented insulin pump therapy refers to the use of an insulin pump in conjunction with a CGM. Insulin delivery is NOT automatically adjusted based on CGM data. Low glucose threshold suspend insulin systems refer to the use of an insulin pump in conjunction with CGM in which insulin delivery can be suspended based on CGM data. Automated insulin delivery systems (also referred to as *closed loop* or *automatic mode*) refer to the use of an insulin pump in conjunction with a CGM in which automatic adjustment of insulin doses are made based on CGM data. These delivery systems still require the entry of food intake either as amount of carbohydrates being eaten or size of meal being consumed.

Nutrition

Balancing the daily meal plan with the dosages of insulin is crucial for maintaining serum glucose concentrations within the target range and avoiding hypoglycemia or hyperglycemia. The content and schedule of meals vary according to the type of insulin regimen used. It is recommended that carbohydrates contribute 50–65% of the total calories, protein 12–20%, and fat less than 30%. Saturated fat should contribute less than 10% of the total caloric intake, and cholesterol intake should be less than 300 mg per 24 hours. High-fiber content is recommended.

Patients using multiple daily injections or the insulin pump can maintain a more flexible meal schedule with regard to the timing of meals and the carbohydrate content. These patients give an injection of insulin before or immediately after each meal with the total dose calculated according to the carbohydrate content of the meal. Further adjustments in the dose can be made based on the measured serum glucose concentration and plans for activity during the day. Children using a twice-a-day combination of intermediate-acting and fast-acting insulins need to maintain a relatively consistent meal schedule so that carbohydrate absorption and insulin action peaks correspond. A typical meal schedule for a patient using this type of regimen involves three meals and three snacks daily. The total carbohydrate content of the meals and snacks should be kept constant.

Long-Term Glycemic Control

Measurements of **glycohemoglobin** or **HbA_{1c}** reflect the average blood glucose concentration over the preceding 3 months and provide a means for assessing long-term glycemic control. HbA_{1c} should be measured four times a year, and the results should be used for counseling of patients. The American Diabetes Association has set HbA_{1c} targets for children at less than 7.5%. Measurements of HbA_{1c} are inaccurate in patients with hemoglobinopathies. Glycosylated albumin or fructosamine can be used in these cases. As CGMs are more widely used, more data on an individual's "time in range" (duration of euglycemia) are available, although the relationship between this and long-term glycemic control or risk of long-term complications is unknown.

Complications

Patients with T1D for more than 3–5 years should receive an annual ophthalmologic examination for retinopathy. Urine should be collected annually for assessment of microalbuminuria, which suggests early kidney dysfunction and indicates a high risk of progression to nephropathy. Treatment with angiotensin-converting enzyme inhibitors may halt the progression of microalbuminuria. In children with T1D, annual cholesterol measurements and periodic assessment of blood pressure are recommended. Early detection of hypertension and hypercholesterolemia with appropriate intervention can help limit future risk of coronary disease.

Other Disorders

Chronic autoimmune lymphocytic thyroiditis is particularly common and can result in hypothyroidism. Because symptoms can be subtle, thyroid function tests should be performed annually. Other disorders that occur with increased frequency in children with T1D include celiac disease, immunoglobulin A deficiency, Addison disease, and peptic ulcer disease.

Hypoglycemia

Hypoglycemia occurs commonly in patients with T1D. For patients in adequate or better control, it is expected to occur on average once or twice a week. Severe episodes of hypoglycemia, resulting in seizures or coma or requiring assistance from another person, occur in 10–25% of these patients per year.

Hypoglycemia in patients with T1D results from a relative excess of insulin in relation to the serum glucose concentration. This excess can be caused by alterations in the dose, timing, or absorption of insulin; alterations of carbohydrate intake; or changes in insulin sensitivity resulting from activity. Defective counter-regulatory responses also contribute to hypoglycemia. Abnormal glucagon responses to falling serum glucose concentrations develop within the first few years of the disease, and abnormalities in epinephrine release occur after a longer duration.

Lack of awareness of hypoglycemia occurs in approximately 25% of patients with diabetes. Recent episodes of hypoglycemia may play a role in the pathophysiology of *hypoglycemia unawareness*; after an episode of hypoglycemia, autonomic responses to subsequent episodes are reduced. A return of symptoms of hypoglycemia can be exhibited in these patients after 2–3 weeks of strict avoidance of hypoglycemic episodes.

Symptoms of hypoglycemia include those resulting from neuroglycopenia (headache, visual changes, confusion, irritability, or seizures) and those resulting from the catecholamine response (tremors, tachycardia, diaphoresis, or anxiety). Mild episodes can be treated with administration of rapidly absorbed oral glucose (glucose gel or tablets or fruit juices). More severe episodes that result in seizures or loss of consciousness at home should be treated with glucagon, which can be given as an injection or intranasally. IV glucose should be given in hospital settings.

Prognosis

Long-term complications of T1D include retinopathy, nephropathy, neuropathy, and macrovascular disease. Evidence of organ damage caused by hyperglycemia is rare in patients with diabetes of less than 5–10 years' duration; diagnosis of secondary disease complications rarely occurs before 10–15 years' duration. Diabetic retinopathy is the leading cause of adult blindness in the United States. Nephropathy eventually occurs in 30–40% and accounts for approximately 30% of all new adult cases of end-stage kidney disease. Neuropathy occurs in 30–40% of postpubertal patients with T1D and leads to sensory, motor, or autonomic deficits. Macrovascular disease results in an increased risk of myocardial infarction and stroke among individuals with diabetes.

Intensive control of diabetes, using frequent blood glucose testing, continuous glucose monitoring, and multiple daily injections of insulin or an insulin pump, can reduce the development or progression of diabetic complications, including a 76% reduction of risk for retinopathy, a 39% reduction in microalbuminuria, and a 60% reduction in clinical neuropathy. For pubertal and adult patients, the benefits of intensive therapy likely outweigh the increased risk for hypoglycemia. For younger patients, in whom the risks for hypoglycemia are greater and the benefits of tight glucose control may be lower, a less intensive regimen may be appropriate.

TYPE 2 DIABETES MELLITUS

Pathophysiology

T2D can occur as the result of various pathophysiologic processes; however, the most common form results from peripheral insulin resistance and compensatory hyperinsulinemia, followed by failure of the pancreas to maintain adequate insulin secretion (see Table 172.1).

Epidemiology

The prevalence of T2D in children is increasing in parallel with childhood obesity and is highest in children of ethnic groups with a high prevalence of T2D in adults, including those of Native American, Hispanic, and African descent. Obesity, metabolic syndrome, ethnicity, and a family history of T2D are risk factors. Autoantibodies to the pancreas are present among some clinically assumed to have T2D, compounding the difficulty in differentiating T1D from T2D at the time of diagnosis.

Clinical Manifestations and Differential Diagnosis

Fasting and postprandial glucose levels for diagnosis of T2D are the same as those for T1D. The diagnosis of T2D may be suspected when polyuria and polydipsia occur in the setting of **metabolic syndrome** (central obesity, hypertension, glucose intolerance, high triglyceride levels, and low high-density lipoprotein cholesterol levels). Differentiating T2D from T1D in children on clinical grounds alone can be challenging. The possibility of T2D should be considered in patients who are obese, have a strong family history of T2D, have other characteristics of metabolic syndrome, or have absence of antibodies to β-cell antigens at the time of diagnosis of diabetes. **Acanthosis nigricans**, a dermatologic manifestation of hyperinsulinism and insulin resistance, presents as hyperkeratotic pigmentation in the nape of the neck and in flexural areas and is noted as a sign in metabolic syndrome (Fig. 172.3). Although ketoacidosis occurs far more commonly in T1D, it also can occur in patients with T2D under conditions of physiologic stress and cannot be used as an absolute differentiating factor. T2D can be confirmed by the evaluation of insulin or **C-peptide** (measurable byproduct of endogenous insulin production) levels after stimulation with oral carbohydrate and in the absence of islet cell autoimmunity.

Therapy

T2D is the result of a combination of insulin resistance, relative insulin deficiency, and a secretory β-cell defect. Asymptomatic patients with mildly elevated glucose values (slightly >126 mg/dL for fasting or slightly >200 mg/dL for random glucose) may be managed initially with lifestyle modifications, including nutrition therapy (dietary adjustments) and increased exercise, which has been shown to decrease insulin resistance. In most children with new-onset, uncomplicated T2D, oral agents are the first line of therapy. Metformin, an insulin secretagogue, and glucagon-like peptide-1 (GLP-1) agonists (liraglutide, exenatide, and dulaglutide) are approved by the U.S. Food and Drug Administration for use in children. Metformin carries the rare side effect of lactic acidosis, occurring mainly in patients with compromised kidney function. The most common side effect of metformin is gastrointestinal upset. A GLP-1 agonist is typically added if monotherapy with metformin fails. If ketonuria or ketoacidosis occur, insulin treatment is necessary to first achieve adequate glycemic control but may be discontinued within weeks with continuation of oral medications. Insulin therapy may be added if therapy with metformin and a GLP-1 agonist fails.

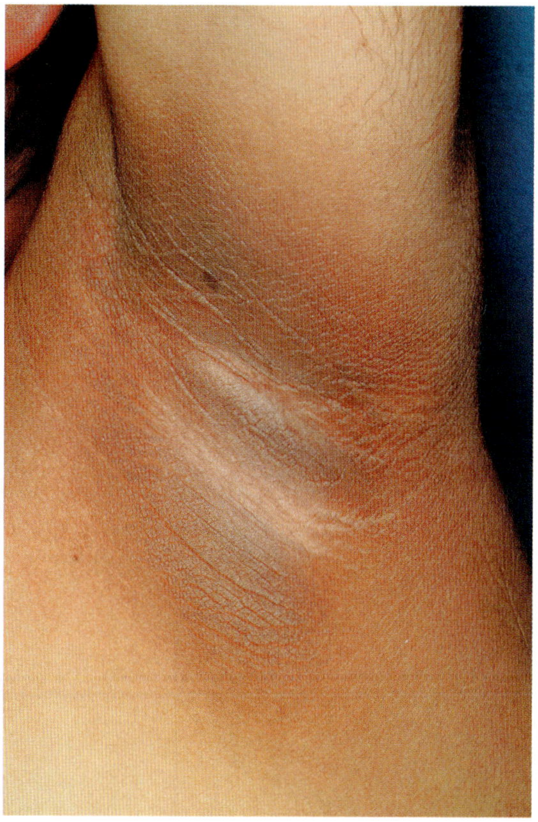

FIGURE 172.3 Acanthosis nigricans. Velvety hyperpigmentation involves the axillae in this patient. (From Paller AS, Mancini AJ. *Hurwitz Clinical Pediatric Dermatology: A Textbook of Skin Disorders of Childhood and Adolescence.* 5th ed. Philadelphia: Elsevier; 2016:Fig. 23–26.)

Because T2D may have a long preclinical course, early diagnosis is possible in patients with metabolic syndrome or other risk factors. Significant lifestyle modifications, such as improved eating habits and increased exercise, have a role in preventing or decreasing the morbidity of T2D. Finally, it is critical to monitor and manage the other components of metabolic syndrome, such as advanced pubertal development, hypertension, hyperlipidemia, nonalcoholic fatty liver disease, and polycystic ovary syndrome in females.

MATURITY-ONSET DIABETES OF YOUTH (MODY)

MODY comprises a group of monogenetic dominantly inherited forms of relatively mild diabetes with onset before age 25 years. Insulin resistance does not occur in these patients; instead, the primary abnormality is an insufficient insulin secretory response to glycemic stimulation. There are multiple forms, but the most common forms are due to pathogenic variants in *hepatocyte nuclear factor (HNF)1α, HNF4α, HNF1β*, and glucokinase genes. Treatment depends on the type and can include the use of sulfonylureas.

PEARLS FOR PRACTITIONERS

See Endocrinology: Pearls for Practitioners at the end of this section.

REVIEW QUESTIONS

Available online.

CHAPTER 173

Hypoglycemia

Hypoglycemia in infancy and childhood can result from a large variety of hormonal and metabolic defects (Table 173.1). Hypoglycemia occurs most frequently in the early neonatal period, often as a result of transient neonatal hyperinsulinemia in infants of diabetic mothers or as a result of inadequate energy stores to meet the disproportionately large metabolic needs of premature or small for gestational age newborns. After the initial 2–3 days of life, hypoglycemia is far less common and is more frequently the result of endocrine or metabolic disorders.

DEFINITION

Clinical hypoglycemia is defined as a plasma glucose (PG) concentration low enough to cause symptoms (usually below 60 mg/dL in children >1 month of life) and/or signs of impaired brain function and improvement of symptoms with glucose administration (Whipple's triad). Brain glucose utilization is reduced at a PG concentration of approximately 55–65 mg/dL. **Autonomic system** (neurogenic) symptoms are perceived at a PG concentration <55 mg/dL. Cognitive function is impaired **(neuroglycopenia)** at a PG concentration <50 mg/dL (Table 173.2).

DIAGNOSIS

While timely treatment is the first priority, diagnosing the etiology of hypoglycemia requires assessment of the metabolic and hormonal regulation of glucose (Fig. 173.1). Frequently, it is difficult to make an accurate diagnosis until one can obtain a *critical sample* of blood and urine at the time of the hypoglycemic episode (Fig. 173.2). In a child with unexplained hypoglycemia, a serum sample should be obtained before treatment for plasma glucose, β-hydroxybutyrate (BOHB), a comprehensive metabolic panel, insulin, C-peptide, free fatty acids (FFAs), lactate, ammonia, cortisol, growth hormone, an acylcarnitine profile, and free and total carnitines. A urine specimen should be obtained for measuring ketones and organic acids. The results of this initial testing can establish whether hormonal causes are responsible and, if not, can provide initial information regarding which types of metabolic disorders are most likely.

CLINICAL MANIFESTATIONS

The symptoms and signs of hypoglycemia result from direct depression of the central nervous system (CNS) owing to lack of energy substrate and the counter-regulatory adrenergic response to low glucose via catecholamine secretion designed to correct hypoglycemia (see Table 173.2). Compared with older children, infants do not usually show adrenergic symptoms. Symptoms of hypoglycemia in newborns and infants may be less obvious and include jitters, hypothermia, hypotonia, poor feeding, lethargy, apnea, bradycardia, and seizures, all due to the deprivation of glucose for normal brain function. Hypothermia, or cold stress, may also exacerbate or induce hypoglycemia in infants by prompting increased metabolic consumption to produce heat. In older children, signs and

TABLE **173.1** Clinical Manifestations and Differential Diagnoses in Childhood Hypoglycemia

				SERUM		EFFECT OF 24–36 HR FAST ON PLASMA					GLYCEMIC RESPONSE TO GLUCAGON		GLYCEMIC RESPONSE TO INFUSION OF	
CONDITION	HYPOGLYCEMIA	URINARY KETONES OR REDUCING SUGARS	HEPATOMEGALY	LIPIDS	URIC ACID	GLUCOSE	INSULIN	KETONES	ALANINE	LACTATE	FED	FASTED	ALANINE	GLYCEROL
Normal	0	0	0	Normal	Normal	↓	↓	↑	↓	Normal	↑	↓		Not indicated
Hyper insulinemia	Recurrent severe	0	0	Normal or ↑	Normal	↓↓	↑↑	↓↓	Normal	Normal	↑	↑		Not indicated
Ketotic hypoglycemia	Severe with missed meals	Ketonuria +++	0	Normal	Normal	↓↓	↓	↑↑	↓↓	Normal	↑	↓↓		Not indicated
Fatty acid oxidation disorder	Severe with missed meals	Absent	0 to + Abnormal liver function test results	Abnormal	↑		Contraindicated				↑	↓		Not indicated
Hypopituitarism	Moderate with missed meals	Ketonuria ++		Normal	Normal	↓↓	↓	↑↑	↓↓	Normal	↑	↓↓	↑	↑
Adrenal insufficiency	Severe with missed meals	Ketonuria ++	0	Normal	Normal	↓↓	↓	↑↑	↓↓	Normal	↑	↓↓	↑	↑
Type 1 glycogen storage disease*	Severe with missed meals	Ketonuria +++†	+++	↑↑	↑↑	↓↓	↓	↑↑	↑↑	↑↑	0	0-↓↓	0	0
Glycogen debrancher	Moderate with fasting	++	++	Normal	Normal	↓↓	↓	↑↑	↓↓	Normal	↑	0-↓↓	↑	↑
Glycogen phosphorylase	Mild-moderate	Ketonuria ++	+	Normal	Normal	↓	↓	↑↑	↓↓	Normal	0-↑	0-↓↓	↑	↑
Fructose-1,6-diphosphatase	Severe with fasting	Ketonuria +++	+++	↑↑	↑↑	↓↓	↓	↑↑	↑↑	↑↑	↑	0-↓↓	↓	↓
Galactosemia	After milk or milk products	0 Ketones(s) +	+++	Normal	Normal	↓	↓	↑	↓	Normal	↑	0-↓↓	↑	↑
Fructose intolerance	After fructose	0 Ketones(s) +	+++	Normal	Normal	↓	↓	↑	↓	Normal	↑	0-↓↓	↑	↑

*Glucose-6-phosphatase deficiency.
†Hepatomegaly may not be present in the newborn.
0, Absence; ↑ or ↓ indicates, respectively, small increase or decrease; ↑↑ or ↓↓ indicates, respectively, large increase or decrease; +++, markedly increased; +, mildly detected ketonuria or hepatomegaly; ++, moderately increased; 0, absence of ketonuria or hepatomegaly.
From Kliegman RM, St. Geme J, eds. Nelson Textbook of Pediatrics. 21st ed. Philadelphia: Elsevier; 2020. (table 111.8).

TABLE 173.2 Symptoms and Signs of Hypoglycemia in Children >1 Month of Age

FEATURES ASSOCIATED WITH EPINEPHRINE RELEASE*	FEATURES ASSOCIATED WITH CEREBRAL GLYCOPENIA
Perspiration	Headache
Palpitations (tachycardia)	Mental confusion
Pallor	Somnolence
Paresthesia	Dysarthria
Trembling	Personality changes
Anxiety	Inability to concentrate
Weakness	Staring
Nausea	Hunger
Vomiting	Convulsions
	Ataxia
	Coma
	Diplopia
	Stroke

*These features and perceptions of the features may be blunted if the patient is receiving β-blocking agents.

symptoms include confusion, irritability, headaches, visual changes, tremors, pallor, sweating, tachycardia, weakness, seizures, and coma.

Sequelae

Failure to recognize and treat severe, prolonged hypoglycemia can result in serious long-term morbidity, including intellectual disability and nonhypoglycemic seizures. Because the greatest development of the brain is in the first year of life, sustained or frequent episodes of hypoglycemia in infants and children can negatively impact brain development and function. Younger infants and patients with more severe or prolonged hypoglycemia are at greatest risk for adverse outcomes. Transient and asymptomatic short-term hypoglycemia has not been found to be associated with these severe sequelae. While the body has a tightly regulated system to prevent hypoglycemia through use of alternative fuels such as ketone bodies, the

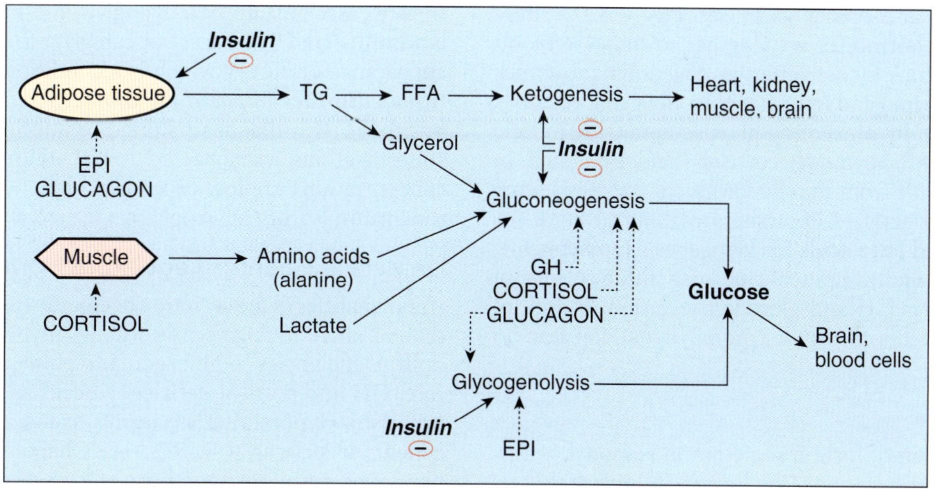

FIGURE 173.1 Regulation of serum glucose. ⊖ represents inhibitions. *EPI*, Epinephrine; *FFA*, free fatty acid; *GH*, growth hormone; *TG*, triglyceride.

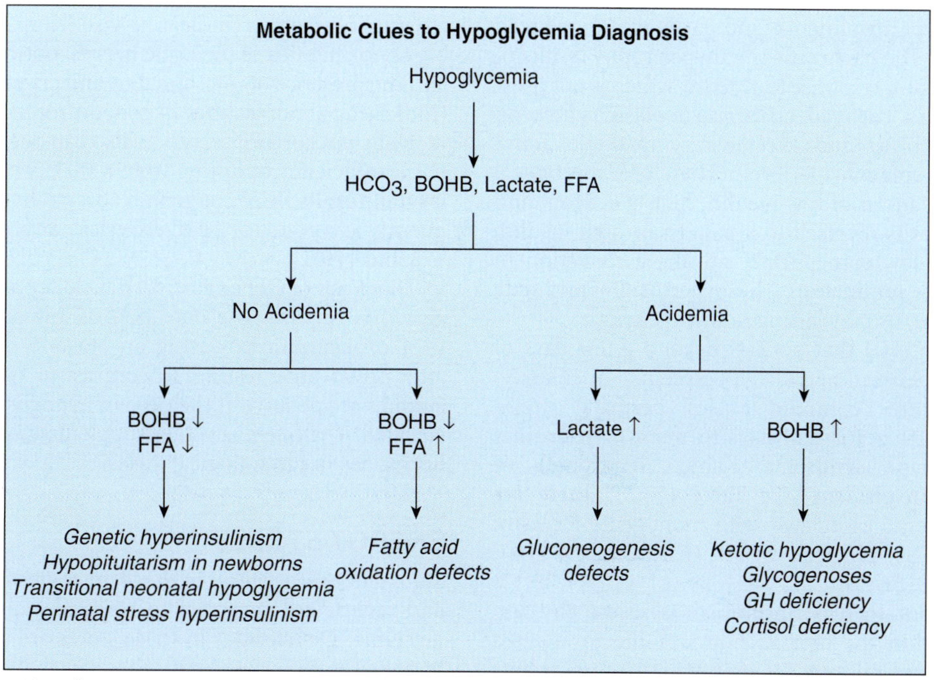

FIGURE 173.2 Algorithm demonstrating an interpretation of a hypoglycemia "critical sample." Serum and urine samples should be obtained when serum glucose is less than 50 mg/dL and after 48 hours of life. *BOHB*, β-hydroxybutyrate; *FFA*, free fatty acids; *GH*, growth hormone; *HCO_3*, bicarbonate. (From Thornton PS, Stanley CA, De Leon DD, et al. Recommendations from the Pediatric Endocrine Society for evaluation and management of persistent hypoglycemia in neonates, infants, and children. *J Pediatr*. 2015;167[2]:238–245.)

ability of a newborn to produce ketone bodies is limited, especially in the presence of hyperinsulinism, which is an inhibitor of hepatic glucose output, lipolysis, and ketogenesis. In addition, although the brain may be able to utilize ketones, glucose remains the best form of energy for CNS function.

PATHOPHYSIOLOGY

See Table 173.3 for the classification of hypoglycemia in infants and children.

Hormonal Signal

Normal regulation of serum glucose concentrations requires appropriate interaction of a number of hormonal signals and metabolic pathways (see Fig. 173.1). In a normal individual, a decrease in serum glucose concentrations leads to a suppression of insulin secretion and increased secretion of the counter-regulatory hormones (growth hormone [GH], cortisol, glucagon, and epinephrine; see Fig. 173.1). These counter-regulatory hormones act together to increase blood glucose concentrations by activating glycogenolytic enzymes (glucagon, epinephrine) and inducing gluconeogenic enzymes (glucagon, cortisol), by preventing glucose uptake by muscle (epinephrine, growth hormone, cortisol), and by aiding in release of amino acids from muscle for gluconeogenesis (cortisol). They will all activate lipolysis, providing glycerol for gluconeogenesis and fatty acids for ketogenesis (epinephrine, cortisol, GH, glucagon). Epinephrine also inhibits insulin release and promotes GH and glucagon secretion. Failure of any of the components of this hormonal signal can lead to hypoglycemia.

Hyperinsulinemia

A lack of suppression of insulin secretion in response to low serum glucose concentrations can occur in infants but is uncommon beyond the neonatal period. Hypoglycemia in infants of diabetic mothers is a common example of this and primarily due to hyperinsulinemia and partly due to reduced glucagon secretion. The pancreatic islet hypertrophy results in a brisk, biphasic insulin response to glucose, which is not present in normal infants. The inadequate rise in plasma glucagon immediately after birth and excessive sympathetic activity may cause low epinephrine levels. Therefore, the typical plasma hormonal pattern of low insulin, high glucagon, and high catecholamines is reversed to a pattern of high insulin, low glucagon, and low epinephrine, causing a reduction in endogenous glucose production. The hyperinsulinemic state is transient, however, usually lasting hours to days.

Hyperinsulinism (HI) that persists beyond a few days of age (persistent hyperinsulinemic hypoglycemia of infancy) can result from three common causes: perinatal stress-related factors (which resolve in days to weeks), syndromes (Beckwith-Wiedemann syndrome, Kabuki syndrome), or **monogenic hyperinsulinism** (see Table 173.3). There are currently several genes associated with monogenic forms of HI *(KCNJ11, HNF4A, HNF1A, UCP2, GCK, HADH, HK1, GLUD1, SLC16A1, ABCC8).*

Hypoglycemia due to hyperinsulinism is severe and frequently occurs within the first 12 hours of life in affected newborns. For older children, hypoglycemia occurs despite frequent feeding (within 1–3 hours of a feed). Glucose requirements are increased, generally requiring a high glucose infusion rate of >10 mg/kg/min. The *diagnosis* of HI in children is supported by suppressed BOHB and FFAs, detectable insulin or C-peptide levels, and glycemic response to glucagon. Diagnosis is most reliably confirmed by a closely monitored provocative fast that ends with a glucagon challenge; this is critical in distinguishing HI from defects in counter-regulatory hormone secretion.

Treatment initially involves the infusion of intravenous (IV) glucose at high rates. HI is managed medically initially with diazoxide (agonist of the sulfonylurea receptor; opens the adenosine triphosphate-sensitive potassium channel and inhibits insulin secretion) and then somatostatin analogs. If hypoglycemia does not improve with IV dextrose and maximum doses of diazoxide and somatostatin analogs, partial or near-total pancreatectomy should be considered to prevent long-term neurological sequelae of hypoglycemia.

Factitious Hyperinsulinemia

In rare cases, insulin or a hypoglycemic-inducing medication is administered by a parent or caregiver to a child to create the appearance of illness, which is a condition referred to as ***factitious disorder imposed on another*** *(Munchausen syndrome by proxy)*. This diagnosis should be suspected if high insulin concentrations are detected (>100 μU/mL) and C-peptide concentrations are low or undetectable, which confirms that the insulin is from an exogenous source.

Defects in Counter-Regulatory Hormones

Abnormalities in the secretion of counter-regulatory hormones that produce hypoglycemia usually involve GH, cortisol, or both. Deficiencies in glucagon and epinephrine secretion are rare. GH and cortisol deficiency occur as a result of hypopituitarism. Hypopituitarism results from a number of different genetic or structural factors (see Chapter 171). Infants with hypopituitarism are often born at expected length and weight but may have midline facial or neurological defects (e.g., cleft lip and palate or absence of the corpus callosum), pendular (roving) nystagmus (indicating visual impairment from possible abnormalities of the optic nerves; optic nerve hypoplasia), and the presence of microphallus and cryptorchidism in males (indicating abnormalities in gonadotropin secretion).

Deficient cortisol secretion also can occur in primary adrenal insufficiency, resulting from a variety of causes. In infants, it often results from congenital adrenal hyperplasia, most frequently as a result of 21-hydroxylase deficiency (see Chapters 178 and 179).

Diagnosis of GH or cortisol deficiency as the cause of hypoglycemia requires the detection of low serum GH and cortisol concentrations during an episode of hypoglycemia or after provocative testing. In contrast to HI, serum and urine ketones are positive at the time of hypoglycemia and FFAs are elevated. *Treatment* involves supplementation of the deficient hormones in physiological doses.

ENERGY STORES

Sufficient energy stores in the form of glycogen, adipose tissue, and muscle are necessary to respond appropriately to hypoglycemia. Deficiencies in these stores are a common cause of hypoglycemia in neonates who are small for gestational age or premature. Beyond the early neonatal period, energy stores

TABLE 173.3 Classification of Hypoglycemia in Infants and Children

NEONATAL TRANSITIONAL HYPOGLYCEMIA

Adaptive

Occurs in first 72 hours of life
Associated with inadequate substrate or immature enzyme function in otherwise normal neonates
Prematurity
Small for gestational age
Normal newborn

Transient Neonatal Hyperinsulinism

Presents at or shortly after birth, but may persist beyond first 72 hours of life
Infant of diabetic mother
IUGR
Perinatal asphyxia
Infant of birth parent with preeclampsia
Rhesus hemolytic disease

NEONATAL, INFANTILE, OR CHILDHOOD PERSISTENT HYPOGLYCEMIA

Congenital Hyperinsulinism

Inactivated K_{ATP} channel pathogenic variants account for approximately 60% of identifiable associated pathogenic variants
ABCC8/KCNJ11/GCK/GDH/HADH/HNF4A/HNF1A/UCP2/SLC16A1/PMM2/HK1/PGM1/FOXA2/CACNA1D/EIF2S3

Others

Postprandial hyperinsulinemic hypoglycemia
Insulinoma
Factitious disorder imposed on another
Exercise-induced hyperinsulinemic hypoglycemia

PRENATAL AND POSTNATAL OVERGROWTH (MACROSOMIA)	
Beckwith-Wiedemann	(11p15)
Sotos	*NSD1* (5q35)
Simpson-Golabi-Behmel	*GPC3* (Xq26), *GPC4* (Xp22)
Perlman	*DIS3L2* (2q37)
POSTNATAL GROWTH FAILURE	
Kabuki	*KMT2D* (12q13), *KDM6A* (Xp11.3)
Costello	*HRAS* (11p15)
CHROMOSOMAL ABNORMALITY	
Mosaic Turner	Loss of X in some cells
Patau	Trisomy 13
CONGENITAL DISORDERS OF GLYCOSYLATION	
Types 1a, 1b, and 1d	*PMM2* (16p13.2), *MPI* (15q24.1), *ALG3* (3q27.1)
Insulin-resistance syndrome (leprechaunism)	*INS* (19p13)
Congenital central hypoventilation syndrome	*PHOX2B* (4p13)

Counter-Regulatory Hormone Deficiency

Panhypopituitarism
Isolated growth hormone deficiency
Adrenocorticotropic hormone deficiency
Addison disease (including congenital adrenal hypoplasia, adrenal leukodystrophy, triple A syndrome, ACTH receptor deficiency, and autoimmune disease complex)
Epinephrine deficiency

Glycogenolysis and Gluconeogenesis Disorders

Glucose-6-phosphatase deficiency (GSD Ia)
Glucose-6-phosphate translocase deficiency (GSD Ib)
Amylo-1,6-glucosidase (debranching enzyme) deficiency (GSD III)
Liver phosphorylase deficiency (GSD VI)
Phosphorylase kinase deficiency (GSD IX)
Glycogen synthetase deficiency (GSD 0)
Fructose-1,6-diphosphatase deficiency
Pyruvate carboxylase deficiency
Galactosemia
Hereditary fructose intolerance

Lipolysis Disorders

Fatty acid oxidation disorders
Carnitine transporter deficiency (primary carnitine deficiency)
Carnitine palmitoyltransferase-1 deficiency
Carnitine translocase deficiency
Carnitine palmitoyltransferase-2 deficiency
Secondary carnitine deficiencies
Very long-, long-, medium-, and short-chain acyl-CoA dehydrogenase deficiency

OTHER ETIOLOGIES

Substrate-Limited Causes

Ketotic hypoglycemia
Poisoning
- Salicylates
- Alcohol
- Oral hypoglycemic agents
- Insulin
- Propranolol
- Pentamidine
- Quinine
- Disopyramide
- Ackee fruit (unripe)—hypoglycin
- Litchi-associated toxin (toxic hypoglycemic syndrome)
- Vacor (rat poison)
- Trimethoprim-sulfamethoxazole (with renal failure)
- L-Asparaginase and other antileukemic drugs

Liver Disease

Reye syndrome (mitochondrial dysfunction)
Hepatitis
Cirrhosis
Hepatoma

AMINO ACID AND ORGANIC ACID DISORDERS

Maple syrup urine disease
Propionic acidemia
Methylmalonic acidemia
Tyrosinosis
Glutaric aciduria
3-Hydroxy-3-methylglutaric aciduria

SYSTEMIC DISORDERS

Sepsis
Cold stress
Carcinoma/sarcoma (secreting—insulinlike growth factor II)
Heart failure
Malnutrition
Malabsorption
Antiinsulin receptor antibodies
Antiinsulin antibodies
Neonatal hyperviscosity
Renal failure
Diarrhea
Burns
Shock
Chiari malformation
Postsurgical complication
Pseudohypoglycemia (leukocytosis, polycythemia)
Excessive insulin therapy of insulin-dependent diabetes mellitus
Factitious disorder imposed on self or other
Nissen fundoplication (dumping syndrome)
Falciparum malaria

ACTH, Adrenocorticotropic hormone; *CoA*, acyl-coenzyme A; *GSD*, glycogen storage disease; *IUGR*, intrauterine growth restriction; K_{ATP}, regulated potassium channel.
Adapted from Kliegman RM, St. Geme J, eds. Nelson Textbook of Pediatrics. *22nd ed. Philadelphia: Elsevier; 2024:Tables 113.3, 113.4, 113.5.*

are usually sufficient to meet the metabolic requirements except in malnourished children.

IDIOPATHIC KETOTIC HYPOGLYCEMIA

A common cause of new-onset hypoglycemia beyond the newborn period is idiopathic ketotic hypoglycemia, usually seen in children between 18 months and 8 years of age. Patients have symptoms of hypoglycemia after a period of prolonged fasting, often in the setting of an intercurrent illness with decreased feeding. Healthy children of similar age can withstand fasting without hypoglycemia developing during the same period, although even children without ketotic hypoglycemia may acquire these features by 36 hr of fasting. Children with this disorder are often thin and small, may have a history of being small for gestational age, and often have a history of transient neonatal hypoglycemia. The etiology of ketotic hypoglycemia may be a defect in any of the processes involved in protein catabolism, oxidative deamination of amino acids, transamination, alanine synthesis, or alanine efflux from muscle. There are no specific diagnostic tests for this disorder.

Treatment involves avoidance of fasting and frequent feedings of a high-protein, high-carbohydrate diet. Patients may require hospitalization for IV glucose infusion if they cannot maintain adequate oral intake during a period of illness.

DISRUPTED METABOLIC RESPONSE PATHWAYS

Maintenance of normal serum glucose concentrations in the fasting state requires glucose production via glycogenolysis and gluconeogenesis and the production of alternative energy sources (FFAs and ketones) via lipolysis and fatty acid oxidation.

Glycogenolysis

Glycogen storage diseases (GSDs) occur in a variety of subtypes that differ in severity (see Chapter 51). Among the subtypes that result in hypoglycemia, the most severe form is glucose-6-phosphatase deficiency, which is characterized by severe hypoglycemia, massive hepatomegaly, growth delay, and lactic acidosis. GSDs are classified into types primarily affecting the liver, the skeletal muscle, or the skeletal and cardiac muscles.

The *diagnosis* of GSD is suggested by a finding of ketotic hypoglycemia, +/– hepatomegaly, +/– muscle weakness. Confirmation of the diagnosis is generally performed with molecular genetic testing; however, there may be instances that would benefit from biopsy of the liver or skeletal muscle, depending on the patient's presentation.

Treatment for the most common types involves frequent high-carbohydrate feedings during the day and feedings of uncooked cornstarch to maintain serum glucose concentrations in some patients. Some GSDs, like GSD type II, can now be treated with enzyme replacement therapy using recombinant alglucosidase alfa, which degrades lysosomal glycogen (Chapter 51).

Gluconeogenesis

Disorders of gluconeogenesis are uncommon and include fructose-1,6-diphosphatase deficiency and phosphoenolpyruvate carboxykinase deficiency. Affected patients exhibit fasting hypoglycemia, hepatomegaly, lactic acidosis, and hyperuricemia. Ketosis occurs, and FFA and alanine concentrations are high. *Treatment* involves frequent high-carbohydrate, low-protein feedings (see Chapter 51).

Fatty Acid Oxidation Disorders

Fatty acid oxidation disorders of ketogenesis include the fatty acid acyl-coenzyme A (CoA) dehydrogenase deficiencies; long-chain, medium-chain, and short-chain acyl-CoA dehydrogenase deficiencies; and hereditary carnitine deficiency. Mild hepatomegaly may be present along with mild hyperammonemia, hyperuricemia, and mild elevations in hepatic transaminases. Episodes of nonketotic hypoglycemia usually occur with prolonged fasting or during episodes of intercurrent illness (see Chapter 54).

Other Metabolic Disorders

Many metabolic disorders can lead to hypoglycemia, including galactosemia, hereditary fructose intolerance, and disorders of organic acid metabolism (see Table 173.3). Hypoglycemia in these disorders is usually a reflection of global hepatic dysfunction secondary to the buildup of hepatotoxic intermediates. Many of these disorders present with low concentrations of ketone bodies because ketogenesis also is affected. The finding of nonglucose-reducing substances in the urine after ingestion of offending substances suggests a diagnosis of galactosemia or hereditary fructose intolerance. *Treatment* requires dietary restriction of the specific offending substances.

MEDICATIONS AND INTOXICATION

Hypoglycemia can occur as an adverse effect of numerous medications (see Table 173.3). Ethanol ingestion also can cause hypoglycemia, especially in younger children, because the metabolism of ethanol results in the depletion of cofactors necessary for gluconeogenesis.

EMERGENCY MANAGEMENT

Acute care of a patient with hypoglycemia who has altered consciousness consists of rapid administration of IV glucose (2 mL/kg of 10% dextrose in water). After the initial bolus, an infusion of IV glucose should provide approximately 1.5 times the normal hepatic glucose production rate (5–6 mg/kg/min in infants, 2–3 mg/kg/min in children). This infusion allows for suppression of the catabolic state and prevents further decompensation in patients with certain metabolic disorders. If adrenal insufficiency is suspected, stress doses of glucocorticoids should be administered.

PEARLS FOR PRACTITIONERS

See Endocrinology: Pearls for Practitioners at the end of this section.

REVIEW QUESTION

Available online.

CHAPTER 174 Short Stature

GROWTH

Normal growth is the final common pathway of many factors, including endocrine, environmental, nutritional, and genetic influences (see Chapter 5). A normal linear growth pattern is good evidence of overall health and can be considered a *bioassay* for the well-being of the whole child. The effects of certain hormones on growth and ultimate height are listed in Table 174.1. Just as various factors influence stature, stature itself influences psychological, social, and potentially economic well-being. Parental concern about the psychosocial consequences of abnormal stature often causes a family to seek medical attention.

Growth Hormone Physiology

Growth hormone (GH) is a 191–amino acid protein secreted by the pituitary in a pulsatile fashion, stimulated by hypothalamic **GH-releasing hormone (GHRH)** and inhibited by **somatostatin** (also known as *somatotropin release–inhibiting factor*), which interact with their individual receptors on the pituitary somatotrope in a noncompetitive manner (Fig. 174.1). In addition, GH secretion is *enhanced* by α-adrenergic stimulation, β-adrenergic stimulation, hypoglycemia, stress, starvation, exercise, early stages of sleep, GH-releasing peptides, sex steroids, thyroxine, glucocorticoids, ghrelin, and clonidine and is *suppressed* by insulin-like growth factor 1 (IGF-1) and hyperglycemia. GH, GHRH, and somatostatin are also modulated by multiple neurotransmitters and neuropeptides, including serotonin, histamine, norepinephrine, dopamine, thyroid-releasing hormone, neuropeptide Y, vasopressin, corticotrophin-releasing hormone, and galanin.

GH stimulates IGF-1 production in the liver along with production of the acid-labile subunit and the IGF-binding protein 3 (IGF-BP3); this forms the complex that delivers IGF-1 to tissue. The anabolic actions of GH are partially mediated through the IGF polypeptides. GH is also capable of stimulating processes independent of IGF activity, including a variety of metabolic effects, such as lipolysis, protein synthesis, and phosphate, water, and sodium retention.

IGF-1 acts primarily as a paracrine and autocrine agent and is most closely associated with postnatal growth. When IGF-1 attaches to its membrane-bound receptor, second messengers are stimulated to change the physiology of the cell and produce growth effects. IGF-1 production is influenced by disease states such as malnutrition, chronic kidney and liver disease, hypothyroidism, and obesity.

IGF-BP3 is measurable in clinical assays and is less influenced by nutrition and age than IGF-1; measuring IGF-1 and IGF-BP3 is useful in evaluating GH adequacy, particularly in infancy and early childhood.

Measurement of Growth

The correct measurement of an infant's length requires one adult to hold the infant's head still and another adult to extend the feet with the soles perpendicular to the lower legs. The use of a recumbent length board, composed of a firm platform, a fixed head plate, and a moveable footplate for reading the measurement, requires two people and is required for accurate length measurement. Marking the position of the head and feet of an infant lying on a sheet of paper on the examining table leads to inaccuracies. True disorders of growth may be missed or false concerns about a disorder of growth in a normal child may be created.

After 2 years of age, the height of a child should be measured in the standing position barefoot against a hard surface. A wall-mounted stadiometer or equivalent device is optimal for the measurement of stature. A decrease of roughly 1.25 cm in height measurement may occur when the child is measured in the standing position rather than in the lying position, leading to the inappropriate referral of many children who appear to be not growing to a subspecialist. Accurate measurements of height (standing) or length (lying down) and weight should be plotted on the Centers for Disease Control and Prevention growth charts for the timely diagnosis of growth disorders (https://www.cdc.gov/growthcharts/cdc-growth-charts.htm).

Measurement of the **arm span** (distance between the tips of the fingers when the patient holds both arms outstretched horizontally while standing against a solid surface) is essential when the diagnoses of Marfan or Klinefelter syndrome,

TABLE 174.1 Hormonal Effects on Growth

HORMONE	BONE AGE	GROWTH RATE	ADULT HEIGHT*
Androgen excess	Advanced	Increased	Diminished
Androgen deficiency	Normal or delayed	Normal or decreased	Increased slightly or normal
Thyroxine excess	Advanced	Increased	Normal or diminished
Thyroxine deficiency	Delayed	Decreased	Diminished
Growth hormone excess	Normal or advanced	Increased	Excessive
Growth hormone deficiency	Delayed	Decreased	Diminished
Cortisol excess	Delayed	Decreased	Diminished
Cortisol deficiency	Normal	Normal	Normal

*Effect in most patients with treatment.

Modified from Underwood LE, Van Wyk JJ. Normal and aberrant growth. In: Wilson JD, Foster DW, eds. Textbook of Endocrinology. 8th ed. Philadelphia: WB Saunders; 1992.

short-limbed dwarfism, or other dysmorphic conditions are considered. The **upper-to-lower segment ratio** is the ratio of the upper segment (determined by subtraction of the measurement from the symphysis pubis to the floor [known as the *lower segment*] from the total height) to the lower segment. A normal term infant has an upper-to-lower ratio of 1.7:1, a 1-year-old has a ratio of 1.4:1, and a 10-year-old has a ratio of 1:1. Untreated conditions of hypogonadism lead to a greatly decreased upper-to-lower ratio in an adult, whereas long-lasting and untreated hypothyroidism leads to a high upper-to-lower ratio in the child.

Endocrine Evaluation of Growth Hormone Secretion

Because concentrations of GH are low throughout the day, except for brief secretory peaks in the middle of the night or early morning, the daytime ascertainment of GH deficiency or sufficiency based on a single determination of a random GH concentration is impossible. Adequacy of GH secretion may be determined by a stimulation test to measure peak GH secretion. A normal response is a vigorous secretory peak after stimulation; the lack of such a peak is consistent with GH deficiency. However, there is a high false-positive rate (on any day, about 10% or more of normal children may not reach the normal GH peak even after two stimulatory tests). Indirect measurements of GH secretion, such as serum concentrations of IGF-1 and IGF-BP3, are considered better screens for GH deficiency.

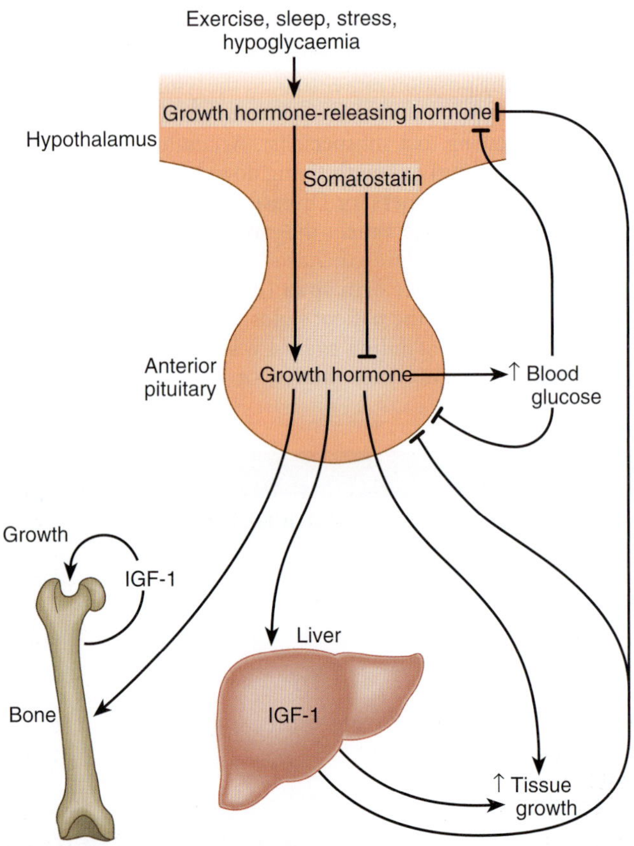

FIGURE 174.1 Growth hormone regulation. *IGF-1,* Insulinlike growth factor 1. (From Hinson J, Raven P. Endocrinology and the reproductive system. In: Court DS, Kadri A, Xiu P, eds. *Medical Sciences.* 4th ed. London: Elsevier; 2025:Fig. 10.14.)

ABNORMALITIES OF GROWTH

Short stature is defined as subnormal height relative to other children of the same gender and age, taking family heights into consideration. It can be caused by numerous conditions (Table 174.2). The Centers for Disease Control and Prevention growth charts use the 3rd percentile of the growth curve as the demarcation of the lower limit. **Growth failure** denotes a slow growth rate regardless of stature. Ultimately, a slow growth rate leads to short stature, but a disease process is detected sooner if the decreased growth rate is noted before the stature becomes short. Plotted on a growth chart, growth failure appears as a curve that crosses percentiles downward and is associated with a height velocity below the 5th percentile of height velocity for age (Fig. 174.2). A corrected midparental, or genetic target, height helps determine whether the child is growing well for the family (see Chapter 6). To determine a range of normal height for the family under consideration, the corrected midparental height is bracketed by 2 standard deviations (SDs), which, for the United States, is approximately 10 cm (4 in.). The presence of a height 3.5 SDs below the mean, a height velocity below the 5th percentile for age, or a height below the target height corrected for midparental height requires a diagnostic evaluation.

Short Stature Caused by Growth Hormone Deficiency

Etiology and Epidemiology

Classic congenital or **idiopathic GH deficiency** occurs in about 1:4,000 to 1:10,000 children. Idiopathic GH deficiency of unidentified specific etiology is the most common cause of both congenital and acquired GH deficiency. Less often, GH deficiency is caused by anatomical defects of the pituitary gland, such as pituitary aplasia or other midline defects (such as septo-optic dysplasia), with variable degrees of deficiency of other pituitary functions. Hereditary forms of GH deficiency that affect pituitary differentiation are the result of heterogeneous defects of the gene for GH, GHRH, or GH receptor. *Classic GH deficiency* refers to very reduced to absent secretion of GH; numerous short children may have intermediate forms of decreased GH secretion. Acquired GH deficiency causing late-onset growth failure suggests the possibility of a **tumor** of the hypothalamus or pituitary causing compression of the area (see Tables 174.2 and 174.3).

Clinical Manifestations

Infants with congenital GH deficiency achieve a normal or near-normal birth length and weight at term, but the growth rate slows after birth, most noticeably after age 2–3 years. These children become progressively shorter for age and tend to have an elevated weight-to-height ratio. Careful measurements in the first year of life may suggest the diagnosis, but most patients elude diagnosis until several years of age. A patient with classic GH deficiency often has a high-pitched voice resulting from an immature larynx. The patient has normal intellectual growth and age-appropriate speech.

A more comprehensive evaluation is warranted in children with one or more of the following features:

- Growth failure—This is suggested if their height has crossed two major height percentile curves (e.g., from above the

TABLE 174.2 Causes of Short Stature

VARIATIONS OF NORMAL

Constitutional (delayed bone age)
Genetic (short familial height)
Idiopathic
Small for gestational age infant (without catch-up growth in first 2 years)

ENDOCRINE DISORDERS

GH deficiency
- *Congenital*
  - Isolated GH deficiency
  - With other pituitary hormone deficiencies
  - With midline defects
  - Pituitary agenesis
  - With gene pathogenic variant
- *Acquired*
  - Hypothalamic/pituitary tumors
  - Langerhans cell histiocytosis
  - CNS infections and granulomas
  - Head trauma (birth and later)
  - Hypothalamic/pituitary irradiation
  - CNS vascular accidents
  - Hydrocephalus
  - Autoimmune
  - Psychosocial short stature (functional GH deficiency)
  - Amphetamine treatment for hyperactivity*

Laron syndrome (increased GH and decreased IGF-1)
Underexpression of growth hormone receptor (normal GH and IGF-2 but decreased IGF-1)
Hypothyroidism
Glucocorticoid excess
- Endogenous
- Exogenous

Diabetes mellitus under poor control
Diabetes insipidus (untreated)
Hypophosphatemic vitamin D–resistant rickets
Virilizing congenital adrenal hyperplasia (tall child, short adult)

SKELETAL DYSPLASIAS

Osteogenesis imperfecta
Osteochondrodysplasias

LYSOSOMAL STORAGE DISEASES

Mucopolysaccharidoses
Mucolipidoses

SYNDROMES OF SHORT STATURE

Turner syndrome (syndrome of gonadal dysgenesis)
Noonan syndrome
Autosomal trisomy 13, 18, 21
Laurence-Moon-Bardet-Biedl syndrome
Prader-Willi syndrome
Autosomal abnormalities
Dysmorphic syndromes (e.g., Russell-Silver or Cornelia de Lange syndrome)
Pseudohypoparathyroidism
SHOX (short-stature homeobox) gene haploinsufficiency

CHRONIC DISEASE

Cardiac disorders
- Left-to-right shunt
- Heart failure

Pulmonary disorders
- Cystic fibrosis
- Asthma (severe steroid-dependent)

Gastrointestinal disorders
- Malabsorption (e.g., celiac disease, cystic fibrosis)
- Disorders of swallowing
- Inflammatory bowel disease

Hepatic disorders
Hematologic disorders
- Sickle cell anemia
- Thalassemia

Kidney disorders
- Renal tubular acidosis
- Chronic uremia

Immunologic disorders
- Connective tissue disease
- Juvenile idiopathic arthritis
- Chronic infection
- AIDS

Hereditary fructose intolerance
Malnutrition
Kwashiorkor, marasmus
Iron deficiency
Zinc deficiency
Anorexia caused by chemotherapy for neoplasms
Cerebral palsy

*Only if caloric intake is severely diminished.
CNS, Central nervous system; *GH*, growth hormone; *IGF*, insulinlike growth factor.
Modified from Styne DM. Growth disorder. In: Fitzgerald PA, ed. Handbook of Clinical Endocrinology. Norwalk, CT: Appleton & Lange; 1986.

25th percentile to below the 10th percentile) or if the child is growing slower than the following rates:
- Age 2 to 4 years—Height velocity less than 5.5 cm/year (<2.2 inches/year)
- Age 4 to 6 years—Height velocity less than 5 cm/year (<2 inches/year)
- Age 6 years to puberty:
  - Height velocity less than 4 cm/year for males (<1.6 inches/year)
  - Height velocity less than 4.5 cm/year for females (<1.8 inches/year)
- Severe short stature (e.g., height ≤−2.5 SD, i.e., 0.6th percentile) or less severe short stature combined with growth failure
- Features concerning for hypothalamic or pituitary dysfunction, either congenital (e.g., hypoglycemia, microphallus, cryptorchidism, visual abnormalities) or acquired (e.g., intracranial tumor, cranial irradiation, or head trauma), with decelerating growth, even if the child's height is within the normal range but deviating from predicted parental percentiles
- Evidence for deficits in other pituitary hormones, either congenital or acquired

If chronic disease or familial short stature are ruled out and routine laboratory testing is normal (Table 174.4), two GH provocative (stimulation) tests are commonly performed (see Table 171.2).

Classic GH-deficient patients do not show an increase in serum GH levels after stimulation. Some patients release GH in response to secretagogue testing but cannot release GH spontaneously during the day or night. Tests for GH secretion are insensitive, not very specific, and fairly

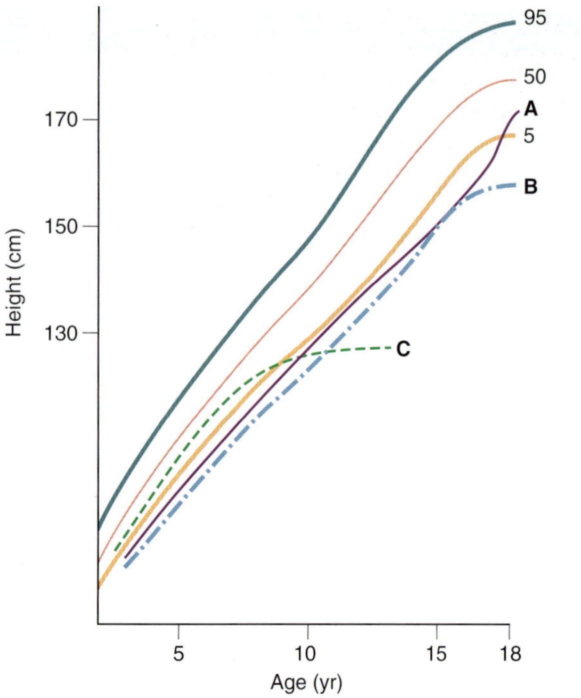

FIGURE 174.2 Patterns of linear growth. Normal growth percentiles (5th, 50th, and 95th) are shown along with typical growth curves for *(A)* constitutional delay of growth and adolescence (short stature with normal growth rate for bone age, delayed pubertal growth spurt, and eventual achievement of normal adult stature); *(B)* familial short stature (short stature in childhood and as an adult); and *(C)* acquired pathological growth failure (e.g., acquired untreated primary hypothyroidism) (see Chapter 5).

variable. In equivocal cases, an operational definition of GH deficiency might be that patients grow significantly faster when administered a normal dose of GH than before treatment.

Treatment

GH deficiency is treated with biosynthetic recombinant DNA-derived GH (rhGH). Dosage is titrated to the growth rate, weight of the patient, and IGF-1 levels. Treatment with GH carries the slightly higher risk of developing idiopathic intracranial hypertension (formerly known as *pseudotumor cerebri*), increased intraocular pressure, slipped capital femoral epiphysis, and worsening of existing scoliosis. Whether these are true side effects of rhGH itself or whether some are related to the rapid growth induced by rhGH remains unknown. Risks and benefits must be weighed with the family and treatment team.

Administration of GH to patients with normal GH responsiveness to secretagogues (**idiopathic short stature**, with height 2.25 SDs or less below the mean) is controversial, but, as noted earlier, diagnostic tests are imperfect; if the patient is growing extremely slowly without alternative explanation, GH therapy is sometimes used. GH is effective in increasing the growth rate and final height in **Turner syndrome**, ***SHOX*** **pathogenic variants**, **chronic kidney failure**, **Noonan syndrome**, and **Prader-Willi syndrome**. Other indications include children born small for gestational age who have not exhibited catch-up growth by 2 years of age.

Other Causes of Short Stature

The factors responsible for postnatal growth are not the same as the factors that mediate fetal growth. **Thyroid hormone** is essential for normal postnatal growth, although a thyroid hormone-deficient fetus achieves a normal birth length; similarly, a GH-deficient fetus has a normal birth length, although in IGF-1 deficiency resulting from GH resistance **(Laron syndrome)**, fetuses are shorter than control subjects. A very rare cause of growth failure, *GH resistance*, is inherited in an autosomal recessive fashion and is caused by abnormal number or function of GH receptors or by a postreceptor defect. Patients have a prominent forehead, hypoplastic nasal bridge, delayed dentition, sparse hair, blue sclerae, delayed bone maturation and osteoporosis, progressive adiposity, hypercholesterolemia, and low blood glucose. They have elevated serum GH concentrations, although serum IGF-1 and IGF-BP3 concentrations are low.

Adequate thyroid hormone is necessary to allow the secretion of GH. Patients with hypothyroidism may appear falsely to be GH deficient; with thyroid hormone repletion, GH secretion normalizes. Gonadal steroids are important in the pubertal growth spurt. The effects of other hormones on growth are noted in Table 174.1.

Nutrition is the most important factor affecting growth on a worldwide basis (see Chapter 28). Growth faltering may develop in the infant as a result of **maternal deprivation** (nutritional deficiency or aberrant psychosocial interaction) or as a result of organic illness (anorexia, nutrient losses through a form of malabsorption, or hypermetabolism caused by hyperthyroidism or other causes). Malnutrition may cause **acquired GH resistance** because serum GH is elevated and IGF-1 is decreased.

Psychological difficulties also can affect growth, as in **psychosocial short stature**, in which the child develops functional temporary GH deficiency and poor growth as a result of psychological abuse; when placed in a different, healthier psychosocial environment, GH physiology normalizes, and growth occurs.

The common condition known as ***constitutional delay*** in growth or puberty (or both) is considered a variation of normal growth, caused by a reduced tempo of physiological development (see Fig. 174.2). Usually, a family member had delayed growth or puberty but achieved a final height consistent with midparental height predictions. The bone age is delayed, but the growth rate remains mostly within the lower limits of normal. Constitutional delay usually leads to a delay in secondary sexual development. **Genetic or familial short stature** (Table 174.3) refers to the stature of a child of short parents who is expected to reach a lower-than-average height that is consistent with parental height.

Phenotypic features suggesting an underlying **chromosomal disorder** can occur in many syndromes. These syndromes may be suspected after assessing arm spans and upper-to-lower segment ratios. Genetic syndromes often combine obesity and decreased height, whereas otherwise normal obese children are usually taller than average and have advanced skeletal development and physical maturation (see Table 174.2). **Prader-Willi syndrome (PWS)** includes fetal and infantile hypotonia, small hands and feet, postnatal acquired obesity with an insatiable appetite, developmental

TABLE 174.3 Differential Diagnoses and Therapy of Short Stature

DIAGNOSTIC FEATURE	HYPOPITUITARISM GH DEFICIENCY*	CONSTITUTIONAL DELAY	FAMILIAL SHORT STATURE	PSYCHOSOCIAL SHORT STATURE	TURNER SYNDROME	HYPOTHYROIDISM	CHRONIC DISEASE
Family history positive	Rare	Frequent	Always	No	No	Variable	Variable
Gender	Both	Males more often affected than females	Both	Both	Female	Both	Both
Facies	Immature or with midline defect (e.g., cleft palate or optic hypoplasias)	Immature	Normal	Normal	Turner facies or normal	Generalized myxedema	Normal
Sexual development	Delayed	Delayed	Normal	May be delayed	Female prepubertal	Usually delayed, may be precocious if hypothyroidism is severe	Delayed
Bone age	Delayed	Delayed	Normal	Usually delayed; growth arrest lines present	Delayed	Delayed	Delayed
Dentition	Delayed	Normal; delay usual	Normal	Variable	Normal	Delayed	Normal or delayed
Hypoglycemia	Variable	No	No	No	No	No	No
Karyotype	Normal	Normal	Normal	Normal	45,X or partial deletion of X chromosome or mosaic	Normal	Normal
Free T_4	Low (with TRH deficiency) or normal	Normal	Normal	Normal or low	Normal: hypothyroidism may be acquired	Low	Normal
Stimulated GH	Low	Normal for bone age	Normal	Possibly low, or high if patient malnourished	Usually normal	Low	Usually normal
Insulinlike growth factor 1	Low	Normal or low for chronologic age	Normal	Low	Normal	Low	Low or normal (depending on nutritional status)
Therapy	Replace deficiencies	Reassurance; sex steroids to initiate secondary sexual development in selected patients	None	Change or improve environment	Sex hormone replacement, GH; oxandrolone may be useful	T_4	Treat malnutrition, organ failure (e.g., dialysis, transplant, cardiotonic drugs, insulin)

Possibly with GnRH, CRH, or TRH deficiency.

CRH, Corticotropin-releasing hormone; *GH*, growth hormone; *GnRH*, gonadotropin-releasing hormone; *T_4*, thyroxine; *TRH*, thyrotropin-releasing hormone.

delay, hypogonadism, and almond-shaped eyes. PWS is caused by a lack of expression of paternally inherited genes in the region of chromosome 15q11.2-q13. The majority of patients (70%) have a deletion of the paternal allele, whereas one-quarter have maternal uniparental disomy (UPD[15q] m). **Laurence-Moon-Bardet-Biedl syndrome** is characterized by retinitis pigmentosa, hypogonadism, and developmental delay with an autosomal dominant inheritance pattern. Laurence-Moon syndrome is associated with spastic paraplegia; Bardet-Biedl syndrome is associated with obesity and polydactyly. **Pseudohypoparathyroidism** leads to short stature and developmental delay with short fourth and fifth digits (Albright hereditary osteodystrophy phenotype), resistance to parathyroid hormone and resultant hypocalcemia, and elevated levels of serum phosphorus. **Turner syndrome** is characterized by a karyotype of 45,XO or by a mosaic karyotype and clinically presents with short stature, shield chest, wide-spaced nipples, wide-carrying angle of the upper extremities, high-arched palate, gonadal failure, kidney dysplasias with normal function, and aortic arch abnormalities. **Noonan syndrome (NS)** has an estimated prevalence of 1 in 1,000 to 1 in 2,500 live births (equal between male and female). It is inherited in an autosomal dominant pattern (one-third of affected children), with two-thirds of the diagnoses caused by de novo pathogenic variants and near complete penetrance but marked clinical heterogeneity. NS is characterized by distinctive facial dysmorphic features, congenital heart defects, chest wall abnormalities (pectus carinatum and/or excavatum), and growth delays. Postnatal delay in growth is accompanied by reduced IGF-1 concentrations but usually normal GH secretion, although GH deficiency has been described in some patients.

The short-stature homeobox containing gene ***(SHOX)*** encodes a homeodomain transcription factor and is a gene implicated in short stature. *SHOX* gene is located on the short arm pseudoautosomal region 1 (PAR 1) of both the X and Y chromosomes. Males and females express two active copies of this gene; it does not become inactivated on the second X chromosome in females. *SHOX* gene is expressed during skeletal development in the fetal period, as well as within the chondrocytes of the epiphyseal growth plate. *SHOX* pathogenic variants have variable phenotypes, including mild-to-severe short stature and mesomelia (shortened forearms and lower legs).

TABLE **174.4** Growth Failure: Screening Tests

TEST	RATIONALE
CBC	*Anemia:* nutritional, chronic disease, malignancy
	Leukopenia: bone marrow failure syndromes
	Thrombocytopenia: malignancy, infection
ESR, CRP	Inflammation of infection, inflammatory diseases, malignancy
Metabolic panel (electrolytes, liver enzymes, BUN)	Signs of acute or chronic hepatic, kidney, adrenal dysfunction; hydration and acid-base status
Carotene, folate, and prothrombin time; celiac antibody panel	Assess malabsorption; detect celiac disease
Urinalysis with pH	Signs of kidney dysfunction, hydration, water and salt homeostasis; renal tubular acidosis
Karyotype	Determines Turner (XO) or other syndromes
Cranial imaging (MRI)	Assesses hypothalamic-pituitary tumors (craniopharyngioma, glioma, germinoma) or congenital midline defects
Bone age	Compare with height age and evaluate height potential
IGF-1, IGF-BP3	Reflects growth hormone status or nutrition
Free thyroxine	Detects MPHD or isolated hypothyroidism
Prolactin	Elevated in hypothalamic dysfunction or destruction, suppressed in pituitary disease

BUN, Blood urea nitrogen; *CBC,* complete blood count; *CRP,* C-reactive protein; *ESR,* erythrocyte sedimentation rate; *IGF-1,* insulinlike growth factor 1; *IGF-BP3,* insulinlike growth factor-binding protein 3; *MPHD,* multiple pituitary hormone deficiency; *MRI,* magnetic resonance imaging.

Diagnosis

If family or other medical history does not provide a likely diagnosis, laboratory screening tests may include a complete blood count, C-reactive protein, creatinine, glucose, electrolytes, bicarbonate, liver function tests, calcium, phosphate, albumin, celiac serologies, thyroxine (T_4), thyroid-stimulating hormone (TSH), IGF-1, and IGFBP-3. A urine study should be performed to assess kidney function and evaluate for renal tubular acidosis. A karyotype may be indicated to rule out **Turner syndrome** in females or in short males with associated genital abnormalities.

A radiograph of the left hand and wrist should be obtained for a bone age evaluation by an expert to estimate the remaining growth potential. Malformations on this radiograph may sometimes point to a skeletal dysplasia (see Table 174.4).

PEARLS FOR PRACTITIONERS

See Endocrinology: Pearls for Practitioners at the end of this section.

REVIEW QUESTIONS

Available online.

CHAPTER 175 Disorders of Puberty

PHYSIOLOGY

The staging of pubertal changes and the sequence of events are discussed in Chapter 66. The onset of puberty is marked by adrenarche and gonadarche. **Adrenarche** results from adrenal maturation and is marked with the appearance of pubic hair; other features include oiliness of hair and skin, acne, axillary hair, and body odor. **Gonadarche** is characterized by increasing secretion of gonadal sex steroids as a result of the maturation of the hypothalamic-pituitary-gonadal axis. These sex steroids differ between males and females, consisting of testosterone from the testes and estradiol and progesterone from the ovaries. In males, physical signs are pubic hair, axillary hair, facial hair, increased muscularity, deeper voice, increased penile size, and increased testicular volume. In females, the physical signs are breast development, development of the female body habitus, increased size of the uterus, and menarche with regular menstrual cycles. The third component is the growth spurt of puberty.

Hypothalamic **gonadotropin-releasing hormone (GnRH)**, produced by cells in the arcuate nucleus, is secreted from the median eminence of the hypothalamus into the pituitary portal system and reaches the membrane receptors on the pituitary gonadotropes to stimulate the production and release of **luteinizing hormone (LH)** and **follicle-stimulating hormone (FSH)** into the circulation.

Numerous genes have been identified that are critical for normal pubertal development and progression. Those include pathogenic variants in (1) the pathway that controls the development or function of GnRH-producing neurons *(KAL1, FGFR1, KISS1R, NELF, PROK2, PROKRR2)*; (2) transcription factors critical for ventromedial hypothalamus and pituitary development (*SF1, DAX1, HESX1, LHX3, SOX2,* or *PROP1*); (3) genes affecting GnRH release and action (*GNRH1* and *GNRHR*); and (4) genes involved in gonadotropin production (*LHβ* or *FSHβ, SF1, DAX1*). Kisspeptin and neurokinin B are neuropeptides that appear to be "gatekeepers of puberty."

In females, FSH stimulates the growth of ovarian follicles and, in conjunction with LH, stimulates production of estradiol by the ovaries. Early in puberty, estradiol stimulates breast development and growth of the skeleton, leading to pubertal growth acceleration. Later in puberty, the interplay between pituitary secretion of FSH and LH and the secretion of estradiol by ovarian follicles leads to ovulation and menstrual cycles, and estradiol leads to fusion of growth plates. In males, LH stimulates the production of testosterone from the Leydig cells; later in puberty, FSH stimulates the development and support of the seminiferous tubules. The gonads also produce the protein inhibin. Both sex steroids and inhibin suppress the secretion of gonadotropins. The interplay of the products of the gonads and GnRH modulates the serum concentrations of gonadotropins. GnRH is released in episodic pulses that vary during development and during the menstrual period. These pulses ensure that gonadotropins are released in a pulsatile manner. With the onset of puberty, the amplitude of the pulses of gonadotropins and, in turn, the sex steroids, increases, first at night and then throughout the day. Adrenarche generally occurs several years earlier than gonadarche and is heralded by increasing circulating dehydroepiandrosterone (DHEA) or androstenedione. Serum DHEA increases years before the appearance of its effects.

The typical developmental sequence in females is **thelarche**, the beginning of adult breast development due to gonadarche, followed closely by **pubarche**, the appearance of pubic hair due to adrenarche, and finally **menarche**, onset of menstruation, 2–3 years later. In males the first typical event is scrotal thinning followed by the enlargement of testes and by the appearance of pubic hair (long diameter of the testis >2.5 cm, volume >4 mL). Most of the enlargement of testes during puberty is the result of seminiferous tubule maturation.

DELAYED PUBERTY

Puberty is delayed when there is no sign of pubertal development by age 13 years in females and 14 years in males living in the United States (Tables 175.1 and 175.2).

Constitutional Delay in Growth and Adolescence

Patients with constitutional delay have delayed onset of pubertal development and significant bone age delay (2 standard deviations below the mean, which is equal to a 1.5- to 2-year delay as a teenager). Usually height gain is below, although fairly parallel to, the normal percentiles on the growth curve. The prepubertal nadir, or deceleration before the pubertal growth spurt, is prolonged or protracted. A family history of delayed puberty in a parent or sibling is reassuring. Spontaneous puberty usually begins in these patients by the time the bone age reaches 12 years in males and 11 years in females. Other causes of delayed puberty must be eliminated before a diagnosis of constitutional delay in puberty is made. Observation and reassurance are appropriate. Adult height normal for the genetic potential is generally attained. In some cases, males may be treated with low-dose testosterone for a few months if the bone age is at least 11–12 years. Treatment is not required for longer than 4–8 months because endogenous hormone production usually ensues. Estrogen treatment has been used in females with constitutional delay because they may, as males often do, jumpstart into puberty with a short course of priming with estrogen. Children who do not initiate endogenous hormone production should be evaluated for other causes of hypogonadism.

Hypogonadotropic Hypogonadism

As a cause of delayed or absent puberty, hypogonadotropic hypogonadism may be difficult to distinguish from constitutional delay (see Tables 175.1 and 175.2). Hypogonadotropic hypogonadism precludes spontaneous entry into gonadarche; adrenarche usually occurs to some degree. Throughout childhood and in early puberty, patients with hypogonadotropic hypogonadism have normal proportions and growth. When

TABLE 175.1 Classification of Delayed Puberty

IDIOPATHIC (CONSTITUTIONAL) (Delayed activation of hypothalamic GnRH pulse generator)
HYPOGONADOTROPIC HYPOGONADISM
CNS disorders
Tumors
Craniopharyngiomas
Germinomas
Other germ cell tumors
Hypothalamic and optic gliomas
Astrocytomas
Pituitary tumors (including MEN-1, prolactinoma)
Other causes
Langerhans histiocytosis
Postinfectious lesions of the CNS
Vascular abnormalities of the CNS
Radiation therapy
Congenital malformations especially associated with craniofacial anomalies
Head trauma
Lymphocytic hypophysitis
Isolated gonadotropin deficiency
Kallmann syndrome (with hyposmia or anosmia; without anosmia)
GnRH receptor pathogenic variant
Congenital adrenal hypoplasia (*DAX1* pathogenic variant)
Isolated LH deficiency
Isolated FSH deficiency
Prohormone convertase 1 deficiency (PCI)
Idiopathic and genetic forms of multiple pituitary hormone deficiencies including *PROP1* pathogenic variant
Miscellaneous disorders
Prader-Willi syndrome
Bardet-Biedl syndrome
Biemond syndrome
CHARGE anomaly
Adrenohypoplasia congenita
Septo-optic dysplasia
Solitary median maxillary incisor syndrome
Börjeson-Forssman-Lehmann syndrome
Gordon Holmes syndrome
Functional gonadotropin deficiency
Chronic systemic disease and malnutrition
Sickle cell disease
Cystic fibrosis
AIDS
Chronic gastroenteric disease
Chronic renal disease
Malnutrition
Eating disorders (anorexia nervosa, bulimia, avoidant/restrictive food intake disorder, etc.)
Psychogenic amenorrhea
Exercise amenorrhea (impaired puberty and delayed menarche in female athletes)
Hypothyroidism
Diabetes mellitus
Cushing disease
Hyperprolactinemia
Marijuana use
Gaucher disease
HYPERGONADOTROPIC HYPOGONADISM
Males
The syndrome of seminiferous tubular dysgenesis and its variants (Klinefelter syndrome)
Other forms of primary testicular failure
Chemotherapy
Radiation therapy
Testicular steroid biosynthetic defects
Sertoli-only syndrome
LH receptor pathogenic variant
Anorchia and cryptorchidism
Trauma/surgery
Females
The syndrome of gonadal dysgenesis (Turner syndrome) and its variants
XX and XY gonadal dysgenesis
Familial and sporadic XX gonadal dysgenesis and its variants
Familial and sporadic XY gonadal dysgenesis and its variants
Aromatase deficiency
Other forms of primary ovarian failure
Premature menopause
Radiation therapy
Chemotherapy
Autoimmune oophoritis
Galactosemia
Glycoprotein syndrome type 1
Resistant ovary
FSH receptor pathogenic variant
LH/hCG resistance
Polycystic ovarian disease
Trauma/surgery
Noonan or pseudo-Turner syndrome
Ovarian steroid biosynthetic defects

CNS, Central nervous system; *FSH*, follicle-stimulating hormone; *GnRH*, gonadotropin-releasing hormone; *hCG*, human chorionic gonadotropin; *LH*, luteinizing hormone.

Modified from Pitteloud N, Papadakis GE, Jacobs AN. Physiology and disorders of puberty. In: Melmed S, Auchus RJ, Goldfine AB, Rosen CJ, Kopp PA, eds. Williams Textbook of Endocrinology. 15th ed. Philadelphia: Elsevier; 2025:Box 23.5.

these patients reach adulthood, they often have an upper-to-lower ratio below the lower limit of normal of 0.9 and an arm span greater than their height due to prolonged time growing.

Isolated Gonadotropin Deficiency

Disorders that can cause hypogonadism include congenital hypopituitarism, such as midline defects, tumors, infiltrative disease (hemochromatosis), and many syndromes, including Laurence-Moon-Bardet-Biedl, Prader-Willi, and Kallmann syndromes. If there is an inability to release gonadotropins but no other pituitary abnormality, the patient has isolated gonadotropin deficiency (almost universally a result of absent GnRH). Patients grow normally until the time of the pubertal growth spurt, when they fail to experience the accelerated growth characteristic of the normal growth spurt. There are more than 30 known pathogenic variants to date that are associated with hypogonadism (*GNRHR*, *FGFR1*, *FGF8*, *NSMF*,

TABLE 175.2 Differential Diagnostic Features of Delayed Puberty

CAUSATIVE CONDITION/ DISORDER	STATURE	PLASMA GONADOTROPINS	GNRH TEST: LH RESPONSE	PLASMA GONADAL STEROIDS	PLASMA DHEAS	KARYOTYPE	OLFACTION
Constitutional delay in growth and puberty	Short for chronologic age, usually appropriate for bone age	Prepubertal, later pubertal	Prepubertal, later pubertal	Prepubertal, later normal	Low for chronologic age, appropriate for bone age	Normal	Normal
HYPOGONADOTROPIC HYPOGONADISM							
Isolated gonadotropin deficiency	Normal, absent pubertal growth spurt	Low	Prepubertal or no response	Low	Appropriate for chronologic age	Normal	Normal
Kallmann syndrome	Normal, absent pubertal growth spurt	Low	Prepubertal or no response	Low	Appropriate for chronologic age	Normal	Anosmia or hyposmia
Idiopathic multiple pituitary hormone deficiencies	Short stature and poor growth since early childhood	Low	Prepubertal or no response	Low	Usually low	Normal	Normal
Hypothalamic-pituitary tumors	Decrease in growth velocity of late onset	Low	Prepubertal or no response	Low	Normal or low for chronologic age	Normal	Normal
PRIMARY GONADAL FAILURE							
Differences in gonadal dysgenesis and variants (e.g., Turner Syndrome)	Short stature since early childhood	High	Hyperresponsive for age	Low	Normal for chronologic age	XO or variant	Normal
Klinefelter syndrome and variants	Normal to tall	High	Hyperresponsive at puberty	Low or normal	Normal for chronologic age	XXY or variant	Normal
Familial XX or XY gonadal dysgenesis	Normal	High	Hyperresponsive for age	Low	Normal for chronologic age	XX or XY	Normal

DHEAS, Dehydroepiandrosterone sulfate; *GnRH*, gonadotropin-releasing hormone; *LH*, luteinizing hormone.
From Pitteloud N, Papadakis GE, Jacobs AN. Physiology and disorders of puberty. In: Melmed S, Auchus RJ, Goldfine AB, Rosen CJ, Kopp PA, eds. Williams Textbook of Endocrinology. 15th ed. Philadelphia: Elsevier; 2025:Table 23.3.

GNRH1, *KISS1*, *KISS1R*, *PROK2*, *PROKR2 TAC3* and its receptor *TACR3*, to name a few), with varying levels of ability to smell.

Kallmann syndrome combines isolated gonadotropin deficiency with disorders of olfaction. There is genetic heterogeneity; some patients have a decreased sense of smell, others have abnormal reproduction, and some have both. Most cases are sporadic, but a number of patients may have pathogenic variants in the *(ANOS1) KAL1* gene at Xp 22.31 (X chromosome). These variants cause the GnRH neurons to remain ineffectually located in the primitive nasal area, rather than migrating to the correct location at the medial basal hypothalamus. Olfactory bulbs and olfactory sulci are often absent on magnetic resonance imaging (MRI).

Abnormalities of the Central Nervous System

Central nervous system (CNS) tumors, including pituitary adenoma, glioma, prolactinoma, or craniopharyngioma, are important causes of gonadotropin deficiency. Craniopharyngiomas have a peak incidence in the teenage years and may cause any type of anterior or posterior hormone deficiency. Craniopharyngiomas usually calcify, eroding the sella turcica when they expand. They may impinge on the optic chiasm, leading to bitemporal hemianopsia and optic atrophy. Other tumors that may affect pubertal development include astrocytomas and gliomas.

Idiopathic hypopituitarism is the congenital absence of various combinations of pituitary hormones. Genes associated with this include *HESX1*, *OTX2*, *TCF7L1*, *SHH*, *GLI2*,

PROP1, POU1F1(PIT1), LHX3, LHX4, TBX19, SOX2, and *SOX3*. Although this disorder may occur in family constellations in X-linked or autosomal recessive patterns, sporadic types of congenital idiopathic hypopituitarism are more common. Congenital hypopituitarism may manifest in a male as a microphallus or hypoglycemia with seizures due to growth hormone (GH) deficiency and gonadotropin deficiency, especially if adrenocorticotropic hormone deficiency occurs as well.

Acquired Causes of Hypogonadotropic Hypogonadism

Decreased gonadotropin function occurs when voluntary dieting, malnutrition, or chronic disease results in weight loss to less than 80% of ideal weight. **Eating disorders** characterized by failure to meet appropriate nutritional needs can be associated with primary or secondary amenorrhea in females and absent or minimal pubertal development depending on the level of weight loss and the age at onset (see Chapter 69). Regaining weight to the ideal level may not immediately reverse the condition. Increased physical activity, even without weight loss, can lead to decreased menstrual frequency and gonadotropin deficiency in **athletic amenorrhea**; when physical activity is interrupted, menstrual function may return. Chronic or systemic illness (e.g., cystic fibrosis, diabetes mellitus, inflammatory bowel disease, or hematological diseases) can lead to pubertal delay or to amenorrhea from hypothalamic dysfunction. **Hypothyroidism** inhibits the onset of puberty and delays menstrual periods. Conversely, severe primary hypothyroidism may lead to precocious puberty.

Hypergonadotropic Hypogonadism

Hypergonadotropic hypogonadism is characterized by elevated gonadotropins and low sex steroid levels resulting from primary gonadal failure. This permanent condition is almost always diagnosed following the lack of entry into gonadarche and is not suspected throughout childhood. Gonadotropins do not increase to greater than normal until shortly before or around the normal time of puberty.

Ovarian failure is diagnosed by elevated gonadotropins. **Turner syndrome** is a common cause of ovarian failure and short stature. The karyotype is classically 45,XO, but other abnormalities of the X chromosome, or mosaicism, are possible. The incidence of Turner syndrome is 1 in 2,000–2,500. The features of Turner syndrome need not be evident on physical examination or by history. The diagnosis must be considered in any female who is short without a contributory history. Patients with other types of gonadal dysgenesis, or galactosemia, as well as patients who have undergone radiation therapy or chemotherapy for malignancy, may develop ovarian failure.

Klinefelter syndrome (seminiferous tubular dysgenesis) is the most common cause of **testicular failure**. The karyotype is 47,XXY, but variants with more X chromosomes are possible. The incidence is approximately 1 in 500–1,000 in males. Testosterone levels may be close to normal, at least until mid-puberty, because Leydig cell function may be spared; however, seminiferous tubular function characteristically is lost, causing infertility. Commonly, LH levels may be normal to elevated, whereas FSH levels are usually more unequivocally elevated. The age of onset of puberty is usually normal, but secondary sexual changes may not progress because of inadequate Leydig cell function.

Primary Amenorrhea

In addition to other diagnoses mentioned, other conditions need to be considered when evaluating females with lack of menses. The Mayer-Rokitansky-Kuster-Hauser syndrome of congenital absence of the uterus occurs in 1 in 4,000–5,000 female births. Anatomical obstruction by imperforate hymen or vaginal septum also presents with normal secondary sexual development without menstruation. The complete syndrome of **androgen insensitivity** includes normal feminization, absence of pubic or axillary hair, and primary amenorrhea. In this syndrome, all Müllerian structures, including ovaries, uterus, fallopian tubes, and upper third of the vagina, are lacking; the karyotype is 46,XY, and patients have intraabdominal testes.

Evaluation

When no secondary sexual development is present after the upper age limits of normal pubertal development, serum gonadotropin levels should be obtained to determine whether the patient has a hypogonadotropic or hypergonadotropic hypogonadism (see Table 175.2). Based on gonadotropin measurements only, the differentiation between constitutional delay in growth and hypogonadotropic hypogonadism is difficult; the gonadotropin levels are low in both conditions. Sometimes observation for months or years is necessary before the diagnosis is confirmed. Ultrasound of the pelvic structures in females would be helpful in the work-up of delayed puberty.

Treatment

If a permanent condition is apparent, replacement with sex steroids is indicated. Females are given titrated doses of transdermal estradiol, low-dose oral ethinyl estradiol, or conjugated estrogens until breakthrough bleeding occurs, at which time cycling is started with a dose for 25 days; on days 20–25, a progestational agent, such as medroxyprogesterone acetate (5 mg), is added to mimic the normal increases in gonadal hormones and to induce a menstrual period. Alternatively, combined estrogen and progesterone agents (oral contraceptives) may be used after breakthrough bleeding occurs. In males, testosterone enanthate or cypionate (50–100 mg monthly with a progressive increase to 100–200 mg) is given intramuscularly once every 4 weeks. This starting regimen is appropriate for patients with hypogonadotropic or hypergonadotropic hypogonadism, and doses are increased gradually to adult levels, often increasing the frequency of injections as needed. Alternatively, patients are transitioned to daily topical testosterone agents to keep levels more consistent. Oral agents are not used due to risk of hepatotoxicity. Patients with apparent constitutional delay in puberty who have, by definition, passed the upper limits of normal onset of puberty may be given a 3- to 6-month course of low-dose, sex-appropriate gonadal steroids to see whether spontaneous puberty occurs. This course of therapy might be repeated once without undue advancement of bone age.

All patients with any form of delayed puberty are at risk for decreased bone density; adequate calcium intake is essential. Patients with hypogonadotropic hypogonadism may be able to achieve fertility by the administration of gonadotropin therapy or pulsatile hypothalamic-releasing hormone therapy administered by a programmable pump on an appropriate schedule.

In patients with Turner syndrome, the goals of therapy include promoting growth with exogenous human GH supplementation and induction of the secondary sexual characteristics and of menses with low-dose cyclic estrogen/progesterone replacement therapy. Patients with Turner syndrome have had successful pregnancies after in vitro fertilization with a donor ovum and endocrine support; however, cardiac risks need to be considered and close counseling and monitoring are recommended.

PRECOCIOUS PUBERTY

Classification

Precocious puberty is classically defined as secondary sexual development occurring before the age of 9 years in males or 8 years in females (Tables 175.3 and 175.4). **Central precocious puberty**, resulting in gonadarche, emanates from premature activation of the hypothalamic-pituitary-gonadal axis (GnRH-dependent). **Peripheral precocious puberty**, gonadarche or adrenarche, does not involve the hypothalamic-pituitary-gonadal axis (GnRH-independent).

TABLE 175.3 Classification of Precocious Puberty

CENTRAL PRECOCIOUS PUBERTY (GnRH-dependent precocious puberty or premature activation of the hypothalamic GnRH pulse generator)
Idiopathic central precocious puberty
CNS tumors
Optic glioma associated with neurofibromatosis type 1
Hypothalamic astrocytoma
Other CNS disorders
Developmental abnormalities including hypothalamic hamartoma of the tuber cinereum
Encephalitis
Static encephalopathy
Brain abscess
Sarcoid or tubercular granuloma
Head trauma
Hydrocephalus
Arachnoid cyst
Myelomeningocele
Vascular lesion
Cranial irradiation
Central precocious puberty after late treatment of congenital virilizing adrenal hyperplasia or other previous chronic exposure to sex steroids
Central precocious puberty caused by pathogenic variants in the following genes: *KISS1R/GPR54, KISS1, MKRN3, DLK1*
PERIPHERAL PRECOCIOUS PUBERTY (Hypothalamic GnRH-independent)
Males
Gonadotropin-secreting tumors
hCG-secreting CNS tumors (e.g., chorioepitheliomas, germinoma, teratoma)
hCG-secreting tumors located outside the CNS (hepatoma, teratoma, choriocarcinoma)
Increased androgen secretion by adrenal or testis
Congenital adrenal hyperplasia (*CYP21* and *CYP11B1* pathogenic variants)
Virilizing adrenal neoplasm
Leydig cell adenoma
Familial male-limited precocious puberty (FMPP) ("testotoxicosis") (autosomal dominant pathogenic variant in *LHCGR* causing gonadotropin-independent precocious Leydig cell and germ cell maturation)
Cortisol resistance syndrome
Females
Ovarian cyst
Estrogen-secreting ovarian or adrenal neoplasm
Peutz-Jeghers syndrome with SCTAT
Both Sexes
McCune-Albright syndrome *(GNAS1)*
Hypothyroidism
Iatrogenic or exogenous exposures (including inadvertent exposure to estrogens in food, drugs, or cosmetics)
VARIATIONS OF PUBERTAL DEVELOPMENT
Premature thelarche
Premature isolated menarche
Premature adrenarche
Adolescent gynecomastia in males
Macroorchidism
CONTRASEXUAL PRECOCITY
Feminization in Males
Adrenal neoplasm
Chorioepithelioma
Testicular neoplasm (Peutz-Jeghers syndrome)
Increased extraglandular conversion of circulating adrenal androgens to estrogen
Iatrogenic (exposure to estrogens)
Virilization in Females
Congenital adrenal hyperplasia
CYP21 deficiency
CYP11B1 deficiency
3β-HSD deficiency
Virilizing adrenal neoplasm (with or without Cushing syndrome)
Virilizing ovarian neoplasm (e.g., arrhenoblastoma)
Iatrogenic (exposure to androgens)
Cortisol resistance syndrome
Aromatase deficiency

3β-HSD, 3β-hydroxysteroid dehydrogenase 4,5-isomerase; *CNS*, central nervous system; *CYP11B1*, 11-hydroxylase; *CYP21*, 21-hydroxylase; *GnRH*, gonadotropin-releasing hormone; *hCG*, human chorionic gonadotropin; *KISS1R/GPR54*, kisspeptin receptor/G protein–coupled receptor 54; *SCTAT*, sex cord tumor with annular tubules.

Modified from Styne DM, Grumbach MM. Physiology and disorders of puberty. In: Melmed S, Polonsky KS, Larsen PR, Kronenberg HM, eds. Williams Textbook of Endocrinology. *13th ed. Philadelphia: Elsevier; 2016:Table 25.25, p. 1163.*

Central Precocious Puberty (GnRH-Dependent Precocious Puberty)

In central precocious puberty, every endocrine and physical aspect of pubertal development is normal but too early; this includes accelerated linear growth velocity, advanced bone age consistent with somatic age, increased sex steroid and pulsatile gonadotropin secretion, and increased response of LH to GnRH. The clinical course of central precocious puberty may wax and wane. Benign precocious puberty is the presumptive diagnosis in individuals who begin puberty early on a **constitutional** or **familial** basis. If no cause can be determined, the diagnosis is idiopathic precocious puberty, which occurs much more often in females than in males. Obese females have earlier adrenarche, and sometimes menarche as well, than average-weight females. Compared with females, males with precocious puberty have a higher incidence of CNS disorders, such as tumors and hamartomas, precipitating the precocious puberty.

Almost any condition that affects the CNS, including hydrocephalus, meningitis, encephalitis, suprasellar cysts, head trauma, epilepsy, and irradiation, can precipitate central precocious puberty and must be considered before other causes of central precocious puberty are diagnosed. **Hamartomas** are nonmalignant tumors of the tuber cinereum with a characteristic appearance on computed tomography or MRI; biopsy is rarely required. The GnRH neurons within the hamartoma secrete GnRH and cause precocious puberty. Although hamartomas are not true neoplasms, they may require neurosurgical attention. The resulting precocious puberty is responsive to medical therapy with GnRH agonists, and surgery is rarely indicated.

GnRH-Independent Precocious Puberty

The most common cause of GnRH-independent precocious puberty, **McCune-Albright syndrome**, is more frequent in females than males and includes precocious gonadarche, a bone disorder with polyostotic fibrous dysplasia, and hyperpigmented cutaneous macules (café-au-lait spots). The precocious gonadarche results from ovarian hyperfunction and sometimes cyst formation, leading to episodic estrogen secretion. This disorder results from a somatic pathogenic variant in *GNAS1*, which arises postconception and impacts the G protein intracellular signaling system (specifically G_{sa}, which leads to unregulated constitutive activation of adenylate cyclase and of cyclic adenosine monophosphate (cAMP) in the absence of trophic hormone stimulation) in the affected cells in ovary, bone, and skin; other endocrine organs may also autonomously hyperfunction for the same reason. Hyperthyroidism, hyperadrenalism, or acromegaly may occur. **Adrenal carcinomas** usually secrete adrenal androgens, such as DHEA; **adrenal adenomas** may virilize a child as a result of the production of androgen or may feminize a child as a result of the production of estrogen.

Males may have precocious gonadarche on the basis of a rare entity called **familial male-limited precocious puberty** (or *testotoxicosis*). This condition, with germ cell maturation caused by an X-limited dominant pathogenic variant in the *LHCGR* gene, produces constitutive activation of the LH receptor that leads to continuous production and secretion of testosterone without requiring LH or human chorionic gonadotropin (hCG).

hCG-secreting tumors stimulate LH receptors and increase testosterone secretion. These tumors may be found in various places, including the ovary (dysgerminomas) and the liver (hepatoblastoma).

Germinomas are noncalcifying hypothalamic or pineal tumors that frequently produce hCG, which may cause sexual precocity in prepubertal males (hCG cross reacts with the LH receptor because of the similarity of structure between LH and hCG). **Optic** or **hypothalamic gliomas** (with or without neurofibromatosis), astrocytomas, and ependymomas may cause precocious puberty by disrupting the negative restraint of the areas of the CNS that normally inhibit pubertal development throughout childhood. These tumors may require radiotherapy, which contributes to a significant risk for hypopituitarism.

Ovarian cysts may occur once or may be recurrent. High serum estrogen values may mimic ovarian tumors. **Congenital adrenal hyperplasia (CAH)** is a cause of virilization in females (see Chapter 179).

Evaluation of Precocious Puberty

The first step in evaluating precocious puberty is to determine which characteristics of normal puberty are apparent (see Chapter 66) and whether estrogen effects, androgen effects, or both are present (see Table 175.4). In females, the estrogen effect manifests as breast development, uterine growth, and, eventually, menarche. Both males and females manifest the androgen effect as adult body odor, pubic and axillary hair, and facial skin oiliness and acne. In males it is also important to note whether the testes are enlarged more than 2.5 cm in length (4 mL volume), which implies gonadarche. If the testes are not enlarged but virilization is progressing, the source of the androgens may be the adrenal glands or exogenous sources.

Laboratory evaluation includes determination of adrenal androgen and sex steroid levels (testosterone/estradiol, dehydroepiandrosterone sulfate [DHEAS]) and baseline gonadotropin concentrations. The inherent nature of gonadotropin secretion is characterized by low secretory rates throughout childhood and pulsatile secretion in adolescents and adults. If baseline gonadotropin values are elevated into the normal pubertal range, central precocious puberty is likely. If baseline gonadotropins are low, however, no immediate conclusion may be drawn as to GnRH-dependent versus GnRH-independent precocious puberty. This distinction often requires the assessment of gonadotropin responsiveness to luteinizing hormone-releasing hormone (LHRH) stimulation. A prepubertal LHRH response is FSH predominant, whereas a pubertal response is more LH predominant. Thyroid hormone determination also is useful because severe primary hypothyroidism can cause peripheral precocious puberty. If there is a suggestion of a CNS anomaly or a tumor (CNS, hepatic, adrenal, ovarian, or testicular), MRI of the brain and pituitary with and without contrast is indicated. MRI of the brain is recommended in patients with the diagnosis of central precocious puberty; however, the yield is generally low in females over age 6. Males as well as young females have a higher risk of CNS lesions as a cause of precocious puberty.

Treatment

Long-acting analogs of GnRH (leuprolide acetate depot, histrelin implant, triptorelin) are the treatment of choice for central

TABLE 175.4 Differential Diagnoses of Precocious Puberty

CAUSATIVE DISORDER	SERUM GONADOTROPIN CONCENTRATION*	LH RESPONSE TO GNRH	SERUM SEX STEROID CONCENTRATIONS	GONADAL SIZE	MISCELLANEOUS
GONADOTROPIN-DEPENDENT					
Central precocious puberty	Pubertal values	Pubertal	Pubertal values of testosterone or estradiol	Normal pubertal testicular enlargement or ovarian and uterine enlargement (by sonography)	MRI scan of brain to rule out CNS tumor or other abnormality; bone scan for McCune-Albright syndrome
GONADOTROPIN-INDEPENDENT					
Males					
Chorionic gonadotropin-secreting tumor in males	High hCG (low LH)	Prepubertal (suppressed)	Pubertal values of testosterone	Slight-to-moderate uniform enlargement of testes	Hepatomegaly suggests hepatoblastoma; MRI scan of brain if chorionic gonadotropin-secreting CNS tumor suspected
Leydig cell tumor in males	Suppressed	Suppressed	Very high testosterone	Irregular, asymmetric enlargement of testes	Testicular US
Familial male-limited precocious puberty	Suppressed	Suppressed	Pubertal values of testosterone	Testes symmetric and >2.5 cm but smaller than expected for pubertal development; spermatogenesis may occur	Familial; probably sex-linked, autosomal dominant trait
Virilizing congenital adrenal hyperplasia	Prepubertal	Prepubertal LH response	Elevated 17-OHP in CYP21 deficiency or elevated 11-deoxycortisol in CYP11B1 deficiency	Testes prepubertal	Autosomal recessive, variable severity/ age of onset; may have salt wasting in CYP21 deficiency or hypertension in CYP11B1 deficiency
Virilizing adrenal tumor	Prepubertal	Prepubertal LH response	High DHEAS, DHEA, and/or androstenedione values	Testes prepubertal	CT or MRI of abdomen
Premature adrenarche	Prepubertal	Prepubertal	Prepubertal testosterone; DHEAS values appropriate for pubic hair stage 2	Testes prepubertal	Onset usually after 6 yr of age; more frequent in brain-injured children
Females					
Granulosa cell tumor (presentation may be similar to that with follicular cysts)	Suppressed	Suppressed	Very high estradiol	Ovarian enlargement on physical examination, MRI, CT, or sonography	Tumor often palpable on abdominal examination
Follicular cyst	Suppressed	Suppressed	Prepubertal to very high estradiol values	Ovarian enlargement on physical examination, MRI, CT, or sonography	Single or repetitive episodes; exclude McCune-Albright syndrome (e.g., perform skeletal survey and inspect skin)
Feminizing adrenal tumor	Suppressed	Suppressed	High estradiol and DHEAS values	Ovaries prepubertal	Unilateral adrenal mass

Continued

TABLE 175.4 Differential Diagnoses of Precocious Puberty—cont'd

CAUSATIVE DISORDER	SERUM GONADOTROPIN CONCENTRATION*	LH RESPONSE TO GNRH	SERUM SEX STEROID CONCENTRATIONS	GONADAL SIZE	MISCELLANEOUS
Nonclassical congenital adrenal hyperplasia	Prepubertal	Prepubertal LH response	Elevated 17-OHP in basal or in corticotropin-stimulated state	Ovaries prepubertal	Autosomal recessive
Premature thelarche	Prepubertal	Prepubertal	Prepubertal or early pubertal estradiol	Ovaries prepubertal	Onset usually before 3 yr of age
Premature adrenarche	Prepubertal	Prepubertal	Prepubertal estradiol; DHEAS values appropriate for pubic hair Tanner stage 2	Ovaries prepubertal	Onset usually after 6 yr of age; more frequent in brain-injured children
Both Sexes					
McCune-Albright syndrome	Suppressed	Suppressed	Sex steroid pubertal; estradiol may be quite high in females	Ovarian enlargement (asymmetrical) on US; slight (usually symmetrical) testicular enlargement	Skeletal survey/ bone scan for polyostotic fibrous dysplasia and skin examination for café-au-lait macules
Primary hypothyroidism	LH prepubertal; FSH may be slightly elevated	Prepubertal; flat FSH, LH response	Estradiol often pubertal	Testicular enlargement; ovaries macrocytic	TSH very high, prolactin mildly elevated; T_4 low

*In supersensitive assays.

17-OHP, 17-hydroxyprogesterone; *CNS*, central nervous system; *CT*, computed tomography; *CYP11B1*, 11-hydroxylase; *CYP21*, 21-hydroxylase; *DHEA*, dehydroepiandrosterone; *DHEAS*, dehydroepiandrosterone sulfate; *FSH*, follicle-stimulating hormone; *GnRH*, gonadotropin-releasing hormone; *hCG*, human chorionic gonadotropin; *LH*, luteinizing hormone; *MRI*, magnetic resonance imaging; T_4, thyroxine; *TSH*, thyrotropin; *US*, ultrasonography.

Modified from Styne DM, Grumbach MM. Physiology and disorders of puberty. In: Melmed S, Polonsky KS, Larsen PR, Kronenberg HM, eds. Williams Textbook of Endocrinology. 13th ed. Philadelphia: Elsevier; 2016:Table 25.41, p. 1196–1197.

precocious puberty. They suppress gonadotropin secretion by downregulating GnRH receptors in the pituitary gonadotropes (Table 175.5), causing gonadal secretion to revert to the prepubertal state. Males with familial male-limited precocious puberty do not respond to GnRH analogs and instead require treatment with a combination of an antiandrogen (an androgen-receptor antagonist, e.g., spironolactone, bicalutamide) and an aromatase inhibitor (e.g., anastrozole), which inhibits the conversion of testosterone to estradiol, thereby slowing further epiphyseal maturation. Patients with precocious puberty from a hormone-secreting tumor require surgical removal, if possible. The precocious puberty of McCune-Albright syndrome is GnRH-independent and unresponsive to therapy with a GnRH analog. Therapy is provided with antiandrogens or antiestrogens, such as tamoxifen or an aromatase inhibitor such as letrozole.

VARIATIONS IN PUBERTAL DEVELOPMENT

Isolated Premature Thelarche (Premature Breast Development)

Benign **premature thelarche** is the isolated appearance of unilateral or bilateral breast tissue in females, usually between ages 6 months to 3 years. The likely cause appears to be an idiopathic subtle over function of the pituitary-ovarian axis, with FSH levels in those females being sustained around the upper end of the prepubertal normal range. FSH response to GnRH is significantly increased, whereas LH is not. Estradiol levels are generally below the level of detection in most standard assays but are significantly elevated according to ultrasensitive assay. Mild estrogenization of the urogenital mucosa is sometimes found but without menarche or discharge. Linear growth acceleration is not generally seen.

Ingestion or dermal application of estrogen-containing compounds must be excluded. Laboratory investigations are not usually necessary, but a pelvic ultrasound study rarely may be indicated to exclude ovarian disease. Females with this condition should be re-evaluated at intervals of 6–12 months to ensure that apparent premature thelarche is not the beginning of progression into precocious puberty. The prognosis is excellent; if no progression occurs, no treatment other than reassurance is necessary.

Gynecomastia

In males, development of breast tissue is termed ***gynecomastia***, and it may occur to some degree in 45–75% of normal early pubertal males (see Chapter 67). Androgens normally are converted to estrogen by aromatization; in early puberty, only modest amounts of androgens are produced, and the estrogen effect can overwhelm the androgen effects at this stage. Later in pubertal development, the androgen production is so great that there is little effect from the estrogen produced by aromatization. Gynecomastia also can suggest the possibility of **Klinefelter syndrome** as puberty progresses. Prepubertal gynecomastia suggests an unusual source of estrogen either from exogenous sources (oral or dermal estrogen administration is possible from contamination of food or ointments) or

TABLE 175.5 Pharmacologic Therapy for Precocious Puberty

DISORDER	TREATMENT	ACTION AND RATIONALE
GnRH-dependent central precocious puberty	GnRH agonists/analogs	Desensitization of gonadotropes; blocks action of endogenous GnRH
GnRH-independent peripheral precocious puberty		
FEMALES		
Autonomous ovarian cysts	Medroxyprogesterone acetate	Inhibition of ovarian steroidogenesis; regression of cyst (inhibition of FSH release)
McCune-Albright syndrome	Medroxyprogesterone acetate*	Inhibition of ovarian steroidogenesis; regression of cyst (inhibition of FSH release)
	Third-generation aromatase inhibitor (e.g., letrozole)	Inhibition of P450 aromatase; decrease serum estradiol and mitigate its effects on skeletal maturation
MALES		
Familial GnRH-independent precocious puberty with premature Leydig cell maturation	Ketoconazole*	Inhibition of CYP17 (mainly 17,20-lyase activity)
	Antiandrogens (flutamide, bicalutamide) and aromatase inhibitor (letrozole or anastrozole)	Blocks effect of androgens on the androgen receptor; reduces conversion of testosterone to estrogen
	Medroxyprogesterone acetate*	Inhibition of testicular steroidogenesis

*If central precocious puberty develops, an LHRH agonist can be added.

CYP17, Cytochrome P450 17α-hydroxylase/17,20-lyase; *FSH*, follicle-stimulating hormone; *GnRH*, gonadotropin-releasing hormone; *LHRH*, luteinizing hormone-releasing hormone.

Modified from Grumbach MM, Kaplan SL. Recent advances in the diagnosis and management of sexual precocity. Acta Paediatr Jpn. 1988;30(Suppl):155.

from endogenous sources (from abnormal function of adrenal gland or ovary or from increased peripheral aromatization).

Isolated Premature Adrenarche (Pubarche)

The isolated appearance of pubic hair before age 6–7 years in females or before age 9 years in males is termed ***premature pubarche***, usually resulting from adrenarche. It is relatively common. If the pubic hair is associated with any other feature of virilization (clitoral or penile enlargement or advanced bone age) or other signs (acne, rapid growth, or voice change), a detailed investigation for a pathological cause of virilization is indicated. Measurements of serum testosterone, 17-hydroxyprogesterone, and DHEAS are indicated to investigate the possibility of CAH. Ultrasound studies may reveal a hyperplastic adrenal gland or a virilizing adrenal or ovarian tumor. Most patients with isolated pubic hair do not have progressive virilization and simply have premature adrenarche *(pubarche)* resulting from premature activation of DHEA secretion from the adrenal gland. The skeletal maturation, as assessed by bone age, may be slightly advanced and the height slightly increased, but testosterone concentrations are normal. DHEAS levels usually are high for prepubertal age but are consistent with Tanner (sexuality maturity rating) stages II and III. In females, those with premature adrenarche may have a 15–20% increased risk of development of irregular menses or polycystic ovarian syndrome later in adolescence.

PEARLS FOR PRACTITIONERS

See Endocrinology: Pearls for Practitioners at the end of this section.

REVIEW QUESTIONS

Available online.

CHAPTER 176
Thyroid Disease

THYROID PHYSIOLOGY AND DEVELOPMENT

Thyrotropin-releasing hormone, a tripeptide synthesized in the hypothalamus, stimulates the release of pituitary **thyroid-stimulating hormone (TSH)**. Pituitary TSH is a glycoprotein that stimulates the synthesis and release of thyroid hormones by the thyroid gland. Thyroid function develops in three stages. At the end of the first trimester, the gland descends from the floor of the primitive oral cavity to its definitive position in the anterior lower neck. The hypothalamic-pituitary-thyroid axis becomes functional in the second trimester. Peripheral metabolism of thyroid hormones matures in the third trimester.

Thyroxine (T_4), **triiodothyronine** (T_3), and TSH do not cross the placenta in significant amounts. Concentrations in fetal serum reflect primarily fetal secretion and metabolism. Maternal thyroid antibodies, iodides (including radioactive iodides), and medications given to mothers to treat hyperthyroidism (methimazole and propylthiouracil) cross the placenta and affect fetal thyroid function. An infant born prematurely or with intrauterine growth restriction may have an interruption of the normal maturational process and appear to have hypothyroidism by standard tests (and newborn screen).

The thyroid gland concentrates iodine and binds it to tyrosine molecules to produce either monoiodotyrosine or diiodotyrosine, with subsequent coupling of two tyrosines, T_4 or T_3. The major fraction of circulating T_3 (approximately two thirds) is derived from peripheral deiodination of T_4 to T_3 but some is produced by the gland itself. The conversion of T_4 to T_3 requires the removal of one iodine from the outer ring of tyrosine; removing an iodine from the inner ring results in reverse T_3, which has little biologic effect. Preferential conversion of T_4 to reverse T_3 rather than T_3 occurs in utero and in all forms of severe illness, including respiratory distress syndrome, fevers, anorexia, and starvation. Conversion from T_4 to T_3 increases immediately after birth and throughout life. T_4 and T_3 are noncovalently bound to a specific serum carrier protein, **thyroxine-binding globulin**, and to a lesser extent, albumin. Only small (<0.02%) fractions of T_4 and T_3 are not bound; free T_4 (as it is converted to free T_3) and free T_3 are biologically active. Free T_3 exerts metabolic effects and negative feedback on TSH release (Fig. 176.1).

Serum TSH increases just after birth but soon decreases to lower values considered normal for later life. T_4 secretion increases after birth as a result of the peak in TSH and because

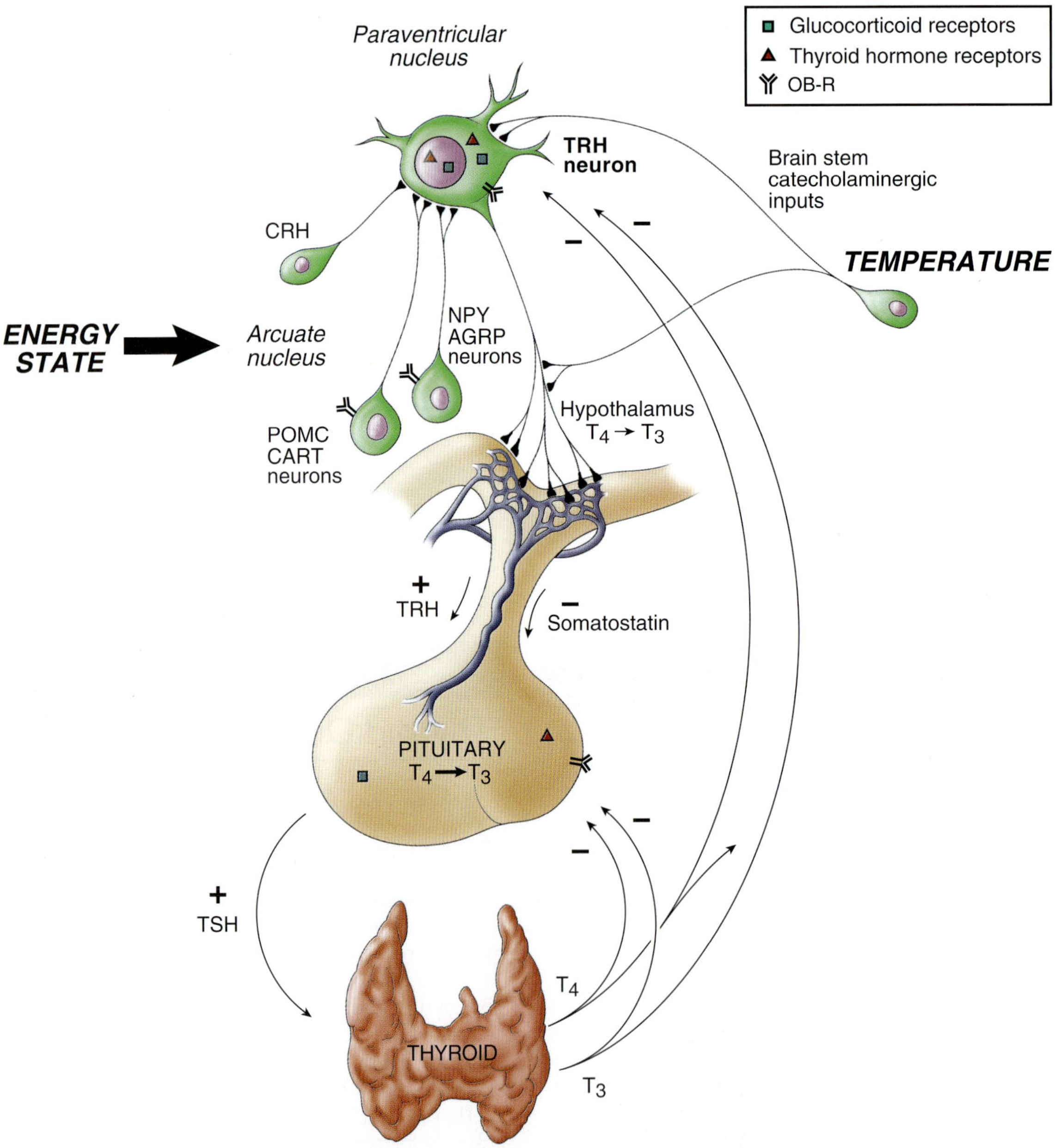

FIGURE 176.1 Interrelationships of the hypothalamic-pituitary-thyroid axis. TSH from the pituitary gland stimulates the secretion of T_4 and T_3 from the thyroid gland. These act at the pituitary gland level to control secretion of TSH by a negative feedback mechanism. In addition, T_4 is metabolized to the potent T_3 within the pituitary gland by a deiodinase. Secretion of TSH is stimulated by TRH from the hypothalamus and inhibited by somatostatin. Thyroid hormone acts at the hypothalamus to stimulate secretion of somatostatin (somatostatin acts as a negative signal to the pituitary secretion of TSH). *AGRP,* Agouti-related peptide; *CART,* cocaine- and amphetamine-regulated transcript; *CRH,* corticotropin-releasing hormone; *NPY,* neuropeptide-Y; *OB-R,* leptin receptor; *POMC,* proopiomelanocortin; T_3, triiodothyronine; T_4, thyroxine; *TRH,* thyrotropin-releasing hormone; *TSH,* thyroid-stimulating hormone. (From Melmed S, Polonsky K, Kronenberg H, et al., eds. *Williams Textbook of Endocrinology.* 10th ed. Philadelphia: Saunders; 2003:101.)

TABLE 176.1 Laboratory Test Results in Various Types of Thyroid Function Abnormalities in Children*

ABNORMALITY	SERUM TOTAL T_4	SERUM FREE T_4	SERUM TSH	SERUM TBG
Primary hypothyroidism	↓	↓	↑	N
Hypothalamic (TRH) tertiary hypothyroidism	↓	↓	↓	N
Pituitary (TSH) secondary hypothyroidism	↓	↓	↓	N
TBG deficiency	↓	N	N	↓
TBG excess	↑	N	N	↑

*TSH may be slightly elevated.
↓, Decreased; ↑, increased; *N*, normal; T_4, thyroxine; *TBG*, thyroxine-binding globulin; *TRH*, thyrotropin-releasing hormone; *TSH*, thyroid-stimulating hormone.

of maturation of thyroid metabolism. It is important to refer to age-adjusted normative data to interpret thyroid function tests properly, whether making a diagnosis of hyperthyroidism or hypothyroidism or when adjusting therapy. Free T_4 is the test of choice because it eliminates the effects of variation in protein binding, which can be substantial.

Table 176.1 summarizes laboratory test results in various types of thyroid abnormalities. In usual circumstances, plasma concentrations of TSH above the normal range indicate primary hypothyroidism, and concentrations below the normal range most often indicate the presence of hyperthyroidism. Thyroid scans with 99m-pertechnetate or 123-I-iodine are occasionally indicated in the evaluation of pediatric thyroid disease. They can be useful in identifying thyroid agenesis or ectopic thyroid tissue.

THYROID DISORDERS

Hypothyroidism

Hypothyroidism is diagnosed by a decreased serum free T_4 and may be the result of diseases of the thyroid gland (primary hypothyroidism), abnormalities of the pituitary gland (secondary), or abnormalities of the hypothalamus (tertiary). Hypothyroidism is congenital or acquired and may or may not be associated with a goiter (Table 176.2).

Congenital Hypothyroidism

Congenital hypothyroidism occurs in approximately 1 in 2,000–4,000 live births and is caused by dysgenesis (agenesis, aplasia, ectopia) or less often dyshormonogenesis (e.g., enzyme defects). Thyroid tissue usually is not palpable in these sporadic nongoitrous conditions. A goiter reflects an inborn error of metabolism in the pathway of iodide incorporation or thyroid hormone biosynthesis or reflects the transplacental passage of antithyroid drugs given to the pregnant person. Routine neonatal screening programs to measure postnatal thyroid function between 24–48 hours of life occur in every state in the United States. States differ regarding if the screening test evaluates TSH, T_4, or both. An immediate confirmatory serum sample should be obtained from any infant having a positive result on a screening test. A low free T_4 and high TSH confirm the finding of primary hypothyroidism.

Isolated secondary or tertiary hypothyroidism occurs in 1 in 100,000 live births; the free T_4 is normal to low, as is the TSH. When tertiary or secondary hypothyroidism is detected, assessment of other pituitary hormones and investigation of pituitary-hypothalamic anatomy via magnetic resonance imaging are indicated. Although not a hypothyroid condition, **congenital thyroxine-binding globulin deficiency** occurs in about 1 in 10,000 live births and is associated with low serum total T_4 concentration, normal TSH, and normal serum free T_4. This is a euthyroid condition and does not require treatment with thyroid hormone because it is merely a binding protein abnormality. It may show X-linked inheritance of a pathogenic variant in the *SERPINA7* gene family.

Clinical manifestations of congenital hypothyroidism in the immediate newborn period usually are subtle but become more evident weeks or months after birth, which is often too late to ensure that there is not a detriment to the infant's

TABLE 176.2 Causes of Hypothyroidism in Infancy and Childhood

AGE GROUP	MANIFESTATION	CAUSE
Newborn	No goiter	Thyroid gland dysgenesis or ectopic location Exposure to iodides TSH deficiency TRH deficiency
	±Goiter	Inborn defect in hormone synthesis* or effect Maternal goitrogen ingestion, including propylthiouracil, methimazole, iodides Severe iodide deficiency (endemic)
Child	No goiter	Thyroid gland dysgenesis Cystinosis Hypothalamic-pituitary insufficiency Surgical after thyrotoxicosis or other thyroid surgery
	Goiter	Hashimoto thyroiditis: chronic lymphocytic thyroiditis Inborn defect in hormone synthesis or effect Goitrogenic drugs, infiltrative (sarcoid, lymphoma)

*Impaired iodide transport, defective thyroglobulin iodination, defective iodotyrosine dehalogenase, or defective thyroglobulin or its coupling to iodotyrosine.
TRH, Thyrotropin-releasing hormone; *TSH*, thyroid-stimulating hormone.

cognitive development. Newborn screening is crucial to make an early diagnosis and initiate thyroid replacement therapy by younger than 1 month of age. Findings at various stages after birth include hypothermia, acrocyanosis, respiratory distress, large fontanelle, abdominal distention, lethargy and poor feeding, prolonged jaundice, edema, umbilical hernia, mottled skin, constipation, large tongue, dry skin, and hoarse cry. Thyroid hormones are crucial for maturation and differentiation of tissues, such as bone and brain. Most thyroid-dependent brain maturation occurs in the first 2–3 years after birth (Table 176.3).

When *treatment* (with levothyroxine) is initiated within the first month, the prognosis for normal intellectual development is excellent. State screening programs usually allow for therapy within 1–2 weeks of birth. If therapy is instituted after 6 months, when the signs of severe hypothyroidism are present, the likelihood of normal intellectual function is markedly decreased. Growth improves after thyroid replacement even in late diagnosed cases. The dose of levothyroxine changes with age; 10–15 mcg/kg/day of levothyroxine is initiated for a newborn with congenital hypothyroidism, and then titrated over time to maintain TSH and T_4 levels within the age-specific normal range. In neonatal hypothyroidism, the goal is to bring the serum free T_4 rapidly into the upper half of the range of normal. Suppression of TSH is not seen and not necessary in all cases because such suppression may lead to excessive doses of levothyroxine.

TABLE 176.3 Symptoms and Signs of Hypothyroidism
ECTODERMAL
Poor growth Dull facies: thick lips, large tongue, depressed nasal bridge, periorbital edema Dry scaly skin Sparse brittle hair Diminished sweating Carotenemia Vitiligo
CIRCULATORY
Sinus bradycardia/heart block Cold extremities Cold intolerance Pallor ECG changes: low-voltage QRS complex
NEUROMUSCULAR
Muscle weakness Hypotonia: constipation, potbelly Umbilical hernia Myxedema coma (carbon dioxide narcosis, hypothermia) Pseudohypertrophy of muscles Myalgia Physical and mental lethargy Developmental delay Delayed relaxation of reflexes Paresthesias (nerve entrapment: carpal tunnel syndrome) Cerebellar ataxia
SKELETAL
Delayed bone age Epiphyseal dysgenesis, increased upper-to-lower segment ratio
METABOLIC
Myxedema Serous effusions (pleural, pericardial, ascites) Hoarse voice (cry) Weight gain Menstrual irregularity Arthralgia Elevated CK Macrocytosis (anemia) Hypercholesterolemia Hyperprolactinemia Precocious puberty in severe cases

CK, Creatine kinase; *ECG*, electrocardiogram.

Acquired Hypothyroidism

The *etiology* of acquired hypothyroidism is presented in Table 176.2. The clinical manifestations may be subtle. Hypothyroidism should be suspected in any child who has a decline in growth velocity, especially if **not** associated with weight loss (see Table 176.3). The most common cause of acquired hypothyroidism in older children in the United States is **lymphocytic autoimmune thyroiditis** (also known as ***Hashimoto thyroiditis***). In many areas of the world, iodine deficiency is the etiology of endemic goiter. The failure of the thyroid gland may be heralded by an increase of TSH before T_4 levels decrease. In contrast to untreated congenital hypothyroidism, acquired hypothyroidism is not a cause of permanent developmental delay.

Hashimoto Thyroiditis

Hashimoto thyroiditis is a common cause of goiter and acquired thyroid disease in older children and adolescents. A family history of thyroid disease is present in 25–35% of patients. The *etiology* is an autoimmune process targeted against the thyroid gland with lymphocytic infiltration and lymphoid follicle and germinal center formation preceding fibrosis and atrophy.

Clinical manifestations include a firm, nontender euthyroid, hypothyroid, or, rarely, hyperthyroid (Hashitoxicosis) diffuse goiter with a pebblelike surface. See Table 176.3 for signs and symptoms, which can be diverse. Onset typically occurs after 6 years of age with a peak incidence in adolescence with a female predominance. Associated autoimmune diseases include celiac disease, type 1 diabetes mellitus, adrenal insufficiency, and hypoparathyroidism. **Autoimmune polyglandular syndrome type I** consists of hypoparathyroidism, Addison disease, mucocutaneous candidiasis, and hypothyroidism. **Autoimmune polyglandular syndrome type II** consists of Addison disease, type 1 diabetes mellitus, and, frequently, hypothyroidism. Trisomy 21 and Turner syndrome are predisposed to the development of autoimmune thyroiditis.

The *diagnosis* may be confirmed by serum antithyroid peroxidase and antithyroglobulin antibodies. Neither biopsy nor thyroid scan is indicated in Hashimoto thyroiditis, although a thyroid scan with reduced uptake may differentiate Hashitoxicosis from Graves disease.

Treatment with thyroid hormone sufficient to normalize TSH and free T_4 is indicated for hypothyroidism in Hashimoto thyroiditis. Patients without manifestation of hypothyroidism require thyroid function testing (serum TSH and free T_4) every 6–12 months to detect the later development of hypothyroidism. Goiter with a normal TSH usually is not an indication for treatment.

Hyperthyroidism

Graves Disease

Most children with hyperthyroidism have Graves disease, the autonomous functioning of the thyroid caused by autoantibodies (thyroid-stimulating immunoglobulins [TSIs]) stimulating the thyroid. The resulting excessive synthesis, release, and peripheral metabolism of thyroid hormones produce the clinical features. Hashimoto thyroiditis and thyrotoxicosis are on a continuum of autoimmune diseases; there is overlap in their immunologic findings.

Antithyroid peroxidase and antithyroglobulin antibodies may be present in thyrotoxicosis, although the values are usually lower than in Hashimoto thyroiditis. Exceptionally high titers of antibodies may indicate the thyrotoxic phase of Hashimoto thyroiditis with the subsequent evolution toward permanent hypothyroidism. In Graves disease, serum free T_4, free T_3, or both levels are elevated, whereas TSH is suppressed. Rare causes of hyperthyroidism include McCune-Albright syndrome, thyroid nodule (often an adenoma), TSH hypersecretion, subacute thyroiditis, and iodine or thyroid hormone ingestion.

Clinical Manifestations

Graves disease presents as hyperthyroidism (Table 176.4) and is about five times more common in females than in males with a peak incidence in adolescence. Personality changes, mood instability, and poor school performance are common initial problems. Tremor, anxiety, inability to concentrate, and weight loss may be insidious and confused with a psychologic disorder until thyroid function tests reveal the elevated serum free T_4 level. In rare cases, serum free T_4 may be near normal, whereas serum T_3 is selectively elevated (T_3 toxicosis). A firm homogeneous goiter is usually present. Many patients complain of neck fullness. Thyroid gland enlargement is best visualized with the neck only slightly extended and with the examiner lateral to the patient. Palpation of the thyroid gland is best performed with the examiner's hands around the neck from the back. The patient swallows so that the examiner can feel and examine the size, consistency, nodularity, and motion of the gland. The examiner should watch the patient swallow to note any discernible enlargement or asymmetry of the thyroid lobes. Auscultation may reveal a bruit over the gland that needs to be differentiated from a carotid bruit.

TABLE 176.4 Clinical Manifestations of Hyperthyroidism

ASSOCIATED CHANGE	SIGN/SYMPTOM
Increased catecholamine effects	Nervousness Palpitations Tachycardia Atrial arrhythmias Systolic hypertension Tremor Brisk reflexes
Hypermetabolism	Increased sweating Shiny, smooth skin Heat intolerance Fatigue Weight loss—increased appetite Increased bowel movement (loose stools) Hyperkinesis
Myopathy	Weakness Periodic paralysis Cardiac failure—dyspnea
Miscellaneous	Proptosis, stare, exophthalmos, lid lag, ophthalmopathy Hair loss Inability to concentrate Personality change (emotional lability) Goiter Thyroid bruit Onycholysis Painful gland* Acute thyroid storm (hyperthermia, tachycardia, altered mental status, high-output heart failure, shock)

**Unusual except in subacute thyroiditis with hyperthyroid phase.*

Treatment

Three treatment choices are available: pharmacologic, radioactive iodine, and surgical.

Medications

Medical therapy to block thyroid hormone synthesis consists of methimazole (0.2–0.5 mg/kg/day with maximum daily dose 30 mg/day) or propylthiouracil (5–7 mg/kg/day divided every 8 hours). Both medications are equally effective; however, propylthiouracil is no longer a first-line therapy secondary to concerns of severe liver injury and acute liver failure. A β blocker, such as propranolol or atenolol, is started if symptoms are severe to control cardiac manifestations and is tapered as the methimazole takes effect. Antithyroid medication is usually continued for 1–2 years because the clinical remission rate is approximately 25% per year (antibodies persist regardless of clinical remission). In patients complying with the treatment regimen, the 2-year course of treatment can be repeated. Medication should suppress thyroid function to normal without the need to add thyroid hormone replacement to normalize serum free T_4. Complications of methimazole are muscle pain, rash, granulocytopenia, and jaundice. The granulocytopenia is an idiosyncratic complication of rapid onset, which is observed only in the early months after institution of antithyroid medication and requires monitoring if febrile illness or pharyngitis develops. If a suppressed white blood cell count is observed, antithyroid therapy must be discontinued. This potentially lethal, rare complication affects 3 in 10,000 users a year. After resolution, the other of the two antithyroid medications can be started because there is usually less than a 50% chance of a similar reaction from the other medication. Iodine administration, which may suppress thyroid function but becomes ineffective in a few weeks, is sometimes used as a preparation for surgery but never for long-term therapy.

Radioiodine

Radioiodine (^{131}I) is slower in exerting therapeutic effects, may require repeated dosing, and is likely to cause permanent hypothyroidism. Hypothyroidism is the desired outcome because it is easier and safer to treat than continued hyperthyroidism. Although studies reveal no long-term consequences, concern remains about possible sequelae in children. Radioiodine given to a pregnant person renders the fetus hypothyroid and is contraindicated.

Surgery

Surgical treatment consists of partial or complete thyroidectomy. Risks associated with thyroidectomy include the use of anesthesia and the possibility that the thyroid removal will be excessive, causing hypothyroidism, or that it will be inadequate, resulting in persistent hyperthyroidism. In addition, keloid formation, recurrent laryngeal nerve palsy, and hypoparathyroidism (transient postoperative or permanent) may occur. Thyroid storm caused by the release of large amounts of preformed hormone is a serious but rare complication. Even with optimal immediate postoperative results, patients may become hypothyroid within 10 years.

Thyroid Storm

Thyroid storm (see Table 176.4) is a rare medical emergency consisting of tachycardia, disorientation, elevated blood pressure, and hyperthermia. Treatment includes reducing the hyperthermia with a cooling blanket and administering a β blocker to control the tachycardia, hypertension, and autonomic hyperfunction symptoms. Iodine may be given to block thyroid hormone release after an antithyroid medication is started. Hydrocortisone may be indicated for relative adrenal insufficiency, and therapy for heart failure includes diuretics and digoxin.

Congenital Hyperthyroidism

This disorder results from transplacental passage of maternal TSIs and may be masked for several days until the short-lived effects of transplacental maternal antithyroid medication wear off (assuming the birth parent was receiving such medication), at which time the effects of TSIs are observed. Irritability, tachycardia (often with signs of cardiac failure simulating cardiomyopathy), polycythemia, craniosynostosis, bone age advancement, poor feeding, and growth faltering are the clinical hallmarks. This condition may be anticipated if the pregnant person is known to be thyrotoxic or has an elevated TSI during the third trimester of pregnancy. Cure of hyperthyroidism before pregnancy (surgery or radioiodine treatment) limits or curtails T_4 production but not the underlying immune disturbance producing TSIs; thus, the infant still may be affected, at least transiently.

Treatment for a severely affected neonate includes methimazole and, as needed, a β blocker to help decrease symptoms. Because the half-life of the immunoglobulin is several weeks, spontaneous resolution of neonatal thyrotoxicosis resulting from transplacental passage of TSIs usually occurs by 2–3 months of age. Observation without treatment is indicated in patients who are minimally affected (see Chapter 58).

NODULES/TUMORS OF THE THYROID

About 2% of children develop solitary thyroid nodules, most of which are benign. Evaluation of a nodule includes thyroid function tests, neck ultrasound, and, if needed, fine-needle aspiration (FNA). Ultrasound guidance may be needed for aspiration of small nodules or those not palpable. Nodules found to be benign on FNA may be monitored through clinical exam and ultrasound.

Carcinoma of the thyroid is rare in children (1% of all pediatric cancers in the 5- to 9-year-old age group and up to 7% of cancers in the 15- to 19-year-old age group). Papillary and follicular carcinomas represent 90% of childhood thyroid cancers. A history of therapeutic head or neck irradiation or radiation exposure from nuclear accidents predisposes a child to thyroid cancer. Carcinoma usually presents as a firm-to-hard, painless, nonfunctional solitary nodule and may spread to adjacent lymph nodes. Rapid growth, hoarseness (recurrent laryngeal nerve involvement), and lung metastasis may be present. If the nodule is solid on ultrasound, is *cold* on radioiodine scanning, and feels hard, the likelihood of a carcinoma is high. Excisional biopsy usually is performed, but FNA biopsy also may be diagnostic.

Treatment includes total thyroidectomy, selective regional node dissection, and radioablation with ^{131}I for residual or recurrent disease. Current recommendations have evolved for use of ^{131}I as research has shown noninvasive follicular thyroid neoplasms with papillary-like features have a low recurrence risk without radioablation. The *prognosis* is usually excellent if the disease is diagnosed early.

Medullary carcinoma of the thyroid may be asymptomatic except for a mass. Diagnosis is based on the presence of elevated calcitonin levels, either in the basal state or after pentagastrin stimulation (difficult to obtain) and histologic examination. This tumor most often occurs with multiple endocrine neoplasia 2a or 2b, possibly in a familial pattern. In some families, the presence of pathogenic variants of the *RET* protooncogene is predictive of the development of medullary carcinoma of the thyroid. The location of the pathogenic variant can help determine when removal of the thyroid is warranted. Genetic screening of other members of the family is indicated after a proband is recognized. Prophylactic thyroidectomy is indicated for the family members with the same pathogenic variant.

PEARLS FOR PRACTITIONERS

See Endocrinology: Pearls for Practitioners at the end of this section.

REVIEW QUESTIONS

Available online

CHAPTER 177

Disorders of Parathyroid Bone and Mineral Endocrinology

PARATHYROID HORMONE AND VITAMIN D

Calcium and phosphate are regulated mainly by diet and three hormones: parathyroid hormone (PTH), vitamin D, and calcitonin. PTH is secreted in response to a decrease in serum ionized calcium level. PTH attaches to its membrane receptor then acts via adenylate cyclase to mobilize calcium from bone into the serum and to enhance fractional reabsorption of calcium by the kidney while inducing phosphate excretion; all increase the serum calcium concentration and decrease serum phosphate. Lack of PTH effect is heralded by low serum calcium in the presence of elevated phosphate for age. PTH stimulates vitamin D secretion by increasing renal 1α-hydroxylase activity and acts indirectly to elevate serum calcium concentration by stimulating the production of 1,25-dihydroxyvitamin D from 25-hydroxyvitamin D. Calcitonin increases the deposition of calcium into bone; in normal states the effect is subtle, but calcitonin may be used temporarily to suppress extremely elevated serum calcium values.

1,25-Dihydroxyvitamin D enhances calcium absorption from the gastrointestinal tract, increasing serum calcium levels and bone mineralization. Vitamin D is derived from exposure of the skin to ultraviolet rays (usually via the sun) or from oral ingestion. It is modified first to 25-hydroxyvitamin D in the liver and then 1α-hydroxylated to the metabolically active form (1,25-dihydroxyvitamin D) in the kidney. The serum concentration of 25-hydroxyvitamin D is a better reflection of vitamin D sufficiency than the measurement of 1,25-hydroxyvitamin D (see Chapter 29).

HYPOCALCEMIA

The clinical manifestations of hypocalcemia result from increased neuromuscular irritability and include muscle cramps, carpopedal spasm (tetany), weakness, paresthesia, laryngospasm, and seizure-like activity. Tetany can be detected by the **Chvostek sign** (facial spasms produced by lightly tapping over the facial nerve just in front of the ear) or by the **Trousseau sign** (carpal spasms exhibited when arterial blood flow to the hand is occluded for 3–5 minutes with a blood pressure cuff inflated to 15 mm Hg above systolic blood pressure). Total serum calcium concentration is usually measured, although a determination of serum ionized calcium, the biologically active form, is preferable. Albumin is the major reservoir of protein-bound calcium. Disorders that alter plasma pH or serum albumin concentration must be considered when circulating calcium concentrations are being evaluated. The fraction of ionized calcium is inversely related to plasma pH; **alkalosis** can precipitate hypocalcemia by lowering ionized calcium without changing total serum calcium. Alkalosis may result from hyperpnea caused by anxiety or from hyperventilation related to physical exertion. Hypoproteinemia may lead to a false suggestion of hypocalcemia because the total serum calcium level is low even though the ionized Ca^{2+} remains normal. It is best to measure serum ionized calcium if hypocalcemia or hypercalcemia is suspected.

Primary hypoparathyroidism causes hypocalcemia but does not cause rickets. The etiology of primary hypoparathyroidism includes the following:

- Congenital malformation (e.g., 22q11 syndrome or other complex syndromes) resulting from developmental abnormalities of the third and fourth branchial arches
- Surgical procedures, such as thyroidectomy or parathyroidectomy, in which parathyroid tissue is removed either deliberately or as a complication of surgery for another goal
- Autoimmunity, which may destroy the parathyroid gland

Pseudohypoparathyroidism (hypocalcemia and hyperphosphatemia) may occur in one of four forms as follows:

- *Type Ia:* an abnormality of the G_{sa} protein linking the PTH receptor to adenylate cyclase; biologically active PTH is secreted in great quantities, but it does not stimulate its receptor
- *Type Ib:* normal phenotype, normal G_{sa} with abnormalities in the production of adenylate cyclase
- *Type Ic:* abnormal phenotype, normal production of adenylate cyclase, but a distal defect eliminates the effects of PTH
- *Type II:* normal phenotype, normal production of adenylate cyclase, with a postreceptor defect, close to type Ib

Pseudohypoparathyroidism is an autosomal dominant condition that may present at birth or later. Pseudohypoparathyroidism is associated with **Albright hereditary osteodystrophy** *(GNAS1)*, with clinical manifestations that include short stature, stocky body habitus, round facies, short fourth and fifth metacarpals, calcification of the basal ganglia, subcutaneous calcification, and developmental delay. Albright hereditary osteodystrophy may be inherited separately so that a patient may have a normal appearance with hypocalcemia or may have the Albright hereditary osteodystrophy phenotype with normal serum calcium, phosphate, PTH, and response to PTH.

Transient neonatal hypocalcemia may occur during the first 3 days after birth when serum calcium concentrations normally decline in response to withdrawal of the maternal calcium supply via the placenta. Sluggish PTH response in a neonate may result in a transient hypocalcemia. Clinically, this most often presents as jittery movements. Neonatal hypocalcemia caused by decreased PTH release is found in infants of mothers with diabetes, hypoparathyroid dysfunction, or after perinatal asphyxia. Normal serum magnesium concentrations are required for normal parathyroid gland function and action. **Hypomagnesemia** may cause a secondary hypoparathyroidism, which responds poorly to therapies other than magnesium replacement. This is the suspected mechanism of neonatal hypocalcemia (and transient, functional hypoparathyroidism) in infants of diabetic mothers.

The *etiology* of hypocalcemia usually can be discerned by combining features of the clinical presentation with determinations of serum ionized calcium, phosphate, alkaline phosphatase, PTH (preferably at a time when the calcium is low), magnesium, and albumin. If the PTH concentration is not appropriately elevated in relation to the low serum calcium, hypoparathyroidism (transient, primary, or caused by hypomagnesemia) is present. Vitamin D stores can be estimated by measuring serum 25-hydroxyvitamin D. Kidney function is assessed by a serum creatinine measurement or determination of creatinine clearance (Table 177.1).

Treatment of severe tetany or seizures resulting from hypocalcemia consists of intravenous calcium gluconate (0.29–0.6 mL/kg of a 10% solution) given slowly over 10 minutes while cardiac status is monitored by electrocardiogram for bradycardia, which can be fatal. Long-term treatment of hypoparathyroidism involves administering vitamin D, preferably as 1,25-dihydroxyvitamin D and calcium. Therapy is adjusted to keep the serum calcium in the lower half of the normal range to avoid episodes of hypercalcemia that might produce nephrocalcinosis and to avoid pancreatitis.

RICKETS

Rickets is defined as decreased or defective bone mineralization in growing children; **osteomalacia** is the same condition

TABLE 177.1 Important Physiologic Changes in Bone and Mineral Diseases

CONDITION	CALCIUM	PHOSPHATE	PARATHYROID HORMONE	25(OH)D
Primary hypoparathyroidism	↓	↑	↓	Nl
Pseudohypoparathyroidism	↓	↑	↑	Nl
Vitamin D deficiency	Nl(↓)	↓	↑	↓
Familial hypophosphatemic rickets	Nl	↓	Nl (sl↑)	Nl
Hyperparathyroidism	↑	↓	↑	Nl
Immobilization	↑	↑	↓	Nl

↓, Low; *↑*, high; *25(OH)D*, 25-hydroxyvitamin D; *Nl*, normal; *sl*, slight.

in adults. The proportion of osteoid (the organic portion of bone) is excessive. As a result, the bone becomes soft and the metaphyses of the long bones widen. In older infants, poor linear growth, bowing of the legs on weight bearing (which can be painful), thickening at the wrists and knees, and prominence of the costochondral junctions (rachitic rosary) of the rib cage occur. At this stage, x-ray findings are diagnostic.

In **nutritional vitamin D deficiency**, calcium is not absorbed adequately from the intestine (see Chapter 29). Low vitamin D intake in infants (especially in exclusively breast-fed infants) may contribute to the development of rickets. Fat malabsorption resulting from hepatobiliary disease (biliary atresia, neonatal hepatitis) or other causes (cystic fibrosis) also may produce vitamin D deficiency because vitamin D is a fat-soluble vitamin. Defects in vitamin D metabolism by the kidney (kidney failure, autosomal recessive deficiency of 1α-hydroxylation, **vitamin D–dependent rickets**) or liver (defect in 25-hydroxylation) also can cause rickets.

In **familial hypophosphatemic rickets**, the major defect is failure of the kidney to adequately reabsorb filtered phosphate so that serum phosphate decreases, and urinary phosphate is high. The *diagnosis* of this disease usually is made within the first few years of life and is typically more severe in males. Multiple pathogenic variants and modes of inheritance have been identified.

The *etiology* of rickets usually can be determined by an assessment of the mineral and vitamin D status (25-hydroxyvitamin D < 8 ng/mL suggests nutritional vitamin D deficiency is the etiology of the child's rickets) (see Table 177.1). Further testing of mineral balance or measurement of other vitamin D metabolites may be required.

Several forms of vitamin D can be used for *treatment* of the different rachitic conditions, but their potencies vary widely. Required dosages depend on the condition being treated (see Chapter 29). Rickets may also be treated with 1,25-hydroxyvitamin D and supplemental calcium. In hypophosphatemic rickets, phosphate supplementation (not calcium) must accompany vitamin D therapy, which is given to suppress secondary hyperparathyroidism. Adequate therapy restores normal skeletal growth and produces resolution of the radiographic signs of rickets. Nutritional rickets is treated with vitamin D given as a single large weekly dose or multiple smaller replacement doses. Surgery may be required to straighten legs in untreated patients with long-standing disease.

PEARLS FOR PRACTITIONERS

See Endocrinology: Pearls for Practitioners at the end of this section.

REVIEW QUESTIONS

Available online

CHAPTER 178

Disorders of Sexual Differentiation

TYPICAL SEXUAL DEVELOPMENT

The various actions and interactions of specific genes, epigenetic influences, transcription factors, and hormones are involved in **sexual development**. Studies from genetics, endocrinology, and neurology support the concept that there are biological foundations to gender identity development. **Gender identity** involves a complex interplay of biological, environmental, and cultural factors.

Disturbances in these processes of gene regulation and gene expression determining fetal gonadal development result in **differences of sex development** (DSD). Approximately 1 in 4,000 infants are estimated to be born with a DSD.

The internal and external genitalia are formed between 6–13 weeks of gestation. Fetal gonad and external genitalia are bipotential and have the capacity to support development of a male or female phenotype (Fig. 178.1). In the presence of a gene called *SRY*, the sex-determining region on the Y chromosome, the primitive fetal gonad differentiates into a testis. The Leydig cells of the testis secrete testosterone, which has direct effects (stimulating development of the Wolffian ducts) but also is locally converted to dihydrotestosterone (DHT) by the 5α-reductase enzyme. DHT causes enlargement, rugation, and fusion of the labioscrotal folds into a scrotum; fusion of the ventral surface of the penis to enclose a penile urethra; and enlargement of the phallus with ultimate development of male external genitalia. Testicular production and secretion of Müllerian-inhibitory substance by Sertoli cells cause the regression and disappearance of the Müllerian ducts and their

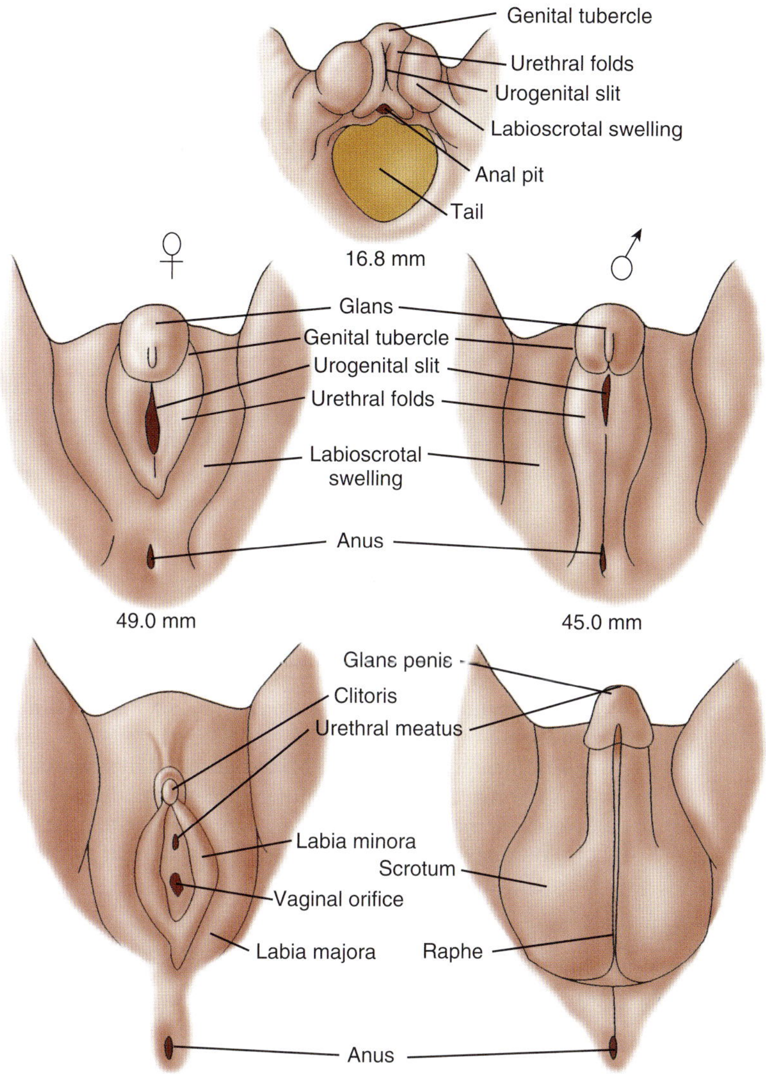

FIGURE 178.1 Differentiation of male and female external genitalia as proceeding from a common embryonic anlage. Testosterone acts at 9–13 weeks of gestation to virilize the bipotential anlage. In the absence of testosterone action, the female phenotype develops. (From Grumbach MM, Conte FA. Disorders of sexual differentiation. In: Wilson JD, Foster DW, eds. *Textbook of Endocrinology*. 8th ed. Philadelphia: WB Saunders; 1990:873; modified from Spaulding MH. The development of the external genitalia in the human embryo. *Contrib Embryol Instit.* 1921;13:69–88.)

derivatives, such as the fallopian tubes and uterus. In the presence of testosterone, the Wolffian ducts develop into the vas deferens, seminiferous tubules, and prostate.

The female phenotype develops unless specific male influences alter development, although *WNT4* and R spondin 1 *(RSPO1)* are also required for development of the ovary. In the absence of fetal testicular secretion of Müllerian-inhibitory substance, a normal uterus, fallopian tubes, and posterior third of the vagina develop out of the Müllerian ducts, and the Wolffian ducts degenerate.

Classification

DSDs are categorized under three main subgroups according to karyotype (XX, XY, and sex chromosome for mosaic karyotypes).

ATYPICAL SEXUAL DEVELOPMENT

46,XX Differences of Sexual Development

Masculinization of the external genitalia of genotypic females (except for isolated enlargement of the clitoris, which can occur from later androgen exposure) is always caused by the presence of excessive androgens during the critical period of development (8–13 weeks of gestation) (Table 178.1). The degree of virilization can range from mild clitoral enlargement to the appearance of a male phallus with a penile urethra and fused scrotum with raphe. Congenital virilizing adrenal hyperplasia is the most common cause of 46,XX DSDs; it is most commonly the result of an enzyme deficiency that impairs synthesis of glucocorticoids, but does not affect androgen production. The impaired cortisol secretion leads to adrenocorticotropic hormone (ACTH) hypersecretion, which stimulates hyperplasia of the adrenal cortex and excessive adrenal production of androgens (see Chapter 179).

46,XY Differences of Sexual Development

Underdevelopment of the male external genitalia occurs because of a relative deficiency of testosterone production or action (see Table 178.1). **Microphallus** is defined as a stretched penile length of less than 2–2.5 standard deviations (SD) below the mean for age. In a full-term newborn male, a stretched penile length of 2–2.5 cm (2.5 SDs below the mean)

TABLE 178.1 Associations of Genital Anomalies

ATYPICAL CHARACTERISTICS	EXAMPLES OF ASSOCIATED DISORDERS
MALE-APPEARING GENITALIA	
Micropenis	Growth hormone or luteinizing hormone deficiency Testosterone deficiency (in 2nd and 3rd trimesters) Partial androgen insensitivity Syndrome (variants in *AR* gene)
Hypospadias (more severe)	Disorders of gonadal development Ovotesticular DSD 46,XX or 46,XY DSD Idiopathic
Impalpable gonads	Anorchia Persistent Müllerian duct syndrome 46,XX DSD with 21- or 11β-hydroxylase deficiency Cryptorchidism
Small gonads	47,XXY, 46,XX DSD Dysgenetic or rudimentary testes
Inguinal mass (uterus or tube)	Persistent Müllerian duct syndrome, dysgenetic testes
FEMALE-APPEARING GENITALIA	
Clitoromegaly	XX with 21- or 11β-hydroxylase or 3β-hydroxy dehydrogenase deficiency Other 46,XX DSD Gonadal dysgenesis, dysgenetic testes, ovotesticular DSD 46,XY DSD Tumor infiltration of clitoris
Posterior labial fusion	As for clitoromegaly
Palpable gonad(s)	Gonadal dysgenesis, dysgenetic testes, ovotesticular DSD 46,XY DSD
Inguinal hernia or mass	As for palpable gonad(s)

AR, Androgen receptor; *DSD*, disorders of sex development.
Modified from Al Remeithi S, Wherrett DK. Disorders of sex development. In: Martin RJ, Fanaroff AA, Walsh MC, eds. Fanaroff & Martin's Neonatal-Perinatal Medicine. *10th ed. Philadelphia: Elsevier; 2015:Table 98.3.*

warrants evaluation. Various degrees of hypospadias (penile or perineal) and associated chordee or ventral binding of the phallus may be present, in addition to unilateral, but more often bilateral, cryptorchidism. Careful inspection for testes in the inguinal canal or labioscrotal folds by palpation or ultrasound is necessary. Rarely, a palpable gonad in the inguinal canal or labioscrotal fold represents a herniated ovary or an ovotestis (ovarian and testicular tissue). Production of testosterone by a gonad implies that testicular tissue is present and that at least some cells carry the *SRY* gene.

Testosterone production can be reduced by specific deficiencies of the enzymes needed for androgen biosynthesis or by dysplasia of the gonads. In the latter, if Müllerian-inhibiting substance production is also reduced, a rudimentary uterus and fallopian tubes are present.

The complete form of **androgen resistance** or **androgen insensitivity syndrome** is the most dramatic example of resistance to hormone action by defects in the androgen receptor. Affected patients have a **46,XY** karyotype, normally formed testes (usually located in the inguinal canal or labia majora), and female external genitalia with a short vagina and no internal Müllerian structures. At the time of puberty, testosterone concentrations increase to normal or above normal male range. Because a portion of the testosterone is normally converted to estradiol in peripheral tissues and the estrogen cannot be opposed by the androgen, breast development ensues at the normal age of puberty without growth of pubic, facial, or axillary hair or the occurrence of menstruation. This condition may demonstrate X-linked recessive inheritance of pathogenic variants of the *XR* gene, but nearly a third of cases are de novo variants.

5α-Reductase deficiency is caused by autosomal recessive inheritance of a pathogenic variant in the *SRD5A2* gene, and it presents at birth with predominantly female phenotype or with ambiguous genitalia, including perineoscrotal hypospadias. The defect is in 5α reduction of testosterone to its metabolite DHT. At puberty, spontaneous secondary male sexual development occurs.

Sex Chromosome and Ovotesticular Differences of Sexual Development

Turner syndrome (most commonly 45,X) and **Klinefelter syndrome** (47,XXY) and their mosaic variants are classified as sex chromosome DSDs. **Mixed gonadal dysgenesis** (45,X; 46,XY) often may present with genital ambiguity, asymmetric external genitalia, and inguinal hernias. There may be virilization on one side and none on the other. Similar findings may be seen with **ovotesticular DSD**.

APPROACH TO THE INFANT WITH GENITAL AMBIGUITY

Ambiguous genitalia in a newborn must be attended to with as little delay as possible and with informed sensitivity to the psychosocial context. The laboratory evaluation required for diagnosis might take days or weeks to complete, delaying the assignment of a sex. Parental choice of name and sex may precede a diagnosis. Beyond infancy and childhood, factors to consider in aiding families on deciding on the sex or rearing include: the most probable adult gender identity, based on the clinical outcomes for the specific DSD type (when available); potential for adult psychosocial and psychosexual function, including fertility potential; degree of virilization as a marker of prenatal androgen exposure; and the family's preferences and expectations, which may be influenced by their sociocultural background. With that, most centers caring for patients with ambiguous genitalia include a behavioral health specialist with a focus on patients and families encountering these issues.

On physical examination, it is essential to note where the urethral opening lies and whether there is fusion of the anterior portion of the labioscrotal folds. Endogenous excessive production of androgen (as in congenital adrenal hyperplasia [CAH]) in a female fetus between weeks 9–13 of gestation leads to ambiguous genitalia. If the vaginal opening is normal and there is no fusion, but the clitoris is enlarged without ventral fusion of the ventral urethra, the patient likely had later exposure to androgens. In a patient with a fully formed scrotum and a normally formed but small penis, the patient likely had normal exposure to and action of androgen during weeks 9–13 of gestation.

The major goal is a rapid identification of any life-threatening disorders (salt loss and shock caused by the salt-losing form of CAH). Although the classic approach to sex assignment has been based on the feasibility of genital reconstruction and potential fertility rather than on karyotype or gonadal histology, the effects of prenatal androgen must be considered. Experts recommend waiting until the child is able to be part of the dialogue regarding gender identity and reconstruction when appropriate. Present management of ambiguous genitalia involves extensive open discussion with parents involving the biology of the infant and the likely prognosis. Treatment should be individualized and managed by a team, including an experienced pediatric endocrinologist, urologist or gynecologist, psychologist, geneticist, and the primary care physician.

Diagnosis

The first step toward diagnosis is to determine whether the findings represent virilization of a genetic female (androgen excess) or underdevelopment of a genetic male (androgen deficiency; see Fig. 178.1). Inguinal gonads that are evident on palpation may be testes and indicate that incomplete development of a male phenotype has occurred; however, ovaries and ovotestes may feel similar. Absence of female internal genitalia (detected by ultrasound) implies that Müllerian-inhibiting substance was present and secreted by fetal testes. Karyotype determination is only one of many factors needed to assist the family in the decision of sex of rearing; the *SRY* gene may be found on chromosomes other than the Y chromosome, and, conversely, a Y chromosome may lack an *SRY* gene (it may have been translocated to an X chromosome, leading to the development of a 46,XX male-XX sex reversal, testicular DSD).

Statistically, most virilized females have CAH; 90% of these females have 21-hydroxylase deficiency. The diagnosis is established by measuring the plasma concentration of 17-hydroxyprogesterone and androstenedione (see Chapter 179), which typically is hundreds of times above the normal range. Other enzymatic defects also may be diagnosed by quantifying circulating levels of the adrenal steroid precursor proximal to the defective enzyme block.

Establishing an accurate diagnosis is more difficult in underdeveloped males. When certain types of adrenal hyperplasia coexist with defects in testicular androgen production, excessive ACTH secretion elevates levels of specific adrenal steroid precursors, allowing a diagnosis. If the defect is restricted to testosterone biosynthesis, the measurement of testosterone and its precursors in the basal state and after stimulation by human chorionic gonadotropin may be required. Patients with normal levels of testosterone either have persistent androgen resistance or have had an interruption of normal morphogenesis of the genitalia. Abnormalities of the sex chromosomes may be associated with incomplete or dysfunctional formation of the gonads, which may be associated with persistence of Müllerian structures.

Treatment

Treatment consists of replacing deficient hormones (cortisol in adrenal hyperplasia or testosterone in a child with androgen biosynthetic defects who will be raised as male), surgical restoration to make the individual look more appropriate for the gender of rearing (with thoughtful discussion), and psychological support of the whole family. Gonads and internal organs discordant for the gender of rearing may be removed; however, delaying permanent surgeries has been the recent mainstay of management. Intraabdominal dysgenetic gonads with Y-genetic material should be removed because **gonadoblastomas** or **dysgerminomas** may develop in the organ. Age at which reconstructive surgery is recommended is controversial; some advocate that surgery not be performed in infancy or early childhood so that the child or young adolescent can be involved in the decision.

PEARLS FOR PRACTITIONERS

See Endocrinology: Pearls for Practitioners at the end of this section.

REVIEW QUESTIONS

Available online.

CHAPTER 179
Adrenal Gland Dysfunction

PHYSIOLOGY

The **adrenal gland** consists of an outer cortex, which is responsible for the synthesis of steroids, and an inner medulla derived from neuroectodermal tissue, which synthesizes catecholamines. The *adrenal cortex* consists of three zones: an outer glomerulosa (end product is the mineralocorticoid, aldosterone, which regulates sodium and potassium balance), a middle fasciculata (end product is cortisol), and an inner reticularis (synthesizes sex steroids). The general scheme of these synthetic steps is shown in Figure 179.1.

Hypothalamic corticotropin-releasing hormone (CRH) stimulates the release of pituitary adrenocorticotropic hormone (ACTH or corticotropin), derived by selective processing from proopiomelanocortin. ACTH governs the synthesis and release of cortisol and adrenal androgens. Primary adrenal insufficiency or cortisol deficiency from any defect in the adrenal gland results in an oversecretion of ACTH; adrenal insufficiency may also occur from ACTH (secondary) or CRH (tertiary) deficiency, resulting in low serum ACTH concentrations and low cortisol. Endogenous (or exogenous) glucocorticoids feedback to inhibit ACTH and CRH secretion. The renin-angiotensin system and potassium regulate aldosterone secretion; ACTH has little effect on aldosterone production except in excess when it may increase aldosterone secretion.

Steroids that circulate in the free form (not bound to cortisol-binding protein transcortin) may cross the placenta from pregnant person to fetus, but ACTH does not. The placenta plays an important role in steroid biosynthesis in utero by acting as a metabolic mediator between pregnant person and fetus. As the fetal CRH-ACTH-adrenal axis is operational in utero, any deficiencies in cortisol synthesis lead to excessive

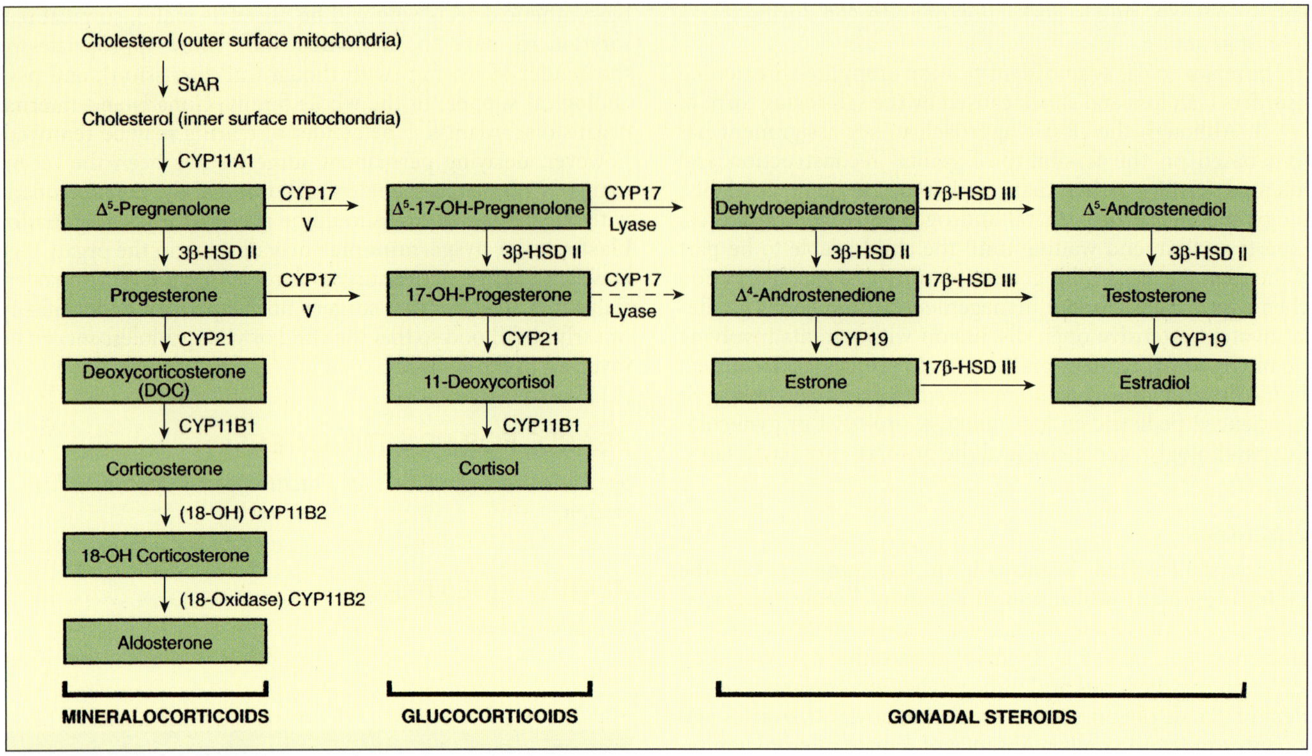

FIGURE 179.1 Diagram of the steroid biosynthetic pathways and the biosynthetic defects that result in congenital adrenal hyperplasia. CYP19 (aromatase) is responsible for the aromatization of androgens into estrogens. 3β-HSD I and 3β-HSD II, 3β-hydroxysteroid dehydrogenase/$\Delta^{4,5}$-isomerase types I and II; CYP21 (P450c21), 21-hydroxylase; 17β-HSD 3, 17β-hydroxysteroid dehydrogenase type 3. (From Melmed S, Polonsky K, Kronenberg H, et al., eds. *Williams Textbook of Endocrinology.* 10th ed. Philadelphia: Saunders; 2003:917.)

ACTH secretion. If a virilizing adrenal enzyme defect is present, such as 21-hydroxylase deficiency, the fetal adrenal gland secretes excess androgens, resulting in a virilized fetus. Normal variation of serum cortisol and ACTH levels leads to values that are high early in the morning and lower at night. This normal diurnal variation may take months to years to fully develop in neonates.

ADRENAL INSUFFICIENCY

The clinical manifestations of inadequate adrenal function result from inadequate secretion or action of glucocorticoids, mineralocorticoids, or both (Table 179.1). In the case of enzyme defects that affect the gonad and the adrenal gland, overproduction or underproduction of potent androgens can occur depending on the site of enzyme blockade (see Fig. 179.1). Progressive prenatal virilization of the external genitalia may occur in genotypic females while incomplete virilization may occur in genotypic males. Ambiguity of the external genitalia is a common manifestation of disordered fetal adrenal enzyme function. Precise *diagnosis* is essential for the prescription of appropriate therapy, long-term outlook, and genetic counseling. In patients with enzyme defects, an elevation in the precursor steroid is present proximal to the enzyme block and is metabolized through remaining normal alternate enzyme pathways, whereas a deficiency of steroids is present subsequent to the block.

The dominant clinical features of **congenital adrenal mineralocorticoid deficiency** are hyponatremia and hyperkalemia, usually developing by 5–7 days after birth but not immediately after birth. Vomiting, dehydration, and acidosis soon follow as does hypotensive shock from glucocorticoid deficiency. Death may occur if the disorder remains undiagnosed and untreated. In females, the ambiguity of the external genitalia is an obvious clue that salt-losing congenital adrenal hyperplasia (CAH) or simple virilizing CAH are potential diagnoses that must be investigated. Because these forms cannot be distinguished clinically, all presentations of ambiguous genitalia should involve evaluation for mineralocorticoid deficiency. In males, 21-hydroxylase deficiency (the most common form of CAH) does not cause abnormal genitalia; although there may be hyperpigmentation of the scrotal skin, this is a subtle sign and can result in delayed diagnosis. In all infants, the diagnosis of adrenal insufficiency may be overlooked or confused with pyloric stenosis. In pyloric stenosis, vomiting of stomach contents results in hypochloremia, low or normal serum potassium, and alkalosis, in contrast to CAH, which has hyponatremia, hyperkalemia, and acidosis. This distinction may be lifesaving in preventing unnecessary investigations or inappropriate therapy.

Not all forms of adrenal hyperplasia present in the newborn period; the spectrum of disorder ranges from severe (classic) to mild (late-onset) or nonclassic. Milder forms may manifest in childhood, adolescence, or even young adulthood (not as glucocorticoid or mineralocorticoid deficiencies, but as androgen excess).

In patients with **congenital adrenal hypoplasia** or **adrenal hemorrhage**, the secretion of all adrenal steroids is low. In contrast, CAH leads to a diagnostic steroid pattern in blood and urine (see Fig. 179.1). Deficiency of 21-hydroxylase is the most common form (95%) and serves as a paradigm for these disorders.

TABLE 179.1 Clinical Manifestations of Adrenal Insufficiency

Ambiguous Genitalia in Certain Conditions
Androgen Excess or Deficiency (Caused by Adrenal Enzyme Defect)
CORTISOL DEFICIENCY
Hypoglycemia Hemodynamic instability with exposure to stress Vasomotor collapse Hyperpigmentation (in primary adrenal insufficiency with excess of adrenocorticotropic hormone) Apneic spells Muscle weakness, fatigue
ALDOSTERONE DEFICIENCY
Hyponatremia Hyperkalemia Vomiting Urinary sodium wasting Salt craving Acidosis Growth faltering Volume depletion Hypotension Dehydration Shock Diarrhea Muscle weakness

21-HYDROXYLASE DEFICIENCY

Classic 21-hydroxylase deficiency occurs in about 1 in 15,000 newborns, and nonclassic occurs in ~1 in 1,000 newborns. Nonclassic CAH may occur with an incidence of 1 in 50 in certain populations (Ashkenazi Jews). The gene for 21-hydroxylase lies on the short arm of chromosome 6; the genotype may be determined in a proband, permitting prenatal diagnosis in a subsequent pregnancy.

Deficient 21-hydroxylase activity (P-450_{c21} deficiency) impairs the conversion of 17-hydroxyprogesterone (17-OHP) to 11-deoxycortisol in the production pathway of cortisol. In the salt-losing form, progesterone to deoxycorticosterone is also impaired in the production pathway of aldosterone. The decreased production of cortisol causes hypersecretion of ACTH, which stimulates the synthesis of steroids immediately proximal to the block and shunting of these to overproduction of androgens. The primary clinical manifestation is the virilization of the external genitalia of the affected genotypically female fetus. The development of the uterus, ovaries, and fallopian tubes is unaffected by the androgens. The degree of virilization varies, ranging from mild clitoromegaly to complete fusion of labioscrotal folds, with severe clitoromegaly simulating a phallus (see Chapter 178). A male infant with this defect appears normal at birth, although penile enlargement may be apparent thereafter. The deficiency in aldosterone, found in about 75% of patients, causes salt wasting with shock and dehydration until the diagnosis is established and appropriate treatment is given.

The treatment of 21-hydroxylase deficiency requires hydrocortisone and fludrocortisone in the case of the salt-losing form. Therapy must be adjusted throughout childhood at regular intervals. Overtreatment will cause growth stunting and weight gain (cushingoid features), whereas undertreatment will cause excessive height gain, skeletal advance, and early-appearance puberty, ultimately jeopardizing adult height potential.

Late-onset CAH is typically noted in childhood or adults. Affected subjects have milder manifestations without ambiguous genitalia, but they may have acne, hirsutism, and, in females, irregular menstrual cycles or amenorrhea. Late-onset CAH in females may be confused with **polycystic ovarian syndrome**.

Biochemical diagnostic studies show elevated levels of serum 17-OHP, the substrate for the defective 21-hydroxylase enzyme activity. In newborns with CAH, the values are elevated 100-fold to a 1,000-fold. In late-onset CAH, an ACTH stimulation test may be necessary to show an abnormally high response of 17-OHP. Serum cortisol and aldosterone levels (in cases of salt wasting) are low and renin levels are high, whereas the testosterone level is elevated because it is derived from 17-OHP.

The goals of *treatment* are to achieve normal linear growth and bone age advancement. Long-term therapy consists of providing glucocorticoids at a dose of approximately 10–15 mg/m^2 per 24 hours in three divided doses of oral hydrocortisone or its equivalent. Mineralocorticoid therapy for children affected by salt wasting consists of fludrocortisone at a dose of 0.05–0.2 mg per 24 hours, often with sodium chloride supplementation in infancy and early childhood. Surgical correction of ambiguous external genitalia may be considered. The adequacy of glucocorticoid replacement therapy is monitored by determining serum concentrations of adrenal precursors, including androstenedione and 17-OHP for 21-hydroxylase deficiency. In addition, the assessment of linear growth and skeletal age, by bone age determination, is required as a reflection of appropriate therapy. To avoid adrenal insufficiency, threefold higher doses of glucocorticoids are given during **stressful states**, such as febrile illness or surgery. Intramuscular hydrocortisone is used in severe emergencies or with illnesses involving emesis. Mineralocorticoid therapy is monitored with serum sodium, potassium, and plasma renin activity levels. Prenatal treatment with dexamethasone to suppress fetal ACTH-induced androgen production can reduce or eliminate the ambiguity of the external genitalia in affected female fetuses, if begun at approximately 7 weeks of gestation; however, this remains controversial as impact on other aspects of the human fetal adrenal axis are unknown.

OTHER ENZYME DEFECTS

Other enzyme defects are rare in contrast to 21-hydroxylase deficiency. In **11-hydroxylase deficiency**, the next most common cause of CAH, virilization occurs with salt retention and hypokalemia as a result of the buildup of deoxycorticosterone, a potent mineralocorticoid (see Fig. 179.1). Hypertension develops as a result of excessive mineralocorticoid production. Table 179.2 summarizes the clinical and biochemical features of adrenal insufficiency in infancy.

ADDISON DISEASE

Addison disease is a rare acquired disorder of childhood, usually associated with autoimmune destruction of the adrenal cortex. It is a form of primary adrenal insufficiency with absence of glucocorticoid and mineralocorticoid.

TABLE **179.2** Clinical and Biochemical Features in Newborn Adrenal Insufficiency

FEATURE	ELECTROLYTE DISTURBANCE*	AMBIGUOUS GENITALIA		SERUM CORTISOL	URINE 11-DEOXYCORTISOL	17-OHP	DHEA	ALDOSTERONE	17-OHCS	17-KS	PREGNANETRIOL
		VIRILIZED FEMALE	UNDERVIRILIZED MALE								
Hypoplasia	Severe	No	No	↓	↓	↓	↓	↓	↓	↓	↓
Hemorrhage	Moderate to severe	No	No	↓	↓	↓	↓	↓	↓	↓	↓
StAR deficiency	Severe	No	Yes	↓	↓	↓	↓	↓	↓	↓	↓
3β-HSD	Severe	Yes	Yes	↓	↓	↓	↑	↓	↓	↑	↓
$P450_{c21}$ deficiency	Absent to severe	Yes	No	↓	↓	↑	↑	↓	↓	↑	↑
Aldosterone synthesis block	Severe	No	No	Nl	Nl	Nl	Nl	↓	Nl	Nl	Nl
Pseudohypo-aldosteronism	Severe	No	No	Nl	Nl	Nl	Nl	↑	Nl	Nl	Nl
$P450_{c11}$ deficiency	None	Yes	No	↓	↑	Nl or ↑	Nl	↓	↑	↑	Nl-slight ↑
$P450_{c17}$ deficiency	†	No	Yes	↓	Nl-↓	↓	↓	Nl-↓	↓	↓	↓
Unresponsiveness to ACTH	†	No	No	↓	Nl-↓	Nl-↓	Nl-↓	Nl-↓	↓	↓	Nl-↓

**Usually manifests after 5 days of age.*

†High normal sodium (Na^+) and low normal to low potassium (K^+).

↓, Decrease; *↑*, increase; *17-KS*, 17-ketosteroid; *17-OHCS*, 17-hydroxycorticosteroid; *17-OHP*, 17-hydroxyprogesterone; *ACTH*, adrenocorticotropic hormone; *DHEA*, dehydroepiandrosterone; *HSD*, hydroxysteroid dehydrogenase; *Nl*, normal; *StAR*, steroid acute regulatory protein.

Clinical manifestations are hyperpigmentation, salt craving, postural hypotension, fasting hypoglycemia, anorexia, weakness, and episodes of shock during severe illness. Subnormal baseline and ACTH-stimulated cortisol values confirm the diagnosis. The presence of hyponatremia, hyperkalemia, and elevated plasma renin activity indicate mineralocorticoid deficiency. Addison disease may occur within the context of autoimmune polyglandular syndromes (APS I and APS II). Other rare causes of adrenal insufficiency include X-linked adrenal leukodystrophy and conditions that affect the hypothalamus-pituitary, whether acquired, such as in craniopharyngioma, or iatrogenic, such as in irradiation for treatment of malignancy.

Replacement *treatment* with 10–15 mg/m^2 per 24 hours of hydrocortisone is indicated, with supplementation during stress at three times the maintenance dosage or the use of intramuscular hydrocortisone. The dose is titrated to allow a normal growth rate. Mineralocorticoid replacement with fludrocortisone is monitored by plasma renin activity along with serum sodium and potassium determinations.

CUSHING SYNDROME

Classic *clinical manifestations* of **Cushing syndrome** in children include progressive central or generalized obesity, marked failure of longitudinal growth, hirsutism, weakness, a nuchal fat pad, acne, striae, hypertension, and often hyperpigmentation when ACTH is elevated. The most frequent cause is long-term administration of exogenous glucocorticoids due to chronic medical conditions. Endogenous causes include adrenal adenoma, carcinoma, nodular adrenal hyperplasia, an ACTH-secreting pituitary microadenoma resulting in bilateral adrenal hyperplasia **(Cushing disease)**, or an extremely rare ACTH-secreting tumor. *Diagnostic tests* include 24-hour urinary cortisol excretion, low-dose dexamethasone suppression test, high-dose dexamethasone suppression test (helps distinguish Cushing syndrome from Cushing disease), and *late evening* salivary cortisol sampling.

Treatment of Cushing syndrome is directed to the etiology and may include excision of adrenal, pituitary, or ectopic ACTH-secreting tumors. Rarely, adrenalectomy is needed to control the symptoms. Parenteral glucocorticoid therapy is necessary during and immediately after surgical treatment to avoid acute adrenal insufficiency.

PEARLS FOR PRACTITIONERS

See Endocrinology: Pearls for Practitioners at the end of this section.

REVIEW QUESTIONS

Available online.

Suggested Readings

Backeljauw PF, Chernausek SD. The insulin-like growth factors and growth disorders of childhood. *Endocrinol Metab Clin North Am.* 2012;41(2):265–282.
Kliegman RM, St. Geme J, eds. *Nelson Textbook of Pediatrics.* 22nd ed. Philadelphia: Elsevier; 2025.
Nimkarn S, Lin-Su K, New MI. Steroid 21 hydroxylase deficiency congenital adrenal hyperplasia. *Pediatr Clin North Am.* 2011;58(5):1281–1300.
Palmert MR, Dunkel L. Clinical practice: delayed puberty. *N Engl J Med.* 2012;366(5):443–453.
Péter F, Muzsnai A. Congenital disorders of the thyroid: hypo/hyper. *Pediatr Clin North Am.* 2011;58(5):1099–1115.
Romero CJ, Nesi-França S, Radovick S. The molecular basis of hypopituitarism. *Trends Endocrinol Metab.* 2009;20(10):506–516.
Schatz DA, Haller MJ, Atkinson MA. Type 1 diabetes. Preface. *Endocrinol Metab Clin North Am.* 2010;39(3):481–667.
Speiser PW, Arlt W, Auchus RJ, et al. Congenital adrenal hyperplasia due to steroid 21-hydroxylase deficiency: an Endocrine Society Clinical Practice Guideline. *J Clin Endocrinol Metab.* 2018;103(11):4043–4088. Erratum in: *J Clin Endocrinol Metab.* 2019;104(1):39–40.
Thornton PS, Stanley CA, De Leon DD, et al. Recommendations from the Pediatric Endocrine Society for Evaluation and Management of Persistent Hypoglycemia in Neonates, Infants, and Children. *J Pediatr.* 2015;167(2):238–245.
Williams RM, Ward CE, Hughes IA. Premature adrenarche. *Arch Dis Child.* 2012;97(3):250–254.

PEARLS FOR PRACTITIONERS

CHAPTER 171

Endocrinology Assessment

- Hormones are produced in a regulated fashion in one cell and then travel through the bloodstream (often bound to binding factors) to a target cell; then, hormones either bind to receptors on the plasma membranes of target cells or are transported into cells to bind to intracellular receptors.
- Hormones generally are regulated in a feedback loop so that the production of a hormone is linked to its effect or its circulating concentration.
- Endocrine disorders generally manifest from one of four ways: excess hormone, deficient hormone, abnormal response of end-organ, gland enlargement.
- The assessment of pituitary function may be determined by measuring some of the specific pituitary hormones in the basal state; other assessments require the measurement after stimulation.

CHAPTER 172

Diabetes Mellitus

- Type 1 diabetes (T1D) is an autoimmune disease and most often presents with hyperglycemia, ketoacidosis, polyuria, and polydipsia.
- T1D is typically treated with multiple daily injections of a short-acting (bolus) insulin and a single dose of long-acting (basal) insulin.
- Preprandial blood glucose target concentrations are 80–130 mg/dL and concentrations before bedtime and overnight are 80–150 mg/dL.
- Treatment of diabetic ketoacidosis (DKA) requires careful management of isotonic fluids, continuous infusions of insulin until acidosis has resolved, and monitoring of blood glucose, electrolytes, and neurologic status.
- Type 2 diabetes (T2D) is associated with obesity and insulin resistance.

- Initial management of T2D in children includes lifestyle modifications including nutrition therapy (dietary adjustments) and increased exercise.
- Metformin (an insulin secretagogue) and select GLP-1 analogs are first-line drugs for the pharmacologic treatment of T2D; they are approved by the U.S. Food and Drug Administration for use in children.
- A goal of $HbA_{1c} < 7.5\%$ is set for children with diabetes (both T1D and T2D) of all ages.
- Diabetes mellitus is a complex chronic illness that requires a team of providers, including an endocrinologist, diabetes educator, nutritionist, and social worker/psychologist, and close interactions with the family for success.

CHAPTER 173
Hypoglycemia

- Hypoglycemia occurs most frequently in the early neonatal period, often as a result of transient neonatal hyperinsulinemia in infants of diabetic mothers or as a result of inadequate energy stores to meet the disproportionately large metabolic needs of premature or small for gestational age newborns.
- Clinical hypoglycemia is defined as a plasma glucose (PG) concentration low enough to cause symptoms and/or signs of impaired brain function.
- The most common causes for congenital hyperinsulinism involve inactivating K_{ATP} channel pathogenic variants.
- The *diagnosis* of hyperinsulinism in children is determined by evaluating markers of inappropriate insulin effects (e.g., suppressed ketogenesis) because plasma insulin concentrations are frequently not clearly elevated.
- Idiopathic ketotic hypoglycemia usually begins at about 18 months of age in thin children and remits by 8 years of age; it presents with symptoms of hypoglycemia after a period of prolonged fasting, often in the setting of an intercurrent illness with decreased feeding.
- The *diagnosis* of glycogen storage disease (GSD) is suggested by hypoglycemia in the setting of hepatomegaly without splenomegaly (although GSD type 0 is not associated with hepatomegaly).
- A *critical sample* of blood and urine at the time of the hypoglycemic episode should be obtained before treatment for plasma glucose, β-hydroxybutyrate (BOHB), a comprehensive metabolic panel, insulin, C-peptide, free fatty acids (FFAs), lactate, ammonia, cortisol, growth hormone, an acyl-carnitine profile, and free and total carnitines. A urine specimen should be obtained for measuring ketones and organic acids.

CHAPTER 174
Short Stature

- Normal growth is the final common pathway of many factors, including endocrine, environmental, nutritional, and genetic influences.
- Insulinlike growth factor-1 (IGF-1) acts primarily as a paracrine and autocrine agent and is most closely associated with postnatal growth, although GH exerts its own metabolic effects.
- Accurate measurements of height (standing) or length (lying down) and weight should be plotted on the Centers for Disease Control and Prevention growth charts for the timely diagnosis of growth disorders.
- Short stature is defined as subnormal height relative to other children of the same sex and age, taking family heights into consideration.
- Marking the position of the head and feet of an infant lying on a sheet of paper on the examining table leads to inaccuracies and may miss true disorders of growth or create false concerns about a disorder of growth in a normal child. Use of a stadiometer or recumbent length board is recommended.
- Adequacy of GH secretion may be determined by a stimulation test to measure peak GH secretion.
- GH deficiency is treated with biosynthetic recombinant DNA-derived GH (rhGH).
- Constitutional delay in growth or puberty (or both) is considered a variation of normal growth, caused by a reduced tempo of physiological development.

CHAPTER 175
Disorders of Puberty

- Pubarche results from adrenal maturation or adrenarche and is marked with the appearance of pubic hair, oiliness of hair and skin, acne, axillary hair, and body odor; gonadarche is characterized by increasing secretion of gonadal sex steroids as a result of the maturation of the hypothalamic-pituitary-gonadal axis.
- Puberty is delayed when there is no sign of pubertal development by age 13 years in females and 14 years in males living in the United States.
- Disorders that can cause hypogonadotropic hypogonadism include congenital hypopituitarism, such as midline defects, tumors, infiltrative disease, and many syndromes, including Laurence-Moon-Bardet-Biedl, Prader-Willi, and Kallmann syndromes.
- Turner syndrome is a common cause of ovarian failure and short stature; Klinefelter syndrome (seminiferous tubular dysgenesis) is the most common cause of testicular failure.
- When no secondary sexual development is present after the upper age limits of normal pubertal development, serum gonadotropin levels should be obtained to determine whether the patient has hypogonadotropic or hypergonadotropic hypogonadism.
- Central precocious puberty, resulting in gonadarche, emanates from premature activation of the hypothalamic-pituitary-gonadal axis (gonadotropin-releasing hormone [GnRH]-dependent); peripheral precocious puberty, gonadarche or adrenarche, does not involve the hypothalamic-pituitary-gonadal axis (GnRH-independent).

- The first step in evaluating precocious puberty is to determine which characteristics of normal puberty are apparent and whether estrogen effects, androgen effects, or both are present; laboratory evaluation includes determination of adrenal androgen and sex steroid levels (testosterone, estradiol, DHEAS [dehydroepiandrosterone sulfate]) and baseline gonadotropin concentrations.
- A prepubertal GnRH response is follicle-stimulating hormone (FSH) predominant, whereas a pubertal response is more luteinizing hormone (LH) predominant.
- Long-acting analogs of GnRH (leuprolide depot, histrelin implant, triptorelin) are the treatment of choice for central precocious puberty; antiandrogens, antiestrogens, and aromatase inhibitors are used for peripheral precocious puberty.
- Most patients with isolated pubic hair do not have progressive virilization and simply have premature adrenarche *(pubarche)* resulting from premature activation of DHEA secretion from the adrenal gland; no treatment is needed.

CHAPTER 176
Thyroid Disease

- Hypothyroidism is common in children, and treatment with levothyroxine is typically initiated when thyroid-stimulating hormone (TSH) is >10 mIU/L.
- Early treatment in congenital hypothyroidism is essential to prevent delayed development.
- Hypothyroidism must be considered in evaluation of short stature, especially if not associated with weight gain.
- Acquired hypothyroidism is an autoimmune disease and may be associated with type 1 diabetes, Addison disease, hypoparathyroidism, or celiac disease.
- Hyperthyroidism is initially treated with pharmacologic therapy. Ablation or surgical removal are long-term permanent treatment options.
- Most thyroid nodules in children and adolescents are benign.

CHAPTER 177
Disorders of Parathyroid Bone and Mineral Endocrinology

- Calcium and phosphate are regulated mainly by diet and three hormones: parathyroid hormone (PTH), vitamin D, and calcitonin.
- Neonatal hypocalcemia has multiple causes depending on timing of onset and is often transient.
- It is essential to make sure both vitamin D and magnesium levels are normal when replacing calcium.
- Hypocalcemia may be associated with multiple nonendocrine disorders and diseases, thus requiring a complete evaluation.

CHAPTER 178
Disorders of Sexual Differentiation

- The first step toward diagnosis of ambiguous genitalia is to determine whether the findings represent virilization of a genetic female (androgen excess) or underdevelopment of a genetic male (androgen deficiency)
- Disorders of sexual development (DSDs) are categorized under three main subgroups according to karyotype (XX, XY, and sex chromosome for mosaic karyotypes).
- Congenital virilizing adrenal hyperplasia is the most common cause of female ambiguous genitalia.
- Although the classic approach to sex assignment has been based on the feasibility of genital reconstruction and potential fertility rather than on karyotype or gonadal histology, the effects of prenatal androgen must be considered; experts recommend waiting until the child is able to be part of the dialogue regarding gender identity and reconstruction when appropriate.
- The major goal at birth is a rapid identification of any life-threatening disorders (salt loss and shock caused by the salt-losing form of congenital adrenal hyperplasia [CAH]).

CHAPTER 179
Adrenal Gland Dysfunction

- The clinical manifestations of inadequate adrenal function result from inadequate secretion or action of glucocorticoids, mineralocorticoids, or both.
- The dominant clinical features of congenital adrenal mineralocorticoid deficiency are hyponatremia and hyperkalemia, usually developing by 5–7 days after birth but not immediately after birth. Deficiency of 21-hydroxylase is the most common form (95%).
- Early diagnosis and treatment of salt wasting congenital adrenal hyperplasia involves replacement therapy with hydrocortisone, fludrocortisone, and saline solution.
- Adrenal insufficiency (Addison disease) is associated with hyperpigmentation, salt craving, postural hypotension, fasting hypoglycemia, anorexia, weakness, and episodes of shock during severe illness.
- Cushing syndrome is commonly a result of chronic use of high-dose oral steroids. Cushing disease is caused by an ACTH-secreting pituitary microadenoma resulting in bilateral adrenal hyperplasia.

SECTION **24**

NEUROLOGY

Rachel J. Gottlieb-Smith | Erin E. Neil Knierbein | Jocelyn Huang Schiller

CHAPTER **180**

Neurology Assessment

A neurologic evaluation, including history, physical examination, and judicious use of ancillary studies, allows the localization and diagnosis of nervous system pathology. The process and interpretation of the neurologic examination varies with age; the newborn is unique, with many transient and primitive reflexes, whereas the examinations of adolescents and adults are similar. Careful evaluations of social, cognitive, language, fine motor, and gross motor skills, and their age-appropriateness, are key.

HISTORY

Gathering neurologic history follows the traditional medical model while focusing on the **pace** and **localization** of the problem and the developmental assessment. The symptom evolution provides clues to the underlying process. Symptoms may evolve in a progressive, static, or episodic fashion. **Progressive** symptoms may present acutely over minutes or hours (e.g., epidural hemorrhage), subacutely over days or weeks (e.g., brain tumor), or slowly over years (e.g., hereditary neuropathies). **Static** neurologic abnormalities are observed early in life and do not change in character over time (e.g., cerebral palsy due to congenital brain abnormalities or prenatal/perinatal brain injury). Intermittent attacks of recurrent, stereotyped episodes often suggest epilepsy or migraine. **Episodic** disorders are characterized by periods of symptoms, followed by partial or complete recovery (e.g., demyelinating diseases).

Careful evaluations of social, cognitive, language, fine motor, and gross motor skills are key to distinguish normal development from isolated or global delays (see Chapter 7). Loss of skills over time **(regression)** is particularly worrisome and may suggest an underlying degenerative disease, emerging autism spectrum disorder, or epileptic encephalopathy.

PHYSICAL EXAMINATION

Observation of the child's appearance, movement, and behavior begins at the start of the encounter. For example, the child may display an unusual posture, abnormal gait, or lack of awareness of the environment.

The brain and skin have the same embryonic origin (ectoderm), so abnormalities of hair, skin, teeth, and nails are associated with congenital brain disorders **(neurocutaneous disorders)** such as neurofibromatosis (NF type 1), in which **café-au-lait macules** (flat, light brown macules) are characteristic. **Facial angiofibromas** (fibrovascular lesions that look like acne on the nose and malar regions), nail fibromas, ash-leaf spots (hypopigmented macules), and Shagreen patches (flesh-colored soft plaques with prominent follicular openings) are commonly seen in older children and adults with **tuberous sclerosis.**

The **head circumference** is measured in its largest occipitofrontal circumference and plotted against standard growth curves (see Chapter 5). **Microcephaly** and **macrocephaly** represent an occipitofrontal circumference two or more standard deviations below or above the mean, respectively, for age and sex. Measurements plotted over time may show an accelerating pattern (e.g., hydrocephalus) or decelerating pattern (e.g., brain injury, degenerative neurologic disorder). The anterior fontanel is slightly depressed and pulsatile when a calm infant is upright. A tense or bulging fontanel may indicate increased intracranial pressure (ICP) but may also be seen in a crying infant. Premature closure of one or more sutures **(craniosynostosis)** results in an unusual shape of the head. Abnormal shape, location, or condition of the face, eyes, nares, philtrum, lips, or ears (dysmorphic features) are found in many genetic syndromes.

A careful **ocular examination** is essential and should include a search for epicanthal folds, coloboma, conjunctival telangiectasias, and cataracts. Direct ophthalmoscopy assesses the optic discs and macula for abnormalities, such as papilledema or a cherry red spot. A complete examination of the retina involves dilating the pupil and indirect ophthalmoscopy.

Examination of the hands and feet may reveal abnormal creases or digits (see Chapters 49 and 202). The neck and spine should be examined for obvious (e.g., myelomeningocele) or subtle (e.g., cutaneous dimples, sinus tracts, hair tufts, subcutaneous lipomas) midline defects. Nervous system abnormalities may result in kyphosis or scoliosis (see Chapter 203).

NEUROLOGIC EXAMINATION OF A NEONATE

The neonatal neurologic examination primarily assesses the function of the basal ganglia, brainstem, and more caudal structures due to immature cortical function.

Mental Status

A healthy newborn infant should have periods of quiet, sustained wakefulness interspersed with sleep. Irritability, lethargy, or more severely depressed consciousness are nonspecific signs of abnormal brain function.

Reflexes

Examination of the **primitive reflexes** provides assessment of the functional integrity of the brainstem and basal ganglia (Table 180.1). Many of these stereotyped motor responses are present at birth. They are symmetric and typically disappear by 4–6 months of age, indicating the normal maturation of descending inhibitory cerebral influences. Asymmetry or persistence of the primitive reflexes may indicate focal brain or peripheral nerve lesions.

Motor Examination and Tone

Posture is the position that a calm infant naturally assumes when placed supine. An infant at 28 weeks of gestation lies with extended extremities. By 32 weeks, there is an increase in tone and flexion of the lower extremities. At 34 weeks, the lower extremities are flexed; the upper extremities are extended. The term infant flexes both lower and upper extremities. **Recoil**, the readiness with which an arm or leg springs back to its original position after passive stretching and release, is essentially absent in very premature infants but is brisk at term. Because of the asymmetric tonic neck reflex, it is essential to maintain the infant's head in a neutral position (facing forward) during assessment of posture and tone. Spontaneous movements of premature infants are slow and writhing; those of term infants are more rapid.

NEUROLOGIC EXAMINATION OF A CHILD

The purpose of the neurologic examination is to localize or identify the region from which the symptoms arise. The mental status and developmental examinations assess cerebral cortex function. The cranial nerve examination evaluates the integrity of the brainstem. The motor examination evaluates upper and lower motor neuron function. The sensory examination assesses the peripheral sensory receptors and their central reflections. Deep tendon reflexes assess upper and lower motor connections.

Mental Status and Developmental Evaluation

Alertness is assessed in infants by observing spontaneous activities, feeding behavior, and visual ability to fix and follow objects. Note responses to tactile, visual, and auditory stimuli. If consciousness is altered, note the response to painful stimuli. Observation of toddlers at play allows a nonthreatening assessment of developmentally appropriate skills. In addition to language function, older children can be tested for reading, writing, numeric skills, fund of knowledge, abstract reasoning, judgment, and memory.

The simplest way to assess intellectual abilities is through language skills. **Language function** is receptive (understanding speech and gestures) and expressive (use of speech and gestures). Abnormalities of language resulting from cerebral

TABLE 180.1 Central Nervous System Reflexes of Infancy

REFLEX	DESCRIPTION	AGE AT APPEARANCE	AGE AT DISAPPEARANCE
Moro	With the infant supine, light pull upward on the arms without lifting the head followed by release of arms (or controlled drop of head) produces sudden extension followed by flexion of the arms and legs.	Birth	3–6 mo
Grasp	Placing finger in palm results in flexing of infant's fingers.	Birth	3–4 mo
Rooting	Tactile stimulus at the side of the mouth causes the mouth to pursue the stimulus.	Birth	3–4 mo
Trunk incurvation (Gallant)	Stroking the skin along the edge of vertebrae produces curvature of the spine with concavity on the side of the stimulus.	Birth	4 mo
Placing	When dorsum of foot is brought into contact with the edge of a surface, infant places foot on the surface.	Birth	4–6 mo
Asymmetric tonic neck	With infant supine, turning of the head results in ipsilateral extension of the arm and leg with flexion of opposite extremities in a "fencing" posture.	Birth	3 mo
Parachute	Infant is suspended face down by the chest. When infant is moved toward a table, the arms extend as if to protect self.	8–10 mo	Never
Babinski	Stroking lateral aspect of sole from heel up results in dorsiflexion of the great toe and fanning of the remaining toes.	Birth	12–18 mo

hemisphere disorders are referred to as aphasias. Anterior, **expressive aphasia** (Broca aphasia) is characterized by sparse, nonfluent language. Posterior, **receptive aphasia** (Wernicke aphasia) is characterized by an inability to understand language, with speech that is fluent but nonsensical. **Global aphasia** refers to impaired expressive and receptive language.

CRANIAL NERVE EVALUATION

The cranial nerve evaluation assesses brainstem integrity but depends on the stage of brain maturation and the ability to cooperate. A colorful toy may capture a young child's attention and permit observation of coordination, movement, and cranial nerve function.

Cranial Nerve I

Smell can be assessed in verbal, cooperative children >2 years of age. Aromatic substances (perfumes, vanilla) should be used instead of volatile substances (ammonia), which irritate the nasal mucosa and stimulate the trigeminal nerve.

Cranial Nerve II

By 2–3 months of age, term newborns in a quiet, awake state follow human faces, lights in a dark room, or large, optokinetic strips. Visual acuity has been estimated to be 20/200 in newborns and gradually matures throughout childhood. Standard visual charts displaying pictures instead of letters can be used to assess visual acuity in toddlers. Peripheral vision is tested by surreptitiously bringing objects into the visual field from behind. A reduced pupillary reaction to light suggests a lesion to the anterior visual pathway (e.g., retina, optic nerves, chiasm). Unilateral lesions are identified by the swinging flashlight test. With an optic nerve abnormality, both pupils constrict when light is directed into the normal eye. When light is swung over to the abnormal eye, both pupils do not constrict or even may dilate inappropriately; this is called an afferent pupillary defect **(Marcus Gunn pupil)**. Interruption of the sympathetic innervation to the pupil produces **Horner syndrome** (ptosis, miosis, and unilateral facial anhidrosis). In this instance, anisocoria (unequal pupils) is more pronounced in a dark room because the affected pupil is unable to dilate appropriately. Lesions of the posterior visual pathway (e.g., lateral geniculate, optic radiations, occipital cortex) have normal pupillary light reactions but are expressed by loss of visual fields.

Cranial Nerves III, IV, and VI

These three cranial nerves control eye movements and are most easily examined with the use of a colorful toy to capture the child's attention. For infants too young to fix and follow, rotating the infant's head assesses the **oculocephalic reflex** (doll's-eye maneuver). If the brainstem is intact, rotating a newborn or comatose patient's head to the right causes the eyes to move to the left and vice versa. In awake, older patients, voluntary eye movements mask the reflex.

Abnormalities of these cranial nerves may cause diplopia (double vision). With unilateral third cranial (oculomotor) nerve palsy, the involved eye deviates down and out (infraducted, abducted), with associated ptosis and a dilated (mydriatic) pupil. Injury to cranial nerve IV (trochlear) causes weakness of downward eye movement with consequent vertical diplopia. Cranial nerve VI (abducens) palsy results in the inability to move the eye laterally. Cranial nerve VI has a long intracranial route within the subarachnoid space; failure of abduction of one or both eyes is a frequent, but nonspecific, sign of increased intracranial pressure.

Cranial Nerve V

The muscles of mastication can be observed as an infant sucks and swallows. The **corneal reflex** tests cranial nerves V ophthalmic division (sensory arc) and VII (motor arc). Facial sensation of light touch can be determined with cotton gauze. Facial sensation can be functionally assessed in an infant by gently brushing the cheek, which will produce the **rooting reflex**.

Cranial Nerve VII

Facial muscles are assessed by observing the face during rest, crying, and blinking if a child is not old enough to voluntarily smile or move the face. Weakness of all unilateral muscles of the face, including the forehead, eye, and mouth, indicates a lesion of the ipsilateral peripheral facial nerve (e.g., **Bell's palsy**). Because the upper third of the face receives bilateral cortical innervation, a lesion of upper motor neurons in the brain (e.g., tumor, stroke, abscess) will result in contralateral weakness of only the lower face and mouth.

Cranial Nerve VIII

Lesions of cranial nerve VIII cause deafness, tinnitus, and vertigo. Normally, alert neonates blink in response to a bell or other abrupt, loud sound. Four-month-old infants turn the head and eyes to localize a sound. Delayed language development or any concerns about hearing should trigger a referral for a formal hearing assessment.

Lesions of the vestibular component of cranial nerve VIII produce symptoms of vertigo, nausea, vomiting, diaphoresis, and nystagmus. Nystagmus is an involuntary beating eye movement with a rapid phase in one direction and a slow phase in the opposite direction. By convention, the direction of the nystagmus is defined by the fast phase and may be horizontal, vertical, or rotatory.

Cranial Nerves IX and X

The gag reflex is brisk at all ages except the very immature neonate. An absent gag reflex suggests a lesion of the brainstem, cranial nerves IX or X, neuromuscular junction, or pharyngeal muscles. Weak, breathy, or nasal speech; a weak suck; drooling; and gagging are additional symptoms of cranial nerve X dysfunction.

Cranial Nerve XI

Observing the infant's posture and spontaneous activity assesses the functions of the trapezius and sternocleidomastoid muscles. Head tilt and drooping of the shoulder suggest lesions involving cranial nerve XI. In later childhood, strength in these muscles can be tested directly.

Cranial Nerve XII

Atrophy and fasciculation (quivering muscle movements that are typically best seen on the lateral aspect of the tongue) usually indicate a lesion of the anterior horn cells (spinal muscular atrophy). Assessment is most reliable when an infant is asleep. The tongue deviates toward the weak side in unilateral lesions.

MOTOR EXAMINATION

Tone

Tone represents the dynamic resistance of muscles to passive stretch. Lower motor neuron and cerebellar lesions produce decreased tone **(hypotonia)**. **Hypertonia** is seen with upper motor neuron or extrapyramidal (e.g., basal ganglia) lesions; upper motor neuron lesions produce spasticity (velocity-dependent increased tone) and extrapyramidal disease often leads to rigidity (increase in resistance present throughout passive movement of a joint).

Bulk

Muscle bulk may be decreased due to disuse or to lower motor neuron or neuromuscular disease. Excessive muscle bulk is seen in rare conditions, such as myotonia congenita; males with Duchenne muscular dystrophy have pseudohypertrophy of the calves.

Strength

In infants, strength is assessed by observation of spontaneous movements. Extremity movements should be symmetric and are best seen when the infant is held supine with one hand supporting the buttocks and one supporting the shoulders. Strength is graded as follows:

5 Normal
4 Weak but able to move against resistance
3 Able to move against gravity but not against resistance
2 Movement in the plane of gravity
1 Muscle contraction but no movement
0 Complete paralysis

Strength in toddlers is assessed by observing functional abilities, such as walking, stooping to pick up an object, and standing up from the floor. An older child should be able to easily reach high above the head, wheelbarrow walk, run, hop, go up and down stairs, and arise from the ground. Cooperative children can undergo individual muscle strength testing. **Gower sign** (child arises from lying on the floor by using arms to climb up legs and body) is a sign of significant proximal weakness. Subtle upper extremity asymmetry can be detected when the child extends arms out in front with the palms upward and eyes closed. The hand on the weaker side cups and begins to pronate and move slowly downward **(pronator drift)**. **Muscle fasciculations** indicate denervation from disease of the anterior horn cell or peripheral nerve.

Coordination

Ataxia is the lack of coordination of movement, which is typically due to a dysfunction of the cerebellar pathways. Watching the child sit or walk assesses truncal stability. Exchanging toys or objects with the child permits assessment of intention tremor and **dysmetria** (errors in judging distance to a target), signs of cerebellar dysfunction. Cooperative children can do repetitive finger or foot tapping to test rapid alternating movements. Cerebellar and corticospinal tract dysfunctions produce slow and irregular alternating movements.

Gait

Watching a child creep, crawl, cruise, or walk is the best global assessment for the motor and coordination systems. Subtle deficits and asymmetries in strength, tone, or balance may be observed. The toddler gait is normally wide based and unsteady. The base of the gait narrows with age. By 6 years, a typical child can walk on the toes or heels and tandem walk (heel to toe). Cerebellar dysfunction results in a broad-based, unsteady gait accompanied by difficulty in executing turns. Corticospinal tract dysfunction produces a stiff, scissoring gait (legs adduct past midline) and toe walking; arm swing is decreased, and the affected arm is flexed across the body. Extrapyramidal dysfunction produces a slow, stiff, shuffling gait with dystonic postures. A waddling gait occurs with hip weakness due to lower motor neuron or neuromuscular disorders. A steppage gait results from weakness of ankle dorsiflexors (e.g., common peroneal palsy).

Reflexes

Deep tendon reflexes can be elicited at any age and are reported on a 5-point scale:

0 Absent
1+ Trace
2+ Normal
3+ Exaggerated reflex, sometimes with spread to contiguous areas (e.g., tapping a patellar reflex and observing an ankle jerk as well)
4+ With **clonus** (rhythmic oscillating stretch reflex)

These reflexes are decreased in lower motor neuron diseases and increased in upper motor neuron disease. In neonates, the normal **Babinski response** (extensor plantar reflex) is an upward movement of the great toe and flaring of the toes on stimulation of the lateral foot. The response may vary and be unreliable in young infants except when asymmetric. By 12–18 months of age the plantar response should consistently be flexor (toes flexing down); extension after this age is a sign of corticospinal tract dysfunction.

SENSORY EXAMINATION

The sensory examination of newborns and infants is limited to observing the behavioral response to light touch or pinprick. Stimulation of a limb should produce a facial grimace. A spinal reflex alone may produce withdrawal movement of a limb. In a cooperative child, the senses of pain, touch, temperature, vibration, and joint position can be tested individually. The cortical areas of sensation must be intact to identify an object placed in the hand **(stereognosis)** or a number written in the hand **(graphesthesia)** or to distinguish between two sharp objects applied simultaneously and closely on the skin **(two-point discrimination)**.

SPECIAL DIAGNOSTIC PROCEDURES

Cerebrospinal Fluid Analysis

Analysis of cerebrospinal fluid (CSF) is essential when central nervous system infection is suspected and provides important clues to other diagnoses (Table 180.2). Differentiating hemorrhagic CSF caused by a traumatic lumbar puncture (LP) from a true subarachnoid hemorrhage may be difficult. In most cases of traumatic LP, the fluid clears significantly as the sequence of tubes is collected. If there is clinical evidence of increased ICP (papilledema, depression of consciousness, focal neurologic deficits), caution must be exercised before performing an LP to limit risk of cerebral herniation. Neuroimaging should be performed and confirmed to be normal before the LP if increased ICP is suspected. If increased ICP is present, it must be treated before an LP is performed.

Electroencephalography

The electroencephalogram (EEG) records electrical activity generated by the cerebral cortex. EEG rhythms mature throughout childhood. There are three key features present: background patterns, behavioral state modulation, and presence or absence of epileptiform patterns. The background varies with age but in general should be symmetric and synchronous between the two hemispheres. Persistent focal slowing suggests an underlying structural abnormality (e.g., brain tumor, abscess, stroke). Diffuse slow wave activity suggests bilateral cerebral involvement (e.g., increased ICP, metabolic encephalopathy). Spikes, polyspikes, and spike-and-wave abnormalities, either in a localized region (focal) or bihemispheric (generalized), suggest an increased risk for seizures.

Electromyography and Nerve Conduction Studies

Electromyography (EMG) and nerve conduction studies (NCSs) assess for abnormalities of the neuromuscular apparatus, including anterior horn cells, peripheral nerves, neuromuscular junctions, and muscles. EMG evaluates the electrical activity of muscle, typically via needle electrodes. NCSs assess the action potential transmission along peripheral nerves.

Neuroimaging

Imaging the brain and spinal cord is accomplished using computed tomography scan (CT) or magnetic resonance imaging (MRI). CT is quick and accessible for emergency purposes but exposes the patient to radiation. For a child with an acute head injury or sudden headache, cranial CT is the study of choice because it can rapidly reveal intracranial hemorrhage, impending herniation, or other large lesions. Advantages to MRI include finer detail and, with different sequences, the ability to detect posterior fossa lesions, subtle cerebral abnormalities, vascular anomalies, low-grade tumors, ischemic changes, and greater detail but with greater expense and time requirement, sometimes requiring general anesthesia for children who are unable to cooperate. For a child with new-onset focal seizures who has returned to baseline, MRI is typically the study of choice because an area of focal cortical dysplasia or other subtle lesions might not be apparent on CT. MRI also provides excellent views of the spinal cord. Fast MRI techniques have been developed to reduce imaging times and are often used in evaluating ventricular size without the need for radiation; it is limited in detection of certain findings such as sinovenous thrombosis and extraaxial hemorrhage. MR angiography and MR venography provide detailed images of major intracranial vasculature structures and assist in the diagnosis of conditions such as stroke, vascular malformations, and cerebral venous sinus thrombosis. Cranial ultrasonography is a noninvasive bedside procedure used to visualize the brain and ventricles of infants with open fontanels (e.g., hydrocephalus, intracranial hemorrhage, or periventricular leukomalacia).

TABLE 180.2 Analysis of Cerebrospinal Fluid

	NORMAL CSF VALUES	
CSF FINDING	**NEWBORN**	**>1 MO OLD**
Cell count*	5–15/mm³	5/mm³
Protein	65–150 mg/dL	<100 mg/dL
Glucose	>2/3 blood glucose or >25 mg/dL	>2/3 blood glucose or >40 mg/dL

CSF CHANGE	SIGNIFICANCE
Increased polymorphonuclear cells and decreased CSF glucose	Bacterial infection Brain or parameningeal abscess Parasitic infection
Increased lymphocytes and decreased CSF glucose	Mycobacterial infection (tuberculosis) Fungal infection Sarcoidosis
Increased lymphocytes and normal CSF glucose	Viral meningitis Postinfectious disease (ADEM) Vasculitis Multiple sclerosis Tumor (although CSF glucose could be low)
Increased CSF protein	Infection Guillain-Barré syndrome Inflammatory disease (ADEM, multiple sclerosis) Leukodystrophy Venous thrombosis Hypertension Spinal block (Froin syndrome)
Decreased glucose without pleocytosis	Common: Hypoglycemia Rare: GLUT-1 deficiency
Bloody CSF	Subarachnoid hemorrhage Subdural hemorrhage Intraparenchymal hemorrhage Hemorrhagic meningoencephalitis (group B *streptococcus*, HSV) CNS trauma Vascular malformation Coagulopathy Traumatic lumbar puncture

**In healthy children, cells present should be lymphocytes. Cell count differs by age and individual. See Thomson et al. Cerebrospinal fluid reference values for young infants undergoing lumbar puncture.* Pediatrics. *2018;141(3):e20173405.*
ADEM, Acute disseminated encephalomyelitis; *CNS,* central nervous system; *CSF,* cerebrospinal fluid; *GLUT-1 deficiency,* glucose transporter type 1 deficiency syndrome; *HSV,* herpes simplex virus.

Genetic Testing

Children with developmental delay, intellectual disability, or other neurologic symptoms are often evaluated with metabolic or genetic testing. State newborn screening results should be reviewed. Specific features of the history or physical examination may point to particular disorders, allowing for targeted genetic or metabolic testing. Chromosomal microarray analysis is a diagnostic test that detects copy number variants (duplications or deletions of chromosome material). Multigene panels typically include sequencing analysis, and sometimes deletion/duplication analysis, of a number of genes associated with particular symptoms. Whole exome sequencing is a broad test involving sequencing of all genes that encode for proteins (exons). Whole genome sequencing expands beyond this and sequences the entire genome, including non–protein-coding regions.

PEARLS FOR PRACTITIONERS

See Neurology: Pearls for Practitioners at the end of this section.

REVIEW QUESTIONS

Available online.

CHAPTER 181

Headache and Migraine

ETIOLOGY AND EPIDEMIOLOGY

Headache is a common symptom among children and adolescents. Primary headaches, such as migraines or tension-type headaches, can cause significant pain but do not require additional evaluation for an underlying cause. Secondary headaches are most often associated with minor illnesses such as upper respiratory infections or sinusitis but may be the first symptom of serious conditions (e.g., meningitis, brain tumors), so a systematic approach is necessary.

CLINICAL MANIFESTATIONS

The temporal pattern (acute, recurrent episodic, chronic progressive, chronic nonprogressive) is useful in the differential diagnosis of headache (Table 181.1).

Tension-type headaches are the most common type of recurrent primary headaches in children and adolescents. Because they are generally mild without associated symptoms, they typically do not disrupt daily activities. The pain is global and squeezing or pressing in character and can last for hours or days. There is no associated nausea or vomiting, and phonophobia or photophobia are uncommon. Headaches can be related to environmental stresses.

Migraine headaches are another common type of recurrent headaches and frequently begin in childhood. Headaches are stereotyped attacks of moderate to severe, pounding or throbbing pain that are aggravated by activity and last 2–72 hours. Associated symptoms include nausea, vomiting, pallor, photophobia, phonophobia, and an intense desire to seek a quiet, dark room for rest. Toddlers may be unable to verbalize the source of their discomfort and exhibit episodes of irritability, sleepiness, pallor, and/or vomiting. An aura can precede or coincide with the headache and typically persists between 5 and 60 minutes. Visual auras are common and consist of spots, flashes, or lines of light that flicker in one or both visual fields. Complex, atypical auras (e.g., hemiparesis, monocular blindness, vertigo, confusion) that are accompanied by a headache warrant careful diagnostic investigation, such as neuroimaging and electroencephalogram.

TABLE 181.1 Four Temporal Patterns of Childhood Headache

Acute: Single episode of pain without a history of such episodes. The "first and worst" headache raises concerns for aneurysmal subarachnoid hemorrhage in adults but is commonly due to febrile illness related to upper respiratory tract infection in children. Regardless, more ominous causes of acute headache (hemorrhage, meningitis, tumor) must be considered.
Acute recurrent: Pattern of attacks of pain separated by symptom-free intervals. Primary headache syndromes, such as migraine or tension-type headache, usually cause this pattern. Recurrent headaches are occasionally due to specific epilepsy syndromes (benign occipital epilepsy), substance use, or recurrent trauma.
Chronic progressive: Implies a gradually increasing frequency and severity of headache. The pathologic correlate is increasing ICP. Causes of this pattern include idiopathic intracranial hypertension, brain tumor, hydrocephalus, chronic meningitis, brain abscess, and subdural collections.
Chronic nonprogressive: Pattern of frequent or constant headache without progression. In chronic migraine or chronic tension-type headache, headaches occur on at least 15 days a month for more than 3 months.

ICP, Intracranial pressure.

Common causes of **secondary headaches** include head trauma, viral illness, and sinusitis. Serious causes of secondary headache include increased intracranial pressure (ICP) caused by a mass (e.g., tumor, vascular malformation) or intrinsic increase in pressure (idiopathic intracranial hypertension). Increased ICP should be suspected if the headache and associated vomiting are worse when lying down or on first awakening, if they awaken the child from sleep, if they remit on arising, or if they are exacerbated by coughing, Valsalva maneuver, or bending over. Papilledema (Fig. 181.1) or focal neurologic deficits should trigger an intensive etiologic investigation.

DIAGNOSTIC STUDIES

For most children, a thorough history and physical examination provide an accurate diagnosis and obviate the need for further testing. Neuroimaging is not necessary to diagnose primary headache disorders. Imaging is warranted, however, if the patient has an abnormal neurologic examination, symptoms of increased ICP, unusual neurologic features during the headache (atypical aura), or progressive worsening of headaches. In these cases, brain magnetic resonance imaging is the study of choice, providing the highest sensitivity for detecting posterior fossa lesions and other, more subtle abnormalities. When the headache has a sudden, severe onset, emergent

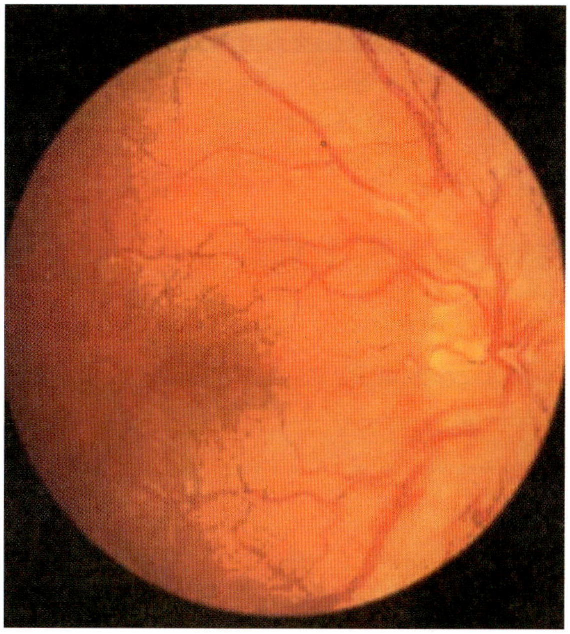

FIGURE 181.1 Papilledema with dilation of the vessels, obliteration of the optic cup, loss of disc margin, and hemorrhages around the disc. (From Kliegman RE, Behrman RM, Jenson HB, eds. *Nelson Textbook of Pediatrics*. 18th ed. Philadelphia: Saunders; 2007:2107.)

computed tomography (CT) can quickly evaluate for intracranial bleeding. If the CT is negative, a lumbar puncture should be performed to measure opening pressure and evaluate for pleocytosis, elevated red blood cells, and xanthochromia as signs of a subarachnoid bleed.

TREATMENT

Treating migraine attacks requires an individually tailored regimen to address the frequency, severity, and disability produced by the headaches. Intermittent symptomatic (abortive) analgesics are the mainstay for treatment of infrequent episodes of migraine. Symptomatic therapy requires early analgesic administration, often accompanied by rest in a quiet, dark room. Nonsteroidal antiinflammatory drugs such as ibuprofen or naproxen sodium are often effective. Because **medication-overuse headaches** may exacerbate primary and secondary headaches, NSAID use should be limited to less than 15 days per month. Hydration and antiemetics are useful adjunctive therapies. If these first-line medications are insufficient, triptan agents may be considered. Triptans, available in injectable, nasal spray, oral disintegrating, and tablet form, are serotonin receptor agonists that can alleviate migraine symptoms promptly. Based on theoretical concerns regarding increased risk for stroke, it is generally recommended that triptans be avoided for patients with hemiplegic migraine or migraine with brainstem aura. Triptan use should be limited to 9 days per month or less to avoid medication-overuse headache.

Children may suffer severe and frequent migraine attacks that disrupt their daily lives. Before initiating daily medications, lifestyle modifications including adequate hydration, regular meals, good sleep hygiene, and routine exercise, as well as identification and management of any precipitating or aggravating influences (e.g., caffeine withdrawal, stress), are beneficial. Other adjunctive treatment options include psychological support, stress management, and biofeedback. Although there are limited data on the effectiveness of nutraceuticals, riboflavin and magnesium may be helpful for migraine prophylaxis with a low side effect profile. Children with more than one disabling headache per week may require **daily preventive agents** to reduce both attack frequency and severity. Preventive medications include tricyclic antidepressants (e.g., amitriptyline, nortriptyline), antiseizure medications (e.g., topiramate, valproic acid), antihistamines (e.g., cyproheptadine), β blockers (e.g., propranolol), and calcium channel blockers (e.g., verapamil). Calcitonin gene-related peptide receptor antagonists are approved for both preventive and abortive migraine therapy in adults but are still being studied in children.

PEARLS FOR PRACTITIONERS

See Neurology: Pearls for Practitioners at the end of this section.

REVIEW QUESTIONS

Available online.

CHAPTER 182
Seizures

A seizure is a transient occurrence of signs or symptoms resulting from abnormal excessive or synchronous neuronal activity in the brain.

ETIOLOGY AND EPIDEMIOLOGY

The differential diagnosis of paroxysmal disorders includes **seizures** and **nonepileptic events** (Table 182.1). Nonepileptic paroxysmal events are often normal or benign phenomena, although some are clinically significant and consequential. A thorough medical history from the patient and primary witnesses is the most reliable tool for establishing the correct diagnosis.

Acute symptomatic seizures are secondary to an acute problem affecting brain excitability, such as electrolyte imbalance or infection (Table 182.2). In the classification of seizures, "symptomatic" refers to seizures that are temporally correlated with an acute neurologic or systemic insult. In contrast, **epilepsy** is defined as recurrent, unprovoked seizures. Epileptic seizures are generally classified as focal, arising from one region of the cortex, or generalized, which arise from both hemispheres simultaneously (Table 182.3). Approximately 4–10% of children experience at least one seizure. The incidence of childhood epilepsy is 1–2%.

FOCAL SEIZURES

Clinical symptoms of focal seizures may include motor (tonic, clonic, myoclonic), sensory, or autonomic abnormalities.

Focal aware seizures (previously termed *simple partial seizures*) arise from a specific anatomic focus and may or may

TABLE 182.1 Paroxysmal Disorders of Childhood

Seizures/epilepsy
Migraine and variants
- Paroxysmal torticollis of infancy
- Benign paroxysmal vertigo
- Cyclic vomiting

Syncope (including vasovagal syncope, cardiac syncope)
Breath-holding spells
Transient ischemic attack
Metabolic disorders
- Hypoglycemia

Sleep disorders (including night terrors, benign sleep myoclonus, narcolepsy)
- Cataplexy

Paroxysmal dyskinesias and other movement disorders
- Tics
- Stereotypies

Shuddering attacks
Sandifer syndrome (gastroesophageal reflux causing paroxysmal stiffening and posturing)
Functional neurologic symptom disorder
Normal behavior
- Neonatal jitteriness
- Daydreaming
- Self-stimulatory behavior

not spread to surrounding brain regions. The location and extent of spread of the seizure focus determine the clinical symptoms.

Focal seizures with impaired awareness (previously termed *complex partial seizures*) can have similar sensorimotor signs but also have associated alteration of consciousness. Although the child may not be completely unresponsive, subtle slowing or alteration of mental status (dyscognitive features) may occur. Along with altered responsiveness, patients may have automatisms or stare during these seizures. **Automatisms** are automatic semipurposeful movements of the mouth (lip smacking, chewing) or extremities (rubbing of fingers, shuffling of feet). Focal seizures that manifest only with autonomic symptoms, such as a feeling of déjà vu during a temporal lobe seizure, can be difficult to recognize.

Focal seizures can spread to involve both cerebral hemispheres and evolve to a bilateral tonic-clonic seizure (previously called a *secondarily generalized seizure*). It is often difficult to distinguish primary generalized tonic-clonic seizures from those that evolved from focal seizures on purely clinical grounds. Clarifying any premonitory symptoms suggestive of an aura can be helpful. This distinction is important because evaluation and treatment for focal or generalized epilepsy syndromes are different.

GENERALIZED SEIZURES

Tonic, **clonic**, and biphasic **tonic-clonic** seizures may occur alone or in association with other seizure types. Typically, the seizure begins abruptly but occasionally is preceded by a series of myoclonic jerks. During a tonic-clonic seizure, consciousness and control of posture are lost, followed by tonic stiffening and upward deviation of the eyes. Loss of bowel or bladder control, pooling of secretions, pupillary dilation, diaphoresis, and hypertension are common. Clonic jerks follow the tonic phase. In the postictal phase, the child might be hypotonic. Irritability and headache are common as the child awakens.

TABLE 182.2 Causes of Seizures

PERINATAL CONDITIONS
Hypoxic-ischemic encephalopathy*
Hemorrhage*
Malformation of cortical development
Intrauterine infection
Trauma
INFECTIONS
Encephalitis*
Meningitis*
Brain abscess
METABOLIC CONDITIONS
Hypoglycemia*
Hypocalcemia
Hypomagnesemia
Hyponatremia
Hypernatremia
Storage diseases
Degenerative disorders
Porphyria
Pyridoxine dependency and deficiency
POISONING
Lead
Medication or substance toxicity
Medication or substance withdrawal
NEUROCUTANEOUS SYNDROMES
Tuberous sclerosis
Neurofibromatosis
Sturge-Weber syndrome
Incontinentia pigmenti
SYSTEMIC DISORDERS
Vasculitis
Systemic lupus erythematosus
Hypertensive encephalopathy
Hepatic encephalopathy
OTHER CAUSATIVE DISORDERS/CONDITIONS
Febrile illnesses*
Accidental trauma*
Child abuse*
Other genetic*
Cryptogenic* (no underlying disorder found)
Increased intracranial pressure
Tumor
Remote brain injury

*Common.

Absence Seizures

Seizures in which the primary clinical feature is staring can be either absence (generalized) or focal seizures. The clinical hallmark of absence seizures is a brief (<15 seconds) loss of awareness accompanied by eyelid fluttering or simple automatisms, such as fumbling with the fingers and lip smacking. The characteristic electroencephalographic (EEG) patterns consist of **generalized 3-Hz spike-and-wave activity**. An absence seizure can often be provoked by **hyperventilation**. Differentiating absence from focal seizures with impaired awareness can be difficult but is essential for appropriate evaluation and treatment (Table 182.4).

Atypical Absence, Myoclonic, and Atonic Seizures

Atypical absence seizures manifest as episodes of impaired consciousness with automatisms, autonomic phenomena, and motor manifestations, such as eye opening, eye deviation, and body stiffening. They are associated with slower EEG discharges (2 Hz) and accompany other seizure types. **Myoclonus** is a sudden jerk of all or part of the body; not all myoclonus is due to epilepsy. Nonepileptic myoclonus may be benign, as in sleep myoclonus, or indicate serious disease. Myoclonic epilepsy usually is associated with multiple seizure types. The underlying disorder producing myoclonic epilepsy may be static (e.g., **juvenile myoclonic epilepsy** [JME]) or progressive and associated with neurologic deterioration (e.g., neuronal ceroid lipofuscinosis). **Myoclonic absence** refers to body jerks that commonly accompany typical or atypical absence seizures. Atonic seizures involve a sudden loss of postural tone that often results in falls and injuries; though typically brief (lasting 1–2 seconds), they can cause significant injury.

TABLE **182.3** Classification of Seizures and Epilepsy Syndromes

FOCAL ONSET
With retained awareness (focal aware seizures) Motor onset (can be automatisms, tonic, clonic, myoclonic, atonic, or epileptic spasms) Nonmotor onset (e.g., autonomic, behavioral arrest, cognitive, emotional, or sensory [such as visual, auditory, olfactory, or gustatory]) With impaired awareness (dyscognitive features) Motor or nonmotor onset (see above) Focal to bilateral tonic-clonic seizures
GENERALIZED ONSET
Motor (can be tonic, clonic, myoclonic, atonic, or epileptic spasms) Nonmotor (absence)
UNKNOWN ONSET
Motor (can be tonic-clonic, epileptic spasms) Nonmotor (behavioral arrest)

Febrile Seizures

Seizures in the setting of fever may be caused by central nervous system infections (meningitis, encephalitis, brain abscess), first presentation of epilepsy triggered by fever, or **febrile seizures**. The latter represents the most common cause of seizures among children between 6 months and 5 years of age, occurring in about 4% of all children. By definition, a febrile seizure occurs in the presence of fever. **Simple febrile seizures** are generalized at onset, last less than 15 minutes, and occur only once in a 24-hour period. If the seizure has focal features, lasts longer than 15 minutes, or recurs within 24 hours, the seizure is referred to as a **complex febrile seizure**.

The prognosis of children with simple febrile seizures is excellent. Although febrile seizures recur in 30–50% of children, intellectual achievements are normal. The risk of subsequent epilepsy is not substantially greater than that of the general population (~2%). Factors that increase the risk for the development of epilepsy include abnormal neurologic examination or development, family history of epilepsy, and complex febrile seizures.

Because simple febrile seizures are brief and the outcome is benign, most children require no treatment. Rectal diazepam can be administered during a seizure to abort a prolonged convulsion; it is appropriate to provide a rescue medication for children with a history of prolonged febrile seizures. Because antiseizure medications have side effects and children with febrile seizures have an excellent prognosis, daily antiseizure medication to prevent febrile seizures is not recommended. Administration of antipyretics during the same fever episode may reduce the risk of recurrence within that illness, but it does not seem to impact febrile seizure recurrence during subsequent fever episodes.

TABLE **182.4** Differentiating Absence Seizures and Focal Seizures With Impaired Awareness

FEATURE	ABSENCE SEIZURE	FOCAL SEIZURE WITH IMPAIRED AWARENESS
Duration	Seconds	Minutes
Provoking maneuver	Hyperventilation Photic stimulation	Variable, but often none
Postictal phase	None (return immediately to baseline)	Confusion, sleepiness
Number of seizures	Many per day	Infrequent (rarely >1/day)
EEG features	Interictal: normal except bursts of generalized spike wave and sometimes occipital intermittent rhythmic delta activity Ictal: 3-Hz generalized spike-wave	Interictal: normal or focal slowing, sharp waves, or spikes Ictal: focal discharges (with or without spread to contiguous regions or the contralateral hemisphere)
Neurologic examination	Normal	Normal, or focal deficits
Neuroimaging	Normal*	Normal, or focal abnormalities (mesial temporal sclerosis, focal cortical dysplasia, neoplasm, encephalomalacia)
First-line treatment	Ethosuximide or valproic acid†	Often levetiracetam, oxcarbazepine, or lamotrigine are used

In the proper clinical context, and with an appropriate EEG, a diagnosis of childhood absence epilepsy can be made without neuroimaging.

†Oxcarbazepine and carbamazepine are relatively contraindicated for children with typical absence epilepsy, because their seizures can be exacerbated by these medications.

EEG, Electroencephalographic.

Psychogenic Nonepileptic Events

Functional neurologic disorders (FNDs) describe when neurologic symptoms occur with no clear underlying disease or neurological pathology. An example of FNDs are **psychogenic nonepileptic events (PNEEs)**. Children with epilepsy may exhibit concurrent PNEE. PNEE semiology typically differs from epileptic seizures. In PNEE, the patient's eyes are often closed and the movements are tremulousness or thrashing. In contrast, during seizures, the eyes are typically open and movements are tonic or clonic. Verbalization and pelvic thrusting are seen more commonly in PNEE, urinary and fecal continence is usually preserved, and injury does not usually occur. If the tongue is bitten, more often the tip of the tongue is injured (as opposed to the sides of the tongue in epileptic seizures). PNEE can often be initiated or terminated by suggestion. An EEG performed during PNEE does not show epileptiform patterns. The diagnosis is critical because appropriate mental health care, and not antiseizure medication, is the crux of treatment. Careful assessment and intervention for social stressors and abuse is a key component of the care of children with PNEE.

EPILEPSY SYNDROMES

Epilepsy syndromes have distinctive EEG and clinical features (age of seizure onset, specific seizure types). Recognition of epilepsy syndromes provides useful information regarding the underlying etiologies that must be considered, treatments that may be helpful (or harmful), and long-term prognostic information. Co-morbid learning difficulties, especially language-based learning disabilities, and attention-deficit/hyperactivity disorder (ADHD) are common. There is no contraindication to treating these children's ADHD with stimulant medication.

Self-limited epilepsy with centrotemporal spikes, also known as childhood epilepsy with centrotemporal spikes or **benign Rolandic epilepsy**, is among the most common epilepsy syndromes and usually begins between ages 5 and 10 years. The seizures typically occur only during sleep or on awakening. Affected children usually have focal motor seizures involving the face and arm (abnormal movement or sensation around the face and mouth, drooling, rhythmic guttural sound, impaired speech and swallowing). Seizures sometimes evolve to bilateral convulsions. The interictal EEG classically demonstrates independent bilateral centrotemporal sharp waves but is otherwise normal. With a classic history, typical EEG, and a normal neurologic examination, the diagnosis can be made with confidence and neuroimaging is not required. Seizures usually respond promptly to antiseizure medication. Intellectual outcome is typically normal, and the epilepsy resolves after puberty.

Childhood absence epilepsy is another common syndrome. Absence seizures typically begin between ages 4 and 10 years and usually resolve by late childhood or adolescence. Neurologic examination is normal, and neuroimaging is not necessary with typical clinical and EEG findings. If absence seizures do not remit, nearly half will go on to develop JME (see later discussion). Ethosuximide is usually the first-choice medication. A subset of patients also has generalized tonic-clonic seizures. For these children, valproic acid is often prescribed because it can prevent both absence and convulsive seizures.

Juvenile myoclonic epilepsy (JME) is the most common generalized epilepsy among adolescents and young adults. Onset is typically in early adolescence with myoclonic jerks (exacerbated in the morning, often causing the patient to drop objects), generalized tonic-clonic seizures, and absence seizures. Seizures usually resolve promptly with antiseizure medication. JME is classically treated with valproic acid; however, there are concerns about side effects and teratogenicity. Levetiracetam has a much lower risk of teratogenicity and is generally well tolerated. As such, levetiracetam is favored, particularly for females because treatment of JME is usually lifelong.

Infantile epileptic spasms syndrome (commonly referred to as **infantile spasms**) involves brief contractions of the neck, trunk, and arm muscles, followed by a phase of sustained muscle contraction lasting less than 2 seconds. Spasms occur most frequently when the child is awakening or going to sleep. Each jerk is followed by a brief period of relaxation with repeated spasms in clusters of variable duration. When flexion of the thighs and crying are prominent, the syndrome may be mistaken for colic or gastroesophageal reflux. **West syndrome** is the triad of infantile spasms, developmental regression, and a dramatically abnormal EEG pattern (**hypsarrhythmia**, a pattern of chaotic high-voltage slow waves, spikes, and polyspikes). The peak age at onset of infantile spasms is 3–8 months. The underlying etiology of the spasms dictates the prognosis. More than 200 different etiologies have been identified, including tuberous sclerosis, malformations of cortical development (e.g., lissencephaly), genetic syndromes (e.g., trisomy 21), acquired brain injury (e.g., stroke, perinatal hypoxic-ischemic encephalopathy), and metabolic disorders (e.g., phenylketonuria). Infants for whom an etiology is determined are classified as having "symptomatic" infantile spasms and are at very high risk for long-term neurodevelopmental difficulties. With advances in genetic testing, few children have infantile spasms of uncertain etiology, but those with uncertain etiology have a somewhat better long-term prognosis.

Infantile spasms are a neurologic emergency because rapid initiation of effective therapy offers the best chance for favorable neurodevelopmental outcomes. First-line treatment options for infantile spasms include adrenocorticotropic hormone, high-dose oral corticosteroids, and vigabatrin. Other antiseizure medications are much less effective. For infants with underlying tuberous sclerosis, vigabatrin is the treatment of choice. For other patients, treatment determinations are made on a case-by-case basis.

Lennox-Gastaut syndrome is a severe epilepsy syndrome with variable age of onset, although most children present before age 5 years. Frequent, multiple seizure types including atonic, focal, atypical absence, and generalized tonic, clonic, or tonic-clonic semiologies characterize the disorder. Many children have underlying brain injury, malformations, or genetic etiologies. The seizures are typically difficult to control, and most patients have significant intellectual disability.

Self-limited (familial) neonatal epilepsy (previously called *benign neonatal convulsions*) is an autosomal dominant genetic disorder (pathogenic variant of *KCNQ2* or *KCNQ3*) linked to abnormal neuronal potassium channels. Otherwise well newborns present with focal seizures toward the end of the first week of life, leading to the other colloquial term, *fifth-day fits*. Response to treatment is generally excellent, and the long-term outcome is typically favorable.

Acquired epileptic aphasia (Landau-Kleffner syndrome) may be linked to pathogenic variants in *GRIN2A* and is characterized by the abrupt loss of previously acquired language in young children. The language disability is an acquired cortical auditory deficit (auditory agnosia). The EEG is highly epileptiform in sleep, the peak area of abnormality often being in the dominant perisylvian region (language areas). This diagnosis should be considered for young patients with clear language regression, because it is potentially treatable with antiepileptic medications.

FEBRILE EPILEPSY SYNDROMES

Some forms of epilepsy are intrinsically linked to fever. **Dravet syndrome** is primarily caused by pathogenic variants in the *SCN1A* gene and is an epileptic encephalopathy with seizures often triggered by high body temperature. **Febrile Infection-Related Epilepsy Syndrome (FIRES)** is prolonged refractory status epilepticus (acute phase, 1–12 weeks) in otherwise healthy children after febrile illness, which is then followed by a chronic phase with refractory seizure activity clustered every 2–4 weeks. There is no known cause and limited treatments.

STATUS EPILEPTICUS

Status epilepticus is a neurologic emergency defined as (1) ongoing seizure activity for 5 or more minutes or (2) repetitive seizures without recovery of consciousness. Status epilepticus carries an approximately 14% risk of new neurologic deficits and 4–5% mortality, both related to the underlying etiology. Etiologies include new-onset epilepsy, drug intoxication, drug withdrawal (especially missed antiseizure medication doses among children with epilepsy), hypoglycemia, electrolyte imbalance, acute head trauma, infectious and autoimmune encephalitis, ischemic stroke, intracranial hemorrhage, metabolic disorders, and hypoxia.

The first priority of treatment is to ensure adequate airway, breathing, and circulation (see Chapter 37). Vital signs should be obtained and oxygen administered as needed. If respirations are inadequate, positive pressure ventilation may be required. Intravenous (IV) access should be obtained, and laboratory evaluation should be undertaken.

Several pharmacologic options exist for management of status epilepticus (Table 182.5). Initial management is with a benzodiazepine and should be administered if the seizure persists longer than 5 minutes. Lorazepam, diazepam, and midazolam are all effective agents and should be given as an adequate single dose (rather than successive smaller doses), which can be repeated one time. IV administration is preferred. When IV access is not available, benzodiazepines may be administered via rectal, intranasal, buccal, or intramuscular routes.

If the seizure does not resolve after two doses of benzodiazepine, a second-line agent must be administered. For newborns, phenobarbital is typically used. For older children, IV fosphenytoin (preferred over phenytoin due to tolerability), levetiracetam, and valproic acid show similar efficacy; lacosamide or phenobarbital may also be considered. If the seizures persist, options include repeating one of the second-line medications or beginning a continuous infusion of midazolam or pentobarbital (with appropriate airway protection, blood pressure support, and strong consideration of video-EEG monitoring to evaluate for ongoing subclinical seizures). If this approach is ineffective, preparations for general anesthesia are undertaken.

TABLE 182.5 Management of Status Epilepticus

STABILIZATION
ABCs (airway, breathing, circulation)
Cardiac monitoring
Oxygen and pulse oximetry
Intravenous access
Immediate laboratory tests
Glucose
Basic metabolic panel—sodium, calcium, magnesium
Antiseizure medication levels
Toxicology studies as appropriate
Complete blood counts, platelets, and differential
PHARMACOLOGIC MANAGEMENT
Benzodiazepine
Lorazepam IV, IM, IN
Diazepam IV, IM, IN, rectal
Midazolam IV, IM, IN, buccal
Standard antiseizure medications
Fosphenytoin IV, IM
Valproic acid IV
Levetiracetam IV
Phenobarbital IV
Lacosamide IV
Continuous infusions
Pentobarbital
Midazolam
General anesthesia

IM, Intramuscularly; *IN*, intranasally; *IV*, intravenous.

LABORATORY AND DIAGNOSTIC EVALUATION

Children with simple febrile seizures who have recovered completely require little or no laboratory evaluation other than studies necessary to evaluate the source of the fever. Outside of simple febrile seizures, it is important to consider possible provoking factors for a first lifetime seizure, such as meningitis, sepsis, head trauma, metabolic abnormalities (including hypoglycemia, hyper- or hyponatremia, and hypocalcemia), and toxins. Laboratory evaluation for a new-onset seizure may include a complete blood count and measurement of glucose, calcium, sodium, potassium, chloride, bicarbonate, urea nitrogen, creatinine, magnesium, and phosphorus, as well as blood or urine toxicology screening. For an otherwise healthy child with a single self-resolved seizure and a normal examination, in the absence of history to suggest a provoking etiology, laboratory evaluation may not be necessary. Children with clinical signs and symptoms of meningitis (e.g., fever, neck rigidity, Kernig sign, Brudzinski sign), or history or physical examination suggestive of intracranial infection, should undergo a lumbar puncture. CSF should be analyzed for cell counts, culture, protein, and glucose levels. In children <18 months old, particularly young infants, the clinical symptoms of meningitis may be subtle. Neonates also may require testing for inborn errors of metabolism, blood ammonia, CSF glycine and lactate, and a clinical trial of intravenous pyridoxine. Evaluation for infections, such as urine and stool cultures, and polymerase chain reactions for herpes simplex virus, cytomegalovirus, and enterovirus should be considered.

The **EEG** is the most useful neurodiagnostic test for distinguishing seizures from nonepileptic paroxysmal disorders and for classifying seizures as having focal or generalized onset. The EEG must be interpreted in the context of the clinical history; some normal children have focal or epileptiform EEG patterns. Conversely, children with seizures may have normal interictal EEGs. When the diagnosis is unclear, EEG with prolonged recordings and simultaneous video monitoring in an attempt to capture a typical event may be necessary.

Magnetic resonance imaging (MRI) is superior to computed tomography (CT) in showing most brain pathology, but in the emergency department setting, CT can be performed rapidly and often shows acute intracranial hemorrhage more clearly than MRI. MRI is unnecessary in patients with primary generalized epilepsies, such as typical childhood absence epilepsy and JME. Lesions (e.g., tumors, arteriovenous malformations, cysts, strokes, gliosis, focal atrophy) may be identified in 25% of patients with other epilepsy types, even when the clinical examination and EEG do not suggest focal features. Identification of some lesions, such as focal cortical dysplasia, hamartoma, and mesial temporal sclerosis, can assist in consideration of surgical treatment of pharmacoresistant epilepsy.

LONG-TERM THERAPY

The decision to institute daily antiseizure medications for a first unprovoked seizure is based on the likelihood of recurrence balanced against the risk of long-term drug therapy. Determination of the recurrence risk is based on the clinical history and neurodiagnostic testing. Absence seizures, infantile spasms, and atonic seizures are universally recurrent at the time of diagnosis, so treatment should be initiated immediately.

The goal of treatment is to maintain an optimal functional state. Medication toxicity should be weighed against the risk of the seizures. Initial drug selection is based on the seizure type (Fig. 182.1). Using a single agent limits toxicity, contains cost, and improves adherence. Approximately 60% of children obtain satisfactory seizure control and minimal side effects with the initial medication. If seizure control is not achieved, despite good adherence, addition of a second medication is considered.

The duration of antiseizure medication treatment varies according to seizure type and epilepsy syndrome. For most children, medications can be weaned off after 2 years without seizures. There are some exceptions. For example, children with JME, progressive myoclonic epilepsy, atypical absence seizures, and Lennox-Gastaut syndrome usually require lifelong treatment. Children who have other neurologic comorbidities, seizures that were initially difficult to control, or persistently epileptiform EEGs are at highest risk for recurrence when therapy is discontinued.

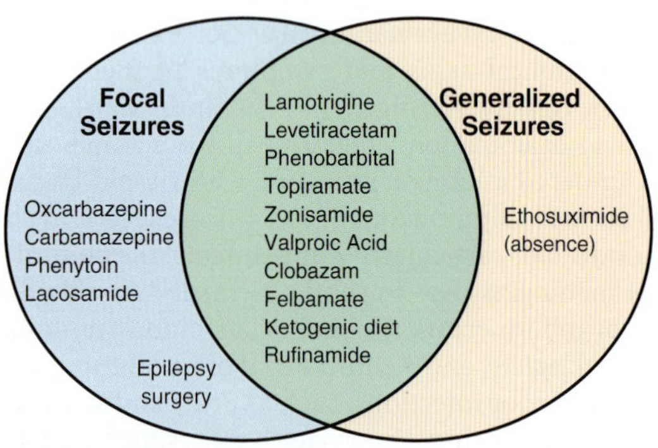

Special circumstances:
1. For absence epilepsy, ethosuximide is the first line treatment.
2. Adrenocorticotropic hormone, oral corticosteroids, or vigabatrin are used to treat infantile spasms.

FIGURE 182.1 Treatment for epilepsy.

There are important safety considerations for people with epilepsy. The risk of drowning is high, so swimming and bathing must only occur under direct adult supervision. Children should use appropriate helmets for sports such as bicycling or ice skating. There is no contraindication to participation in contact sports, but scuba diving, hang gliding, and free climbing are not safe for people with epilepsy. Each country and individual states have specific laws regarding driving for people with epilepsy. Most require a period of seizure freedom before driving.

PEARLS FOR PRACTITIONERS

See Neurology: Pearls for Practitioners at the end of this section.

REVIEW QUESTIONS

Available online.

CHAPTER 183
Weakness and Hypotonia

Weakness is a decreased ability to voluntarily move muscles. This may be generalized or localized to one aspect of the body. Hypotonia is a state of low muscle resistance to movement. Hypotonia can be associated with weakness but in some cases is present with normal motor strength. The differential diagnosis for weakness is extensive (Table 183.1).

ETIOLOGY

Weakness and hypotonia may be due to disorders of **upper** or **lower motor neurons**. Upper motor neurons originate in the cerebral motor cortex; their axons form the corticospinal tract and end in the spinal cord, controlling voluntary motor activity. The anterior horn cells, their motor roots, peripheral motor nerves, neuromuscular junctions, and muscles represent the lower motor neurons and muscle units. Maintenance of normal strength, tone, and coordination requires integrated communication throughout this complex system, including the cerebral cortex, thalamus, basal ganglia, cerebellum, brainstem, and spinal cord.

CLINICAL MANIFESTATIONS

Weakness caused by upper motor neuron disease differs from weakness produced by lower motor units (Table 183.2). Dysfunction of the upper motor neuron causes loss of voluntary control but not total loss of movement because motor nuclei of the basal ganglia, thalamus, and brainstem have tracts that produce simple or complex stereotyped patterns of movement. The corticospinal tract permits fine motor activity and is best tested

TABLE 183.1 Disorders Causing Weakness in Infants and Children

ANATOMIC REGION	CORRESPONDING DISORDERS
Central nervous system—brain	Brain tumor Trauma (accidental, nonaccidental) Infection (meningitis, encephalitis, abscess, congenital infection) Ischemia (arterial or venous) Hemorrhage Demyelinating disease (ADEM, MS) Metabolic disease (leukodystrophy; inborn error of metabolism; mitochondrial encephalomyopathy, lactic acidosis, and strokelike episodes) Degenerative disease Hemiplegic migraine Toxins Electrolyte disorders Functional neurologic symptom disorder
Central nervous system—spinal cord	Transverse myelitis Neuromyelitis optica spectrum disorder (NMOSD) tumor Abscess Trauma Infarction Myelomeningocele Tethered cord
Anterior horn cell	Spinal muscular atrophy Poliomyelitis Acute flaccid myelitis (AFM)
Peripheral nerve	Guillain-Barré syndrome Hereditary motor sensory neuropathy Tick paralysis Bell palsy
Neuromuscular junction	Myasthenia gravis (juvenile, transient neonatal, congenital) Botulism
Muscle	Muscular dystrophies (Duchenne, Becker, limb-girdle) Myotonic dystrophies Congenital myopathies Metabolic myopathies Dermatomyositis Polymyositis Myositis/rhabdomyolysis

ADEM, Acute disseminated encephalomyelitis; *MS*, multiple sclerosis.

by fine movements of the distal extremities. In the acute phase, upper motor neuron disorders cause hypotonia and decreased deep tendon reflexes. Over time, however, spasticity and hyperreflexia develop. A central lesion usually results in weakness that is more pronounced in the flexors of the lower extremities than in the extensors, so affected patients tend to be spastic with legs extended and adducted. In the upper extremities, the extensors are weaker than flexors, so elbows and wrists are flexed.

TABLE 183.2 Clinical Distinction Between Upper Motor Neuron and Lower Motor Neuron Lesions

CLINICAL SIGN	UPPER MOTOR NEURON (CORTICOSPINAL TRACT)	LOWER MOTOR NEURON (NEUROMUSCULAR)
Tone	Increased (spastic)	Decreased
Reflexes	Increased	Decreased
Babinski reflex	Present	Absent
Atrophy	Possible from disuse	Common and usually more prominent
Fasciculations	Absent	Possible

Damage to the spinal cord leaves residual simple, stereotyped reflex movements coordinated by local spinal reflexes below the level of the lesion.

Destruction of the lower motor neuron, the final common pathway producing muscle activity, leads to hypotonia and absence of movement. Function is best tested by measuring the strength of individual muscle groups or, in a young child, by observing the ability to perform functional tasks requiring particular muscle groups (walk up or down stairs, rise from the ground, walk on toes or heels, raise the hands above the head, squeeze a ball). With lower motor neuron disorders, atrophy and fasciculations are common and deep tendon reflexes are typically decreased or absent.

DISEASE OF THE UPPER MOTOR NEURON

Etiology and Epidemiology

Tumors, trauma, central nervous system (CNS) infections, stroke, demyelinating syndromes (such as multiple sclerosis, transverse myelitis, acute disseminated encephalomyelitis [ADEM]), metabolic diseases, and neurodegenerative diseases may injure the brain or spinal cord, producing an upper motor neuron pattern of weakness coupled with increased deep tendon reflexes, spasticity, and extensor plantar responses (Babinski sign). In neonates, weakness with upper motor neuron patterns may be caused by congenital infections (see Chapter 65), developmental brain anomalies, hemorrhage, stroke, hypoxia, genetic syndromes, metabolic/electrolyte disturbances, or toxic exposure.

The distribution of weakness depends on the location of the lesion. A tumor in the left frontal region may produce a right hemiparesis. A brainstem glioma may produce a slowly progressive quadriparesis.

Acute disseminated encephalomyelitis (ADEM) is an acute, inflammatory demyelinating disorder that may affect infants and children after a febrile illness. Children may present with a variety of symptoms and signs including monocular vision loss (e.g., acute optic neuritis), hemiparesis, ataxia, seizures, headache, weakness, or dysphagia. The pathophysiology mimics that of multiple sclerosis, except children with ADEM also have encephalopathy. Although multiple sclerosis is most commonly diagnosed in adulthood, childhood cases have been increasingly recognized. ADEM and multiple sclerosis exacerbations are treated with high-dose steroids. Physical and occupational therapies are often helpful.

Acute spinal cord lesions, such as infarction or compression, may produce a **flaccid, areflexic paralysis** that mimics lower motor neuron disease. The hallmarks of spinal cord disease are a sensory level and a motor level of impairment, disturbance of bowel and bladder function, and local spinal pain or tenderness. Patients may be bradycardic and hypotensive due to neurogenic shock. A child who exhibits an acute or subacute flaccid paraparesis is most likely to have an acute cord syndrome or Guillain-Barré syndrome. Acute cord syndrome may be due to a spinal cord injury causing compression, contusion or shear injury to the cord, ischemia, tumors (e.g., neuroblastoma, lymphoma, sarcoma), or space-occupying infections such as epidural abscesses. In addition to neurologic deficits, patients with epidural abscesses often have fever and spinal pain. Compression of the cord may require immediate neurosurgical management to preserve vital function. Other causes of weakness localized to the spine are **transverse myelitis**, an acute postinfectious demyelinating disorder of the spinal cord that is treated with high-dose steroids and **neuromyelitis optica spectrum disorder** (NMOSD), causing demyelination of the optic nerve and spinal cord.

DISEASES OF THE LOWER MOTOR NEURON

Neuromuscular disease affects component(s) of the lower motor neuron unit. The distribution of muscle weakness can point toward specific diseases (Table 183.3).

TABLE 183.3 Topography of Neuromuscular Diseases

LOCATION	CLINICAL SYNDROMES/ DISORDERS
Proximal muscle weakness	Muscular dystrophy (Duchenne/Becker/limb-girdle) Spinal muscular atrophy Myopathies/dermatomyositis/ polymyositis
Distal limb weakness	Polyneuropathy (Guillain-Barré syndrome) Hereditary motor sensory neuropathy Myotonic dystrophy Distal myopathy
Ophthalmoplegia and limb weakness	Myasthenia gravis Botulism Myotonic dystrophy Congenital myotubular myopathy Miller Fisher variant of Guillain-Barré syndrome
Facial and bulbar weakness	Myasthenia gravis Botulism Polio Miller Fisher variant of Guillain-Barré syndrome Myotonic dystrophy Congenital myopathy Facioscapulohumeral dystrophy

Spinal Muscular Atrophy

Etiology

Progressive degeneration of anterior horn cells is the key manifestation of spinal muscular atrophy (SMA), a genetic disease with signs and symptoms that may begin in intrauterine life or any time thereafter. Over half of patients have a severe infantile form (SMA type 1/**Werdnig-Hoffmann disease**). Other forms include a late infantile and more slowly progressive form (SMA type 2/**Kugelberg-Welander syndrome**) and a more chronic, juvenile form (SMA type 3). SMA is one of the most frequent autosomal recessive diseases, with a carrier frequency of 1 in 50.

Clinical Manifestations

The earlier in life the signs develop, the more severe the progression. Infants with SMA type 1 present in early infancy with severe hypotonia, generalized weakness, and facial involvement. Infants have normal cognitive, social, and language skills and sensation. **Fasciculations** are best identified by inspecting the tongue when the child is asleep. Deep tendon reflexes are absent. With disease progression, breathing patterns change. Weak intercostal muscles and a relatively stronger diaphragm result in a collapsed chest wall (bell-shaped chest) and prominent abdominal movements with rapid, shallow breathing. In an extremely weak child, respiratory compromise leads to atelectasis, pulmonary infection, and death. Without treatment, most infants with SMA type 1 die within the first 2 years. Early detection and early therapeutic intervention facilitated by universal state newborn screening in the United States have altered the natural history of this disease.

Laboratory and Diagnostic Studies

The diagnosis of SMA is made by genetic testing, most commonly linked to a pathogenic variant in the *SMN1* gene. Creatine phosphokinase (CK) may be normal or mildly elevated.

Treatment

Three disease-modifying therapies are available: nusinersen, an antisense oligonucleotide given by intermittent intrathecal injections; onasemnogene abeparvovec, a gene therapy administered as a one-time intravenous infusion; and risdiplam, a small molecule given as a daily oral medication. Clinical trials have shown motor benefits and widespread administration of these medications in clinical practice demonstrate a change in the trajectory of the disease. Preventive care is directed toward minimizing contractures, preventing scoliosis, optimizing nutrition, and avoiding infections. Many patients benefit from early use of noninvasive ventilation to reduce infections. Respiratory infections are managed early and aggressively with preventative pulmonary hygiene and antibiotics. The use or nonuse of artificial ventilation and tube feedings must be individualized for each patient in each stage of the illness.

Acute Flaccid Myelitis

Another cause of weakness is **acute flaccid myelitis (AFM)**, a rapid-onset flaccid weakness with gray matter involvement of the spine, sometimes with cranial nerve impairment, occurring 1–2 weeks after a febrile viral illness. Multiple viral infections have been associated with AFM, including enterovirus D68 and A71. Clinically, this presents similarly to **poliomyelitis**, an infectious cause of life-threatening paralysis in children precipitated by viral destruction of anterior horn cells in the brainstem and spinal cord, although polio virus has not been isolated from individuals affected by AFM. Lesions of the spinal cord are best delineated with magnetic resonance imaging (MRI).

Peripheral Neuropathy

There are many peripheral nerve diseases in childhood, but the most classic presentations are Guillain-Barré syndrome, chronic inflammatory demyelinating polyneuropathy (CIDP), hereditary motor sensory neuropathy (HMSN), and tick paralysis. Peripheral neuropathies due to diabetes mellitus, alcoholism, chronic renal failure, exposure to toxins, vasculitis, and neoplasm are common in adults but rare in children.

Guillain-Barré Syndrome

Guillain-Barré syndrome is an immune-mediated, heterogeneous peripheral neuropathy syndrome with several variants, the most common being **acute inflammatory demyelinating polyradiculoneuropathy (AIDP)**. AIDP classically occurs about 10 days after a respiratory or gastrointestinal infection (e.g., *Mycoplasma pneumoniae* or *Campylobacter jejuni*). It is the most common cause of acute flaccid paralysis in children. A cranial nerve variant of Guillain-Barré syndrome called the **Miller Fisher variant** manifests with ataxia, partial ophthalmoplegia, and areflexia.

The characteristic symptoms of AIDP are areflexia, flaccidity, and symmetric ascending weakness. Progression can occur rapidly, in hours, or more indolently over weeks. Typically, symptoms start with numbness or paresthesia in the hands and feet, then a heavy, weak feeling in the legs. Weakness ascends to involve the arms, trunk, and bulbar muscles (tongue, pharynx, larynx). Deep tendon reflexes are absent even when strength may be relatively preserved. Objective signs of sensory loss are usually minor compared with the dramatic weakness, but many patients experience pain. Bulbar and respiratory insufficiency may progress rapidly. Dysfunction of autonomic nerves can lead to hyper- or hypotension, tachycardia or bradycardia, urinary retention or incontinence, or stool retention. This polyneuropathy can be difficult to distinguish from acute spinal cord syndrome. Loss of arm reflexes, absence of a sensory level, and lack of spinal tenderness point toward Guillain-Barré syndrome.

The cerebrospinal fluid in Guillain-Barré syndrome is sometimes normal early in the illness but classically shows elevated protein levels without significant pleocytosis (albuminocytologic dissociation). MRI with gadolinium may reveal enhancement of the spinal nerve roots. Electromyography (EMG) and nerve conduction velocity are not always required but can provide corroborative diagnostic evidence and prognostic indicators.

Children in early stages of the disease should be admitted to the hospital to monitor pulmonary and cardiac functions. Those with moderate, severe, or rapidly progressive weakness should be treated in an intensive care unit. Endotracheal intubation is required by patients with impending respiratory failure or an inability to clear secretions. Most patients are treated initially with intravenous immunoglobulin (IVIG). Plasma exchange is an alternative option. Physical, occupational, and speech therapies are mainstays of treatment.

The illness usually resolves spontaneously, albeit slowly; 80% of patients recover normal function within 1–12 months. Twenty percent of patients are left with mild to moderate residual weakness.

Chronic Inflammatory Demyelinating Polyneuropathy

A small minority of patients who initially present with Guillain-Barré syndrome will have a relapsing course and will ultimately be diagnosed with CIDP. CIDP is an immune-mediated peripheral neuropathy typically presenting as both proximal and distal weakness in an episodic, relapsing-remitting pattern. Patients may also experience sensation changes such as numbness, tingling, or pain. The diagnosis is clinical, although EMG or nerve biopsy may confirm the diagnosis. The mainstays of treatment for CIDP are IVIG, glucocorticoids, and plasmapheresis.

Hereditary Motor Sensory Neuropathy

HMSN (also called **Charcot-Marie-Tooth disease** [CMT]) is a group of inherited, progressive, distal peripheral nerve diseases. Motor components generally dominate the clinical picture, with sensation and autonomic functions affected later. Some subtypes present with severe symptoms starting in infancy, whereas other forms may have milder symptoms. It is possible to have more than one type of HMSN if a child inherits more than one disease-causing genetic variant.

Most often, complaints begin in the preschool to early adolescent years, with weakness of the ankles and frequent tripping. Examination shows **pes cavus deformity of the feet** (high-arched feet), bilateral weakness of foot dorsiflexors, and normal sensation despite occasional complaints of paresthesia. Progression of HMSN is slow, extending over years and decades. Eventually, patients may develop weakness and atrophy of the entire lower legs and hands with mild to moderate sensory loss in the hands and feet. There is variable severity between types of HMSN and even within families affected by the same type. Some patients never have more than a mild foot deformity, loss of ankle reflexes, and electrophysiologic abnormalities. Others in the same family may need to use a wheelchair and have difficulties performing everyday tasks with their hands.

HMSN can be characterized by demyelination (e.g., CMT1) or axonal (e.g., CMT2) damage. Specific genetic testing is available for many subtypes of HMSN. Specific treatment for HMSN is not available, but braces that maintain the feet in dorsiflexion can maintain function and reduce the risk of injury.

Tick Paralysis

Tick paralysis produces an acute lower motor neuron pattern of weakness, clinically similar to Guillain-Barré syndrome. An attached female tick releases a toxin, similar to botulism, blocking neuromuscular transmission. Affected patients present with a severe generalized flaccid weakness, including ocular and bulbar paralysis. A methodic search for an affixed tick, particularly in hairy areas, must be made in any child with acute weakness. Removal of the tick results in a prompt return of motor function.

Myasthenia Gravis

There are different conditions called myasthenia. Each has a different mechanism. These include juvenile myasthenia gravis seen in late infancy and childhood, transient neonatal myasthenia seen after birth, and congenital myasthenic syndrome seen in infancy through childhood.

Juvenile Myasthenia

Juvenile myasthenia gravis is an autoimmune condition. Most commonly, antibodies block the acetylcholine receptors (AChRs) at the neuromuscular junction, decreasing the number of effective receptors, which results in rapid fatigability of striated muscle; other types of autoantibodies exist. The cardinal feature of myasthenia gravis is fluctuating skeletal muscle weakness. Rapid fatigue of muscles distinguishes myasthenia from other neuromuscular disorders, with progressive worsening over the day or with repetitive activity and improvement after rest. Although myasthenia can produce weakness in any muscle group, variable ptosis, diplopia, ophthalmoplegia, and facial weakness are typical presenting symptoms. There can be any degree of involvement. In some children, the disease never advances beyond ophthalmoplegia and ptosis **(ocular myasthenia)**. Others may have a progressive and potentially life-threatening illness that involves all musculature, including that of respiration and swallowing. Treatment includes pyridostigmine (an acetylcholinesterase inhibitor) and, depending on severity, various forms of immunosuppression.

Transient Neonatal Myasthenia Gravis

A transient myasthenic syndrome develops in the first hours to days after birth in neonates born to birth parents with myasthenia gravis related to maternal anti-AChR antibodies. Almost all infants born to birth parents with myasthenia have maternal anti-AChR antibodies, but only 10–20% will develop signs. Signs include weak facial movements, poor feeding, hypotonia, respiratory difficulty, and variable extremity weakness; ptosis and ophthalmoplegia can also occur but are less common. Neonates with transient myasthenia gravis require cholinesterase inhibitors and supportive care for a few days to weeks until the weakness remits. Importantly, these neonates can have symptoms of transient neonatal myasthenia gravis even if the birth parent does not have current symptoms of myasthenia gravis.

Congenital Myasthenic Syndromes

A variety of rare disorders of the neuromuscular junction have been reported that are not autoimmune mediated. The congenital myasthenic syndromes (CMS) are due to pathogenic gene variants in the components of the neuromuscular junction (more than half of cases caused by variants of the *CHRNE* gene). They typically present in infancy with hypotonia, extremity weakness, ptosis, facial diplegia, and sometimes ophthalmoplegia, although symptoms can present throughout childhood. Respiratory function and feeding may be compromised. Children with CMS usually have lifelong disability. Treatment of CMS depends on the type; some types can respond to pyridostigmine or other drugs that improve neuromuscular junction function, whereas other types can be exacerbated by pyridostigmine.

Diagnostic Studies

Autoimmune myasthenia is most commonly diagnosed through the combination of clinical symptoms and antibody testing. The majority of individuals have antibodies to the AChR, although some have antibodies to other components of the neuromuscular junction. Nerve conduction studies classically reveal an electrodecrement with 3-Hz repetitive stimulation. An ice pack test (applying an ice pack to a closed eyelid) may lead to transient improvement in ptosis, but this can be difficult to interpret.

Infant Botulism

Infant botulism results from intestinal infection by *Clostridium botulinum*, which produces a neurotoxin that blocks presynaptic cholinergic transmission. Young age and the absence of competitive bowel flora predispose infants to this disease. Infants may ingest dust, soil, or food (e.g., honey, poorly canned foods) contaminated with spores. The progressive neuromuscular blockade ranges from mild to severe. Infants typically present with constipation and poor feeding. Hypotonia and weakness develop progressively, along with cranial nerve dysfunction manifested by decreased gag reflex, diminished eye movements, decreased pupillary contraction, and ptosis. Autonomic dysfunction can result in fluctuations in heart rate and blood pressure. Severely affected infants may develop respiratory failure. The diagnosis is made by detecting *C. botulinum* spores and toxin in stool samples. Therapy with botulism immune globulin should be administered as soon as the diagnosis is suspected. With prompt treatment and respiratory and supportive care, the prognosis is good.

Muscular Dystrophy

Muscular dystrophies are a group of genetic muscle diseases characterized by progressive myofiber degeneration and the gradual replacement of muscle by fibrotic tissue.

Etiology

Duchenne muscular dystrophy (DMD) is an X-linked disorder (Xp21) that arises from a pathogenic genetic variant in the dystrophin gene. It is the most common muscular dystrophy; approximately 1 in 3,500 males is affected. **Becker muscular dystrophy** also involves the dystrophin gene but is associated with more mild symptoms due to a semifunctional dystrophin protein.

Clinical Manifestations

Typically, at about 2–3 years of age, males with DMD develop a waddling gait and an inability to run properly. Some have an antecedent history of mild delay in attaining motor milestones or poor head control during infancy. Examination shows firm pseudohypertrophy of the calves and mild to moderate proximal leg weakness with a hyperlordotic, waddling gait. The child typically arises from a lying position on the floor by using the arms to climb up the legs and body **(Gower sign)**. By 12 years of age, most males are not walking and use a wheelchair full time. Other manifestations include cardiomyopathy, scoliosis, respiratory decline, and variable cognitive and behavioral dysfunction. In the past, most people with DMD died in their 20s or early 30s, usually as a result of progressive respiratory decline or cardiac dysfunction; life expectancy may increase with current therapies.

Laboratory and Diagnostic Studies

Serum CK levels are always markedly elevated. Diagnosis is established by testing for a pathogenic variant in the dystrophin gene. Approximately one third of cases represent sporadic genetic changes. Prenatal genetic testing is possible, and newborn screening for elevated CK is available in some states.

Treatment

Chronic oral steroid therapy delays motor disability and improves longevity by preventing cardiac and pulmonary decline, even after a male stops ambulating. Supportive care includes physical therapy, bracing, proper wheelchairs, and treatment of cardiac dysfunction and sleep-related hypoventilation. Several exon-skipping medications are Food and Drug Administration (FDA) approved. They are indicated for use with specific dystrophin variants; one version of gene therapy, administered via intravenous infusion of a microdystrophin protein, is approved by the FDA.

Myotonic Dystrophy

Etiology and Epidemiology

Myotonic dystrophy (often abbreviated DM in reference to its Greek name, *dystrophia myotonica*) is the second most common muscular dystrophy and the most common form to present in adulthood. An autosomal dominant disease, DM is caused by progressive expansion of a triplet repeat, CTG, in the DM protein kinase gene. Presentation is roughly correlated with the number of CTG repeats: higher repeats result in more severe symptoms and younger age of onset. The disease is characterized by genetic anticipation in which each generation presents with an increased number of CTG repeats and therefore earlier and more severe symptoms.

Clinical Manifestations

Although DM most typically presents in adulthood, it can present at any age. Clinical features of childhood-onset "classic" DM include slowly progressive facial and distal extremity weakness as well as **myotonia**. Myotonia is delayed muscle relaxation after contraction. When patients grasp onto an object, they have difficulty releasing their grasp and may appear to peel their fingers away slowly. The facial appearance is characteristic, with hollowing of muscles around temples, jaw, and neck; ptosis; facial weakness; and drooping of the lower lip. Not only is the striated muscle affected but smooth muscle of the gastrointestinal tract and cardiac muscle are involved. Patients have variable arrhythmias, endocrinopathies, immunologic deficiencies, hypoventilation during sleep, and cataracts. Most patients with DM have intellectual disability, and those with congenital DM are more severely impacted.

A severe **congenital myotonic dystrophy** can appear in infants of genetic parents with DM because of rapid expansion of the CTG repeat length. Infants are immobile and hypotonic, with ptosis, absence of sucking and Moro reflexes, poor feeding, and respiratory difficulties. Often, weakness and atony of uterine smooth muscle during labor lead to associated hypoxic ischemic encephalopathy and its sequelae, which make the clinical diagnosis more difficult. The presence of congenital contractures, clubfoot, or a history of poor fetal movements indicates intrauterine neuromuscular disease. Individuals with congenital DM often make significant gains in terms of motor skills, and many children eventually ambulate independently.

Other Forms of Childhood Muscle Disease

Congenital muscular dystrophies (CMDs) refer to a group of genetically determined conditions that present in infancy or early childhood. The most common subtypes include merosin-deficient CMD, Ullrich CMD, and the dystroglycanopathies. The characteristic clinical features include hypotonia, extremity weakness, delayed motor development, and congenital contractures. Contractures and scoliosis are often progressive and severely worsen; respiratory status diminishes with age. An elevated CK is typical. Diagnosis is established through genetic testing; very rarely muscle biopsy is utilized.

Emery-Dreifuss muscular dystrophy (EDMD), also known as humeroperoneal muscular dystrophy, typically begins in childhood. Patients may experience early contractures, slowly progressive humeroperoneal muscle weakness or wasting, and cardiac disease with conduction defects and arrhythmias. EDMD is associated with mild elevations of serum CK levels and abnormal electrocardiograms (ECGs). There are no disease-specific modifying therapies for EDMD; early placement of defibrillators in patients with abnormal ECGs reduces the incidence of sudden death.

Several forms of **limb-girdle muscular dystrophy** (LGMD) have been described. Most are inherited in an autosomal recessive pattern, but autosomal dominant forms exist as well. Depending on the subtype of LGMD, presentation can be throughout childhood. LGMD primarily affects muscles of the hip and shoulder girdles. Distal muscles may later become weak and atrophic; some forms are more likely to have progressive cardiac and respiratory failure.

Facioscapulohumeral dystrophy is an autosomal dominant myopathy. Weakness first appears in the facial and shoulder girdle muscles. Shoulder weakness results in the characteristic observation of scapular winging, which can often be asymmetric. Patients have mild ptosis, a decrease in facial expression, inability to pucker the lips or close eyes during sleep, neck weakness, difficulty in fully elevating the arms, and thinness of upper arm musculature (i.e., deltoid muscles).

Congenital myopathies (CMs) are a group of nondystrophic muscle disorders that, like CMDs, most typically present in infancy with hypotonia and weakness. Additional signs and symptoms include congenital contractures, hip subluxation/dislocation, small/atrophic muscles, thin body habitus, and characteristic facial appearance (the "myopathic facies" appears expressionless with sunken cheeks, ptosis, and inability to move the corners of the mouth). Symptoms are often nonprogressive or only slowly progressive, although children often have severe lifelong disabilities including severe scoliosis, respiratory failure, and weakness for which they use wheelchairs. Histopathologic subtypes are distinguished by characteristic features on muscle biopsy, the most common being nemaline myopathy, centronuclear myopathy, and core myopathy. More commonly genetic testing is used for diagnosis. No specific therapies currently exist for any CM subtype.

Metabolic Myopathies

Glycogen storage disease type II (Pompe disease) and muscle carnitine deficiency are discussed in Chapters 51 and 54, respectively. **Several mitochondrial myopathies** may present with hypotonia, ophthalmoplegia, and progressive weakness, but the phenotype of these disorders is broad (see Chapter 56). **Endocrine myopathies**, including hyperthyroidism, hypothyroidism, hyperparathyroidism, and Cushing syndrome, are associated with proximal muscle weakness (see Chapters 176, 177, and 179). **Periodic paralysis** due to familial forms of hypokalemia or hyperkalemia produces episodic weakness.

Laboratory and Diagnostic Studies

For most muscular dystrophies and myopathies, the diagnosis is usually established based on laboratory and genetic testing. If the diagnosis is unclear, muscle biopsy may be needed.

Malignant Hyperthermia

Malignant hyperthermia is a life-threatening syndrome precipitated by exposure to anesthetic agents in patients with a genetic predisposition. Calcium accumulation within skeletal muscles leads to sustained muscle contraction, cellular hypermetabolism, and anaerobic metabolism. These effects can lead to rhabdomyolysis with resulting hyperkalemia, myoglobinuria, and arrhythmia. Hypermetabolism leads to hypercarbia, tachycardia, and hyperthermia. Patients with Duchenne muscular dystrophy, central core myopathy, and other myopathies are susceptible. Some patients may report a family history of unexplained death during anesthesia. Widespread organ dysfunction and disseminated intravascular coagulation may occur. Treatment consists of discontinuation of anesthetic agents, dantrolene, and cooling. In patients without a known predisposing neuromuscular condition, genetic testing is recommended to identify potential pathogenic variants in *RYR1, CACNA1S,* or *STAC3.*

NEONATAL AND INFANTILE HYPOTONIA

The clinical distinction between upper and lower motor neuron disorders in infants is less evident because incomplete myelination of the developing nervous system limits expression of many cardinal signs, such as spasticity. The two critical clinical points are whether the child is weak and the presence or absence of deep tendon reflexes. Hypotonia and weakness coupled with depressed or absent deep tendon reflexes suggest a neuromuscular disorder. A stronger child with brisk reflexes suggests an upper motor neuron source for the hypotonia. Causes of neonatal weakness are outlined earlier.

Hypotonia Without Significant Weakness (Central Hypotonia)

Some infants who appear to move well when supine in their cribs are floppy when handled or moved. When lifted, their heads flop, they slip through at the shoulders, do not support weight on their legs, and form an inverted U in prone suspension **(Landau posture)**. When placed prone as neonates, they may lie flat with extended arms and legs. Passive tone is decreased, but reflexes are normal. Hypotonia may be associated with significant cerebral disease or may be a benign phenomenon that is outgrown. The most common cause of hypotonia is hypoxic-ischemic encephalopathy (see Chapter 63).

Prader-Willi syndrome (PWS) presents with severe neonatal hypotonia, profound feeding problems leading to growth faltering, and small hands and feet; males also present with a small penis, small testicles, and cryptorchidism. Severe hyperphagia and obesity develop in early childhood. Approximately 60–70% of affected individuals have an interstitial deletion of paternal chromosome 15q11q13. PWS and trisomy 21 are the most common genetic causes of neonatal hypotonia.

Infants who have a connective tissue disorder, such as **Ehlers-Danlos syndrome**, **Marfan syndrome**, or familial laxity of the ligaments, may exhibit marked passive hypotonia, ligamentous laxity, and increased skin elasticity. They have normal strength and cognition and achieve motor and mental milestones normally. They may have peculiar postures of the feet or unusual gaits.

STROKE IN CHILDHOOD

Etiology

The incidence of pediatric stroke is 2.5–10 per 100,000 children and is higher among neonates, approaching the incidence in elderly patients. A wide spectrum of conditions can produce stroke in childhood (Table 183.4). Pediatric strokes may be **arterial ischemic stroke** (AIS), **hemorrhagic stroke**,

TABLE **183.4** Causes of Stroke in Childhood

ARTERIAL ISCHEMIC STROKE
Vasculopathies • Idiopathic arterial stenosis • Vasculitis (primary, autoimmune, or infectious; may be focal or diffuse) • Arterial dissection (traumatic or spontaneous) • Moyamoya disease Cardiac • Cyanotic congenital heart disease • Valvular disease • Patent foramen ovale • Arrhythmias • Cardiomyopathy • Infective endocarditis Hematologic • Sickle cell anemia • Iron-deficiency anemia • Hypercoagulable state Hereditary prothrombotic states (factor V Leiden) Acquired prothrombotic states (antiphospholipid antibodies) Prothrombotic medications (oral contraception)
CEREBRAL SINOVENOUS THROMBOSIS
Hematologic • Hypercoagulable states (see above) • Iron-deficiency anemia • Severe dehydration Infections • Meningitis • Otitis media • Mastoiditis Systemic disease • Leukemia • Inflammatory bowel disease • Nephrotic syndrome Trauma
HEMORRHAGIC STROKE
Head trauma (accidental or abusive) Vascular malformations • Arteriovenous malformations • Cerebral aneurysms Brain tumor Vasculitis Moyamoya disease

or **cerebral sinovenous thrombosis** (CSVT). AIS is focal brain infarction that results from occlusion of the arteries in the brain. The most common causes are vasculopathies (including inflammatory and noninflammatory arteriopathies) and cardioembolic infarcts due to congenital heart disease, sickle cell anemia, or coagulation disorders. Coagulation disorders also increase the risk of CSVT (the occlusion of venous structures in the brain), which can result in ischemia and, sometimes, hemorrhage as the cerebral venous pressure rises. CSVT can also be caused by infections or dehydration. Hemorrhagic strokes (HS) may be intraparenchymal (primary or secondary bleeding after AIS or CSVT) or due to subarachnoid hemorrhage. The most common causes of HS are vascular malformations, head trauma, and vasculitis.

Clinical Manifestations

The acute onset of focal neurologic deficits in a child is stroke until proven otherwise. Symptoms may be subtle and nonspecific, which can lead to a delay in diagnosis. AIS typically presents with acute, focal neurologic deficits. Hemiparesis is most common, but visual, speech, sensory, or balance deficits may be present. Focal seizures and headaches are more common in children with AIS than in adults. Neonatal AIS most often presents with acute symptomatic focal seizures (typically in the first day of life) or encephalopathy.

Symptoms of CSVT may progress more gradually and be more variable and nonspecific than AIS. In CSVT, acute focal deficits may occur or the child may have progressive signs of elevated intracranial pressure, including headache, papilledema, diplopia (most often from cranial nerve VI palsy), seizures, lethargy, or confusion.

HS tends to present acutely, with a sudden "thunderclap" headache. HS may also present with loss of consciousness, nuchal rigidity, focal deficits, or seizures and can be rapidly fatal.

Some early-life strokes are not recognized until later in life, when an infant or child presents with hemiplegia. Such congenital hemiplegia becomes increasingly apparent as infants develop; they may use one side of the body less, have early handedness, or ignore one side of the body or aspects of the environment. Neuroimaging reveals an area of encephalomalacia in the contralateral cerebral hemisphere that is the residual effect of a prior stroke. The area of encephalomalacia may predispose the child to epilepsy. The details of the child's intrauterine, labor, delivery, and postnatal history are often unremarkable, so the timing of the stroke typically remains uncertain.

Differential Diagnosis

There are many conditions that mimic pediatric stroke, most of which are more common than AIS, HS, or CSVT. Some of these mimics are benign (e.g., migraine, functional neurologic disorder, musculoskeletal abnormalities), but others require specific, prompt diagnosis and treatment (e.g., transient postictal weakness, intracranial infection, inflammatory disease of the central nervous system, tumor, posterior reversible leukoencephalopathy syndrome).

Diagnostic Tests and Imaging

On initial presentation, acute neuroimaging is necessary. A noncontrast head computed tomography (CT) scan is highly sensitive to acute HS and can reveal larger, mature AIS, but acute, nonhemorrhagic stroke may not be seen on routine CT. Therefore MRI with diffusion-weighted imaging is required for most presentations. Fast MRI technology may be used to obtain limited images without need for sedation in young children. Angiography by magnetic resonance angiography (MRA) or CT angiography is used to confirm arterial occlusion in AIS and can identify underlying arteriopathy, vascular malformations, and aneurysms. Perfusion imaging has been used in adults to identify a penumbra (tissue at risk but not yet infarcted), but its role is not yet clear in children. Diagnosis of CSVT requires a high clinical suspicion and purposeful imaging of the cerebral venous system by magnetic resonance or CT venography. If clinical assessment does not reveal the cause of the stroke, a complete laboratory investigation should be undertaken promptly based on suspected etiologies (see Table 183.4). Many children with AIS have more than one predisposing factor, so identifying one risk factor does not obviate the need for a complete evaluation.

Treatment

Treatment must focus on limiting secondary neuronal injury and prevention of future strokes. Neuroprotection by maintaining normal body temperature, normal blood pressure, normal glucose, and stopping seizures is essential. There are limited data regarding the safety and efficacy of emergency thrombolysis with medications or mechanical thrombectomy in children, but these may be considered in discussion with pediatric stroke experts. Anticoagulants (IV heparin, subcutaneous low molecular weight heparin, oral warfarin) and platelet antiaggregants (aspirin) are used for secondary stroke prevention in some instances. For those with acute, progressive CSVT, anticoagulation is the mainstay of therapy. Long-term rehabilitation programs are required for most survivors.

PEARLS FOR PRACTITIONERS

See Neurology: Pearls for Practitioners at the end of this section.

REVIEW QUESTIONS

Available online.

CHAPTER 184

Ataxia and Movement Disorders

ATAXIA

Ataxia is the inability to make accurate, smooth, and coordinated movements. **Truncal ataxia** reflects disturbances of the midline cerebellar vermis (e.g., medulloblastoma, acute postinfectious cerebellar ataxia, ethanol intoxication). **Appendicular ataxia** reflects disturbances of the ipsilateral cerebellar hemisphere (e.g., pilocytic astrocytoma). Ataxias may be acute or chronic. The most common causes of acute ataxia in childhood are postinfectious acute cerebellar ataxia and drug intoxications. Discrete lesions within the posterior fossa, tumors (e.g., medulloblastoma, ependymoma, cerebellar astrocytoma), cerebellar abscess, demyelinating diseases, acute labyrinthitis, strokes, and hemorrhages may cause ataxia. Other causes include benign paroxysmal vertigo, head trauma, seizures, postictal states, migraine, paraneoplastic opsoclonus-myoclonus syndrome associated with neuroblastoma, and inborn errors of metabolism. Congenital disorders also may produce chronic, nonprogressive ataxia. There are several inherited ataxia syndromes (Table 184.1).

Clinical Manifestations

Signs of ataxia include a broad-based, unsteady gait; difficulty sitting (truncal ataxia); and **dysmetria** (over- or undershooting of the target due to abnormal distance perception). An intention tremor worsens as the arm/hand approaches the target. Some children may be perceived as clumsy. Classically, these signs stem from disorders of the cerebellar pathways, but peripheral nerve lesions causing loss of proprioceptive inputs to the cerebellum (e.g., Guillain-Barré syndrome) may present with similar findings. In addition, weakness may intensify or mimic ataxia, so strength must be assessed, along with coordination.

Etiologies

Drug intoxication is the most common cause of acute ataxia among children. Overdosage of any sedative-hypnotic agent can produce acute ataxia and lethargy, but ataxia without lethargy usually results from intoxication with ethanol or antiseizure medications. Over-the-counter cough syrups (e.g., dextromethorphan), essential oils (e.g., tea tree), and other toxins (e.g., pesticides) may also cause ataxia. It is important to ask about any medications, substance use, or other toxins to which the child may have access. Treatment is supportive.

Postinfectious acute cerebellar ataxia may occur 1–3 weeks following varicella, infectious mononucleosis, mild respiratory or gastrointestinal viral illnesses, or other infections. The pathogenesis is uncertain and may represent a direct viral infection of the cerebellum or, more likely, an autoimmune response precipitated by the viral infection and directed at the cerebellar white matter. Symptoms begin abruptly, causing truncal ataxia, unsteady gait, and frequent falls. Dysmetria of the arms, dysarthria, nystagmus, vomiting, and irritability may be prominent. Symptoms, which may be severe enough to prevent standing or sitting, usually peak within 2 days, then stabilize and resolve over several weeks. CSF examination sometimes shows a mild lymphocytic pleocytosis or mild elevation of protein content. Brain magnetic resonance imaging may reveal cerebellar enhancement. Treatment is generally supportive. If children do not improve within several weeks, evaluation for an alternative etiology of ataxia (e.g., tumor, opsoclonus-myoclonus syndrome) should be considered.

Difficulty walking with a severe staggering gait is one manifestation of **acute labyrinthitis**, but the diagnosis is usually clarified by the associated symptoms of a severe sense of spinning dizziness (vertigo), nausea and vomiting, and associated signs of pallor, sweating, and nystagmus.

Brain tumors are the second most common neoplasm in children (see Chapter 158). About 50% arise from within the

TABLE 184.1 Causes of Ataxia

BRAIN TUMORS
Medulloblastoma*
Pilocytic astrocytoma*
Ependymoma
Brainstem glioma
PARANEOPLASTIC DISEASE
Neuroblastoma (opsoclonus-myoclonus-ataxia)
INFECTIOUS DISORDERS
Encephalitis (including brainstem encephalitis)*
Meningitis
Labyrinthitis*
Cerebellar abscess
POSTINFECTIOUS DISORDERS
Acute cerebellar ataxia (acute postinfectious cerebellitis)*
Guillain-Barré syndrome*
MIGRAINOUS DISORDERS
Migraine with brainstem aura (previously called basilar migraine)*
Benign paroxysmal vertigo*
TRAUMA
Concussion/postconcussion syndrome*
Cerebellar hemorrhage
Cerebellar contusion
TOXIC INGESTIONS*
Ethanol
Antiseizure medications
Antihistamines
Benzodiazepines
Carbon monoxide
Inhalants
Other substance use
VASCULAR DISORDERS
Cerebellar hemorrhage or infarction
Vertebral artery dissection
DEMYELINATING DISORDERS
Acute disseminated encephalomyelitis
Multiple sclerosis
STRUCTURAL OR CONGENITAL DISORDERS
Cerebellar hypoplasia
Vermal aplasia
Dandy-Walker malformation
Arnold-Chiari malformation
Hydrocephalus
HEREDITARY ATAXIC DISORDERS
Episodic ataxia
Friedreich ataxia
Ramsay Hunt syndrome
Spinocerebellar ataxia 1 and 2
Ataxia-telangiectasia
GENETIC AND METABOLIC DISORDERS
Metachromatic leukodystrophy
Adrenoleukodystrophy
Maple syrup urine disease
Hartnup disease
GM2 gangliosidosis (juvenile)
Refsum disease
Vitamin E deficiency
Leigh disease
Wilson disease
Abetalipoproteinemia

*Common.

posterior fossa. Tumors that arise in the posterior fossa or brainstem produce progressive ataxia with headache that may be acute or gradual in onset. There is a progressive worsening over days to months, typically with associated signs and symptoms of elevated intracranial pressure. The ataxia and dysmetria may result from primary cerebellar invasion or from obstruction of the CSF pathways (e.g., cerebral aqueduct) with resultant hydrocephalus. The most common tumors in this region include medulloblastoma, ependymoma, pilocytic astrocytoma, and brainstem glioma.

Rarely, a **neuroblastoma**, located in the adrenal medulla or anywhere along the paraspinal sympathetic chain in the thorax or abdomen, is associated with degeneration of cerebellar Purkinje cells and the development of severe ataxia, dysmetria, irritability, myoclonus, and opsoclonus (see Chapter 159). An immunologic reaction directed toward the tumor may be misdirected to attack Purkinje cells and other neuronal elements. The myoclonic movements are irregular, lightning-like movements of a limb or the head. Opsoclonus is a rapid, multidirectional, conjugate movement of the eyes, which suddenly dart in random directions. The presence of **opsoclonus-myoclonus** in a child should prompt a vigorous search for an occult neuroblastoma.

Ataxia-telangiectasia, an autosomal recessive genetic disorder of the *ATM* gene, causes a degenerative ataxia. Affected patients present with ataxia around age 2 years, progressing to loss of ambulation by adolescence. In mid-childhood, telangiectasias are evident over the sclerae, nose, ears, and extremities. Abnormalities in immune function and greatly increased risk of lymphoreticular tumors result in early death.

Friedreich ataxia is a progressive, autosomal recessive disorder. Children present in the late elementary school years with ataxia, dysmetria, dysarthria, diminished proprioception and vibration sense, absent deep tendon reflexes, and nystagmus. Most develop hypertrophic cardiomyopathy and skeletal abnormalities (e.g., high-arched feet, hammer toes, kyphoscoliosis).

Several rare **inborn errors of metabolism** can present with intermittent episodes of ataxia and somnolence. These include Hartnup disorder, maple syrup urine disease, mitochondrial disorders, abetalipoproteinemia, and vitamin E deficiency (see Chapter 50).

MOVEMENT DISORDERS

Movement disorders or **dyskinesias** are a diverse group of entities associated with abnormal excessive, exaggerated, chaotic, or explosive movements of voluntary muscles. They are generally the result of abnormalities of the extrapyramidal system including the basal ganglia. Movement disorders in children are typically **hyperkinetic** (increased movement). The abnormal movements are activated by stress and fatigue and often, but not always, disappear in sleep. They are typically diffuse and migratory (e.g., chorea) but may be isolated to specific muscle groups (e.g., segmental myoclonus, palatal myoclonus).

Chorea is a hyperkinetic, rapid, unsustained, irregular, purposeless movement that seems to flow from one body part to another. Affected patients may demonstrate difficulty keeping the tongue protruded or maintaining grip (milkmaid grip). Patients often attempt to incorporate the involuntary movements into more purposeful movements, which make them appear fidgety. Choreiform movement disorders may be autoimmune/parainfectious, infectious, genetic, structural, metabolic, or toxic in origin (Table 184.2). The movements may occur alone or as part of a more extensive disorder (e.g., Sydenham chorea, Huntington chorea, systemic lupus erythematosus, encephalitis).

Athetosis is a hyperkinetic, slow, coarse, writhing movement that is most pronounced in the distal muscle groups. Athetosis is seen frequently in combination with chorea (choreoathetosis). It may be seen in virtually all the disorders mentioned as causes of chorea. Many children with mixed forms of cerebral palsy have spasticity and choreoathetosis.

Dystonia is characterized by abnormally sustained muscle contraction, causing twisting motions (torsion spasm) and repetitive movements or abnormal postures, usually associated with basal ganglia or thalamic lesions. Cerebral palsy is the most common cause of dystonia among children, but

TABLE 184.2 Causes of Movement Disorders

CHOREA
Autoimmune/parainfectious (e.g., acute rheumatic fever,* systemic lupus erythematosus)
Infectious (e.g., HIV, neurosyphilis, encephalitis)
Genetic (e.g., Huntington disease, ataxia-telangiectasia)
Structural (e.g., stroke, neoplasm)
Metabolic/toxic (e.g., hepatic/kidney failure, hyperthyroidism)
Drug induced
ATHETOSIS
Cerebral palsy*
Kernicterus
Hypoxic-ischemic encephalopathy
Drug induced
DYSTONIA
Acute dystonic reaction*
Cerebral palsy*
Metabolic disorders (e.g., Wilson disease)
Tardive dyskinesia
Inherited primary dystonias
TREMOR
Physiologic*
Essential tremor*
Drugs/toxins* (e.g., caffeine, bronchodilators, amphetamines, tricyclic antidepressants)
Hereditary, degenerative (e.g., Huntington disease, Wilson disease)
Stroke
Metabolic (e.g., hyperthyroidism, hepatic encephalopathy, electrolyte disturbances)
Psychogenic tremor
MYOCLONUS
Benign*
Epilepsy
Infection
Toxin
Metabolic encephalopathies
Autoimmune encephalitis
TICS*
Provisional (transient) tic disorder
Chronic motor tic disorder
Tourette syndrome

*Common.

many genetic variants have been implicated in primary dystonias. Antipsychotics and antiemetics can produce **acute dystonic reactions**, typically involving the face and neck with torticollis, retrocollis, tongue protrusions, and oculogyric crises (eye rotation). Treatment is with anticholinergics and/or antihistamines.

Tardive dyskinesia is usually associated with chronic antipsychotic drug use and presents with characteristic facial involvement (tongue thrusting, chewing).

Tremor is a hyperkinetic, rhythmic, oscillatory movement caused by simultaneous contractions of antagonistic muscles. The amplitude and frequency are regular. In children, tremor is usually due to a physiologic tremor or essential tremor. Essential tremor is the most common movement disorder in adults; half report onset in childhood. Other causes of tremor include thyrotoxicosis, hypoglycemia, or drugs (e.g., caffeine, bronchodilators, amphetamines, tricyclic antidepressants).

Myoclonus is a hyperkinetic, brief contraction of a muscle group, resulting in a sudden jerk. Myoclonus may be caused by seizures or by other etiologies (see Chapter 182). Myoclonus is distinguished from tremor in that it is a simple contraction of an agonist muscle, whereas tremor is a simultaneous contraction of agonist and antagonist muscles. Myoclonus is seen as a manifestation of various epilepsies and infectious, toxic, autoimmune, and metabolic encephalopathies. Benign myoclonus is commonly observed during sleep and may be particularly pronounced in neonates.

Tics are rapid, purposeless, involuntary, stereotyped movements and typically involve the face, eyes, shoulder, and arm. Examples of simple motor tics include blinking, nose twitching, and extremity jerking. Complex motor tics are more orchestrated movements, including head shaking, gesturing, or jumping. Phonic tics may be simple (e.g., grunting, throat clearing) or complex (e.g., uttering words, phrases). Approximately 25% of children have transient tics. Most tic disorders in children are transient and not intrusive into the child's life but may be a source of parental anxiety. Although it was previously thought that tics could be unmasked by stimulant agents, this has not been validated in controlled studies. Persistent motor tics (lasting >12 months) combined with phonic tics are characteristic of **Tourette syndrome**, a chronic tic disorder that usually begins before age 12 years. The pathophysiology underlying tics is unknown, but a family history of tics is commonly elicited. Comorbid features, such as obsessive-compulsive disorder and attention-deficit/hyperactivity disorder, are present in half of children with Tourette syndrome (see Chapters 13 and 19). Tic disorders are clinical diagnoses, and neurodiagnostic studies have limited value. Many children with tic disorders or Tourette syndrome are unperturbed by their tics and require no therapy. Others may benefit from psychological support, including the first-line therapy, Comprehensive Behavioral Intervention for Tics (CBIT), and sometimes pharmacologic therapy, typically with α-adrenergic receptor agonists (e.g., clonidine, guanfacine) or neuroleptics (e.g., pimozide, aripiprazole, risperidone). Chronic tic disorders wax and wane regardless of intervention and most often improve substantially or resolve entirely by late adolescence.

PEARLS FOR PRACTITIONERS

See Neurology: Pearls for Practitioners at the end of this section.

REVIEW QUESTIONS

Available online.

CHAPTER 185

Altered Mental Status

Altered mental status refers to a wide range of nonspecific symptoms indicating a change in brain function from the patient's baseline. This can include confusion, disorientation, alteration in consciousness, decreased awareness, or agitation.

DISORDERS OF CONSCIOUSNESS

Etiology

In childhood, the most common causes of altered mental status are toxins, hypoxia-ischemia (e.g., cardiac arrest, near-drowning), metabolic alterations, infections, and structural etiologies (e.g., masses, head trauma) (Table 185.1). Seizures (e.g., postictal state, nonconvulsive status epilepticus) are also a common cause of altered consciousness. A detailed history and physical examination usually provide sufficient clues to differentiate among the major diagnostic categories producing coma. In most clinical situations, the cause of coma is readily identified.

Intoxication and ingestion are common causes of acute alteration of consciousness. A subacute course of somnolence progressing to difficulty arousing from a deep sleep (stupor) over hours suggests drug intoxication or organ system failure (e.g., kidney, liver) producing a metabolic encephalopathy. A thorough history must be taken to search for the offending agent (see Chapter 44). Medications and toxins in the home should be reviewed. Toddlers are naturally curious and explore with oral behaviors, putting them at risk for ingestions. A history of social stressors, depression, substance disorder, or other mental health issues raises concern for self-inflicted injury or toxic ingestion.

Metabolic derangements, particularly **hypoglycemia**, can give rise to episodes of lethargy, confusion, seizures, or coma. Disturbances of blood chemistries (e.g., glucose, sodium, calcium, bicarbonate, blood urea nitrogen, ammonia) may produce depressed mental status, as can hypoxemia and cerebral ischemia (inadequate cerebral perfusion). Metabolic disorders are suggested by spontaneous fluctuations in the level of consciousness, tremors, myoclonus, asterixis, visual and tactile hallucinations, and deep coma with preservation of pupillary light reflexes. Care must be taken to investigate background medical conditions that may produce a decline in consciousness (e.g., diabetes mellitus, leukemia, kidney failure, liver disease). Acute metabolic or toxic disorders usually produce a hypotonic, limp state, but hypertonia, rigidity, or posturing can be seen in some causes of coma (e.g., hypoglycemia, hepatic encephalopathy, short-acting barbiturates).

CNS infection usually causes abrupt alteration of mental status, although viral meningoencephalitis (particularly herpes simplex virus) can present with subacute alterations in mental status. The presence of fever, petechiae, chills, and diaphoresis suggests infection. Prodromal photophobia and pain

TABLE 185.1 Causes of Altered Mental Status and Diagnostic Approach

CAUSES
Infection/Inflammation
Meningitis Encephalitis (e.g., herpes simplex virus, arboviruses) Brain abscess or subdural empyema HIV Tuberculosis meningitis Toxic shock syndrome Postinfectious (e.g., acute disseminated encephalomyelitis) Autoimmune encephalitis
Trauma
Abusive head trauma Hemorrhage (e.g., epidural, subdural, subarachnoid) Brain contusion Concussion Diffuse axonal injury
Toxins (Intoxication or Withdrawal)
Ethanol Opioids Barbiturates Antihistamines Antiseizure medications Iron Acetaminophen Benzodiazepines Lead poisoning Synthetic cannabinoids
Hypoxia-Ischemia
Near-drowning Post–cardiopulmonary arrest (e.g., cardiac arrhythmia, obstructive cardiomyopathy) Carbon monoxide intoxication Perinatal asphyxia Strangulation
Epilepsy
Subclinical (or nonconvulsive) status epilepticus Postictal states
Stroke
Arterial ischemic stroke Cerebral sinovenous thrombosis Hemorrhage
Increased Intracranial Pressure
Brain tumor Cerebral edema Hydrocephalus
Migraine
Systemic Disorders
Gastrointestinal (e.g., intussusception) Vasculitis (e.g., systemic lupus erythematosus) Hepatic failure Hypertensive encephalopathy Mitochondrial disorders Endocrine disorders (e.g., adrenal insufficiency, thyroid disorders) Kidney disorders (e.g., uremia) Demyelinating disorders (e.g., multiple sclerosis, ADEM) Thiamine deficiency (Wernicke encephalopathy)

(Continued)

TABLE 185.1 Causes of Altered Mental Status and Diagnostic Approach—cont'd

Metabolic Derangements
Hypoglycemia Hyperglycemia or rapid correction Hyponatremia or rapid correction Hypernatremia or rapid correction Hyperosmolality or rapid correction Hypercapnia Hyperammonemia Inborn errors of metabolism
DIAGNOSTIC APPROACH

Routine laboratory testing
  Glucose
  Sodium, potassium, calcium, magnesium, chloride, bicarbonate, BUN, creatinine, AST, ALT, blood gases, ammonia, TSH
  Blood, urine analyses for toxic substances
  Blood, urine cultures if infection suspected

Neuroimaging
  Head CT
  Brain MRI, MRA, MRV
CSF analysis (if no evidence for increased intracranial pressure on neuroimaging)
  Opening pressure
  White and red blood cell counts, protein, glucose
  Culture (±viral PCR testing)
Electrodiagnostic studies
  EEG
Skeletal survey
Ophthalmologic examination
Secondary laboratory testing (if cause remains unknown)
Lead level, pyruvate, lactate, serum amino acids, urine organic acids, acylcarnitine profile

ADEM, Acute disseminated encephalomyelitis; *ALT*, alanine aminotransferase; *AST*, aspartate aminotransferase; *BUN*, blood urea nitrogen; *CSF*, cerebrospinal fluid; *CT*, computed tomography; *EEG*, electroencephalogram; *MRI/MRA/MRV*, magnetic resonance imaging/angiography/venography; *PCR*, polymerase chain reaction; *TSH*, thyroid-stimulating hormone.

on movement of the head or eyes are symptoms of meningeal irritation. Preceding symptoms, such as abdominal pain, diarrhea, sore throat, conjunctivitis, cough, or rash, point toward viral encephalitis or post infectious syndrome as the cause of the altered consciousness.

Structural processes, such as hemorrhage, acute hydrocephalus, or stroke, can cause sudden depressed consciousness in children. An evolution of headache and morning vomiting suggests increased ICP. A gradual fading of alertness or declining school performance over preceding weeks suggests an expanding intracranial mass, subdural hematoma, or chronic infection.

Episodic alteration or depression of consciousness with full recovery is usually due to seizure, migraine, syncope, or metabolic abnormality (e.g., hypoglycemia). Consciousness can be impaired during seizures or in the postictal state. Nonconvulsive status epilepticus (generalized or focal) can directly impair consciousness and is a common complicating factor for infants and children with acute neurologic disorders (e.g., head trauma, meningitis, stroke, following convulsive status epilepticus). **Migraine with brainstem aura** (formerly known as basilar migraine) can last hours and be accompanied by decreased consciousness, ataxia, vertigo, impaired hearing, tinnitus, dysarthria, or diplopia; headache may precede or follow the neurologic signs.

Syncope is one of the most common causes of abrupt, episodic loss of consciousness. Neurocardiogenic syncope, cardiac arrhythmia, or obstructive cardiomyopathy can cause recurrent episodes of loss of consciousness. Two thirds of children with syncope have irregular, myoclonic movements as they lose consciousness (anoxic seizures), which must be distinguished from epilepsy (unprovoked seizures). Children with unexplained syncope require a complete cardiac evaluation (see Chapter 141).

Clinical Manifestations

Consciousness is a cortical function that allows for awareness of self and environment (place, time). **Arousal** represents the system that initiates and maintains consciousness and is mediated by the reticular activating system (RAS), which extends from the pons through the midbrain to the hypothalamus and thalamus. Acute changes in consciousness vary in degree from mild lethargy and confusion to deep coma. **Lethargic** patients have difficulty maintaining an aroused state. Patients who are **obtunded** have decreased arousal but are responsive to stimuli. **Stupor** is a state of responsiveness to pain but not to other stimuli. **Coma** is a state of unresponsive unconsciousness and is caused by dysfunction of the cerebral hemispheres bilaterally, the bilateral thalami, and/or the brainstem.

Breathing patterns may provide important clues to the neurologic localization and etiology of the depressed consciousness. A low respiratory rate may be associated with CNS depressants or increased ICP. Tachypnea may be due to hypoxia, metabolic acidosis, or fever but in more ominous situations may be due to brainstem herniation. Systemic diseases such as sepsis, ingestions, or cardiac failure may lead to hypotension and shock. Hypotension may also result from severe traumatic brain injury (TBI) or spinal cord injury. Hypertension may be due to increased ICP.

Body posture at rest and after noxious stimulation can indicate the anatomic level responsible for the alteration of consciousness. Posturing in response to noxious stimulation indicates more serious neurologic conditions. **Decorticate posturing** consists of rigid extension of the lower extremities, flexion and supination of the arms, and fisting of the hands. It indicates bilateral cortical or subcortical abnormalities or herniation, with preserved brainstem function. **Decerebrate posturing** (rigid extension and internal rotation of the upper and lower extremities) is associated with herniation with midbrain compression or toxic-metabolic abnormalities. These postures may be symmetric or asymmetric. A structural cause is most likely when posturing is asymmetric, whereas symmetric posturing may suggest an underlying toxic-metabolic etiology.

Recognition of the signs associated with increased intracranial pressure and the major herniation syndromes can be lifesaving if emergent neuroimaging and treatment are initiated. Papilledema or paralysis of cranial nerves III (dilated "blown" pupil, eye deviated down and laterally) or VI (unable to move eye laterally) in a patient with depressed consciousness is strong evidence of elevated ICP, a medical and neurosurgical emergency. **Herniations** can occur under the falx, through the tentorial notch, or into the foramen magnum (Table 185.2). **Uncal herniation** implies displacement of one mesial temporal lobe over the tentorial edge, producing a unilateral third nerve palsy and hemiparesis (which can be ipsilateral due to compression of the contralateral cerebral peduncle or contralateral if the uncus compresses the ipsilateral peduncle). Another type of transtentorial herniation, **central herniation**, occurs when both temporal lobes and the diencephalon (thalamus and hypothalamus) herniate through the tentorium. A progressive loss of consciousness accompanied by miosis, decorticate posturing, and Cheyne-Stokes respirations (rhythmic waxing and waning of respiratory amplitude) suggests incipient transtentorial herniation. Late findings include decerebrate posturing and **Cushing triad** (bradycardia, irregular respirations, hypertension).

Laboratory and Diagnostic Imaging

Physical examination searches for clues as to the cause of altered consciousness, such as unusual odors, needle puncture sites, trauma, dehydration, or organ system failure. The glucose level should also be checked immediately because hypoglycemia is a rapidly treatable cause of altered mental status. The **Glasgow Coma Scale** (see Table 41.1) can be used to assess unresponsive patients regarding their best verbal and motor responses and eye opening to stimulation with scores ranging from 3 to 15 points.

Testing the structures immediately adjacent to the reticular system is essential. Changes in pupillary response generally suggest midbrain lesions, though pontine lesions can cause pinpoint pupils. In comatose patients, eye movements are observed or elicited with the **oculocephalic vestibular**

TABLE 185.2 Herniation Syndromes

LOCATION	ETIOLOGY	DESCRIPTION	CLINICAL FINDING(S)
Transtentorial Unilateral (uncal) or bilateral	Supratentorial mass lesions, diffuse brain swelling, focal edema, or acute hydrocephalus	Downward displacement of supratentorial brain tissue into infratentorial compartment (below tentorium), compressing the cerebral peduncles, midbrain, third cranial nerve, and posterior circulation	Headache Altered consciousness Dilated ipsilateral pupil Cranial nerve III palsy Hemiparesis Decerebrate posturing Cushing triad Respiratory arrest
Subfalcine	Increased pressure in one hemisphere (mass, focal edema)	Brain tissue displaced under the falx cerebri, compressing the anterior cerebral artery	Weakness, bladder incontinence, coma
Foramen magnum	Cerebellar mass or edema	Downward displacement of cerebellar tonsils, compressing the medulla and upper spinal cord	Bradycardia, bradypnea, hypertension, death

reflexes (doll's-eye maneuver) (see Chapter 180). If the oculocephalic responses are not elicited or are unclear, the **oculovestibular response** (cold caloric stimulation) is elicited by flushing cold water into the external ear canal. In a comatose patient, cold water irrigation into the ear canal elicits a tonic eye deviation toward the irrigated ear if the brainstem is functioning.

Further evaluation is guided by the history and physical examination. Computed tomography (CT) remains the preferred imaging technique in emergency situations because it can be performed rapidly, and it accurately identifies intracranial acute hemorrhages, large space-occupying lesions, edema, and shifts of the midline. The initial head CT scan is done without contrast to identify blood and calcifications. Contrast can be administered to identify inflammatory and neoplastic lesions but is not usually required for identification of major lesions.

Examination of the CSF may establish the cause of the alteration of consciousness. Lumbar puncture (LP) in a patient with elevated ICP can result in transtentorial herniation, so neuroimaging must be performed before the LP if elevated ICP is suspected. The presence of red blood cells in the CSF may suggest primary subarachnoid hemorrhage, parenchymal hemorrhage, hemorrhagic infection (e.g., herpes simplex virus), or trauma from the procedure causing bleeding into the subarachnoid space. White blood cells in the CSF usually denote infectious meningitis or meningoencephalitis but may also be associated with autoimmune disorders or parainfectious syndromes. Elevated CSF protein is seen in patients with meningeal inflammation, tumors, or white matter diseases, whereas abnormal CSF glucose levels are also markers of infection and inflammation (e.g., neurosarcoidosis).

Treatment

Clinicians should rapidly consider causes of unresponsiveness that could easily and quickly be reversed (see Table 185.1). If trauma or immersion injuries are suspected, neck manipulation should be avoided until cervical spine imaging excludes vertebral fracture or subluxation. The most common cause of long-term morbidity in a patient with depressed consciousness is hypoxia; therefore airway, breathing, and circulation are addressed first.

Beyond supportive measures, the etiology of altered mental status determines the treatment. Ingestions may necessitate charcoal administration, forced diuresis, dialysis, or specific antidotes (see Chapter 44). Infections are treated with appropriate antibiotics or antiviral agents (see Chapters 101 and 102). If mental status changes are due to increased ICP, acute medical interventions (e.g., osmotic agents, a trial of hyperventilation, and elevating the head of the bed to 30 degrees) must be instituted, emergent neuroimaging performed, and urgent neurosurgical consultation obtained. Structural brain lesions may necessitate medical treatment of increased ICP or surgical excision.

Prognosis

The outcome of altered mental status relates to many variables, including etiology. Intoxication typically carries a good prognosis, whereas herniation carries a poor prognosis. Other prognostic factors include the duration of coma and the age of the patient; children have better outcomes than adults. Complete recovery from coma of several days' duration after head trauma is possible in children; however, many survivors of prolonged coma remain in an unresponsive wakefulness syndrome (partial arousal but without awareness) or have severe neuropsychiatric disability.

INCREASED INTRACRANIAL PRESSURE

Etiology

When the cranial sutures are fused, the skull becomes a rigid container enclosing a fixed volume, including the brain (80–85%), CSF (10–15%), and blood (5–10%). The exponential relationship between the volume within a closed container and pressure results in a massive increase in ICP as intracranial volume increases. The brain accommodates increased ICP initially by expelling CSF and blood from the intracranial compartment into the spinal subarachnoid space. When the limits of this accommodation are reached, the brain itself begins to shift in response to the continuing elevation of ICP. Brain shifts may cause herniations across the dural extensions or skull barriers (see Table 185.2).

The most common causes of increased ICP include mass lesions, hydrocephalus, cerebral edema due to trauma or infection, and idiopathic intracranial hypertension (formerly known as pseudotumor cerebri) (Tables 185.3 and 185.4).

Mass lesions (e.g., brain tumor, abscess, hemorrhage) may produce increased ICP not only by virtue of large size but by blockage of CSF pathways leading to hydrocephalus, blockage of venous outflow, or creation of vasogenic cerebral edema. Brain abscesses usually present as mass lesions producing focal neurologic signs and increased ICP. Symptoms of infection, such as fever, malaise, anorexia, and stiff neck, may be subtle or absent. Children with chronic cardiac or pulmonary

TABLE 185.3 Causes of Increased Intracranial Pressure

MASS EFFECT
Hydrocephalus
Hemorrhage
Tumor
Abscess
Cyst
Inflammatory mass
Arterial ischemic stroke with edema
Cerebral sinovenous thrombosis
DIFFUSE EDEMA
Hypoxic-ischemic injury
Trauma
Infection
Meningitis
Encephalitis
Hypertension
Metabolic derangement or toxin
Hyponatremia
Diabetic ketoacidosis
Dialysis disequilibrium syndrome
Mitochondrial disorders
Fulminant hepatic encephalopathy
Pulmonary insufficiency with hypercarbia
Lead intoxication
Idiopathic intracranial hypertension (pseudotumor cerebri)
Medications
Withdrawal of long-term steroid administration
Endocrinologic disturbance

TABLE 185.4 Causes of Hydrocephalus

PATHOGENIC MECHANISM	ETIOLOGIC DISORDER/ CONDITION
Obstruction of CSF pathways	Intraventricular foramina (Monro) obstruction Parasellar mass (craniopharyngioma, germinoma, pituitary tumor) Intraventricular tumor (ependymoma) Tuberous sclerosis with subependymal giant cell astrocytoma Aqueduct of Sylvius (cerebral aqueduct) obstruction/ stenosis Midbrain or pineal region tumor Impaired flow from the fourth ventricle foramina of Luschka and Magendie Dandy-Walker malformation Arnold-Chiari malformation Bone lesions of the cranial base (achondroplasia, rickets) Postinfectious or postinflammatory Posthemorrhagic
Overproduction of CSF	Choroid plexus papilloma
Defective reabsorption of CSF (extraventricular obstruction or communicating hydrocephalus)	Hypoplasia of the arachnoid villi Postinfectious or posthemorrhagic destruction of arachnoid villi or subarachnoid fibrosis Extensive cerebral sinovenous thrombosis

CSF, Cerebrospinal fluid.

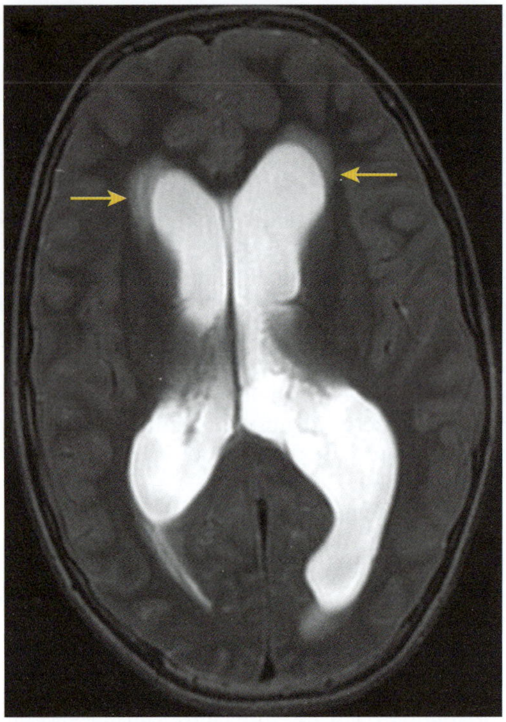

FIGURE 185.1 Axial T2 image shows moderate dilation of the lateral ventricles with periventricular seepage *(yellow arrows)* suggestive of obstructive hydrocephalus. (From Camargo A, Kanekar S. Neuroimaging in pediatric headache. *Neurol Clin.* 2022;40[3]:679–698. Fig 5A.)

disease may embolize infected material to the brain, predisposing them to brain abscesses. Brain tumors in children are most often located in the posterior fossa and can result in elevated ICP due to obstruction of CSF flow through the cerebral aqueduct and fourth ventricle. Brain tumors and abscesses can both result in vasogenic edema, which further increases ICP.

Hydrocephalus is the abnormal accumulation of CSF in the ventricles due to the obstruction of CSF flow anywhere along its course (see Table 185.4, Fig. 185.1). CSF is continuously produced by the choroid plexus within the lateral, third, and fourth ventricles. CSF circulates through the ventricular systems and is then absorbed, predominantly by the arachnoid villi into the large dural sinuses. **Obstructive hydrocephalus** is caused by a block before the CSF flows to the subarachnoid space, usually within the fourth ventricle or at the level of the aqueduct. Congenital hydrocephalus can result from CNS malformations, intrauterine infection, intraventricular hemorrhage, pathogenic genetic variants, trauma, and teratogens. Acquired hydrocephalus may be caused by CNS infections, brain tumors, or hemorrhage. Impairment of CSF flow within the subarachnoid space or impairment of absorption is known by the misnomer "communicating hydrocephalus," where there is actually extraventricular obstruction of CSF flow. Hydrocephalus caused by overproduction of CSF without true obstruction is seen in choroid plexus papillomas, which account for 2–4% of childhood intracranial tumors. Hydrocephalus from congenital abnormalities or due to an intracranial mass is typically characterized by a slowly evolving syndrome of increased ICP extending over weeks or months.

Bacterial meningitis may produce increased ICP by several mechanisms including blockage of CSF pathways, cytotoxic cerebral edema, increase in cerebral blood flow, or multifocal cerebral infarctions (see Chapter 101). Most children with bacterial meningitis can undergo LP safely because the brain swelling is diffuse and distributed evenly throughout the brain and spinal CSF compartments. A few patients with meningitis, however, develop transtentorial herniation within a few hours of LP. Focal neurologic signs, poorly reactive pupils, and decorticate or decerebrate posturing are contraindications to LP in a patient with suspected bacterial meningitis.

Idiopathic intracranial hypertension (formerly known as pseudotumor cerebri) is a cause of increased ICP with normal brain imaging. Patients exhibit a daily debilitating headache associated with diplopia, abducens palsy, transient visual obscurations, and papilledema. If untreated, permanent visual field loss may develop. The syndrome has been associated with ingestion of medications (e.g., tetracycline, vitamin A, oral contraceptive agents) and endocrine disturbances (e.g., thyroid disease, Addison disease). Most commonly, this condition is idiopathic and affects children who are otherwise well with rapid weight gain and obesity being a predisposing factor. Weight loss and cessation of triggering medications are mainstays of treatment. Additional treatment with acetazolamide, another diuretic, or topiramate may be necessary. Infrequently, chronic papilledema from persistent idiopathic intracranial hypertension produces visual impairment, and more aggressive management is required (e.g., optic nerve fenestration) to preserve visual function.

Clinical Manifestations

The symptoms and signs of increased ICP include headache, vomiting, lethargy, irritability, altered consciousness, third and sixth nerve palsies, strabismus, diplopia, and papilledema. Classically, headaches related to increased ICP worsen with time as the disease progresses and with maneuvers that increase ICP such as lying down (nocturnal headaches or upon awakening), bending over, coughing, or Valsalva maneuvers. Specific signs of increased ICP in the infratentorial compartment (posterior fossa) include stiff neck and head tilt. Focal neurologic deficits reflect the site of the lesion that is producing the increased ICP and may include hemiparesis from supratentorial lesions or ataxia and cranial nerve palsies from infratentorial lesions. Critically increased ICP may result in herniation syndromes, as discussed earlier. In addition, the **Cushing triad** of elevated blood pressure, bradycardia, and irregular respirations is a late sign of critically elevated ICP. Infants who have an open fontanel may present with less specific symptoms such as irritability, lethargy, and poor feeding. Specific signs of increased ICP in infants consist of a bulging fontanel, suture diastasis, distended scalp veins, a persistent downward deviation of the eyes ("sunsetting"), and rapid growth of head circumference. Manifestations of increased ICP may evolve slowly when there is slow growth of a mass or incomplete obstruction allowing for transependymal absorption of CSF into the veins. On the other hand, symptoms may develop rapidly in the setting of acute intracranial hemorrhage or abrupt CSF obstruction.

Laboratory and Diagnostic Studies

The cause of increased ICP is determined by brain imaging with either CT or magnetic resonance imaging (MRI). CT is rapid, readily available, and provides clear visualization of an acute hemorrhage, dilated ventricles, or mass lesions. Diffuse brain swelling produced by hypoxic-ischemic injury, meningitis, encephalitis, metabolic abnormalities, or toxins may be better delineated by MRI. MRI is also superior to CT for visualizing the posterior fossa and cortical contusions. To avoid radiation from head CT, many centers now use limited sequences to allow for a rapid MRI without sedation as an initial screen for acute causes of elevated ICP. LP is the diagnostic test for infection and for documentation of elevated ICP (essential for patients with idiopathic intracranial hypertension). However, LP may be contraindicated in the setting of an intracranial mass lesion or clear hydrocephalus because withdrawal of CSF can change pressures between the intracranial compartments and promote brainstem shifts and herniation. Idiopathic intracranial hypertension is diagnosed when direct measurement of ICP with a manometer during LP reveals elevated ICP in the absence of other CSF or imaging abnormalities.

Treatment of Elevated Intracranial Pressure

The treatment of acute increased ICP should be carried out in an intensive care setting with continuous monitoring and vigilant attention to vital signs. The first goal is stabilization of the cardiopulmonary status. Once the child is stabilized, the head is placed at midline, and the head of the bed is elevated to 30 degrees. Indications for endotracheal intubation include refractory hypoxia, hypoventilation, Glasgow Coma Score of 8 or less, loss of airway protective reflexes, and acute herniation requiring controlled hyperventilation. Slight hyperventilation to a $Paco_2$ not lower than 35 mm Hg produces rapid, but transient, reduction in ICP by cerebral vasoconstriction, leading to decreased cerebral blood volume. More aggressive hyperventilation may cause cerebral ischemia and is only indicated if there are clinical signs of acute herniation. Three percent saline or mannitol may be used acutely to produce an osmotic shift of fluid from the brain to the plasma. A ventricular catheter may be used to monitor the ICP continuously and to remove CSF. In refractory cases, a pentobarbital-induced coma reduces pressure by severely suppressing cerebral metabolism. The antiinflammatory effects of corticosteroids may be helpful in the management of vasogenic edema associated with tumors and abscesses. Because acute interventions such as hyperventilation, osmotic therapies, and barbiturates can have negative impacts on systemic and cerebral perfusion and have only transient effects on ICP, they must be used judiciously.

Vasopressor drugs may be necessary to maintain adequate arterial blood pressure and cerebral perfusion pressure. Serum electrolytes and osmolarity should be monitored because of risk of the syndrome of inappropriate antidiuretic hormone or cerebral salt wasting (see Chapter 34). Maintaining normoglycemia may have a positive impact on outcomes. Other supportive measures include controlling agitation, fever, and seizures.

All treatments for increased ICP are temporary measures intended to prevent herniation until the underlying disease process either is treated or resolves spontaneously. Timely intervention can prevent or reverse cerebral herniation. Complete neurologic recovery is possible, but rare, after signs of transtentorial or foramen magnum herniation have begun. When these signs are complete, however, with bilaterally dilated, unreactive pupils, absent eye movements, and flaccid quadriplegia, recovery is no longer possible.

Treatment specific to hydrocephalus may be medical or surgical, depending on the etiology. After subarachnoid hemorrhage or meningitis, the flow or absorption of CSF may be transiently impaired. In this circumstance, the use of medication that decreases CSF production, such as acetazolamide, may be beneficial. Surgical management consists of removing the obstructive lesion, placing a shunt, or both. A shunt consists of tubing extending usually from a lateral ventricle to the peritoneal cavity (**ventriculoperitoneal shunt**). Shunts carry the hazards of infection or sudden occlusion with signs and symptoms of acute hydrocephalus.

TRAUMATIC BRAIN INJURY

Following head injury, children may have immediate depression of consciousness and neurologic deficits or may be completely alert without any immediate signs of neurologic injury. Most serious trauma results from motor vehicle crashes, sports, recreation-related injuries, and violence. Head trauma may result in concussion, post-traumatic intracranial hemorrhage, skull fractures, or cranial nerve or cervical spine injuries. Head injury, or other injuries, with associated retinal hemorrhages in infants and young children should raise the suspicion of nonaccidental head trauma (see Chapter 21).

Concussion

Concussion is the process in which traumatic forces on the brain result in the rapid onset of short-lived neurologic impairment that typically resolves spontaneously. In some cases, however, symptoms and signs may evolve over minutes to hours, so patients should not be left alone following the injury. Patients may have signs or symptoms in one or more domain: somatic (headache), cognitive (slowed reaction times, poor attention, amnesia), emotional (lability, irritability), sleep disturbance (drowsiness), or physical signs (loss of consciousness). A child athlete with any features of a concussion should be evaluated by a licensed health care provider onsite or be referred to a physician. Acute symptoms usually reflect a functional disturbance rather than structural injury, and no abnormalities are seen on standard imaging. If the child appears well after several hours and is discharged home, parents should be instructed to call their physician for any change in alertness, orientation, or neurologic functioning. An increase in somnolence, headache, or vomiting is cause for concern and evaluation for potential emergent neuroimaging. Most concussions resolve within 10 days, although the recovery may be slower in children, and in a small percentage of cases the symptoms are prolonged. Physical and cognitive rest are the cornerstones of initial concussion management, with subsequent gradual return to school and physical activities (Table 185.5). Repeated concussions, especially within a short time frame (days or weeks), carry a significant risk of permanent brain injury **(second impact syndrome)**.

Traumatic Intracranial Hemorrhage

Head trauma can result in epidural, subdural, parenchymal, and subarachnoid intracranial hemorrhages, as well as brain contusions (Table 185.6). Symptoms include headache, vomiting, lethargy, decreased consciousness, and seizures. The classic presentation of **epidural hemorrhages** involves a lucid interval: following the primary brain injury, a child has a decreased level of consciousness and then returns to normal for several hours before developing rapidly progressive neurologic symptoms. When associated with neurological decompensation, prompt evacuation of the epidural hematoma is the primary therapy. **Subdural hemorrhages** may result from direct trauma or rotational forces from vigorous shaking

TABLE 185.5 Protocol for Return to Sport After Concussion

Return to play protocol follows a stepwise progression with each step taking ≥24 hr. The athlete should continue to the next level if asymptomatic at the current level.

1. Back to regular activities such as school
2. Light aerobic exercise such as walking or stationary cycling for 5–10 minutes; no weightlifting
3. Moderate activity such as jogging, brief running, moderate-intensity stationary biking, moderate-intensity weightlifting (less than their prior weightlifting routine)
4. Heavy, noncontact physical activity such as sprinting/running, regular weightlifting routine, noncontact sport-specific drills
5. Practice and full contact
6. Competition

TABLE 185.6 Syndromes of Post-Traumatic Intracranial Hemorrhage

SYNDROME	CLINICAL AND RADIOLOGIC CHARACTERISTICS	TREATMENT
Epidural	Onset over minutes to hours Lucid interval followed by progressive neurologic deficits Lens-shaped extracerebral hemorrhage compressing brain	Medical treatment of elevated intracranial pressure, if needed Surgical evacuation or observation Prognosis good with prompt treatment, otherwise poor
Acute subdural	Onset over hours Focal neurologic deficits Crescentic extracranial hemorrhage compressing brain	Medical treatment of elevated intracranial pressure, if needed Surgical evacuation Prognosis guarded
Chronic subdural	Onset over weeks to months Anemia, macrocephaly Seizures, vomiting Crescentic, low-density mass on CT	Subdural taps or subdural shunt as necessary Prognosis can be good
Intraparenchymal	Depressed consciousness Focal neurologic deficits ± Additional multiple contusions	Medical treatment of elevated intracranial pressure, if needed Possible surgical decompression depending on site; otherwise, supportive care Prognosis guarded
Subarachnoid	Stiff neck Worst headache of life Late hydrocephalus	Supportive care Medical treatment of elevated intracranial pressure, if needed Prognosis variable
Contusion	Focal neurologic deficits Brain swelling with transtentorial herniation CT findings: multifocal low-density areas with punctate hemorrhages	Medical treatment of elevated intracranial pressure Prognosis guarded

CT, Computed tomography.

(abusive head trauma). In neonates and infants with open fontanels, signs and symptoms may be absent or nonspecific. **Subarachnoid hemorrhages** classically present as a sudden, severe headache due to rupture of an intracranial aneurysm. Brain **contusions** are areas of bruising with associated localized ischemia, edema, and mass effect.

Skull Fractures

Skull fractures may present with localized swelling and pain, subcutaneous bleeding over the mastoid process **(Battle sign)** or around the orbit **(raccoon eyes)**, blood behind the tympanic membrane **(hemotympanum)**, or CSF leak from the nose (rhinorrhea) or ear (otorrhea). Skull fractures may be linear, diastatic (spreading the suture), depressed (an edge displaced inferiorly), or compound (bone fragments breaking the skin surface). Linear, diastatic, and minimally depressed fractures necessitate no specific treatment, but imaging is indicated to evaluate for associated intracranial hemorrhages. If the depression is >0.5–1 cm, surgical elevation of bone fragments and repair of associated dural tears are generally recommended. Compound fractures or penetrating injuries necessitate emergent surgical debridement and tetanus prophylaxis. The risk of associated brain contusion and early seizures is high in compound fractures.

CSF leak occurs when a skull fracture tears adjacent dura, creating communications between the subarachnoid space and the nose, paranasal sinuses, mastoid air cells, or ear. Clear fluid that leaks from the nose or ear after head trauma is presumed to be CSF until proved otherwise. The presence of air within the subdural, subarachnoid, or ventricular space also indicates a dural tear and open communication between the nose or paranasal sinuses and brain. In most cases, the dura heals spontaneously when the patient's head is kept elevated. Patients with CSF leaks are at risk for the development of meningitis or extradural abscesses. If the leak persists or recurs or if meningitis develops, the dura is surgically repaired. **Cranial nerve palsies**, secondary to a laceration or contusion of the cranial nerves, may result from a skull fracture and may be transitory or permanent.

Other Complications of Head Trauma

Cervical spine injuries must be suspected in any unconscious child, especially if bruises are present on the head, neck, or back. In conscious children, findings of neck or back pain, burning or stabbing pains radiating to the arms, paraplegia, quadriplegia, or asymmetric motor or sensory responses of arms or legs suggest spinal cord injury. Cervical spine injury (displaced or fractured vertebra) may result in complete transection of the cord with spinal shock, loss of sensation, and flaccid paralysis. A contused cord (without vertebral abnormality) may present in a similar manner. Any patient with a clinical or radiological abnormality of the spine requires immediate spine immobilization, cardiopulmonary stabilization, and neurosurgical consultation.

Post-traumatic seizures are divided into one of two patterns: early post-traumatic seizures (including immediate seizures) and post-traumatic epilepsy. Immediate seizures occur within seconds of the injury and are presumed to reflect a direct mechanical stimulation to the cortex. The prognosis is excellent, and likelihood of later epilepsy is negligible. Early post-traumatic seizures occurring within the first week of the head injury are likely the result of a localized area of cerebral contusion or edema. The long-term prognosis for these seizures is also quite favorable. Post-traumatic epilepsy arises more than a week after the trauma and most likely indicates an area of cortical gliosis or scarring that will be a source for long-term epilepsy. These patients often require long-term antiseizure medication.

Transient neurologic disturbances may develop a few minutes after head trauma and last for minutes to hours before clearing. The most common symptoms are cortical blindness and confusional states, but hemiparesis, ataxia, or any other neurologic deficit may appear. These symptoms may represent a trauma-triggered migraine in susceptible children. Care must be exercised to exclude intracranial pathology.

Evaluation and Treatment

Children who have loss of consciousness or amnesia following a head injury should be evaluated in an emergency department. High-risk patients include those with persistent depressed or decreasing level of consciousness, focal neurologic signs, penetrating skull injury, depressed skull fractures, or worsening symptoms. Because patients with intracranial hemorrhage may progressively deteriorate and require immediate neurosurgical care, these patients warrant care in a skilled trauma center. The **Glasgow Coma Scale** is a valuable tool for monitoring the course of patients after trauma for signs of deterioration (see Table 41.1). The observation period varies with the severity of the injury and may include hospitalization.

Immediate management of severe injuries includes ensuring an appropriate airway, breathing, and circulation. Neuroimaging with CT or MRI and cervical spine radiographs are obtained emergently. Patients with intracranial hemorrhage may require emergent surgical intervention for decompression and drainage of the blood collection. Increased ICP may require monitoring, placement of a ventricular drain, and aggressive medical management, including intubation and ventilation, osmotic therapy, and sedation.

Neuroimaging is not necessary for uncomplicated concussions but should be employed whenever suspicion of structural intracranial lesion exists. Drowsiness, headache, and vomiting are common after head trauma. They are not, by themselves, of concern if consciousness is preserved, the clinical trend is one of improvement, and results of the neurologic examination are normal. Children are especially susceptible to somnolence after head trauma but should be easily arousable. If symptoms worsen or persist for >1–2 days, neuroimaging may be indicated to evaluate for intracranial hemorrhage or cerebral edema.

Prognosis

Children with mild TBI (without subsequent neurologic deficits) have a favorable long-term prognosis, and late sequelae are rare. Children with moderate TBI usually make good recoveries even when neurologic signs persist for weeks. Long-term sequelae may include headaches, poor memory, slowing of motor skills, decline in cognitive skills, behavioral alterations, or attention deficits. Language function, especially in a young child, frequently makes a good recovery. Rehabilitation programs with physical therapy, behavioral management, and appropriate education may be necessary.

Coma lasting for weeks after head trauma may be compatible with a good outcome, although the risk of late sequelae is significant. Poor prognostic signs include a Glasgow Coma

Scale score below 4 on admission without improvement in 24 hours, absent pupillary light reflexes, and persistent extensor plantar reflexes. Extracranial trauma also contributes to the morbidity of these patients (e.g., aspiration pneumonia, acute respiratory distress syndrome, sepsis, emboli). Children with TBI who experience acute cerebral swelling may improve gradually or may remain in an unresponsive wakefulness syndrome. Maximal recovery may take weeks or months. Patients who remain in an unresponsive wakefulness syndrome for months after head injury are unlikely to improve.

PEARLS FOR PRACTITIONERS

See Neurology: Pearls for Practitioners at the end of this section.

REVIEW QUESTIONS

Available online.

CHAPTER 186

Neurodegenerative Disorders

Children typically acquire developmental milestones in a variable but predictable sequence (see Chapter 7). Rarely, children present with stagnation of development or frank loss of previously acquired skills. The **neurodegenerative disorders** encompass a large heterogeneous group of diseases that result from specific genetic and biochemical defects and varied unknown causes. Neurodegenerative disorders can present at any age. Clinical phenotypes vary, but neurologic deterioration may be demonstrated as loss of speech, vision, hearing, and intellectual or motor abilities, sometimes in concert with seizures, feeding difficulties, and intellectual disability. Progression may be slow over many years or may lead to death in early childhood.

HEREDITARY AND METABOLIC DEGENERATIVE DISEASES

Degenerative diseases may affect gray matter **(neuronal degenerative disorders)**, white matter **(leukodystrophies)**, both gray and white matter, or specific focal regions of the brain. Early seizures and intellectual impairment mark gray matter disorders, whereas upper motor neuron signs and progressive spasticity are the hallmarks of white matter disorders. Neuroimaging, usually with brain magnetic resonance imaging (MRI), is recommended, with specific genetic or metabolic testing considered depending on the result. Many neurodegenerative illnesses result from enzymatic disorders within subcellular organelles, including lysosomes, mitochondria, and peroxisomes. Therefore, for any patient with a degenerative neurologic condition of unknown cause, leukocytes or skin fibroblasts may be harvested for measurement of a standard battery of lysosomal, peroxisomal, and mitochondrial enzymes (see Chapters 55 and 56). An overnight EEG may be considered for patients with unexplained cognitive, language, or motor regression to evaluate for significant epileptiform activity meeting criteria for developmental and/or epileptic encephalopathy with spike-wave activation in sleep (previously called electrical status epilepticus in sleep), an EEG finding that can be associated with regression.

Sphingolipidoses

The sphingolipidoses are characterized by intracellular storage of lipid substrates resulting from defective catabolism of the cell membrane sphingolipids. Nearly all are inherited in an autosomal recessive pattern. In most cases, there are several forms of these diseases, and the tempo of disease progression reflects the amount of residual enzyme activity. The infantile forms are generally the most severe, usually presenting in the first or second year of life with rapid disease progression; affected individuals have virtually no normal enzyme activity. Juvenile and chronic forms manifest somewhat later in childhood or even adulthood and have a less fulminant disease course because there is some residual enzyme activity.

Classic **Niemann-Pick disease** (type A) is caused by a deficiency of sphingomyelinase and should be suspected in infants who exhibit the combination of hepatosplenomegaly, developmental delay, interstitial lung disease, and **retinal cherry red spots**. The ganglion cells of the retina and macula are distended and appear as a large area of white surrounding a small red fovea that is not covered by ganglion cells. Cognitive regression, hypotonia, and jaundice are also noted within the first year of life. Genetic testing reveals biallelic pathogenic variants in either *NPC1* or *NPC2*. Enzyme replacement therapy is available.

Although the most common form of **Gaucher disease** is an indolent illness of adults, there is a rapidly fatal infantile form featuring severe neurologic involvement caused by deficiency of the enzyme glucocerebrosidase. Glucosylceramide accumulates in the liver, spleen, and bone marrow leading to hepatosplenomegaly and cytopenias. The characteristic neurologic signs are opisthotonos (arching of the trunk), spasticity, trismus (difficulty opening mouth), eye movement abnormalities, and bulbar signs including difficulty swallowing. Gaucher disease inheritance is autosomal recessive with pathogenic variants found on the *GBA* gene from both parents.

Tay-Sachs disease (GM_2 gangliosidosis) is caused by deficiency of hexosaminidase A and results in the accumulation of GM_2 ganglioside in cerebral gray matter and cerebellum. Infants are typically normal, except for a marked startle response, until 6 months of age, when they develop listlessness, irritability, hyperacusis, cognitive regression, and retinal cherry red spots. Within months, blindness, convulsions, spasticity, and opisthotonos develop. Tay-Sachs disease inheritance is autosomal recessive with pathogenic variants found on the *HEXA* gene from both parents.

Metachromatic leukodystrophy (MLD) is a lipidosis caused by deficiency of arylsulfatase resulting from pathogenic variants of the *ARSA* gene, resulting in demyelination of the central nervous system (CNS) and peripheral nervous system. Children with the late-infantile form present between 1 and 2 years of age. After a period of normal development, progressive gait ataxia, spasticity, optic atrophy, intellectual deterioration, and absent reflexes occur. Diagnostic testing reveals increased CSF protein (a sign of CNS demyelination) and slowing of motor nerve conduction velocity (a sign of peripheral demyelination). Older school-age children with the juvenile form of MLD may present with gradual onset of behavior difficulties and declining academic abilities, followed by gait difficulties, clumsiness, slurred speech, and, sometimes, seizures. Hematopoietic stem cell transplantation may be considered for eligible patients, and ex vivo gene therapy has also been approved for use in the United States.

Krabbe disease (globoid cell leukodystrophy) is caused by a deficiency of galactocerebrosidase resulting from pathogenic variants of the *GALC* gene. Demyelination of the CNS and peripheral nervous system results in upper and lower motor neuron signs. Individuals with the infantile form (85–90% of cases) appear to be normal during the first months of life. Symptoms begin by 6 months of age and include extreme irritability, hyperpyrexia, vomiting, seizures, hypertonia, and blindness. Hematopoietic stem cell transplantation during infancy may be a treatment option.

Neuronal Ceroid Lipofuscinoses

The **neuronal ceroid lipofuscinoses** (NCLs) (also known as ***Batten disease***) are a group of inherited, neurodegenerative lysosomal storage disorders resulting from pathogenic variants in *CLN1–CLN14* genes; they are clinically characterized by progressive vision loss, seizures, declining cognitive abilities, motor deterioration, and early death. More than 10 different types have been characterized, including infantile, late-infantile, and juvenile types. Enzyme replacement therapy is available for NCL type 2 (*CLN2* disease).

Adrenoleukodystrophy

The adrenoleukodystrophies (ALDs) are a group of X-linked neurodegenerative disorders that are often associated with adrenocortical insufficiency. ALD is caused by accumulation of very long chain fatty acids in neuronal and adrenal tissue (see Chapter 179) and is diagnosed by abnormal very long-chain fatty acid testing. The most common leukodystrophy is **classic X-linked adrenoleukodystrophy**, caused by a pathologic variant in the *ABCD1* gene. X-linked ALD is recommended to be part of each state's newborn screening panel in the United States. Males present between ages 5 and 15 years with academic difficulties, behavioral disturbances, and gait abnormalities, progressing to seizures, spasticity, ataxia, and swallowing difficulties. Brain MRI demonstrates a classic pattern of symmetric abnormal white matter signal in the parietal-occipital regions, with contrast enhancement at the margins. Symptomatic adrenocortical insufficiency with fatigue, vomiting, and hypotension develops in 20–40% of patients with X-linked ALD. ALD should be considered in any male with primary adrenocortical insufficiency, even in the absence of clear-cut neurologic abnormalities. Patients with early stages of cerebral disease can be treated with allogeneic hematopoietic cell transplantation; if that is not an option, autologous hematopoietic cell transplantation with ex vivo gene therapy may be considered.

Mucopolysaccharidoses

Mucopolysaccharidoses (MPSs) are caused by defective lysosomal hydrolases resulting in the accumulation of glycosaminoglycans (formerly known as mucopolysaccharides) within lysosomes (see Chapter 55). There are several types of MPS, the most common being type I **(Hurler syndrome)**, type II **(Hunter syndrome)**, and type III **(Sanfilippo syndrome)**. Both MPSI and MPSII are recommended to be part of each state's newborn screening panel in the United States. Signs and symptoms are usually not present at birth with the exception of the more severe forms of MPS type VII. Most types present within the first few years of life, but some of the more attenuated forms can present as late as adolescence to early adulthood. The clinical manifestations are variable and include coarse facies, short stature, kyphoscoliosis, hepatosplenomegaly, cardiovascular abnormalities, corneal clouding, and neurologic involvement. Children with the severe form of Hurler syndrome appear normal during the first 6 months of life and then develop the characteristic skeletal and neurologic features. Intellectual disability, spasticity, deafness, and optic atrophy are progressive. Hydrocephalus frequently occurs because of obstruction to CSF flow by thickened leptomeninges. Treatment options for certain types of MPS include enzyme replacement therapy or hematopoietic cell transplantation.

Mitochondrial Disorders

Mitochondrial diseases represent a clinically heterogeneous group of disorders that fundamentally share a disturbance in oxidative phosphorylation (adenosine triphosphate synthesis; see Chapter 56). Symptoms may include hypotonia, developmental delay, seizures, hearing loss, optic nerve atrophy, progressive external ophthalmoplegia, and/or myopathy, including cardiomyopathy. Abrupt symptoms are often manifest concurrent with periods of physiologic stress such as febrile illness or fasting. Mitochondrial DNA is inherited from the mother; specific genetic diagnoses are often difficult to identify because several different gene variants can cause the same disease, single variants can have multiple phenotypes, and analysis of mitochondrial protein function is technically demanding.

Specific syndromes include **MELAS** (mitochondrial encephalomyopathy, lactic acidosis, and strokelike episodes); **MERRF** (myoclonic epilepsy with ragged red fibers), which can also manifest as combinations of dementia, sensorineural hearing loss, optic nerve atrophy, peripheral neuropathy, and occasionally cardiomyopathy with Wolff-Parkinson-White syndrome; and **NARP** (neuropathy, ataxia, and retinitis pigmentosa).

Subacute necrotizing encephalomyelopathy, or **Leigh disease**, is a neuropathologically defined, degenerative, inherited CNS disease primarily involving the periaqueductal region of the brainstem, caudate, and putamen. Symptoms usually begin before 2 years of age and consist of hypotonia, feeding difficulties, respiratory irregularity, weakness of extraocular movements, and ataxia. Blood and CSF lactate and pyruvate levels are elevated. Several alterations of mitochondrial function produce this clinical syndrome.

Rett Syndrome

Rett syndrome is a neurodevelopmental disorder that classically affects females. Typically, development appears normal during the first 6–18 months of life, but this is followed by developmental regression, loss of purposeful hand movements, loss of verbal communication skills, gait apraxia, and stereotypic repetitive hand movements that resemble washing, wringing, or clapping of the hands. Affected females also develop acquired microcephaly. Episodic apnea and/or hyperpnea, peripheral vasomotor disturbances, growth retardation, abnormal muscle tone, and prolonged QTc interval often occur. The developmental regression plateaus and stabilizes, but seizures, spasticity, and kyphoscoliosis develop. The etiology is a change on an X chromosome gene coding for methyl-CpG-binding protein 2 *(MECP2)* transcription factor. Males with *MECP2* variants usually do not survive to delivery but can present with severe neonatal encephalopathy, seizures, microcephaly, abnormal tone, and respiratory insufficiency. Trofinetide is a disease-modifying therapy for Rett syndrome.

Degenerative Diseases With Focal Manifestations

Some neurodegenerative disorders have predilections to target specific regions or systems within the neuraxis and produce symptoms referable to the affected region.

Wilson disease is an autosomal recessive inborn error of copper metabolism caused by pathogenic variants in the *ATP7B* gene, resulting in copper deposition in several organs. Abnormal copper deposition produces cirrhosis in the liver, a characteristic green-brown (Kayser-Fleischer) ring in the peripheral cornea, and neuronal degeneration, predominantly in the cerebellum and basal ganglia in the CNS. Neurologic symptoms characteristically begin in the early teenage years with dysarthria, dysphasia, drooling, fixed smile, tremor, and dystonia. Psychiatric manifestations such as depression, personality change, or declining school performance may precede hepatic or neurologic symptoms. Serum ceruloplasmin levels are low. MRI shows abnormalities of the basal ganglia. Treatment is with a copper-chelating agent, such as oral penicillamine.

ACQUIRED ILLNESSES MIMICKING DEGENERATIVE DISEASES

Children with poorly controlled epilepsy may be continuously in either an ictal or a postictal state and may appear stuporous because of their epileptic encephalopathy. Antiseizure medications that are sedating or affect mood, memory, motivation, or attention may contribute to the lack or loss of developmental abilities and school failure.

Chronic drug use or overuse (e.g., sedatives, tranquilizers, anticholinergics) can cause progressive confusion, lethargy, and ataxia. Intoxications with heavy metals, such as lead, may cause chronic learning difficulties or may present acutely with irritability, listlessness, anorexia, and pallor, progressing to fulminant encephalopathy. Vitamin deficiency of thiamine, niacin, vitamin B_{12}, and vitamin E can produce encephalopathy, peripheral neuropathy, and ataxia.

Congenital and acquired hypothyroidism impairs cognition and slows developmental progress. Unrecognized congenital hypothyroidism produces irreversible damage if it is not treated immediately after birth (see Chapter 176).

Structural brain diseases, such as hydrocephalus and slow-growing tumors, may cause slowly progressive cognitive decline and other focal deficits. Certain indolent brain infections, such as measles (causing subacute sclerosing panencephalitis), rubella (German measles), syphilis, and some fungal infections, cause neurologic deterioration over months and years. Congenital HIV infection causes failure of normal development and regression of acquired skills.

Psychiatric disorders, such as depression and severe psychosocial deprivation in infancy, can give rise to apathy and failure to attain developmental milestones (see Chapter 21). Children with autism spectrum disorder may go through a phase of developmental stagnation or disintegration at about 12–18 months of age after a period of early normal milestones. Depression in older children can lead to blunting of affect, social withdrawal, and poor school performance, which raise the question of encephalopathy or dementia.

PEARLS FOR PRACTITIONERS

See Neurology: Pearls for Practitioners at the end of this section.

REVIEW QUESTION

Available online.

CHAPTER 187

Neurocutaneous Disorders

The skin, teeth, hair, nails, and brain are derived embryologically from ectoderm. Abnormalities of these surface structures may indicate abnormal brain development. Neurofibromatosis (types 1 and 2), tuberous sclerosis, Sturge-Weber syndrome, von Hippel-Lindau disease, and ataxia-telangiectasia are the most common neurocutaneous disorders.

NEUROFIBROMATOSIS TYPE 1

Etiology

Neurofibromatosis type 1 (NF1), also known as **von Recklinghausen disease**, is an autosomal dominant disorder with an incidence of approximately 1 in 3,000. It is caused by pathogenic variants of the *NF1* gene, which codes for a tumor suppressor gene, neurofibromin. Neurofibromin is a major negative regulator of a key signal transduction pathway, the Ras pathway. Genetic changes result in increased downstream mitogenic signaling. Somatic mosaicism, in which an abnormality in one copy of the *NF1* gene is present in some cells but not others, indicates a postzygotic genetic change and is called **segmental neurofibromatosis**.

Clinical Manifestations

The cardinal features of neurofibromatosis are café-au-lait spots, axillary or inguinal freckling, cutaneous neurofibromas, and iris hamartomas (Lisch nodules). **Café-au-lait spots** are present in more than 90% of patients who have NF1 (Fig. 187.1). They typically appear in the first few years of life and increase in number and size over time. The presence of six or more café-au-lait spots larger than 5 mm in a prepubescent child suggests the diagnosis.

Neurofibromas are composed of various combinations of Schwann cells, fibroblasts, mast cells, and vascular elements. Dermal neurofibromas are nearly universal and consist of discrete, small, soft lesions that lie within the dermis and

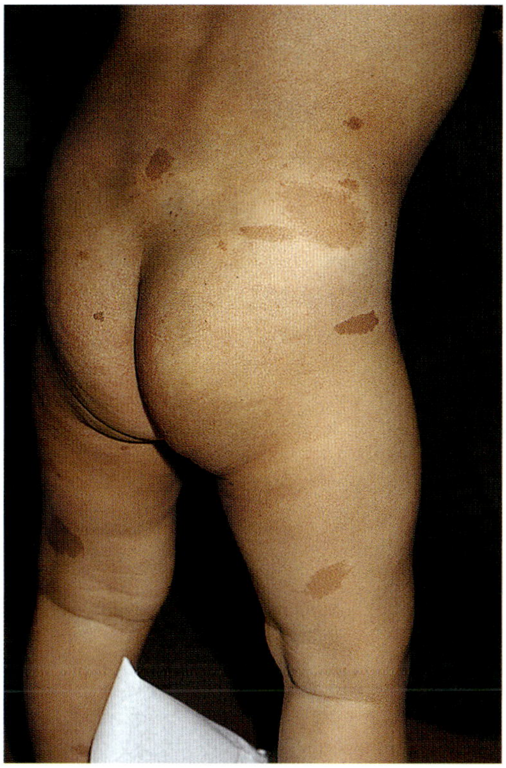

FIGURE 187.1 Café-au-lait macules. (From Eichenfield LF, Frieden IJ, Esterly NB. *Textbook of Neonatal Dermatology*. Philadelphia: Saunders; 2001:372.)

epidermis. They rarely cause any symptoms but can cause significant cosmetic concerns. Neurofibromas may also be situated within viscera or along blood vessels and peripheral nerves. Plexiform neurofibromas are large, occasionally nodular, subcutaneous lesions that lie along the major peripheral nerve trunks. They often cause symptoms including pain, weakness, and invasion of adjacent viscera, bone, or spinal cord. Surgical treatment may be attempted, but results are often unsatisfactory. Mitogen-activated protein kinase (MEK) inhibitors have been used to treat symptomatic or inoperable tumors.

Common complications are learning disability, scoliosis, seizures, and cerebral vasculature abnormalities (e.g., moyamoya). Other tumors that occur in NF1 are optic nerve gliomas, astrocytomas of the brain and spinal cord, and malignant peripheral nerve tumors. T2-weighted magnetic resonance images (MRIs) reveal hyperintense lesions (focal areas of high signal intensity), commonly in the subcortical white matter, basal ganglia, cerebellum, and brainstem, that are distinctive for the disease. They are benign and often disappear in adulthood.

Genetic counseling is an essential component of care. Although it is an autosomal dominant disorder, spontaneous somatic genetic changes account for 30–50% of cases.

Neurofibromatosis Type 2

Neurofibromatosis type 2 (NF2) is an autosomal dominant disorder with an incidence of 1 in 25,000. Half the cases have no family history. The *NF2* gene is a tumor suppressor gene, and disease results in neurologic, eye, and skin lesions. NF2 predisposes patients to multiple intracranial and spinal tumors, including bilateral acoustic schwannomas, schwannomas of other cranial and spinal nerves, meningiomas, and gliomas. Posterior capsular or cortical cataracts are common, and skin lesions include plaque-like lesions, subcutaneous nodules, and cutaneous schwannomas. Lisch nodules, café-au-lait spots, and axillary freckling (seen in NF1) are not features of NF2.

TUBEROUS SCLEROSIS COMPLEX

Etiology

Tuberous sclerosis complex (TSC), an autosomal dominant disorder, is characterized by hamartomas in many organs, especially the brain, eyes, skin, kidneys, and heart. The incidence is 1 in 10,000 births. Two thirds of cases are sporadic and thought to represent new genetic changes. Variants affecting either the *TSC1* or *TSC2* genes cause tuberous sclerosis. The *TSC1* and *TSC2* genes encode distinct proteins, hamartin and tuberin, which are widely expressed in the brain and result in constitutive activation of the protein kinase mTOR (mammalian target of rapamycin), leading to the formation of numerous benign tumors (hamartomas).

Clinical Manifestations

TSC is an extremely heterogeneous disease with variable expression and a wide clinical spectrum varying from normal intelligence without seizures to severe intellectual disability with refractory epilepsy and autism, often within the same family. People with TSC may have retinal lesions (retinal hamartomas, white depigmented patches) and brain lesions (cortical tubers, subependymal nodules, hydrocephalus). **Tubers** in the cerebral cortex are areas of dysplasia that, in combination with other microscopic areas of abnormal development, are responsible for the symptoms of intellectual disability and epilepsy. TSC is one of the most common causes of infantile spasms; in this context, the infantile spasms often respond to treatment with vigabatrin. **Subependymal nodules** are hamartomas that may mutate into a growth phase and become **subependymal giant cell astrocytomas (SEGAs)**, causing obstruction of cerebrospinal fluid outflow and resultant hydrocephalus. SEGAs can be treated with everolimus, an mTOR inhibitor, which also can be used for patients with TSC as an adjunctive treatment for epilepsy. Some children with SEGAs require surgical resection.

Extracerebral manifestations include typical skin findings of hypomelanotic macules **(ash leaf spots)**, which are easiest to visualize under a Wood ultraviolet lamp and are apparent in infancy. Facial angiofibromas (formerly referred to as adenoma sebaceum) appear as small red nodules over the nose and cheeks that are sometimes confused with acne. **Shagreen patches** are elevated, rough plaques of skin with a predilection for the lumbar and gluteal regions that develop in late childhood or early adolescence. **Cardiac rhabdomyomas** are largest during prenatal life and infancy and are rarely symptomatic. Occasionally, they may cause arrhythmias or cardiac outflow obstruction. Renal angiomyolipomas may undergo malignant transformation. Interstitial pulmonary disease (pulmonary lymphangioleiomyomatosis) also affects adults with TSC.

STURGE-WEBER SYNDROME

Sturge-Weber syndrome is sporadic (not inherited) and is caused by a somatic mosaic variant of the *GNAQ* gene. It is characterized by abnormal blood vessels **(angiomas)** of the leptomeninges overlying the cerebral cortex in association with an ipsilateral facial **port-wine stain** involving the ophthalmic division of the trigeminal nerve (forehead and upper eyelid) and, often, glaucoma. The port-wine stain, also known as nevus flammeus, is due to an ectasia of superficial venules and may have a much more extensive and even bilateral distribution. Not all children with a facial port-wine stain have Sturge-Weber syndrome.

MRI with contrast demonstrates leptomeningeal angioma and white matter abnormalities thought to be due to chronic hypoxia and atrophy. Seizures are the most common associated neurologic abnormality, occurring in most patients. Many children with Sturge-Weber syndrome are intellectually normal, and seizures are well controlled with standard antiseizure medications. However, progressive ischemia of the underlying brain develops in some children with Sturge-Weber syndrome, resulting in hemiparesis, hemianopia, intractable focal epilepsy, cognitive impairment, or strokelike events. Hemispherectomy may be pursued for individuals with unilateral disease whose seizures are difficult to control, both to control the epilepsy and to preserve cognitive and motor development. Low-dose aspirin may result in improved perfusion and thereby reduce strokelike events and seizures. Pulse dye laser surgery is a therapeutic option for cosmetic management of the facial nevus flammeus. Expert ophthalmologic management of glaucoma is required. Endocrinology evaluations are also necessary, because these patients often have growth hormone deficiency and/or hypothyroidism.

PEARLS FOR PRACTITIONERS

See Neurology: Pearls for Practitioners at the end of this section.

REVIEW QUESTIONS

Available online.

CHAPTER 188

Congenital Malformations of the Central Nervous System

Central nervous system malformations include disorders of spinal cord and neural tube formation, structure specification (e.g., neuronal migration, gray matter), brain growth and size, and skull growth and shape.

The precursor of the nervous system is the neural plate of the embryonic ectoderm, which develops at 18 days of gestation. The neural plate gives rise to the neural tube, which forms the brain and spinal cord, and neural crest cells, which form the peripheral nervous system, meninges, melanocytes, and adrenal medulla. The neural tube begins to form on day 22 of gestation. The rostral end forms the brain, and the caudal region forms the spinal cord. The lumen of the neural tube forms the ventricles of the brain and the central canal of the spinal cord. Most brain malformations are produced by a variety of injuries occurring during a vulnerable period of gestation. Precipitating factors include genetic and metabolic abnormalities; congenital infections; and exposure to irradiation, certain drugs, and maternal illness during pregnancy.

CONGENITAL ANOMALIES OF THE SPINAL CORD

Etiology and Clinical Manifestations

Defective closure of the caudal neural tube at the end of week 4 of gestation results in anomalies of the lumbar and sacral vertebrae or spinal cord called **spina bifida**. These anomalies range in severity from clinically insignificant defects of the L5 or S1 vertebral arches to major malformations, leaving the spinal cord uncovered by skin or bone on the infant's back. The latter severe defect, called a **myelomeningocele**, may result in flaccid paralysis and loss of sensation in the legs and incontinence of bowel and bladder, with the extent and degree of neurologic deficit dependent on the location of the myelomeningocele. In addition, affected children usually have an associated **Chiari type II malformation** (downward displacement of the cerebellar tonsils and medulla), resulting in hydrocephalus and weakness of face and swallowing. In a **meningocele**, the spinal canal and cystic meninges are exposed on the back, but the underlying spinal cord is anatomically and functionally intact. In **spina bifida occulta**, the skin of the back is apparently intact but defects of the underlying bone or spinal canal are present. Meningoceles and spina bifida occulta may be associated with a lipoma, dermoid cyst, or tethering of the cord to a thick filum terminale. A dimple or tuft of hair may be present over the affected area. Patients may also have an associated dermoid sinus, an epithelial tract extending from the skin surface to the meninges; this increases the risk of meningitis. Patients with spina bifida occulta or meningocele may have weakness and numbness in the feet that can result in recurrent ulcerations, or difficulties controlling bowel or bladder function that may result in recurrent urinary tract infections, reflux nephropathy, and renal insufficiency.

Diagnostic Studies

Myelomeningocele in the fetus is suggested by an elevated α-fetoprotein (AFP) in the pregnant person's blood and confirmed by ultrasound, with greater sensitivity beginning in the second trimester. After birth, screening ultrasound may be used with magnetic resonance imaging to confirm underlying spinal abnormalities.

Treatment and Prevention

Neonates with myelomeningocele must undergo operative closure of the open spinal defects (fetal or postnatal surgery) and often require treatment of hydrocephalus by placement of a ventriculoperitoneal shunt. Compared to postnatal surgery, fetal surgery prior to 26 weeks of gestation to close the myelomeningocele reduces the need for CSF shunting and improves motor development. Toddlers and children with lower spinal cord dysfunction require physical therapy, bracing of the lower extremities, and intermittent bladder catheterization.

In the absence of associated brain anomalies, most survivors have normal intelligence, but learning problems and epilepsy are more common than in the general population.

Spina bifida can be prevented in many cases by **folate** supplementation for the pregnant person. Because the defect occurs so early in gestation, all people who could get pregnant are advised to take oral folic acid daily.

CONGENITAL MALFORMATIONS OF THE BRAIN

Defective closure of the rostral neural tube produces anencephaly or encephaloceles. Neonates with **anencephaly** have a rudimentary brainstem or midbrain but no cortex or cranium. This is rapidly fatal after delivery. Patients with **encephalocele** usually have a skull defect and exposure of meninges alone or meninges and brain. The recurrence risk in subsequent pregnancies for either cranial or spinal neural tube defects is 3–4%. Within a family, an anencephalic birth may be followed by the birth of a child affected with a lumbosacral myelomeningocele. The inheritance of neural tube defects is polygenic.

Agenesis of the corpus callosum may be partial or complete and may occur in an isolated fashion or in association with other anomalies of cellular migration. **Dandy-Walker malformation** is diagnosed on the basis of the classic triad: complete or partial agenesis of the cerebellar vermis, cystic dilation of the fourth ventricle, and enlarged posterior fossa. There may be associated hydrocephalus, absence of the corpus callosum, and neuronal migration abnormalities. Intelligence may be normal or impaired, depending on the degree of associated cerebral dysgenesis.

Holoprosencephaly represents varying degrees of failure of the forebrain (prosencephalon) to divide into two distinct cerebral hemispheres. Holoprosencephaly is often associated with midline facial defects (hypotelorism, cleft lip, cleft palate). This anomaly may be isolated or associated with a genetic disorder. The prognosis for infants with severe (alobar) holoprosencephaly is uniformly poor, but those with milder forms (semilobar, lobar) may have less severe neurologic outcomes. Holoprosencephaly can be seen in children with trisomy 13 and trisomy 18.

Hydranencephaly is a condition in which the brain presumably develops normally but then is destroyed by an intrauterine, probably vascular, insult. The result is virtual absence of the cerebrum with an intact skull. The thalamus, brainstem, and some occipital cortex are typically present. Children may have a normal external appearance at the time of birth but do not achieve developmental milestones.

Macrocephaly and Microcephaly

Macrocephaly represents a head circumference above the 97th percentile and may be the result of **macrocrania** (increased skull thickness), **hydrocephalus** (enlargement of the ventricles; see Chapter 185), or **megalencephaly** (enlargement of the brain). Diseases of bone metabolism or hypertrophy of the bone marrow causes macrocrania. Megalencephaly may be the result of a significant disorder of brain development or an accumulation of abnormal metabolic substances (Table 188.1). Most often, however, macrocephaly is a familial trait of no clinical significance. If the child is developmentally normal but has macrocephaly, plotting the parents' head circumference on a growth chart can provide reassurance and help to avoid unnecessary neurodiagnostic testing.

TABLE 188.1 Common Causes of Macrocephaly

Macrocrania (increased skull thickness)
Achondroplasia
Hypochondroplasia
Fragile X syndrome
Osteopetrosis
Chronic, severe anemia
Hydrocephalus (enlargement of the ventricles; Chapter 185)
Masses
Cysts
Arteriovenous malformations
Subdural fluid collections/hematoma
Neoplasm
Megalencephaly (enlargement of the brain)
Embryologic disorder causing abnormal proliferation of brain tissue (e.g., neurofibromatosis, tuberous sclerosis)
• Accumulation of abnormal metabolic substances (e.g., Krabbe disease, mucopolysaccharidoses)
Benign causes
Benign extracerebral collections of infancy
Familial macrocephaly

Microcephaly represents a head circumference below the 3rd percentile. A myriad of syndromes and metabolic disorders are associated with microcephaly, some of which are hereditary (Table 188.2). In most instances, a small head circumference is a reflection of a small brain. Brain growth is rapid during the perinatal period, and any insult (e.g., infectious, metabolic, toxic, vascular) sustained during this period or during early infancy is likely to impair brain growth and result in microcephaly. Rarely, a small head is the result of premature closure of one or more skull sutures, called **craniosynostosis**. In patients with craniosynostoses, the shape of the head depends on which of the major sutures has prematurely closed (e.g., metopic, coronal, sagittal, lambdoid). To accommodate the growing brain, compensatory skull growth occurs parallel to the affected suture. This diagnosis is readily made by the abnormal shape of the skull. Posterior plagiocephaly caused by craniosynostosis may be confused with positional plagiocephaly (skull flattening related to pressure on one side of the head). Positional plagiocephaly has increased, in part because of supine sleep positioning recommendations. As a rule, macrocephaly and microcephaly raise a concern about cognitive ability, but head circumference alone should never be used to establish a prognosis for intellectual development.

Disorders of Neuronal Migration

Many malformations result from the failure of normal migration of neurons from the periventricular germinal matrix zone to the cortical surface at 1–5 months of gestation. Multiple malformations may exist in the same patient. Neurologic development with these anomalies varies and depends on the type and extent of the malformation. Many children with disorders of neuronal migration have treatment-resistant epilepsy.

Schizencephaly is characterized by clefts within the cerebral hemispheres that extend from the cortical surface to the ventricular cavity. Unilateral clefts can cause isolated congenital hemiparesis, whereas bilateral schizencephaly causes spastic quadriparesis and associated intellectual disability. Affected individuals are at high risk for focal epilepsy.

TABLE 188.2 Common Causes of Microcephaly

PRIMARY MICROCEPHALY
Genetic microcephalies*
Trisomy 21
Trisomy 13
Trisomy 18
Angelman syndrome
Prader-Willi syndrome
Smith-Lemli-Opitz syndrome
Cornelia de Lange syndrome
Rett syndrome
CNS malformation
Holoprosencephaly
Encephalocele
Hydranencephaly
CNS migrational disorder
Lissencephaly
Schizencephaly
Pachygyria
Polymicrogyria
SECONDARY (ACQUIRED) MICROCEPHALY
Infections (congenital)
Rubella
Cytomegalovirus
Toxoplasmosis
Syphilis
HIV
Zika virus
Infections (noncongenital)
Meningitis
Encephalitis
Stroke
Toxic
Radiation exposure—fetal
Fetal alcohol syndrome
Maternal phenylketonuria
Hypoxic-ischemic or other severe brain injury
Periventricular leukomalacia
Severe chronic illness resulting in poor nutrition
Craniosynostosis totalis

*Genetic microcephalies are nearly always present at birth, with the exception of Rett syndrome.
CNS, Central nervous system.

A severe defect in cortical migration, **lissencephaly**, results in a smooth brain without sulcation (agyria). The normal six-layered cortex does not develop. Affected children have difficult-to-control seizures and profound developmental delay. This anomaly most commonly is part of a genetic disorder, which may be X-linked (*DCX* variants) or caused by de novo autosomal dominant pathogenic variants in *LIS1*. In **pachygyria**, the gyri are few in number and too broad. In **polymicrogyria**, the gyri are too many and too small. Sometimes pachygyria and polymicrogyria affect an entire hemisphere, producing enlargement of that hemisphere and a clinical syndrome of severe, medically intractable seizures that begin in early infancy. **Gray matter heterotopias** are abnormal islands within the central white matter of neurons that have never completed the migratory process.

PEARLS FOR PRACTITIONERS

See Neurology: Pearls for Practitioners at the end of this section.

REVIEW QUESTIONS

Available online.

Suggested Readings

Ahmed MI, Iqbal M, Hussain N. A structured approach to the assessment of a floppy neonate. *J Pediatr Neurosci*. 2016;11(1):2–6.

Aylward SC, Reem RE. Pediatric Intracranial Hypertension. *Pediatr Neurol*. 2017;66:32–43.

Blackburn J, Parnes M. Tics, tremors and other movement disorders in childhood. *Curr Probl Pediatr Adolesc Health Care*. 2021;51(3):100983.

Ferriero DM, Fullerton HJ, Bernard TJ, et al. Management of Stroke in Neonates and Children: A Scientific Statement From the American Heart Association/American Stroke Association. *Stroke*. 2019;50(3):e51–e96.

Gelineau-Morel RN, Zinkus TP, Le Pichon JB. Pediatric Head Trauma: A Review and Update. *Pediatr Rev*. 2019;40(9):468–481.

Klein J, Koch T. Headache in Children. *Pediatr Rev*. 2020;41(4):159–171.

Korf BR, Bebin EM. Neurocutaneous Disorders in Children. *Pediatr Rev*. 2017;38(3):119–128.

Patra KP, Lancaster JD, Hogg J, Carpenter JS. Pediatric MRI of the brain: a primer. *Pediatr Rev*. 2014;35(3):106–111.

Piña-Garza J, James K. *Fenichel's Clinical Pediatric Neurology: A Signs and Symptoms Approach*. 8th ed. Philadelphia: Saunders; 2019.

Sandoval Karamian AG, DiGiovine MP, Massey SL. Neonatal Seizures. *Pediatr Rev*. 2024;45(7):381–393.

Specchio N, Wirrell EC, Scheffer IE, et al. International League Against Epilepsy classification and definition of epilepsy syndromes with onset in childhood: Position paper by the ILAE Task Force on Nosology and Definitions. *Epilepsia*. 2022;63(6):1398–1442.

PEARLS FOR PRACTITIONERS

CHAPTER 180

Neurology Assessment

- The pediatric neurologic examination varies with age; the newborn is unique, with many transient and primitive reflexes, which provide assessment of the functional integrity of the brainstem and basal ganglia.
- Careful evaluations of social, cognitive, language, fine motor and gross motor skills and their age-appropriateness are key in the neurologic assessment of children.
- Watching a child creep, crawl, cruise, or walk is the best global assessment for the motor and coordination systems.

CHAPTER 181

Headache and Migraine

- There are four temporal patterns of childhood headache: acute, acute recurrent, chronic progressive, and chronic nonprogressive.
- Additional investigation is warranted for headaches in the presence of an abnormal neurologic exam (especially papilledema), signs or symptoms of increased intracranial pressure, atypical headache, progressive chronic headache, or "worst headache of my life."

- Symptoms of increased intracranial pressure include early morning vomiting or headache that wakes the child from sleep.

CHAPTER 182

Seizures

- Focal aware seizures (previously termed *simple partial seizures*) arise from a specific anatomic focus.
  - Clinical symptoms include motor (tonic, clonic, myoclonic), sensory, or autonomic abnormalities, but consciousness is preserved.
- Focal seizures with impaired awareness (previously termed *complex partial seizures*) can have similar sensorimotor signs but also have associated alteration of consciousness.
- The clinical hallmark of absence seizures is a brief (<15 seconds) loss of awareness accompanied by eyelid fluttering or simple automatisms, such as fumbling with the fingers and lip smacking. Childhood absence epilepsy usually begins between 4 and 10 years of age.
- Children with febrile seizures have an excellent prognosis; daily antiseizure medication to prevent febrile seizures is not recommended.
- Infantile spasms are clusters of brief contractions of the neck, trunk, and arm muscles, followed by a phase of sustained muscle contraction lasting less than 2 seconds. Rapid initiation of effective therapy offers the best chance for favorable neurodevelopmental outcomes.
- Initial management of status epilepticus is with a benzodiazepine and should begin if the seizure persists longer than 5 minutes.
  - If the seizure does not resolve after two doses of benzodiazepines, a second-line agent must be administered, typically phenobarbital for newborns and infants and intravenous fosphenytoin, valproic acid, levetiracetam, or lacosamide for older children.
- Psychogenic nonepileptic events (PNEE) are a type of functional neurologic disorders (FND).
  - Children with epilepsy may also have concurrent PNEE.
  - Careful assessment and intervention for abuse, as well as other social stressors, is a key component of the care of children with PNEE.

CHAPTER 183

Weakness and Hypotonia

- Weakness is a decreased ability to voluntarily and actively move muscles; hypotonia is a state of low muscle resistance to movement.
- An upper motor neuron pattern of weakness with increased deep tendon reflexes, spasticity, and extensor plantar responses may be caused by tumors, traumatic brain injury, infections, stroke, demyelinating syndromes, spinal cord trauma or mass, metabolic diseases, or neurodegenerative diseases.
- A lower motor neuron pattern of weakness has decreased muscle tone, decreased or absent reflexes, and sometimes fasciculations.
- Acute spinal cord lesions, such as infarction or compression, may produce a flaccid, areflexic paralysis that mimics lower motor neuron disease. Lesions of the spinal cord are best delineated with magnetic resonance imaging.
- Spinal muscular atrophy is a genetic disease characterized by progressive degeneration of anterior horn cells, which results in weakness.
- Guillain-Barré syndrome (acute inflammatory demyelinating polyradiculoneuropathy) is a postinfectious autoimmune peripheral neuropathy that can occur after an infection and is the most common cause of acute flaccid paralysis in children. It presents with areflexia, flaccidity, and symmetric ascending weakness.
- Muscular dystrophies are characterized by progressive myofiber degeneration and the gradual replacement of muscle by fibrotic tissue. Duchenne muscular dystrophy is the most common muscular dystrophy.
- The acute onset of focal neurologic deficits in a child is stroke until proven otherwise.
  - The most common causes of pediatric stroke are vasculopathies, infection, cardioembolic infarcts due to congenital heart disease, sickle cell anemia, coagulation disorders, dehydration, and head trauma.

CHAPTER 184

Ataxia and Movement Disorders

- The most common causes of acute ataxia in childhood are postinfectious acute cerebellar ataxia and drug intoxications.
- Movement disorders in children are typically hyperkinetic.
- Tics are rapid, purposeless, involuntary, stereotyped movements and typically involve the face, eyes, shoulder, and arm. Approximately 25% of children have transient tics.
- A child who is unsteady and has erratic eye movements may have opsoclonus-myoclonus syndrome and should be evaluated for occult neuroblastoma.

CHAPTER 185

Altered Mental Status

- In childhood, the most common causes of coma are toxins, infections, head trauma, hypoxia-ischemia (e.g., cardiac arrest, near-drowning), and seizures.
- Computed tomography is the preferred head imaging technique in emergency situations because it can be performed rapidly without sedation and accurately identifies acute hemorrhages and mass lesions.
- Cerebral herniation is a medical emergency. Signs include altered mental status, signs of increased intracranial pressure (ICP) with dilated pupil or miosis, hemiparesis, decorticate or decerebrate posturing, and irregular respirations.

- Lumbar puncture may be contraindicated in the setting of an intracranial mass lesion or clear hydrocephalus because withdrawal of cerebrospinal fluid (CSF) can change pressures between the intracranial compartments and promote brainstem shifts and herniation.
- Head trauma may result in concussion, post-traumatic intracranial hemorrhage, skull fractures, cranial nerve, or cervical spine injuries.
  - Concussion is the rapid onset of short-lived neurologic impairment that typically resolves spontaneously.
    - Symptoms may include headache, slowed reaction times, emotional lability, drowsiness, loss of consciousness, or amnesia.
  - Epidural, subdural, parenchymal, and subarachnoid intracranial hemorrhages can occur following head trauma.
    - Intracranial bleeding accompanied by neurologic deterioration requires prompt assessment for likely evacuation of the blood.

CHAPTER 186

Neurodegenerative Disorders

- Neurodegenerative disorders encompass a large heterogeneous group of diseases that result from specific genetic and biochemical defects and varied unknown causes.
  - Neuronal degenerative disorders affect gray matter.
    - Early signs are seizures and intellectual impairment.
  - Leukodystrophies affect white matter.
    - Early signs include upper motor neuron signs and progressive spasticity.
- Mitochondrial diseases represent a clinically heterogeneous group of disorders in oxidative phosphorylation.
  - Abrupt symptoms often manifest during physiologic stress (e.g., febrile illness, fasting).

CHAPTER 187

Neurocutaneous Disorders

- Abnormalities of skin, teeth, hair, and nails may indicate abnormal brain development, because all are derived from ectoderm.

CHAPTER 188

Congenital Malformations of the Central Nervous System

- Central nervous system malformations include disorders of the spinal cord, neural tube formation, structure specification (neuronal migration), brain growth, and skull growth and shape.
  - Spina bifida is the defective closure of the caudal neural tube and ranges in severity from insignificant defects of vertebral arches to myelomeningocele.
    - An elevated α-fetoprotein in the pregnant person's blood suggests myelomeningocele in the fetus.
    - Children with myelomeningocele often have an associated Chiari type II malformation.
- Defective closure of the rostral neural tube produces anencephaly or encephalocele.
- Holoprosencephaly represents varying degrees of failure of the forebrain to divide into two distinct cerebral hemispheres.
- Hydranencephaly is a condition in which the brain presumably develops normally but is destroyed by an intrauterine, probably vascular, accident.
- Schizencephaly and lissencephaly are disorders or neuronal migration that result in abnormal neurologic development and often are associated with treatment-resistant epilepsy.

SECTION 25

DERMATOLOGY

Hsi Yen | Yvonne E. Chiu

CHAPTER 189

Dermatology Assessment

Approximately one in three Americans has at least one recognizable skin disorder at any time. The most common diagnoses in children include atopic dermatitis, seborrheic dermatitis, acne vulgaris, verruca vulgaris, molluscum contagiosum, and impetigo.

HISTORY

The age of the patient, onset, duration, progression, associated cutaneous symptoms (pain, pruritus), previous treatments, and associated systemic signs or symptoms (fever, malaise, weight loss) are important clues. Obtaining an accurate description of the original lesion improves diagnostic accuracy. Patients often do not consider over-the-counter remedies, especially topical medications, as treatment, so it is important to inquire about these treatments specifically as they may alter the appearance of a rash. Other important information includes a history of allergies, environmental exposures, travel history, previous treatment, affected contacts, and family history.

PHYSICAL EXAMINATION

A careful examination of the skin requires a visual and tactile assessment. Examination of the skin over the entire body must be performed systematically. Mucous membranes, hair, nails, and teeth should also be assessed as they are all ectodermal in origin and may be involved in cutaneous disorders.

COMMON MANIFESTATIONS

A descriptive nomenclature of skin lesions helps with generating a differential diagnosis and with communication between health care providers. Determination of the primary lesion and secondary change is the cornerstone of dermatologic diagnosis. A **primary lesion** is defined as the basic lesion that arises de novo and is most characteristic of the disease process (Table 189.1). Primary lesions may not be present on a patient at the time of presentation, as some are altered by time or external factors such as medication applied, secondary infection, or physical manipulation (e.g., scratching). A search for the primary lesion often proves worthwhile and focuses the differential diagnosis to a category of lesion that is specific for the underlying diagnosis. On occasion, two different types of primary lesions may be present. Inquiring about prior photographs can be crucial for making a diagnosis when primary lesions are minimal or absent. **Secondary lesions** result from the evolution of the primary lesion due to external factors or temporal effects; these may be seen in the absence of a primary lesion (Table 189.2).

The color, texture (e.g., rough, smooth), configuration (e.g., annular, serpiginous, linear), location, and distribution (e.g., localized, widespread, symmetric, dermatomal, blaschkoid) of the lesion should be recorded.

INITIAL DIAGNOSTIC EVALUATION AND TESTS

A thorough history and physical examination are usually sufficient for diagnosis because of the visibility of the skin. Adjunctive tests at the time of examination include potassium hydroxide (KOH) examination for fungal infections, skin scrapings for scabies, cytologic examination (Tzanck test) for herpesvirus and varicella-zoster virus infection, and Wood light examination for various cutaneous infections (e.g., yellowish-orange fluorescence of tinea versicolor), depigmentation (e.g., vitiligo), or hypopigmentation (e.g., ash leaf macules of tuberous sclerosis). A skin biopsy, either shave or punch, may be performed to help with the diagnosis, and both can be in-office procedures for the appropriate pediatric patient. Occasionally, supporting laboratory or imaging studies are necessary.

TABLE 189.1 Primary Skin Lesions

LESION	DESCRIPTION	FIGURE
Macule	Flat, nonpalpable lesion <1 cm in diameter	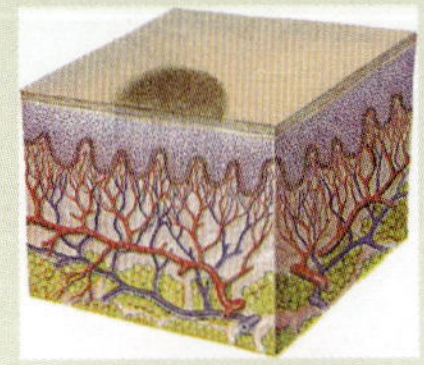
Patch	Similar to macule, but >1 cm in diameter	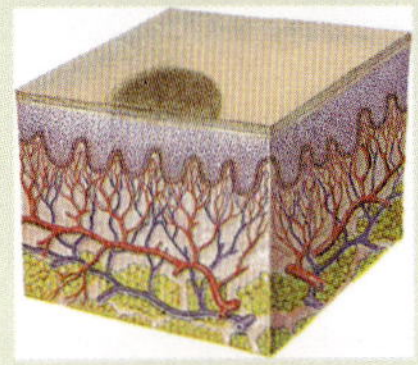
Papule	Elevated, solid lesion <1 cm in diameter	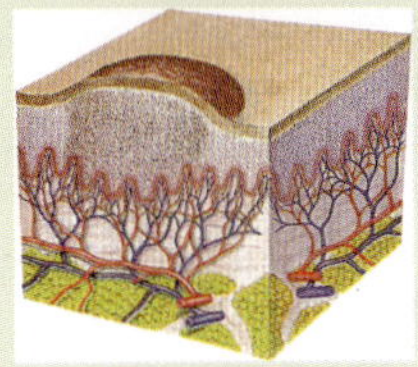
Plaque	Similar to papule, but >1 cm in diameter; has a flat and broad surface, in contrast to a nodule	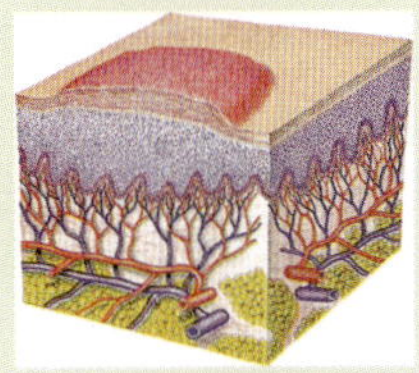
Nodule	Similar to papule, but >1 cm in diameter; has a rounded surface, in contrast to a plaque	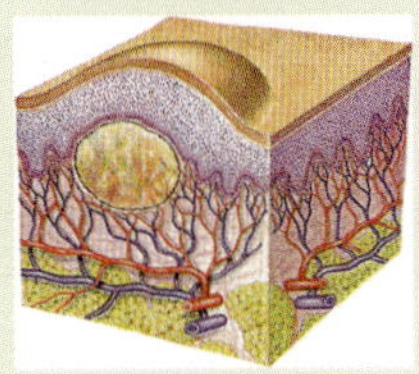
Tumor	Similar to nodule, but implies a neoplastic growth rather than an inflammatory process	
Vesicle	Fluid-filled (usually clear or straw-colored) epidermal lesion	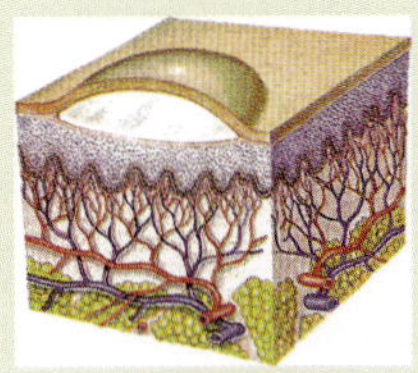
Bulla	Similar to vesicle, but >1 cm in diameter	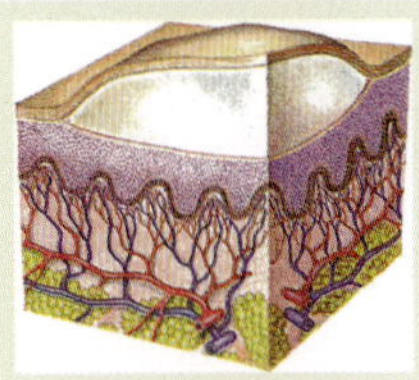
Pustule	Pus-filled epidermal lesion, which often is surrounded by erythema	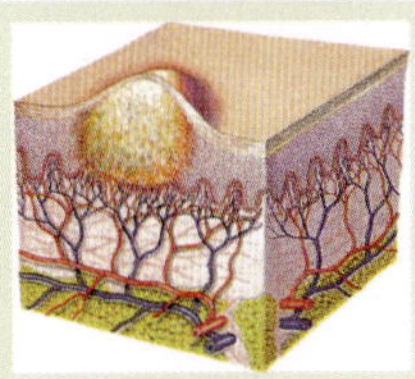
Purpura	Red-purple macule or papule resulting from extravasated blood into the skin; does not blanch with pressure	
Petechia	Similar to purpura, but less than a few millimeters in diameter	
Ecchymosis	Larger, hemorrhagic patch or plaque resulting from extravasated blood	

(Continued)

TABLE 189.1 Primary Skin Lesions—cont'd

LESION	DESCRIPTION	FIGURE
Wheal (hive)	Pink, edematous papules and plaques that vary greatly in size and configuration; characterized by transient nature, with individual lesions resolving within 24 hours	
Telangiectasia	Collection of small, superficial red blood vessels	
Milia	Superficial, white, small epidermal keratin cysts	
Comedone	Plug of keratin and sebum within the orifice of a hair follicle, which can be open (blackhead) or closed (whitehead); characteristic lesion of acne vulgaris	
Cyst	Papule or nodule with an epidermal lining and filled with solid material	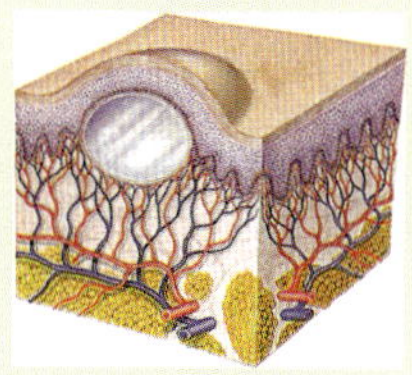

Modified from Black JM, Hawks JH. Medical-Surgical Nursing: Clinical Management for Positive Outcomes, 8e. Philadelphia: Saunders, 2009.

TABLE 189.2 Secondary Skin Lesions

LESION	DESCRIPTION	FIGURE
Scale	Results from abnormal keratinization; may be fine or sheetlike	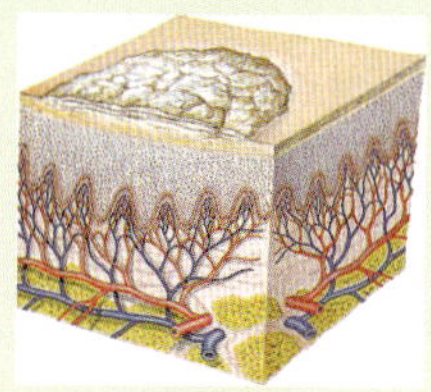
Crust	Dried collection of serum and cellular debris	
Erosion	Shallow depression with loss of the superficial epidermis	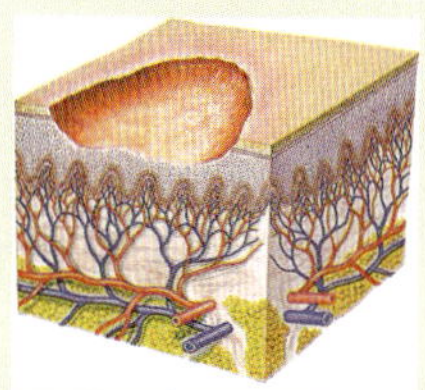
Ulcer	Deeper depression with loss of the entire epidermis into dermis; heals with scarring	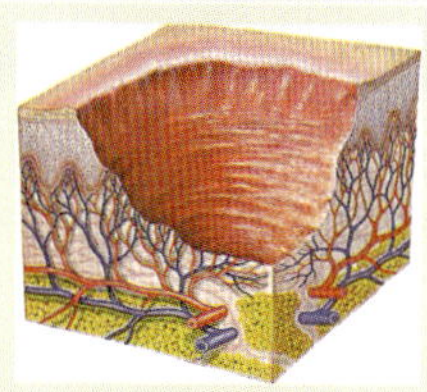
Atrophy	Thinning of epidermis (surface appears shiny and translucent) or dermis (skin is depressed with epidermis intact)	
Scar	Thickened, firm, and discolored collection of connective tissue that results from dermal damage; initially pink, but lightens with time	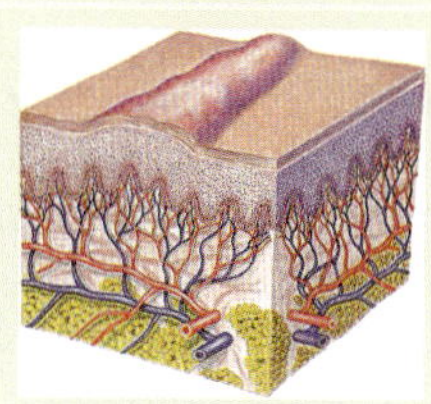
Sclerosis	Circumscribed or diffuse hardening of skin	

(Continued)

TABLE 189.2 Secondary Skin Lesions—cont'd

LESION	DESCRIPTION	FIGURE
Lichenification	Accentuated skin lines/markings that result from thickening of the epidermis due to rubbing	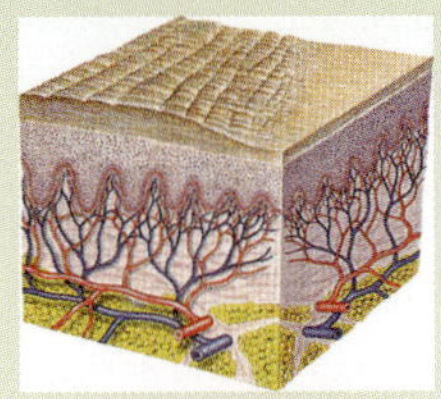
Excoriation	Superficial linear erosion that is caused by scratching	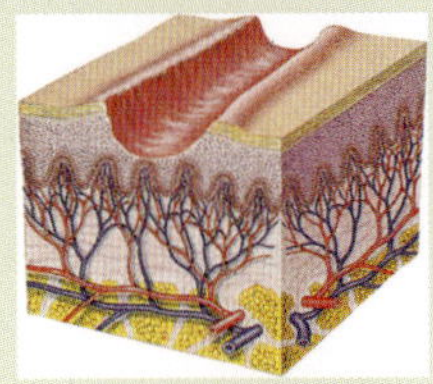
Fissure	Linear break within the skin surface that usually is painful	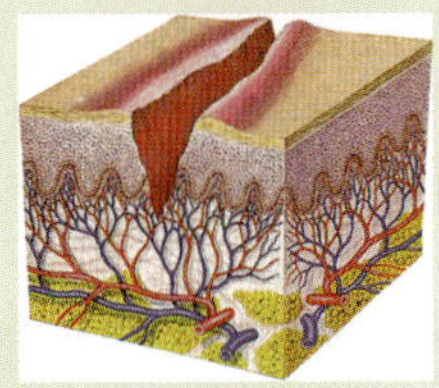

From Black JM, Hawks JH. Medical-Surgical Nursing: Clinical Management for Positive Outcomes, 8e. Philadelphia: Saunders, 2009.

PEARLS FOR PRACTITIONERS

See Dermatology: Pearls for Practitioners at the end of this section.

REVIEW QUESTIONS

Available online

CHAPTER 190

Acne Vulgaris

ETIOLOGY

Acne vulgaris (or acne) is a chronic inflammatory disorder that affects areas with the greatest concentration of sebaceous glands, such as the face, chest, and back. Sex, age, and environmental and genetic factors are all contributory to the pathology of acne. Stress may trigger acne through hormonal imbalances. Certain dietary choices may also contribute to acne (e.g., high glycemic diet, low-fat/skim milk intake).

Acne is caused by chronic inflammation of the pilosebaceous unit (hair follicle with an associated sebaceous gland). The primary event in all acne lesions is the development of the **microcomedone**, which results from the obstruction of the hair follicle with keratin, increased sebum production from sebaceous glands, and overgrowth of normal skin flora, leading to pilosebaceous occlusion and enlargement. Androgens are a potent stimulus of the sebaceous gland. The subsequent inflammatory component and pustule formation result from proliferation of *Cutibacterium acnes*, a commensal organism of the skin. The pathogenesis of acne involves various components: increased sebum production, follicular hyperkeratosis, bacterial proliferation, and inflammation. Effective treatment focuses on minimizing these factors.

EPIDEMIOLOGY

Acne is the most common skin disorder in adolescents, occurring in up to 85% of teenagers. The incidence is similar across sexes, although males often are more severely affected. Acne may begin as early as 6–8 years of age and may continue into adulthood. Mid-childhood acne between 1–6 years of age may be a sign of hyperandrogenism and requires an endocrine evaluation.

CLINICAL MANIFESTATIONS

Acne primarily affects areas with increased sebaceous gland density, such as the face, upper chest, and back. Superficial plugging of the pilosebaceous unit results in noninflammatory, small (1- to 2-mm) **open (blackhead)** and **closed (whitehead) comedones**. Rupture of a comedone into adjacent dermis and proliferation of *C. acnes* induce an inflammatory response and development of inflammatory **papules** and **pustules** (Fig. 190.1). Larger, skin-colored or red cysts and nodules represent progressive inflammation and **cystic acne**. Increased and persistent inflammation, especially with rupture of a deep cyst, increases the risk of scarring.

The diagnosis of acne can be made by the presence of characteristic lesions, and it is important to note that presentation with mixed morphologies is common (e.g., both comedonal and papulopustular lesions). Laboratory studies and imaging studies are not necessary to diagnose acne. Screening tests may be necessary if there are signs of hyperandrogenism due to *polycystic ovarian syndrome* (irregular menses, hirsutism, insulin resistance) or an underlying androgen-secreting tumor (irregular menses, hirsutism, deepening voice, clitoromegaly).

TREATMENT

The mainstay of acne treatment includes topical agents that have comedolytic, antibacterial, and/or antiinflammatory properties. Creams, lotions, gels, foams, and solutions are available. Gels and solutions are commonly used; these agents tend to be drying and may not be as well tolerated. Creams and lotions are better tolerated but may be less effective than the corresponding gel or solution. Twice daily face washing and moisturizer use should also be part of a patient's acne skin care routine.

The comedolytic agents (salicylic acid, tretinoin, adapalene, tazarotene) produce superficial desquamation and, subsequently, relieve follicular obstruction. They are a cornerstone of first-line therapy. The topical retinoids (tretinoin, adapalene, tazarotene, trifarotene) are vitamin A derivatives. They decrease keratin and sebum production and have some antiinflammatory and antibacterial activity. Topical antimicrobials (benzoyl peroxide, dapsone) and topical antibiotics (erythromycin, clindamycin) are antiinflammatory and inhibit *C. acnes* proliferation. Erythromycin efficacy has decreased as *C. acnes* is almost always resistant to this antibiotic, and it should no longer be used. Topical antibiotics should be combined with an antimicrobial, such as benzoyl peroxide, to prevent the development of resistance, and topical antibiotic monotherapy should be avoided. Combination therapy of a topical comedolytic agent and a topical antimicrobial is more effective than either agent alone for inflammatory acne. A triple regimen consisting of a topical retinoid, topical antimicrobial, and topical antibiotic can be utilized.

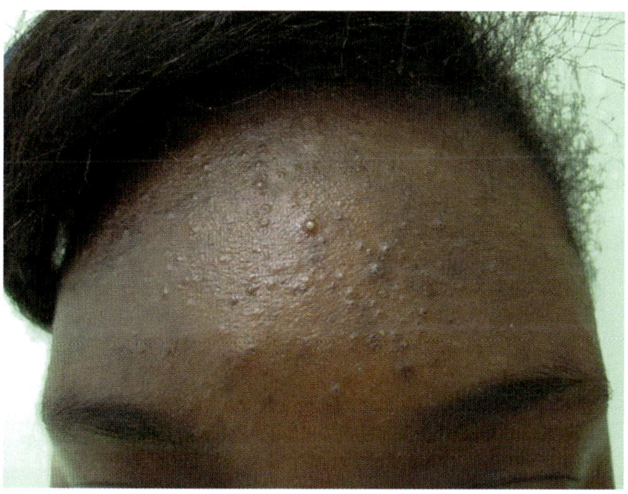

FIGURE 190.1 Forehead acne with comedones, papules, and pustules.

Oral antibiotics are added for moderate-to-severe acne but should always be used in combination with a topical regimen. Tetracyclines such as doxycycline and minocycline are the most effective antibiotics because of their significant antiinflammatory activity but should not be used in children 8 years of age and younger. Oral antibiotic courses should be limited to 3 months and should be combined with a topical regimen.

For recalcitrant, severe nodulocystic, or scarring acne, oral isotretinoin may be instituted. Isotretinoin, an oral analog of vitamin A, normalizes follicular keratinization, reduces sebum production, and decreases 5α-dihydrotestosterone formation and androgen receptor–binding capacity. A course of isotretinoin is the only medication that can permanently alter the course of acne and induce a durable remission. Isotretinoin therapy requires careful patient selection, pretreatment counseling, and laboratory monitoring and should be used only by providers familiar with the medication and monitoring requirements. It is teratogenic and must not be used immediately before or during pregnancy. Other adverse effects include dry skin, cheilitis, musculoskeletal pain, hepatitis, and elevated lipids. Patients in the United States are required to enroll in the iPLEDGE safety program for isotretinoin prescription.

For females, hormonal agents can also be considered for acne therapy. These include the estrogen-containing combined oral contraceptives and oral spironolactone.

COMPLICATIONS

Acne has significant and frequently devastating effects on an adolescent's body image and self-esteem. The psychosocial impact of acne should not be underestimated and does not necessarily correlate with the severity of disease. Scarring may result in permanent morbidity.

PROGNOSIS

Classically, acne lasts 3–5 years, although some individuals may have a longer duration of 15–20 years. Only treatment with isotretinoin may alter the natural course of acne. Acne lesions often heal with temporary postinflammatory erythema and hyperpigmentation. Depending on the severity, chronicity, and depth of involvement, pitted, atrophic, or hypertrophic scars may develop. **Cystic acne** has the highest incidence of scarring because rupture of a deep cyst induces the greatest inflammation, although scarring may be caused by milder pustular or even comedonal acne.

PREVENTION

Comedogenic hair and skin products should be avoided because they exacerbate preexisting acne. There are no effective means for preventing acne, although a low-milk or low-glycemic diet may improve acne. Repetitive cleansing with soap and water or use of astringents or abrasives removes only surface lipids; their use makes the skin appear less oily but does not prevent formation of microcomedones and may paradoxically worsen acne.

PEARLS FOR PRACTITIONERS

See Dermatology: Pearls for Practitioners at the end of this section.

REVIEW QUESTIONS

Available online.

CHAPTER 191

Atopic Dermatitis

ETIOLOGY

Atopic dermatitis is a chronic inflammatory disease with no known cure; it is associated with significant psychosocial morbidity and decreased health-related quality of life. For some individuals, atopic dermatitis is the skin manifestation of atopy accompanied by asthma and allergic rhinitis.

Atopic dermatitis manifests with a defective skin barrier, reduced innate immune responses, and exaggerated immune responses to allergens and microbes. Both genetic predisposition and environmental factors play a role in the development of atopic dermatitis. Genes such as *FLG* that are associated with skin barrier dysfunction and inflammation have been linked with atopic dermatitis. Inflammatory mediators involved include predominantly T helper (Th) cells, with the Th2 pathway implicated early in acute lesions and a Th1 predominance found in chronic lesions. Langerhans cells, immunoglobulin (Ig) E, and eosinophils play a prominent role, as well as other inflammatory mediators. Environmental and contact allergens, infections, irritants, extremes of temperature, sweat, and lack of humidity can exacerbate the condition, as can scratching or rubbing. Triggers can vary from individual to individual.

EPIDEMIOLOGY

Atopic dermatitis is the most common skin disease in children, with an estimated prevalence of up to 20% of children. Atopic dermatitis occurs more frequently in non-White children, urban areas, and higher socioeconomic classes. Prevalence is lower in areas where industrial pollution is less and where eosinophil-mediated infections such as helminthic infections are endemic.

Patients generally have a family history of atopy. Children with atopic dermatitis are predisposed to the development of asthma and allergic rhinitis, referred to as the *atopic march.* Asthma develops in up to half of children with atopic dermatitis, and allergic rhinitis develops even more frequently. Food allergies commonly coexist in children with atopic dermatitis but are a rare cause of atopic dermatitis itself.

CLINICAL MANIFESTATIONS

Atopic dermatitis is a chronic, relapsing skin disease characterized by xerosis, pruritus, and characteristic skin findings. The condition generally improves with age and remits in adulthood, although some childhood cases will continue into adulthood.

Characteristic lesions of atopic dermatitis are erythematous papules or plaques with ill-defined borders and overlying scale or hyperkeratosis. Weeping may be present in acute stages, which then develops into yellow crust. Lesions can be secondarily excoriated and result in hemorrhagic crusting and lichenification in older lesions. Formation of fissures is common in both acute and chronic lesions. Temporary hypo- and hyperpigmentation can be seen after lesions resolve, but atopic dermatitis is not usually scarring unless secondary features become severe (e.g., secondary infection or scratching).

Characteristic locations vary with the age of the patient. Infantile atopic dermatitis affects the face and extensor surfaces of the extremities and is often generalized. Childhood lesions predominate in flexural surfaces (antecubital and popliteal fossae), wrists, ankles, hands, and feet (Fig. 191.1). The adult phase occurs after puberty and manifests in the flexural areas, including the neck, as well as predominant involvement on the face, hands, fingers, toes, upper arms, and back.

Secondary bacterial infection, most commonly with *Staphylococcus aureus* or less commonly with *Streptococcus pyogenes*, is a common complication. Patients can develop disseminated skin infections with viruses such as herpes simplex virus (HSV; eczema herpeticum), varicella-zoster virus, coxsackievirus (eczema coxsackium), smallpox virus (eczema vaccinatum), and molluscum contagiosum. Atopic skin is more susceptible to fungal infections as well. Signs of concomitant infection include acute worsening of disease in an otherwise well-controlled patient, resistance to standard therapy, fever, and presence of pustules, fissures, punched out erosions, or exudative or crusted lesions (Fig. 191.2). Eczema herpeticum and eczema vaccinatum can be life threatening if not treated.

LABORATORY AND IMAGING STUDIES

Diagnosis of atopic dermatitis is based on clinical signs and symptoms. Skin biopsy findings are generally characteristic but not exclusively diagnostic and can overlap with other skin conditions. Peripheral blood eosinophilia and elevated IgE levels can be found but are not specific and not routinely obtained. Skin prick testing or measurement of specific IgE antibody levels can detect sensitization to food and environmental allergens, although false-positive findings occur.

DIFFERENTIAL DIAGNOSIS

The differential diagnosis of atopic dermatitis is extensive, but a history of a relapsing pruritic condition in the setting of atopy and skin lesions in a characteristic distribution is typical.

The lesions of **seborrheic dermatitis** have circumscribed and well-defined borders. The scale or hyperkeratosis is thicker, greasy, and yellowish. The distribution of seborrheic dermatitis is different from that of atopic dermatitis, involving the scalp, eyebrows, nasolabial region, upper chest, and back. The two conditions occasionally coexist, especially in infants.

Psoriasis tends to localize on the elbows, knees, lower back, and scalp. The lesions of psoriasis on exposed surfaces are salmon colored at the base with an overlying thick, silver scaling hyperkeratosis. They are generally very well-demarcated, oval or round, thick plaques.

Allergic contact dermatitis has a distribution limited to one area of the body corresponding to contact with the

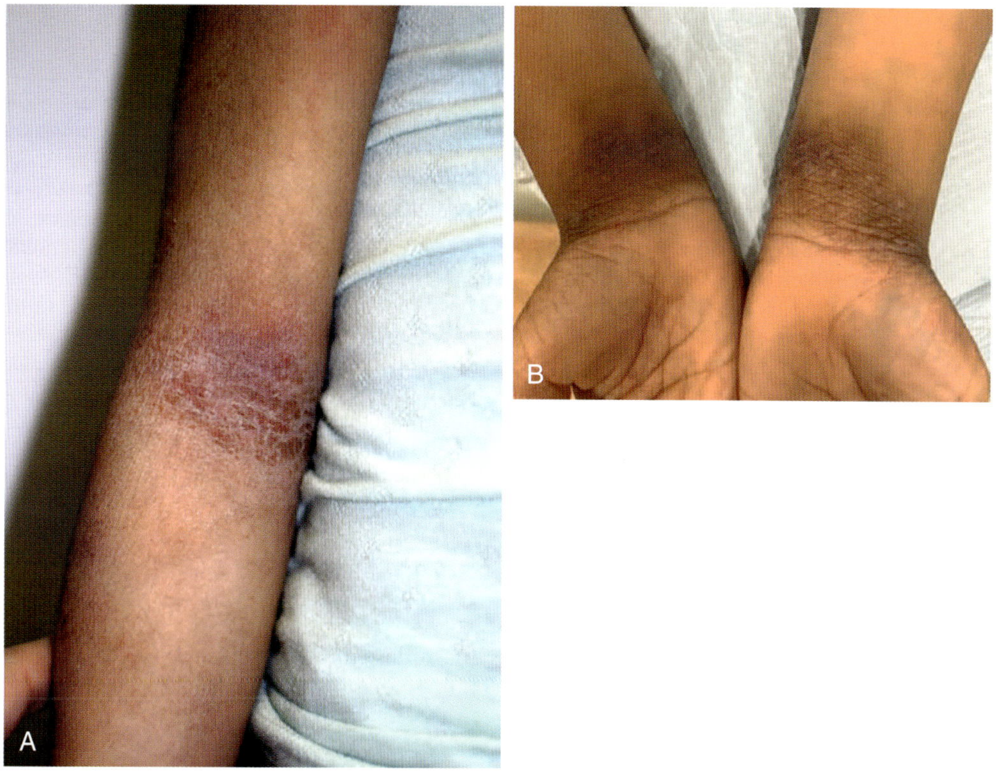

FIGURE 191.1 **(A)** Atopic dermatitis (arm). **(B)** Atopic dermatitis (wrists). Erythema may be harder to appreciate in darker skin tones.

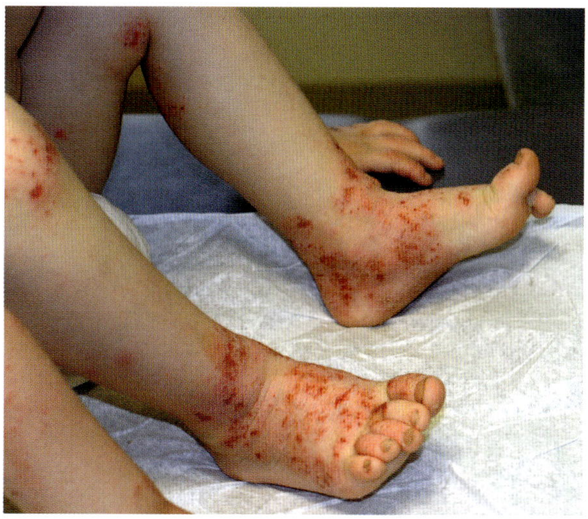

FIGURE 191.2 Atopic dermatitis with *Staphylococcus* superinfection.

allergen. The lesions generally make well-demarcated, bizarre, linear, square, or angulated shapes corresponding to the source. **Nickel dermatitis** is common and results from contact sensitization to nickel in metals. It occurs in characteristic locations such as the periumbilical area (where metal from pant buttons rubs against skin), on the ear lobule or neck (where earrings contact skin), circumferentially around the neck (where necklaces contact skin), and under rings or wristbands. Patients with atopic dermatitis can have concomitant contact dermatitis as well.

TREATMENT

Ideal therapy for atopic dermatitis includes three main components: frequent liberal use of bland moisturizers to restore the skin barrier, avoidance of triggers of inflammation, and use of topical antiinflammatory medication to affected areas of skin when needed. Control of pruritus and secondary infection should be addressed on an individual basis. If topical therapy and these measures are inadequate, systemic therapy with immunomodulatory agents or ultraviolet (UV) light therapy may be indicated.

Daily, short baths with warm but not hot water are generally recommended. A moisturizing cream or ointment should be applied to the entire body immediately afterwards to trap moisture. Application of topical medications is also most effective immediately after bathing. Additional information for patients and families can be found at the website of the National Eczema Association (http://www.nationaleczema.org).

Common triggers of inflammation in atopic dermatitis include rubbing or scratching; saliva; contact with acidic foods, soaps and detergents, wool or other harsh materials; fragranced products; sweat; highly chlorinated pools; low humidity; tobacco smoke; dust mites; animal dander; environmental pollens; and molds. Exposure to these triggers should be limited whenever possible. Infections that are unrelated to skin disease, such as an upper respiratory infection, can also exacerbate atopic dermatitis. Food allergy is commonly seen in patients with atopic dermatitis but presents with urticaria or anaphylaxis rather than exacerbation of the atopic dermatitis.

Topical corticosteroids are the mainstay of antiinflammatory therapy for atopic dermatitis and are an effective and safe treatment when used appropriately. Hundreds of topical corticosteroids are available and are classified according to strength from class I (highest potency) to VII (lowest potency). Potency varies according to the steroid molecule (active ingredient), and, for a given ingredient, strength can vary according to relative concentration and vehicle base. Enhanced penetration occurs in areas of thinner stratum corneum (face), natural occlusion (flexures such as axillae and groin), with external occlusion (diapers or bandages), in areas of open skin (excoriations), and with heat or hydration. Use of wet wraps with topical corticosteroid application takes advantage of this principle of heat and hydration for enhanced penetration for recalcitrant lesions. Class I and II steroids are avoided in young children and in areas of enhanced penetration.

Corticosteroids are available in different vehicles. In general, ointments are preferred because of their increased efficacy, occlusive nature, and tolerability. Creams may be slightly less effective for a given steroid ingredient but may be more cosmetically acceptable for some patients or in warmer climates. Lotions may cause more irritation and are generally less potent. Sprays, foams, solutions, oils, and gels can be especially useful for hair-bearing areas like the scalp. Creams, lotions, sprays, solutions, and gels can be particularly irritating when applied to atopic skin and should generally be avoided on areas of skin with secondary excoriations and erosions.

Topical corticosteroids should be used in conjunction with adequate skin care, such as avoiding triggers of inflammation and frequent application of moisturizers. Twice-daily application of corticosteroids is recommended. The goal is to limit the need for antiinflammatory medications and thereby avoid the potential for adverse effects. Local side effects such as skin atrophy, striae, and acne are related to corticosteroid potency, site of application, and duration of application. While hyper- or hypopigmentation can rarely result from topical corticosteroid use, pigmentation changes are much more likely to be caused by inflammation secondary to atopic dermatitis itself. Systemic side effects of adrenal suppression or Cushing syndrome can result with application of a potent topical corticosteroid to large surface areas or occluded areas at risk of enhanced penetration.

Topical immune modulators such as calcineurin inhibitors (tacrolimus and pimecrolimus), phosphodiesterase-4 inhibitors (crisaborole and roflumilast), and Janus kinase inhibitor (ruxolitinib) may be part of the treatment regimen for atopic dermatitis. There is no potential for skin atrophy; these agents are particularly useful for facial, axillary, or genital lesions. These topical immune modulators are currently approved for intermittent therapy as second-line treatments for mild-to-moderate atopic dermatitis.

Sedating antihistamines (e.g., diphenhydramine, hydroxyzine) have only mild effect on pruritus but can decrease sleeplessness due to scratching during the night. A dose before bedtime is most effective. Additional daytime doses can be added on an individual basis as needed. Nonsedating antihistamines are of limited benefit in controlling the pruritus of atopic dermatitis.

Short-term administration of systemic corticosteroids is rarely indicated for cases of severe disease due to the risk of rebound flare following withdrawal. Long-term and frequent repeated courses should be avoided to prevent adverse effects such as growth restriction and adrenal insufficiency.

UV phototherapy with narrowband UVB can be an option for moderate-to-severe cases in older children. Phototherapy is administered two to three times weekly until improvement is seen and then is tapered or discontinued once the acute flare has resolved. More frequent use of phototherapy in children is hindered by requirements for frequent office visits, ability to cooperate with standing in a phototherapy booth while wearing protective goggles, and risk of long-term skin damage, including the theoretic potential for skin cancer development with excessive UV light exposure.

Systemic immunosuppressants such as cyclosporine, methotrexate, azathioprine, or mycophenolate mofetil can be effective therapies for atopic dermatitis in severe cases. Increasingly, biologic agents and small molecule inhibitors are used to treat moderate-severe atopic dermatitis. Dupilumab, a monoclonal IgG4 antibody that inhibits interleukin-4 (IL-4) and IL-13, is an injectable biologic used to treat atopic dermatitis in children. Other injectable biologics include tralokinumab, lebrikizumab, and nemolizumab. Oral Janus kinase inhibitors, such as abrocitinib and upadacitinib, are also systemic treatment options.

COMPLICATIONS

There is increased risk for bacterial, viral, and fungal skin infections due to an impaired skin barrier, a decrease in innate immune proteins in the skin, and maladaptive secondary immune responses.

Secondary impetigo with *S. aureus* is the most common secondary skin infection found in atopic dermatitis, followed by group A streptococcus infection. Infection manifests with pustules, erythema, crusting, flare of disease, or lack of response to previously adequate antiinflammatory therapy. Localized lesions can be treated with topical mupirocin. Widespread and generalized lesions require oral antibiotic therapy, most commonly with a first-generation cephalosporin such as cephalexin. Methicillin-resistant *S. aureus* infection is increasingly common, and antibiotic therapy should be tailored based on local resistance rates and patient factors. Diagnosis of superinfection may be made clinically, but a superficial bacterial culture can confirm the diagnosis and provide antimicrobial susceptibilities. Treatment should include a concomitant atopic skin care routine including the continued use of topical corticosteroids. Although secondary skin infection with *S. aureus* is common, progression to cellulitis or septicemia is unusual. Rarely, intravenous antibiotics may be required. Children with colonization and frequent infections may benefit from dilute bleach baths two to three times weekly; one-fourth to one-half cup of household bleach is added to a half-full or full bathtub. Intranasal treatment with topical mupirocin can also be used to treat *S. aureus* colonization.

Eczema herpeticum (Kaposi varicelliform eruption) is a serious, infectious complication in atopic dermatitis. After HSV infection, an eruption of multiple pruritic, vesiculopustular lesions occurs in a disseminated pattern, both within plaques of atopic dermatitis and on normal-appearing skin. These characteristically rupture and form crusted umbilicated papules and punched-out hemorrhagic erosions (Fig. 191.3). Irritability, anorexia, and fever can also be seen. Systemic and central nervous system disease have been reported. Bacterial superinfection of eroded areas of the skin often occurs. Diagnosis can be made rapidly from a scraping of the skin lesion stained with Giemsa or Wright stain (Tzanck test) looking for multinucleated giant cells, although these are not highly sensitive. Vesicle fluid can also be sent for polymerase chain

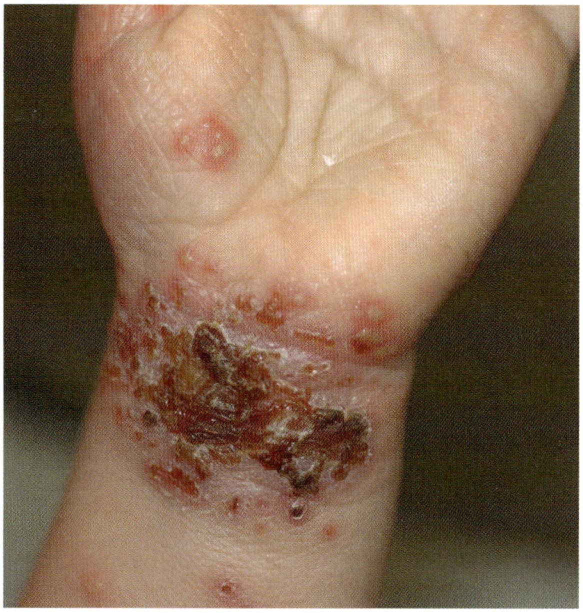

FIGURE 191.3 Eczema herpeticum (hand).

reaction detection of HSV DNA or rapid direct fluorescent antibody testing, both of which are faster and more sensitive than viral culture. Laboratory confirmation of infection is important because similar clinical manifestations can occur with bacterial infections. Treatment of severe cases requires intravenous acyclovir, while milder cases can be managed with oral acyclovir or valacyclovir.

The psychosocial impact of atopic dermatitis can be significant. There is often significant detrimental impact on quality of life; lack of sleep from pruritus, resulting in irritability and fatigue; and limitations on participation in sports. Significant time, as well as financial strain, is involved in caring for a child with atopic dermatitis. Management should address these potential issues and provide adequate anticipatory guidance.

PROGNOSIS

Atopic dermatitis frequently remits during childhood and is much less common after puberty. The condition is generally most severe and widespread in infancy and early childhood. Relapse of disease in adults can occur and commonly manifests as face or hand dermatitis. Patients with atopic dermatitis can also develop asthma and allergic rhinitis. Asthma is commonly associated with more severe skin disease.

PREVENTION

Individual flares of atopic dermatitis can be prevented by avoiding triggers of inflammation and can be lessened with frequent moisturizer application. There is conflicting evidence on exclusive breastfeeding and hydrolyzed formula in decreasing atopic dermatitis frequency or severity. There is no convincing evidence that an antigen-avoidance diet in pregnant or lactating mothers prevents the development of atopic disease. For infants with atopic dermatitis, early introduction of highly allergenic foods is recommended to decrease the frequency of food allergy.

PEARLS FOR PRACTITIONERS

See Dermatology: Pearls for Practitioners at the end of this section.

REVIEW QUESTIONS

Available online.

CHAPTER 192

Contact Dermatitis

ETIOLOGY AND EPIDEMIOLOGY

Inflammation in the top layers of the skin, caused by direct contact with a substance, is divided into two subtypes: irritant contact dermatitis and allergic contact dermatitis. **Irritant contact dermatitis** is observed after the skin surface is exposed to an irritating chemical or substance. Contact dermatitis may occur in any age, and females are more frequently affected than males. **Allergic contact dermatitis** is a cell-mediated immune reaction, also called *type IV* or *delayed-type hypersensitivity*. The antigens, or haptens, involved in allergic contact dermatitis readily penetrate the epidermis and are bound by Langerhans cells, the antigen-presenting cells of the skin. The hapten is presented to T lymphocytes, and an immune cascade follows.

CLINICAL MANIFESTATIONS

Irritant contact dermatitis is characterized by ill-defined, scaly, pink or red patches and plaques (Fig. 192.1) localized to skin surfaces that are exposed to the irritant. Irritant contact dermatitis is observed frequently on the dorsal surfaces of the hands, often from repeated handwashing or exposure to irritating chemicals.

Diaper dermatitis is a common problem in infants and most commonly is a form of irritant contact dermatitis. The dermatitis is caused by irritation from urine and feces, affecting the perianal region and the buttocks while sparing the protected groin folds and other occluded areas. Secondary infection by *Candida albicans* or bacterial pathogens may complicate diaper dermatitis.

Allergic contact dermatitis may be acute (such as *Rhus* dermatitis) or chronic (such as nickel dermatitis). Acute lesions are bright pink, pruritic patches, often in linear or sharply marginated, bizarre configurations. Within the patches are clear vesicles and bullae (Fig. 192.2). Signs and symptoms of the disease may be delayed for 7–14 days after exposure if the individual has not been sensitized previously. On re-exposure, symptoms begin within hours and are usually more severe. The eruption may persist for weeks and can spread beyond the site of initial exposure. Chronic lesions are pink, scaly, pruritic plaques, often mimicking atopic dermatitis. Even intermittent exposure can result in a persistent dermatitis.

LABORATORY STUDIES

The diagnosis of allergic contact dermatitis is established by clinical presentation and history of exposure to a recognized

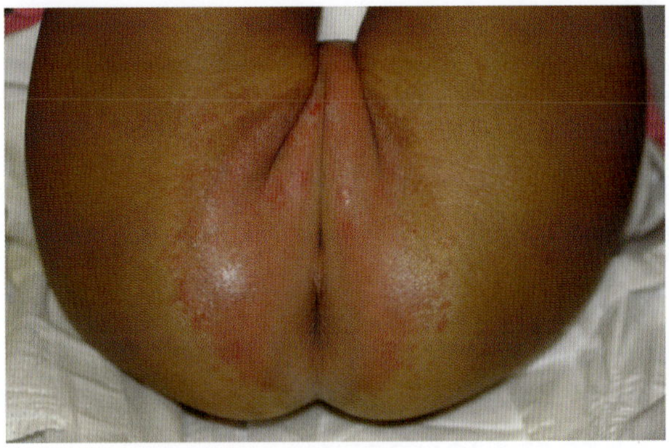

FIGURE 192.1 Irritant diaper dermatitis.

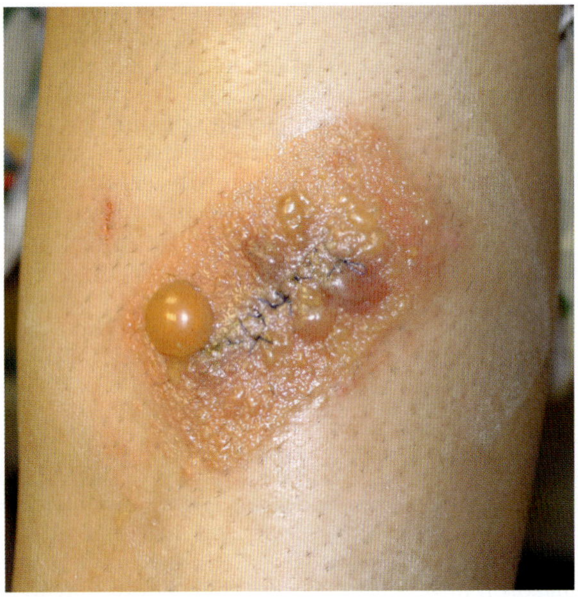

FIGURE 192.2 Allergic contact dermatitis to tincture of benzoin.

irritant or allergen. Skin-prick testing and serum immunoglobulin E levels are not helpful in determining the cause of allergic contact dermatitis. Patch testing may be used to determine the allergen causing the reaction in difficult cases.

DIFFERENTIAL DIAGNOSIS

The distribution and appearance of the dermatitis and a detailed exposure history are the most useful diagnostic tools. Involvement of the lower legs and distal arms suggests exposure to plants of the *Rhus* species (poison ivy or poison oak), especially when linear configurations of lesions are present. Dermatitis of the ears (earrings), wrist (bracelet or watch), or periumbilical region (belt buckle or pant buttons) suggests a metal allergy to nickel. Topical antibiotics (neomycin) and fragrances (soaps, perfumes, cosmetics) are frequent causes of allergic contact dermatitis.

Diaper rashes caused by *Candida* are quite common. Irritant contact dermatitis primarily affects the prominent, exposed surfaces; *Candida* primarily affects intertriginous areas. The two often present simultaneously, as secondary *Candida* infection may complicate irritant dermatitis.

Psoriasis, seborrheic dermatitis, and Langerhans cell histiocytosis can also present with an erythematous rash in the diaper area. Referral to a dermatologist should be considered for any child with a severe rash or with a diaper rash that does not respond to conventional therapy.

TREATMENT

Topical corticosteroids are effective in treatment of allergic and irritant contact dermatitis. High-potency corticosteroids, and even short courses of oral corticosteroids, may be necessary for severe reactions of allergic contact dermatitis. Oral antihistamines can be helpful to control itching.

Treatment of candidal diaper dermatitis consists of topical nystatin or topical azole antifungals. Low-potency topical corticosteroids are frequently used in addition to topical antifungal therapy to treat the irritant component of the diaper dermatitis when present concomitantly.

COMPLICATIONS

In addition to superinfection of diaper dermatitis by *C. albicans*, bacterial superinfection may complicate any form of contact dermatitis. This is especially common if the skin barrier is no longer intact due to blistering or scratching.

PREVENTION

Every effort should be made to identify the trigger of allergic or irritant contact dermatitis; with allergic contact dermatitis, re-exposure often leads to increasingly severe reactions.

PEARLS FOR PRACTITIONERS

See Dermatology: Pearls for Practitioners at the end of this section.

REVIEW QUESTIONS

Available online.

CHAPTER 193

Seborrheic Dermatitis

ETIOLOGY

Seborrheic dermatitis is a common, chronic inflammatory disease that has different clinical presentations at different ages. Seborrheic dermatitis presents in infants as cradle cap or dermatitis in the intertriginous areas of the axillae, groin, antecubital and popliteal fossae, and umbilicus. In adolescents, the most common presentation is dandruff. The pathogenesis of seborrheic dermatitis is unclear, but it is theorized that there is an abnormal inflammatory response to commensal *Malassezia* species in sebum-rich areas. Areas prone to seborrheic dermatitis include the scalp, eyebrows, eyelids, nasolabial folds, external auditory canals, and posterior auricular folds.

CLINICAL MANIFESTATIONS

Seborrheic dermatitis in infants begins during the first month and persists during the first year of life. It is also called ***cradle cap*** because of the thick, greasy, waxy, yellow-white scaling and crusting of the scalp (Fig. 193.1). Greasy, scaly, erythematous, nonpruritic patches and plaques may extend to the face and posterior auricular folds, sometimes involving the flexural folds or even the entire body. Diaper and intertriginous areas can have sharply demarcated, shiny, erythematous patches with minimal scale. Hypopigmentation may persist after the inflammation has faded. The eruption is usually asymptomatic, which helps differentiate it from infantile atopic dermatitis, which is pruritic.

Classic seborrheic dermatitis during adolescence is localized to the scalp. The mild form is commonly known as ***dandruff***, a fine, white, dry scaling of the scalp with minor itching. Additional findings of seborrheic dermatitis vary, from diffuse scaling to focal areas of thick, oily, yellow crusts with underlying erythema. The external auditory canals, eyebrows, eyelids, and intertriginous areas may be involved as well. Pruritus may be minimal or severe.

LABORATORY AND IMAGING STUDIES

Laboratory studies and imaging studies are not necessary to diagnose seborrheic dermatitis. Fungal cultures and potassium hydroxide studies may be necessary to help differentiate seborrheic dermatitis of the scalp from tinea capitis (see Chapter 99).

DIFFERENTIAL DIAGNOSIS

Seborrheic dermatitis in an infant may be difficult to differentiate from atopic dermatitis and in some cases may represent an overlap. In an adolescent, seborrheic dermatitis of the scalp and psoriasis of the scalp may have very similar clinical findings; it can be very difficult to differentiate the two disorders, especially if there are no other cutaneous findings to provide additional clues. Intractable, severe, generalized seborrheic dermatitis could suggest Langerhans cell histiocytosis.

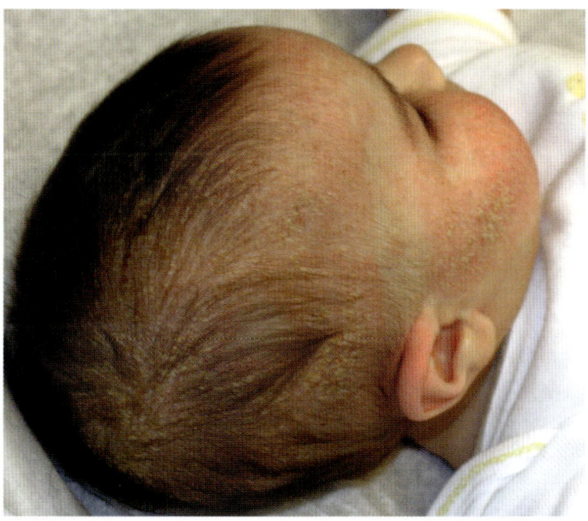

FIGURE 193.1 Seborrheic dermatitis (cradle cap).

TREATMENT

Seborrheic dermatitis of the scalp is usually asymptomatic and generally does not require treatment. Minor amounts of scale can be removed easily by regular shampooing. For infants with cradle cap, mineral oil may be gently massaged into the scalp and left on for a few minutes before gently brushing out the scale and shampooing. Shampooing with ketoconazole, zinc pyrithione, selenium sulfide, coal tar, or salicylic acid shampoos can treat scalp scale. Seborrheic dermatitis with inflamed lesions responds rapidly to treatment with low-potency steroids two times daily.

The response to treatment is usually rapid. Secondary bacterial infection can occur but is uncommon. Intractable disease and other complications warrant further evaluation for other etiologies.

PROGNOSIS

Cradle cap is self-limited and resolves during the first year of life. Seborrheic dermatitis does not cause permanent hair loss. For teenagers, continued use of an antiseborrheic shampoo is often required for control of dandruff.

PREVENTION

Frequent shampooing, especially with early signs of seborrheic dermatitis, may help prevent progression.

OTHER PAPULOSQUAMOUS DERMATOSES

Pityriasis Rosea

Pityriasis rosea is a benign, self-limited eruption that may occur at any age, with peak incidence during adolescence. A solitary 2- to 5-cm, pink, oval patch with central clearing, the so-called ***herald patch***, is the first manifestation of the eruption. The herald patch is found on the trunk or proximal thigh and is often misdiagnosed as fungal or eczematous in origin. One to 2 weeks later, a generalized eruption occurs on the torso and proximal extremities. Multiple 0.5- to 2-cm, oval to oblong, red or tan macules with a fine scale are characteristically arranged parallel to skin tension lines (Christmas tree pattern). Rarely, the eruption may have an inverse distribution involving the axillae and groin or a papular or papulovesicular appearance. Mild prodromal symptoms may be present with the appearance of the herald patch, and pruritus is present in 25% of cases. The eruption lasts 4–14 weeks, with gradual resolution. Residual hyperpigmentation or hypopigmentation can take additional months to clear. Treatment is unnecessary, though pruritus can be managed with oral antihistamines, phototherapy, and low-potency topical corticosteroids.

Psoriasis

Psoriasis is a common papulosquamous condition characterized by well-demarcated, erythematous, scaling papules and plaques. Psoriasis occurs at all ages, including infancy, with onset during childhood in 30% of cases. The disease is characterized by a chronic and relapsing course, although spontaneous remissions can occur. Infections (especially *Streptococcus pyogenes*), stress, trauma, and medications may cause disease exacerbations. Various subtypes of psoriasis exist. The most common variety is **plaque psoriasis (psoriasis vulgaris)**, which can be localized or generalized. The lesions consist of round, well-demarcated, pink to red plaques measuring 1–7 cm with micaceous scale, which is distinctive in its thick, silvery appearance (Fig. 193.2) with pinpoint bleeding points revealed on removal of the scales **(Auspitz sign)**. The lesions of psoriasis have a distinctive distribution involving the extensor aspect of the elbows and knees, posterior occipital scalp, periumbilical region, lumbosacral region, and intergluteal cleft. Children often have facial lesions involving the superomedial aspect of the eyelids. Nail plate involvement is common and includes pitting, onycholysis, subungual hyperkeratosis, and oil spots (reddish brown macular discoloration beneath the nail plate). **Guttate** (numerous small papules and plaques diffusely distributed predominantly on the torso and proximal extremities) (Fig. 193.3), **erythrodermic** (covering large body surface areas), **inverse** (moist red patches affecting body folds), and **pustular** forms of psoriasis may occur. Children with psoriasis are at increased risk for several comorbidities, including obesity, hypertension, hyperlipidemia, metabolic syndrome, diabetes mellitus, depression, and anxiety.

The **treatment** for psoriasis is topical corticosteroids. Due to the risk of atrophy, striae, and telangiectases, especially when potent corticosteroid preparations are administered long term, the goal is to use the least potent corticosteroid necessary. Topical vitamin D analogs, calcineurin inhibitors, salicylic acid, and tar preparations are useful adjuvants to topical corticosteroids. Nonsteroidal topical agents such as roflumilast are also effective. Phototherapy with narrowband ultraviolet B light can be useful as secondary therapy in older children. Extensive plaque or guttate, erythrodermic, and pustular psoriasis may necessitate systemic treatments. Systemic therapies include methotrexate, cyclosporine, and acitretin; the benefit of more targeted biologic therapies has become increasingly recognized, including tumor necrosis factor-α antagonists and interleukin (IL)-12, IL-23, and IL-17 inhibitors. Disease triggers such as infection or medications should be identified and removed. Treatment of psoriasis with oral corticosteroids can induce psoriasis flare after withdrawal and should be avoided as monotherapy.

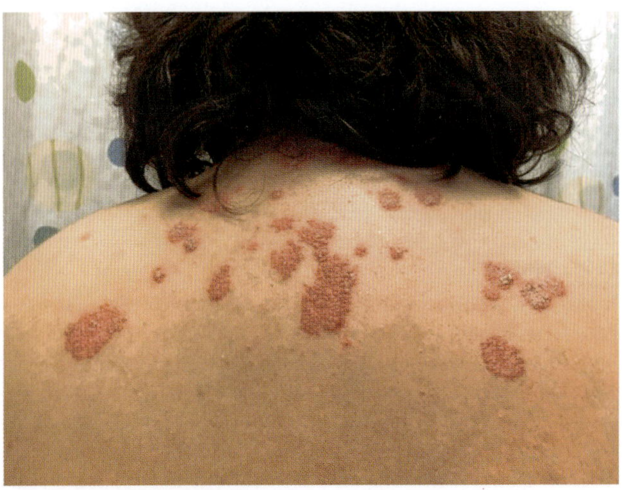

FIGURE 193.2 Plaque psoriasis (back).

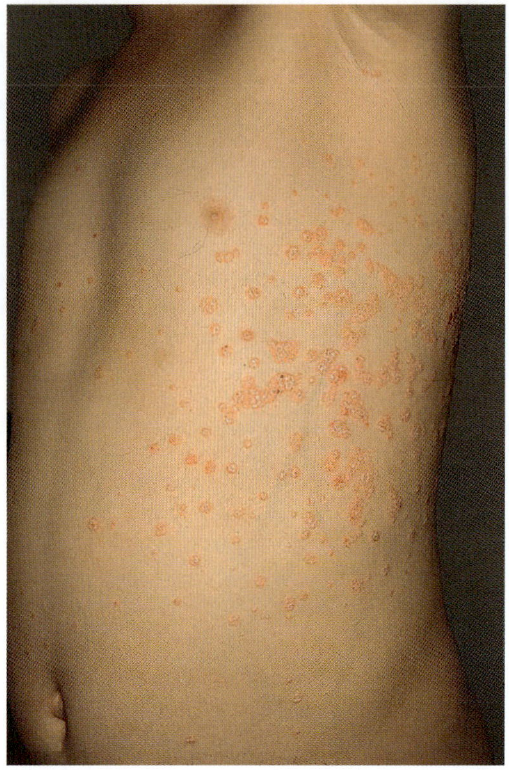

FIGURE 193.3 Guttate psoriasis (trunk). (From Herbst RA, Hoch O, Kapp A, Weiss J. Guttate psoriasis triggered by perianal streptococcal dermatitis in a four-year-old boy. *J Am Acad Dermatol.* 2000;42[5 Pt 2]:885–887.)

PEARLS FOR PRACTITIONERS

See Dermatology: Pearls for Practitioners at the end of this section.

REVIEW QUESTIONS

Available online.

CHAPTER 194
Pigmented Lesions

Birthmark is a term that describes congenital anomalies of the skin. It should not be used as a definitive diagnosis because congenital skin lesions vary greatly in their appearance and prognosis. The differential diagnoses of various birthmarks are listed in Table 194.1.

DERMAL MELANOCYTOSIS

The most frequently encountered pigmented lesion is **dermal melanocytosis**, which occurs in 70–95% of Black, Hispanic, Asian, and Native American infants and in approximately 5% of White infants. Dermal melanocytosis is a congenital lesion caused by entrapment of melanocytes in the dermis during their migration from the neural crest into the epidermis. Although

TABLE 194.1 Common Birthmarks

COLOR/LESION	BIRTHMARK	LOCATION	OTHER FEATURES
Brown/macule or patch	Café-au-lait macule	Variable	May be associated with genetic syndromes
Brown (<40 cm)/patch or plaque	Congenital melanocytic nevus	Variable	Low risk of melanoma
Brown (>40 cm)/patch or plaque	Giant congenital melanocytic nevus	Trunk most common	Risk of melanoma and neuromelanosis
Brown or skin colored/plaque	Epidermal nevus	Variable, trunk and neck	May enlarge with time
Red/patch	Port-wine stain (nevus flammeus)	Variable, face most common	May be associated with Sturge-Weber syndrome or overgrowth syndromes
Red/patch	Salmon patch (nevus simplex)	Glabella, eyelids, nape of neck	Improves or resolves with time
Red/papule or plaque	Infantile hemangioma	Variable	May be associated with liver hemangiomas, airway hemangiomas, and PHACE syndrome
Gray-blue/patch	Dermal melanocytosis	Lower trunk (dermal melanocytosis); face (nevus of Ota); posterior shoulder (nevus of Ito)	Nevus of Ota may be associated with ocular pigmentation
Blue-purple/plaque	Venous, lymphatic, or mixed malformation	Variable	Intermittent swelling and pain
Yellow-orange/plaque	Nevus sebaceus	Head and neck	Malignant and benign tumors may arise within
Yellow-orange/papule	Juvenile xanthogranuloma	Head and neck most common	Spontaneously involutes
Yellow-brown/papule or plaque	Mastocytoma	Variable	Spontaneously involutes
Hypertrichosis/plaque	Smooth muscle hamartoma	Trunk	
Hypertrichosis/tumor	Plexiform neurofibroma	Trunk most common	Associated with neurofibromatosis type 1
White/patch	Nevus anemicus	Variable	Blanched patch with surrounding redness and telangiectasia
White/patch	Nevus depigmentosus	Variable	

PHACE, Posterior fossa malformations, Hemangiomas, Arterial anomalies, Coarctation of aorta and cardiac defects, and Eye abnormalities.

most of these lesions are found in the lumbosacral area, they also occur at other sites, such as the buttocks, flank, extremities, and (rarely) the face (Fig. 194.1). Single or multiple poorly demarcated, gray-blue patches up to 10 cm in size may be present. Most lesions gradually disappear during early childhood; aberrant lesions in unusual sites are more likely to persist.

CAFÉ-AU-LAIT MACULES

Café-au-lait macules are pigmented macules or patches that may be present in a newborn but more often develop during childhood (Fig. 194.2); they range in color from very light brown to a chocolate brown. Up to five café-au-lait macules are found in 1.8% of newborns and 25–40% of healthy children and have no significance. Children with six or more café-au-lait macules (0.5 cm in diameter before puberty or >1.5 cm in diameter after puberty), especially when accompanied by **axillary or inguinal freckling**, should be evaluated carefully for additional stigmata of neurofibromatosis type 1. Other disorders also associated with café-au-lait macules include the other forms of neurofibromatosis, Legius syndrome, McCune-Albright syndrome, Noonan syndrome, and Russell-Silver syndrome.

CONGENITAL MELANOCYTIC NEVI

Approximately 1–6% of newborns have **congenital melanocytic nevi**. Lesions are categorized based on their anticipated diameter in adulthood, with small lesions generally defined as less than 1.5 cm, medium 1.5–20 cm, large 20–40 cm, and giant more than 40 cm. Small and medium congenital melanocytic nevi may resemble café-au-lait macules initially, but darker pigmentation, variegated speckles, textural changes, and elevation develop with time and help to differentiate these lesions (Fig. 194.3). Thick, dark, coarse hair frequently is associated with congenital melanocytic nevi. These lesions vary in site and size but are most often solitary. Small and medium-size congenital melanocytic nevi pose a very slightly increased

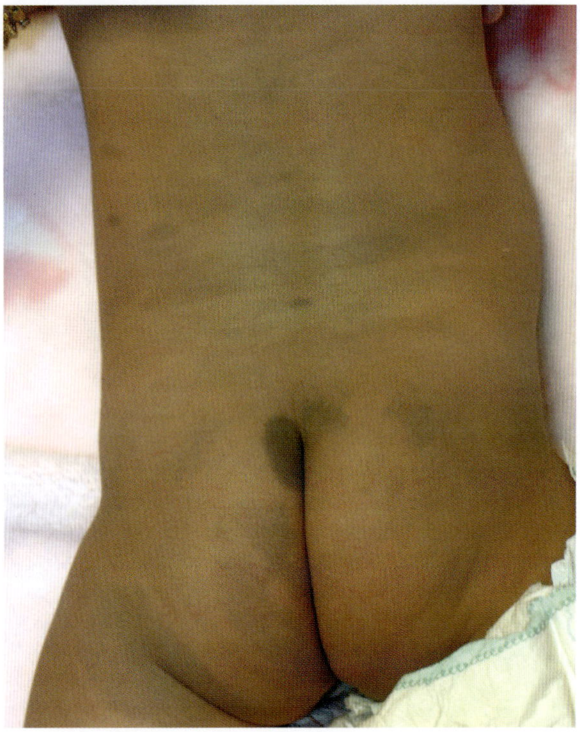

FIGURE 194.1 Dermal melanocytosis (back and buttock).

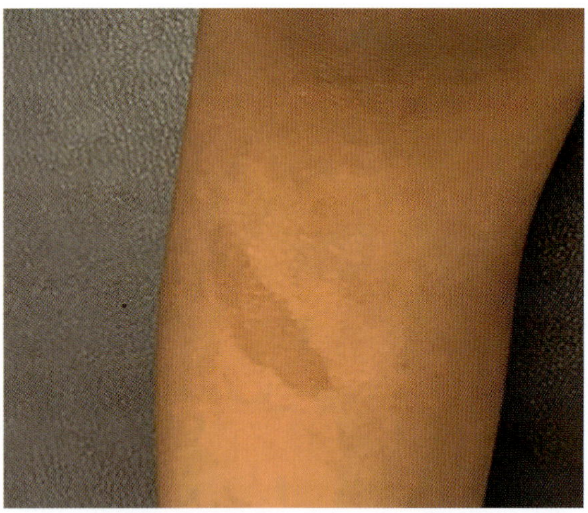

FIGURE 194.2 Café-au-lait macule (leg).

risk for the development of malignant melanoma, usually during adulthood, with risk proportional to the size of the nevus. Surgical removal may be considered to improve the cosmetic appearance or to reduce the likelihood of malignant transformation in difficult-to-monitor lesions, although some patients and physicians elect for observation. Excisional biopsy is indicated when malignant change is suspected.

GIANT CONGENITAL MELANOCYTIC NEVI

Giant congenital melanocytic nevi are defined as nevi that would be 40 cm or more in size in adulthood. These lesions

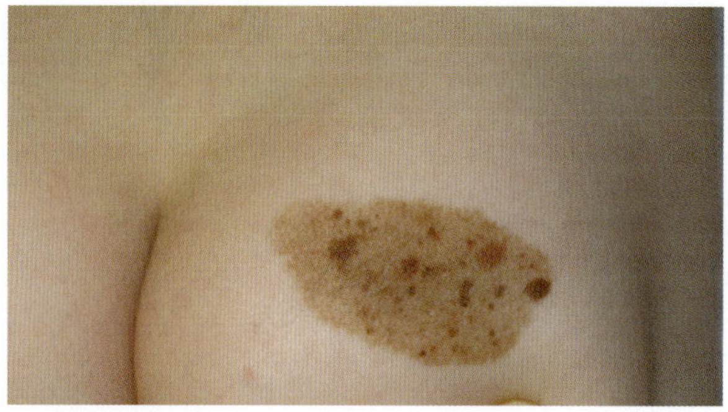

FIGURE 194.3 Congenital melanocytic nevus (buttock).

appear as color variegated, light brown-to-black patches or plaques, sometimes with additional smaller macules and papules **(satellite nevi)**. The affected skin may be smooth, nodular, or leathery. Prominent, dark hypertrichosis is often present. **Neuromelanosis**, the presence of melanocytes in the central nervous system, may be associated with giant congenital melanocytic nevi, referred to as *neurocutaneous melanocytosis*. Affected patients may be asymptomatic or have hydrocephalus and seizures; in symptomatic patients, death often results during early childhood. **Malignant melanoma** develops in approximately 2–10% of patients with giant congenital melanocytic nevi, in either the cutaneous lesion or the neural melanocytes. In contrast to small and medium-sized congenital melanocytic nevi, melanoma is more likely to develop within the first 10 years of life. Surgical excision may be considered for resectable lesions. The use of tissue expansion techniques has greatly improved the capability for surgical removal of large lesions.

ACQUIRED MELANOCYTIC NEVI

Acquired melanocytic nevi are common skin lesions. Melanocytic nevi may occur at any age; the lesions develop most rapidly in prepubertal children and teenagers. Melanocytic nevi are well-delineated, round-to-oval, brown macules and papules. Lesions are most common on the face, upper torso, and arms. Family history, fair skin, and sun exposure are considered major risk factors. Biopsy should be considered when there is presence of irregular pigmentation, rapid growth, bleeding, or a change in configuration or borders. Malignant melanoma is rare in childhood; there is an alarming increase in incidence in adolescence, especially in those who use indoor tanning. Education of parents and children regarding the risks of sun exposure, appropriate sun protection, and recognition of concerning changes is important.

PEARLS FOR PRACTITIONERS

See Dermatology: Pearls for Practitioners at the end of this section.

REVIEW QUESTIONS

Available online.

CHAPTER 195
Vascular Anomalies

Vascular anomalies can be divided into two major categories: tumors and malformations. Vascular tumors are characterized by hypercellularity, proliferation, and growth. Vascular malformations are developmental defects derived from the capillary, venous, arterial, or lymphatic vessels with a lesser degree of proliferation and growth. Differentiating between these entities is important because they have different prognoses and clinical implications.

VASCULAR TUMORS

Infantile Hemangiomas

Infantile hemangiomas are the most common soft tissue tumors of infancy, occurring in approximately 4–5% of infants. Hemangiomas occur predominantly in females (3:1) and have an increased incidence in low birthweight infants. They range from a few millimeters to several centimeters in diameter and are usually solitary; 20% of affected children have multiple lesions. Hemangiomas are not present at birth but then appear as a small red macule or pale white macule or patch with telangiectasia (precursor lesions). When the tumor proliferates, it assumes its most recognizable form as a bright red, lobulated plaque or nodule (superficial type) (Fig. 195.1). Hemangiomas that lie deeper in the skin are soft masses with a subtle blue discoloration (deep type). Hemangiomas can sometimes have both a superficial and a deep component (mixed type).

Approximately 65% have precursor lesions present at birth; the rest develop in the first weeks of life. Superficial hemangiomas reach their maximal size by 5 months with the most rapid growth occurring before 8 weeks of life, but deep hemangiomas may grow for longer. Hemangiomas then undergo slow, spontaneous involution, which takes 1–10 years.

Despite the benign nature of most cutaneous hemangiomas, there may be the risk of functional compromise or permanent disfigurement, depending on the location and extent. Ulceration, the most frequent complication, can be painful and increases the risk of infection, hemorrhage, and scarring. Areas frequently associated with complications include the periocular region, lip, nasal tip, beard, face (large lesions), groin, and buttocks. **Periorbital hemangiomas** pose considerable risk to vision and should be monitored carefully. Amblyopia can result from the hemangioma, causing obstruction of the visual axis or pressure on the globe, resulting in astigmatism. If there is any concern, the patient should have urgent evaluation by an ophthalmologist as treatment may be indicated to prevent blindness. **Subglottic hemangiomas** manifest as hoarseness and stridor; progression to respiratory failure may be rapid. Symptomatic airway hemangiomas develop in more than 50% of infants with extensive facial hemangiomas on the chin and jaw (beard distribution); any infant with a beard hemangioma should be urgently referred for laryngoscopy. Multiple cutaneous hemangiomas (diffuse hemangiomatosis) may be associated with hepatic hemangiomas. Liver ultrasound is recommended to evaluate for hepatic hemangiomas in infants who have at least five cutaneous hemangiomas. **Segmental cervicofacial hemangiomas** may be associated with **PHACE syndrome**, characterized by **P**osterior fossa malformations, **H**emangiomas, **A**rterial anomalies, **C**oarctation of aorta and cardiac defects, and **E**ye abnormalities. Magnetic resonance imaging (MRI) and magnetic resonance angiography of the head, neck, and aortic arch, as well as echocardiogram and ophthalmology evaluation are recommended for all infants with a segmental cervicofacial hemangioma. **Lumbosacral hemangiomas** suggest an occult spinal dysraphism with or without anorectal and urogenital anomalies **(LUMBAR syndrome)**. MRI of the spine is indicated in all patients with large midline cutaneous hemangiomas in the lumbosacral area.

Some hemangiomas do not necessitate medical intervention and involute spontaneously. Treatment may be indicated if there is functional impairment, ulceration, or potential for cosmetic disfigurement. It is important to note that even after hemangioma involution, more than half of patients have sequelae, which can include residual fibrofatty tissue, redundant skin, anetodermic skin, or telangiectasia. If complications arise and treatment is warranted, oral propranolol or topical timolol are the mainstays of therapy.

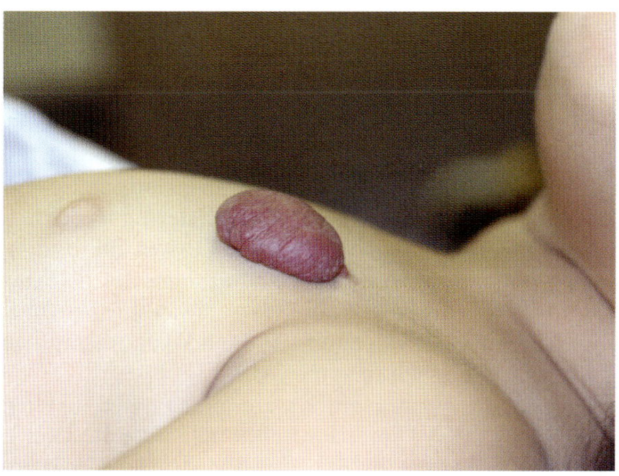

FIGURE 195.1 Superficial type infantile hemangioma (chest).

Pyogenic Granuloma

A pyogenic granuloma is an acquired, benign vascular tumor commonly seen in children. Initially, the lesions appear as friable, granulation tissue-like, pink-red papules that often arise after minor trauma, growing rapidly over a period of weeks into a 2- to 10-mm, bright red, vascular, often pedunculated papule. They may occur anywhere on the body, but the head, neck, and upper extremities are most affected. When traumatized, these lesions may bleed profusely, often requiring emergent medical attention. Surgical excision is the most definitive treatment option, although pulsed dye laser, cryosurgery, electrodesiccation, and topical β blockers can be useful.

VASCULAR MALFORMATIONS

Port-Wine Stain

Port-wine stains (nevus flammeus, capillary malformation) are malformations of the superficial capillaries of the skin that arise due to a somatic mosaic pathogenic variant in genes such as *GNAQ* or *GNA11*. These lesions are present at birth, permanent in nature, and grow with the child. A port-wine stain may be localized to any body surface, but facial lesions are the most common. They are pink or red macules and patches in infancy (Fig. 195.2). With time, they darken to a purple or *port-wine* color and may develop a pebbly or slightly thickened surface. Vascular blebs may form within the lesions and become symptomatic or bleed. The most successful treatment modality is the pulsed dye laser, which can result in 80–90% improvement in these lesions after a series of treatment sessions and can help the patient avoid future complications associated with vascular dilation. Treatment is more effective if started in infancy.

Most port-wine stains occur as isolated defects and are not syndromic. Overgrowth of underlying soft tissues, muscle, and bone can occur depending on which cell lines harbor the somatic variant. Affected patients often need surgical maxillofacial intervention for malalignment that develops. Rarely, port wine stains may suggest ocular defects or specific neurocutaneous syndromes.

Sturge-Weber syndrome, caused by somatic variants in *GNAQ* and *GNA11*, may occur with a facial port-wine stain associated with an adjacent leptomeningeal capillary-venous malformation of the brain and eye. The facial port-wine stain is usually in the cutaneous distribution of the first branch of the trigeminal nerve. Other features include seizures, contralateral hemiparesis, ipsilateral intracortical calcification, and frequent ocular manifestations such as buphthalmos, glaucoma, angioma of the choroid, hemianoptic defects, and optic atrophy. Anticonvulsant therapy and neurosurgical procedures may be required in some patients. Glaucoma can occur in association with port-wine stains located on the eyelid, even in the absence of Sturge-Weber syndrome, and these patients need lifelong monitoring of ocular pressures. **Klippel-Trénaunay syndrome** is characterized by the triad of capillary and venous malformations, venous varicosities, and hyperplasia of the soft tissues—and often bone—of the involved area. The lower limb is most affected. Klippel-Trénaunay syndrome is now recognized to be due to somatic pathogenic variants in the *PIK3CA* gene and considered part of the *PIK3CA*-related overgrowth spectrum of disease. A port-wine stain overlying the spine may rarely be a marker of spinal dysraphism or an intraspinal vascular malformation.

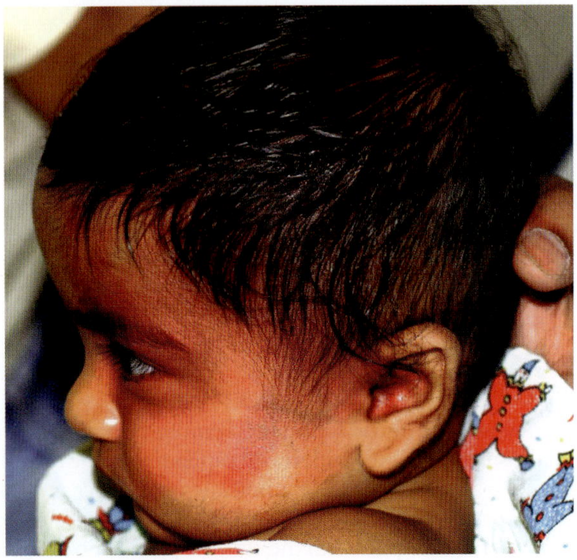

FIGURE 195.2 Port-wine stain (face).

Nevus Simplex

A nevus simplex (salmon patch, stork bite, angel's kiss) is a vascular birthmark that is present in up to 80% of newborns. They are light pink or red, irregular patches resulting from dilation of dermal capillaries and are usually found on the nape of the neck, eyelids, and glabella. Most of the facial lesions fade by 1 year of age, but lesions on the neck may persist for life.

PEARLS FOR PRACTITIONERS

See Dermatology: Pearls for Practitioners at the end of this section.

REVIEW QUESTIONS

Available online.

CHAPTER 196

Erythema Multiforme, Reactive Infectious Mucocutaneous Eruption, Stevens-Johnson Syndrome, and Toxic Epidermal Necrolysis

Erythema multiforme (EM), reactive infectious mucocutaneous eruption (RIME), Stevens-Johnson syndrome (SJS), and toxic epidermal necrolysis (TEN) are acute hypersensitivity reactions characterized by cutaneous and mucosal necrosis. These syndromes represent a hypersensitivity reaction to a precipitating cause, usually infectious organisms or medications. These disorders are not all a spectrum of the same disease process; EM and RIME are distinct from the SJS/TEN spectrum of disease. The differential diagnoses of vesiculobullous eruptions are listed in Table 196.1.

ERYTHEMA MULTIFORME

EM is a common, self-limiting, acute hypersensitivity syndrome characterized by the abrupt onset of round, deep red, well-demarcated macules and papules with a dusky gray or bullous center. The size may vary, but most lesions are approximately 1 cm in diameter. The classic **target lesion** consists of three concentric rings: The outermost is red, the intermediate is paler pink or white, and the center is a dusky red or purple blister (Fig. 196.1). These lesions can progress to edematous plaques or bullae. If blistering occurs, it is circumscribed and involves less than 10% of the body surface area. Cutaneous lesions are symmetrically distributed and commonly involve acral areas such as the hands, feet, elbows, and knees. Involvement of the ocular, oral, and genital mucosa can be seen in some cases.

Most EM cases in children are precipitated by herpes simplex virus (HSV) infection, although the infection may no longer be apparent by the time EM develops. Symptomatic treatment is usually sufficient. Oral antihistamines help

TABLE 196.1 Vesiculobullous Eruptions

ENTITY	CLINICAL CLUES
INFECTIOUS	
Bacterial	
Staphylococcal scalded skin syndrome	Generalized, tender erythema Perioral crusting and radial fissures Nikolsky sign Occasionally associated with underlying infection such as osteomyelitis, septic arthritis, pneumonia Desquamation and moist erosions observed, especially in intertriginous regions More common in children <5 yr of age
Bullous impetigo	Localized blisters from staphylococcal infection
Viral	
Herpes simplex	Grouped vesicles on erythematous base May be recurrent at same site—lips, eyes, cheeks, hands Reactivated by fever, sunlight, trauma, stress
Varicella	Crops of vesicles on erythematous base ("dewdrops on rose petal") Highly contagious May see multiple stages of lesions simultaneously Associated with fever
Herpes zoster	Grouped vesicles on erythematous base limited to one or several adjacent dermatomes May be varicella vaccine associated Usually unilateral Burning, pruritus
Hand-foot-mouth syndrome (coxsackievirus infection)	Prodrome of fever, anorexia, sore throat Few oval blisters in acral distribution Shallow, oral erosions on erythematous base in oral mucosa Highly infectious Peak incidence in late summer and in fall
HYPERSENSITIVITY	
Erythema multiforme	Target lesions on acral sites May have involvement of mucosal surfaces Associated with herpes simplex virus infection
Reactive infectious mucocutaneous eruption	Prodrome of fever and cough Severe mucositis of 2+ mucosal surfaces Scarce/absent rash Associated with *Mycoplasma pneumonia*, *Chlamydophila pneumonia*, or viral respiratory infection
Stevens-Johnson syndrome and toxic epidermal necrolysis	Prodrome of fever, headache, malaise, sore throat, cough, vomiting, diarrhea Macules and atypical targets that coalesce and progress into extensive and diffuse erythema with blistering Extensive epidermal necrosis with mucosal involvement (hemorrhagic erosions of lips) Frequently related to medications (e.g., sulfonamides, anticonvulsants, allopurinol) Nikolsky sign
EXTRINSIC	
Contact dermatitis	Irritant or allergic Distribution dependent on the irritant or allergen Distribution helpful in identifying cause
Insect bites	Occur occasionally following flea or mosquito bites May be hemorrhagic bullae Often in linear or irregular clusters Very pruritic
Burns	Irregular shapes and configurations May be suggestive of nonaccidental trauma Bullae with second- and third-degree injuries
Friction	Usually on acral surfaces May be related to footwear Often activity-related
MISCELLANEOUS	
Maculopapular cutaneous mastocytosis	Red-brown macules and papules; bullous lesions are rare Darier sign Lesions appear in infancy and spontaneously resolve in childhood
Miliaria crystallina	Monomorphous 1- to 2-mm superficial vesicles occurring in crops Rupture spontaneously Intertriginous areas, especially neck and axillae
Hereditary: epidermolysis bullosa, incontinentia pigmenti, epidermolytic hyperkeratosis	
Autoimmune: linear immunoglobulin A disease, bullous pemphigoid, dermatitis herpetiformis	

Modified from Nopper AJ, Rabinowitz LG. Rashes and skin lesions. In: Kliegman RM, ed. Practical Strategies in Pediatric Diagnosis and Therapy. *Philadelphia: WB Saunders; 1996.*

suppress pruritus, stinging, and burning. The use of systemic corticosteroids may be considered for severe mucosal disease. Antiviral medications targeting HSV do not alter the course of the EM, although children with recurrent EM may be candidates for prophylactic antivirals. The prognosis is excellent, with most lesions lasting no more than 2 weeks. Healing occurs without scarring.

REACTIVE INFECTIOUS MUCOCUTANEOUS ERUPTION

RIME is a disorder characterized by a respiratory illness prodrome including fever and cough, severe mucositis (most often involving at least two mucosal surfaces), and a scarce-to-absent rash (Fig. 196.2). When present, the rash associated with RIME is most often targetoid, but varying morphologies have been described. In contrast to SJS/TEN, which is caused by medications, RIME is caused by infection with *Mycoplasma pneumoniae*, *Chlamydophila pneumoniae*, or respiratory viruses such as rhinovirus, enterovirus, influenza, parainfluenza, and human metapneumovirus. While most patients with RIME fully recover, the disorder can be associated with sepsis requiring monitoring and treatment in an intensive care unit. Ocular and urogenital complications can occur as the result of the mucosal ulceration and subsequent scarring. Subcutaneous etanercept injection and systemic corticosteroids are treatment options for severe cases.

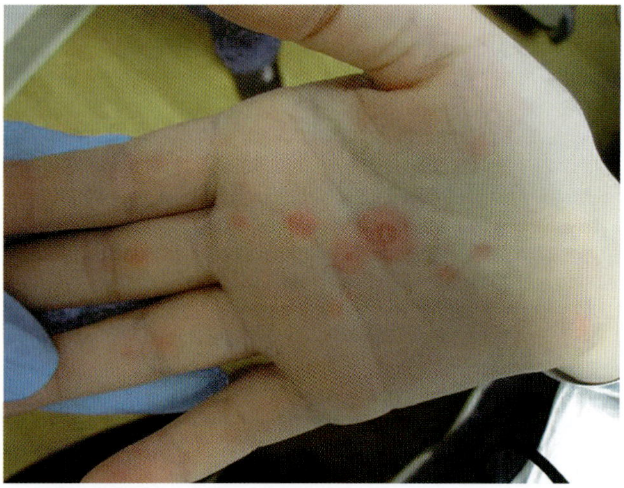

FIGURE 196.1 Target lesions of erythema multiforme. (Courtesy Dr. Kristen Holland.)

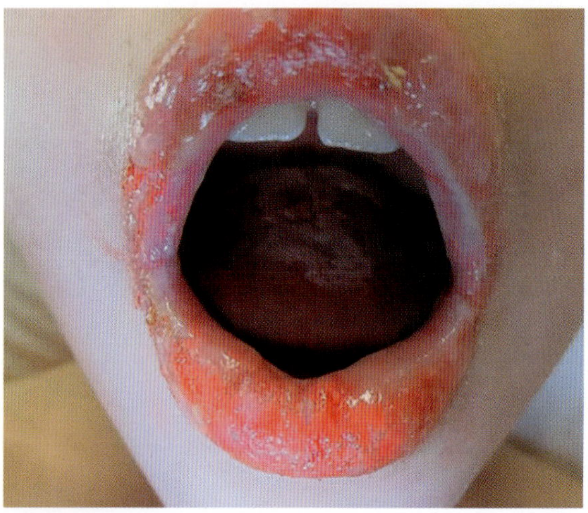

FIGURE 196.2 Ulceration of the lips and tongue in reactive infectious mucocutaneous eruption.

STEVENS-JOHNSON SYNDROME AND TOXIC EPIDERMAL NECROLYSIS

SJS, TEN, and SJS/TEN overlap are severe disorders thought to represent the same disease continuum. They are usually preceded by a prodrome of fever, malaise, and upper respiratory symptoms 1–14 days before the onset of cutaneous lesions. Red macules appear suddenly and tend to coalesce into large patches, with a predominant distribution over the face and trunk (Fig. 196.3). Atypical targets may be present, causing diagnostic confusion initially with EM, although the atypical targets lack the characteristic three zones. Skin lesions evolve rapidly into bullae and areas of necrosis. SJS is defined as epidermal detachment of less than 10% of the body surface area, SJS/TEN overlap has 10–30%, and TEN has greater than 30% body surface area involvement.

Any mucosal surface may be involved. The upper and lower lips are generally swollen and bright red with erosions and hemorrhagic crusts. The remainder of the oral mucosa may also be involved. Early in the disease process, there is bilateral conjunctival injection; this usually progresses to conjunctival erosions. There may be erosions of the penile, vaginal, or perianal mucosa. Urogenital, esophageal, and tracheal surfaces may be involved in severe cases.

Medications are the most common triggers of SJS/TEN in children, including nonsteroidal antiinflammatory drugs, sulfonamides, anticonvulsants, and antibiotics. Infections may be precipitating factors in some cases, and the relationship to RIME in these situations is controversial.

SJS/TEN can occur at any age. The diagnosis of SJS/TEN is clinical; confusion with EM, RIME, Kawasaki disease, and bacterial toxin-mediated diseases (scarlet fever, toxic shock syndrome, and staphylococcal scalded skin syndrome) may occur. Patients with Kawasaki disease may also have conjunctival injection and hyperemia of the mucous membranes;

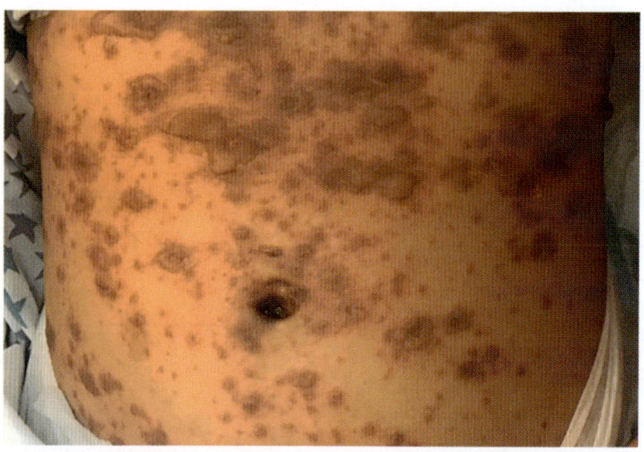

FIGURE 196.3 Toxic epidermal necrolysis secondary to lamotrigine or risperidone; both medications were started simultaneously. (Courtesy Dr. Beth Drolet.)

necrosis of the mucosal surfaces does not occur, and blistering, erosions, and severe crusting are not observed. The mucosal changes of staphylococcal scalded skin syndrome are minor, and the blistering of the skin is more superficial and favors intertriginous regions.

SJS/TEN is a serious illness with a mortality rate as high as 37% for severe cases of TEN. Prompt discontinuation of the offending agent is key; additional treatment may include systemic corticosteroids, intravenous immunoglobulin, cyclosporine, and etanercept. A multidisciplinary care team is often necessary. Sepsis is the major cause of morbidity and mortality, so meticulous wound care is crucial, with stringent surveillance for cutaneous infections and use of antibiotics as warranted. Parenteral or nasogastric feeding should be instituted early to accelerate the healing process, and monitoring of fluid and electrolyte status is critical. Ocular complications are a major cause of long-term morbidity, making early involvement of an ophthalmologist important.

PEARLS FOR PRACTITIONERS

See Dermatology: Pearls for Practitioners at the end of this section.

REVIEW QUESTIONS

Available online.

CHAPTER 197

Cutaneous Infestations

Arthropods are common in the environment. Although many can bite or sting humans, only a few infest humans. Mites are the most common, parasitizing humans and animals by burrowing into the skin and depositing eggs within the skin.

SCABIES

Scabies is caused by the mite *Sarcoptes scabiei*. The female mite burrows into the epidermis and deposits her eggs, which hatch in 3–4 days. The disease is highly contagious, as infested humans do not manifest the typical signs or symptoms for 3–4 weeks, facilitating transmission. An immunocompetent person with scabies harbors less than 15 mites.

The clinical presentation varies depending on the age of the patient, duration of infestation, and immune status of the patient. Severe and paroxysmal itching is the hallmark, with complaints of itching that is frequently worse than the eruption would suggest. Most children exhibit an eczematous eruption composed of red, excoriated papules and nodules. The classic linear papule or burrow is often difficult to find. Distribution is the most diagnostic finding; the papules are found in the axillae, umbilicus, groin, penis, wrist, instep of the foot, and web spaces of the fingers and toes (Fig. 197.1). Infants infested with scabies have diffuse erythema, scaling, and pinpoint papules, along with pustules, vesicles, and nodules. The face and scalp are usually involved in infants but are spared in adults and older children. Nodular lesions may represent active infection or prolonged hypersensitivity lesions following resolution of infestation. Immunocompromised or neurologically impaired individuals may develop a severe form of the disease known as ***crusted scabies***, with infestation of up to 2 million live mites at one time.

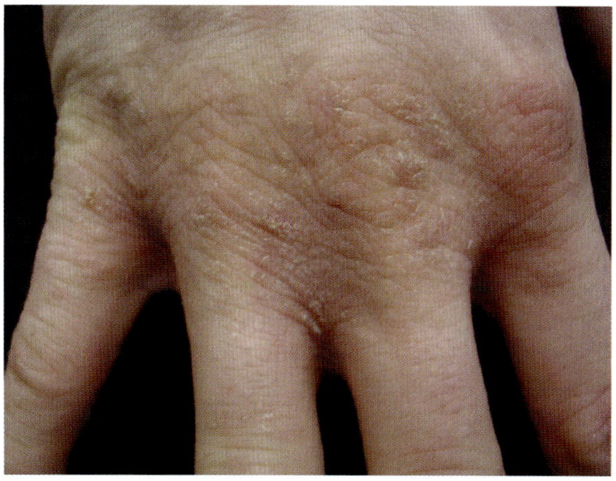

FIGURE 197.1 Scabies (hand).

The diagnosis of scabies can be confirmed by microscopic visualization of the mite, eggs, larvae, or feces in scrapings of papules or burrows examined under oil immersion. Skin biopsy is rarely necessary but may be useful if lesions have become nodular.

Curative treatment is achieved by permethrin 5% cream applied to the entire body and left on for 12 hours. Because permethrin is not effective against the eggs, the treatment should be repeated 1 week later to kill any subsequently hatched larvae. All household members and close contacts should be treated simultaneously, even if asymptomatic. Bed linens, towels, and clothes worn for the previous 2 days before treatment should be machine-washed in hot water and machine-dried using high heat; heat is the most effective scabicide. Items that are not washable may be dry-cleaned or placed in a sealed plastic bag for 7 days.

Secondary bacterial infection may occur but is uncommon. In contrast to the pediculoses, scabies is not a vector for infections. Pruritus may persist for 7–14 days after successful therapy because of a prolonged hypersensitivity reaction, which does not indicate treatment failure. Inadequate treatment or reinfestation should be suspected if new lesions develop after treatment. Combination treatment with topical permethrin and oral ivermectin is indicated for crusted scabies.

PEDICULOSES

Three species of lice infest humans: *Pediculus humanus capitis*, the **head louse**; *Pthirus pubis*, the **pubic louse** or **crab louse**; and *Pediculus humanus humanus* (also known as *Pediculus humanus corporis*), the **body louse**. Lice are wingless insects 2–4 mm in length that cannot fly or jump. Transmission usually occurs by direct contact with another infested individual. Indirect spread through contact with fomites or personal belongings (e.g., hairbrushes, combs, caps) is much less frequent.

Pediculosis differs from scabies infestation in that the louse resides on the hair or clothing and intermittently feeds on the

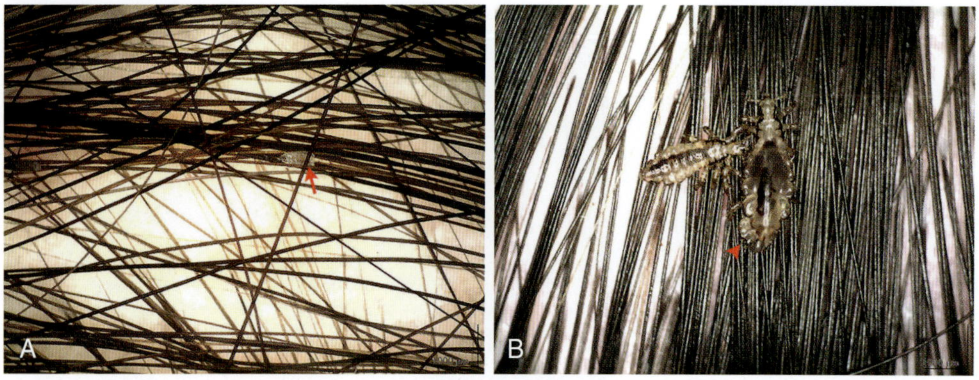

FIGURE 197.2 Nit *(red arrow)* and adult lice *(red arrowhead)* in pediculosis (scalp hair). (From Zhong YH, Li XY, Fan YM. Two copulatory lice with a harasser on scalp hair. *Int J Infect Dis.* 2024;138:19–20.)

host by piercing the skin. The *bite* causes small urticarial papules and itching. Head lice live close to the skin and may live for 30 days, depositing 100–400 eggs as **nits** on hair shafts, usually within 6 mm of the scalp (Fig. 197.2).

Head lice are seen most frequently in early school-age children. Head lice infestations are unrelated to hygiene and are not more common among children with long hair or with dirty hair. It is estimated that 6–12 million persons in the United States and 1–3% of persons in developed countries are infested with head lice each year.

Pubic lice are transmitted by sexual contact. Their presence in children may be a sign of child abuse. Body lice are evidence of poor hygiene, such as infrequent washing and clothing changes.

Itching is the primary symptom. Pediculosis capitis usually causes pruritus behind the ears or on the nape of the neck or a crawling sensation in the scalp. Pediculosis pubis usually causes pruritus in the groin. Eyelash involvement in children may cause crusting and blepharitis. Pediculosis corporis causes pruritus that, because of repeated scratching, may result in lichenification or secondary bacterial infection. Excoriations and crusting, with or without associated regional lymphadenopathy, may be present.

Infestation with the head louse may be asymptomatic and has little morbidity. The diagnosis can be confirmed by visualizing a live louse. A fine-toothed comb to trap lice is more effective than simply looking at the hair. Wet combing is more time consuming, but dry combing produces static that may propel the lice away from the comb.

Nits represent the outer casing of the louse ova. Viable nits have an intact operculum (cap) on the nonattached end and a developing louse within the egg. **Brown nits** located on the proximal hair shaft suggest active infestation. **White nits** located on the hair shaft 4 cm or farther from the scalp indicate previous infestation. Because nonviable nits can remain stuck in the hair for weeks to months after an infestation has resolved, most children with nits do not have active lice infestation.

The treatment of head lice is variable because of resistance to several established options. Topical permethrin (1%) and pyrethrin-based products (0.17–0.33%) (pyrethroids) are over-the-counter options, but drug resistance is prevalent. Malathion (0.5%) lotion, benzyl alcohol (5%) lotion, spinosad (0.9%) suspension, and ivermectin (0.5%) lotion may be used as alternatives for resistant cases. As 20–30% of eggs may survive one treatment, a second treatment should be applied in 1 week.

To reduce the risk of reinfestation, everyone in the family should be checked for head lice and treated if live lice are found. Bed linens, towels, and clothes worn for the previous 2 days before treatment should be machine-washed in hot water and machine-dried using high heat. Items that are not washable may be dry-cleaned or placed in a sealed plastic bag for 2 weeks. Brushes and combs should be soaked in dish detergent or rubbing alcohol for 1 hour. Rugs, furniture, mattresses, and car seats should be vacuumed thoroughly.

Manual removal of nits after treatment is not necessary to prevent spread. Children treated for head lice should return to school immediately after completion of the first effective treatment or first wet combing, regardless of the presence of remaining nits. There is no evidence that *no nit* or *nit-free* policies reduce transmission of head lice. If required for return to school, nit removal is best achieved by wetting the hair and combing with a fine-toothed metal comb.

Excoriations can become secondarily infected with skin bacteria, usually *Staphylococcus* and *Streptococcus*. The body louse functions as a vector for potentially serious infectious diseases, including **epidemic typhus**, caused by *Rickettsia prowazekii*; **louse-borne relapsing fever**, caused by *Borrelia recurrentis*; and **trench fever**, caused by *Bartonella quintana*. These louse-borne infections are rare in the United States. In contrast to body lice, head lice and pubic lice are not associated with transmission of other infections.

PEARLS FOR PRACTITIONERS

See Dermatology: Pearls for Practitioners at the end of this section.

REVIEW QUESTIONS

Available online.

Suggested Readings

Eichenfield LF, Frieden IJ, Mathes EF, Zaenglein AL, eds. *Neonatal and Infant Dermatology*. 3rd ed. Philadelphia: Saunders; 2015.

Eichenfield LF, Krakowski AC, Piggott C, et al. Evidence-based recommendations for the diagnosis and treatment of pediatric acne. *Pediatrics*. 2013;131(suppl 3):S163–S186.

Eichenfield LF, Tom WL, Chamlin SL, et al. Guidelines of care for the management of atopic dermatitis: section 1. Diagnosis and assessment of atopic dermatitis. *J Am Acad Dermatol*. 2014;70(2):338–351.

Eichenfield LF, Tom WL, Berger TG, et al. Guidelines of care for the management of atopic dermatitis: section 2. Management and treatment of atopic dermatitis with topical therapies. *J Am Acad Dermatol*. 2014;71(1):116–132.

Krowchuk DP, Frieden IJ, Mancini AJ, et al. Clinical Practice Guideline for the Management of Infantile Hemangiomas. *Pediatrics*. 2019;143(1):e20183475.
Paller AS, Mancini AJ. *Hurwitz Clinical Pediatric Dermatology*. 5th ed. Philadelphia: Elsevier; 2015.
Reynolds RV, Yeung H, Cheng CE, et al. Guidelines of care for the management of acne vulgaris. *J Am Acad Dermatol*. 2024;90(5):1006.e1–1006.e30.
Torrelo A, ed. *Schachner and Hansen's Pediatric Dermatology*. 5th ed. New Delhi: Jaypee Brothers; 2023.
Zaenglein AL, Pathy AL, Schlosser BJ, et al. Guidelines of care for the management of acne vulgaris. [published correction appears in J Am Acad Dermatol. 2020 Jun;82(6):1576.] *J Am Acad Dermatol*. 2016;74(5). 945–73. e33.

PEARLS FOR PRACTITIONERS

CHAPTER 189
Dermatology Assessment

- Common cutaneous conditions in pediatrics include atopic dermatitis, seborrheic dermatitis, acne vulgaris, verruca vulgaris, molluscum contagious, and impetigo.
- Obtaining a thorough history including the age of the patient, onset, duration, progression, associated cutaneous symptoms (pain, pruritus), previous treatments, and associated systemic signs or symptoms (fever, malaise, weight loss) is important.
- Characterizing and describing the primary and secondary skin lesions is important for diagnosis and communication with other health care providers.

CHAPTER 190
Acne Vulgaris

- Acne vulgaris is the most common skin condition in adolescents.
- The pathogenesis of acne involves increased sebum production, hyperkeratosis, bacterial proliferation, and inflammation. Treatment is aimed at decreasing these factors.

CHAPTER 191
Atopic Dermatitis

- Atopic dermatitis is the most common chronic skin disease in children and is associated with allergic rhinitis, asthma, and food allergies. Both genetic and environmental factors play a role in the development of atopic dermatitis.
- Treatment of atopic dermatitis is aimed at decreasing inflammation.
- Complications of atopic dermatitis include secondary impetigo and eczema herpeticum.

CHAPTER 192
Contact Dermatitis

- Contact dermatitis occurs when the skin is directly exposed to irritating chemicals or substances (irritant contact dermatitis) or allergens in predisposed individuals (allergic contact dermatitis).
- Diaper dermatitis is a common type of irritant contact dermatitis from urine and feces, frequently complicated by secondary candida and bacterial infections. Differential diagnosis for diaper dermatitis includes psoriasis, seborrheic dermatitis, and Langerhans cell histiocytosis. Referral to a pediatric dermatologist should be made in recalcitrant, difficult-to-treat cases.
- Treatment of contact dermatitis is generally avoidance of irritating substances and allergens as well as topical corticosteroids.

CHAPTER 193
Seborrheic Dermatitis

- Seborrheic dermatitis is a common, chronic inflammatory disease that presents as cradle cap or dermatitis in intertriginous areas in infants and dandruff in adolescents.
- The pathogenesis of seborrheic dermatitis is unclear, but it is theorized that there is an abnormal inflammatory response to commensal *Malassezia* species in sebum-rich areas.
- Treatment for seborrheic dermatitis is generally not needed, but oils, shampoos, and topical steroids can be used if needed.
- Pityriasis rosea is a benign, self-limited eruption that starts with a herald patch, which precedes a generalized eruption on the torso and extremities in a Christmas tree pattern.
- Psoriasis is a common papulosquamous disorder with various subtypes, including plaque-type (psoriasis vulgaris), guttate, erythrodermic, and pustular psoriasis.
- Treatments for psoriasis include topical corticosteroids, topical vitamin D analogues, salicylic acid, tar preparations, phototherapy, systemic immunosuppressants, and biologics.

CHAPTER 194
Pigmented Lesions

- Dermal melanocytosis is the most frequently encountered pigmented lesion. The gray-blue lesions are found in the lumbosacral area, buttocks, flank, extremities, or (rarely) the face.
- Café-au-lait macules are light brown pigmented macules or patches that can be found in normal newborns and children.

- Children with six or more café-au-lait macules (0.5 cm in diameter before puberty or >1.5 cm in diameter after puberty), especially when accompanied by axillary or inguinal freckling, should be evaluated carefully for additional stigmata of neurofibromatosis type 1.
- Other disorders also associated with café-au-lait macules include the other forms of neurofibromatosis, Legius syndrome, tuberous sclerosis, McCune-Albright syndrome, Noonan syndrome, and Russell-Silver syndrome.
- There is an increased risk of neuromelanosis and malignant melanoma when congenital melanocytic nevi are giant (>40 cm in length in adulthood).

CHAPTER 195
Vascular Anomalies

- Infantile hemangiomas are the most common soft tissue tumors of infancy and present as superficial, deep, or mixed types.
  - They undergo spontaneous involution after a rapid growth phase.
  - They should be treated if symptomatic and/or if they pose risks that can lead to functional compromise or permanent disfigurement, in which case oral propranolol and topical timolol are the mainstays of therapy.
  - Even after involution, more than half of hemangiomas have sequelae that include residual fibrofatty tissue, redundant skin, anetodermic skin, or telangiectasia.
- Infantile hemangiomas can have visceral involvement and be associated with other underlying anomalies.
  - Evaluation for airway hemangiomas should be undertaken in infants with a cutaneous hemangioma in a beard distribution.
  - Evaluation with echocardiogram, MRI/MR angiography of the head, neck, and aortic arch, and ophthalmology exam should be performed in infants with large segmental infantile hemangiomas of the head at risk for PHACE syndrome.
  - Large lumbosacral hemangiomas should be investigated with magnetic resonance imaging (MRI) of the spine to evaluate for LUMBAR syndrome.

CHAPTER 196
Erythema Multiforme, Reactive Infectious Mucocutaneous Eruption, Stevens-Johnson Syndrome, and Toxic Epidermal Necrolysis

- Erythema multiforme (EM) is a common, self-limiting, acute hypersensitivity syndrome characterized by the abrupt onset of target lesions in an acral distribution.
  - EM can be precipitated by infections (most commonly herpes simplex virus) or medications.
- Reactive infectious mucocutaneous eruption (RIME) is characterized by a prodrome with fever and cough, severe mucositis (most often involving at least two mucosal surfaces), and a scarce-to-absent rash. RIME is caused by infection with *Mycoplasma pneumoniae, Chlamydophila pneumoniae*, or respiratory viruses.
- Stevens-Johnson syndrome (SJS), toxic epidermal necrolysis (TEN), and SJS/TEN overlap are severe, life-threatening disorders thought to represent the same disease continuum. They are precipitated by medications.
  - SJS is defined as epidermal detachment of <10% of the body surface area; SJS/TEN overlap has 10–30%; and TEN has >30% body surface area involvement.

CHAPTER 197
Cutaneous Infestations

- Scabies is caused by the mite *Sarcoptes scabiei.*
  - Curative treatment for scabies is achieved by a 12-hour (overnight) application of permethrin 5% cream applied to the entire body and repeated in 1 week. All household members and close contacts should be treated for scabies simultaneously, even if asymptomatic.
- Household treatment for scabies and pediculosis includes machine washing (in hot water) and machine drying (using high heat) all bed linens, towels, and clothes worn in the previous 2 days. Items that are not washable may be dry-cleaned or placed in a sealed plastic bag for 7 days (scabies) or 14 days (pediculosis).

ORTHOPEDICS

Kevin D. Walter

CHAPTER 198

Orthopedic Assessment

Providers should understand the growth and development of the musculoskeletal system as well as common orthopedic terms (Table 198.1). It is also important to recognize common mechanisms for congenital and acquired orthopedic disorders (Table 198.2).

TABLE 198.1 Common Orthopedic Terminology

Abduction	Movement away from midline
Adduction	Movement toward or across midline
Apophysis	Bone growth center that has a muscular insertion but is not considered a growth plate (e.g., tibial tubercle)
Arthroscopy	Surgical exploration of a joint using an arthroscope
Arthroplasty	Surgical reconstruction of a joint
Arthrotomy	Surgical incision into a joint; an "open" procedure
Deformation	Changes in limb, trunk, or head due to mechanical force
Dislocation	Displacement of bones at a joint
Disruption	Normally developing structure that is destroyed, removed, or stops developing
Equinus	Plantar flexion of the forefoot, hindfoot, or entire foot
Femoral anteversion	Increased angulation of the femoral head and neck with respect to the frontal plane
Malformation	Defect in development that occurs during fetal life (e.g., syndactyly)
Osteotomy	Surgical division of a bone
Pes cavus	High medial arch of the foot
Pes planus	Flat foot
Rotation, internal	Inward rotation (toward midline)
Rotation, external	Outward rotation (away from midline)
Subluxation	Incomplete loss of contact between two joint surfaces
Tibial torsion	Rotation of the tibia in an internal or external fashion
Valgus/valgum	Angulation of a bone or joint in which the apex is toward the midline (e.g., knock-knee)
Varus/varum	Angulation of a bone or joint in which the apex is away from the midline (e.g., bowlegs)

(Continued)

TABLE 198.2 Mechanisms of Common Pediatric Orthopedic Problems

CATEGORY	MECHANISM	EXAMPLE(S)
CONGENITAL		
Malformation	Teratogenesis <12 wk of gestation	Spina bifida
Disruption	Amniotic band constriction	Extremity amputation
	Fetal varicella infection	Limb scar/atrophy
Deformation	Neck compression	Torticollis
Dysplasia	Abnormal cell growth or metabolism	Osteogenesis imperfecta Skeletal dysplasias
ACQUIRED		
Infection	Pyogenic-hematogenous spread	Septic arthritis, osteomyelitis
Inflammation	Antigen-antibody reaction Immune mediated	Systemic lupus erythematosus Juvenile idiopathic arthritis
Trauma	Mechanical forces, overuse	Child abuse, sports injuries, unintentional injury, fractures, dislocations, tendinitis
Tumor	Primary bone tumor	Osteosarcoma
	Metastasis to bone from other site	Neuroblastoma
	Bone marrow tumor	Leukemia, lymphoma

GROWTH AND DEVELOPMENT

The ends of the long bones contain a much higher proportion of cartilage in the skeletally immature child than in an adult (Figs. 198.1 and 198.2). The high cartilage content allows for a unique vulnerability to trauma and infection, particularly in the metaphysis.

The physis is responsible for the longitudinal growth of the long bones. Articular cartilage allows for enlargement of the ends of the bone and accounts for growth of smaller bones, such as the tarsals. The periosteum provides for circumferential growth. Trauma, infection, nutritional deficiency (e.g., rickets), inborn errors of metabolism (e.g., mucopolysaccharidoses), and other disorders (e.g., renal tubular acidosis, hypothyroid) may affect each of the growth processes and produce distinct aberrations.

DEVELOPMENTAL MILESTONES

Neurologic maturation, marked by achievement of developmental motor milestones, is important for normal musculoskeletal development (see Section 2—Growth and Development). A neurologic disorder may cause a secondary musculoskeletal abnormality (e.g., extremity contractures in Duchenne muscular dystrophy). Thus, normal motor development must be included in the definition of a normal musculoskeletal system.

Infants

In utero positioning of the fetus may affect the angular and torsional alignment (temporary or permanent) of the skeletal system, especially of the lower extremity (Fig. 198.3). A newborn has externally rotated hips and commonly has pes planus and genu varum. The flexed posture of an infant usually becomes neutral within the first 4–6 months. The foot is often flat and tucked under at birth, with the ankle inverted and the forefoot adducted when compared with the hindfoot. A provider must be able to straighten the lateral border of the foot, even while in dorsiflexion, for this to be considered secondary to in utero positioning.

While the head and neck may also be distorted by in utero positioning, the spine and upper extremities are less likely to be affected. By the age of 3–4 years, the effects of in utero positioning have usually resolved.

Gait

Normal gait has a stance phase and a swing phase. Each leg should have symmetric timing during each phase. The stance phase represents 60% of the gait and begins with foot contact (usually the heel strike) and ends with the toe-off. During the swing phase (40%), the foot is off the ground. The gait cycle is the interval between stance phases on the same limb.

Toddlers will generally walk independently by 18 months of age. Their externally rotated gait is usually inconsistent, characterized by short, rapid steps, and does not have the reciprocal arm swing. Gait coordination improves over time, with a normal gait usually achieved by the time a child enters elementary school.

Limping Child

The differential diagnoses for a limping child are often categorized by age and presence or absence of a painful limp (Table 198.3). The gluteus medius muscle stabilizes the pelvis during the stance phase, preventing the pelvis from dropping toward the leg in swing phase. An **antalgic gait** is a painful limp; the stance phase and stride of the affected limb are shortened to decrease the discomfort of weight bearing on the affected limb. The **Trendelenburg gait** has a normal stance phase but excessive swaying of the trunk. A **waddling gait** causes bending of the trunk toward the stance phase leg and is caused by weakness in the hip girdle and upper thigh.

Toe walking is a common parental concern in early walkers. A provider should evaluate any child older than 3 years of age who still toe walks. Although this is most likely habit, a neuromuscular disorder (e.g., cerebral palsy, tethered cord), Achilles tendon contracture (heel cord tightness), or a leg-length discrepancy should be considered.

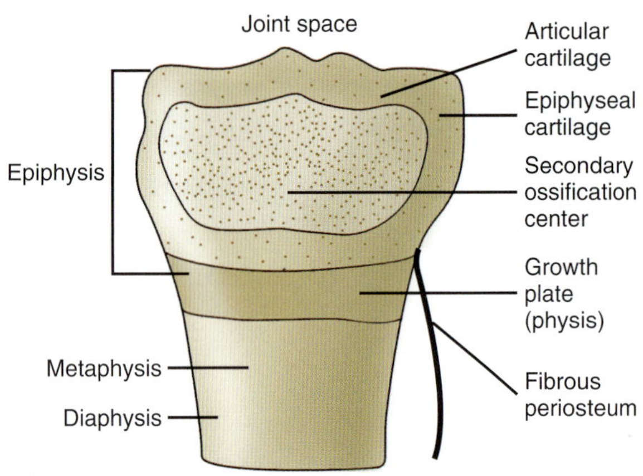

FIGURE 198.1 Schematic of long bone structure.

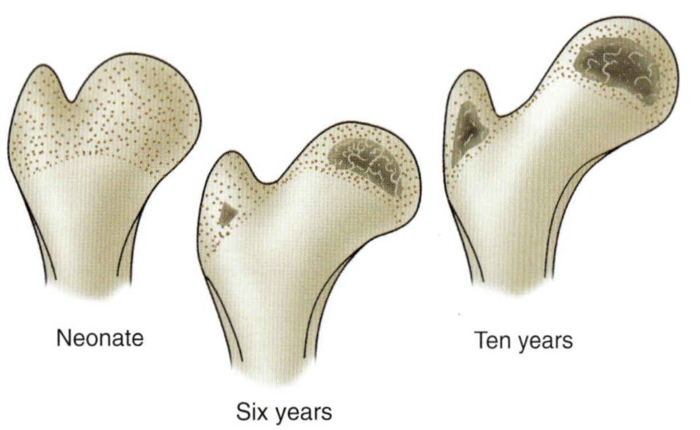

FIGURE 198.2 The ends of long bones at various ages. Lightly stippled areas represent cartilage composition, and heavily darkened areas are zones of ossification. (From Tachjidan MO. *Congenital Dislocation of the Hip*. New York: Churchill Livingstone; 1982:105.)

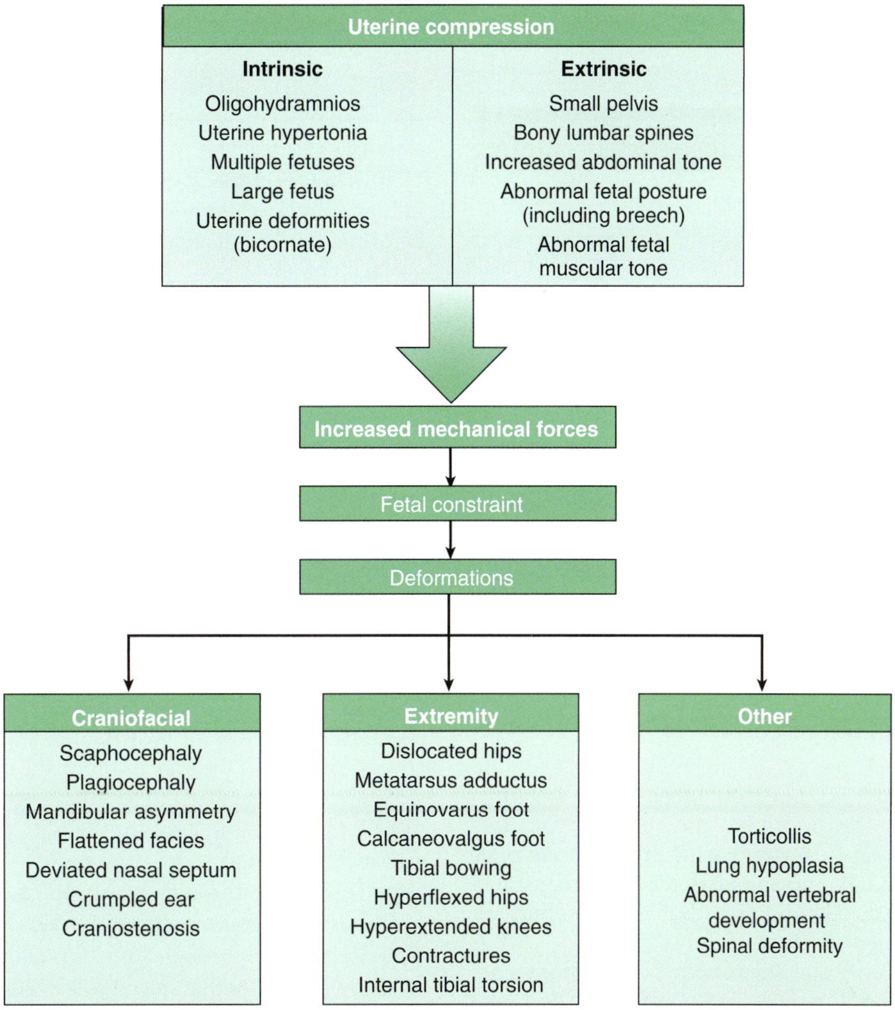

FIGURE 198.3 Deformation abnormalities resulting from uterine compression.

TABLE **198.3** Differential Diagnoses of Limping in Children

AGE GROUP	DIAGNOSTIC CONSIDERATIONS	AGE GROUP	DIAGNOSTIC CONSIDERATIONS
Early walker: 1–3 yr of age	*Painful limp* Septic arthritis and osteomyelitis Transient monoarticular synovitis Occult trauma ("toddler's fracture") Spondylodiscitis Malignancy *Painless limp* Developmental dysplasia of the hip Neuromuscular disorder Cerebral palsy Lower extremity length inequality	Adolescent: 11 yr of age to maturity	*Painful limp* Septic arthritis, osteomyelitis, myositis Trauma Rheumatologic disorder Slipped capital femoral epiphysis: acute, unstable Malignancy *Painless limp* Slipped capital femoral epiphysis: chronic; stable Developmental dysplasia of the hip: acetabular dysplasia Lower extremity length inequality Neuromuscular disorder
Child: 3–10 yr of age	*Painful limp* Septic arthritis, osteomyelitis, myositis Transient monoarticular synovitis Trauma Rheumatologic disorders Juvenile idiopathic arthritis Spondylodiscitis Malignancy *Painless limp* Developmental dysplasia of the hip Legg-Calve-Perthes disease Lower extremity length inequality Neuromuscular disorder Cerebral palsy Muscular dystrophy (Duchenne)		

PEARLS FOR PRACTITIONERS

See Orthopedics: Pearls for Practitioners at the end of this section.

REVIEW QUESTIONS

Available online.

CHAPTER 199

Fractures

Fractures account for 10–15% of all childhood injuries. The anatomic, biomechanic, and physiologic differences in children account for unique fracture patterns and management. Understanding fracture terminology helps improve communication with specialists (Table 199.1).

The pediatric skeleton has a higher proportion of cartilage and a thicker, stronger, and more active periosteum capable of producing a larger callus more rapidly than in an adult. The thick periosteum may decrease the rate of displaced fractures and helps stabilize fractures. With a higher proportion of cartilage, the skeletally immature patient can withstand more force before deformation or fracture than adult bone. As children mature into adolescence, the rate of healing slows and approaches that of adults.

PEDIATRIC FRACTURE PATTERNS

Buckle or **torus fractures** occur after compression of the bone; the bony cortex does not truly break. These fractures will typically occur in the metaphysis and are stable fractures that heal in approximately 4 weeks with immobilization. A common example is a fall onto an outstretched arm causing a buckle fracture in the distal radius; removable wrist splints are effective for management of these fractures.

Complete fractures occur when both sides of bony cortex are fractured. This is the most common fracture and may be classified as comminuted (broken into >3 pieces), oblique, transverse, or spiral, depending on the direction of the fracture line.

Greenstick fractures occur when a bone is angulated beyond the limits of plastic deformation. The bone fails on the tension side and sustains a bend deformity on the compression side. The force is insufficient to cause a complete fracture (Fig. 199.1).

Bowing fractures demonstrate no fracture line evident on radiographs, but the bone is bent beyond its limit of plastic deformation. This is not a true fracture but will heal with periosteal reaction.

TABLE 199.1 Useful Fracture Terminology

Complete	The bone fragments separate completely
Incomplete	The bone fragments are still partially joined
Linear	A fracture line that is parallel to the bone's long axis
Transverse	A fracture line that is at a right angle to the bone's long axis
Oblique	A fracture line that is diagonal to the bone's long axis
Spiral	A twisting fracture with diagonal line
Comminution	A fracture that results in several fragments
Compaction	The bone fragments are driven into each other
Angulation	The fragments of bone are at an angle to each other
Rotation	The fracture fragments rotated on each other when the bone broke
Shortening	The fractured ends of the bones overlap
Open	A fracture in which the bone has pierced the skin

Physeal Fractures

Fractures involving the growth plate constitute about 20% of all fractures in the skeletally immature patient. These fractures are twice as common in males. The peak incidence is 13–14 years in males and 11–12 years in females. The distal radius, distal tibia, and distal fibula are the most common locations.

Traumatic forces to an extremity may be transmitted to the physis, which is not as biomechanically strong as the metaphysis. The physis may fracture with mechanisms of injury that may cause sprains in the adult. The growth plate is most susceptible to torsional and angular forces.

Physeal fractures are described using **Salter-Harris classification**, which allows for prognostic information regarding premature closure of the growth plate and poor functional outcomes. The higher the type number, the more likely the patient will have complications. There are five main types (Fig. 199.2):

Type I: transverse fracture through the physis; growth disturbance is unusual

Type II: fracture through a portion of the physis and metaphysis; most common type of Salter-Harris fracture (75%)

Type III: fracture through a portion of the physis and epiphysis into the joint that may result in complication because of intraarticular component and because of disruption of the growing or hypertrophic zone of the physis

Type IV: fracture through the metaphysis, physis, and epiphysis with a high risk of complication

Type V: a crush injury to the physis with a poor functional prognosis

Types I and II fractures can often be managed by closed reduction and do not require perfect alignment. A major exception is the type II fracture of the distal femur, which is associated with a poor outcome unless proper anatomic

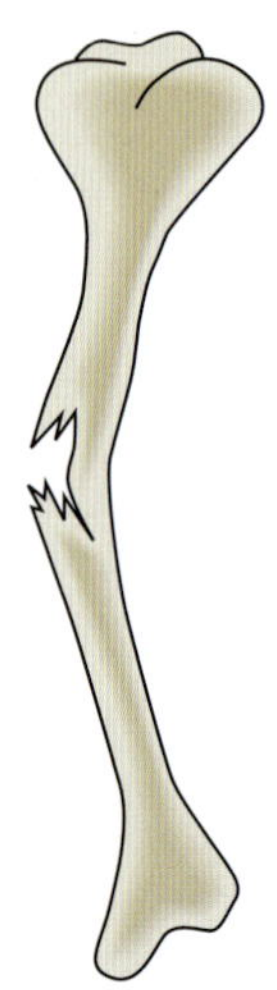

FIGURE 199.1 The greenstick fracture is an incomplete fracture. (Modified from White N, Sty R. Radiological evaluation and classification of pediatric fractures. *Clin Pediatr Emerg Med*. 2002;3:94–105.)

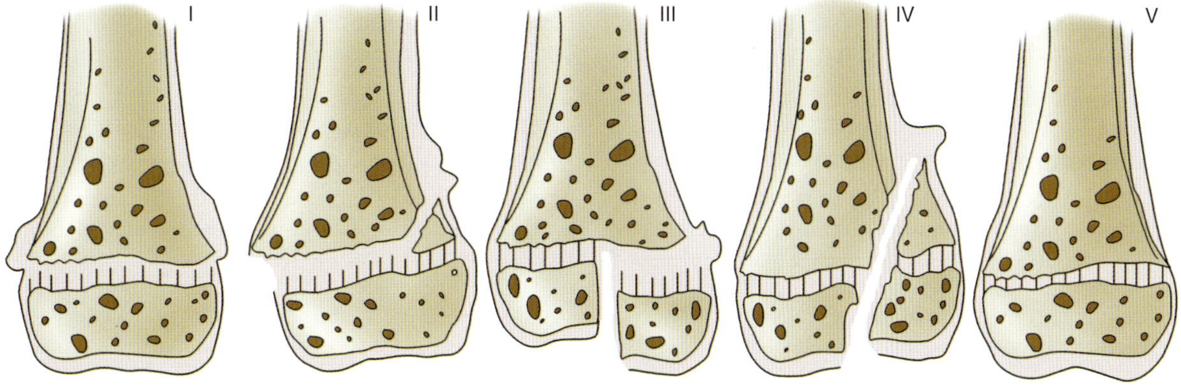

FIGURE 199.2 The types of growth plate injury as classified by Salter and Harris. See text for descriptions of types I to V. (From Salter RB, Harris WR. Injuries involving the epiphyseal plate. *J Bone Joint Surg Am*. 1963;45:587–622.)

alignment is obtained. Types III and IV fractures require anatomic alignment for successful treatment. Type V fractures are rare and often result in premature closure of the physis.

MANAGEMENT OF PEDIATRIC FRACTURES

The majority of pediatric fractures can be managed with closed methods. Some fractures need closed reduction to improve alignment. Approximately 4% of pediatric fractures require internal fixation. Patients with open physes are more likely to require internal fixation if they have one of the following fractures:

- Displaced epiphyseal fractures
- Displaced intraarticular fractures
- Fractures in a child with multiple injuries
- Open fractures
- Unstable fractures

The goal of internal fixation is to improve and maintain anatomic alignment. This is usually done with Kirschner wires, Steinmann pins, and cortical screws with subsequent external immobilization in a cast until healing is satisfactory. After healing, the hardware is frequently removed to prevent incorporation into the callus and prevent physeal damage.

External fixation without casting may be necessary for pelvic fractures causing hemodynamic instability. Fractures associated with soft tissue loss, burns, and neurovascular damage may benefit from external fixation.

SPECIAL CONCERNS

Remodeling

Fracture remodeling occurs because of a combination of periosteal resorption and new bone formation. Many pediatric fractures do not need perfect anatomic alignment for proper healing. Younger patients have greater potential for fracture remodeling. Fractures that occur in the metaphysis, near the growth plate, may undergo more remodeling. Fractures angulated in the plane of motion also remodel very well. Intraarticular fractures, angulated or displaced diaphyseal fractures, rotated fractures, and fracture deformity not in the plane of motion tend not to remodel as well.

Overgrowth

Overgrowth occurs in long bones as the result of increased blood flow associated with fracture healing. Femoral fractures in children younger than 10 years of age will frequently overgrow 1–3 cm. This is the reason end-to-end alignment for femur and long-bone fractures may not be indicated. After 10 years of age, overgrowth is less of a problem, so end-to-end alignment is recommended.

Progressive Deformity

Fractures and injuries to the physis can result in premature closure. If it is a partial closure, the consequence may be an angular deformity. If it is a complete closure, limb shortening may occur. Commonly affected locations are the distal femur and the distal and proximal tibia.

Neurovascular Injury

Fractures and dislocations may damage adjacent blood vessels and nerves. The most common location is the distal humerus (supracondylar fracture) and the knee (dislocation and physeal fracture). It is necessary to perform and document a careful neurovascular examination distal to the fracture (pulse, sensory, and motor function).

Compartment Syndrome

Compartment syndrome is an orthopedic emergency that results from hemorrhage and soft tissue swelling within the tight fascial compartments of an extremity. This can result in muscle ischemia and neurovascular compromise unless it is surgically decompressed. The most common sites are the lower leg (tibial fracture) and arm (supracondylar fracture).

Swollen and tight compartments and pain with passive stretching are present. Affected patients have severe pain not well controlled with prescribed medication. If not promptly identified and treated, patients may develop decreased sensation in the dermatomes supplied by the nerves located in the compartment or decreased perfusion of the extremity. Sometimes compartment syndrome may happen underneath a cast and may occur when a cast is applied too tightly; for this reason, many casts are split on each side (bivalved) in the postreduction period to allow room for swelling. It is important to educate all patients with fractures on the signs of compartment syndrome and ensure that they realize it is an emergency.

Toddler's Fracture

This is an oblique fracture of the distal tibia without a fibula fracture. There is often no significant trauma. Patients are usually 1–3 years old but can be as old as 6 years and present with limping and pain with weight bearing. There may be minimal swelling and pain. Initial radiographs do not always show the fracture. If symptoms persist, a repeat x-ray in 7–10 days may be helpful; an oblique view on x-ray may also show the fracture.

Child Abuse

Child abuse must always be considered in the differential diagnosis of a child with fractures, especially in younger children (see Chapter 21). Common fracture patterns that should increase the index of suspicion include multiple fractures in different stages of radiographic healing, metaphyseal corner fractures (caused by twisting and shaking), fractures too severe for the history, or fractures in nonambulatory infants. Although spiral fractures of long bones were historically considered pathognomonic for abuse, they are also seen in nonabuse situations.

When there is concern for child abuse, providers should report to child protective services and the child should undergo a full evaluation. A thorough and well-documented physical examination should focus on soft tissue injuries, the cranium, and a funduscopic examination for retinal hemorrhages or detachment. Skeletal survey radiographs may be helpful in identifying other fractures. If suspicious fractures are identified, careful evaluation should be performed to rule out metabolic bone disease (e.g., osteogenesis imperfecta).

PEARLS FOR PRACTITIONERS

See Orthopedics: Pearls for Practitioners at the end of this section.

REVIEW QUESTIONS

Available online.

CHAPTER 200

Hip

The hip is a ball (femoral head) and socket (acetabulum) joint that is important for skeletal stability. The femoral head and acetabulum are interdependent for normal growth and development. The femoral neck and head, which contain the capital femoral epiphysis, are intraarticular. The blood supply to this region is unique because the blood vessels are extraosseous and lie on the surface of the femoral neck, entering the epiphysis peripherally. Thus, the blood supply to the femoral head is vulnerable to trauma, infection, and other damage that may increase intraarticular pressure. Damage to the blood supply can lead to **avascular necrosis** and permanent deformity of the hip.

DEVELOPMENTAL DYSPLASIA OF THE HIP

In developmental dysplasia of the hip (DDH), the hips may be dislocated or dislocatable at birth. The femoral head and acetabulum develop from the same mesenchymal cells; by 11 weeks of gestation, the hip joint is formed. There are two types of DDH: teratologic and typical. **Teratologic dislocations** occur early in utero and are usually associated with neuromuscular disorders (e.g., spina bifida, arthrogryposis). **Typical dislocations** occur in the neurologically normal infant and can occur before or after birth. The true incidence of DDH is unknown, but it may be as high as 1.5 cases per 1,000 infants.

Etiology

Newborn infants have ligamentous laxity that, if significant enough in the hip, may lead to spontaneous dislocation and then reduction of the femoral head. Persistence of this spontaneous pattern can lead to pathologic changes, such as flattening of the acetabulum, muscle contractures that limit motion, and joint capsule tightening. The left hip is affected three times as often as the right hip, possibly because of in utero positioning.

Physiologic risk factors for DDH include a generalized ligamentous laxity, perhaps from maternal hormones that are associated with pelvic ligament relaxation (estrogen and relaxin). Female infants are at higher risk (9:1); family history is positive in 20% of all patients with DDH.

Other risk factors include breech presentation, firstborn child (60%), oligohydramnios, and intrauterine and postnatal infant positioning. In breech presentations, the fetal pelvis is situated in the maternal pelvis. This can increase hip flexion and limit overall fetal hip motion, causing further stretching of the already lax joint capsule and exposing the posterior aspect of the femoral head. The altered relationship between the acetabulum and femoral head causes abnormal acetabular development. Postnatal positioning of the hips in a tight swaddle with the hips adducted and extended can displace the hip joint.

Congenital muscular torticollis, metatarsus adductus, and clubfoot are associated with DDH. An infant with any of these three conditions should receive a careful examination of the hips.

Clinical Manifestations

Every newborn requires a screening physical examination for DDH; further evaluation through at least the first 18 months of life is part of the physical examination for toddlers. DDH evolves over time, so the examination may change as the patient ages. The examination starts with inspection for asymmetric thigh and gluteal folds with the hips and knees flexed. A relative shortening of the femur with asymmetric skinfolds is a positive **Galeazzi sign** and indicates DDH. Range of motion should be assessed with the pelvis stabilized and the child supine on the examining table, not in the parent's lap (Fig. 200.1). Hip abduction should easily reach or exceed 75 degrees; limitations may indicate contractures associated with DDH.

The **Barlow test** attempts to dislocate an unstable hip (Fig. 200.2). The examiner should stabilize the infant's pelvis with one hand and grasp the abducted and flexed thigh in the

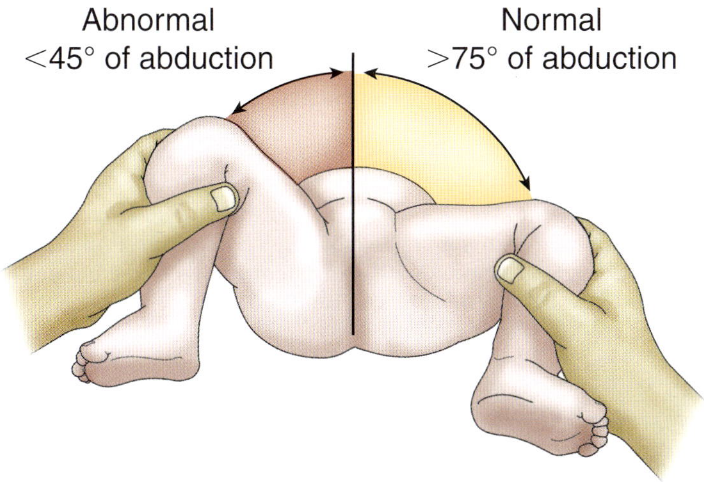

FIGURE 200.1 Normal and abnormal hip abduction. With the infant supine, flex the hips to 90 degrees, and fully abduct the hips. Normal abduction is >75 degrees, and an angle <45 degrees is abnormal.

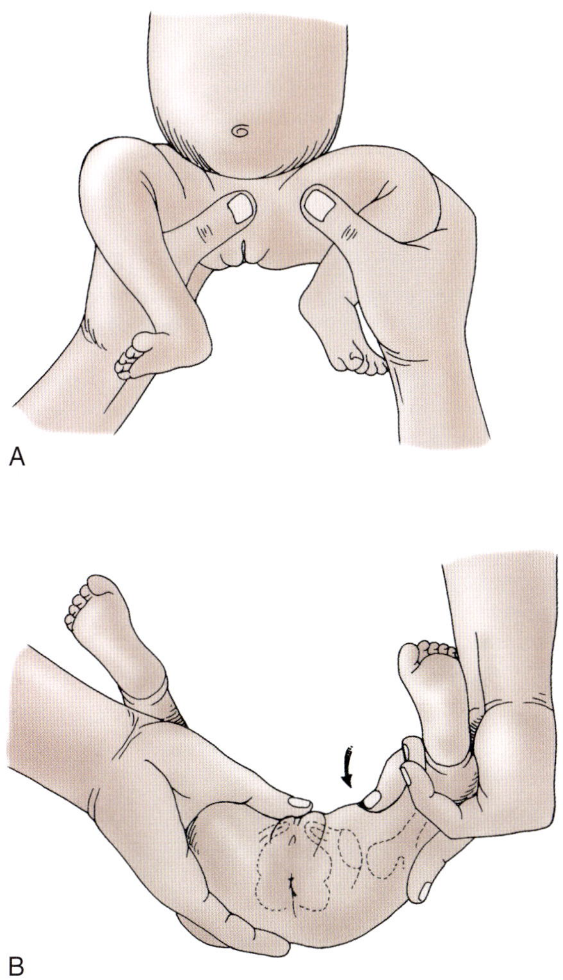

FIGURE 200.2 Barlow (dislocation) test. Reverse of Ortolani test. If the femoral head is in the acetabulum at the time of examination, the Barlow test is performed to discover any hip instability. **(A)** The infant's thigh is grasped as shown and adducted with gentle downward pressure. **(B)** Dislocation is palpable as the femoral head slips out of the acetabulum. Diagnosis is confirmed with the Ortolani test.

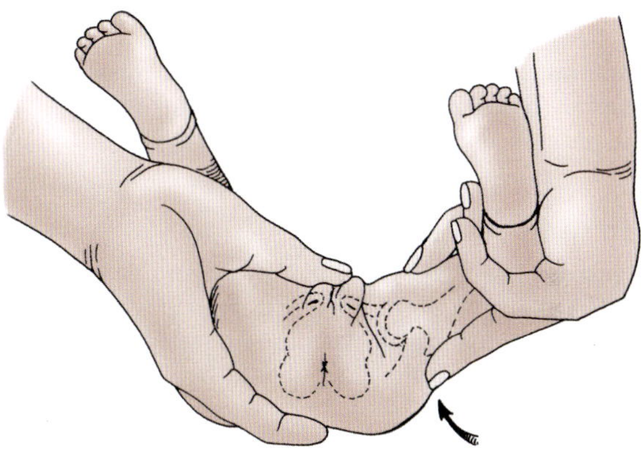

FIGURE 200.3 Ortolani (reduction) test. With the infant relaxed and content on a firm surface, the hips and knees are flexed to 90 degrees. The hips are examined one at a time. The examiner grasps the infant's thigh with the middle finger over the greater trochanter and lifts the thigh to bring the femoral head from its dislocated posterior position to opposite the acetabulum. Simultaneously, the thigh is gently abducted, reducing the femoral head in the acetabulum. In a positive finding, the examiner senses reduction by a palpable, nearly audible *clunk*.

other hand. The hip should be flexed to 90 degrees. Next, begin to adduct the hip while applying a posterior force to the anterior hip. A hip that can be dislocated in this method is readily felt (clunk feeling) and is a positive test. It may reduce spontaneously once the posterior force is removed, or the examiner may need to perform the Ortolani test.

The **Ortolani test** attempts to reduce a dislocated hip (Fig. 200.3). The examiner should stabilize the pelvis and hold the leg in the same method as for the Barlow test. The infant's hip should be in 90 degrees of flexion. Abduct the hip while applying anterior pressure to the lateral thigh over the greater trochanter. A positive test is the palpable reduction of the dislocation, which may be felt (clunk). After 2 months of age, the hip may develop muscular contractures, preventing positive Ortolani tests.

These tests should be performed with only gentle force and done one hip at a time. The test may need to be repeated multiple times, as they can be difficult to interpret. A click, which is not pathologic, may occur from breaking the surface tension of the hip joint or snapping gluteal tendons.

Bilateral fixed dislocations present a diagnostic dilemma because of the symmetry on exam. The **Klisic test** is useful in this situation; it is done by placing the third finger over the greater trochanter and the index finger over the anterior superior iliac spine, then drawing an imaginary line between the two. The line should point to the umbilicus in a normal child. However, in a dislocated hip, the greater trochanter is elevated, which causes the line to project lower (between the umbilicus and pubis). This test is helpful in identifying bilateral DDH, which can otherwise be difficult to diagnose because of the symmetry found on examination.

Older children with unrecognized DDH may present with limping. A patient with increased lumbar lordosis and a waddling gait may have an unrecognized bilateral DDH.

Radiologic Evaluation

Ultrasound is used for initial evaluation of infants with DDH and should be done for females with a positive family history or breech presentation in both sexes. Ultrasound should be obtained after 6 weeks of age in the absence of abnormal examination findings to avoid confusion with physiologic laxity. Because the femoral head doesn't begin to ossify until 4–6 months of age, plain radiographs can be misleading until patients are older. Plain radiographs are the imaging study of choice once the child reaches 6 months of age.

Treatment

The treatment of DDH is individualized and depends on the child's age at diagnosis. The goal of treatment is a stable reduction that results in normal growth and development of the hip. If DDH is suspected, the child should be sent to a pediatric orthopedic specialist.

The **Pavlik harness** is an effective treatment up to 6 months of age. It provides hip flexion to just over 90 degrees and limits adduction to no more than neutral. This positioning redirects the femoral head toward the acetabulum. The hip must be reduced within 1–2 weeks of beginning the Pavlik harness, although the infant will need more time in the device. The Pavlik harness is successful in treating approximately 95% of dysplastic or subluxated hips and 80% successful for treatment of true dislocations. Persistently dislocated hips should not remain in a Pavlik harness for more than 2 weeks for fear of iatrogenic acetabular damage. Patients failing the Pavlik harness warrant treatment with a rigid abduction orthosis.

Children over 6 months or those who have failed nonoperative treatment should undergo closed reduction using a hip spica cast. This is done under general anesthesia; reduction is evaluated with an intraoperative arthrogram then confirmed by postoperative computed tomography or magnetic resonance imaging (MRI). If closed reduction fails, open reduction is indicated. Patients over 18 months of age may require a pelvic and femoral osteotomy.

Complications

The most important and severe complication of DDH is iatrogenic avascular necrosis of the femoral head. This can occur from excessive flexion or abduction during positioning of the Pavlik harness or hip spica cast. Infants under 6 months of age are at highest risk. Pressure ulcers can occur with prolonged casting. Redislocation or subluxation of the femoral head and residual acetabular dysplasia can occur.

TRANSIENT MONOARTICULAR SYNOVITIS

Transient synovitis, also known as ***toxic synovitis***, is a common cause of limping in children. It is a diagnosis of exclusion because **septic arthritis** and **osteomyelitis** of the hip must be excluded (see Chapters 118 and 119).

Etiology and Epidemiology

The etiology of transient synovitis is uncertain; possible causes are viral illnesses and nonspecific inflammatory reactions. Approximately 70% of children diagnosed with transient synovitis have an upper respiratory tract viral infection in the preceding 7–14 days. Biopsies may reveal nonspecific synovial hypertrophy. Hip joint aspirations, when necessary, are negative for bacterial culture or signs of bacterial infection.

The mean age at onset is 6 years, with a range of 3–8 years. It is twice as common in male children.

Clinical Manifestations and Evaluation

There is an acute onset of pain in the groin/hip, anterior thigh, or knee. Irritation of the obturator and femoral nerves can cause referred pain in the thigh and knee when the pathology is at the hip. Patients with transient synovitis are often afebrile, walk with a painful limp, and have normal-to-minimally elevated white blood cell count (WBC), C-reactive protein (CRP), and erythrocyte sedimentation rate (ESR) compared with bacterial diseases of the hip (Table 200.1). Table 198.3 lists the differential diagnoses of a limping child.

Anteroposterior and frog-leg radiographs of the hip are usually normal. Ultrasonography may reveal a joint effusion. Presence of an effusion along with refusal to bear weight, fever, or elevated WBC, ESR, or CRP should prompt evaluation for septic arthritis with a joint aspiration that is sent for Gram stain, bacterial culture, and cell count; MRI is also indicated under these circumstances.

TABLE **200.1** Differences Between Bacterial Infection and Transient Synovitis

BACTERIAL INFECTION*	TRANSIENT SYNOVITIS
Elevated joint fluid WBC count	Joint fluid WBC count <15,000 cells/mm^3
Fever—temperature >38.5°C	Afebrile
Leukocytosis	Normal WBC count
ESR >20 mm/hr	Normal ESR and CRP
Refusal to walk	Painful limp
Hip held in external rotation, abduction, and flexion	Hip held normally
Severe pain and tenderness	Moderate pain and mild tenderness

**Examples: Septic arthritis, osteomyelitis of hip*
CRP, C-reactive protein; *ESR,* erythrocyte sedimentation rate; *WBC,* white blood cell.

Treatment

The mainstay of treatment for transient synovitis is bed rest and minimal weight bearing until the pain resolves. Nonsteroidal antiinflammatory medication is usually sufficient to decrease pain. Limiting strenuous activity and exercise for 1–2 weeks following recovery is helpful. Follow-up will help ensure that there is no deterioration. Lack of improvement necessitates further evaluation for more serious disorders.

LEGG-CALVE-PERTHES DISEASE

Etiology and Epidemiology

Legg-Calve-Perthes disease (LCPD) is idiopathic **avascular necrosis (osteonecrosis)** of the capital epiphysis of the femoral head. The etiology is unclear, but it is likely caused by an interruption of the blood supply to the capital femoral epiphysis. There may be an associated hypercoagulable state (e.g., factor V Leiden).

LCPD commonly presents in patients 3–12 years of age, with a mean age of 7 years. It is four to five times more common in males.

Clinical Manifestations

Patients may not present for several weeks because of minimal discomfort; the classic presentation is a child with an atraumatic, painless limp. There may be mild or intermittent hip/groin, anterior thigh, or knee pain. Decreased internal rotation and abduction with some discomfort, thigh muscle spasm, and anterior thigh muscular atrophy may be present. Patients have delayed bone age.

Radiologic Evaluation

Anteroposterior and frog-leg radiographs of both hips are usually adequate for diagnosis and management. It is necessary to document the extent of the disease and follow its progression. MRI is helpful to diagnose early LCPD.

Treatment and Prognosis

LCPD is usually a self-limited disorder that should be followed by a pediatric orthopedist. Initial treatment focuses on pain control and restoration of hip range of motion. The goal of treatment is prevention of complications, such as femoral head deformity and secondary osteoarthritis (OA).

Containment is important in treating LCPD; the femoral head is contained inside the acetabulum, which acts like a mold for the capital femoral epiphysis as it reossifies. Nonsurgical containment uses abduction casts and orthoses, and surgical containment is accomplished with osteotomies of the proximal femur and pelvis.

The short-term prognosis is determined by the magnitude of the femoral head deformity after healing has completed. It is improved by early diagnosis, good follow-up, and compliance with the treatment plan. Older children and children with a residual femoral head deformity are more likely to develop OA. The incidence of OA in patients who developed LCPD after 10 years of age is close to 100%; it is negligible in children with onset before 5 years of age. Patients between 6 and 9 years of age have a risk of OA of less than 40%.

SLIPPED CAPITAL FEMORAL EPIPHYSIS

Etiology and Epidemiology

Slipped capital femoral epiphysis (SCFE) is an adolescent hip disorder that is an orthopedic emergency. The incidence is 10.8 per 100,000, and it is slightly higher in males. Approximately 20% of patients with SCFE will have bilateral involvement at presentation, and another 20–40% may progress to bilateral involvement. The average age is 10–16 years, with a mean of 12 years in males and 11 years in females. Additional risk factors for SCFE include obesity, trisomy 21, and endocrine disorders (e.g., hypothyroidism, pituitary tumor, growth hormone deficiency).

Classification

SCFE is classified as stable or unstable. Unstable patients refuse to ambulate even with crutches. Stable patients have an antalgic gait. SCFE can also be characterized as acute (symptoms <3 weeks) or chronic (symptoms >3 weeks). Acute-on-chronic SCFE occurs when more than 3 weeks of symptoms are accompanied by an acute exacerbation of pain and difficulty/inability to bear weight.

Clinical Manifestation

The presentation is variable, based on severity and type of slip. Patients will often report hip, thigh, or knee pain; limp or inability to ambulate; and decreased hip range of motion. There may or may not be a traumatic event. *Any knee pain mandates an examination of the hip, as hip pathology can cause referred pain to the anterior thigh and knee along the femoral or obturator nerves.* The patient usually holds the affected extremity in external rotation. As the hip is flexed, it will progressively externally rotate (obligate external rotation). There is usually a limitation of internal rotation, but there may also be a loss of flexion and abduction. If the patient can bear weight, it is typically an antalgic gait with the affected leg in external rotation. It is important to examine both hips given the high rate of bilateral involvement.

Radiologic Evaluation

Anteroposterior and frog-leg radiographs are indicated. Patients with known SCFE or with a high index of suspicion *should not* undergo frog-leg lateral radiographs. Instead, a cross-table lateral radiograph reduces the risk of iatrogenic progression. The earliest sign of SCFE is blurring or widening of the physis without slippage **(preslip condition)**. Klein's line, a straight line drawn along the superior cortex of the femoral neck (Fig. 200.4), is helpful in assessing the anteroposterior radiograph for SCFE. The slippage can be classified radiographically as type I (0–33% displacement), type II (34–50%), or type III (>50%). The likelihood of complications increases with degree of displacement.

Treatment

Patients with SCFE should be immediately made non–weight bearing and referred to a pediatric orthopedist. The goal is to prevent further slippage, enhance physeal closure, and minimize complications, which is usually accomplished with

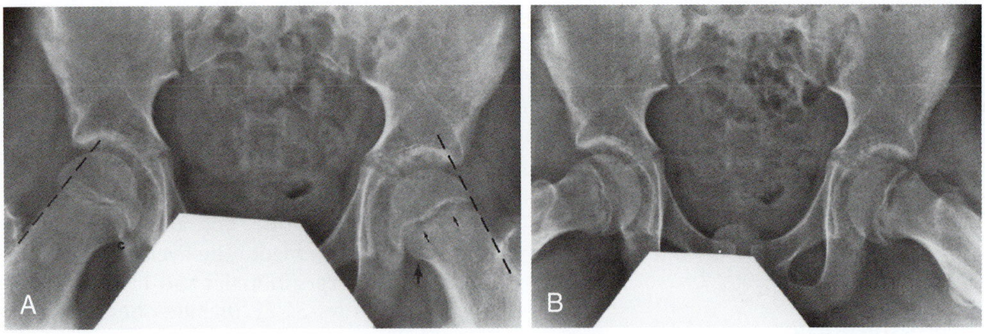

FIGURE 200.4 Slipped capital femoral epiphysis. **(A)** Anteroposterior radiograph reveals a widened physis *(small arrows)* and decreased height of the epiphysis on the left. In addition, there is loss *(large arrow)* of the Capener triangle (c) (normal double density of the medial metaphysis superimposed on the posterior acetabular rim on right) and an abnormal lateral femoral neck line (normal on right). **(B)** Frog, lateral view confirms the inferomedial position of the slipped capital femoral epiphysis. (From Blickman H. *Pediatric Radiology, The Requisites.* 2nd ed. St. Louis: Mosby; 1998:244.)

internal fixation in situ with a single cannulated screw. More severe cases may require surgical hip dislocation and reduction to realign the epiphysis. There is controversy surrounding the prophylactic fixation of the nonaffected side. Assessment for endocrine disorders is important, particularly in children outside the range of 10–16 years of age.

Complications

The two most serious complications of SCFE are **chondrolysis** and **avascular necrosis.** Chondrolysis is destruction of the articular cartilage. It is associated with more severe slips and with intraarticular penetration of operative hardware. This can lead to severe OA and disability. Avascular necrosis occurs when there is a disruption of the blood supply to the capital femoral epiphysis. This usually happens at the time of injury but may occur during forced manipulation or reduction of an unstable slip. Avascular necrosis may occur in up to 50% of unstable SCFEs and may lead to OA.

PEARLS FOR PRACTITIONERS

See Orthopedics: Pearls for Practitioners at the end of this section.

REVIEW QUESTIONS

Available online.

CHAPTER 201

Lower Extremity and Knee

Torsional (in-toeing and out-toeing) and **angular** (physiologic bowlegs and knock knees) variations in the legs are common reasons that parents seek medical attention for their child. Most of these concerns are physiologic and resolve with normal growth. Understanding the natural history allows providers to reassure the family and to identify nonphysiologic disorders that necessitate further intervention. Physiologic disturbances are referred to as *variations*; pathologic disturbances are called *deformities*.

TORSIONAL VARIATIONS

The femur is internally rotated (anteversion) about 30 degrees at birth, decreasing to about 10 degrees at maturity. The tibia begins with up to 30 degrees of internal rotation at birth and can decrease to a mean of 15 degrees at maturity.

Torsional variations do not cause a limp or pain. Unilateral torsion raises the index of suspicion for a neurologic (hemiplegia) or neuromuscular disorder.

In-Toeing

Femoral Anteversion

Internal femoral torsion and femoral anteversion are the most common causes of in-toeing in children 2 years or older (Table 201.1). The rotation is maximal between 4 and 6 years of age and then decreases. It occurs twice as often in females. Many cases are associated with generalized ligamentous laxity. The etiology of femoral anteversion is likely congenital and is common in individuals with abnormal sitting habits such as *W-sitting*.

Clinical Manifestations

The family may give a history of W-sitting, and there may be a family history of similar concerns when the parents were younger. The child may have *kissing kneecaps* due to increased internal rotation of the femur. While walking, the entire leg will appear internally rotated, and with running, the child may appear to have an *egg-beater* gait where the lower legs circle laterally during the swing phase. The flexed hip will have internal rotation increased to 80–90 degrees (normal 60–70 degrees) with corresponding external rotation limitation to about 10 degrees. Radiographic evaluation is usually not indicated.

Internal Tibial Torsion

Internal (medial) tibial torsion is the most common cause of in-toeing in a child younger than 2 years old. When it is the result of in utero positioning, it may be associated with metatarsus adductus (see Chapter 202).

Clinical Manifestations

The child will present with a history of in-toeing. **Thigh-foot angle** (Fig. 201.1) is used to measure the degree of tibial torsion. The patient lies prone with the knee flexed to 90 degrees.

TABLE 201.1 Common Causes of In-Toeing and Out-Toeing

IN-TOEING	OUT-TOEING
Internal femoral torsion or anteversion Internal tibial torsion Metatarsus adductus Talipes equinovarus (clubfoot) Developmental dysplasia	External femoral torsion or retroversion External tibial torsion Calcaneovalgus feet Hypermobile pes planus (flatfoot) Slipped capital femoral epiphysis

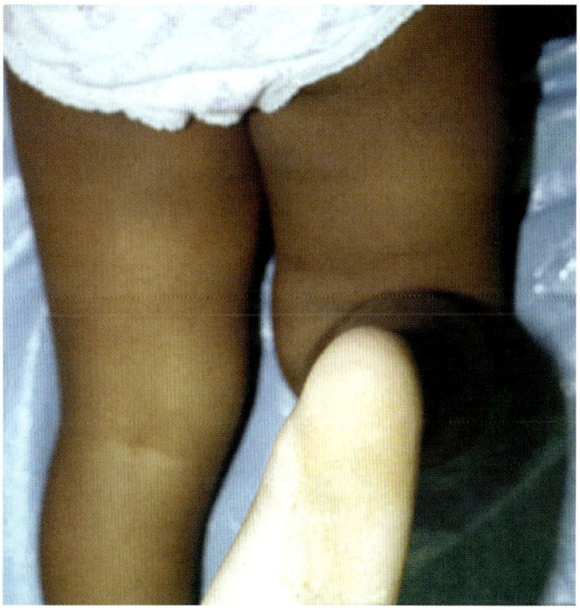

FIGURE 201.1 Thigh-foot angle measurement. The thigh-foot angle is useful for assessment of tibial torsion. The patient lies prone, with knees flexed to 90 degrees. The long axis of the thigh is compared to the long axis of the foot to determine the thigh-foot angle. Negative angles are associated with internal tibial torsion, and positive angles are associated with external tibial torsion.

The long axis of the foot is compared with the long axis of the thigh. An inwardly rotated foot represents internal tibial torsion and is measured as a negative angle. If follow-up is warranted, measurements should be taken at each visit.

Treatment of In-Toeing

It is critical to identify patients who have pathologic reasons for in-toeing and provide reassurance and follow-up to document improvement for patients with femoral anteversion and internal tibial torsion. Correction may not occur until 7–8 years of age, so it is important to inform families of the appropriate timeline. Braces (Denis Browne splint) do not improve or hasten outcomes. Surgical intervention because of functional disability or cosmetic appearance is needed in less than 1% of patients.

Out-Toeing

External Tibial Torsion

External tibial torsion is the most common cause of out-toeing and may be associated with a calcaneovalgus foot (see Chapter 202). This is often related to in utero positioning. It may improve over time, but because the tibia rotates externally with age, external tibial torsion can worsen. It may be an etiologic factor for patellofemoral pain syndrome, especially when combined with femoral anteversion. Thigh-foot angle is used to measure external tibial torsion. Treatment is usually observation and reassurance, but patients with functional disability and cosmetic concerns may benefit from surgical intervention.

ANGULAR VARIATIONS

The majority of patients who present with knock-knees **(genu valgum)** or bowlegs **(genu varum)** are normal variations (Fig. 201.2). Infants are born with maximum genu varum. The lower extremity straightens out around 18 months of age, then typically progresses to maximal genu valgum around 4 years. Further growth and development usually end with the legs straight to a slight genu valgum in adulthood.

It is important to inquire about family history and assess overall height. A child who is 2 standard deviations below the normal height curve with angular deformities may have skeletal dysplasia. Dietary history should be obtained, as rickets (see Chapter 29) may cause angular deformities. For genu valgum, measure the intermalleolar distance (distance between the two medial malleoli at the ankles with the knees touching). Measure intercondylar distance (the distance between the medial femoral condyles at the knee with the medial malleoli touching) for genu varum. These measurements should be followed to track improvement or progression. For accurate radiographic measurement, it is important to have the patella, not the feet, facing forward. In the child with external tibial torsion, having the feet facing forward gives the false appearance of bowlegs.

Genu Valgum

Physiologic knock-knees are most common in 3–4 year olds and usually resolve between 5–8 years of age. Patients with asymmetric genu valgum or severe deformity may have

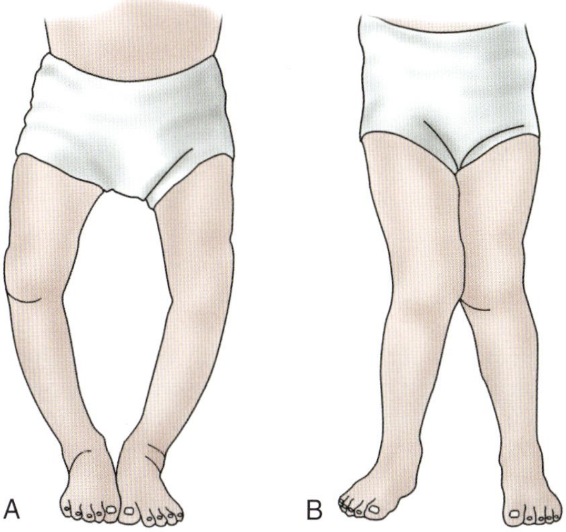

FIGURE 201.2 Bowleg and knock-knee deformities. **(A)** Bowleg deformity. Bowlegs are referred to as *varus angulation* (genu varum) because the knees are tilted away from the midline of the body. **(B)** Knock-knee or valgus deformity of the knees. The knee is tilted toward the midline. (From Scoles P. *Pediatric Orthopedics in Clinical Practice*. Chicago: Year Book Medical Publishers; 1982:84.)

underlying disease causing their knock-knees (e.g., renal osteodystrophy, skeletal dysplasia). Treatment is usually reassurance; however, surgical intervention may be indicated for severe deformities, gait dysfunction, pain, and cosmesis.

Genu Varum

Physiologic bowlegs are most common in children older than 18 months with symmetric genu varum. This generally improves as the child approaches 2 years of age. The most important consideration for genu varum is differentiating between physiologic genu varum and Blount disease (tibia vara).

Tibia Vara (Blount Disease)

Tibia vara is the most common pathologic disorder associated with genu varum. It is characterized by abnormal growth of the medial aspect of the proximal tibial epiphysis, resulting in a progressive varus deformity. Blount disease is classified according to age of onset:

- Infantile (1–3 years)
- Juvenile (4–10 years)
- Adolescent (>11 years)

Late-onset Blount disease is less common than infantile disease. The etiology is unknown but is thought to be secondary to growth suppression from increased compressive forces across the medial knee. There may also be a genetic component.

Clinical Manifestations

Infantile tibia vara is more common in children who are early walkers (prior to 12 months) and those who are overweight. Nearly 80% of infantile Blount disease is bilateral. It is usually painless. Patients will often have significant internal tibial torsion and lower extremity leg-length discrepancy (LLD). There may also be a palpable medial tibial metaphyseal beak.

Late-onset Blount disease (encompassing both juvenile and adolescent forms) is more common in markedly obese patients or patients with a rapid weight gain. Only 50% of juvenile onset cases have bilateral involvement; adolescent Blount disease is usually unilateral. The initial presentation is often painful bowlegs. Late-onset Blount disease is usually not associated with palpable metaphyseal beaking, significant internal tibial torsion, or significant LLD.

Radiologic Evaluation

Weight-bearing anteroposterior and lateral radiographs of both legs are necessary for the diagnosis of tibia vara. Fragmentation, wedging, and metaphyseal beak deformities of the proximal medial tibia are the major radiologic features of infantile Blount disease. In late-onset Blount disease, the medial deformity may not be as readily noticeable. It can be very difficult to tell the difference between physiologic genu varum and infantile Blount disease on radiographs in patients younger than 2 years of age.

Treatment

Treatment of Blount disease should begin immediately. In children younger than 3 years of age with a mild deformity, orthotics to unload the medial compressive forces can be used, but compliance with this regimen can be difficult. Most cases of Blount disease require surgical management. Patients older than 4 years, patients with moderate-to-severe deformity, and patients with mild deformity that fails orthotic treatment should undergo surgical intervention. Proximal tibia/fibula osteotomy or distal femur osteotomy or epiphysiodesis (surgical physeal closure) are the usual procedures.

LEG-LENGTH DISCREPANCY

LLD may be due to differences in the femur, tibia, or both bones. The majority of the lower extremity growth comes from the distal femur (38%) and the proximal tibia (27%) physes. The differential diagnosis is extensive, but common causes are listed in Table 201.2.

Measuring Leg-Length Discrepancy

Clinical measurements using bony landmarks (anterior superior iliac spine to medial malleolus) are inaccurate. Measuring the LLD through imaging is more accurate. The **teleroentgenogram** is a single radiograph of both legs that can be done in very young children. Historically, in older patients, the **orthoradiograph** (three slightly overlapping exposures of the hips, knees, and ankles) or the **scanogram** (three standard radiographs of the hips, knees, and ankles with a ruler next to the extremities) has been used. **Computed tomography (CT) scanogram** is an accurate measure of LLD but also has the highest radiation exposure. Technology known as ***EOS/slot scanning*** is an extremely accurate, reduced-radiation alternative to CT scan. The measured discrepancy is followed using Moseley and Green-Anderson graphs.

Treatment

Treating LLD is complex. The physician must take into account the estimated adult height, discrepancy measurements, skeletal

TABLE 201.2 Common Causes of Leg-Length Discrepancy

Congenital	Coxa vara Clubfoot Hypoplasia
Developmental	Developmental dysplasia of the hip Legg-Calve-Perthes disease
Neuromuscular	Hemiplegia Cerebral palsy
Infectious	Physeal injury secondary to osteomyelitis
Tumors	Fibrous dysplasia Physeal injury secondary to irradiation or neoplastic infiltration Overgrowth
Trauma	Physeal injury with premature closure Malunion (shortening of extremity) Overgrowth of healing fracture
Syndromes	Neurofibromatosis Beckwith-Wiedemann syndrome KTS PROS: *PIK3CA* related (vascular malformation) overgrowth spectrum including KTS

KTS, Klippel-Trenaunay syndrome.

maturity, and psychologic aspects of the patient and family. LLD greater than 2 cm usually requires treatment. Shoe lifts can be used, but they often cause psychosocial problems and may make the shoes heavier and less stable. Surgical options include shortening of the longer extremity, lengthening of the shorter extremity, or a combination of the two procedures. Discrepancies less than 5 cm are treated by epiphysiodesis of the affected side, and discrepancies greater than 5 cm are treated by lengthening. Use of removable implants, which permit growth modulation without permanent impact on growth plates, has allowed for early and more accurate treatment.

KNEE

The knee joint is constrained by soft tissues rather than the usual geometric fit of articulating bones. The medial and lateral collateral ligaments as well as the anterior and posterior cruciate ligaments maintain knee stability. Weight and force transmission crosses articular cartilage and the meniscus. The patellofemoral joint is the extensor mechanism of the knee and a common site of injury in the adolescent (Fig. 201.3).

Knee effusion, or intraarticular swelling, is a common sign of injury. When the fluid accumulates rapidly after an injury, it is usually a hemarthrosis (blood in the joint) and may indicate a fracture, ligamentous disruption (often the anterior cruciate ligament [ACL]), or meniscus tear. Unexplained knee effusion may occur with arthritis (e.g., septic, Lyme disease, viral, postinfectious, juvenile idiopathic arthritis, systemic lupus erythematosus). It may also occur as a result of overactivity and hypermobile joint syndrome (ligamentous laxity).

Discoid Lateral Meniscus

Each meniscus is normally semilunar in shape; but rarely the lateral meniscus will be disk shaped. A normal meniscus is attached at the periphery and glides anteriorly and posteriorly with knee motion. The discoid meniscus is less mobile and may tear more easily. When there is inadequate posterolateral attachment, the discoid meniscus can displace anteriorly with knee flexion, causing an audible click. Most commonly, patients are asymptomatic for years before presenting in late childhood or early adolescence after an injury with knee pain and swelling. The anteroposterior radiographs can show increased joint space and a squared-off appearance of the lateral femoral condyle; magnetic resonance imaging (MRI) can confirm the diagnosis. Treatment is usually arthroscopic excision of tears and reshaping of the meniscus.

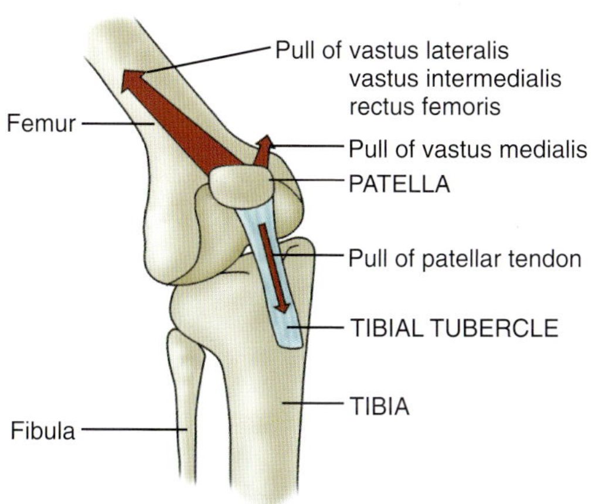

FIGURE 201.3 Diagram of the knee extensor mechanism. The major force exerted by the quadriceps muscle tends to pull the patella laterally out of the intercondylar sulcus. The vastus medialis muscle pulls medially to keep the patella centralized. (Modified from Smith JB. Knee problems in children. *Pediatr Clin North Am.* 1986;33:1439.)

Popliteal Cyst

A popliteal cyst **(Baker cyst)** is commonly seen in the middle childhood years. The cause is the distension of the gastrocnemius and semimembranous bursa along the posteromedial aspect of the knee by synovial fluid. In adults, Baker cysts are associated with meniscus tears. In childhood, the cysts are usually painless and benign; they may be associated with juvenile idiopathic arthritis. They often spontaneously resolve, but it may take several years. Knee radiographs are normal. The diagnosis can be confirmed by ultrasound or MRI. Treatment is reassurance; aspiration or surgical excision is indicated only for progressive cysts or cysts that cause disability.

Osteochondritis Dissecans

Osteochondritis dissecans (OCD) occurs when an area of bone near the articular cartilage suffers a vascular insult and may separate from the adjacent bone. It most commonly affects the lateral aspect of the medial femoral condyle. Patients may complain of knee pain or swelling. The lesions can be seen on anteroposterior, lateral, and tunnel view radiographs. MRI is needed to determine the extent of the injury. In young patients with intact articular cartilage, the lesion will often revascularize and heal with crutch use and rest from activities. This healing process often takes several months and requires serial radiographic imaging to document healing. With increasing skeletal maturity, the risk for articular cartilage damage and separation of the bony fragment increases. Older patients are more likely to need surgical intervention. Patients of any age with a fracture through the articular cartilage are unlikely to improve without surgical intervention. Patients with OCD should be referred to a specialist.

Osgood-Schlatter Disease

Osgood-Schlatter disease is a common cause of knee pain at the insertion of the patellar tendon on the tibial tubercle. The stress from a contracting quadriceps muscle is transmitted through the developing tibial tubercle, which can cause microfractures and apophysitis. It usually occurs after a growth spurt and is more common in males. The age at onset is typically at 11 years for females and 13–14 years for males.

Patients will present with pain during and after activity and often have tenderness and local swelling over the tibial tubercle. Radiographs may be necessary to rule out infection, tumor, or avulsion fracture.

Rest and activity modification are paramount for treatment. Medication and icing may provide pain control. Treatment centers on rest from offending activity and rehabilitation exercises, particularly lower extremity flexibility and strengthening exercise programs. The course is usually benign, but symptoms frequently last 1–2 years. Complications can include bony enlargement of the tibial tubercle and avulsion fracture of the tibial tubercle.

Patellofemoral Disorders

The patellofemoral joint is a complex joint that depends on a balance between restraining ligaments of the patella, muscular forces around the knee, and alignment for normal function. The interior surface of the patella has a V-shaped bottom that moves through a matching femoral groove called the *trochlea*. When the knee is flexed, the patellar ligaments and the majority of the quadriceps muscular forces pull the patella laterally. The vastus medialis muscle counteracts the lateral motion, pulling the patella toward the midline. Problems with function of this joint usually result in anterior knee pain.

Patellofemoral pain syndrome (PFPS), also known as *idiopathic anterior knee pain* or "*runner's knee*," is particularly prevalent in adolescent female athletes. The patient will present with anterior knee pain that worsens with activity, going up and down stairs, and soreness after sitting in one position for an extended time. There is usually no associated swelling. The patient may complain of a grinding sensation under the kneecap. Palpating and compressing the patellofemoral joint with the knee extended elicits pain. Patients often have weak hip musculature and/or poor lower extremity flexibility. Radiographs are rarely helpful but may be indicated to rule out other diagnoses such as OCD.

Treatment is focused on correcting the biomechanical problems that are causing the pain. A rehabilitation exercise program emphasizing hip girdle and vastus medialis strengthening with lower extremity stretching can be helpful. Activity modification, ice, and antiinflammatory medication may also be helpful. Persistent cases should be referred to a specialist.

One must exclude **recurrent patellar subluxation** and **dislocation** when evaluating a patient with PFPS. Acute traumatic dislocation will usually cause significant pain, swelling, and disability. Patients with recurrent dislocations often have associated ligamentous laxity, genu valgum, and femoral anteversion. The initial treatment is nonoperative and may involve a brief period of immobilization, followed by an aggressive physical therapy program designed to strengthen the quadriceps and improve function of the patellofemoral joint. Continued subluxation or recurrent dislocation is considered failure of this treatment plan, and surgical repair is usually necessary.

Anterior Cruciate Ligament Tears

Increased sports participation and intensity of training have led to increased prevalence of pediatric ACL injuries, especially in females. The majority of ACL tears occur as noncontact injuries; patients often report a twisting injury to their knee, feeling a pop, and a sudden onset of pain. Exam is significant for a positive Lachman test. The Lachman test is performed when an anteriorly directed force is applied to the proximal tibia (Fig. 201.4); a firm end-point is felt with an intact ACL, while a torn ACL will have an indistinct end-point. The anterior drawer test and lateral pivot shift test may also be used to assess for ACL injury. Radiographs should be obtained to rule out other

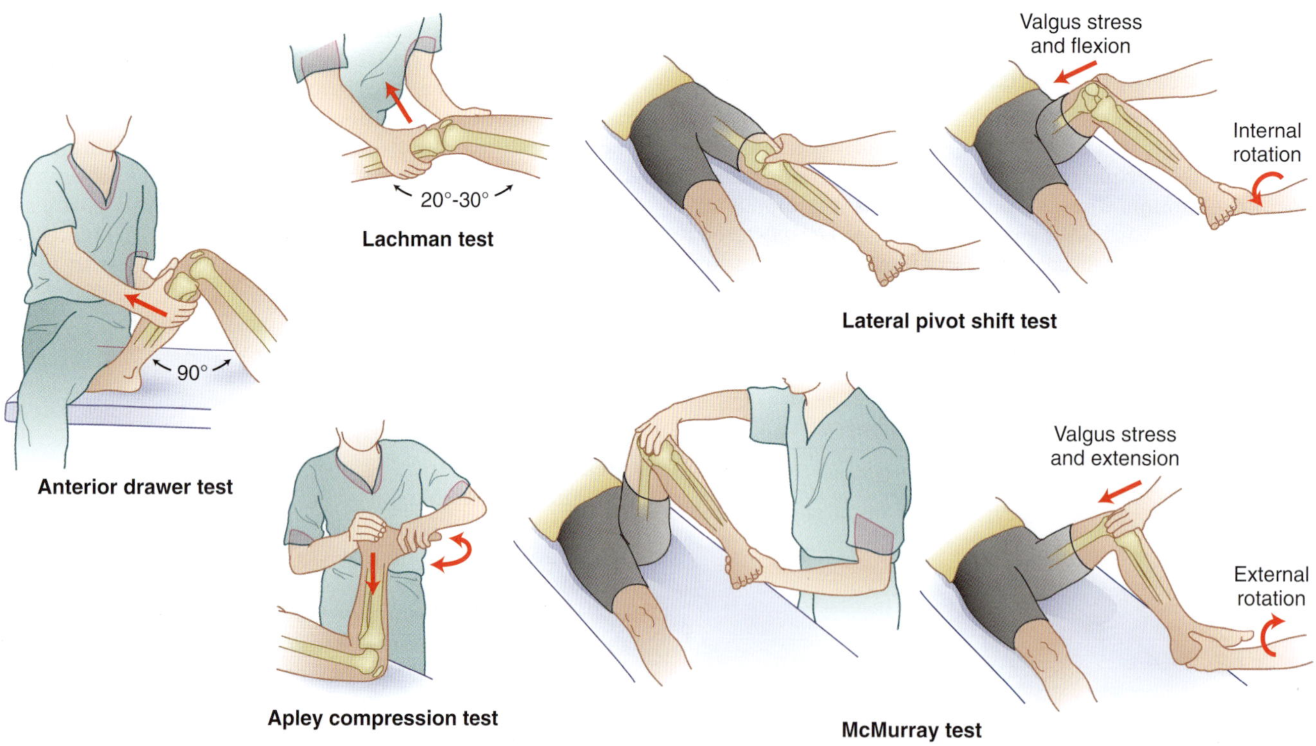

FIGURE 201.4 Select knee examination maneuvers. The Lachman test, performed to detect anterior cruciate ligament (ACL) injuries, is conducted with the patient supine and the knee flexed 20–30 degrees. The anterior drawer test detects ACL injuries and is performed with the patient supine and the knee in 90 degrees of flexion. The lateral pivot shift test is performed with the patient supine, the hip flexed 45 degrees, and the knee in full extension. Internal rotation is applied to the tibia while the knee is flexed to 40 degrees under a valgus stress (pushing the outside of the knee medially). The Apley compression test, used to assess meniscal integrity, is performed with the patient prone and the examiner's knee over the patient's posterior thigh. The tibia is externally rotated while a downward compressive force is applied over the tibia. The McMurray test, used to assess meniscal integrity, is performed with the patient supine and the examiner standing on the side of the affected knee. (From Landry GL, Watson AM. Management of musculoskeletal injury. In: Kliegman RM, St. Geme J, eds. *Nelson Textbook of Pediatrics.* 22nd ed. Philadelphia: Elsevier; 2025:Fig. 728.12.)

injuries, but MRI is ultimately needed for diagnosis. Treatment is generally surgical, although the technique varies, and special care is needed when the patient has open physes at the knee.

Other common knee injuries in adolescent athletes include **medial collateral ligament (MCL) tears and sprains** and **meniscus tears**. MCL injuries often result after a direct blow to the outside of the knee or, less commonly, by forceful twisting. Meniscus tears tend to occur with injuries that involve twisting of the knee. Symptoms for both MCL and meniscus injuries include knee pain and swelling, but patients with meniscus tears may also report a "locking" or "popping" sensation. A McMurray or Apley compression test may be used to evaluate for meniscus injuries (Fig. 201.4). As with ACL injuries, MRI is ultimately needed to confirm diagnosis. Mild injuries may respond to conservative measures, but many meniscus tears in adolescents require surgical intervention.

PEARLS FOR PRACTITIONERS

See Orthopedics: Pearls for Practitioners at the end of this section.

REVIEW QUESTIONS

Available online.

CHAPTER 202

Foot

In newborns and non–weight-bearing infants, the difference between posturing and deformity is important. Posturing is the habitual position in which the infant holds the foot; passive range of motion is normal. Deformity produces an appearance similar to posturing, but passive motion is restricted. Most pediatric foot disorders are painless. Foot pain is more common in older children (Table 202.1).

TABLE 202.1 Differential Diagnoses of Foot Pain by Age

AGE GROUP	DIAGNOSTIC CONSIDERATIONS
0–6 years	Poorly fitting shoes Fracture Puncture wound Foreign body Osteomyelitis Cellulitis Juvenile idiopathic arthritis Hair tourniquet Dactylitis Leukemia
6–12 years	Poorly fitting shoes Trauma (fracture, sprain) Juvenile idiopathic arthritis Puncture wound Sever disease Accessory tarsal navicular bone Hypermobile flatfoot Tarsal coalition Oncologic (Ewing sarcoma, leukemia)
12–18 years	Poorly fitting shoes Stress fracture Trauma (fracture, sprain) Foreign body Ingrown toenail Metatarsalgia Plantar fasciitis Achilles tendinopathy Accessory ossicles (navicular, os trigonum) Tarsal coalition Avascular necrosis of metatarsal (Freiberg infarction) or navicular (Kohler disease) Plantar warts

CLUBFOOT (TALIPES EQUINOVARUS)

A clubfoot deformity involves the entire leg, not just the foot. It affects 1 in 1,000 newborns and is bilateral in one-half of cases. The tarsals in the affected foot are hypoplastic with the talus most affected. The muscles of the limb are hypoplastic because of the abnormal tarsal interactions, which leads to a generalized limb hypoplasia, mainly affecting and shortening the foot. There is usually atrophy of the calf musculature.

Etiology

Family history is important. Clubfoot can be congenital or teratologic. Although congenital clubfoot (75% of all cases) is usually an isolated abnormality, every infant should also be assessed for developmental dysplasia of the hip. Teratologic clubfoot is associated with a neuromuscular disorder, such as myelomeningocele, arthrogryposis, or other syndromes. Positional foot deformities that occur due to abnormal positioning in utero must be differentiated from clubfoot as they typically resolve without treatment in the early months of life.

Clinical Manifestations

The diagnosis is seldom confused with other disorders (Fig. 202.1). The presence of clubfoot should prompt a careful search for other abnormalities. The infant will have midfoot cavus, forefoot adduction, hindfoot equinus and varus, and varying degrees of rigidity. All are secondary to the abnormalities of the talonavicular joint. Calf atrophy and foot shortening are more noticeable in older children.

Radiologic Evaluation

In infants, radiographs and advanced imaging are rarely necessary for assessment because their tarsals have incomplete or absent ossification. The navicular ossifies at about 3 years of age for females and 4 years for males. As children age, radiographs can be used to follow the tibial calcaneal and lateral talocalcaneal angles and to assess navicular positioning.

Treatment

The goal of treatment is to correct the deformity and preserve mobility and function. The gold standard for the treatment of clubfoot is the Ponseti method of serial casting. Treatment includes a percutaneous tenotomy of the Achilles tendon to help correct the equinus deformity near the end of casting. An abduction brace is initiated after casting and is an essential part of the treatment of clubfoot. Children who are unable

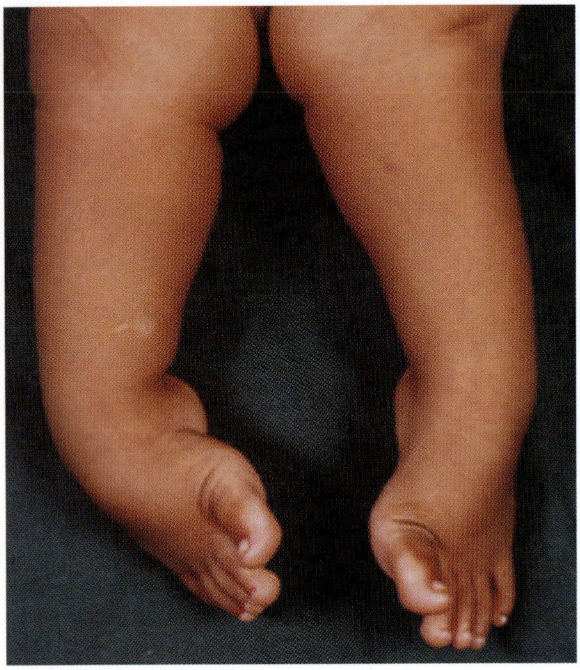

FIGURE 202.1 Clinical picture demonstrating clubfoot deformity. (From Kliegman RM, Behrman RE, Jenson HB, et al., eds. *Nelson's Textbook of Pediatrics.* 18th ed. Philadelphia: Saunders; 2007:2778.)

to achieve good compliance with bracing recommendations demonstrate high rates of recurrence with the need for further casting or surgery.

The two most common procedures performed for recurrent clubfoot are a repeat Achilles lengthening and a tibialis anterior tendon transfer. Rarely, more aggressive surgical procedures may need to be done. Complications of untreated clubfoot include severe disability. Complications of treated clubfoot include recurrence and stiffness.

METATARSUS ADDUCTUS

Metatarsus adductus is the most common foot disorder in infants. It is characterized by a convexity of the lateral foot (Fig. 202.2) and is caused by in utero positioning. It is bilateral in half of cases. It is more common in first-born children because of the smaller primigravid uterus. Two percent of infants with metatarsus adductus have developmental dysplasia of the hip.

Clinical Manifestations

The forefoot is adducted and sometimes supinated, but the midfoot and hindfoot are normal. The lateral border of the foot is convex, while the medial border is concave. Normal ankle dorsiflexion and plantar flexion differentiate this deformity from clubfoot. With the midfoot and hindfoot stabilized, the deformity can be pushed beyond a neutral position (into abduction). Older children may present with an in-toeing gait.

Treatment

True metatarsus adductus resolves spontaneously over 90% of the time without treatment, so reassurance is all that is needed. Metatarsus adductus that does not improve within 2 years needs evaluation by a pediatric orthopedist.

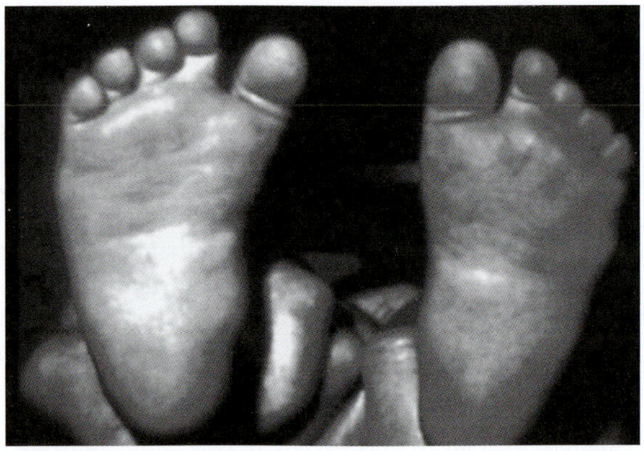

FIGURE 202.2 Clinical picture of metatarsus adductus with a normal foot on opposite side. (From Kliegman RM, Behrman RE, Jenson HB, et al., eds. *Nelson's Textbook of Pediatrics.* 18th ed. Philadelphia: Saunders; 2007:2777.)

Persistent cases may benefit from serial casting or bracing and possibly surgery. The deformity is not associated with a disability.

It is important to differentiate among metatarsus adductus, **metatarsus varus**, and **skewfoot**. Metatarsus varus looks like metatarsus adductus, but it is an uncommon rigid deformity that will need serial casting. Skewfoot is an uncommon deformity that is characterized by hindfoot plantar flexion, midfoot abduction, and forefoot adduction, giving the foot a Z or serpentine appearance. This needs to be managed very carefully with serial casting and surgery to help reduce the risk of disability in adulthood.

CALCANEOVALGUS FOOT

The calcaneovalgus foot is another common foot disorder in newborns that is secondary to in utero positioning. It is characterized by a hyperdorsiflexed foot with forefoot abduction and heel valgus, but it is not a rigid deformity like congenital vertical talus. It is usually unilateral and is often associated with developmental dysplasia of the hip. Simulated weight-bearing radiographs may be necessary for questionable diagnoses. The calcaneovalgus foot will appear normal or have flexible hindfoot valgus.

This disorder requires no treatment beyond reassurance. Parents can be taught passive stretching exercises for their infant's foot. Most affected infants realign by 2 years. A calcaneovalgus foot can be associated with bowing of the tibia, which resolves spontaneously, but a leg length discrepancy may persist.

HYPERMOBILE PES PLANUS (FLEXIBLE FLATFOOT)

Hypermobile or pronated feet are seen in 15% of adults. The child with flatfeet is usually asymptomatic and has no activity limitations. Newborn and toddler flatfoot are the result of ligamentous laxity and fat in the medial longitudinal arch. This is called ***developmental flatfoot*** and usually improves by 6 years of age. In older children, flatfoot is typically the result of generalized ligamentous laxity or tightness of the Achilles tendon, and there is often a positive family history. Hypermobile flatfoot can be thought of as a normal variant.

Clinical Manifestations

In the non–weight-bearing position, the older child with a flexible flatfoot will have a medial longitudinal arch. When weight bearing, the foot pronates (arch collapse) with varying degrees of hindfoot valgus. Subtalar motion (essentially all ankle motion except plantar and dorsiflexion) is normal and allows varus positioning of the hindfoot on heel rise. Any loss of subtalar motion may indicate a rigid flatfoot, which can be related to tarsal coalition or neuromuscular disorders (cerebral palsy). Radiographs of hypermobile flatfeet are usually not indicated.

Treatment

Hypermobile pes planus cannot be diagnosed until after 6 years of age; before that, it is developmental pes planus. Reassurance that this is a normal variant is very important. Patients who are symptomatic with activity may require education on proper, supportive footwear, orthotics/arch supports, and heel cord stretching.

TARSAL COALITION

Patients with tarsal coalition will usually present with a **rigid flatfoot** (loss of inversion and eversion at the subtalar joint). Coalition is produced by a congenital fusion or failure of segmentation of two or more tarsal bones. The attachment may be fibrous, cartilaginous, or osseous. Tarsal coalition can be unilateral or bilateral and will often become symptomatic in early adolescence with progressive ossification of the tarsal bones. The most common forms of tarsal coalition are **calcaneonavicular** and **talocalcaneal**.

Clinical Manifestations

Presentation will depend on the location of the coalition. Talocalcaneal coalitions will usually present with hindfoot pain, which may radiate laterally because of peroneal muscle spasm. Calcaneonavicular coalitions can also present with dorsolateral pain over the site of the coalition. Symptoms are exacerbated by activity, and young athletes can present with frequent ankle sprains. There is a familial component. Pes planus is usually present in both weight-bearing and non–weight-bearing positions. There is usually a loss of subtalar motion, and passive attempts at joint motion may produce pain.

Radiologic Evaluation

Anteroposterior, lateral, and oblique radiographs should be obtained, but they may not always clearly identify the disorder. The oblique view often identifies the calcaneonavicular coalition. Computed tomography (CT) is the gold standard for diagnosis of tarsal coalition. Even patients with obvious calcaneonavicular coalition on plain radiographs should have a CT scan to rule out a second coalition.

Treatment

Coalitions that are asymptomatic (the majority) do not need treatment. Nonoperative treatment for patients with pain consists of cast immobilization for a few weeks and foot orthotics. The symptoms will often return with a return to physical activities, necessitating surgery. Surgical excision of the coalition and soft tissue interposition to prevent reossification can be very effective.

CAVOVARUS FOOT

Cavovarus foot is characterized by increased height of the medial longitudinal arch **(high arch)** and frequently hindfoot varus. It can be classified as physiologic or neuromuscular. Most patients with physiologic cavovarus foot are asymptomatic and have a family history of similar foot deformity. A thorough neurologic examination on all patients with a cavovarus foot is important. Patients with painful high arches have a high risk of neurologic (tethered cord) and neuromuscular disease, and there is a strong association with **Charcot-Marie-Tooth disease**, a familial neuropathy. Unilateral cavovarus foot deformity should raise concern for an underlying intraspinal anomaly, while bilateral disease suggests an underlying muscle or neurologic cause. The underlying disorder should be treated first to halt progression. Nonoperative treatment using orthotics is usually not helpful. Progressive, symptomatic cavovarus foot will likely need surgical reconstruction.

IDIOPATHIC AVASCULAR NECROSIS

Kohler disease (tarsal navicular) and **Freiberg disease** (head of the second metatarsal) are uncommon and due to avascular necrosis. Patients will present with pain at the affected site with activity and weight bearing. Infection, fracture, and neoplasm should be excluded. Treatment consists of immobilization and activity restriction. The majority of patients will improve upon subsequent revascularization and reformation of bone.

SEVER DISEASE (CALCANEAL APOPHYSITIS)

Sever disease is a common cause of heel pain among active young people. The mean age of presentation for females is 9 years of age and 11–12 years for males. Approximately 60% of cases are bilateral. Sever disease is caused by the traction forces of the calf musculature through the Achilles tendon at the calcaneal apophysis, causing microfracture. As the child ages and the apophysis closes, the pain disappears.

Clinical Manifestations

The common presentation is a young athlete who develops heel pain with activity that decreases with rest. Swelling is rare, but limping may be associated with Sever disease. The child will have pain on palpation of the posterior calcaneus and often tight heel cords. Radiographs are rarely indicated, but with persistent pain radiographs help to exclude infection or tumor.

Treatment

Activity modification, icing, and antiinflammatory medications can be helpful. A program designed to improve heel cord flexibility and overall ankle strength may decrease symptoms. Heel elevation using heel wedges or heel cups can be helpful.

TOE DEFORMITIES

Curly toes are the most common congenital deformity of the lesser toes. The third, fourth, and fifth toes are most commonly affected. Curly toes are characterized by flexion at the proximal

TABLE 202.2 Disorders Associated With Syndactyly and Polydactyly*

POLYDACTYLY	SYNDACTYLY
Ellis-van Creveld syndrome	Apert syndrome
Rubinstein-Taybi syndrome	Carpenter syndrome
Carpenter syndrome	Cornelia de Lange syndrome
Meckel-Gruber syndrome	Holt-Oram syndrome
Polysyndactyly	Orofaciodigital syndrome
Trisomy 13	Poland syndrome
Orofaciodigital syndrome	Polysyndactyly
	Trisomy 21
	Trisomy 13
	Trisomy 18

There are many syndromes associated with polydactyly and syndactyly; these are partial lists.

interphalangeal joint with lateral rotation of the toe. It is caused by contractures of the flexor digitorum brevis and longus tendons. Some curly toes will spontaneously resolve by 3–4 years of age. Persistent deformity may be treated with surgical tenotomy.

Polydactyly (extra toes) is usually found on the initial newborn physical examination. When the extra toe is adjacent to the fifth toe and attached by only a stalk of soft tissue or skin, simple ligation or amputation is effective. When the deformity involves the great toe or middle toes, or when the extra digit has cartilage or bone, delayed surgical intervention is indicated. **Syndactyly** occurs when there is fusion of toes, creating a webbed appearance. It is usually a benign cosmetic problem. Both syndactyly and polydactyly may be associated with malformation syndromes (Table 202.2).

PEARLS FOR PRACTITIONERS

See Orthopedics: Pearls for Practitioners at the end of this section.

REVIEW QUESTIONS

Available online.

CHAPTER 203

Spine

SPINAL DEFORMITIES

A simplified classification of the common spinal abnormalities scoliosis and kyphosis is presented in Table 203.1.

TABLE 203.1 Classification of Spinal Deformities

SCOLIOSIS
Idiopathic
Infantile
Juvenile
Adolescent
Congenital
Failure of formation
Wedge vertebrae
Hemivertebrae
Failure of segmentation
Unilateral bar
Bilateral bar
Mixed
Neuromuscular
Neuropathic diseases
Upper motor neuron disease
Cerebral palsy
Spinocerebellar degeneration
Friedreich ataxia
Syringomyelia
Spinal cord tumor
Spinal cord trauma
Lower motor neuron disease
Myelodysplasia
Poliomyelitis
Spinal muscular atrophy
Charcot-Marie-Tooth disease
Myopathic diseases
Duchenne muscular dystrophy
Arthrogryposis
Other muscular dystrophies
Syndromes
Neurofibromatosis
Marfan syndrome
Compensatory
Leg-length inequality
KYPHOSIS
Postural kyphosis (flexible)
Scheuermann disease
Congenital kyphosis

Modified from the Terminology Committee of the Scoliosis Research Society, 1975.

Clinical Manifestations

Most patients will present for evaluation of an asymmetric spine, which is usually pain free. A complete physical examination is necessary for any patient with a spinal deformity because the deformity can indicate an underlying disease. The back is examined from behind (Fig. 203.1). First, the levelness of the pelvis is assessed. Leg-length discrepancy produces pelvic obliquity, which often results in **compensatory scoliosis**. When the pelvis is level, the spine is examined for symmetry and spinal curvature with the patient upright. Cutaneous lesions (hemangioma, skin dimple, or hair tuft) should be noted. The spine should be palpated for areas of tenderness.

The patient is then asked to bend forward with the hands directed between the feet **(Adams forward bend test)**. The examiner should inspect for asymmetry in the spine. The presence of a thoracic prominence on one side in this position is the hallmark for scoliosis. The area opposite the thoracic prominence is usually depressed because of spinal rotation. Scoliosis is a *rotational malalignment* of one vertebra on another, resulting in rib elevation in the thoracic spine and paravertebral muscle elevation in the lumbar spine. With the patient still in the forward flexed position, inspection from the side can reveal the degree of forward curvature. A sharp forward angulation in the thoracolumbar region indicates a **kyphotic deformity**. It is important to examine the skin for café-au-lait

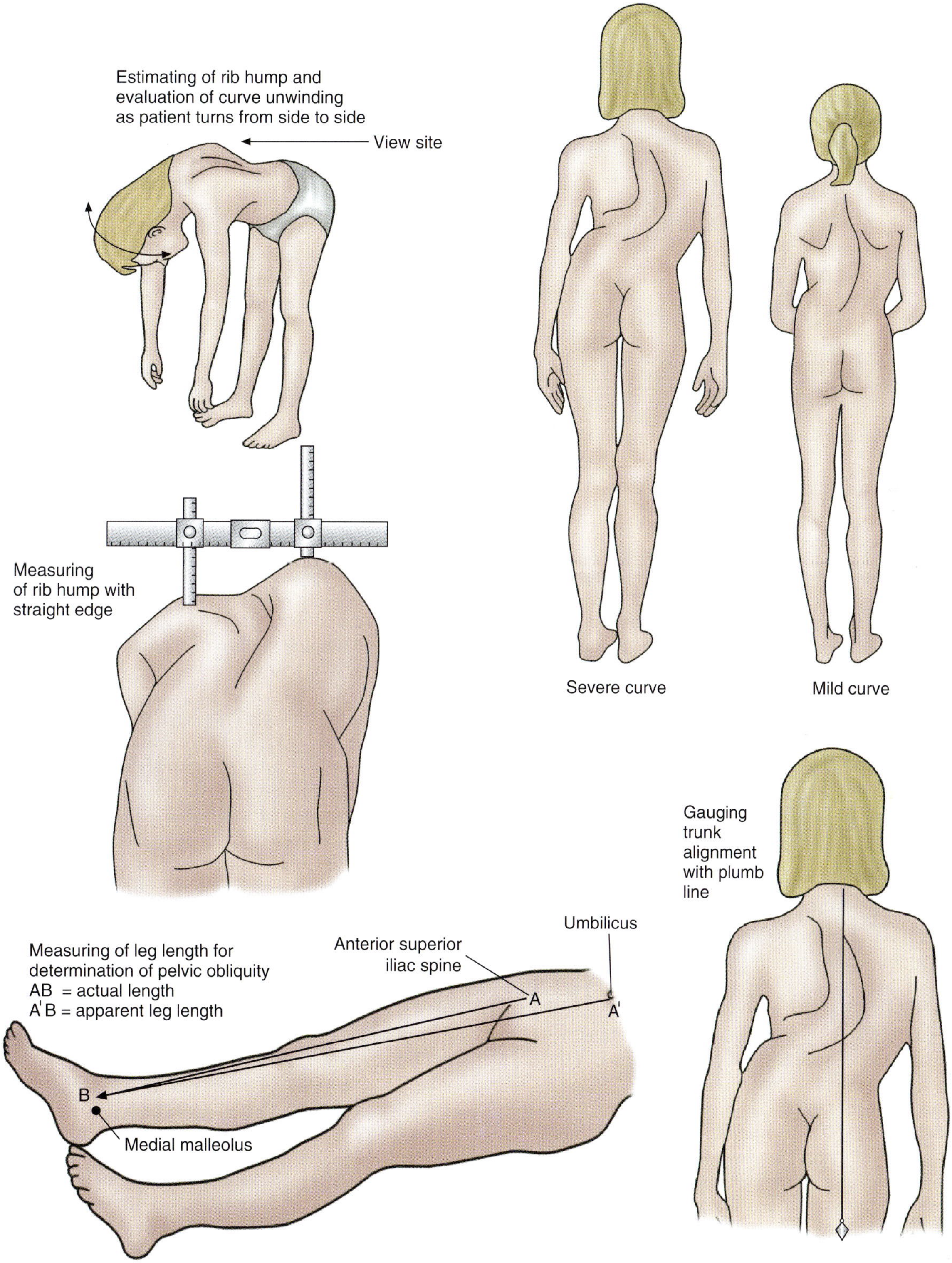

FIGURE 203.1 Clinical evaluation of a patient with scoliosis.

spots (**neurofibromatosis**), hairy patches, and nevi (**spinal dysraphism**). Abnormal extremities may indicate skeletal dysplasia, whereas heart murmurs can be associated with Marfan syndrome. It is essential to do a full neurologic examination to determine whether the scoliosis is idiopathic or secondary to an underlying neuromuscular disease and to assess whether the scoliosis is producing any neurologic sequelae.

Radiologic Evaluation

Initial radiographs should include a posteroanterior and lateral standing film of the entire spine. The entire pelvis including iliac crests should be visible to help determine skeletal maturity. The degree of curvature is determined by the Cobb angle, which is measured from the most tilted or end vertebra of the curve superiorly and inferiorly (Fig. 203.2). Imaging

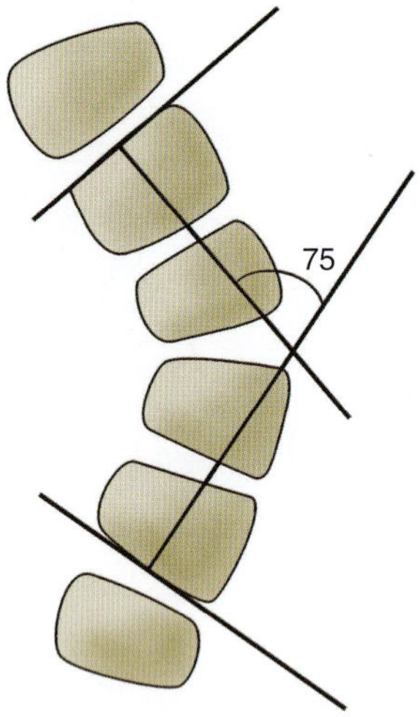

FIGURE 203.2 Cobb method of scoliotic curve measurement. Determine the end vertebrae of the curve: They are at the upper and lower limits of the curve and tilt most severely toward the concavity of the curve. Draw two perpendicular lines, one from the bottom of the lower body and one from the top of the upper body. Measure the angle formed. This is the accepted method of curve measurement according to the Scoliosis Research Society. Curves of 0–20 degrees are mild; 20–40 degrees, moderate; and greater than 40 degrees, severe.

modalities such as slot scanning (e.g., EOS®) provide the ability to obtain accurate measurements with lower radiation.

SCOLIOSIS

Alterations in normal spinal alignment that occur in the anteroposterior plane are termed *scoliosis*. Most scoliotic deformities are idiopathic. Scoliosis may also be congenital, neuromuscular, or compensatory from a leg-length discrepancy.

Idiopathic Scoliosis

Etiology and Epidemiology

Idiopathic scoliosis is the most common form of scoliosis. It occurs in healthy, neurologically normal children. Approximately 20% of patients have a positive family history. The incidence is slightly higher in females than males, and the condition is more likely to progress and require treatment in females. There is some evidence that progressive scoliosis may have a genetic component as well.

Idiopathic scoliosis can be classified into three categories: **infantile** (birth–3 years), **juvenile** (4–10 years), and **adolescent** (>11 years). Idiopathic adolescent scoliosis is the most common cause (80%) of spinal deformity. The right thoracic curve is the most common pattern. Juvenile scoliosis is uncommon but may be underrepresented because many patients do not seek treatment until they are adolescents. In any patient younger than 11 years of age, there is a greater likelihood that scoliosis is *not* idiopathic.

Clinical Manifestations

Idiopathic scoliosis is a painless disorder 70% of the time. A patient with pain requires careful evaluation. Any patient presenting with a *left-sided thoracic curve* has a high incidence of intraspinal pathology (syrinx or tumor). Evaluation of the spine with magnetic resonance imaging (MRI) is indicated in these cases.

Treatment

Treatment of idiopathic scoliosis is based on the skeletal maturity of the patient, the size of the curve, and whether the spinal curvature is progressive or nonprogressive. Initial treatment for scoliosis is likely observation with repeat radiographs to assess for progression. No treatment is indicated for nonprogressive deformities. Risk factors for curve progression include curve location and curve magnitude. Females are five times more likely to progress than males. Younger patients are more likely to progress than older patients. Physical therapy can help reduce discomfort but has not been proven to reliably reduce the spinal curvature.

Typically, curves under 25 degrees are observed. Progressive curves between 20 and 50 degrees in a skeletally immature patient are treated with bracing. A radiograph in the orthotic device is important to evaluate correction. Curves greater than 50 degrees usually require surgical intervention.

Congenital Scoliosis

Abnormalities of the vertebral formation during the first trimester may lead to structural deformities of the spine that are evident at birth or early childhood. Congenital scoliosis can be classified as follows (Fig. 203.3):

- Partial or complete failure of vertebral formation (wedge vertebra or hemivertebra)
- Partial or complete failure of segmentation (unsegmented bars or block vertebra)
- Mixed

More than 60% of patients have other associated abnormalities, such as VACTERL association (vertebral defects, imperforate anus, cardiac anomalies, tracheoesophageal fistula, renal anomalies, limb abnormalities such as radial agenesis) or Klippel-Feil syndrome. Kidney anomalies occur in 20–40% of children with congenital scoliosis, with renal agenesis being the most common; 6% of children have a silent, obstructive uropathy suggesting the need for evaluation with ultrasonography. Congenital heart disease occurs in about 12% of patients. **Spinal dysraphism** (tethered cord, intradural lipoma, syringomyelia, diplomyelia, and diastematomyelia) occurs in approximately 20% of children with congenital scoliosis. These disorders are frequently associated with cutaneous lesions (e.g., hypertrichosis, lipoma, dermal sinus) on the lumbosacral region and abnormalities of the legs and feet (e.g., cavus foot, neurologic changes, calf atrophy). MRI is indicated in evaluation of spinal dysraphism.

The risk of spinal deformity progression in congenital scoliosis is variable and depends on the growth potential of the malformed vertebrae. A unilateral unsegmented bar typically progresses, but a block vertebra has little growth potential. About 75% of patients with congenital scoliosis will show some progression that continues until skeletal growth is complete, and about 50% will require some type of treatment. Progression can be expected during periods of rapid growth (<2 years and >10 years).

Treatment of congenital scoliosis hinges on early diagnosis and identification of progressive curves. Orthotic treatment is not helpful in congenital scoliosis. Early spinal surgery should be performed once progression has been documented. This can help prevent major deformities. Patients with large curves that cause thoracic insufficiency should undergo surgery immediately.

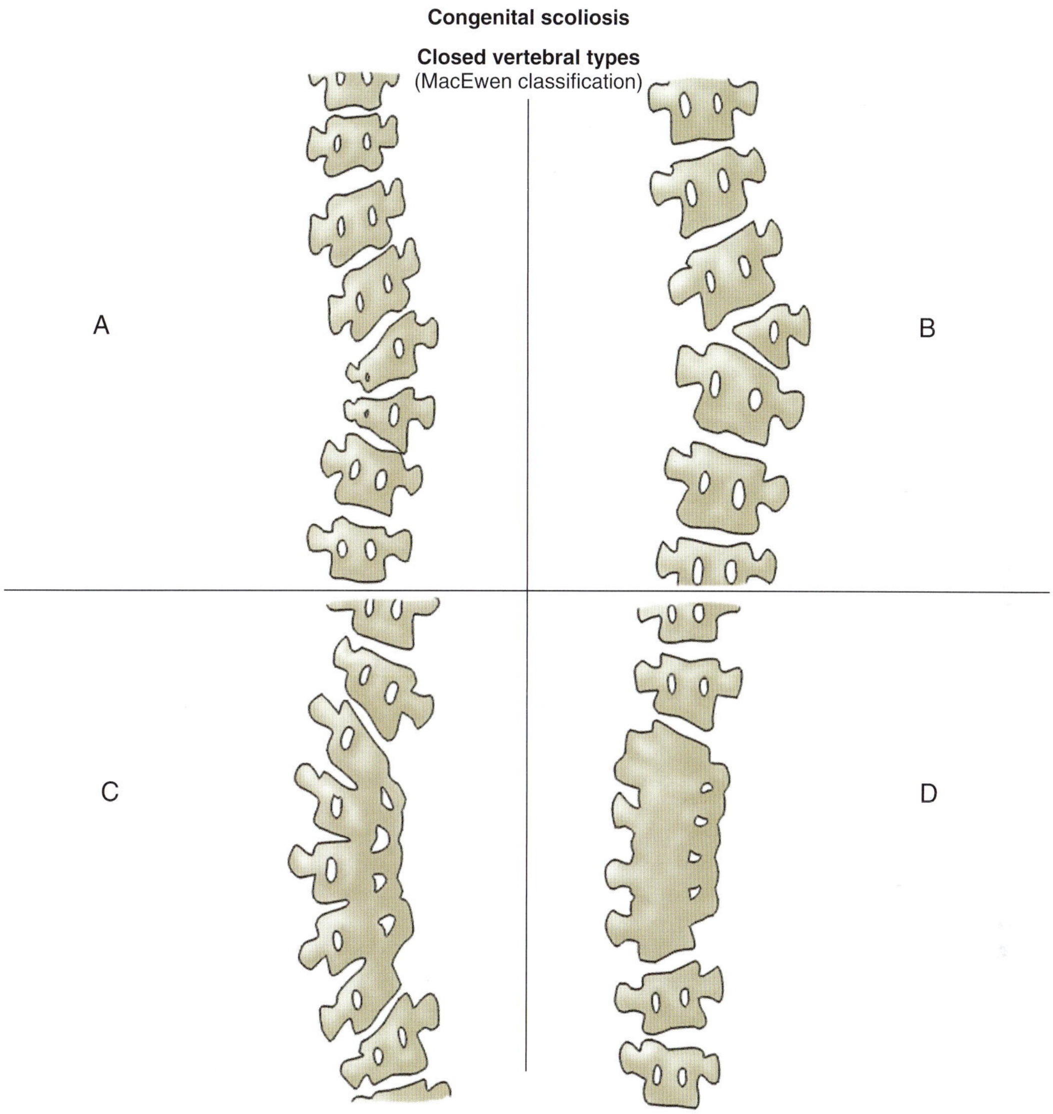

FIGURE 203.3 Types of closed vertebral and extravertebral spinal anomalies that result in congenital scoliosis. **(A)** Partial unilateral failure of formation (wedge vertebra). **(B)** Complete unilateral failure of formation (hemivertebra). **(C)** Unilateral failure of segmentation (congenital bar). **(D)** Bilateral failure of segmentation (block vertebra).

Neuromuscular Scoliosis

Progressive spinal deformity is a common and potentially serious problem associated with many neuromuscular disorders, such as cerebral palsy, Duchenne muscular dystrophy, spinal muscular atrophy, and spina bifida. Spinal alignment must be part of the routine examination for a patient with neuromuscular disease. Once scoliosis begins, progression is usually continuous. The magnitude of the deformity depends on the severity and pattern of weakness, whether the underlying disease process is progressive, and the amount of remaining musculoskeletal growth. Nonambulatory patients have a higher incidence of spinal deformity than ambulatory patients. In nonambulatory patients, the curves tend to be long and sweeping, produce pelvic obliquity, involve the cervical spine, and also produce restrictive lung disease. If the child cannot stand, then a supine or seated anteroposterior radiograph of the entire spine, rather than a standing posteroanterior view, is indicated.

The goal of treatment is to prevent progression and loss of function. Nonambulatory patients are more comfortable and independent when they can sit in a wheelchair without external support. Progressive curves can impair sitting balance, which affects quality of life. Pulmonary dysfunction may be seen with collapse of the spine, which causes the pelvis to impinge on the rib cage. Orthotic treatment is usually ineffective in neuromuscular scoliosis. Surgical intervention may be necessary with frequent fusion to the pelvis.

Compensatory Scoliosis

Adolescents with a leg-length discrepancy (see Chapter 201) may have a positive screening examination for scoliosis. Before correction of the pelvic obliquity, the spine curves in the same direction as the obliquity. However, with identification and correction of any pelvic obliquity, the curvature should resolve, and treatment should be directed at the leg-length discrepancy. Thus, it is important to distinguish between a structural and compensatory spinal deformity.

KYPHOSIS

Kyphosis refers to a round-back deformity or to increased angulation of the thoracic or thoracolumbar spine in the sagittal plane. Kyphosis can be postural, structural (Scheuermann kyphosis), or congenital.

Postural Kyphosis

Postural kyphosis is secondary to poor posture. It is voluntarily corrected in the standing and prone positions. The patient may also have increased lumbar lordosis. Radiographs are usually unnecessary if the kyphosis fully corrects. If not, radiographs will reveal no vertebral abnormalities. Treatment, if needed, is aimed at improving the child's posture.

Scheuermann Kyphosis

Scheuermann disease is the second most common cause of pediatric spinal deformity. It occurs equally in males and females. The etiology is unknown, but there may be hereditary factors. Scheuermann kyphosis is differentiated from postural kyphosis on physical examination and by radiographs.

A child with Scheuermann disease cannot correct the kyphosis with standing or lying prone. When viewed from the side in the forward flexed position, children with Scheuermann disease will have an abrupt angulation in the mid to lower thoracic region (Fig. 203.4), and patients with postural kyphosis show a smooth, symmetric contour. In both conditions, lumbar lordosis is increased. However, half of patients with Scheuermann disease will have atypical back pain, especially with thoracolumbar kyphosis. The classic radiologic findings of Scheuermann kyphosis include the following:

- Narrowing of disk space
- Loss of anterior height of the involved vertebrae producing wedging of 5 degrees or more in at least three consecutive vertebrae

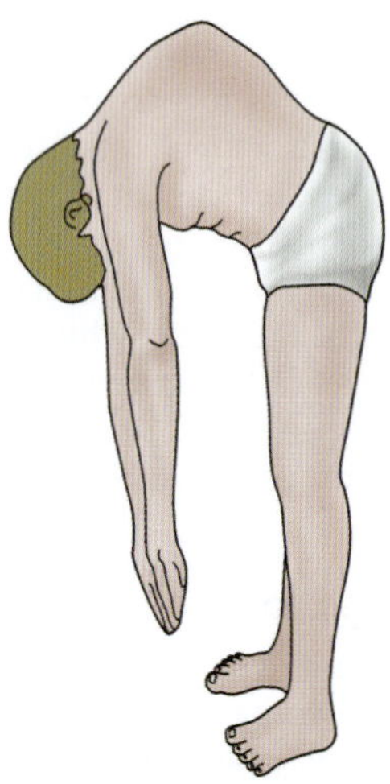

FIGURE 203.4 Note the sharp break in the contour of a child with kyphosis. (From Behrman RE, ed. *Nelson Textbook of Pediatrics*. 14th ed. Philadelphia: WB Saunders; 1992.)

- Irregularities of the vertebral end plates
- Schmorl nodes (disk material herniating into adjacent vertebral bodies)

Treatment of Scheuermann kyphosis is similar to idiopathic scoliosis. It is dependent on the degree of deformity, skeletal maturity, and the presence or absence of pain. Nonoperative treatment begins with bracing and physical therapy to help alleviate any discomfort. Surgical fusion is done for patients who have completed growth, have a severe deformity, or have intractable pain.

Congenital Kyphosis

Congenital kyphosis is a failure of the formation of all or part of the vertebral body (with preservation of posterior elements) or failure of anterior segmentation of the spine, or both. Severe deformities are found at birth and tend to rapidly progress. Progression will not cease until the end of skeletal growth. A progressive spine deformity may result in neurologic deficit. Treatment of congenital kyphosis is often surgical.

TORTICOLLIS

Etiology and Epidemiology

Congenital muscular torticollis is usually first identified in newborns because of a head tilt. This type of torticollis is typically secondary to a shortened sternocleidomastoid muscle and may result from in utero positioning or birth trauma. Acquired torticollis may be related to upper cervical spine abnormalities or central nervous system pathology (mass lesion). More commonly, it can occur in older children secondary to muscle injury or inflammation (potentially secondary to lymphadenitis with respiratory infections), local head or neck infection (e.g., streptococcal pharyngitis or retropharyngeal abscess), or dystonic reactions.

Clinical Manifestations and Evaluation

Infants with muscular torticollis have the ear tilted toward the clavicle on the ipsilateral side. The face will look upward toward the contralateral side. There may be a palpable swelling or fibrosis in the body of the sternocleidomastoid shortly after birth, which is often the precursor of a contracture. Congenital muscular torticollis is associated with skull and facial asymmetry (**plagiocephaly**) and developmental dysplasia of the hip.

For children presenting with acquired torticollis outside of infancy, a thorough head and neck exam as well as a neurologic exam should be completed. Further imaging may be indicated to rule out a nonmuscular etiology with anteroposterior and lateral radiographs or, in some cases, computed tomography (CT) scan or MRI of the head and neck.

Treatment

Treatment of muscular torticollis is aimed at increasing the range of motion of the neck and correcting the cosmetic deformity. Stretching exercises of the neck can be very beneficial for infants. Surgical management is indicated if patients do not improve with adequate stretching exercises in physical therapy. Postoperative physical therapy is needed to decrease the risk of recurrence. Treatment in patients with acquired torticollis secondary to underlying disorders should target the causative disorder.

BACK PAIN IN CHILDREN

Etiology and Epidemiology

Back pain in the pediatric population should always be approached with care. In contrast to the high prevalence of mechanical back pain in adults, back pain in children may be the result of organic causes, especially in preadolescents. Back pain lasting longer than a week requires a detailed investigation. In the pediatric population, approximately 85% of children with back pain for greater than 2 months have a specific lesion: 33% are post-traumatic (spondylolysis, occult fracture), 33% are developmental (kyphosis, scoliosis), and 18% have an infection or tumor. In the remaining 15%, the diagnosis is undetermined.

Clinical Manifestations and Management

The history must include the onset and duration of symptoms. The location, character, and radiation of pain are important. Neurologic symptoms (muscle weakness, sensory changes, gait disturbance, and bowel or bladder dysfunction) must be reviewed. Medical history and family history should be obtained with a focus on back pain, rheumatologic disorders, and neoplastic processes. The review of systems should include detailed questions on overall health, fever, chills, recent weight loss, and recent illnesses. Physical examination should include a complete musculoskeletal and neurologic evaluation. Spinal alignment, range of motion, areas of tenderness, and muscle spasm should be noted. **Red flags** for childhood back pain include persistent or increasing pain, systemic findings (e.g., fever, weight loss), neurologic deficits, bowel or bladder dysfunction, young age (<4 years is strongly associated with tumor), night waking, pain that restricts activity, and a painful left thoracic spinal curvature.

Anteroposterior and lateral standing films of the entire spine with consideration for bilateral oblique views of the affected area should be obtained. Secondary imaging with CT scan or MRI is often necessary for diagnosis. MRI is very useful for suspected intraspinal pathology. Laboratory studies, such as a complete blood count, erythrocyte sedimentation rate (ESR), C-reactive protein (CRP), and specialized testing for juvenile idiopathic arthritis and ankylosing spondylitis, may be indicated.

The differential diagnosis of pediatric back pain is extensive (Table 203.2). Treatment depends on the specific diagnosis. If serious pathology has been ruled out and no definite diagnosis has been established, an initial trial of physical therapy with close follow-up for re-evaluation is recommended.

TABLE 203.2 Differential Diagnoses of Back Pain

INFECTIOUS DISEASES
Spondylodiscitis (most common before the age of 6 yr) Vertebral osteomyelitis (pyogenic or tuberculous) Spinal epidural abscess Pyelonephritis
RHEUMATOLOGIC DISEASES
Juvenile idiopathic arthritis Reactive arthritis Ankylosing spondylitis Psoriatic arthritis Inflammatory bowel disease
DEVELOPMENTAL DISEASES
Scheuermann kyphosis Scoliosis (left thoracic) Spondylolysis Spondylolisthesis Syringomyelia
TRAUMATIC AND MECHANICAL ABNORMALITIES
Hip and pelvic abnormalities (sacroiliac joint dysfunction) Herniated nucleus pulposus (intervertebral disk) Overuse injuries (facet syndrome) Vertebral stress fractures (spondylolysis, spondylolisthesis) Vertebral compression fracture (steroid, sickle cell anemia) Upper cervical spine instability (atlantoaxial instability)
NEOPLASTIC DISEASES
Primary vertebral tumors (osteogenic sarcoma) Metastatic tumor (neuroblastoma) Primary spinal tumor (astrocytoma) Bone marrow malignancy (leukemia, lymphoma) Benign tumors (eosinophilic granuloma, osteoid osteoma)
OTHER
Conversion disorder Juvenile osteoporosis Pancreatitis

SPONDYLOLYSIS AND SPONDYLOLISTHESIS

Etiology and Epidemiology

Spondylolysis is a defect in the pars interarticularis. **Spondylolisthesis** refers to bilateral defects with anterior slippage of the superior vertebra on the inferior vertebra. About 5% of children develop mental spondylolysis by 6 years of age. It is most common in adolescent athletes, especially those involved in sports that involve repetitive back extension. Gymnasts, divers, football interior linemen (extension while blocking), soccer players (extension while shooting), and basketball players (extension while rebounding) are examples of athletes at higher risk. The most common location of spondylolisthesis is L5 on S1, followed by L4 on L5.

Spondylolisthesis is classified according to the degree of slippage:

- Grade 1: less than 25%
- Grade 2: 25–50%
- Grade 3: 50–75%
- Grade 4: 75–99%
- Grade 5: complete displacement or spondyloptosis

Clinical Manifestations

Patients will often complain of an insidious onset of low back pain persisting over 2 weeks. The pain tends to worsen with activity and improve with rest. There may be some radiation of pain to the buttocks, but it is rare to have radicular pain. A loss of lumbar lordosis may occur due to muscular spasm. Pain is present with extension of lumbar spine and with palpation over the lesion. Patients with spondylolisthesis may have a palpable *step-off* at the lumbosacral area. A detailed neurologic examination should be done especially because spondylolisthesis can have nerve root involvement.

Radiologic Evaluation

Anteroposterior and lateral radiographs of the spine should be obtained, with consideration for oblique views. The oblique views may show the classic *Scotty dog* findings associated with spondylolysis. The lateral view will allow measurement of spondylolisthesis. Unfortunately, plain radiographs do not regularly reveal spondylolysis, so advanced imaging may be needed. The most helpful form of advanced imaging among CT, single photon emission CT, or MRI continues to be debated. MRI should be considered in patients with neurologic deficits.

Treatment

Spondylolysis

Painful spondylolysis requires activity restriction. Bracing is controversial but may help with pain relief. Patients benefit from an aggressive physical therapy plan to improve lower extremity flexibility and increase core strength and spinal stability. There is evidence that some patients with an acute spondylolysis can achieve bony union and that these patients have a decreased incidence of low back pain and degenerative change in the low back as they age when compared with spondylolysis patients with nonunion. Rarely, surgery is indicated for intractable pain and disability.

Spondylolisthesis

Patients with spondylolisthesis require periodic evaluation for progression of their slippage. Treatment of spondylolisthesis is based on grading:

- Grade 1: Same treatment as spondylolysis. Failure of nonoperative management may lead to surgical fusion.
- Grade 2: Trial of nonoperative management, but if the slippage is progressing, surgical intervention may be needed. Any patient with neurologic symptoms requires surgical intervention.
- Grades 3–5: Spinal fusion is usually required to prevent further slippage or damage.

SPONDYLODISCITIS

Discitis may begin as an intervertebral disk space infection that may also be associated with an adjacent vertebral osteomyelitis (see Chapter 118). The most common organism is *Staphylococcus aureus*. The infection can occur at any age but is more common in patients under 6 years of age.

Clinical Manifestations

Children may present with back pain, abdominal pain, pelvic pain, irritability, and refusal to walk or sit. Fever is an inconsistent symptom. The child typically holds the spine in a straight or stiff position, generally has a loss of lumbar lordosis due to paravertebral muscular spasm, and refuses to flex the lumbar spine. The white blood cell count is normal or elevated; the ESR and CRP are usually high.

Radiologic Evaluation

Radiographic findings vary according to the duration of symptoms before diagnosis. Anteroposterior, lateral, and oblique radiographs of the lumbar or thoracic spine will typically show a narrow disk space with irregularity of the adjacent vertebral body end plates. In early cases, MRI may be helpful in identifying subtle abnormalities before plain radiographs. MRI can define the extent of disk space, vertebral bone, or epidural space involvement.

Treatment

Intravenous antibiotic therapy is the mainstay of treatment. Blood cultures may occasionally be positive and identify the infectious agent. Aspiration and needle biopsy are reserved for children who are not responding to empiric antibiotic treatment. Symptoms should resolve rapidly with antibiotics, but patients will still require a total of 4–6 weeks of treatment. Conversion from intravenous to oral antibiotics should be considered once the patient shows clear clinical improvement. Pain control can be obtained with medications and temporary orthotic immobilization of the back.

PEARLS FOR PRACTITIONERS

See Orthopedics: Pearls for Practitioners at the end of this section.

REVIEW QUESTIONS

Available online.

CHAPTER 204

Upper Extremity

SHOULDER

The shoulder actually comprises four joints:

- Glenohumeral joint (commonly referred to as the *shoulder joint*)
- Acromioclavicular joint
- Sternoclavicular joint
- Scapulothoracic joint

The glenohumeral joint has minimal geometric stability because the relatively small glenoid fossa articulates with the proportionately larger head of the humerus. The low level of intrinsic stability allows for a large range of motion. The rotator cuff muscles help give the glenohumeral joint more stability. The scapulothoracic movement also expands the range of motion of the shoulder, but like the glenohumeral joint, it requires strong, coordinated musculature to function efficiently.

Sprengel Deformity

Sprengel deformity is the congenital elevation of the scapula. There are varying degrees of severity; it is typically unilateral. There is restricted scapulothoracic motion (especially with abduction), so most of the shoulder motion is through the glenohumeral joint. There is usually associated hypoplasia of the periscapular muscles. Sprengel deformity is often associated with webbing of the neck and low posterior hairline. There is an association with congenital syndromes, such as Klippel-Feil anomaly, so a thorough history and examination are necessary. Mild forms with a cosmetic deformity and small loss of shoulder motion do not need surgical correction. Severe forms may have a bony connection (omovertebral) between the scapula and lower cervical spine. Moderate and severe forms may need surgical repositioning of the scapula in early childhood to improve cosmesis and function.

Clavicular Fractures

Clavicle fractures may be seen in neonates as a result of birth injury (see Chapter 57) or in childhood with falls or direct trauma to the clavicle. Fractures most commonly occur in the distal third of the clavicle. In the case of a posteriorly displaced medial clavicle fracture, computed tomography may be necessary to evaluate great vessels. A simple sling for 3–6 weeks, followed by rest and radiographs to assess healing, is often effective. Surgery is uncommon but may be indicated for older adolescents with significant shortening or displacement, skin tenting, or neurovascular compromise.

Brachial Plexus Injuries

Obstetric brachial plexus palsy is discussed in Section 11. **Brachial plexopathy** is an athletic injury, commonly referred to as a ***stinger*** or ***burner***. The symptoms are often likened to a *dead arm*. There is pain (often burning), weakness, and numbness in a single upper extremity. There are three mechanisms of injury:

- Traction caused by lateral flexion of the neck away from the involved upper extremity
- Direct impact to the brachial plexus at Erb point, a site at the upper trunk of the brachial plexus located 2–3 cm above the clavicle.
- Compression caused by neck extension and rotation toward the involved extremity

Symptoms are always unilateral and should resolve within 15 minutes. It is paramount to assess the *cervical spine* for serious injury. Bilateral symptoms, lower extremity symptoms, persistent symptoms, and recurrent injury are all signs of more serious injury requiring a more extensive work-up. Athletes may return to activity if there are no red flags on history or physical examination and the athlete has full pain-free range of motion and strength in the neck and affected extremity.

Glenohumeral Dislocation

Shoulder dislocation is uncommon in childhood but becomes more frequent in adolescence. Patients that sustain a dislocation at a younger age are more likely to have recurrence. Anterior dislocation is the most common. If assessment of the neurovascular status of the affected extremity reveals any compromise, urgent reduction is needed to prevent further complications. Several techniques may be used to reduce anterior shoulder dislocations including the traction-countertraction technique (Fig. 204.1) and the Stimson maneuver. Patients will need radiographs to assess for fractures of the glenoid (Bankart lesion) and humeral head (Hill-Sachs lesion). Most patients will require a brief period of protection in a sling or shoulder immobilizer. As symptoms resolve, rehabilitation should focus on a gentle range-of-motion program, followed by an aggressive strengthening program. Recurrence rate may be nearly 90% for contact sport athletes, so there is controversy surrounding early surgical intervention at the first dislocation; surgical intervention is needed for repeat dislocations.

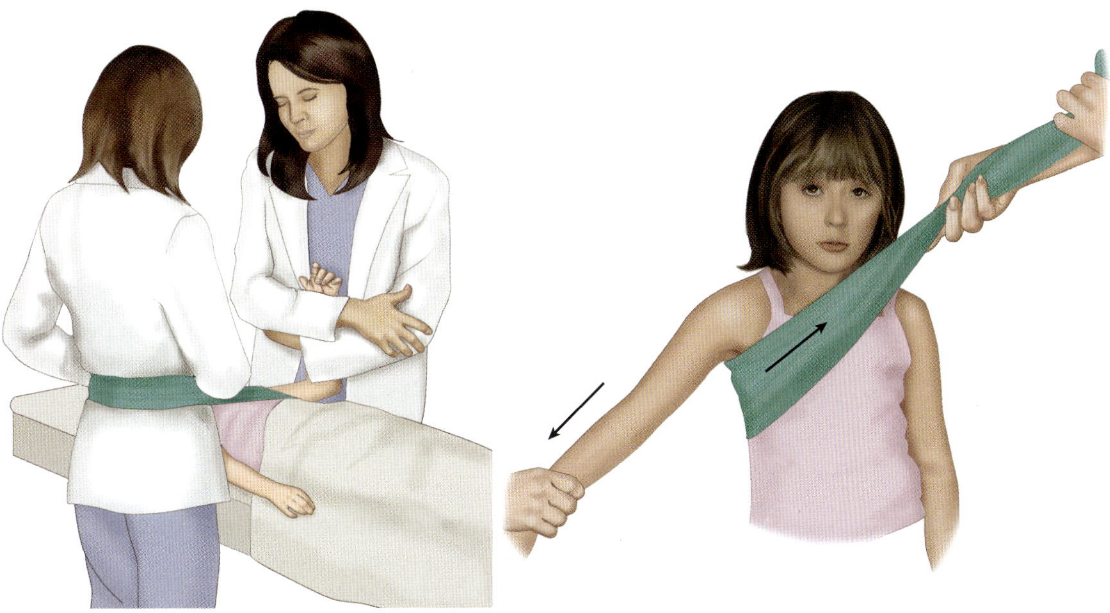

FIGURE 204.1 Traction-countertraction technique for reduction of glenohumeral dislocation. Longitudinal traction is applied through the arm and forearm, with the arm abducted and the elbow flexed. Gentle internal and external rotation will help reduce the humeral head. (From Herring JA, ed. *Tachdjian's Pediatric Orthopaedics*. 6th ed. Philadelphia: Elsevier; 2022:Fig. 29.17.)

Overuse Injuries

The incidence of overuse injuries is increasing because of increased year-round athletic participation as well as higher intensity levels during training. Soft tissue overuse injuries are inflammatory responses in tendons and bursae that are subjected to repetitive motions and trauma (e.g., rotator cuff tendinitis in swimmers). These injuries are more common in adolescents than younger children. Bony injury such as stress injury, physeal fracture, and apophysitis must be ruled out before making the diagnosis of a soft tissue overuse injury. Overuse injuries in the shoulder can be provoked by joint laxity.

Patients often present with discomfort that worsens with activity over the affected area. Physical examination usually reveals tenderness to palpation and often weakness of the associated muscles due to pain. It is important to assess for glenohumeral stability. Radiographs may be indicated for acute trauma or when symptoms are not improving. Treatment consists of activity modification, icing, antiinflammatory medication, and a physical therapy program aimed at improving strength, flexibility, and posture.

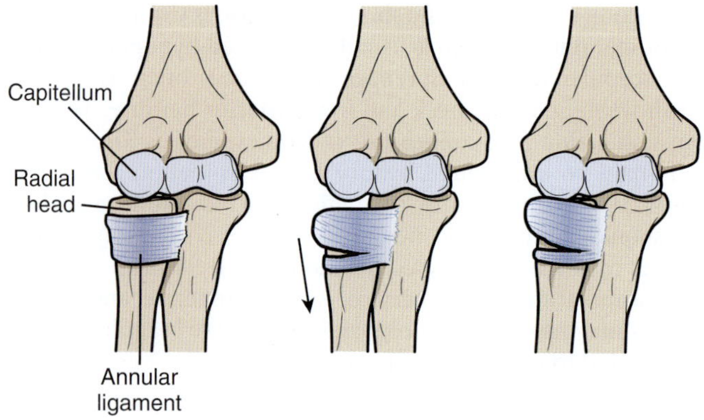

FIGURE 204.2 Nursemaid's elbow. Illustration depicting subluxation of the radial head inferior to the annular ligament, with interposition of the ligament to the radiocapitellar joint space. This entity is sometimes in the differential in the setting of upper extremity injury in a small child. Radiographs are negative and serve only to exclude the presence of bony injury when the diagnosis is not clear. (From Swenson DW, Walters MM. Musculoskeletal imaging. In: Walters MM, Robertson RL, eds. *Pediatric Radiology: The Requisites.* 4th ed. Philadelphia: Elsevier; 2017:Fig. 7.102.)

Proximal Humeral Epiphysiolysis

Proximal humeral epiphysiolysis, often referred to as ***Little League shoulder***, commonly occurs in 9–14-year-olds who participate in overhead (e.g., tennis, volleyball) and throwing sports, particularly baseball pitchers. It is a stress injury that can progress to a fracture (epiphysiolysis) of the proximal humeral physis. Most patients present with pain during or after throwing. There may be tenderness to palpation over the proximal humerus; however, if the athlete has been resting for a few days, examination may be normal. Consider bilateral radiographs for comparison of the physis. There may be widening of the proximal humeral physis in the affected arm, but the imaging may also be normal. Treatment is rest from the offending activity (typically for 6–8 weeks), followed by a rehabilitation program designed to improve strength in the shoulder girdle. Pitchers should also be encouraged to follow USA Baseball youth pitching guidelines.

ELBOW

The elbow consists of three articulations:

- Ulnar-humeral joint
- Radial-humeral joint
- Proximal radioulnar joint

Collectively, these joints produce a hinge-type joint that allows for supination (palm up) and pronation (palm down) positioning of the hand. The elbow has excellent bony stability, and the musculature around the elbow primarily produces flexion and extension.

Radial Head Subluxation

Radial head subluxation is more commonly known as ***nursemaid's elbow***. Because the radial head is not as bulbous in infants and young children, the annular ligament that passes around it can partially slip off the radial head with traction forces (Fig. 204.2). The subluxation is usually caused by a quick pull on the extended elbow when a child is forcefully lifted by the hand or when the child falls while holding hands with an adult. After a subluxation, the child usually holds the hand in a pronated position and will refuse to use the hand or move the elbow. Hyperpronation of the distal forearm will usually reduce the injury with a palpable or audible click; moving the hand into the supinated position while applying pressure to the radial head (known as *supination-flexion*) is another effective reduction method. Radiographs are not usually necessary unless reduction cannot be obtained or there is concern for fracture (swelling and bruising). Once the injury is reduced, the child will begin using the arm again without complaint. Parents should be educated about the mechanism of injury and encouraged to avoid that position. There is a high rate of recurrence for this injury. The problem generally resolves with maturation, but some children with high recurrence rates may benefit from casting or, rarely, surgical intervention.

Panner Disease

Panner disease is an osteochondrosis of the capitellum (lateral portion of distal humeral epiphysis) that occurs spontaneously in late childhood, usually prior to 10 years of age. Clinical features include elbow pain, decreased range of motion, and tenderness to palpation over the capitellum. Radiographs reveal an irregular epiphysis at the capitellum. Treatment is activity restriction and follow-up radiographs to demonstrate spontaneous reossification of the capitellum over several months. There is usually no need for further treatment or imaging studies. This is not to be confused with osteochondritis dissecans of the capitellum, which usually will occur in adolescents involved with throwing sports.

Throwing Injuries in the Elbow

The elbow is especially vulnerable to throwing injuries in the skeletally immature athlete. These occur from excessive and repetitive tension forces across the radial aspect of the elbow and compression forces across the lateral aspect of the elbow. These injuries are commonly known as ***Little League Elbow***.

Although this injury is most common in baseball players, it also occurs in football quarterbacks and tennis players. Patients will usually complain of pain over the medial elbow with throwing that may last for a few days afterward. There may be associated swelling and lateral or posterior elbow pain. Radiation of pain may be secondary to ulnar neuropathy. There may be a flexion contracture of the affected elbow. Palpation often reveals bony tenderness. Ulnar (medial) collateral ligament stability should be assessed. Radiographs should include the contralateral elbow for comparison. Radiographic findings in Little Leaguer's elbow can vary and may include normal anatomy, medial humeral epicondyle apophyseal avulsion fracture, osteochondritis dissecans of the capitellum, radial head abnormalities, and foreign bodies in the elbow. Magnetic resonance imaging may be helpful.

Treatment depends on the underlying diagnosis but always includes pain control and rest from activity. *Classic Little League elbow* refers to medial humeral epicondyle apophysitis. These athletes benefit from rest, ice, antiinflammatory medication, and a physical therapy program aimed at upper body strengthening. Throwing mechanics and USA Baseball pitching guidelines should be reviewed. Switching players to a lower throwing position (e.g., first base) after rehabilitation to avoid pitching for the remainder of the season can be helpful.

WRIST AND HAND

Multiple small joints, a delicately balanced intrinsic muscle system, a powerful extrinsic muscle system, dense sensory innervation, and specialized skin combine to make the hand highly mobile. The extrinsic muscles originate in the forearm, and the intrinsic muscles are located in the hand and coordinate small, delicate movements. The movements of opening the hand, extending and spreading the fingers, and then clenching the hand into a fist require coordinated function of the intrinsic and extrinsic muscles. Tenderness of direct palpation of the bones raises the concern for fracture. **Scaphoid fracture** is the most common carpal bone fracture in the pediatric population and can be difficult to visualize on radiographs. Treatment of nondisplaced fractures requires immobilization in a thumb spica cast, whereas displaced fractures require surgical intervention. **Salter-Harris fractures of the distal radius** are also very common. In young gymnasts, there is increased risk for injury at the distal radial physis from repetitive impact and upper extremity weight bearing. This overuse injury is commonly called ***gymnast's wrist*** and requires absolute rest from impact and weight bearing to prevent premature closure of the growth plate.

Ganglion cysts are synovial fluid-filled cysts about the wrist. The most common location is the dorsum of the wrist near the radiocarpal joint, followed by the volar radial aspect of the wrist. The defect is in the joint capsule, which allows synovial fluid into the soft tissues with wrist use, where it can become walled off with fibrous tissue. Often, in skeletally immature patients, the process is benign and disappears over time. Large ganglion cysts or cysts that are painful and interfere with function may require more aggressive management. Aspiration and steroid injection into the cyst may be helpful, but many will recur. Surgical excision will remove the tract that attaches to the wrist joint and is usually curative.

Finger Abnormalities

Polydactyly (extra digits) occurs in simple and complex variants (see Table 202.2). Skin tags and digit remnants that occur near the metacarpophalangeal joint of the fifth digit and thumb that do not have palpable bones or possess voluntary motion are categorized as simple. These may be excised or ligated in the nursery. Complex deformities should be referred to a pediatric hand surgeon for amputation. **Syndactyly** (fused digits) is concerning because of the possibility of shared structures and the tethering effects on bone growth (see Table 202.2). All patients with syndactyly should be referred for treatment options.

Trigger thumb and **trigger finger** are secondary to isolated thickening of the flexor tendons. As the thickened nodule enlarges, it may catch in a bent position, then snap or *trigger* straight as it passes through the first pulley that anchors the tendon. Ultimately, as it enlarges, it cannot pass through at all and produces a flexion deformity at the interphalangeal joints. The nodule may be palpable near the metacarpophalangeal joint. Children with these issues should be referred for surgical correction.

PEARLS FOR PRACTITIONERS

See Orthopedics: Pearls for Practitioners at the end of this section.

REVIEW QUESTIONS

Available online.

CHAPTER 205

Benign Bone Tumors and Cystic Lesions

Benign bone tumors and cystic lesions are common in childhood. Some represent fibrous dysplasia. Others are benign bone cysts (unicameral) or benign bone tumors (osteoid osteoma). Subacute osteomyelitis **(Brodie abscess)** and eosinophilic granulomas are lesions not associated with abnormal bone or cartilage growth. Some of these lesions can produce pain, limp, and pathologic fractures. Others can be incidental findings on radiographs. The prognosis is usually excellent. Brief differential diagnoses of bone tumors and their management are listed in Table 205.1. Malignant bone tumors are discussed in Section 21.

TABLE 205.1 Benign Bone Tumors and Cysts

DISEASE	CHARACTERISTICS	RADIOGRAPHIC FINDINGS	TREATMENT	PROGNOSIS
Osteochondroma (osteocartilaginous exostosis)	Common; distal metaphysis of femur, proximal humerus, proximal tibia; painless, hard, nontender mass	Bony outgrowth, sessile or pedunculated	Excision, if symptomatic	Excellent; malignant transformation rare
Multiple hereditary exostoses	Osteochondroma of long bones; bone growth disturbances	As above	As above	Recurrences common
Osteoid osteoma	Pain relieved by NSAIDs; femur and tibia; found predominantly in males	Dense sclerosis surrounds small radiolucent nidus, <1 cm	As above. Radiofrequency ablation may also be used	Excellent
Osteoblastoma (giant osteoid osteoma)	As above, but more destructive	Osteolytic component; size >1 cm	Excision or curettage	Excellent
Enchondroma	Tubular bones of hands and feet; pathologic fractures, swollen bone; Ollier disease if multiple lesions are present	Radiolucent diaphyseal or metaphyseal lesion; may calcify	Excision or curettage if symptomatic or large	Excellent; malignant transformation rare
Nonossifying fibroma	Silent; rare pathologic fracture; late childhood, adolescence	Incidental radiographic finding; thin sclerotic border, radiolucent lesion	None or curettage with fractures	Excellent; heals spontaneously
Eosinophilic granuloma	Age 5–10 yr; skull, jaw, long bones; pathologic fracture; pain	Small, radiolucent without reactive bone; punched-out lytic lesion	Biopsy, excision rare; irradiation	Excellent; may heal spontaneously
Brodie abscess	Insidious local pain; limp; suspected as malignancy	Circumscribed metaphyseal osteomyelitis; lytic lesions with sclerotic rim	Surgical debridement; antibiotics	Excellent
Unicameral bone cyst (simple bone cyst)	Metaphysis of long bone (femur, humerus); pain, pathologic fracture	Cyst in medullary canal, expands cortex; fluid-filled unilocular or multilocular cavity	Curettage; steroid injection into lesion	Recurrence in 50%; some heal spontaneously
Aneurysmal bone cyst	As above; contains blood, fibrous tissue	Expands beyond metaphyseal cartilage	Curettage, bone graft	Recurrence in 20%

NSAIDs, Nonsteroidal antiinflammatory drugs.

PEARLS FOR PRACTITIONERS

See Orthopedics: Pearls for Practitioners at the end of this section.

REVIEW QUESTIONS

Available online.

Suggested Readings

Brenner JS, Watson A, Council on Sports Medicine and Fitness. Overuse Injuries, Overtraining, and Burnout in Young Athletes. *Pediatrics.* 2024;153(2):e2023065129.

Herring JA, ed. *Tachdjian's Pediatric Orthopedics.* 6th ed. Philadelphia: Elsevier; 2021.

Kliegman RM, St. Geme J, eds. *Nelson Textbook of Pediatrics.* 22nd ed. Philadelphia: Elsevier; 2025.

Krabak BJ, Brooks MA, eds. *The Youth Athlete: A Practitioner's Guide to Providing Comprehensive Sports Medicine Care.* Philadelphia: Elsevier; 2023.

Miller MD, DeLee Thompson SR, eds. *Drez and Miller's Orthopaedic Sports Medicine: Principles and Practices.* 5th ed. Philadelphia: Elsevier; 2019.

Payares-Lizano M. The limping child. *Pediatr Clin North Am.* 2020;67(1):119–138.

Shipman SA, Helfand M, Moyer VA, et al. Screening for developmental dysplasia of the hip: a systemic literature review for the U.S. Preventive Services Task Force. *Pediatrics.* 2006;117:e557–e576.

Wenger DR, Pring ME, Rang M, eds. *Rang's Children's Fractures.* 3rd ed. Philadelphia: Lippincott Williams & Wilkins; 2005.

PEARLS FOR PRACTITIONERS

CHAPTER 198
Orthopedic Assessment

- Orthopedic "basics" for developmental milestones
  - Sit independently at 6 months
  - Pull to stand at 10 months
  - Cruising at 12 months
  - Walk at 18 months
- Lower extremity angular variants
  - Genu varum (bowlegs) at birth and begin to straighten out by 18 months
  - Genu valgum (knock-knees)—maximum at 4 years old and resolves by 5–8 years of age
  - Pathologic genu varum: Blount disease (tibia vara) and rickets
- Differential diagnosis for the limping child
  - Painful
    - Septic arthritis, osteomyelitis, discitis
    - Transient monoarticular synovitis
    - Toddler's fracture or trauma
    - Malignancy
    - Rheumatologic disorders in older children
    - Acute slipped capital femoral epiphysis (SCFE) in adolescents
  - Painless
    - Development dysplasia of the hip
    - Neuromuscular disorder
    - Leg-length inequality
    - Legg-Calve-Perthes disease in older children
    - Muscular dystrophy in older children
    - Chronic, stable SCFE in adolescents

CHAPTER 199
Fractures

- Unique features of pediatric bone
  - Bone has higher collagen content (tend to undergo plastic deformation before complete fracture)
  - Thicker periosteum (aids healing and can stabilize fracture after reduction)
  - Greater ability to remodel a deformity
  - Possible overgrowth following long-bone fractures (especially femur)
- Salter-Harris fracture classification for growth plate fractures
  - Type I—transverse through physis
  - Type II—through physis into metaphysis
  - Type III—through physis into epiphysis (joint)
  - Type IV—through both metaphysis and epiphysis
  - Type V—crush to the physis
  - Types III–V have higher rates of postinjury growth arrest
- Always assess neurovascular status distal to an injury
- Signs/symptoms of acute compartment syndrome producing neurovascular injury
  - Early findings: pain out of proportion to the injury, pain with passive stretch or muscle contraction
  - Later findings: pallor, pulselessness, paresthesia, poikilothermy (cold)
  - Most common sites at risk: supracondylar humerus fracture and tibia fracture

CHAPTER 200
Hip

- Development dysplasia of the hip
  - Risk factors: first born, female, breech, family history, oligohydramnios
  - Associated lesions include congenital torticollis, metatarsus adductus, and clubfoot
  - Ortolani test: reduces dislocated hip
  - Barlow test: dislocates unstable hip
  - Imaging: ultrasound <6 months of age, x-ray >6 months of age
  - Treatment: Pavlik harness <6 months of age, spica cast or surgery >6 months or failed Pavlik harness
- Legg-Calve-Perthes disease
  - Avascular necrosis of the femoral head
  - Classic presentation is painless limp in elementary school-aged male
  - Mean age: 7 years
  - Delayed treatment increases risk of arthritis
- Transient monoarticular synovitis often follows a recent viral illness by 1–2 weeks
  - Typically afebrile
  - Labs: normal to minimally elevated white blood cell (WBC), erythrocyte sedimentation rate (ESR), and C-reactive protein (CRP)
- Septic arthritis has elevated WBC, ESR, CRP, and elevated joint fluid cell count
  - Usually febrile and hold hip in flexion and external rotation
- Slipped capital femoral epiphysis
  - Mean age is 12 years in males and 11 years in females
  - Risk factors: adolescent, obese, trisomy 21, endocrine disorder
  - May present as isolated hip or knee pain
  - Hip held externally rotated, especially when moved into hip flexion
  - Treat as orthopedic emergency—non–weight-bearing and immediate referral

CHAPTER 201
Lower Extremity and Knee

- Apophysitis
  - Osgood-Schlatter disease at tibial tubercle
  - Sever disease at posterior calcaneus
  - Treat with rest, stretching, and ice; counsel family that symptoms may last for about 2 years
  - Usually no long-term complications
- Rotational variants
  - Internal tibial torsion is the most common cause of in-toeing in children <2 years of age
  - Internal femoral torsion (anteversion) may be seen in children with W-sitting positions
  - Unilateral rotational anomalies have higher association with neurologic or neuromuscular disorders
- Acute swelling of the knee joint after injury may indicate a hemarthrosis (ACL tear or meniscus tear)
  - Lachman test to assess for ACL tear
  - McMurray test to assess for meniscus tear
- Patellofemoral pain syndrome is anterior knee pain that worsens with activity such as going up and down stairs
  - Treatment focuses on a rehabilitation program to improve flexibility and strength and correct biomechanics

CHAPTER 202
Foot

- Clubfoot (talipes equinovarus) may be congenital or teratologic
  - Treatment involves Ponseti serial casting, percutaneous heel cord lengthening, and bracing
- Metatarsus adductus is a common foot disorder in infants, resolving spontaneously in >90% of infants
- Flat feet/Pes planus
  - Hypermobile pes planus involves pronated feet associated with generalized ligamentous laxity in children >6 years of age
  - Rigid flat foot should be evaluated for tarsal coalition
- A cavovarus foot (high arch) is associated with Charcot-Marie-Tooth disease (genetic neuropathy) and other spinal disorders (e.g., tethered cord)

CHAPTER 203
Spine

- Scoliosis
  - Coronal curvature is >10 degrees
  - Adams forward bend test shows rotational deformity/asymmetry
  - Congenital scoliosis has abnormal bony morphology
  - Neuromuscular scoliosis is associated with underlying neurologic disorder
  - Idiopathic scoliosis—no clear etiology
  - Treatment
    - Observation: <25 degrees
    - Bracing: 20–50 degree curve or if progressing
    - Spinal fusion surgery: >50 degrees
- Kyphosis
  - Postural—normal bony structure
  - Scheuermann kyphosis
    - >5 degree anterior wedging on three consecutive vertebral bodies
    - Treat with bracing if skeletally immature; observation or surgical correction if skeletally mature
- Congenital—abnormal bony structure that often requires bracing or surgery to treat

CHAPTER 204
Upper Extremity

- Brachial plexus injury
  - At birth, differential diagnoses include clavicle or humerus fracture
  - Athletic "stingers" are unilateral upper extremity injuries that resolve within a few minutes
    - Bilateral symptoms and lower extremity symptoms should be concerning for more severe spine injury
- Radial head subluxation (nursemaid's elbow)
  - Mechanism—pulling the outstretched arm of a child
  - Treatment is reduction, usually with supination of forearm and flexion of elbow or hyperpronation
- Complex polydactyly and syndactyly require surgical correction
- Nondisplaced scaphoid fractures require a thumb spica cast, while displaced fractures may need surgical correction

CHAPTER 205
Benign Bone Tumors and Cystic Lesions

- Often found incidentally; management depends on specific diagnosis but prognosis is usually excellent

INDEX

Page numbers followed by "*f*" indicate figures and "*t*" indicate tables.

B

C

D

E

F

G

H

M

N

O

P

Q

R

S

W

X

Y

Z